ONCOLOGY 1970

Being the Proceedings of the Tenth International Cancer Congress

ONCOLOGY 1970

ONCOLOGY 1970

Being the Proceedings of the

Tenth International Cancer Congress

Volume I

A. Cellular & Molecular Mechanisms of Carcinogenesis

B. Regulation of Gene Expression

Edited and Prepared for Publication

under the Direction of:

R. LEE CLARK, M.D., M.Sc. (Surg.), D.Sc. (Hon.)
*President, The University of Texas M. D. Anderson Hospital
and Tumor Institute at Houston
and Chairman, National Organizing Committee of the
Tenth International Cancer Congress*

RUSSELL W. CUMLEY, Ph.D.
*Editor and Head, Department of Publications,
The University of Texas M. D. Anderson Hospital and Tumor Institute at Houston*

JOAN E. McCAY, M.A.
*Managing Editor and Supervisor of Publications, Department of Publications,
The University of Texas M. D. Anderson Hospital and Tumor Institute at Houston*

MURRAY M. COPELAND, M.D., D.Sc. (Hon.)
*Professor of Surgery (Oncology), The University of Texas M. D.
Anderson Hospital and Tumor Institute at Houston
and Secretary General, Tenth International Cancer Congress*

With the Cooperation of the
Officials of the Tenth International Cancer Congress

YEAR BOOK MEDICAL PUBLISHERS · INC.
35 EAST WACKER DRIVE · CHICAGO

281924

Library of Congress Catalog Card Number: 70-150262

International Standard Book Number: 0-8151-1764-7

Acknowledgments

The following members of the Department of Publications of The University of Texas M. D. Anderson Hospital and Tumor Institute at Houston participated in the editing and preparation of this volume for publication:

Associate Editor

DOROTHY M. BEANE, B.A.

Assistant Editors

SUSAN BIRKEL, B.A.	DEBORAH L. KENSEL, B.A.
LYNDA G. BURGNER	JUDITH WIBLE LETTENEY, B.A.
JANINA M. ELY, A.B.	M. LUCINDA MARINIS, B.A.
SHIRLEY J. HARTMAN, B.B.A.	DEBORAH L. RYLANDER, M.A.
PAMELA HESTER	DIANE SHOQUIST, B.A.
BARBARA E. JOHNSON, B.A.	KATHLEEN S. YACUZZO, B.S.

Acknowledgment is made of the kind services of Dr. Clifton D. Howe, Associate Director for Clinics and Chief of Clinics, Dr. Darrell N. Ward, Head, Department of Biochemistry, and Dr. Felix L. Haas, Head, Department of Biology, The University of Texas M. D. Anderson Hospital and Tumor Institute at Houston for their assistance in arranging the contents of the volumes. The help of Miss Donna McCormick and Mrs. Marilyn Cavanagh of the Congress' Secretariat is gratefully acknowledged.

OFFICIALS OF THE
TENTH INTERNATIONAL CANCER CONGRESS

President: DR. WENDELL M. STANLEY

Vice Presidents:

DR. R. LEE CLARK, *President, The University of Texas M. D. Anderson Hospital and Tumor Institute at Houston*

DR. KENNETH M. ENDICOTT, *Director, Bureau of Health Professions Education and Manpower Training, National Institutes of Health*

DR. SIDNEY FARBER, *American Cancer Society, Inc.*

DR. JAMES F. HOLLAND, *American Association for Cancer Research*

DR. CARL G. BAKER, *Acting Director, National Cancer Institute, National Institutes of Health*

Secretary General: DR. MURRAY M. COPELAND

Treasurer: MR. E. DON WALKER

National Organizing Committee of the Congress

Chairman: DR. R. LEE CLARK

Honorary Chairman: THE HONORABLE JOHN B. CONNALLY, Former Governor of Texas

Members:

DR. WERNER H. KIRSTEN, *American Association for Cancer Research*

DR. RICHARD P. MASON, *American Cancer Society*

DR. HAROLD W. WALLGREN, *American Cancer Society*

DR. JOHN J. TRENTIN, *American Association for Cancer Research*

DR. FRANK L. HORSFALL, JR., *National Cancer Institute*

DR. DONALD P. SHEDD, *National Cancer Institute*

DR. DAVID A. WOOD, *American Association of Cancer Institutes*

Chairman, Program Committee: DR. CHARLES HEIDELBERGER

Chairman, Local Organizing Committee: DR. CLIFTON D. HOWE

Honorary Chairman, Local Organizing Committee: MR. THEODORE N. LAW

Ex-Officio Members (Members, USA National Committee of the International Union Against Cancer and National Academy of Sciences):

DR. MURRAY M. COPELAND, Chairman	DR. JAMES A. MILLER
DR. W. RAY BRYAN	DR. GREGORY O'CONOR
DR. R. LEE CLARK	DR. H. MARVIN POLLARY
DR. EMIL FREI, III	DR. JOHN S. SPRATT, JR.
DR. JAMES T. GRACE, JR.	DR. C. CHESTER STOCK
DR. CHARLES HEIDELBERGER	DR. ALTON I. SUTNICK
DR. FRANK L. HORSFALL, JR.	DR. SHIELDS WARREN
DR. LLOYD W. LAW	MR. FRANCIS J. WILCOX

MR. W. ARMIN WILLIG

Program Committee of the Congress

Chairman: DR. CHARLES HEIDELBERGER

Members:

DR. MALCOLM A. BAGSHAW	DR. ROBERT W. MILLER
DR. EMIL FREI, III	DR. RICHMOND PREHN
DR. ROALD GRANT*	DR. JONATHAN RHODES
DR. FELIX HAAS	DR. FRANK SCHABEL
DR. ROY HERTZ	DR. JOHN J. TRENTIN
DR. WERNER KIRSTEN	DR. GEORGE WEBER
DR. PAUL KOTIN	DR. R. LEE CLARK, Ex-Officio
DR. JAMES A. MILLER	DR. MURRAY M. COPELAND, Ex-Officio

In Appreciation

Special contributions in support of the Tenth International Cancer Congress have been made by the following:

AMERICAN CANCER SOCIETY, INC. (NEW YORK)

AMERICAN CANCER SOCIETY, TEXAS DIVISION

MR. AND MRS. JAMES A. ELKINS, JR.

CALOUSTE GULBENKIAN FOUNDATION

MR. AND MRS. HUB HILL

HUMBLE OIL AND REFINING CO.

MR. AND MRS. THEODORE N. LAW

LEUKEMIA SOCIETY OF AMERICA, INC.

EDWARD MALLINCKRODT, JR. FOUNDATION

NATIONAL CANCER INSTITUTE OF THE NATIONAL INSTITUTES OF HEALTH, U. S. DEPARTMENT OF HEALTH, EDUCATION AND WELFARE

SID W. RICHARDSON FOUNDATION

MR. AND MRS. LLOYD H. SMITH

STATE OF TEXAS

THE UNIVERSITY OF TEXAS M. D. ANDERSON HOSPITAL AND TUMOR INSTITUTE AT HOUSTON

THE UNIVERSITY CANCER FOUNDATION OF THE UNIVERSITY OF TEXAS M. D. ANDERSON HOSPITAL AND TUMOR INSTITUTE AT HOUSTON

MRS. HARRY C. WIESS

We are especially indebted to the CALOUSTE GULBENKIAN FOUNDATION which provided funds and support for the publication of the Proceedings of the Tenth International Cancer Congress.

---

* Deceased

OFFICIALS OF THE
INTERNATIONAL UNION AGAINST CANCER

President: PROFESSOR N. N. BLOKHIN (USSR)

President-Elect: DR. W. U. GARDNER (USA)

Past-President: SIR ALEXANDER HADDOW (UK)

Vice Presidents:

Africa: DR. V. A. NGU (Nigeria)
Asia: DR. K. OOTA (Japan)
Europe: DR. P. BUCALOSSI (Italy)
Europe: DR. O. COSTACHEL (Romania)
Latin America: DR. M. GAITAN YANGUAS (Colombia)
North America: DR. G. T. PACK* (USA)
Oceania: DR. R. E. J. TEN SELDAM (Australia)

Secretary General: DR. R. M. TAYLOR (Canada)

Treasurer: DR. P. LOUSTALOT (Switzerland)

Chairmen of Commissions:

Commission on Clinical Oncology: DR. P. DENOIX (France)
Commission on Cancer Control: DR. E. C. EASSON (UK)
Commission on Epidemiology and Prevention: DR. J. HIGGINSON (France)
Commission on Experimental Oncology: DR. R. J. C. HARRIS (UK)
Commission on Fellowships and Personnel Exchange: DR. W. U. GARDNER (USA)

Elected Members:

DR. T. ANTOINE (Australia)	DR. B. S. HANSON (Australia)
DR. O. MÜHLBOCK (The Netherlands)	DR. A. I. RAKOV (USSR)
DR. E. RAVENTOS (Chile)	DR. I. BERENBLUM (Israel)
DR. H. L. STEWART (USA)	DR. M. M. COPELAND (USA)
DR. P. N. WAHI (India)	DR. M. J. DARGENT (France)
DR. E. BARAJAS VALLEJO (Mexico)	DR. A. GRAFFI (GDR)
DR. E. PEDERSEN (Norway)	DR. B. E. GUSTAFSSON (Sweden)
	DR. J. F. MURRAY (South Africa)	

Committee on International Congresses:

Chairman: PROFESSOR N. N. BLOKHIN (USSR)

Members:

DR. M. M. COPELAND (USA)	DR. R. J. C. HARRIS (UK)
DR. P. DENOIX (France)	DR. J. HIGGINSON (France)
DR. E. C. EASSON (UK)	DR. K. OOTA (Japan)
DR. W. U. GARDNER (USA)	DR. R. M. TAYLOR (Canada)

* Deceased

Foreword

THE TENTH INTERNATIONAL Cancer Congress, held in Houston, Texas, U.S.A., May 22 through May 29, 1970, was attended by 6,018 physicians and scientists from throughout the world. Of these, 1,957 participated in the sessions. The speakers, representing 72 different countries, presented 1,740 papers; abstracts of 1,342 proffered papers appeared in the book of *Abstracts,* copies of which were distributed at the Congress. The remaining 398 papers appear *in toto* in the five volumes comprising this set of Proceedings. These 1,740 papers were virtually all of the papers submitted for presentation; less than a dozen titles were rejected. Consequently, one might reasonably assume that these papers and abstracts comprise a comprehensive survey of the international status of the science and art of oncology as it existed in the spring of 1970.

The papers, speeches, and lectures may be divided into seven general groups:

1. Congress Ceremonies
2. Preliminary Special Sessions of the Congress
3. Main Congress Panels
4. Postgraduate Course Panels
5. Proffered Paper Sessions
6. Rapporteur Reports
7. The Harold Dorn Lecture

The sequence in which these various presentations were made, their authors, and the organization of the Congress may be found in the *Program* of the Tenth International Cancer Congress (Library of Congress Card Catalogue No. 42-43259). The members of the Congress, i.e. those who registered at the meeting, and the names and addresses of most of the persons who presented papers may be found in the *Members* of the Tenth International Cancer Congress (Library of Congress Card Catalogue No. 73-124104). Abstracts of papers presented at the Proffered Paper Sessions (No. 5 in the general groups listed above) are contained in the *Abstracts* of the Tenth International Cancer Congress (Library of Congress Card Catalogue No. 70-12413). All three of these volumes were published by The Medical Arts Publishing Co., 1603 Oakdale St., Houston, Texas, U.S.A. 77004.

The papers published in the 5 volumes comprising the published proceedings include the Congress Ceremonies (No. 1 in the above list), the Preliminary Special Sessions (No. 2), the Main Congress Panels (No. 3), the Postgraduate Course Panels (No. 4), the Rapporteur Reports (No. 6), and The Harold Dorn Lecture (No. 7). The papers have not been published in the order in which they were given at the Congress, since during the Congress several presentations occurred simultaneously. Rather, in these volumes, the papers, including the Rapporteur Reports and The Harold Dorn Lecture, have been assembled into groups of related subject matter.

Because of the overwhelming number of citations contained in the reference lists submitted by the authors, it was not possible to verify the citations or to complete those submitted in abbreviated form. Therefore, the reference lists have been published in much the same way in which they were received. In the few instances in which no reference list was submitted, or when the list was excessively lengthy, an editorial note has been added, directing the reader to apply directly to the author for a list of the literature cited.—Editors.

Table of Contents

Tenth International Cancer Congress Ceremonies

OPENING ADDRESSES

N. N. BLOKHIN: *President, International Union Against Cancer*. Dr. Blokhin opened the Tenth International Cancer Congress by welcoming the members and participants to the Congress, and by expressing his acknowledgment of the endeavors of the National Organizing Committee and appreciation of the contributors to the funding of the Congress. He expressed his belief in the continuing success of the International Union Against Cancer through the cooperative efforts of all of the nations represented, in basic research, patient care, and educational programs directed toward the goal of cancer control.

Due to a technical failure of the recording equipment employed at the Congress, the full text of Dr. Blokhin's address is not available.

SIR ALEXANDER HADDOW: *Past President, International Union Against Cancer*. Dr. Lee Clark, Professor Blokhin, Dr. Stanley, Professor Yoshida, Dr. Gardner, Members of the Union, Members of the Congress, Ladies and Gentlemen:

This Tenth International Congress is uniquely welcome to all from our constituent nations beyond these shores, in providing—at long last—a fit opportunity to extend to the United States of America, and indeed to the entire American people, our heartfelt appreciation of the scale and generosity of that vital support which they have lavished upon our Union and upon cancer research throughout the world, over the past generation and more.

The last International Cancer Congress to be held in the United States took place at St. Louis in 1947, under the presidency of Dr. E. V. Cowdry. At that time the affairs of the Union were in parlous disarray, partly due to the War, and from every aspect, financial and otherwise. At St. Louis in 1947 we were accordingly required to reach a clear decision, whether to abandon the Union as no longer viable, or, to resolve to redeem it, to restore it, and to enable it to flourish in its true function. In deciding upon the latter course of action, we were influenced by two main factors: first, our great respect for the pioneer labors of Professor Maisin of Belgium, who from the inauguration of the

1

Union in 1933 had striven valiantly and almost singlehandedly, to keep it alive—usually with little encouragement and on occasion with positive discouragement; and second, our realization that abandonment of the Union would render it excessively difficult, or perhaps indeed impossible, to re-establish and recreate the venture. The decision was taken with Dr. Cowdry's guidance, and although many years were still required to bring the new policy to fruition, no one looking back can doubt that the decision was both timely and wise, leading to a Union capable of interpreting our problems on a truly international scale. What I wish to impress upon you, and what you already very well know, is the evident fact that nothing of this gratifying development would have been possible but for far-sighted American benevolence, expressed not only through governmental channels, especially through the National Institutes of Health of the Public Health Service, but also through a public generosity conveyed mainly through the medium of the American Cancer Society, but in addition by a host of other agencies.

It is my desire and aspiration—I think well-known—that the functions of our Union should not be construed in any narrow fashion, nor be limited to our primary objective, however noble that may be. I have in mind the almost insensible and pervasive effects which international congresses of this kind can focus on the conduct of human relations. Although not our purpose and not our intention, such influences were especially powerful (even if unexpected) during the Moscow Congress of 1962, when we all sensed the reality of a community between our nations which, as a contribution toward peace, however unconscious, made us rejoice. As Professor Blokhin himself has said, surely nothing other than benefit can flow from the meeting together in common cause of scientists of differing political persuasions or, indeed, of none.

In comparison with the great scientific unions of the world, it is certain we possess an advantage, in that our object is not merely scientific but also medical and humane. Let us continue to cherish this prospect for all the good it brings.

Secondly am I persuaded that our Union must adopt its true posture again not narrowly but in proper relation to the entire spectrum of scientific endeavor. In England as in the United States and doubtless in other countries, recent years have witnessed a great debate on scientific priorities, especially between the demands of space exploration and of the more earthbound sciences. I have always taken the view that we have here a quite false confrontation, and that there is nothing antithetic between them. Pursuing this line, I have ever been impressed by the case of the illustrious Ramon y Cajal, who with his own hands delineated the microstructure of the nervous system. To this day, in the Cajal Museum in Madrid one may see the master's desk, his simple microscope, his histological stains, his pencils and his notebooks. Yet apart from his unique talents as microscopist, Cajal also became famous as a gifted astronomer and in the corner of the same room one may still see his astronomical telescope. In a special way this preserves for me, and doubtless many others, as in a moral or exemplar, the unity of Nature from the incomprehensible depths of the universe to the infinitely small structures and dimensions of the living cell—a unity of which our Union remains a part and must seek to uphold.

This is the last occasion on which I shall address the Union and the Congress, certainly in any official capacity. I wish, therefore, to extend to both my grateful thanks for so many kindnesses, and for their confidence in me over these years. I wish to congratulate dear Professor Blokhin upon his own Presidency, and on the eve of his inauguration cannot do better than to wish Dr. Gardner and his wife Katherine all that joy and satisfaction which fell to my own lot in the conduct of the Union.

God bless our Union and its great cause; God bless this city of Houston; God bless our hosts; God bless America!

TOMIZO YOSHIDA: *President, Ninth International Cancer Congress.* Mr. Governor of the State of Texas, Mr. President of the International Union Against Cancer, Dr. Blokhin, Mr. President of the Congress, Dr. Wendell Stanley, Distinguished Guests, Ladies and Gentlemen:

Four years ago it was my very great privilege, as President of the Ninth International Cancer Congress, to welcome to Tokyo over 4,000 oncologists from all over the world.

Today, on behalf of all those who came to our shores, it is my pleasure to address a message of cheer and of good will to our American hosts and to you all, members and associate members of the Tenth International Cancer Congress.

This splendid Ceremony is a unique occasion for the International Union Against Cancer. Indeed, it marks the Tenth International Cancer Congress held under its auspices and also—within a few days—the thirty-fifth anniversary of its foundation in Paris on the 4th of May 1935.

I bring to you every good wish for a successful Congress. May this meeting be a turning point in the worldwide campaign against cancer.

R. LEE CLARK: *Chairman, National Organizing Committee.* More has been learned about the molecular biology of cancer in the past 20 years than in the previous 20 centuries. This has not resulted in the better care of the cancer patient at the community level—which appears at a virtual standstill. Progress has been made in the understanding of the uncontrolled growth of cancers through research in fields such as molecular biology, cytogenetics, virology, and immunology. With the information gleaned in laboratories, it has been possible to exercise some control over the milieu of the growing cell by such procedures as the manipulation of hormones, cell metabolism, the enhancement or suppression of immunologic responses, and by chemotherapy. New accesses to improved care are being opened with examination of the mechanisms of cell replication and DNA elaboration, and the understanding of the role of the genetic messages in chromosome structure and cellular destiny. These and the results of other investigations will eventually solve most of the problems of control or cure of cancer in man.

However, it is difficult to predict the amount of time necessary for the discovery and widespread utilization of this needed knowledge. We must, therefore, also concentrate our efforts and attention on what can be done now. Of great importance is the solution to problems of the delivery of better health care with the technics presently available to us. With more refined technics for prevention and early diagnosis, and more knowledge of environmental factors which influence the development of carcinogenic conditions, leading to increasingly widespread education of the general public, we can no longer fail to recognize the vital and immediate need for the addition of specialty training in oncology.

The most essential factor in the delivery of comprehensive care for the cancer patient is the team approach. Heretofore, in the development of medicine in the United States, the attitude has been that a Board-qualified general surgeon had knowledge of all surgical problems and, therefore, of cancer problems also. This assumption has proved to be one of the greatest drawbacks to the betterment of the care of the cancer patient. Too often the opportunity to cure has been lost through inept surgical therapy or by aggressive operations applied with no real understanding of the specific and unique factors encountered with cancer.

Radiotherapy in many countries has frequently been delivered by men with knowledge of diagnostic radiology but little or no understanding of the natural course or extent of cancerous disease, or of the special knowledge required in the application of radiation energy in the control of neoplastic disease.

The pathologist especially trained and interested in cancer pathology and its clinical interpretation is an invaluable and indispensable participant in the care of the cancer patient. There are too few centers where there is a primary interest in cytology and frozen-section surgical diagnosis, backed up by an ultrafine structure interpretation.

The internist has been invaluable in the diagnostic phase of cancer care and in providing supportive measures during surgical and radiation therapy. In addition, in the past ten years the roles of cancer chemotherapist and hemotherapist have evolved as a medical specialty. This field is of great significance now as regards the palliation of the patient with disseminated malignant disease and, for the future, offers our greatest hope for cure.

A majority of the internists qualified in this field acquired their expertise through the National Cancer Chemotherapy Study Programs in this and other countries. Even so, there is a greater shortage of oncologically oriented physicians in internal medicine than in any of the other medical specialties. No community is adequately staffed with these specially trained internists, and many groups interested in cancer have no internist associated with them.

The psychologist, psychiatrist, and physiatrist are available to the cancer patient in only a very few cancer centers.

With respect to cancer care, there is no longer a place in medicine for the single physician except in cancer detection. The oncologic team is the only answer to better treatment. Proper treatment must be administered in an environment in which decisions regarding long-term management and rehabilitation are made after review of the manifestations of the particular disease in the individual patient. As curative regimens for cancer, be they surgical therapy, radiotherapy, chemotherapy, or a combination of these, are usually radical in application, it is essential that the initial treatment be the proper treatment, effectively administered and followed up. If our present knowledge of proper cancer therapy can be applied in such a manner by a medical team trained in oncology, the financial investment in care of the cancer patient can be reduced considerably and a more productive and longer existence for the patient will result.

The late Dr. Charles H. Mayo (1865-1939) once wrote; "There are two objects of medical education: To heal the sick and to advance the science." (Collected papers of the Mayo Clinic and Mayo Foundation 18:1093, 1926.) We must begin now to insist that our physicians in specialty training receive additional training in oncology, as this knowledge is acquired only by long study and careful application under supervision in a multidisciplinary setting. Only in this manner will we "advance the science" to better heal the sick.

When we have individuals who, in addition to the classic basic medical education, are trained for full-time oncologic work, we will be able to achieve maximum results with the current knowledge. In a very short time, we could increase our five-year survivals by an appreciable percentage, 50 per cent or more.

During this Tenth International Cancer Congress of the International Union Against Cancer, the hundreds of fine presentations will point eloquently to the future possibilities for scientific advances toward cancer prevention, cure, and control. But let us not lose sight of the progress which has been made in the last decade or so which we are obligated to utilize more effectively by the oncologic team approach. While our research laboratories are working so diligently toward the eventual total control and cure of all cancer patients, we have within our grasp the means to enhance the quality and duration of existence of cancer patients NOW, a goal we believe all physicians must subscribe to as they grow to appreciate this opportunity.

WELCOMING ADDRESS

The Honorable SPIRO T. AGNEW

Vice President of the United States of America

Mr. Chairman, Distinguished Members, and Guests:

On behalf of the President, I bid our eminent visitors welcome to the United States of America and extend sincere wishes for a productive and successful congress. We recognize and deeply value the honor you do us by holding this meeting in our country.

You gather here from all parts of the world, joined in a common cause to free man of one of the grim threats to his existence. You represent diverse social and political ways of life and yet you have succeeded in working together, in reasoning together, in exchanging information freely, and in recognizing and enunciating common goals. Your success is vital to all of us, not only because of the improvement in the human condition that the eradication of cancer would achieve, but also because of the example you set.

If we can succeed in working together for the elimination of cancer, why can we not succeed in other areas of human endeavor—in our striving for world peace, in our desire to reverse the insidious course which befounds our environment in our desire to free men to develop to their ultimate capacities with dignity?

Today, we are told that the promising results of research indicate that viruses play an important role in the development of cancer. However, we also are discovering that other factors act as stimuli to activate the conditions induced by viruses. Moreover, it is quite likely that these stimuli are to be found in our environment. Thus, the causal factors of cancer may reside to a significant degree in the surroundings in which we live. The problem of identifying the damaging elements in our environment and of mitigating their effects is one of the critical challenges of our era. We are threatened with the destruction of much that we have created, if we remain ignorant of, or oblivious to, environmental hazards, which appear to be growing with extraordinary rapidity. As in all human endeavors, we need balance. In this case, we need to reconcile the indirect dangers of a rapidly developing technology with the requirements of modern society. We need to perfect the mechanisms by which national and international policies are formulated. To achieve that difficult end, this country is now strongly committed to advancing the quality of life at home and to cooperating with other countries to solve environmental problems of an international nature. Each of our nations is confronted by enormous problems, and our mutual efforts to solve them cooperatively are in their infancy. The difficulty cannot be over-estimated, since we are only beginning to learn how to deal with these challenges at the national level. But we recognize the need and the moral obligation of all countries to share their experience and knowledge so that people every-where can benefit.

As one country learns to cope more successfully with a particular problem, and another country achieves the same progress in relation to a different problem, these capacities must be made known for the benefit of all. In essence, this is a problem of the transfer of technology from one society to another. It involves the transfer of technology from countries with highly developed skills in certain areas to countries with less developed skills. These exchanges have begun, but must be accelerated by a sense of urgency, a sense of commitment, and greater imagination in creating new mechanisms and new institutions to deal with our new problems. One important example of such a new com-mon effort to deal with environmental degradation is the President's initiative within NATO. This initiative, like his renunciation of bio-logical warfare as an offensive weapon, is a clear example of his sincere desire to cope with the practicalities of inherent environmental dan-gers.

At the occasion of the twentieth anniversary of NATO last April he said: "The industrial nations share no challenge more urgent than that of bringing 20th century man and his environment to terms with one another—of making the world fit for man, and helping man learn how to remain in harmony with his rapidly changing world."

At that time he proposed the establishment of the Committee on the Challenges of Modern Society, CCMS, to focus experience in tech-nological transfer and high-level political consultation, which has char-acterized NATO over the last decade, on the common and widespread problems of pollution and social blight.

The preservation of our environment and the maintenance of the quality of life has become one of the vital issues of this generation. The health benefits of clean air and clean water and of a society free of the danger inchoate in a rapidly developing technology are goals which all free nations share in common. These problems, like cancer, re-spect no boundary and require the highest attention on the part of the leaders of all governments.

The CCMS has embarked upon an innovative approach to assist in-ternational technological transfer in the environmental field. It has utilized the concept of "pilot projects," headed by countries which are most advanced in specific fields. These pilot projects place the respon-sibility upon such countries to devise methods by which their advances can be transferred and made useful in other countries. Right now the CCMS is working on the problems of air and water pollution, road safety, regional planning, sea pollution, human motivation, and disaster relief. The goal in each of these fields is concrete action to up-grade the capability of all countries to deal with these threats to our common environment.

I believe that it is imperative that we seek more diligently for new methods to improve the transfer of knowledge and technology. The organization under whose auspices this congress is being held, the International Union Against Cancer, represents some seventy nations of the world, and is a successful example of such efforts. The International Agency for Cancer, which includes countries from east and west, and which has initiated world-wide studies of the factors in our environment which relate to human cancer, is another example. Such efforts deserve continuing and expanded support from every direction.

There is also a need to share advances in the organization and management of health services. Quite obviously, the world's population is served best when the results of basic research can be applied most quickly to patient care or programs of preventive medicine.

I am told that in my country, under conditions as they exist today, we cure approximately one out of every three cancer patients. I am told too that if our current approaches to the delivery of medical care were improved, it might be possible to increase the cure rate to one out of every two patients with cancer. To achieve this, individuals must have greater access to physicians, physicians must be better trained to recognize cancer in its early stages, and highly sophisticated care centers must be available to patients once the disease is recognized. There is much that we need to do to achieve this goal; but even if we did achieve it, it would still be only a partial solution.

Observers of existing techniques in medical care find that it is expensive, poorly distributed, and in need of resourceful innovation and systematic improvement. There is no doubt in my mind that a country with the organizational and developmental capacity to send a man to the moon can also apply managerial and design technology to improve its systems for the delivery of medical care. I find, however, a tendency in my country to look mainly to the government to solve this problem. In some of the countries represented here today, the central government has assumed complete responsibility for the provision of medical care, and I am sure that as we Americans turn to improvement of our own system, we will benefit by an examination of their experience. However, I feel that a totally governmental response is not in our national character. The improvement of medical care is a problem in which the private and public sectors must join together, with the Federal government acting primarily as a catalyst, to accelerate significant change. The President and his Secretary of Health, Education and Welfare are meeting this challenge. They have proposed new legislation to modify Federal support for health care in such a way as to encourage private efforts to improve systems for the delivery of care. We have created a National Center for Health Service, Research and Development in the Delivery of Health Care to explore the path before us. There are those who believe that the simple solution of allocating additional funds will alleviate many of the difficulties. I doubt this. We are spending $12.3 billion a year in Medicare and Medicaid programs alone. Ironically, some economists now claim that this investment is aggravating the medical care problem by increasing the disparity between supply and demand. Money alone is not an answer, and unfortunately, in this period of our nation's economy, unlimited sums of money are not available for all the social causes crying out for support. I believe, however, that we could make significantly better use of the Federal funds now allocated for the delivery of medical care. For solutions to this problem, I am hopeful that the medical profession, our institutions of learning, and government will follow the example set by the organization meeting here today. We must and can join in common cause to see to it that our knowledge and skills reach all patients unimpeded by deficiencies in medical care delivery systems.

As I have noted, even if we improved our system for the delivery of medical care, in the field of cancer it would only bring us halfway toward our goal. It will be primarily from biomedical research that we can glean the information needed to take us the full distance. President Nixon has indicated his full understanding of the value of basic research to our national life. He believes that research is "an investment in the future." He has pointed out that today's basic research leads to tomorrow's treatment and prevention of disease, and that such treatment or prevention not only relieves human misery but also saves billions of dollars which can then be reinvested in improvements in the delivery system. Despite the economic stringency of our time, we will nevertheless make every effort to continue the important work which men like you are doing. Our proposed Federal investment in health research in 1971 will be higher than it ever has been. We recognize that even more money could be utilized for increased support, not just for the study of cancer, but for the broad spectrum of research as well, since no one can really predict the particular field of study that will give rise to tomorrow's treatment for a specific disease. As soon as our economy permits it, we hope to provide even greater support.

I have been talking about tangible contributions made to the nation and to the world by research. I would like to add an intangible one. I call it "the contagiousness of excellence." As a former student of chemistry, I believe I can claim some insight into the standards and philosophy of scientific research. It allows for no false values, no hypocrisy, no cant. An observation is valid or not valid; supported by evidence, or unsupported. A theory either stands the test of further research or falls. The hallmark of research is a quality of thought, a quality of effort which, if spread to other areas of our daily lives, would have a most salutary effect. In times of political and economic difficulty, long-term values are often displaced by short-term ones. We cannot afford to lose the excitement of excellence which permeates the best examples of biomedical research.

I find another virtue in the pursuit of science, namely, as a channel into which the youth of a nation can pour its impressive drive to create a better world. Although I in no way challenge their right and indeed their obligation to make their voices heard responsibly in the corridors of political power, I would draw their attention to the challenges of the laboratories of science as well. I urge more young men and women to join in the difficult but challenging course of action exemplified by the activities of every individual at this meeting. The solution to the problem of cancer will take diligent research, long-term investment of time and energy, an optimistic faith that the problem can be solved, and a dedication to the improvement of human life. Is this not what our youth are demanding, and is this not a proper battle for them to join? Like most adults and young people, I am a fervent supporter of your goals, your values, and your methods. It is my wish that working together we can all contribute to the alleviation of man's suffering.

I propose that the nations of this world, plagued by many ills—some of our own making, some born of nature—that these nations, which occupy only a very small portion of the universe, declare the next ten years to be the Decade Against Disease. Let us join in any manner open to us—by increasing the exchange of information, by joining in co-operative research projects, by avoiding unnecessary duplication of unusual and expensive facilities, by examining the health hazards in our environment, by committing funds when we can, and most important, by rising above narrow self-interest—let us join together in a determined venture to make life and health one birthright of all children born from this day on regardless of nationality, race or religious beliefs.

Thank you for allowing me one opportunity to share the spirit of this congress with you.

ANNOUNCEMENTS AND RESOLUTIONS ADOPTED BY THE COUNCIL

ROBERT M. TAYLOR, *Secretary-General*

International Union Against Cancer

ANNOUNCEMENT 1: *Awards of Merit*

The Council of the Union has created a merit award to be given to individuals who have served the Union with distinction as members of the Council and who have retired.

At the meeting of the Council on May 20, the members gave unanimous approval to the recommendation of the Honors and Awards Committee that the following receive awards of merit:

Dr. E. V. Cowdry	USA
Professor Sir Alexander Haddow	UK
Dr. H. Hamperl	Fed. Rep. of Germany
Dr. J. R. Heller	USA
Dr. V. R. Khanolkar	India
Dr. L. Kreyberg	Norway
Dr. A. Lacassagne	France
Dr. J. H. Maisin	Belgium
Dr. O. Mühlbock	The Netherlands
Dr. P. R. Peacock	UK
Dr. M. J. Shear	USA
Dr. H. L. Stewart	USA
Dr. T. Yoshida	Japan

ANNOUNCEMENT 2: *Members Elected to the Council*

At the General Assembly the following retired from membership on the Council:

Dr. T. Antoine	Austria
Dr. A. Graffi	German Democratic Republic
Dr. I. Berenblum	Israel
Dr. O. Mühlbock	The Netherlands
Dr. E. Raventos	Chile
Dr. H. L. Stewart	USA
Dr. P. N. Wahi	India

In their place the following were elected:

Dr. P. Bucalossi	Italy
Dr. S. Eckhardt	Hungary
Dr. E. Grossmann	Venezuela
Dr. P. Loustalot	Switzerland
Dr. K. Oota	Japan
Dr. C. Heidelberger	USA
Dr. N. Trainin	Israel
Dr. T. Yamamoto	Japan

ANNOUNCEMENT 3: *Vice Presidents*

At the meeting of the Council which followed the General Assembly, the following were elected as Vice-Presidents of the Union:

Africa	Dr. C. Quenum	Dakar
Asia	Dr. K. Shanmugaratnam	Singapore
Europe	Dr. E. Hecker	Fed. Rep. Germany
	Dr. Hanna Kolodziejska	Poland
Latin America	Dr. R. A. Estevez	Argentina
North America	Dr. M. M. Copeland	USA
Oceania	Dr. D. Metcalf	Australia

ANNOUNCEMENT 4: *Eleventh International Cancer Congress*

Mr. President, the Council has given consideration to the time and place of meeting of the Eleventh International Cancer Congress. It had been concluded that it should be held in Europe, and gracious invitations had been received from a number of countries.

I am pleased to announce that the invitation of Italy has been accepted and that the next Congress will be held in the historic city of Florence in September 1974.

> Dr. P. Bucalossi, of Milano, President of the Congress.
> Dr. U. Veronesi, also of Milano, Vice-President of the Congress.

ANNOUNCEMENT 5: *Resolutions of Gratitude*

I. The Council of the International Union Against Cancer expresses its gratitude to the Honorable John B. Connally, former Governor of the State of Texas, and the Honorary Chairman of the National Organizing Committee, to Mr. Frank Erwin, Chairman of the Board of Regents, and to Dr. Harry H. Ransom, Chancellor of The University of Texas System, and to the members of their staffs for the warmth of the reception given to members of the Congress, and delegates of the member organizations of the Union.

II. On behalf of the members and associate members of this Congress, the Council of the International Union Against Cancer congratulates the President, Dr. Wendell M. Stanley, for its success.

The Council offers its gratitude to the members of the National Organizing Committee and, in particular, to Dr. R. Lee Clark, Chairman of the Committee and President of The University of Texas M. D. Anderson Hospital and Tumor Institute at Houston, to Dr. Murray M. Copeland, Secretary General of the Congress, and to the members of his Secretariat under the direction of Miss Donna McCormick on the excellence of the arrangements which made possible this gathering, and which contributed so importantly to its success.

The Council expresses its appreciation and its admiration to Dr. C. Heidelberger and to the members of the Program Committee for having implemented the new design of the Congress format with such competence and vigor.

The Council also makes special mention of the efforts of the local Organizing Committee under the Chairmanship of Dr. Clifton D. Howe.

III. The Council places on record the appreciation of the Union to those whose contributions provided the means of organizing this Congress. They include the Legislature of the State of Texas, the National Cancer Institute, the American Cancer Society (New York), and the Texas Division of the American Cancer Society, The University of Texas M. D. Anderson Hospital and Tumor Institute at Houston, the University Cancer Foundation of The University of Texas, the Calouste Gulbenkian Foundation, the Leukemia Society of America, the Edward Mallinckrodt, Jr. Foundation, and the Sid W. Richardson Foundation.

The Council also records its appreciation of the generosity of Mrs. Harry C. Wiess, Mr. and Mrs. Theodore N. Law, Mr. and Mrs. Lloyd H. Smith, Mr. and Mrs. James A. Elkins, Jr., and Mr. and Mrs. Hub Hill.

CLOSING ADDRESSES

WILLIAM U. GARDNER: *Incoming President, International Union Against Cancer.* As I accept this gavel of office, let me be the first to welcome you, Professor Blokhin, to your position as Past President of the UICC as a member of the Executive Committee.

Dr. Blokhin's extensive experience is respected and will be of great value to us in the UICC in the years to come. I hope that I may be worthy of my predecessors, Professor Blokhin, Sir Alexander Haddow, and Professor Maisin, who are on this stage at this time. I believe that many who participate in the programs of the International Congresses are not aware of what the Union does between the Congresses.

The Congresses and their arrangements, under the auspices of the Union, are predominately the responsibility of the hosting country, or institutions, or organizations therein. They are high points and they occur every four years, in recent years. The work of the Union, however, continues between Congresses, and I think it might be appropriate here to mention some of this. It is largely conducted by Commissions and by Committees. I will introduce the Chairmen of the Commissions and ask them to stand and be recognized so that you may know them. A nucleic Commission begins to function at this Congress. This Commission on the Social Campaign and Organization has Mr. Frank Wilcox, USA, Chairman. Two other Commission chairmen replace former chairmen—the Commission on Fellowships and Personnel Exchange: Dr. Henry Isliker, Switzerland, Chairman. The Commission on Epidemiology: Dr. Gregory T. O'Conor, USA, Chairman. Three other Commission chairmen continue for second terms: Commission on Clinical Oncology: Dr. Pierre Denoix, France, Chairman. Commission on Cancer Control: Dr. E. C. Easson, U.K., Chairman. Commission on Experimental Oncology: Professor R. J. C. Harris, U.K., Chairman.

These are the men who directed the work and arranged the programs of the Union. Those of you who have seen the UICC booths on the exhibit floor have seen some of the results of the activities of these Commissions and their committees in the published monographs and/or the technical reports that have appeared there.

Other members of the Executive Committee are Dr. C. Schmidt, Treasurer, FRG; Sir William Kilpatrick, who is not with us today, Australia, Chairman of the Finance Committee; Dr. Prosper Loustalot and Dr. M. Dargent of France, our electorate from the Executive Committee to the Council.

I shall deliberately overlook one of the important members of the Executive Committee at this time; we will hear more from him later. All of these Commissions and the offices are assisted by the Director of the Geneva Office, Dr. J. F. Delafresnaye and his able staff. Since the office is located in Switzerland, we might say that these are the people who keep the Union ticking between Congresses, and intercongress meetings.

Now during this Congress, we have heard much of transformation, usually transformation from the normal to the malignant state; a change inside is usually by some agent. A transformation has occurred in Houston. After a certain research-oriented surgeon emerged from the Air Force Medical Corps in 1946, he began on August 1, 1946, a transformation of a house called The Oaks, and as I have been told, some army barracks that were at that time serving as a cancer detection center or cancer hospital into what we know as the M. D. Anderson complex. It is obvious that this institution has grown expansively, that it has even metastasized and the agent has emerged to be President of The University of Texas M. D. Anderson Hospital and Tumor Institute at Houston, one of the largest hospitals in one of the largest cancer institutes in the USA.

R. LEE CLARK: *Chairman, National Organizing Committee.* Thank you, Dr. Gardner. I have mixed emotions at this time. We are at the beginning of the second half of the pain-pleasure syndrome. We have had our pains in preparing for the Congress, but now we are going to enjoy it very much in retrospect. It has been wonderful to have all of you here, and I want to say how much Dr. Doll's talk has contributed to this program (see Dorn Lecture, Volume V). I will leave the Congress with new perspectives. If we follow through with all of Dr. Doll's suggestions, it will decrease cancer incidence a great deal—he has given us vital information on how to prevent cancer, if we can carry these recommendations through to their conclusion.

I have been fortunate to be permitted to be the Chairman of the National Organizing Committee, and to work with Dr. Blokhin from Russia and President of the UICC, and Dr. Gardner, an American who now is assuming the Presidency of the UICC, and to have the strength and backing of Dr. Wendell Stanley in making this Congress possible.

In addition, we wish to remind you that we have had the support of the National Academy of Sciences, with President Phil Handler. Over the last four years they have supplied us with the working arrangement of the National Academy of Sciences and its assurance of international cooperation.

To the American Committee of the UICC who appointed me Chairman of the National Organizing Committee of the Congress, my thanks, particularly for your help in making this program the success that it might be; and to Former Governor John Connally for accepting the honorary chairmanship and for working with Mayor Welch in organizing the Houston Salute to the Congress, for which we are most grateful.

Governor Preston Smith also declared this Cancer Week in Texas, and hence we have had excellent support from local individuals and press, who enjoyed their own participation in an international conference.

We are also grateful to the members of the local Organizing Committee, with Dr. Howe as Chairman, for planning the entertainment. The Ladies' Entertainment Committee did an extraordinary job. To Drs. Martin and Jesse, and the many other people who have aided us, we extend our thanks with gratitude. Dr. Scott has done an enormous job in co-ordinating the press and communications coverage. Dr. Charles Heidelberger has done an incredible job in personally reviewing every paper before it was placed on the program. Last, but most certainly not the least, is our thanks to the office of the Secretary General, from which we could have had no greater aid than that provided by Dr. Copeland and his Executive Assistant, Donna McCormick, and their total staff.

Finally, I would like to express my pleasure that Florence has been selected for the next meeting—a city that has been, perhaps, the heartbeat and mind in changing from the medieval period of lack of science to a period of its advancement.

For this reason I look with good faith and anticipation toward the Congress meeting in Florence where hopefully we will report on concrete victories in the war against cancer.

MURRAY M. COPELAND: *Secretary General, Tenth International Cancer Congress.* As secretary general of the Tenth International Cancer Congress of the UICC, I salute you on this final day of the Congress.

On behalf of the officials of the National Organizing Committee, the Program Committee, and all others who have contributed to the preparations for the Congress, I extend you a poignant farewell.

It has been our privilege and pleasure to have you as guests and as participants in the Tenth Congress. May the rapport of friendship and understanding generated at this meeting continue in the years ahead and enhance the deliberations necessary for planning future programs and meetings of the Union.

An organization's stature can be measured by a twofold norm—its ideals and the effort expended to achieve them. Both have their root source in the leadership and the sense of values which such an organization possesses. Of full stature then, is our great organization which, blessed by scholarly leadership and fully conscious of the humanitarian needs in the field of cancer control, stimulates a broad spectrum of activities in cancer education, research, and improved diagnosis and treatment of the cancer patient.

In closing, I should like to offer an expression of hope that the discoveries of a mass of curiously related information which have unfolded at an ever-accelerating rate will ultimately mark the end of some of mankind's cruelest diseases, and liberate the mind to travel further and further into unexplored regions, at least as exciting and full of promise as the frontiers now beckoning beyond the distant stars.

WENDELL M. STANLEY: *President, Tenth International Cancer Congress.* Let me congratulate you, Doctor Gardner, on your ascendancy to the Presidency of the International Union Against Cancer. Your years of experience in international medical affairs will enable you to provide effective leadership. Doctor Blokhin, your warm, friendly personality and great and effective leadership make you a difficult President to follow but in Doctor Gardner you have an able successor. Let me first say how much I appreciate the high honor of being selected to be President of this Tenth International Cancer Congress, a Congress which has been such an outstanding success due largely to the hard work and cooperation of hundreds of men and women. I suspect that I was selected to be President as a representative from basic biomedical science, an area which has contributed so much recently to advance our knowledge of cancer. Although I have worked in the basic biomedical area most of my life, my training was recognized, not by an M.D. but by the Ph.D. Thus, although custom has been temporarily changed, the basic biomedical sciences have been recognized.

Now I am not a stranger to Houston for I have been coming here two or three times a year for well over twenty years, in one capacity or another. I remember seeing the gleam in Lee Clark's eyes many, many years ago. The magnificent M. D. Anderson Hospital and Tumor Institute is one result—an organization equal to any in the world and one which has meant life and hope to so many. Another result is this Tenth International Cancer Congress. Now I know that you will not expect me to summarize the events of the Congress—especially the 1800 or so scientific contributions. But I do feel some comments are in order. First, the organization of this Congress differed from those of previous years —mainly by the two and one-half days of Preliminary Special Sessions and by the Postgraduate Course Panels. During the first, 108 distinguished experts from all parts of the world described the latest advances in four specialized areas of basic and clinical biomedical science, namely (1) Regulation of Gene Expression in Normal and Cancer Cells; (2) Cancer Therapy: Experimental Models and Clinical Trials; (3) Cellular and Molecular Mechanisms of Carcinogenesis; and (4) Trends in the Diagnosis and Management of Cancer. Then four dedicated, especially knowledgeable and brave men, Drs. George Weber, Joseph Burchenal, Robert J. C. Harris, and Pierre Denoix, undertook the difficult task of evaluating this material. They succeeded admirably and made splendid presentations to the entire Congress on Tuesday morning. Insofar as I have been able to ascertain from conversations with colleagues in the basic sciences and in the clinical and teaching areas, this procedure, as well as the Postgraduate Course Panels, was an outstanding success. The Program Committee, with the patient and very able Charles Heidelberger as Chairman, which was responsible for this departure from custom, should be especially comforted and pleased by the result.

I listened to dozens of the hundreds of proffered papers and I must say golden nuggets of useful information turned up in the usual and in unexpected places. I learned that through careful investigative work and innumerable clinical trials during the past few years, we are now ready to battle cancer in its diverse forms with several clinically effective chemical agents. In some cases the cure rates have risen to as high as 80 per cent, a figure approaching perfection in a biological world. Immune mechanisms and immunotherapy are now better understood and the latter is being used effectively. And, of course, the surgeon and the radiotherapist have continued their steady improvement of treatment procedures so that, all in all, we are closely approaching the cure of one out of two cancer patients instead of one out of three.

But, as anticipated by the Program Committee, it is in the basic biomedical sciences, and especially in virology, that the greatest and most important advances have been made. Here the audiences have been large and attentive and the golden nuggets of useful knowledge have been many indeed, so many, in fact, that I cannot possibly do justice to them at this time. But I cannot resist quoting two sentences from the talk I gave just one week ago at the opening of the Preliminary Special Sessions. "It is obvious that an understanding of the mechanism involved in one type of transformation is close at hand. Perhaps via the use of temperature-sensitive viral mutants the door will soon be opened." Well, today, Ladies and Gentlemen, one week later we know the door has been opened. In two or more laboratories viral transformation has been traced down to a single gene or gene product—and the activity of this gene is not necessary for the multiplication of the viral genome. In another case, transformation was accompanied by a change in the carbohydrate synthesized at the cell membrane or by the exposure of a previously hidden carbohydrate site. And in another situation, the elimination of an amino acid from the nutrient medium of certain transformed human cells resulted in a great burst of growth of a previously hidden virus. Studies of membranes and of membrane components are assuming greater importance than ever before. More and more I am becoming convinced—as I stated many years ago—that viruses, chemical carcinogens and radiation have a common target, the DNA of the host cell and even perhaps the DNA of one certain pair of chromosomes in the case of man. We should assume an integrated approach to this common problem. But I still believe that the viruses continue to provide by far the best experimental approach. Integration, semipermanent or readily reversible, of part or all of the information of a virus with the DNA of the host is now an accepted way of life, with all of the consequences and implications which derive therefrom. Truly, molecular biology can be expected to provide very important and useful information in the immediate future.

Now let me pay tribute to the International Union Against Cancer, and our hosts, the National Academy of Sciences and The University of Texas M. D. Anderson Hospital and Tumor Institute at Houston. Also to the National Organizing Committee of the Congress, the Local Organizing Committee and the Secretariat, all of whom deserve much credit for the success of the scientific program and local arrangements. We are all greatly indebted to the United Nations Postal Administration for issuing two "Fight Cancer" stamps on the opening day of the Congress. The special films, exhibits, daily newspaper, and Congress T.V. program were greatly appreciated by all. Although my occupation at the scientific programs prevented my attendance at any of the programs for ladies, my wife tells me that these programs were most outstanding. Homes and hearts were opened to Congress guests from all over the world, and the weather has generally been good to us. The hospitality and organization were magnificent—so on behalf of all participants including my wife—a warm and sincere "Thank you" to the Ladies Entertainment Program Committee. The tours and special events such as the Rodeo, the plays at the Alley Theatre, and the Symphony in this beautiful and functional Jones Hall last evening were great and have served to provide warm, pleasant, lasting memories for hundreds upon hundreds of visitors from this and 70 other countries of the world. As Doctor Blokhin has already said, this Congress has been not only the largest but also the best. Thanks are due to our Houston hosts and to participants from all over the world. I now extend best wishes to all of you as you return to home and work, having benefitted greatly by participation in this Tenth International Cancer Congress. I look forward to seeing you at the next Congress four years hence in Florence, Italy. I now have the duty and the honor to declare the Congress is officially closed.

FAREWELL MESSAGE TO CONGRESS PARTICIPANTS

R. LEE CLARK: *Chairman, National Organizing Committee.* William Hazlitt, 19th century English essayist, said, "When a thing ceases to be a subject of controversy, it ceases to be a subject of interest." You may not fully agree with this man who seemed to thrive on controversy, but it is true that we have a full measure of healthy controversy and a high level of interest in cancer treatment and in cancer research. The third aspect of the cancer troika, that of the need for the exchange and dissemination of information for the education of all, elicits almost total agreement, as has been so eloquently demonstrated during this Congress.

I am sure all of us are most grateful for an opportunity once again to meet, discuss, teach, and learn, and to be united in our efforts to reduce the scourge of cancer to a manageable level, as has been done throughout most of the world with plague, smallpox, poliomyelitis, and other diseases which have killed or maimed human beings in frightening numbers.

We are grateful to each of you for your contributions, cooperation, and good will. We wish you Godspeed on the return to your homes and to your work.

Part A

CELLULAR AND MOLECULAR MECHANISMS OF CARCINOGENESIS

1

Reactive Forms of Chemical Carcinogens: Interactions with Tissue Components

Historical Review and Perspectives

ELIZABETH C. MILLER

*McArdle Laboratory for Cancer Research, University of Wisconsin,
Madison, Wisconsin, USA*

THIS SESSION on the reactive forms of chemical carcinogens occurs in the year of the fortieth anniversary of the first report on the induction of tumors with a pure chemical, i.e., the demonstration by Kennaway and Hieger[42] of the induction of skin tumors in the mouse upon application of 1,2,5,6-dibenzanthracene. Only three years later, the carcinogenic activity of the first of the visceral carcinogens was reported by Yoshida,[109] who had observed the carcinogenicity of o-aminoazotoluene for the liver of the rat. Soon after, Hueper and his associates[37] demonstrated that 2-naphthylamine, previously implicated as a urinary bladder carcinogen for man,[12] was carcinogenic for the urinary bladder of the dog. The succeeding years have seen studies on the mechanism of action of these and many other chemical carcinogens develop on a broad international basis.

In recent years, it has become increasingly apparent that many chemical carcinogens are not active as such, but require conversion in vivo to metabolites which are the ultimate carcinogenic forms. Thus, much of the specificity of certain chemical carcinogens for particular species and particular tissues now appears to be a function of the amounts of the ultimate carcinogenic metabolites which are available to the tissues as a consequence of metabolic activation in situ or of transport from sites of activation or both. Furthermore, deductions as to the nature of the ultimate carcinogenic metabolite (s) for a number of carcinogenic chemicals are now possible on the basis of the in vitro and in vivo reactivities of known and probable metabolites of the carcinogens, from the structures of the protein- and nucleic acid-bound derivatives in tumor-susceptible tissues, and from correlations between the amounts of these macromolecule-bound carcinogens and the likelihood of tumor development under a variety of conditions.

Although much emphasis has been placed on the classes of chemical carcinogens as separate entities, more recent studies indicate that these distinctions are not of fundamental importance, since the ultimate reactive forms of most, if not all, chemical carcinogens appear to be similar in that they are strong electrophiles, i.e., compounds with electron-deficient atoms. The finding that most or all ultimate chemical carcinogens are strong electrophiles (see below) provides a unified view of the in vivo reactivity of the structurally diverse chemical carcinogens. It also predicts some uniformity in the sites on the cellular macromolecules which are susceptible to their attack. Furthermore, it is probable that these strong electrophiles will attack nucleophilic sites in a somewhat indiscriminate manner and that the positions substituted will depend in part on the accessibility of various nucleophilic sites to the electrophile. This accessibility will be determined by such factors as the solubility and half-life of the electrophile, the amounts and natures of competing nucleophiles, and the presence of membranes or structural conformations which may protect certain nucleophilic sites.

Alkylating Agents and Potential Alkylating Agents

The most obvious examples of carcinogens which are electrophilic reactants are the alkylating agents (Figure 1-1). These compounds are electrophilic reactants per se, and their nonenzymatic reactivity under physiologic conditions with nucleophilic sites in proteins and nucleic acids has been well documented.[2, 31, 51, 81, 86, 90] Furthermore, where the reactions of the alkylating agents have been studied in vivo, the observed reactions have been those which also occur in vitro, as exemplified by the studies of Brookes and Lawley[2] with sulfur mustard, of Boutwell and his associates[3] and Colburn and Boutwell[13, 14] with β-propiolactone, and of Swann and Magee[99, 100] with dimethyl sulfate, methyl methanesulfonate and ethyl methanesulfonate.

Another large group of chemical carcinogens are converted to alkylating agents in vivo, and their reactivity and carcinogenicity appear to be referable to the derived alkylating agents. One group of potential alkylating agents is the carcinogenic aliphatic nitrosamides which, as shown by Schoental,[88] react readily with sulfhydryl groups at neutral pH (Figure 1-2). This reaction yields monoalkylnitrosamines, which decompose spontaneously to carbonium ions or alkyl diazonium ions, and the latter derivatives then alkylate available nucleophilic

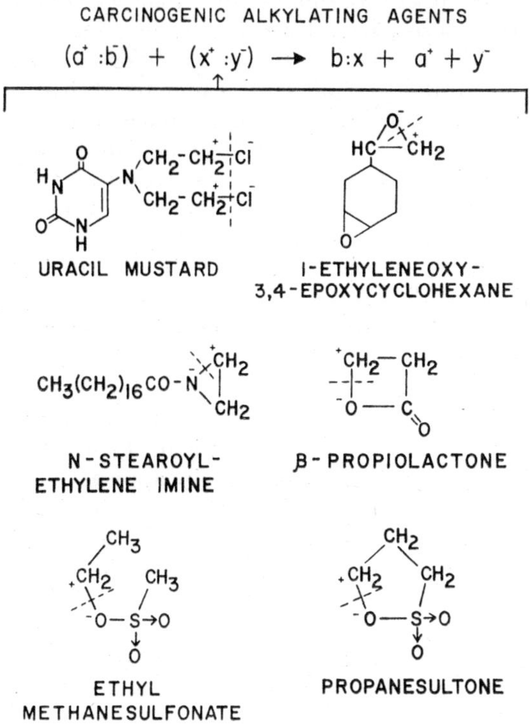
CARCINOGENIC ALKYLATING AGENTS
(a⁺ :b⁻) + (x⁺ :y⁻) → b:x + a⁺ + y⁻
URACIL MUSTARD
I-ETHYLENEOXY-3,4-EPOXYCYCLOHEXANE
N-STEAROYL-ETHYLENE IMINE
β-PROPIOLACTONE
ETHYL METHANESULFONATE
PROPANESULTONE

FIGURE 1-1.—The structures of some carcinogenic alkylating agents and the principal mechanism by which they react with nucleophiles.

sites.[52, 57, 59] In view of the ubiquitous occurrence of sulfhydryl groups in living cells, it is not surprising that tumors develop in a wide variety of tissues and species after administration of nitrosamides, as shown especially by Druckrey et al.[21, 22] Similarly, as studied especially by Magee and his associates,[58, 59] the carcinogenicity of many dialkylnitrosamines for a variety of tissues is apparently mediated by enzymatic

FIGURE 1-2.—The activation of monoalkylnitrosamides by reaction with sulfhydryl groups and the activation of dialkylnitrosamines by enzymatic oxidation to intermediates which yield alkyl carbonium ions. E. R. = endoplasmic reticulum.

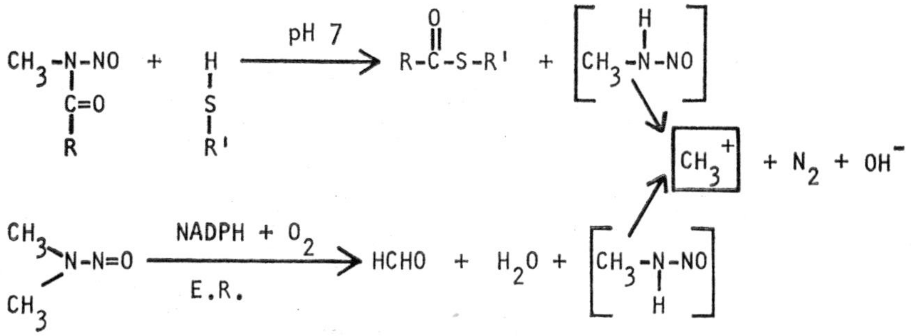
pH 7
NADPH + O2
E.R.
HCHO + H2O +
+ N2 + OH⁻

oxidative dealkylation to monoalkylnitrosamines and the decomposition of the latter to alkylating derivatives. Likewise, as demonstrated recently by Preussmann and his associates,[79, 80] the carcinogenic unsymmetrical dialkyltriazenes and the carcinogenic symmetrical hydrazo-, azo-, and azoxydialkanes are converted by the mixed function oxidases of the endoplasmic reticulum to unstable intermediates which decompose to alkyl carbonium ions (Figure 1-3). Alkylation in vivo has been observed with a number of these potential alkylating agents.[48, 53, 58] With these carcinogens which are activated by the mixed function oxidases, the levels of these enzyme systems in the various tissues and the ease of oxidation of the alkyl groups would appear to be critical factors in determining the sites and extents of alkylation and, consequently, the carcinogenic potencies and tissue specificities of the compounds.

The reactive electrophilic derivatives of these and other carcinogens which are potential alkylating agents are summarized in Figure 1-4. Thus, the carcinogenic activity and reactivity of cycasin appear to depend on its hydrolysis by β-glucosidases, especially those of the intestinal bacteria, to methylazoxymethanol which, probably via a methyl carbonium ion, methylates nucleic acids under physiologic conditions.[44, 49, 61] Likewise, the administration of the hepatocarcinogen ethionine to rats results in the ethylation of hepatic protein, RNA, and, possibly to a small extent, DNA.[25, 27, 73, 74, 85, 92] S-Adenosylethionine is formed in vivo and is probably an intermediate in these ethylation reactions, although the data of Ortwerth and Novelli[74] suggest that other intermediates may also be involved.

Certain of the pyrrolizidine alkaloids have long been known for their

FIGURE 1–3.—The activation of carcinogenic dialkyltriazenes and azoxyalkanes via enzymatic oxidative dealkylation to intermediates which yield alkyl carbonium ions. E. R. = endoplasmic reticulum.

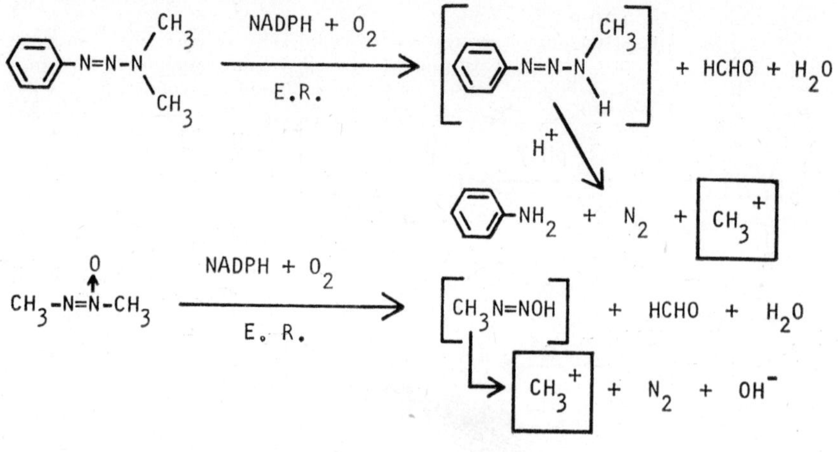

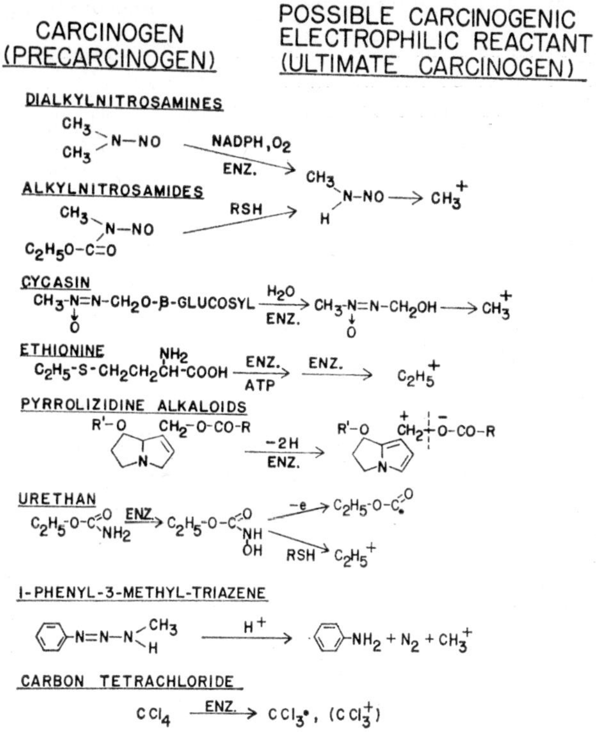

FIGURE 1–4.—Some ultimate carcinogenic electrophilic reactants that may be derived in vivo from various potential alkylating agents.

strong hepatotoxic and hepatocarcinogenic activity.[87] While these compounds have weak alkylating activity per se,[16] the recent studies of Mattocks[63] and of Culvenor et al.[17] indicate that their biologic activity and reactivity are dependent on dehydrogenation in vivo to pyrrole derivatives with strong alkylating activity.

The derivatives responsible for the reactivity and carcinogenicity of urethan and its N-hydroxy metabolites have not been elucidated. However, the finding of Boyland and Williams[9] of the carboxyethylation of cytosine in hepatic RNA of mice administered urethan and the finding of S-ethyl and of S-carboxyethyl cysteine derivatives after administration of urethan[8] suggest that the carboxyethyl-free radical and the ethyl carbonium ion are plausible intermediates. Likewise, the incorporation of ^{14}C or ^{36}Cl from labeled carbon tetrachloride into tissue proteins[83, 84] suggests that the trichloromethyl carbonium ion and the corresponding free radical may be metabolic intermediates of this hepatocarcinogen. Evidence for the formation of the free radical in vivo comes from the recent finding of hexachlorethane as a metabolite of carbon tetrachloride.[28]

Electrophilic Derivatives of Other Chemical Carcinogens

In many cases, such as those which involve the aromatic amines and amides, the natures of the ultimate reactive and carcinogenic form (s) have not been apparent from the structures of the administered carcinogens and have been deduced from other data. The first step in the activation of the aromatic amines and amides is now generally recognized to be N-hydroxylation, a reaction which was first demonstrated in our laboratory in studies on the metabolism of the versatile carcinogen 2-acetylamino-fluorene (AAF) (Figure 1-5).[15] N-Hydroxy-AAF was deduced to be a proximate carcinogenic form of AAF since it is formed in animals susceptible to the carcinogenic action of AAF, it is more carcinogenic than the parent compound at the usual sites of tumor induction, and it is carcinogenic at local sites (i.e., the subcutaneous injection site, the site of application to the skin, and the forestomach on feeding) where AAF is inactive.[66, 67, 68, 70] Furthermore, although N-hydroxy-AAF is not itself appreciably reactive with nucleophilic sites in proteins and nucleic acids,[39, 64, 65] administration of N-hydroxy-AAF gives rise to larger amounts of protein- and nucleic acid-bound fluorene derivatives in the rat liver than does the administration of AAF.[1, 18, 46, 60] Studies with other aromatic amines and amides provide strong support for the thesis that N-hydroxylation is an activation step for most, if not all, aromatic amines and amides.[34, 35, 70, 82]

FIGURE 1-5.—The metabolism of AAF to the proximate carcinogen N-hydroxy-AAF.

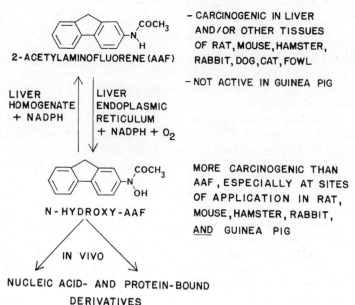

2-ACETYLAMINOFLUORENE (AAF)

– CARCINOGENIC IN LIVER AND/OR OTHER TISSUES OF RAT, MOUSE, HAMSTER, RABBIT, DOG, CAT, FOWL

– NOT ACTIVE IN GUINEA PIG

LIVER HOMOGENATE + NADPH

LIVER ENDOPLASMIC RETICULUM + NADPH + O_2

N-HYDROXY-AAF

MORE CARCINOGENIC THAN AAF, ESPECIALLY AT SITES OF APPLICATION IN RAT, MOUSE, HAMSTER, RABBIT, AND GUINEA PIG

IN VIVO

NUCLEIC ACID- AND PROTEIN-BOUND DERIVATIVES

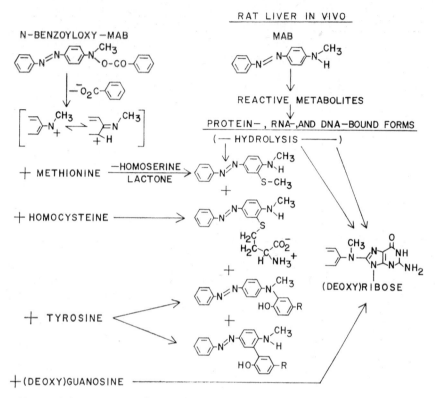

FIGURE 1-6.—Nonenzymatic reactions of the synthetic ester N-benzoyloxy-MAB with various tissue nucleophiles and the formation of the same derivatives on hydrolysis of the hepatic proteins and nucleic acids of rats administered the hepatic carcinogen MAB.

Esterification of the N-hydroxy group appears to hold at least one of the keys to the further activation of these N-hydroxy amines and amides to their ultimate reactive forms.[70, 71] The possible role of esterification was first apparent from the reactivity of synthetic esters of N-hydroxy-AAF and of N-hydroxy-N-methyl-4-aminoazobenzene with tissue nucleophiles, as compared to the inappreciable reactivity of the parent compounds under the same conditions.[54, 55, 56, 64, 65, 76] Furthermore, hydrolysis of the liver proteins and nucleic acids of rats administered the liver carcinogens N-hydroxy-AAF or N-methyl-4-aminoazobenzene yields products identical to those formed by nonenzymatic reaction of the esters with tissue nucleophiles.[18, 40, 45, 46, 54, 55, 69, 70, 89]

This situation is exemplified in Figure 1-6 for derivatives of the hepatocarcinogen N-methyl-4-aminoazobenzene (MAB). Thus, reaction of the synthetic benzoic acid ester of N-hydroxy-MAB (N-benzoyloxy-MAB) with methionine yields a methionyl derivative which decomposes readily to give 3-methylmercapto-MAB, or which, on de-methylation, would yield 3-homocysteinyl-MAB.[54, 56, 76] N-Benzoyloxy-MAB also reacts with tyrosine to yield two derivatives in which the 3-position of tyrosine is attached to the amino nitrogen or to the 3-position of MAB.[55] These two methionine and the two tyrosine derivatives of MAB are each released by hydrolysis of the liver proteins from rats administered MAB (Figure 1-5).[54, 55, 89] Similarly, reaction of N-ben-zoyloxy-MAB with guanine-containing compounds yields derivatives in which the amino nitrogen of MAB is apparently attached to the 8-position of the guanine residue.[69] Further, the ribo and deoxyribo deriva-tives of the guanyl-MAB can be isolated, respectively, from hydrolysates of the liver RNA and DNA of rats injected with MAB.[69] Thus, the re-active derivative (s) of MAB which are formed in vivo have the same reactivity properties as an ester of N-hydroxy-MAB. Furthermore, while MAB is carcinogenic in rats only in the liver where it can be metabolically activated, the synthetic reactive ester N-benzoyloxy-MAB is carcinogenic at the site of subcutaneous injection.[77]

Study of the fluorene derivatives revealed a similar situation (Figure 1-7). Thus, the synthetic sulfuric and acetic acid esters of N-hydroxy-AAF react readily at pH 7 to yield methionyl derivatives which de-compose readily to 1- and 3-methylmercapto-AAF;[18, 56] 1- and 3-meth-ylmercapto-AAF are also liberated on degradation of the liver protein from rats administered N-hydroxy-AAF.[18] The esters of N-hydroxy-AAF also react with guanine-containing compounds to yield derivatives in which the 8-position of guanine is substituted by the amide nitrogen

FIGURE 1-7.—Nonenzymatic reactions of esters of the hepatic carcinogen N-hydroxy-AAF with guanosine, deoxyguanosine, and methionine, and the formation of the same products on hydrolysis of the hepatic nucleic acids and proteins of rats admin-istered N-hydroxy-AAF.

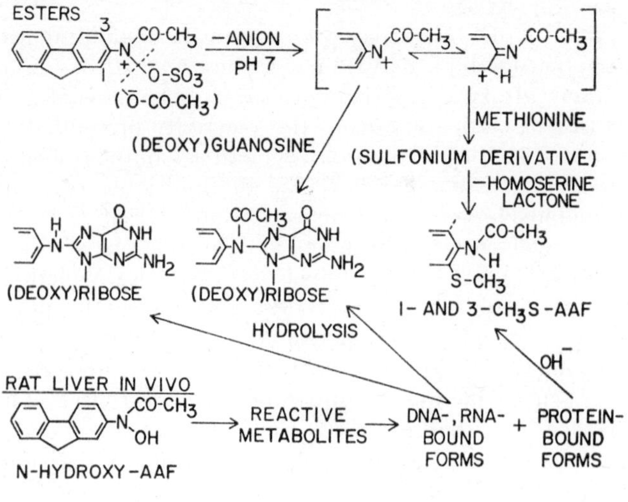

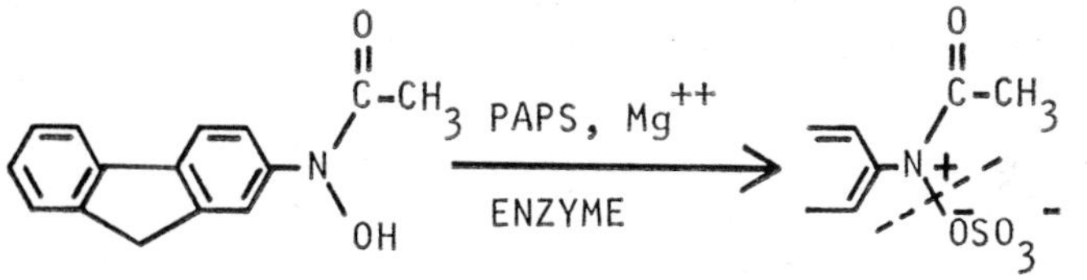

		Liver N-HO-AAF sulfotransferase activity (units)	Liver tumors with N-HO-AAF
Rats,	M	23	+++++
	M, thyroidect.	6	+
	M, hypophysect.	10	+
	F	5	++
Hamsters,	M	<1	+
Mice,	M	<1	+
Guinea pigs,	M	<1	-

FIGURE 1–8.—The enzymatic formation of the sulfuric acid ester of N-hydroxy-2-acetylaminofluorene (N-HO-AAF) by hepatic sulfotransferase(s) and the correlation between this hepatic sulfotransferase activity and susceptibility to liver tumor induction by N-hydroxy-AAF.

of AAF.[48] Furthermore, administration of AAF or N-hydroxy-AAF to rats yields guanyl derivatives in the liver RNA and DNA identical to those obtained by reaction of the esters of N-hydroxy-AAF with the nucleic acids as well as the corresponding 2-aminofluorene derivatives.[40, 45, 46, 70]

Studies in our laboratory[18, 19] and by King and Phillips[43] have shown that the rat liver contains sulfotransferase (s) which transfer the sulfonate group from 3′-phosphoadenosine-5′-phosphosulfate (PAPS) to N-hydroxy-AAF to yield the very reactive electrophilic sulfuric acid ester (Figure 1-8). Our studies showed that the levels of these hepatic sulfotransferase (s) for N-hydroxy-AAF parallel the susceptibility of the liver to hepatic carcinogenesis by N-hydroxy-AAF and the levels of protein-bound methionyl derivatives after administration of N-hydroxy-AAF.[18] Thus, male rats, which are much more susceptible to hepatic carcinogenesis by N-hydroxy-AAF than are female rats, have a several-fold higher level of hepatic sulfotransferase (s) for N-hydroxy-AAF. Hypophysectomy or thyroidectomy, both of which largely protect the male rat against N-hydroxy-AAF-induced hepatocarcinogenesis, cause a considerable decrease in the level of hepatic sulfotransferase activity for N-hydroxy-AAF. Similarly, the livers of various rodents which are much less susceptible to N-hydroxy-AAF-induced carcinogenesis than rat liver have much lower levels of sulfotransferase (s) for N-hydroxy-AAF.

Further evidence that the sulfuric acid ester of N-hydroxy-AAF is a reactive form in vivo was obtained in experiments in which, following the studies of Büch and his associates,[11] p-hydroxyacetanilide was administered to rats to deplete the sulfate pool. With the prior administration of p-hydroxyacetanilide, the levels of protein-, RNA-, and DNA-bound fluorene derivatives formed from N-hydroxy-AAF were depressed to about one half of the control levels, and the administration of sulfate ions largely counteracted this inhibitory effect of p-hydroxyacetanilide.[20] Weisburger et al.[105] have recently presented similar evidence for the importance of the sulfuric acid ester of N-hydroxy-AAF in hepatocarcinogenesis. Administration of acetanilide strongly inhibits the hepatocarcinogenic effect of N-hydroxy-AAF, and this inhibition was partially prevented when sodium sulfate was fed in the diet with the N-hydroxy-AAF and acetanilide. Thus, the sulfuric acid ester of N-hydroxy-AAF appears to be the principal reactive and carcinogenic metabolite of N-hydroxy-AAF in the liver, but the roles of other metabolites in the liver and, especially, in other tissues require much further study.

Various possible and probable strong electrophilic derivatives of other carcinogens are shown in Figure 1-9. 4-Nitroquinoline-1-oxide, itself an electrophile, is reduced enzymatically in the liver and subcutaneous tissue[61, 97] to the more carcinogenic derivative 4-hydroxyaminoquinoline-1-oxide.[23, 91] Synthetic esterification of the latter compound converts it to an electrophile which reacts readily with several nucleic acid bases[24] and, by analogy with the in vivo esterification of N-hydroxy-AAF, provides a model for its metabolic activation. Similarly, recent data from Brown et al. suggest that the carcinogenicity of 3-hydroxyxanthine and guanine-7-N-oxide[10, 98] may be mediated by in vivo esterification of these hydroxylamines. Thus, synthetic esters of 3-hydroxyxanthine react readily with a variety of nucleophiles,[108] some of the products of these reactions (8-chloro- and 8-methylmercaptoxanthine) are excreted in the urine of rats administered 3-hydroxyxanthine,[96] and 3-hydroxyxanthine can be enzymatically esterified by rat liver preparations.[95]

Another type of strong electrophile, the phenyl diazonium cation, is liberated under physiologic conditions from the carcinogen nitrosophenylurea, and may be an essential intermediate in its biologic activity.[78]

The details of the metabolism of the polycyclic aromatic hydrocarbons to carcinogenic and macromolecule-binding derivatives have received intensive study by Gelboin[30] and by Boyland, Grover, and Sims.[4-7, 32, 33] Both groups of investigators have shown that the hydrocarbons are metabolized by the mixed function oxidases of the endoplasmic reticulum to derivatives which react with proteins and nucleic acids; the epoxides appear to be one of the most likely candidates for the reactive electrophilic intermediate. However, other possible intermediates, such as the radical cations which have been studied in model

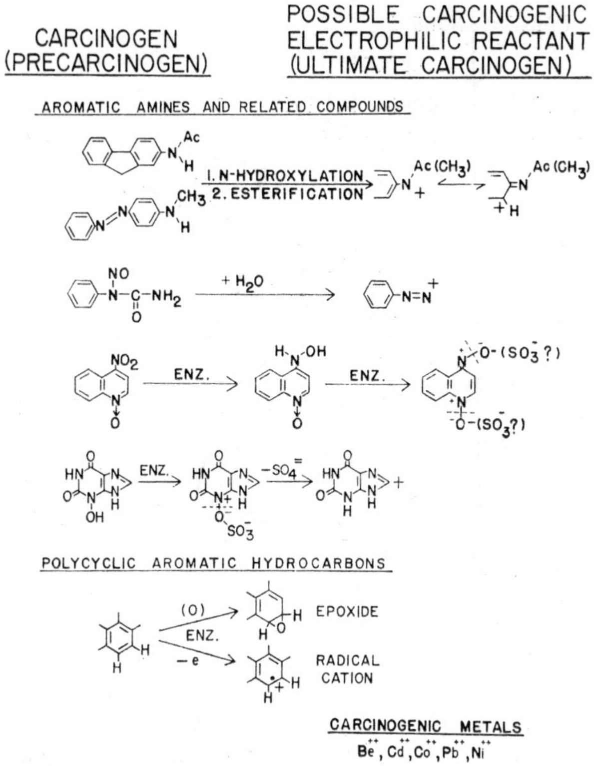

FIGURE 1–9.—Some possible ultimate carcinogenic electrophilic reactants that may be formed in vivo from various aromatic carcinogens. The cationic forms of several carcinogenic metals are also shown.

systems by Wilk et al.,[106, 107] Ts'o et al.,[103] Fried and Schumm,[29] and Morreal et al.[72] are also attractive theoretical possibilities.

Finally, it should be recognized that the ionic forms of carcinogenic metals are, like the alkylating agents, electrophilic reactants per se.

Mechanisms of Action

Thus, in 1970, chemical carcinogens seem much more similar, one to another, than they did even a few years ago. Regardless of the structure of the compound administered, it is likely that all or nearly all chemical carcinogens yield electrophilic reactants in vivo and that these electrophilic derivatives are the ultimate carcinogenic agents (Figure 1-10). It seems axiomatic that these ultimate carcinogens induce neoplasia through interaction with one or more cellular constituents; at the present time it appears most likely that the interactions leading to neoplasia involve DNA, specific RNAs, specific proteins, or

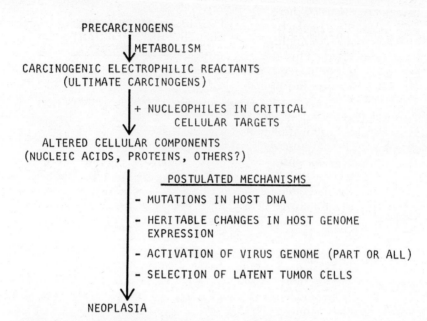

FIGURE 1–10.—Some postulated mechanisms by which ultimate carcinogenic electrophilic reactants may induce neoplasia.

combinations thereof. Thus, at least theoretically, alteration in any of these informational macromolecules could, through genetic or epigenetic means, give rise to new permanent or quasipermanent lines of cells with the altered growth potentials and growth controls which characterize tumor cells.

Since several chemical carcinogens are known to react with cellular DNA in vivo, the possibility that the replication of such altered DNA gives rise to somatic mutations which lead to neoplasia is theoretically attractive. This model of chemical carcinogenesis has been the basis of considerable research and is considered in this symposium by Dr. Lawley[50] (see pages 38-46, this volume).

Heritable changes in genome expression provide another method for the development and perpetuation of clones of cells with altered growth characteristics. Thus, quasipermanent alterations in genome expression are generally considered to be the basis of normal cellular differentiation. Models from phage and bacterial systems[41, 101] suggest that the various cell types may result from the selective transcription of DNA as determined by the interactions of specific proteins with the DNA.[75] Alterations in proteins which regulate the transcription of the DNA would be expected to alter the specificity of these critical interactions and thus to give rise to cells in which the transcription of the DNA is different from that of the cells of origin. It is in this context that the effects of chemical carcinogens on the proteins of the target tissues, as discussed here by Dr. Terayama,[102] (see pages 58-71, this volume) are particularly relevant. Specific models by which alterations in RNA molecules might cause changes in genome expression have not been formulated. This subject is discussed at this symposium by Dr. Weinstein[104] (see pages 47-57, this volume) and has also been reviewed recently by Sueoka and Kano-Sueoka.[96]

Activation of latent oncogenic viral genomes by treatment with a chemical carcinogen is another possible mechanism for the induction of tumors.[36, 38] Activation could consist of transcription of an integrated, previously untranscribed viral genome and would be akin to the alterations in transcription of the host genome outlined above. Alternatively, treatment with a chemical carcinogen might cause release of the virus from the integrated state and the synthesis of infectious virus.

Finally, as emphasized here by Dr. Farber[26] (see pages 72-75, this volume), the change from apparently normal cell populations to clones of tumor cells may involve intermediate clones of hyperplastic cells which are more prone to the neoplastic conversion than are the normal cells of origin. This more complex model may require successive changes in one or more of the macromolecules and may involve more than one of the models discussed here. Furthermore, the administration of certain chemical carcinogens may alter the capacity of the host for preventing or controlling the proliferation of hyperplastic or neoplastic cells, and thus indirectly stimulate the development of tumors.[77]

In spite of the considerable knowledge on the interactions of chemical carcinogens with macromolecules of target tissues, there are still no data which permit a decision with regard to the mechanism(s) by which any chemical carcinogen causes tumors to develop. Attainment of this insight into the molecular mechanisms of chemical carcinogenesis must be a major goal for all of us in this field.

References

1. Barry, E. J., D. Malejka-Giganti, and H. R. Gutmann: Chemico-Biol. Interac., 1:139, 1969.
2. Brookes, P., and P. D. Lawley: Biochem. J., 77:478, 1960.
3. Boutwell, R. K., N. H. Colburn, and C. C. Muckerman: Ann. N. Y. Acad. Sci., 163:751, 1969.
4. Boyland, E., and P. Sims: Biochem. J., 84:571, 1962.
5. Boyland, E., and P. Sims: Biochem. J., 91:493, 1964.
6. Boyland, E., and P. Sims: Biochem. J., 95:788, 1965.
7. Boyland, E., and P. Sims: Biochem. J., 97:7, 1965.
8. Boyland, E., and R. Nery: Biochem. J., 94:198, 1965.
9. Boyland, E., and K. Williams: Biochem. J., 111:121, 1969.
10. Brown, G. B., K. Sugiura, and R. M. Cresswell: Cancer Res., 25:986, 1965.
11. Büch, H., W. Rummel, K. Pfleger, C. Eschrich, and N. Texter: Arch. Pharmakol. Exp. Pathol., 259:276, 1968.
12. Clayson, D. B.: Chemical Carcinogenesis. Little, Brown, and Co., Boston, 1962, 467 pp.
13. Colburn, N. H., and R. K. Boutwell: Cancer Res., 28:642, 1968.
14. Colburn, N. H., and R. K. Boutwell: Cancer Res., 28:653, 1968.
15. Cramer, J. W., J. A. Miller, and E. C. Miller: J. Biol. Chem., 235:885, 1960.

16. Culvenor, C. C. J., A. T. Dann, and A. T. Dick: Nature, 195:570, 1962.
17. Culvenor, C. C. J., D. T. Downing, J. A. Edgar, and M. V. Jago: Ann. N. Y. Acad. Sci., 163:837, 1969.
18. DeBaun, J. R., E. C. Miller, and J. A. Miller: Cancer Res., 30:577, 1970.
19. DeBaun, J. R., J. Y. Rowley, E. C. Miller, and J. A. Miller: Proc. Soc. Exp. Biol. Med., 129:268, 1968.
20. DeBaun, J. R., J. Y. R. Smith, E. C. Miller, and J. A. Miller: Science, 167:184, 1970.
21. Druckrey, H., R. Preussmann, and S. Ivankovic: Ann. N. Y. Acad. Sci., 163:672, 1969.
22. Druckrey, H., R. Preussmann, S. Ivankovic, D. Schmähl, J. Afkham, G. Blum, H. D. Mennel, M. Muller, P. Petropoulos, and H. Schneider: Zeitschr. Krebsforsch., 69:103, 1967.
23. Endo, H., and F. Kume: Gann, 56:261, 1965.
24. Enomoto, M., K. Sato, E. C. Miller, and J. A. Miller: Life Sci., 7:1025, 1968.
25. Farber, E.: Adv. Cancer Res., 7:383, 1963.
26. Farber, E., and S. M. Epstein: Assessment at tissue and cellular level. In: Oncology, 1970, Vol. I. A. Cellular and Molecular Mechanisms of Carcinogenesis. B. Regulation of Gene Expression. (Proceedings of the 10th International Cancer Congress). Year Book Medical Publishers, Inc., Chicago, 1971, pp. 72-75.
27. Farber, E., J. McConomy, B. Franzen, F. Marroquin, G. A. Stewart, and P. N. Magee: Cancer Res., 27:1761, 1967.
28. Fowler, J. S. L.: Brit. J. Pharmacol., 36:181P, 1969.
29. Fried, J., and D. E. Schumm: J. Amer. Chem. Soc., 89:5508, 1967.
30. Gelboin, H. V.: Cancer Res., 29:1272, 1969.
31. Goldschmidt, B. M., T. P. Blazej, and B. L. Van Duuren: Tetraded. Let., 1968, p. 1583.
32. Grover, P. L., and P. Sims: Biochem. J., 110:159, 1969.
33. Grover, P. L., and P. Sims: In Press.
34. Gutmann, H. R., S. B. Galitski, and W. A. Foley: Cancer Res., 27:1443, 1967.
35. Gutmann, H. R., D. S. Leaf, Y. Yost, R. E. Rydell, and C. C. Chen: Cancer Res. In Press.
36. Huebner, R. J., and G. J. Todaro: Proc. Nat. Acad. Sci. USA, 64:1087, 1969.
37. Hueper, W. C., F. H. Wiley, and H. D. Wolfe: J. Ind. Hygiene Toxicol., 20:46, 1938.
38. Igel, H. J., R. J. Huebner, H. C. Turner, P. Kotin, and H. L. Falk: Science, 166:1624, 1969.
39. Irving, C. C., R. A. Veazey, and J. T. Hill: Biochim. Biophys. Acta, 179:189, 1969.
40. Irving, C. C., R. A. Veazey, and L. T. Russell: Chemico-Biol. Interac., 1:19, 1969.
41. Jacob, F., and J. Monod: J. Molec. Biol., 3:318, 1961.
42. Kennaway, E. L., and I. Hieger: Brit. Med. J., 1:1044, 1930.
43. King, C. M., and B. Phillips: Science, 159:1351, 1968.
44. Kobayashi, A., and H. Matsumoto: Arch. Biochem., 110:373, 1965.
45. Kriek, E.: Biochim. Biophys. Acta, 161:273, 1968.
46. Kriek, E.: Chemico-Biol. Interac., 1:3, 1969.
47. Kriek, E., J. A. Miller, U. Juhl, and E. C. Miller: Biochemistry, 6:177, 1967.
48. Kruger, F. W., R. Preussmann, and N. Niepelt: Abstracts, Xth Internat. Cancer Congr., 1970, p. 4.
49. Laqueur, G. L., and M. Spatz: Cancer Res., 28:2262, 1968.
50. Lawley, P. D.: DNA as target of chemical carcinogens. In: Oncology, 1970, Vol. I. A. Cellular and Molecular Mechanisms of Carcinogenesis. B. Regulation of Gene Expression. (Proceedings of the 10th International Cancer Congress). Year Book Medical Publishers, Inc., Chicago, 1971, pp. 38-46.
51. Lawley, P. D., and P. Brookes: Biochem. J., 89:127, 1963.
52. Lawley, P. D., and C. J. Thatcher: Biochem. J., 116:693, 1970.
53. Lijinsky, W., and A. E. Ross: J. Nat. Cancer Inst., 42:1095, 1969.
54. Lin, J.-K., J. A. Miller, and E. C. Miller: Biochemistry, 7:1889, 1968.

55. Lin, J.-K., J. A. Miller, and E. C. Miller: Biochemistry, 8:1573, 1969.
56. Lotlikar, P. D., J. D. Scribner, J. A. Miller, and E. C. Miller: Life Sci., 5:1263, 1966.
57. Loveless, A.: Nature, 223:206, 1969.
58. Magee, P. N., and J. M. Barnes: Adv. Cancer Res., 10:163, 1967.
59. Magee, P. N., and R. Schoental: Brit. Med. Bull., 20:102, 1964.
60. Marroquin, F., and E. Farber: Cancer Res., 25:1262, 1965.
61. Matsumoto, H., and H. H. Higa: Biochem. J., 98:20c, 1966.
62. Matsushima, T., I. Kobuna, F. Fukuoka, and T. Sugimura: Gann, 59:247, 1968.
63. Mattocks, A. R.: Nature, 217:723, 1968.
64. Miller, E. C., U. Juhl, and J. A. Miller: Science, 153:1125, 1966.
65. Miller, E. C., P. D. Lotlikar, J. A. Miller, B. W. Butler, C. C. Irving, and J. T. Hill: Molec. Pharmacol., 4:147, 1968.
66. Miller, E. C., J. A. Miller, and M. Enomoto: Cancer Res., 24:2018, 1964.
67. Miller, E. C., J. A. Miller, and H. A. Hartmann: Cancer Res., 21:815, 1961.
68. Miller, J. A., J. W. Cramer, and E. C. Miller: Cancer Res., 20:950, 1960.
69. Miller, J. A., J.-K. Lin, and E. C. Miller: Proc. Amer. Ass. Cancer Res., 11:56, 1970.
70. Miller, J. A., and E. C. Miller: Prog. Exp. Tumor Res., 11:273, 1969.
71. Miller, J. A., and E. C. Miller: In: The Jerusalem Symposia on Quantum Chemistry and Biochemistry, Vol. I, Physico-Chemical Mechanisms of Carcinogenesis (E. D. Bergmann and B. Pullman, eds.), The Israel Academy of Sciences and Humanities, Jerusalem, 1969, pp. 237-261.
72. Morreal, C. E., T. L. Dao, K. Eskins, C. L. King, and J. Dienstag: Biochim. Biophys. Acta, 169:224, 1969.
73. Orenstein, J. M., and W. H. Marsh: Biochem. J., 109:697, 1968.
74. Ortwerth, B. J., and G. D. Novelli: Cancer Res., 29:380, 1969.
75. Pitot, H. C., and C. Heidelberger: Cancer Res., 23:1694, 1963.
76. Poirier, L. A., J. A. Miller, E. C. Miller, and K. Sato: Cancer Res., 27:1600, 1967.
77. Prehn, R. T.: J. Nat. Cancer Inst., 32:1, 1964.
78. Preussmann, R., H. Druckrey, and Bücheler: Zeitschr. Krebsforsch., 71:63, 1968.
79. Preussmann, R., H. Druckrey, S. Ivankovic, and A. v. Hodenberg: Ann. N. Y. Acad. Sci., 163:697, 1969.
80. Preussmann, R., A. v. Hodenberg, and H. Hengy: Biochem. Pharmacol., 18:1, 1969.
81. Price, C. C., G. M. Gaucher, P. Koneru, R. Shibakawa, J. R. Sowa and M. Yamaguchi: Biochim. Biophys. Acta, 166:327, 1968.
82. Radomski, J. L., and E. Brill: Science, 167:992, 1970.
83. Rao, K. S., and R. O. Recknagel: Exp. Molec. Path., 10:219, 1969.
84. Reynolds, E. S.: J. Pharmacol. Exp. Ther., 155:117, 1967.
85. Rosen, L.: Biochem. Biophys. Res. Comm., 33:546, 1968.
86. Ross, W. C. J.: Biological Alkylating Agents. Butterworth, London, 1962, 232 pp.
87. Schoental, R.: Bull. World Health Org., 29:823, 1963.
88. Schoental, R.: Nature, 192:670, 1961.
89. Scribner, J. D., J. A. Miller, and E. C. Miller: Biochem. Biophys. Res. Comm., 20:560, 1965.
90. Shapiro, R.: Ann. N. Y. Acad. Sci., 163:264, 1969.
91. Shirasu, Y.: Proc. Soc. Exp. Biol. Med., 118:812, 1965.
92. Stekol, J. A.: Adv. Enzymol., 25:369, 1963.
93. Stekol, J. A.: In: Transmethylation and Methionine Biosynthesis (S. K. Shapiro and F. Schlenk, eds.), The University of Chicago Press, Chicago, 1965, pp. 231-248.
94. Stöhrer, G., and G. B. Brown: Science, 167:1622, 1970.
95. Stöhrer, G., E. Corbin, and G. B. Brown: Proc. Amer. Ass. Cancer Res., 11:76, 1970.
96. Sueoka, N., and T. Kano-Sueoka: Prog. Nucl. Acid Res. Molec. Biol., 10:23, 1970.
97. Sugimura, T., K. Okabe, and H. Endo: Gann, 56:489, 1965.
98. Sugiura, K., M. N. Teller, J. C. Parham, and G. B. Brown: Cancer Res., 30:184, 1970.

99. Swann, P. F., and P. N. Magee: Biochem. J., 110:39, 1968.
100. Swann, P. F., and P. N. Magee: Abstracts, Xth Internat. Cancer Congr., Houston, Texas, 1970, p. 3.
101. Szybalski, W., K. Bøvre, M. Fiandt, A. Guha, Z. Hradecna, S. Kumar, H. A. Lozeron, V. M. Maher, H. J. J. Nijkamp, W. C. Summers, and K. Taylor: J. Cell. Physiol., (Suppl. 1) 74:33, 1969.
102. Terayama, H.: Protein as target of reactive forms. In: Oncology, 1970, Vol. I. A. Cellular and Molecular Mechanisms of Carcinogenesis. B. Regulation of Gene Expression. (Proceedings of the 10th International Cancer Congress). Year Book Medical Publishers, Inc., Chicago, 1971, pp. 58-71.
103. Ts'o, P. O. P., S. A. Lesko, and R. S. Umans: In: The Jerusalem Symposia on Quantum Chemistry and Biochemistry, Vol. I. Physico-Chemical Mechanisms of Carcinogenesis (E. D. Bergmann and B. Pullman, eds.), Israel Academy of Sciences and Humanities, Jerusalem, 1969, p. 106.
104. Weinstein, I. B., and D. Grunberger: RNA as the target of reactive forms of chemical carcinogens. In: Oncology, 1970, Vol. I. A. Cellular and Molecular Mechanisms of Carcinogenesis. B. Regulation of Gene Expression. (Proceedings of the 10th International Cancer Congress). Year Book Medical Publishers, Inc., Chicago, 1971, pp. 47-57.
105. Weisburger, J. H., R. S. Yamamoto, P. H. Grantham, and E. K. Weisburger: Proc. Amer. Ass. Cancer Res., 11:82, 1970.
106. Wilk, M., and W. Girke: In: The Jerusalem Symposia on Quantum Chemistry and Biochemistry. Vol. I, Physico-Chemical Mechanisms of Carcinogenesis (E. D. Bergmann and B. Pullman, eds.), Israel Academy of Sciences and Humanities, Jerusalem, 1969, p. 91.
107. Wilk, M., and U. Hoppe: Liebigs Ann. Chem., 727:81, 1969.
108. Wölcke, U., N. J. M. Birdsall, and G. B. Brown: Tetrahed. Let., 10:785, 1969.
109. Yoshida, T.: Trans. Japan Pathol. Soc., 23:636, 1933.

DNA as Target of Chemical Carcinogens

P. D. LAWLEY

Chester Beatty Research Institute, Institute of Cancer Research, Royal Cancer Hospital, London, England

THE CONCEPT that some form of chromosome damage is involved in carcinogenesis began with the work of von Hansemann in the late nineteenth century. The indication that chemical carcinogenesis occurs in man originated with Pott a century earlier. As examples of recent discussions of chemical causation of human cancer, Boyland[1] and Case[2] may be quoted.

TABLE 1–1.—POSITIVE CORRELATIONS BETWEEN TUMOR-PRODUCING ABILITY AND BINDING TO DNA OF TARGET TISSUES IN VIVO

AGENT	MATERIAL TREATED	INVESTIGATORS
Polycyclic aromatic hydrocarbons	Mouse skin	Brookes and Lawley (1964)[8]
Aminoazo dyes	Rat liver	Dingman and Sporn (1967)[38]
4-Nitroquinoline-1-oxide and derivatives	Rat hepatoma	Matsushima, Kobuna and Sugimura (1967)[39]
β-propiolactone and related alkylating agents	Mouse skin	Colburn and Boutwell (1968)[7]
N-hydroxy-N-2-fluorenyl-acetamide (effects of various pretreatments)	Rat liver	Matsushima and Weisburger (1969)[40]

Kennaway's discovery of pure chemical carcinogens was made in the late 1920s, about 10 years before Auerbach and Robson showed that mustard gas was mutagenic (this compound has recently been established[3] as a carcinogen in man). Interest in DNA as a target of chemical carcinogens is thus a natural development from work extending back to the earliest days of cancer research. For a recent discussion of the relevance of mutational theories to human cancer, see Burch.[4] Recent biochemical evidence[5] consistent with the concept that damage to DNA is involved in carcinogenesis in man has come from studies of the DNA repair enzymes for removal of UV-induced lesions in cellular DNA; these enzymes were found to be deficient in skin cells from xeroderma pigmentosum patients. It is possible, therefore, that DNA repair enzymes may be an early "line of defense" of the body against carcinogens.

At about the time of the previous International Cancer Congress, Brookes[6] reviewed available evidence for reactions of carcinogens with DNA in vivo. Since then, several studies[7, 38, 39, 40] have shown posi-

TABLE 1–2.—MUTAGENESIS BY CARCINOGENS IN METAZOAN CELLS

AGENT	MATERIAL TREATED	MUTATIONS	INVESTIGATORS
EMS MNNG	Chinese hamster ovary cells CHO/Pro⁻	pro⁻ → pro⁺ pro⁻ → pro⁻ gly⁻	Kao and Puck (1968)[11]
EMS MMS MNNG	Chinese hamster cells V79-122D1	glu⁻ → glu⁺ azgˢ → azgʳ azgʳ → azgˢ	Chu and Malling (1968)[41]
Aflatoxin benzo(a)pyrene MMS TEM, etc.	Male Swiss mice (CD-1)	Dominant lethals (deciduomata)	Epstein and Shafner (1968)[42]
Aromatic hydrocarbons and amines	Drosophila melanogaster testis	Minutes and bobbed	Fahmy and Fahmy (1969, 1970)[12, 43]

tive correlations between tumor-producing ability of carcinogens and their binding to DNA, following the earlier work of Brookes and Lawley[8] on binding of polycyclic aromatic hydrocarbons to cellular constituents of mouse skin. These are summarized in Table 1-1.

The biologic effects of reactions of chemical agents with DNA in cells which then proceed to division are expected to include cytotoxicity, with an enhanced frequency of mutation in survivors. Early work by Strong[9] (using mice) and by Demerec[10] (using *Drosophila*) on mutagenesis by chemical carcinogens was not generally regarded as conclusive. But with the revived interest in this field, several positive reports[11, 41-44] from work involving treatments of metazoan cells have appeared (Table 1-2). Whether somatic mutations induced by carcinogens could account for tumor initiation is unknown, as in the nature of the supposed heritable alterations in proteins (or perhaps RNA) which would be required to release cells from mitotic control. Fahmy and Fahmy[12] have reported that in *Drosophila* aromatic carcinogens induce mutations at specific loci coding for ribosomal and transfer RNA; it would clearly be of interest to know whether such specificity would be found in mammalian cells. When we consider the mechanisms involved in the induction of mutations in diploid cells by chemical carcinogens, the work of Zimmerman[13, 45] and co-workers, using both aliphatic and aromatic carcinogens in yeast, is notable in stressing the importance of induced mitotic recombination and gene conversion; these are very likely the result of errors in the DNA repair processes.

Apart from the mutagenic effects of chemical attack on cellular DNA, the possibility that such reactions could liberate carcinogenic viral DNA (or perhaps proviral DNA) should not be ignored. The relevant molecular mechanisms are not known, but possibilities which have been considered include release of DNA from chromosomes[14] and derepression of proviral DNA coding for viral RNA.[15] In either case, the initiating event might well be that the presence of chemically modified DNA in the cell stimulates the action of repair enzymes.

It must be admitted, therefore, that at present little is known about the biologic effects of carcinogens that can result from their reaction with target DNA. But the available evidence is not inconsistent with the possibility that such effects may include tumor initiation, and suggests that the DNA repair enzyme systems may play a part in this process.

Returning to the supposed preinitiation stage in the scheme for carcinogenesis, i.e. the activation of carcinogens leading to their attack on the cellular target, some advance has been made concerning the relationships between modes of activation and modes of reaction with DNA (the volume edited by Bergmann and Pullman[16] is a notably valuable recent compilation of reports relevant to this topic). The identification of certain reactive sites in DNA has, in turn, led to suggested molecular mechanisms for mutagenesis.

Here the alkylating agents have proved a useful starting point, since they offer the advantage of relative chemical simplicity.

Alkylating agents are expected to react with nucleophilic groups, and it is now well known[17] that the N-7 atom of guanine is generally the most reactive group of this type in DNA. However, if alkylating agents react through the SN 1 mechanism, following the concepts attributable to Ingold, it may be expected that a wider spectrum of groups could be attacked than when the bimolecular SN 2 mechanism operates exclusively, including some groups of relatively low nucleophilicity. Among the alkylating carcinogens, the alkylnitrosamides are expected to react at least in part through the SN 1 mechanism, since they are activated via formation of unstable alkyldiazonium ions; ethyl methanesulfonate is expected to react proportionately more through the SN 1 mechanism than is methyl methanesulfonate.

The recent important work of Loveless and Hampton[18] has stimulated reconsideration of the possible biologic significance of these concepts. Briefly, the mutagenic potency of ethyl methanesulfonate and of N-methyl- and N-ethyl-N-nitrosoureas, when tested using extracellular treatment of T2 bacteriophage, was contrasted with the lack of mutagenesis in this system with methyl methanesulfonate. Loveless[19] then went on to show a possibly significant difference in the reactions of the two groups of agent with deoxyguanosine—the mutagens, but not the nonmutagen, attacked the extranuclear O-6 atom of this nucleoside. Subsequently, reaction at this site in DNA of mammalian cells treated with the mutagen and carcinogen N-methyl-N'-nitro-N-nitrosoguanidine was demonstrated.[20]

Since the mutations obtained are likely to be of the "transition" type caused by mispairing of bases during replication of DNA, the contribution of the mispairing of O^6-methylguanine with thymine shown in Figure 1-11 seems a satisfactory mechanism. It will be noted

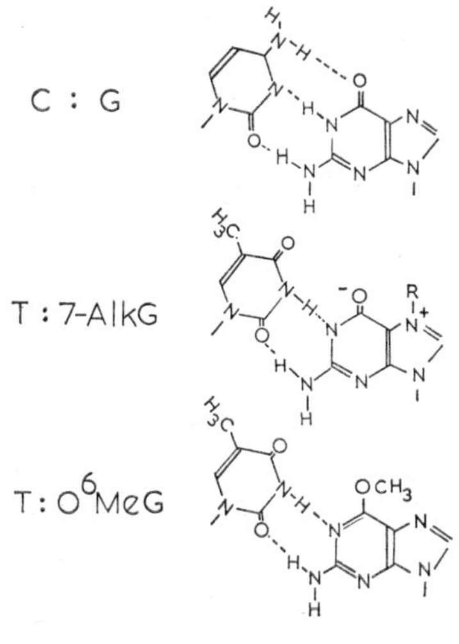

C : G

FIGURE 1–11.—Normal and anomalous base pairs in replicating DNA: C, cytosine; G, guanine; 7-AlkG, 7-alkylguanine; O^6MeG, 2-amino-6-methoxypurine; T, thymine.

T : 7-AlkG

T : O^6MeG

that alkylation at O-6 "fixes" the configuration of the modified guanine residue in the hydrogen-bonding region in the anomalous form previously suggested[21, 46] to occur occasionally for the ionized form of 7-substituted guanine residues.

An interesting outcome of this work has been a positive correlation between ability of a series of alkylating agents to induce supposed transition mutations (Loveless and Hampton) and ability to induce tumors in a target tissue (kidney of rats);[22, 47] in this latter test, again methyl methanesulfonate was negative, while ethyl methanesulfonate and the methylnitrosourea were positive. However it should be noted that methyl methanesulfonate can induce tumors in other tissues, notably in brain.[22, 47] In all cases, alkylation of DNA of target tissues was found. One therefore concludes that the ability of carcinogens to react with DNA in vivo does not always correlate positively with their carcinogenic potency, but the precise chemical nature of the reactions with DNA may be significant.

Another case where this relationship appeared to fail was reported by Warwick,[23, 48] who found binding of the previously supposed noncarcinogen 2-methyl-4-dimethylaminoazobenzene to rat liver DNA; however, the lack of carcinogenic potency of this compound could be overcome by partially hepatectomizing the treated animals. This may be an indication, therefore, that binding of a carcinogen to DNA of a target tissue potentiates tumor initiation but not necessarily tumor promotion, which depends on proliferation of initiated cells.

The nature of the products of reaction between the metabolically activated azo dyes and DNA in vivo does not yet appear to have been specified, but for another important carcinogenic aromatic amine, 2-acetylaminofluorene, the major reactive site in DNA, as revealed by the work of Kriek[24, 49] and the Millers,[25] is the C-8 atom of guanine. This is generally regarded as one of the centers in DNA reactive towards electrophilic agents; the ultimate carcinogen[25] is probably a reactive ester of the N-hydroxylated amine. It has also been shown[26] that reactive derivatives of this type, derived from both 2-acetylaminofluorene and N-methyl-4-aminoazobenzene, will react with transforming DNA in vitro and induce mutations therein. These mutations were reported to be spontaneously reversible and therefore appeared to be of the transition type.

A review of the reactivity of the C-8 position of guanine nucleotides has been given by Hoffmann and Müller,[27] who mentioned further possible biologic consequences of reactions at this site in DNA: inhibition of DNA replication or of transcription and interference with binding to DNA of repressor molecules. They also noted that a small yield of 8-methylguanine was obtained from reaction of diazomethane with DNA in vitro. Thus, whether attack at the C-8 atom of guanine residues in vivo could be a reaction common to aromatic car-

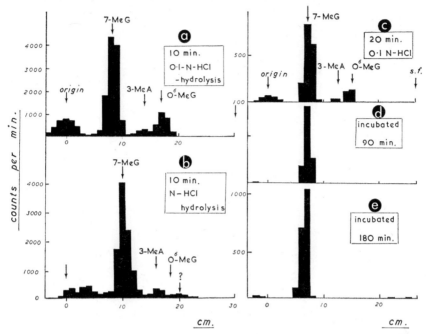

FIGURE 1–12.—Specific excision of methylation products from DNA of *E. coli* B/r after treatment with the mutagen and carcinogen *N*-methyl-*N'*-nitro-*N*-nitrosoguanidine. *a* DNA isolated after 10 min treatment of cells with MNNG-[C^3H_3], 6mM hydrolyzed with 0.1 N-HCl, 70°, 20 min, i.e. conditions known not to demethylate O^6-methylguanine (a-amino-6-methoxypurine). *b* DNA as in *(a)*, but hydrolyzed with N-HCl, 1 hr, 100°, i.e. conditions known to demethylate O^6-methylguanine. *c* DNA isolated after 20 min treatment of cells, in concentrated suspension, with [^{3}H]MNNG, 0.6mM. *d* DNA isolated from a portion of cells treated as in *(c)*, then diluted into growth medium and incubated at 37° for 90 min. *e* As for *(d)*, but 180-min incubation. Hydrolysates of DNA were chromatographed on Whatman 3MM paper using isopropanol-cone, NH_3-H_2O, 7:2:1, by volume, as solvent.

Arrows denote positions of marker bases visualized under 253.7 nm UV light:-

7-MeG, 7-methylguanine,

3-MeA, 3-methyladenine,

O^6-MeG, 2-amino-6-methoxypurine,

cinogens, and to those alkylating agents that are activated through alkyldiazonium ions, remains an interesting possibility.

The evident diversity of products of reaction between carcinogens and DNA prompts consideration of whether the various products differ in their ease of enzymatic excision from cellular DNA. Lawley and Brookes[28] found that, in mustard gas-treated *Escherichia coli*, cross-links induced in DNA were more readily excised than monoalkylated guanine. In cultured mammalian cells treated with this agent, it was found by Roberts, Brent, and Crathorn[29] that some excision occurred, and Reid and Walker[30] reported that cross-links were removed. This type of study is clearly more difficult to carry out using in vivo conditions, and few detailed reports have appeared. Craddock[31] concluded that the evidence for enzymatic excision of 7-methylguanine from liver DNA of rats treated with dimethylnitrosamine was not positive, since the observed rate of loss could be accounted for in terms of chemical hydrolytic depurination.

In view of the possibility that the O^6-methylguanine residue is a potential mutagenic lesion, it is of some interest to report[32] that this group can be excised from DNA of *E. coli* cells treated with the mutagen and carcinogen *N*-methyl-*N*'-nitro-*N*-nitrosoguanidine. The major methylation product 7-methylguanine remained in the cellular DNA during the relatively short period (less than 90 min) sufficing for removal of other methylation products (Figure 1-12). However, it should be noted that the relatively slow rate of hydrolytic removal of this base would be expected to continue, and thus to generate depurinated sites in DNA, known from previous studies with bacteriophage[33] to constitute lesions preventing replication of DNA.

It will thus be of interest to investigate whether similar specific excisions of monoalkylated and other groups can take place in mammalian cells. There is already evidence that the time course of binding of several carcinogens, including aromatic hydrocarbons,[21, 46] azo dyes,[23, 34, 48] and the aromatic amine *ortho*-aminoazotoluene[35] in vivo, follows a characteristic pattern in which only a part of the bound carcinogen persists for long times; but the dependence of this phenomenon on the nature of the reaction products in DNA, if any, is not known. A further possibility concerns the variation of efficiency of excision with type of tissue, leading to the speculation that organotropy might result from such differences.

In conclusion, therefore, it appears that, if the considerations briefly outlined here do prove to be significant in the molecular mechanisms of chemical carcinogenesis, some factors may emerge as offering possibilities for obviating cancer caused by such causes. First, activation of carcinogens in vivo might be modified[36] to permit detoxication but without the side effect of reaction with DNA in certain tissues. Second, if such reaction cannot be prevented, the removal of the potential lesions from DNA might be stimulated. If the supposed initiation stage in cells cannot be avoided, further defensive measures would fall into the categories of opposing the effects designated promotion and progression, presumably involving hormonal and immunologic mechanisms.

With regard to the question whether the supposed early action of carcinogens on DNA as a significant target could be detected in vivo, it may be mentioned that in studies with animals, the detection of even the gross over-all reactions of carcinogens with cellular DNA required isotopically labeled carcinogens of quite high specific radioactivity; for example, it has been calculated[37] that, using conventional procedures, a tritium-labeled carcinogen at a specific radioactivity of 1,000 mCi/m mole would be detectable bound to cellular DNA at a level of about one molecule in 8×10^7 DNA nucleotide units; or at about 200 molecules in the total cellular DNA. It remains possible, however, that, in the whole animal, early effects subsequent to chemical damage to DNA, such as specific modes of degradation of DNA, might be more easily detected than its initial chemical modification.

In summary, therefore, there now exists a good deal of evidence indicating that chemical attack on DNA in vivo may be a significant factor in the early stages of the carcinogenic process. It is hoped that this brief review of some aspects of this question may serve to indicate areas where further investigations will be fruitful.

References

1. Boyland, E.: In: Aktuelle Probleme aus dem Gebiet der Cancerologie II. Springer-Verlag, Berlin, 1968, p. 1.
2. Case, R. A. M.: Proc. Roy. Soc. Med., 62:1061, 1969.
3. Wada, S., M. Miyanishi, Y. Nishimoto, S. Kambe, and R. W. Miller: Lancet, 1: 1161, 1968.
4. Burch, P. R. J.: Nature, 225:512, 1970.
5. Setlow, R. B., J. D. Regan, J. German, and W. L. Carrier: Proc. Nat. Acad. Sci. USA, 64:1035, 1969.
6. Brookes, P.: Cancer Res., 26:1944, 1966.
7. Colburn, N. H., and R. K. Boutwell: Cancer Res., 28:653, 1968.
8. Brookes, P., and P. D. Lawley: Nature, 202:781, 1964.
9. Strong, L. C.: Brit. J. Cancer, 3:97, 1949.
10. Demerec, M.: Brit. J. Cancer, 2:114, 1948.
11. Kao, F.-T., and T. T. Puck: Proc. Nat. Acad. Sci. USA, 60:1275, 1968.
12. Fahmy, O. G., and M. J. Fahmy: Nature, 224:1328, 1969.
13. Zimmermann, F. K., and R. Schwaier: Molec. Gen. Genet., 100:63, 1967.
14. Yamafuji, K.: Enzymologia, 27:217, 1964.
15. Huebner, R. J., and G. J. Todaro: Proc. Nat. Acad. Sci. USA, 64:1087, 1969.
16. Bergmann, E., and B. Pullman, eds.: Physico-Chemical Mechanisms of Carcinogenesis. Jerusalem Symposia on Quantum Chemistry and Biochemistry, I. Israel Academy of Sciences and Humanities, Jerusalem, 1969.
17. Lawley, P. D.: Progr. Nucleic Acid Res. Molec. Biol., 5:89, 1966.
18. Loveless, A., and C. L. Hampton: Mutation Res., 7:1, 1969.
19. Loveless, A.: Nature, 223:206, 1969.
20. Lawley, P. D., and C. J. Thatcher: Biochem. J., 116:693, 1970.
21. Lawley, P. D., and P. Brookes: Nature, 192:1081, 1961.
22. Swann, P. F., and P. N. Magee: Nature, 223:974, 1969.

23. Warwick, G. P.: Europ. J. Cancer, 3:227, 1967.
24. Kriek, E.: Biochem. Biophys. Res. Comm., 20:793, 1965.
25. Miller, J. A., and E. C. Miller: In: Physico-chemical Mechanisms of Carcinogenesis. Jerusalem Symposia on Quantum Chemistry and Biochemistry, I (E. Bergmann and B. Pullman, eds.), Israel Academy of Sciences and Humanities, Jerusalem, 1969, p. 237.
26. Maher, V. M., E. C. Miller, J. A. Miller, and W. Szybalski: Molec. Pharmacol., 4:411, 1968.
27. Hoffmann, H. D., and W. Müller: In: Physico-chemical Mechanisms of Carcinogenesis. Jerusalem Symposia on Quantum Chemistry and Biochemistry, I (E. Bergmann and B. Pullman, eds.), Israel Academy of Sciences and Humanities, Jerusalem, 1969, p. 183.
28. Lawley, P. D., and P. Brookes: Nature, 206:480, 1965.
29. Roberts, J. J., T. P. Brent, and A. R. Crathorn: In: The Interactions of Drugs and Sub-cellular Components (P. N. Campbell, ed.), J. and A. Churchill, Ltd., London, 1968.
30. Reid, B. D., and I. G. Walker: Biochim. Biophys. Acta, 179:179, 1969.
31. Craddock, V. M.: Biochem. J., 111:497, 1969.
32. Lawley, P. D., and D. J. Orr: Unpublished data.
33. Brookes, P., and P. D. Lawley: Biochem. J., 89:138, 1963.
34. Warwick, G. P., and J. J. Roberts: Nature, 213:1206, 1967.
35. Lawson, T. A., and D. B. Clayson: In: Physico-chemical Mechanisms of Carcinogenesis. Jerusalem Symposia on Quantum Chemistry and Biochemistry, I (E. Bergmann and B. Pullman, eds.), Israel Academy of Sciences and Humanities, Jerusalem, 1969, p. 226.
36. Gelboin, H. V.: In: Physico-chemical Mechanisms of Carcinogenesis. Jerusalem Symposia on Quantum Chemistry and Biochemistry, I (E. Bergmann and B. Pullman, eds.), Israel Academy of Sciences and Humanities, Jerusalem, 1969, p. 175.
37. Brookes, P., and P. D. Lawley: In: Chemical Mutagens: Principles and Methods for Their Detection. In press.
38. Dingman, C. W., and M. B. Sporn: Cancer Res., 27:938, 1967.
39. Matsushima, T., I. Kobuna, and T. Sugimura: Nature, 216:508, 1967.
40. Matsushima, T., and J. H. Weisburger: Chemico-Biol. Interact., 1:211, 1969.
41. Chu, E. H. Y., and H. V. Malling: Proc. Nat. Acad. Sci. USA, 61:1306, 1968.
42. Epstein, S. S., and H. Shafner: Nature, 219:385, 1968.
43. Fahmy, O. G., and J. J. Fahmy: Mutation Res., 9:239, 1970.
44. Fahmy, O. G., and J. J. Fahmy: Cancer Res. In press.
45. Zimmermann, F. K.: Z. Krebsforsch., 72:65, 1969.
46. Brookes, P., and P. D. Lawley: J. Cell. Comp. Physiol., 64 (Suppl. 1):111, 1964.
47. Swann, P. F., and P. N. Magee: Biochem. J., 110:39, 1969.
48. Warwick, G. P.: In: Physico-chemical Mechanisms of Carcinogenesis. Jerusalem Symposia on Quantum Chemistry and Biochemistry, I (E. Bergmann and B. Pullman, eds.), Israel Academy of Sciences and Humanities, Jerusalem, 1969, p. 218.
49. Kriek, E.: Chemico-Biol. Interact. 1:1, 1969.

RNA as the Target of Reactive Forms of Chemical Carcinogens

I. BERNARD WEINSTEIN AND DEZIDER GRUNBERGER

Institute of Cancer Research and Department of Medicine,
Columbia University College of Physicians and Surgeons,
Francis Delafield Hospital, New York, New York, USA

Introduction

A FUNDAMENTAL BIOLOGIC PROPERTY of cancer is that once the process is established, the neoplastic state is relatively stable in the sense that, with rare exceptions which are discussed elsewhere,[1] the progeny of tumor cells are usually tumor cells.

Since 1914, when Boveri first proposed the somatic mutation theory of cancer, there has been a tendency to interpret this stable aspect of the neoplastic trait as evidence that neoplastic transformation involves a permanent and irreversible change in the genetic material (DNA) of the cell. I want to emphasize, however, that despite extensive genetic and biochemical studies, there is no direct evidence for the somatic mutation theory of cancer or for a difference in information content between normal and tumor cell DNA. Since the normal process of differentiation leads to the derivation of cell lines with highly unique patterns of gene expression which become stabilized and are transmitted to progeny cells, it is conceivable that certain tumors (and perhaps all tumors in their initial stages) represent aberrations in differentiation which do not involve permanent changes in the host DNA. The following facts are consistent with this concept: (1) tumor cells display gross aberrations in the expression of genes related to fetal development and differentiation,[1] suggesting that the defect is not confined to the control of cell replication; (2) the high efficiency in conversion of normal cells to tumor cells, achieved during in vitro carcinogenesis,[2, 3] is not consistent with conventional mutagenesis or genetic selection; and (3) the increasing number of examples of the reversion of tumor cells towards normalcy.[1] The biochemical mechanisms underlying the normal control of gene expression during differentiation are poorly understood, but it is clear that they do not operate via somatic mutation.[4] It is important, therefore, in considering mechanisms by which exogenous agents produce cancer, to keep our minds open to the possibility that they do so by changing the cytoplasmic environment of a cell in a way which induces an altered and self-sustaining pattern of gene expression.

In view of these considerations, we have focused our attention on the possibility that cellular RNAs are critical targets during chemical carcinogenesis. We believe that RNAs are particularly likely candidates in view of the central role of mRNA in conveying genetic messages from nucleus to cytoplasm, the key roles which tRNA and rRNA occupy in translation and protein synthesis, as well as evidence that certain aspects of cell regulation and differentiation are normally exerted at the level of translation, rather than transcription.[1]

Modifications of tRNA

There is, as a matter of fact, extensive evidence that several carcinogens have the capacity to react with RNA, either in vivo or in vitro, to an extent which is equal to or greater than their capacity to react with DNA (Table 1-3).[5, 6] Qualitative and quantitative changes in the tRNA population of mammalian cells accompany normal differentiation as well as neoplastic transformation.[1] It was, therefore, of particular interest to us that several carcinogens appear to preferentially attack the tRNA fraction of the target tissue.[5-8] The specificity and functional effects of this modification were first demonstrated in collaborative studies done with Dr. Emanuel Farber.[7] We found that liver tRNA obtained from rats which were fed the hepatic carcinogen ethionine for one month, which is prior to the emergence of tumors, was deficient in a minor leucine tRNA. We were unable to detect a loss of amino acid acceptance capacity for several other tRNAs. These findings have been confirmed by Novelli.[9] More recently, we also analyzed the distribution of ^{14}C in liver RNAs 12 to 18 hr after in vivo administration of either ^{14}C-labeled 2-acetylaminofluorene (AAF)

TABLE 1–3.—BINDING OF CARCINOGENS TO NUCLEIC ACIDS IN VIVO

COMPOUND	TISSUE	EXTENT OF INTERACTION* DNA	EXTENT OF INTERACTION* RNA	BINDING RATIO RNA/DNA
Ethionine	Liver	3×10^7	6×10^4	500
AAF	Liver	4×10^5	1×10^5	4
DEN	Liver	—	4×10^2	1-2
DAB	Liver	2×10^5	3×10^4	7
DMBA	Skin	2×10^5	5×10^5	0.5
BP	Skin	3×10^5	6×10^4	5
β-Propiolactone	Skin	1×10^5	6×10^4	1.5

* Nucleotides/mole of carcinogen
"RNA," with ethionine and AAF is tRNA; with DAB it is rRNA; with the others it is total RNA
Modified from Farber, E.[5]

TABLE 1–4.—AMINO ACID ACCEPTANCE CAPACITY
OF *E. coli* tRNA AFTER TREATMENT WITH
N-ACETOXY-AAF (1.5 × 10⁻³M)

| AMINO ACID | AMINO ACID ACCEPTANCE ($\mu\mu$MOLES/ASSAY SYSTEM) | | |
	Control tRNA	AAF tRNA	% of Control*
Arginine	35	12	34
Lysine	17	9	52
Leucine	63	36	57
Isoleucine	15	9	60
Threonine	19	12	62
Glycine	17	11	62
Histidine	6	4	63
Phenylalanine	18	12	65
Proline	17	12	69
Aspartic	20	15	74
Tyrosine	21	17	80
Serine	9	8	88
Methionine	45	41	91
Valine	37	51	136

* Acceptance AAF tRNA × 100/Acceptance control tRNA.
All tRNAs were tested at a limiting concentration, i.e. 0.61 A₂₆₀ units/0.1 ml assay system. For additional details see Fink et al.[12]

or *N*-hydroxy-AAF and found that the tRNA fraction has two to three times the specific activity of 5S, 18S or 28S RNA.[8] Similar results were obtained by Henshaw and Hiatt[10] and by Irving.[11] Fractionation studies indicated that AAF reacts in vivo with several rather than a single species of tRNA, though the amino acid specificity of the species attacked remains to be determined. Our kinetic studies indicated that the drug binds primarily to preformed species of RNA and that most of the modified tRNA and ribosomal RNAs turn over with a T ½ of about five days, which is the same as that in normal liver.[8]

We have also asked the question, does the binding of AAF to tRNA selectively alter the functional properties of specific tRNAs?[12] For these studies we employed the in vitro reaction originally developed by Miller et al.,[13] in which the nucleic acid is reacted at neutral pH with the derivative *N*-acetoxy-AAF. This leads to the covalent attachment of the AAF residue to the 8-position of guanosine, thereby yielding the same type of modification as that which occurs in vivo. The acceptance capacity for 14 amino acids of control tRNA and tRNA previously reacted with 1.5 × 10⁻³M *N*-acetoxy-AAF is indicated in Table 1-4. The activity of arginine and lysine tRNAs was inhibited about 50%; there was a lesser inhibition or no inhibition for several other tRNAs, and there was actual stimulation of valine tRNA acceptance, when com-

TABLE 1-5.—CODON RESPONSE OF AAF tRNA

| TEMPLATE | AMINOACYL-tRNA BOUND TO RIBOSOMES | |
	Control tRNA	AAF tRNA
[14]C-Lys-tRNA		$\Delta\mu\mu$moles
Poly A	1.58	0.61
Poly (A,G) (3:1)	2.06	0.45
		$\mu\mu$moles
None	0.28	0.21
[14]C-Phe-tRNA		$\Delta\mu\mu$moles
Poly U	2.80	2.55
		$\mu\mu$moles
None	0.14	0.27

E. coli control tRNA and *E. coli* tRNA previously reacted with
N-acetoxy-AAF (1.5×10^{-3}M) were charged with the indicated [14]C-
amino acids and tested at comparable concentrations in the ribosomal
binding assay. Details of the assay system are described by Fink et al.[12]

pared to equivalent amounts of control tRNA. In contrast to the selective effects obtained with 1.5×10^{-3}M N-acetoxy-AAF, when the
tRNA was reacted with high concentrations (10^{-2}M) of drug, there
was extensive inactivation of the acceptance capacity of tRNA for all
amino acids.

The functional properties of AAF-tRNA with respect to ribosomal
binding and codon response are indicated in Table 1-5. When AAF
tRNA was aminoacylated with lysine, both the poly A and the poly AG
stimulated ribosomal binding of this tRNA were less than 40% of that
obtained with control lysyl-tRNA. Conversely, no significant difference
between AAF and control tRNA was observed in the binding of phenylalanyl-tRNA stimulated by poly U.

The above studies indicate that the attachment of AAF to tRNA
impairs the ability of certain tRNAs to accept amino acids, and also
produces impairment in the function of specific tRNAs during ribosomal binding and codon recognition. The specificity of these effects
probably relates to differences in the reactivity of individual guanosine
residues in tRNAs, and to whether these residues occupy functionally
important regions of the tRNA. We are currently analyzing this problem by determining which guanosine residue (s) are labeled with
AAF, when a purified species of tRNA[Fmet] is reacted with ^{14}C-labeled
N-acetoxy-AAF and then sequentially degraded enzymatically. Our
preliminary results suggest that guanosine residues in single-stranded
"loops" of tRNA may be the most susceptible to AAF modification.[23]
I will return to the implications of this finding later.

Modification of Oligonucleotides and Polymers with AAF

In the course of protein synthesis, the specificity of translation depends on base pairing between a nucleotide region of tRNA, the anti-

TABLE 1-6.—THE EFFECT OF AAF MODIFICATION OF POLYNUCLEOTIDES UPON THEIR STIMULATION OF ^{14}C-AMINOACYL-tRNA BINDING TO RIBOSOMES

POLYNUCLEOTIDE	^{14}C-AMINOACYL-tRNA BOUND							
	VALYL- (12.2 pmol)		LYSYL- (17 pmol)		PHENYLALANYL- (6.5 pmol)		ISOLEUCYL- (13.4 pmol)	
(0.1 A$_{260}$ nm)	pmol	Δpmol	pmol	Δpmol	pmol	Δpmol	pmol	Δpmol
None	0.35	—	0.67	—	0.68	—	0.96	—
GUU	1.70	1.35	—	—	0.62	−0.06	0.83	−0.13
AAF-GUU	0.36	0.01	—	—	0.53	−0.15	0.75	−0.21
AAG	—	—	1.46	0.79	—	—	—	—
AAG-AAF	—	—	0.66	0.01	—	—	—	—
poly (U,G)	5.87	5.52	—	—	4.26	3.58	0.87	−0.09
poly (U,G-AAF)	3.44	3.09	—	—	4.32	3.64	0.69	−0.30
poly (U,A)	—	—	—	—	—	—	2.53	1.57

The incubation mixture (0.05 ml) contained 0.10 M Tris-acetate (pH 7.2), 0.05 M KCl, 0.03 M magnesium acetate, and 2-2.5 A$_{260}$ units of *E. coli* ribosomes. ^{14}C-aminoacyl-tRNA, trinucleotides, and polymers were added as specified in the Table. Incubation was carried out at 24°C for 20 min, and samples processed and counted as described by Grunberger et al.[15]

codon, and a corresponding triplet of nucleotides (the codon) in mRNA. In contrast to certain other types of chemical modifications, the presence of an AAF residue on the 8 position of guanosine would not be expected to interfere directly with hydrogen bonding and base pairing. Our results with AAF modified tRNA led us to suggest that the observed changes in biologic activity might be caused by a conformational change in the nucleic acid.[12] We then simplified the analysis of this problem by examining the functional properties of certain oligonucleotides and polymers, previously modified with N-acetoxy-AAF, in a ribosomal binding assay, and also obtained information on the conformation of AAF-containing oligonucleotides by examining their circular dichroism (CD) spectra. Later during this Congress, Grunberger will present these results in detail;[14] therefore, I will only briefly summarize these findings.

By reaction with N-acetoxy-AAF, AAF was covalently linked to guanosine residues in several oligonucleotides and in poly (U,G). The products were repurified and their base compositions determined by ribonuclease T$_2$ digestion and thin-layer chromatography. The functional properties of some of these materials, when tested in the ribosomal binding assay, are indicated in Table 1-6. Whereas ^{14}C-valyl-tRNA recognized the unmodified GUU codon, there was no response of ^{14}C-valyl-tRNA to the AAF-containing triplet. AAF modification of G in AAG also led to complete inactivation of the ability of this triplet to stimulate ribosomal binding of ^{14}C-lysyl-tRNA. These results indicate that modification of G in either the 5′ or 3′ end of the triplet totally inhibits the normal template activity of that triplet. There remained the possibility that the AAF-modified G in codons might behave as adenosine or uridine, during base pairing, and thereby produce miscoding during the recognition process. To test this, we measured the effect of modified GUU on the stimulation of ^{14}C-Ile-tRNA (normal codon, AUU), and of modified GUU on the stimulation of ^{14}C-Phe-tRNA (normal codon, UUU), binding to ribosomes. The results in Table 1-6 demonstrate that neither GUU nor AAF-GUU were recognized by either Ile- or Phe-tRNA. It appears, therefore, that AAF modification of G leads to inactivation rather than mistaken base pairing. Binding of *Escherichia coli* ^{14}C-valyl-tRNA to ribosomes by poly (U,G)-AAF was lower than that obtained with unmodified poly (U,G) and the decrease, approximately 40%, corresponded to the extent of G modification by AAF (Table 1-6). The stimulatory effect of poly (U,G) on the binding of ^{14}C-phenylalanyl-tRNA to ribosomes is caused by sequences of UUU. Modification of G residues in this polymer should, therefore, not alter its stimulation of phenylalanyl-tRNA binding to ribosomes. Results in Table 1-6 confirm this, thus indicating that the AAF modification is specific and does not result in total inactivation of the polymer.

Since binding of tRNA to codons and ribosomes represents only one step in the translation process, it was also important to assay the behavior of AAF modified polymers during polypeptide chain formation. For these reasons we tested the ability of poly (U,G), previously modified with AAF, to direct the incorporation of ^{14}C-valine and ^{14}C-phenylalanine into protein employing the S-30 extract from *E. coli*. Poly (U,G), in which 40% of the G residues were modified by AAF, was completely inactive in stimulating the incorporation of ^{14}C-valine into protein (Table 1-7). In contrast to the results obtained in the ribosomal binding assay (Table 1-6), the modified poly (U,G) was also greatly impaired in terms of its ability to stimulate the incorporation of ^{14}C-phenylalanine into protein (Table 1-7).

There are two possible explanations for the lack of incorporation of both valine and phenylalanine into protein in the presence of modified poly (U,G): (1) the modified polymer is not bound to ribosomes and

TABLE 1-7.—EFFECT OF AAF MODIFICATION OF
POLY (U,G) UPON STIMULATION OF AMINO ACID
INCORPORATION INTO PROTEIN

| POLYMER | ^{14}C-AMINO ACID INCORPORATION (Δpmol/assay) | |
	Valine	Phenylalanine
Poly (U,G)	18	45
Poly (U,G)-AAF	1	1.5

Assays systems contained 0.1 ml of the S-30 fraction of *E. coli*, the indicated ^{14}C-amino acid, and 5 mμmoles base residues of either poly (U,G) or poly (U,G) in which 40% of the G residues were modified with AAF. Remaining details of the incorporation system have been described previously.

therefore cannot direct protein synthesis; or (2) the modified polymer is bound to ribosomes, but since modified G residues are not recognized by tRNA, translation and polypeptide chain growth are terminated each time reading comes to a modified G. The first explanation can be excluded because poly (U,G)-AAF was active in stimulating phenylalanyl-tRNA binding to ribosomes, so we know that the modified polymer is bound to ribosomes. The second explanation, therefore, applies and is quite plausible, since the relatively high content of modified G residues would permit the synthesis of only short chains of polyphenylalanine which would escape precipitation with trichloracetic acid. Further studies are in progress to verify this explanation.

CD Spectra of AAF-Modified Oligomers

The results of the codon recognition experiments suggest that nucleotide sequences containing AAF-substituted guanosine residues may undergo substantial conformational changes as a result of the AAF substitution. Accordingly, we have studied the influence of AAF substitution on the CD spectra of several oligonucleotides. These studies were done in collaboration with James Nelson and Charles Cantor.[15]

Figure 1-13 presents the molar ellipticity, $[\theta]$, as a function of wave-

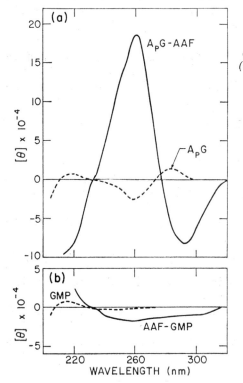

FIGURE 1-13.—Circular dichroism curves of: (a) ApG, and ApG-AAF; (b) GMP and AAF-GMP.

length, for the compounds: GMP, ApG, and their corresponding AAF-substituted derivatives. The dichroism of GMP itself is fairly weak, and there is little optical activity at wavelengths greater than 270 nm. AAF-GMP, however, has a relatively strong negative dichroism in the spectral region of 240 to 310 nm. Since AAF has a high extinction coefficient in this region, it is likely that the strong dichroism of AAF-GMP at these wavelengths results from optical activity induced in AAF by covalent attachment to guanosine. The CD spectrum of AAF-GMP is also much different from that of guanosine at lower wavelengths (200 to 240 nm). Of particular interest are the striking changes in the spectrum of ApG produced by AAF-substitution. The strength of the CD observed for this substituted dinucleoside is an order of magnitude greater than that observed for either unsubstituted ApG or the substituted monomer. The spectacularly large bands in ApG-AAF probaby arise from a strong interaction of AAF with the adjacent adenine residue. Qualitatively similar changes in CD spectra were induced when the G residues of UpG were modified with AAF, though the strength of the dichroism was less than that obtained with ApG-AAF, thus indicating that AAF interacts less strongly with an adjacent U residue than with an adjacent A residue. AAF modification of guanosine residues present in GpA and GpU also affected the CD spectra of these dinucleosides, but the changes were qualitatively different and considerably less intense than those noted when the modified residue was at the 3′ end (right side) of the dinucleoside. It appears, therefore, that the nature of the conformational change induced by AAF is greatly influenced by the base composition and sequence of the local region of the nucleic acid in which modification occurs. We are currently extending this analysis to larger oligonucleotides and polymers.

Discussion

Our results indicate that modifications of nucleic acids with the carcinogen AAF produce major conformational changes in these molecules. The CD spectral data, together with a study of molecular models of AAF-modified dinucleoside phosphates, suggest that the most probable conformational change is a rotation of the modified guanosine about the glycosidic bond, followed by stacking of AAF with the neighboring base on the 5′ side of the substituted guanine (see Grunberger et al.[15] and Figure 1-14). This seems likely for two reasons. First, attachment of AAF to the 8-position of guanine is sterically hindered, if the guanosine remains in the normal "anti" conformation, with torsion angle values of $\phi CN \sim -30°$.[16] However, rotation about the glycosidic bond to torsional angles $\phi CN \sim +50°$ to 150° will relieve this hindrance (Figure 1-14). This conclusion is analogous to that reached with 8-bromoguanosine[17, 18] in which X-ray diffraction studies do indicate a "syn" conformation,[19] presumably related to the bulky sub-

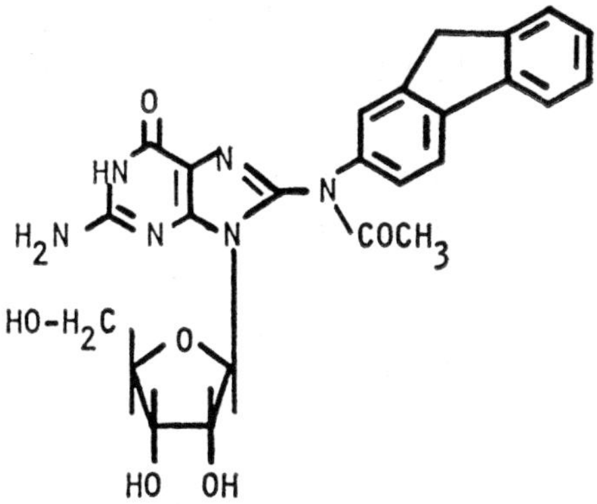

FIGURE 1–14.—Schematic representation of AAF-GMP. In contrast to the normal configuration of GMP, the guanine base has been rotated approximately 180° about the N(9)=C(1′) bond to minimize steric hindrance with the bulky AAF residue.

stituent on the 8-position. Second, the CD data suggest that AAF strongly interacts with the neighboring base. This is quite reasonable, since a large hydrocarbon like AAF should exhibit a strong tendency to stack with nonpolar bases. These conformational changes would result in decreased base stacking between guanine and the adjacent base with a change in the orientation of the two dinucleoside bases with respect to each other. These changes have important implications, because it is reasonable to assume that similar events occur at sites of AAF substitution in coding triplets such as ApApG and GpUpU. Such changes would make it difficult for the normal hydrogen bonding sites of the respective bases along the nucleotide chain to become sufficiently aligned, with respect to orientation and distance, to effect binding to complementary sites on the anticodon of tRNA. A similar effect would also be expected for higher molecular weight polynucleotides. In fact, the substitution of AAF on guanine residues of natural nucleic acids could alter the base-stacking properties of the polymer over a considerable distance.

Our findings may also bear on the types of conformational changes which occur with covalent attachment of other aromatic carcinogens to nucleic acids. The recent exciting discovery of. the Millers[20] that N-methyl-4-aminoazobenzene, like AAF, attaches covalently to the 8-position of guanosines in RNA and DNA, leads us to suggest that this modification may also involve an "anti" to "syn" conformational change, as well as base stacking between the ring systems of the carcinogen and adjacent bases. Lesko et al.[21] have recently described covalent attachment of benzopyrene to guanosine residues in nucleic acids. If this modification also turns out to be a substitution on the 8-position, then our model may extend to the polycyclic carcinogens. Thus the conformational changes described by us with AAF may provide a unifying principle for understanding the action of aromatic amine and polycyclic carcinogens, just as the hypothesis of Lawley and Brookes[22] provides a framework for explaining the effects of substitution of the 7-position of guanosine by alkylating carcinogens.

The relationship of our findings to the carcinogenic activity of aromatic amines is not known at the present time. It is apparent that the conformational changes in nucleic acids produced by AAF could profoundly alter the biologic properties of cellular DNA as well as RNA. The relative susceptibility of specific guanosine residues to AAF modification, as well as the effects of base sequence on the type of conformational distortion which occurs, might play an important role in determining the biologic specificity of this carcinogen. If attack on the DNA is the critical event, then a conformational change would be more likely to produce small deletions rather than single base changes during DNA replication. A conformational change in specific regions of the DNA might also impair the transcription of certain genetic loci. With respect to RNA, the presence of an AAF residue on tRNA would be expected to distort the conformation of that region of the molecule, thereby altering interaction with amino-acyl-tRNA synthetases, codons, and/or ribosomes. It is not known whether AAF interacts with messenger RNAs in vivo, but the present results with synthetic codons suggest that if this does occur, then it would inhibit their function in protein synthesis. These, as well as additional effects on cellular RNAs, might, as I suggested at the beginning of this paper, lead to rather widespread disturbances in the translation apparatus, with secondary consequences with respect to cell differentiation, regulation, and autonomy.[1]

Acknowledgments

This research was supported by U. S. Public Health Service Research Grant No. R10 CA-02332 from the National Cancer Institute and the Alma Toorock Memorial for Cancer Research.

I. Bernard Weinstein is a Career Scientist of the Health Research Council of the City of New York (I-190).

References

1. Weinstein, I. B.: Modifications in transfer RNA during chemical carcinogenesis. In: Genetic Concepts and Neoplasia (The University of Texas M. D. Anderson Hospital and Tumor Institute at Houston, 23rd Annual Symposium on Fundamental Cancer Research 1969). The Williams and Wilkins Co., Baltimore, Maryland, 1970, pp. 380-408.
2. Berwald, Y., and L. Sachs: *In vitro* transformation of normal cells to tumor cells by carcinogenic hydrocarbons. J. Nat. Cancer Inst., 35:641, 1965.
3. Mondal, S., and C. Heidelberger: In vitro malignant transformation by methylcholanthrene of the progeny of single cells derived from C3H mouse prostate. Proc. Nat. Acad. Sci. USA, 65:219, 1970.

4. Gurdon, J. B.: Nuclear transplantation and cell differentiation. Cell Differentiation (CIBA Foundation Symposium) . Little, Brown & Co., Boston, 1967, p. 65.
5. Farber, E.: Biochemistry of carcinogenesis. Cancer Res., 28:1859, 1968.
6. Ortwerth, B. Y., and G. D. Novelli: Studies on the incorporation of L-ethionine-ethyl-1-^{14}C into the transfer RNA of rat liver. Cancer Res., 23:380, 1969.
7. Axel, R., I. B. Weinstein, and E. Farber: Patterns of transfer RNA in normal rat liver and during hepatic carcinogenesis. Proc. Nat. Acad. Sci. USA, 58:1255, 1967.
8. Agarwal, M. K., and I. B. Weinstein: Modification of RNA by chemical carcinogens. II. *In vivo* reaction of N-acetylaminofluorene with rat liver RNA. Biochemistry, 9:503, 1970.
9. Novelli, G. D., B. J. Ortwerth, U. Del Monte, and L. Rosen: Studies on the alkylation of rat liver transfer RNA by the hepatocarcinogen, ethionine. In: Genetic Concepts and Neoplasia (The University of Texas M. D. Anderson Hospital and Tumor Institute at Houston, 23rd Annual Symposium on Fundamental Cancer Research, 1969). The Williams and Wilkins Co., Baltimore, Maryland, 1970, pp. 409-426.
10. Henshaw, E. C., and H. H. Hiatt: Binding of fluorenylacetamide to rat liver ribonucleic acid (RNA) *in vivo* (Abstract). Proc. Amer. Ass. Cancer Res., 4:27, 1963.
11. Irving, C. C., R. A. Veazey, and R. F. Williard: On the significance and mechanism of the binding of 2-acetylaminofluorene and N-hydroxy-2-acetylaminofluorene to rat-liver ribonucleic acid *in vivo*. Cancer Res., 27:720, 1967.
12. Fink, L. M., S. Nishimura, and I. B. Weinstein: Modifications of RNA by chemical carcinogens. I. *In vitro* modification of transfer RNA by N-acetoxy-2-acetylaminofluorene. Biochemistry, 9:496, 1970.
13. Miller, E. C., Y. Juhl, and J. A. Miller: Nucleic acid guanine reaction with the carcinogen N-acetoxy-2-acetylaminofluorene. Science, 153:1125, 1966.
14. Grunberger, D., and I. B. Weinstein: Effect of 2-acetylaminofluorene (AAF) binding to guanosine on coding properties of ribopolynucleotides and triplets (Abstract). Xth Internat. Cancer Congr., Houston, Texas, 1970, p. 613.
15. Grunberger, D., J. H. Nelson, C. R. Cantor, and I. B. Weinstein: Coding and conformational properties of oligonucleotides modified with the carcinogen N-2-acetylaminofluorene. Proc. Nat. Acad. Sci. USA. In press.
16. Donohue, J., and K. N. Trueblood: Base pairing in DNA. J. Molec. Biol., 2:363, 1960.
17. Kapuler, A. M.: Dissertation. The Rockefeller University, 1969.
18. Michelson, A.: Personal communication.
19. Tavale, S. S., and H. M. Sobell: Crystal and molecular structure of 8-bromo-guanosine and 8-bromoadenosine, two purine nucleosides in the *syn* conformation. J. Molec. Biol., 48:109, 1970.
20. Miller, J. A., J.-K. Lin, and E. C. Miller: N-(guanosin-8-YL)- and N-(deoxyguanosin-8-YL)-N-methyl-4-aminoazobenzene: Degradation products of hepatic RNA and DNA from rats administered N-methyl-4-aminoazobenzene (MAB). Proc. Amer. Ass. Cancer Res., 11:56, 1970.
21. Lesko, S. A., H. D. Hoffman, P. O. P. Tsó, and V. M. Maher: Interaction and Linkage of Polycyclic Hydrocarbons to Nucleic Acids. In: Progress in Molecular and Submolecular Biology (F. Hahn, ed.), Springer Verlag, Berlin-Heidelberg, New York, Vol. 2. In Press.
22. Lawley, P. D., and P. Brookes: Molecular mechanisms of the cytotoxic action of difunctional alkylating agents and of resistance to this action. Nature, 206:480, 1965.
23. Fujimura, D. Grunberger, and I. B. Weinstein: Unpublished data.

Protein as Target of Reactive Forms

HIROSHI TERAYAMA

Zoological Institute, Faculty of Science, University of Tokyo, Tokyo, Japan

SINCE THE CHEMICAL BINDING of carcinogenic aminoazo dyes to rat liver proteins in vivo, reported for the first time by Miller and Miller in 1947,[1] similar binding of many other chemical carcinogens to cellular proteins in target tissues has been confirmed.[2-5] The phenomenon of carcinogen-protein interactions has been proved to be well correlated with the various carcinogenic parameters such as specificity of susceptibility of tissues or species to any carcinogen, carcinogenic potency of the agent, as well as effects of nutritional or hormonal conditions,[6] and it has been one of the primary concerns of many cancer researchers who are interested in the molecular basis of chemical carcinogenesis. Recently, however, the interaction of carcinogens with nucleic acids has also been evidenced in many cases of chemical carcinogenesis.

Consequently, two distinctly different lines of thought have been advanced with respect to the molecular mechanism of chemical carcinogenesis. One is the mutation theory, which emphasizes some alterations in the DNA molecules themselves as a real cause of neoplastic transformation of the cell. Another is a theory postulating some alterations in the regulatory mechanism in the expression of genetic information in the cell, which has nothing to do with direct changes in the DNA molecule. The latter view also seems to be intimately related with the mechanism of tissue differentiation during developmental stages, and it goes without saying that the binding of carcinogens to some specific cellular proteins seems to be of the utmost significance. In fact, more and more evidence has been accumulated in the area of cell biology, indicating that the nuclear-cytoplasmic interaction is not a one-way process, but cytoplasmic alterations may affect the nuclear activity and possibly in an apparently irreversible manner. Although some hypothetical models[7, 8] based on the carcinogen-protein binding have been postulated to explain the quasi-irreversible nature of neoplastic transformation of the cell, the experimental evidence does not seem to have been accumulated sufficiently. Nevertheless, our knowledge concerning the chemical structure of carcinogen-protein binding, possible reactive forms of carcinogens in vivo, and the nature of cellular proteins involved in the carcinogen binding has increased tremendously in a recent few years. Aminoazo dye is one of the chemical carcinogens which has been investigated most enthusiastically and most extensively with respect to these points.

For this reason and others, I wish to present the latest information which has been obtained in this particular group of carcinogens instead of discussing the matter of carcinogen-protein interactions in a more general manner. An oriental proverb says, "To know one is to begin to know all."

Methods and Materials

All the aminoazo dyes were purified by chromatography on alumina before use. Dyes were given to male Wistar rats of about 200 g body weight either by a single large-dose administration (40 mg dye dissolved in olive oil, intragastrically) or by a continuous feeding technique (0.06% dye in the semisynthetic diet, ad libitum). In the first group, the rats were killed 40 hr later when the dye-protein binding in the liver reached the maximum level; and in the second group, the rats were killed after certain periods of feeding (two weeks, one month, three months, etc.).

Polar dyes were prepared according to the method of Terayama et al.[9] Hydrolysis of liver proteins by pronase was sometimes repeated or done with a great excess of the enzyme in order to achieve the maximal hydrolysis of proteins. Extraction of polar dye with n-butanol, washing of polar dye in 2N HCl with ethylacetate, and purification of polar dye by successive chromatography on silica gel and Amberlite CG-50 (H+) were performed as usual.[9] Fractionation of polar dye into components was achieved by paper chromatography (Tōyō filter paper No. 51A) or cellulose thin-layer chromatography (Avicel SF). As solvent, usually either an aqueous phase of n-propanol:n-butanol:water (1:4:5 v/v) or an acetone:water (1:3 v/v) mixture was used. Sometimes a two-dimensional (ascending) method was adopted.

N-Methyl,N-benzoyloxy-4-aminoazobenzene (N-benzoyloxy-MAB) was prepared from MAB and benzoylperoxide according to Poirier et al.[10] The reaction of N-benzoyloxy-MAB with proteins or amino acids was done in an aqueous solution at neutral pH by adding a methanolic solution of the reactive form of dye dropwise. In the case of cystein or tyrosine, 0.3N KOH was added dropwise until the amino acid was almost dissolved, and then a methanolic solution containing N-benzoyloxy-MAB was added. The reaction was carried out at 37 C overnight. After the reaction, proteins were washed successively with acetone and ethanol and subjected to pronase hydrolysis. In the case of amino acids, the whole reaction mixture was evaporated under reduced pressure, and the residue was dissolved in 2N HCl and washed with ethylacetate, followed by silica gel and Amberlite CG-50 (H+) chromatography.

Chromatography of rat liver cell sap proteins on CM-cellulose was done by using a 2 × 26 cm column, except in the case of hepatoma cell sap for which a 1 × 20 cm column was used. Elution was done by running 0.01M Tris-HCl buffer, pH 7.0, 0.02M NaCl in the same buffer, and 0.05M NaCl in the same buffer stepwise. Gel filtration was done by using a 2.8 × 62 cm column of Sephadex G-100 (sometimes G-200) and washing was done by running 0.05M Tris-HCl buffer, pH 7.5 containing 0.1M KCl. Fractions were collected every 5.5 ml effluent in both chromatographies. Proteins were assayed by the method of Lowry et al., and arginase was assayed by the method of Van Slyke and Archibald.[11] Protein-bound dye was estimated by the spectrophotometric method in concentrated formic acid. The molar extinction coefficient at the maximum Q band of 4×10^4 was adopted for the calculation of the amount of protein-bound dye. Molecular weights of dye-binding proteins were estimated from elution volumes in Sephadex G-100 (or G-200) gel filtration.

Chemical Structure of Dye-Protein Binding

Studies on the chemical structure of aminoazo dye-protein binding have to start with the isolation of chemically pure polar dye components which consist of one mole dye and one mole amino acid. Usually several polar dye spots can be detected on chromatograms. For instance, on the chromatogram of cellulose thin layer using a mixture of acetone:water (1:3 v/v) as solvent, P3, P2a', P2a, P4, P1, P2b, Po, and Po' are detected in the order of increasing Rf values. P3 seems to consist of three or four subcomponents (P3a, P3b, P3c, and P3d). These polar dyes are not all independent entities. For instance, the change like P2b—P1—one of P3 subcomponent or P2a—another subcomponent of P3 has been reported.[9] It should also be noted that all of these polar dye components cannot always be well separated from each other in a single chromatographic system. More important is that the distribution or the pattern of polar dye components may also vary greatly, depending upon the experimental conditions including the material of polar dye source. For instance, the whole liver cell sap prepared 40 hr after a single large dose of 3'-Me-DAB administration gave P2b, P1, and P2a as major polar dye components, while the whole liver cell sap prepared from one month 3'-Me-DAB fed rats gave P4 and Po as major polar dye components. Such a change in the polar dye pattern seems to be explained as the result of alteration of dye-binding proteins in the rat liver cell sap, as will be discussed below.

Among the polar dye components, P2b and P1 have been investigated most extensively because P2b can be obtained as the largest component among polar dyes prepared from 40 hr 3'-Me-DAB rat liver and can be separated well from other components by paper chromatography.[12, 13] Upon rechromatographing P2b, a small portion of P1 is always accompanied. Treatment of P2b with H_2O_2 yielded P1 and P3 with large yields.[9] Therefore, P1 and P3 were considered as oxidized derivatives of P2b. The involvement of sulfur-containing amino acid in

P2b has been proved by two different micromethods, i.e. the sodium azide reaction[14] and the H_2PtCl_- and KI test.[15] The latter test was performed on the paper chromatogram of the $SnCl_2$ reduction product of the polar dye (P2b, P1). Meanwhile, Scribner et al.[16] suggested the involvement of methionyl residue in the dye-protein binding by the finding that the nonpolar dye, 3-methylmercapto-N-methyl-4-aminoazobenzene, is released by alkali at room temperature from the extracted but nonheated liver proteins of rats fed MAB or DAB. The implication was substantiated in our laboratory by the finding that ^{35}S-methionine but not ^{35}S-cystine is incorporated into P2b and P1, and that Raney Ni reduction of the polar dye yields α-aminobutyric acid instead of alanine.[17] Using [14]C N-methyl-labeled MAB or DAB, it has been confirmed that one N-methyl carbon is retained in the polar dye.[17, 18] Subsequently, data obtained in the Millers' laboratory,[19] and later also in our laboratory,[20] with isotopic MAB-containing N-methyl groups labeled with ^{14}C and ^{3}H, showed that the N-methyl group of MAB is retained in the polar dye as an intact form.[19] The latest synthetic approach confirmed that P2b has a structure of 3-(homocystein-S-yl)-MAB, and P1 is a sulfoxide derivative of it.[21] Thus the chemical structure of the major polar P2b and its S-oxygenated derivative P1 have been elucidated mainly as the results of elaborate works performed in the laboratories in Tokyo and Madison. Recently, the involvement of tyrosine in the polar dye components (P2a and P2a′ in our nomenclature; Pla and Plb in Millers' nomenclature) have also been reported in the two laboratories.[22, 23] Ketterer et al.[24] suggested the involvement of cystein residue in the polar dye derived from a basic dye-binding protein in the rat liver.

As to the amino acid-binding site in the aminoazo dye moiety, both the position 3 and the 4-amino nitrogen seem to be relevant. By the nitrous acid test of Terayama,[12, 13] many of the polar dye components derived from DAB, MAB, etc. (N-alkylated aminoazo dyes) showed a secondary amino group as an auxochromic group. In these polar dyes, N-methyl (alkyl) has been shown to be retained as an intact form,[19] and therefore the amino acid binding site cannot be at the 4-amino nitrogen. However, along with improvement in the isolation of polar dye, the presence of polar dye components having a tertiary amino group has been confirmed.[19, 22] In this case, the amino acid binding site seems to be the 4-amino group. Lin et al.[22] have reported that one tyrosine-derived polar dye (Pl-a) corresponds to this category. However, it might be concluded in general that in the case of N-alkylated aminoazo dyes having no orthosubstituent(s), for instance DAB, MAB, 3′-Me-DAB, 3′-Me-MAB, etc., the binding of dye to amino acid residue in protein occurs preferentially at position 3, although binding at the 4-amino group takes place to a small extent. On the contrary, in the case of aminoazo dyes which have no N-alkyl but have an orthosubstituent, for instance 2′,3-dimethyl-4-aminoazobenzene (orthoaminoazotoluene:o-AT), it has been shown by us[25, 26] that the amino acid binding takes place preferentially at the 4-amino group. In this case, the original aminoazo dye has a primary amino group, but the polar dye prepared from the liver of rats given o-AT has a secondary amino group. Methionine has been shown to be involved in the o-AT-protein binding in vivo.[25] The polar dye having an N-S bridge, as assumed by Terayama et al., for the o-AT polar dye is characterized by its lability and readily liberates nonpolar dye even by treatment in alkaline solution. Recently, model compounds for the o-AT polar dye have been synthesized in our laboratory, and good agreement between the model compounds and the natural o-AT polar dye has been observed with respect to spectral characteristics and chromatographic behavior, as well as readiness to liberate nonpolar dye, o-AT.[26]

In the case of aminoazo dyes having both N-alkyls and orthosubstituents like N,N-dimethyl-3,5-dimethyl-4-aminoazobenzene (3,5-diMe-DAB), it has been shown in our laboratory[25] that the dye is bound to protein in a fashion similar to o-AT after it has been completely N-demethylated. The polar dye obtained from the liver of rats given 3,5-diMe-DAB had a secondary amino group and readily yielded a nonpolar dye, 3,5-dimethyl-4-aminoazobenzene.

As to the reactive form of carcinogenic 2-acetylaminofluorene (AAF), the N-hydroxy derivative was presented by Miller et al.[27] In the case of aminoazo dyes, first N,N-dimethyl-4-aminoazobenzene-N-oxide (DAB-N-oxide) was suggested as a reactive intermediate metabolite by Terayama.[28, 29] This compound prepared from DAB and benzoyl peroxide is rather soluble in water, and induces hepatomas if given in drinking water and a few local tumors if given subcutaneously.[29] DAB-N-oxide was proved to be readily transformed into N-demethylated products (MAB, AB), 3-hydroxylated products (3-HO-DAB, 3-HO-MAB), as well as deoxygenated product (DAB) in the presence of a catalytic amount of heme compounds. The addition of amino acids or proteins to the reaction mixture gave dye-bound derivatives from which polar dyes were prepared.[28] Subsequently, however, the Wisconsin group proposed N-acyloxy-MAB as a reactive form of DAB or MAB.[10] The N-oxygenated product of AB is N-hydroxy-AB which was found in rat urine after AB administration in the form of glucuronide conjugate, but the N-hydroxy-AB was not so reactive.[30] N-Benzoyloxy-MAB prepared from MAB and benzoyl peroxide was shown to react with proteins and a few amino acids such as methionine, tyrosine, tryptophane, and cystein, and even with nucleic acids in an aqueous solution at neutral pH.[10]

N-Benzoyloxy-MAB has been prepared in our laboratory also, and the reactions of it with amino acids (Met, Tyr, Try, CySH), as well as with proteins, were investigated. The methionine polar dye thus synthesized gave two spots on paper and on cellulose thin-layer chromatograms at the same places as P2b and P1, respectively, in addition to a minor spot similar to Po'. The tyrosine polar dye also gave two major spots having Rf values similar to P2a' and P2b and a minor spot similar to P2a. The cystein polar dye gave a major spot having Rf also similar to P2a' and two minor spots resembling P4 and Po, respectively, while tryptophane polar dye gave three spots, two of which were near P2a and one near P1. The lowest Rf spot of both cystein and tryptophane polar dyes was violet in color in HCl. Other polar dyes were pink in HCl except P1 (orange red).

According to the recent report of Lin et al.[22] the tryptophane and cystein polar dyes could not be detected in the natural polar dye prepared from the liver of rats after a single large dose of 3'-Me-DAB. However, this does not exclude the possibility that these amino acid-derived polar dyes can be detected in the polar dye prepared from liver of rats given 3'-Me-DAB under different conditions, because, as will be shown later, the polar dye pattern is quite different under experimental conditions.

In order to investigate whether the in vivo interaction of carcinogenic aminoazo dye with proteins can be reflected well in the in vitro reaction of proteins with N-benzoyloxy-MAB, considered a reactive form or its analogue, we investigated the in vitro reaction of N-benzoyloxy-MAB with the rat liver cell sap, the rat serum, and bovine albumin, respectively. After the reaction, proteins were washed repeatedly with acetone and ethanol and then hydrolyzed with a large excess of pronase. The polar dye thus prepared was purified by HCl-ethylacetate extraction and chromatography on silica gel as well as on Amberlite CG-50 (H⁺) and finally subjected to cellulose thin-layer chromatography using acetone:water (1:3 v/v) as solvent. The rat liver cell sap reacted with N-benzoyloxy-MAB and gave many spots corresponding to P2a', P2b, P1, Po', P4 and P2a in the order of abundance. These polar dye components have been found also in the polar dye prepared from 3'-Me-DAB -40 hr rat liver cell sap. The only difference was the rather high yield of P2a' in the in vitro preparation. The rat liver cell sap reacted with N-benzoyloxy-MAB in vitro was dialyzed against 0.01 M Tris-HCl buffer, pH 7.0, and the soluble supernate obtained by centrifugation of the dialysate was then treated at 55° for 3 min followed by centrifugation. The supernate was subjected to chromatography on CM-cellulose. An elution pattern similar to that obtained for 40 hr 3'-Me-DAB rat liver cell sap (see below) was observed. Analysis of protein-bound dye revealed that it was predominantly located in the preliminary eluate, i.e. fraction I, in accordance with the in vivo results of single, large-dose administration experiments. The gel filtration of this fraction I revealed that almost 95% of protein-bound dye is located in the first peak (I-a) corresponding to 17×10^4 mol wt protein. In the case of rat serum or bovine serum albumin reacted with N-benzoyloxy-MAB in vitro, polar dyes corresponding to P2a', P2a, and P4 were obtained. In fact, the serum is only one extrahepatic tissue where dye-protein binding is detected in vivo and serum albumin is known as the dye-receptor.[31, 32] The serum of rats given 3′-Me-DAB (single large dose or continuous feeding) gave P2a′ solely as a major spot, and none of the methionine-derived polar dyes (P2b and P1) was detected. The above results, therefore, seem to indicate that the in vitro reaction of N-benzoyloxy-MAB mimics the possibly occurring reactions in rats given the carcinogenic aminoazo dye (3′-Me-DAB, etc.). The results of the present investigation also suggest that it is the nature of proteins which determines the type of dye-binding, as evidenced by means of polar dye pattern.

Nature of the Dye-Binding Proteins in the Rat Liver Cell Sap

As to the nature of carcinogenic aminoazo dye-binding proteins in the rat liver cell sap, Sorof et al.[33] first reported that most of the dye-binding proteins in the liver cell sap of rats given 3′-Me-DAB for a few weeks can be separated into a specific narrow band by zonal electrophoresis of the cell sap in pH 8.6 veronal buffer. This slowly migrating band was named "slow h_2" fraction and seemed to consist of proteins of a somewhat basic nature. Recently, they found that the arginase activity is localized in this fraction. Arginase has been known as an entity of the liver cell sap factor inhibiting the proliferation of cultured cells, and it is deleted in hepatomas. Based on these considerations, they proposed an idea that the liver arginase or its subunit might be a target protein for the reactive forms of carcinogenic aminoazo dye.[34] Sorof et al.[35] also indicated the presence of two other dye-binding proteins in the cell sap which were separated in the "slow g" fraction and rapidly moving "a" fraction, though the content of protein-bound dye in these minor fractions was much less than that in the "slow h_2" fraction under the experimental condition used by them (18 to 20 days, 3′-Me-DAB feeding). Whitcutt et al.[36] were the first who tried to isolate the dye-binding proteins from the rat liver by means of chromatographic techniques, and they found that the dye-binding proteins were recovered in the preliminary eluate by chromatography on DEAE-cellulose (pH 7.9). This fraction was subjected to starch-gel electrophoresis (pH 8.5) and divided into eight minor components. The protein-bound dye was observed in only one of them. These data by Whitcutt et al.[36] and Sorof et al.[33] indicate that the major dye-binding protein in the rat liver cell sap is very specific and of little basic nature. Recently, Ketterer et al.,[37] using a single large dose administration technique, investigated the isolation of dye-binding protein from the rat liver. However, they cut off almost two thirds of the dye-bound proteins from the rat liver cell sap by the pH 4.5 precipitation in the presence of Ca^{+2} and Cu^{+2} and NaCl before proceeding to chromatographic isolation of dye-binding proteins. This procedure might be useful for isolation of dye-binding proteins of basic nature, but apparently they have lost the major dye-binding proteins of nonbasic nature. Thus they isolated a basic dye-binding protein of about 4.5×10^4 mol wt and having Ip of 8.4. In addition to this protein, they reported the presence of two low molecular weight (1.4×10^4) dye-binding proteins having Ip near neutrality. According to Sorof et al.,[38] the molecular weight as determined by Sephadex G-200 gel filtration technique of the dye-binding protein in the slow h_2 fraction is in the range of 6-8×10^4. In addition to this, they also indicated the presence of minor dye-binding proteins having mol wt of 3-4×10^4 and 1-1.5×10^4, respectively.

In the present study, we have first investigated the dye-binding proteins in liver cell sap prepared from rats killed 40 hr after a single large dose of 3'-Me-DAB or 2-Me-DAB, and the results were compared with those obtained with the liver cell sap of rats fed a 3'-Me-DAB-containing diet for certain periods (two weeks, one month, three months, etc.).

The rat liver cell sap was prepared from 30% liver homogenate in 0.25 M sucrose by centrifugation at $105,000 \times g$ for 2 hr. The cell sap was then treated at 55° C for three min. By this treatment, almost 90% of the cell sap proteins were removed as insoluble precipitates in the case of single large-dose experiments, while the portions of heat-precipitable proteins decreased in the case of prolonged dye feeding.

Since the protein-bound dye and the arginase activity were retained almost completely in the heat-stable supernate, this thermal treatment seems to be an efficient purification process. The heat-treated cell sap was dialyzed against 0.01 M Tris-HCl buffer, pH 7.0, and the dialysate was subjected to chromatography on CM-cellulose equilibrated with the same buffer, and stepwise elution was performed.

In the case of a single large dose of 3'-Me-DAB, nearly one half of the total protein-bound dye was recovered in the preliminary eluate (fraction I), about 11% in a fraction eluted by 0.02 M NaCl (fraction IV), 2% in the first band eluted by 0.05 M NaCl (fraction VI), and 4% in the second band eluted by 0.05 M NaCl (fraction VII). The dye-binding proteins in fraction I seemed to be heterogenous. By saturating fraction I with ammonium sulfate, 70% of the protein-bound dye was recovered in the precipitates while the rest remained in the supernate. By adjusting pH at 5.0, 30% of the protein-bound dye was recovered in the precipitate while 70% remained in the supernate. Gel filtration of the saturated ammonium sulfate precipitate showed almost 90% of the protein-bound dye in the first peak eluted near the void volume, while gel filtration of the corresponding supernate showed a majority of the protein-bound dye only in the last protein peak. Gel filtration of pH 5 supernate revealed that the protein-bound dye can be divided into two peaks: 20% in the first peak and 50% in the last one. The whole fraction I, without being subjected to differential precipitation, gave a similar result. Ratio of dye bound to the large molecular weight protein (I-a) to that bound to the lower molecular weight protein (I-b) was approximately 3. At this stage of purification the specific dye-binding was 7.8 mμmole dye/mg protein in I-a and 5.7 mμmole dye/mg protein in I-b. The molecular weights of I-a and I-b were estimated as 17×10^4 and 1.2 to 1.5×10^4, respectively. Thus specific dye-binding as expressed in terms of mole dye/mole protein is 1.3 for I-a and 0.07 for I-b. The high specific dye-binding value of I-a suggests that this non-basic dye-binding protein is almost completely modified in the liver of rats 40 hr after 40 mg 3'-Me-DAB administration. Electrophoresis on cellulose acetate strips in different pH buffers indicated that I-a at this stage of purification consists of two molecular species of proteins, and azo dye is bound to one major protein band having Ip near 5.2.

Fraction IV, which was eluted by 0.02 M NaCl, contains the second largest portion of protein-bound dye. The dye-binding protein in fraction IV was completely recovered in 60% saturated ammonium sulfate precipitates, and gel filtration of the precipitated protein revealed that the dye-binding protein is predominantly in the first peak corresponding to a $16\text{-}17 \times 10^4$ mol wt. At this stage of purification, the IV dye-binding protein showed the specific dye-binding value of 9 mμ-mole/mg protein or 1.4 mole dye/mole protein. Electrophoresis at pH 8.6 indicated that it still consists of two molecular species of protein, but dye is bound only to one major protein band which migrates slightly to the anodic side.

Fraction VII was subjected to gel filtration in the same manner. The dye-binding proteins seemed to be divided into the first and the third (the last) bands which corresponded to molecular weights of 16×10^4 and 4×10^4, respectively. The specific dye-binding of the first band protein (VII-a) was 1.0 mole dye/mole protein and that of the third band protein (VII-b) was 0.01 mole dye/mole protein, respectively, at this stage of purification. The analysis of fraction VI has not yet been completed. The electrophoresis of VII-a showed that the dye-bound protein did not migrate at pH 8.6.

In one method for determining which of these dye-binding proteins found in 40 hr 3'-Me-DAB rat liver cell sap might have some special connection to the carcinogenic mechanism, 2-Me-DAB, known as non-carcinogenic but able to bind to liver protein exceptionally, was given to rats. The heat-treated cell sap was subjected to chromatography on CM-cellulose in the same manner. The result was quite interesting. 2-Me-DAB was shown to be bound predominantly to fraction IV. Of the total protein-bound dye, 53% was in this fraction, while only 6% was detected in fraction I. The protein-bound dye was also detected in fractions VI and VII, but to the extent similar to the case of 3'-Me-DAB (6 and 7%, respectively). Thus it seems that the dye-binding to fraction IV seemed to be less specific, as compared with the binding to fraction I with respect to carcinogenesis. The binding of carcinogenic aminoazo dye to fraction I has not been reported before. The main

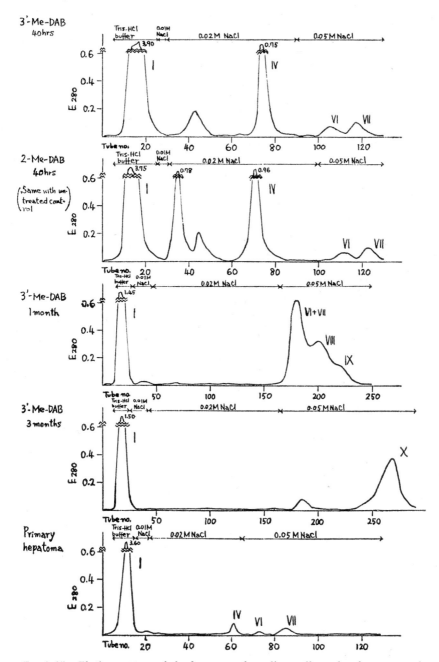

Fig. 1–15.—Elution pattern of the heat-treated rat liver cell sap by chromatography on CM-cellulose.

reason for this is that the investigations hitherto have been performed on the liver cell sap of rats fed a 3'-Me-DAB-containing diet for a few weeks. Only Ketterer et al.[32] have investigated the cell sap shortly after a single large dose of 3'-Me-DAB, but they abandoned this nonbasic dye-binding protein by the pH 4.5 precipitation. As described above, the polar dye from fraction IV gave only P2a' spot, while that from fraction I showed the polar dye pattern similar to that of the whole liver cell sap (P2b, P1, and P2a as major components).

In the second series of investigation, the chromatographic analysis of heat-treated liver cell sap of rats fed a 3'-Me-DAB-containing diet for different periods has been performed. Although the study has not yet been finished, I wish to present some of the results obtained to date. Quite interestingly, the elution pattern of proteins as well as the localization of protein-bound dye were entirely different from those observed for a single large-dose administration. As to the elution pattern of the heat-treated cell sap proteins, a marked decrease of fraction I and almost complete loss of fraction IV should be mentioned. At the same time, the appearance of more basic dye-binding proteins such as fractions VIII, IX, and X in the cell sap seems to deserve special attention. These new protein fractions appeared to be eluted from CM-cellulose by 0.05 M NaCl (pH 7.0) further behind fractions VI and VII which are present in normal as well as 40 hr 3'-Me-DAB rat liver cell sap. All of these basic proteins seem to belong to Sorof's "slow h_2" fraction because they may not be separated by electrophoresis at pH 8.6. The analysis of protein-bound dye revealed that only 11% of the total protein-bound dye is localized in fraction I, 30% in fractions VI + VII, and 30% and 20% in the new, more basic fractions VIII and IX, respectively, in the case of one-month 3'-Me-DAB-fed rat liver. In the three-month 3'-Me-DAB-fed rat liver, the change in the distribution of protein-bound dye was more dramatic. Only 1% was in fraction I, and a majority amounting to 80% was in another new fraction, X. Sephadex gel filtration of fraction I revealed that the dye-binding to I-a disappeared more rapidly than to I-b.

Hepatomas induced by a long-term 3'-Me-DAB feeding have been investigated in the same manner, but no protein-bound dye was detected in any of the fractions separated by chromatography on CM-cellulose.

The CM-cellulose chromatographic elution patterns of proteins in the heat-treated rat liver cell saps prepared under different conditions are illustrated in Figure 1-15. Distributions of protein-bound dye among the CM-cellulose chromatographic fractions are summarized in Table 1-8, and some of the molecular parameters of isolated dye-binding proteins are summarized in Table 1-9.

As to the identification of arginase with any one of the dye-binding proteins as described above, we may comment briefly as follows. Although arginase (in the 55 C, three-min heated liver cell sap) was

TABLE 1–8.—PERCENTAGE DISTRIBUTION OF PROTEIN-BOUND DYE AMONG CM-CELLULOSE CHROMATOGRAPHIC FRACTIONS

Liver Cell Sap Sample	Fr. I (I-A:I-B)		Fr. IV	Fr. VI	Fr. VII	Fr. VIII	Fr. IX	Fr. X	Total Recovery %
40 h 40 mg 3'-Me-DAB	41	(3:1)	11	2	4	N.D.	N.D.	N.D.	69
40 h 40 mg 2-Me-DAB	6		53	6	7	N.D.	N.D.	N.D.	88
1 month 3'-Me-DAB diet	11	(1:2)	0	30		30	20	N.D.	101
3 month 3'-Me-DAB diet	1	(1:6)	0	0	0	7	7	76	91
Induced hepatoma	0		0	0	0	0	0	0	—

shown to be scattered among several fractions such as I, IV, VI, and VII, suggesting the polymorphism of arginase or interaction with cellular components, the major portion of it (70% of the total activity) was recovered in the last two fractions, VI and VII. However, the gel filtration of fraction VII clearly separated the arginase activity from the dye-binding protein. The dye-binding protein in fraction VII was eluted as the first peak (VII-a) and the third peak (VII-b), corresponding to the molecular weights of 16×10^4 and 4×10^4, respectively, while the arginase activity was eluted as the second peak, corresponding to the molecular weight of 13×10^4. During the course of the present investigations, it has been noticed that the arginase activity of the rat liver cell sap decreased shortly after onset of feeding, but then

TABLE 1–9.—ISOLATED DYE-BINDING PROTEINS AND THEIR CHARACTERISTICS

Nomenclature of Dye-Binding Proteins	Electrolytic Nature (Ip)	Mol. Weight ($\times 10^{-4}$)	Specific Dye-Binding (mole dye/mole protein) (Extl. cond.)		Approx. Conc. in the Total Cell Sap Proteins (%)
I-a	non-basic (5.2)	17	1.3	(40 h, 3'-Me-DAB)	0.5
I-b	non-basic	1.2-1.5	0.07	(40 h, 3'-Me-DAB)	0.7
IV	slightly basic (8.2)	16-17	1.4	(40 h, 3'-Me-DAB)	0.05
VII-a	more basic	16	1.0	(40 h, 3'-Me-DAB)	0.01
VII-b	more basic	4	0.01	(40 h, 3'-Me-DAB)	0.2
VIII	more basic	6.8	1.0	(1 month, 3'-Me-DAB)	0.4
XI	more basic	17	1.2	(1 month, 3'-Me-DAB)	0.4

started to increase again and even became much higher than the normal level. The arginase activity either in the normal liver cell sap or in the cell sap from 40 hr 3'-Me-DAB rat was rather stable and no serious loss of activity was observed during 55 C, three min treatment as well as chromatographic procedures, while the arginase activity in the liver cell sap of rats fed 3'-Me-DAB for one month or three months seemed to be more labile, and the increasing loss of activity was observed during the purification processes. It should be mentioned that the stability of dye-binding proteins did not seem to be much altered in contrast to arginase.

To investigate whether the nonbasic dye-binding protein, I-a, is actually detected during the course of chemical carcinogenesis, rabbits were immunized against I-a used as an antigen in the complete Freund adjuvant, and the antisera thus obtained have been reacted with the normal rat liver cell sap, one-month dye-fed rat liver cell sap, primary hepatoma, and ascites hepatoma cell saps. By means of Ouchterlony and immunoelectrophoretic techniques, it has been confirmed that I-a antigen is present in the normal rat liver, greatly reduced in the one-month dye-fed rat liver, and deleted in the two hepatomas.

Discussion

The results presented in this paper seem to indicate that the dye-binding proteins present primarily in the normal liver cell sap not only can be deleted but also can be replaced by another dye-binding protein appearing in succession during the course of the chemical carcinogenesis. It has already been demonstrated[39] that the amount of dye-protein binding increases with the period of dye-feeding, reaches a maximal level at a certain period of dye-feeding, then starts to decline, and appears to be maintained at a constant level later on. Apparently some dramatic changes take place around the time of maximal binding, occurring after two to three weeks' feeding of 3'-Me-DAB, as evidenced also in the present study by means of dye-binding protein analysis. Since the discovery of the dye-protein binding in vivo, the aminoazo dye-binding to "slow h_2" protein has attracted the scientific concern of many investigators. However, the present study has indicated that the nonbasic protein in the rat liver cell sap, especially I-a, is the most efficient azo dye receptor and is the dye-binding protein which seems to be deleted during an early period of dye-feeding relevant to the initiation stage. Further investigations on the biochemical as well as biologic activities of these dye-binding proteins isolated in the present study seem to be of utmost importance.

Acknowledgments

The author acknowledges with gratitude the many contributions by the following dedicated co-workers who made the findings described here possible: Mr. T. Sugimoto, Dr. M. Matsumoto, and Dr. I. Kimura.

References

1. Miller, E. C., and J. A. Miller: Cancer Res., 7:468, 1947.
2. Miller, E. C., and J. A. Miller: Cancer Res., 12:547, 1952.
3. Weisburger, E. K., J. H. Weisburger, and H. P. Morris: Arch. Biochem. Biophys., 43:474, 1953.
4. Miller, E. C.: Cancer Res., 10:232, 1950.
5. Wiest, W. G., and C. Heidelberger: Cancer Res., 13:250, 1953.
6. Miller, J. A., and E. C. Miller: Adv. Cancer Res., 1:339, 1953.
7. Pitot, H. C., and C. Heidelberger: Cancer Res., 23:1964, 1963.
8. Terayama, H., and M. Sasada: Gann, 59:51, 1968.
9. Terayama, H.: Methods in Cancer Research (H. Busch, ed.), Vol. 1, 1967, p. 399.
10. Poirier, L. A., J. A. Miller, E. C. Miller, and K. Sato: Cancer Res., 27:1600, 1967.
11. Van Slyke, D. D., and R. M. Archibald: J. Biol. Chem., 165:293, 1946.
12. Terayama, H., and M. Takeuchi: Gann, 53:293, 1962.
13. Hanaki, H., and H. Terayama: Gann, 53:285, 1962.
14. Feigl, F.: Spot Tests in Organic Analysis (R. E. Oesper, tr.), Elsevier, 5th ed., 1958.
15. Winegard, H. M., and G. Toennies: Science, 108:506, 1948.
16. Scribner, J. D., J. A. Miller, and E. C. Miller: Biochim. Biophys. Res. Comm., 20:560, 1965.
17. Higashinakagawa, T., M. Matsumoto, and H. Terayama: Biochim. Biophys. Res. Comm., 24:811, 1966.
18. Terayama, H., A. Hanaki, and M. Ishidate: Gann, 51:383, 1960.
19. Lin, J.-K., J. A. Miller, and E. C. Miller: Biochim. Biophys. Res. Comm., 29:1040, 1967.
20. Matsumoto, M., and H. Terayama: Chemico-Biol. Interac., 2. In press.
21. Lin, J.-K., J. A. Miller, and E. C. Miller: Biochemistry, 7:1889, 1968.
22. Lin, J.-K., J. A. Miller, and E. C. Miller: Biochemistry, 8:1573, 1969.
23. Matsumoto, M., and H. Terayama: Chemico-Biol. Interac., 1:73, 1969/1970.
24. Ketterer, B., and L. Christodoulides: Chemico-Biol. Interac., 1:173, 1969/1970.
25. Matsumoto, M., H. Takata, and H. Terayama: Gann, 59:231, 1968.
26. Matsumoto, M., and H. Terayama: Chemico-Biol. Interac., 2. In press.
27. Cramer, J. W., J. A. Miller, and E. C. Miller: J. Biol. Chem., 235:885, 1960.
28. Terayama, H.: Gann, 54:195, 1963.
29. Terayama, H., and H. Orii: Gann, 54:455, 1963.
30. Sato, K., L. A. Poirier, J. A. Miller, and E. C. Miller: Cancer Res., 26:1678, 1966.
31. Kusama, K.: Nippon Kagaku Zassi, 81:763, 1960.
32. Dijkstra, J., and H. M. Griggs: Proceedings of the IX International Cancer Congress, 1966, p. 183.
33. Sorof, S., P. P. Cohen, E. C. Miller, and J. A. Miller: Cancer Res., 11:383, 1951.
34. Sorof, S., E. M. Young, L. Luongs, V. Kish, and J. J. Freed: Wistar Symp. Monogr., 7:25, 1967.
35. Sorof, S., E. M. Young, M. M. McCue, and P. L. Fetterman: Cancer Res., 23:864, 1963.
36. Whitcutt, J. M., D. A. Sutton, and J. R. Nunn: Biochem. J., 75:557, 1960.
37. Ketterer, B., P. Ross-Mansell, and J. K. Whitehead: Biochem. J., 103:316, 1967.
38. Sorof, S.: Jerusalem Symp. Quant. Chem. Biochem., 1:208, 1969.
39. Miller, E. C., J. A. Miller, R. W. Sapp, and G. M. Weber: Cancer Res., 9:336, 1949.

Assessment at Tissue and Cellular Level

EMMANUEL FARBER AND
SHELDON M. EPSTEIN

*Department of Pathology, University of Pittsburgh
School of Medicine, Pittsburgh, Pennsylvania, USA*

WORK DURING the past 10 years or so in several laboratories around the world has clearly established that chemical carcinogens interact chemically with various tissue components. Some carcinogens, the so-called "direct-acting," appear to be the ultimate carcinogen per se and seem to require no prior biologic conversion to a "proximate" or ultimate carcinogen. Other carcinogens, the "indirect-acting," appear to require conversion to one or more active derivatives before they are able to interact with tissue components. The details of these metabolic conversions are now being clarified in several laboratories and some have already been discussed by the previous speakers.

Following the initial discovery of protein interaction by the Millers, it seemed as if many of the chemical carcinogens would react only with some cellular proteins. However, more recent work has clearly shown that we are dealing with a surfeit of interactions—we seem to have many more than we need. As already presented in the preceding four papers, carcinogens interact with DNA, RNA, and protein. Some also interact with glycogen. Very likely, other more complex polysaccharides as well as possibly lipids, may also be active sites for interaction. Do all of the various interactions play some role in the development of cancer, or only certain one or ones? This now becomes one of the most challenging questions in carcinogenesis today.

It appears to us that there are at least two ways to approach this problem—one we might call "prospective" and one "retrospective," borrowing the terminology of the epidemiologist. The prospective approach would attempt to establish a one-to-one correlation between a single interaction and the ability to induce cancer. Conceivably, through the use of different species of animals or cell types or by the use of compounds designed to competitively or noncompetitively suppress all but one of the interactions, it might become possible to establish a one-to-one correlation. In this case, the end point could be presence or absence of malignant neoplasia. This is an approach which might entice some talented organic chemists with a biologic interest to come into cancer research.

The retrospective approach looks backward from a result to a cause. By examining from different points of view a consequence of the administration of a carcinogen, can one rationally select the relevant alterations and discard the others? A prejudged example of this is DNA and somatic mutation. If one could be certain that the essential change in neoplastic transformation lies in the information content of the chromosomal genetic apparatus, it would be logical to focus exclusive or major attention on the DNA. This judgment seems to have been made already by many workers. However, the judgment is premature, since the biologic aberration of the malignant neoplastic cell may reflect only a change in information expression and not in information content. If such be the case, altered highly selective proteins or RNA or even polysaccharides or lipids may play important roles in the carcinogenic process.

Basic to any analysis of carcinogenesis is the establishment of the cell populations involved. Are we dealing with the direct transformation of an initial cell population into a malignant neoplastic one? If so, the relatively long latent period between the cessation of the administration of the carcinogen and the appearance of cancer is the time required for growth of a committed transformed cell. This presupposes that a cancer cell can arise from a nonneoplastic precursor cell in the absence of growth or cell proliferation. There is virtually no evidence to support this hypothesis.

Are we dealing with a sequence of changes, an early one being nonmalignant semiautonomous growth of another cell population which is the precursor for the cancer cell? This appears to be valid in many systems—liver, skin, mammary gland, several endocrine glands, melanomas, stomach, etc. It may turn out that the carcinogen must have two essential properties: (1) to alter some one or more key cellular macromolecules in such a manner as to leave a lasting impression, and (2) to stimulate some altered cells to proliferate so as to fix or imprint the change and to allow it to become magnified. The next stage, the malignant transformation, would no longer require the carcinogen but would occur with a reasonably high probability given the first two changes.

Let us look briefly at one such system which, although early in its development, has already given us some new insight into carcinogenesis in the liver.

The new proliferating cell population in the liver has been called the hyperplastic nodule (HLN). After years of dietary manipulation, we have finally been able to develop a reasonably satisfactory model for looking at this stage in liver carcinogenesis.

Using three different hepatic carcinogens, 2-acetylaminofluorene (AAF), ethionine or aflatoxin B_1, we are able to induce large HLN in well over 50% of rats. These nodules persist for many weeks after the carcinogen is removed from the diet. They are being examined during this time and not while the carcinogen is still being administered.

This new cell population has lost or acquired whatever is necessary to set in motion growth in vivo and in vitro under conditions in which the original surviving cell population does not. For example, in vivo, the nodules show slow progressive growth with a considerably elevated labeling index with thymidine. In vitro, the nodule shows growth under conditions in which the surrounding liver does not. The growth is different than that of liver cancer. Using several criteria, the cells appear to be liver cells. Unlike cancer, they do not have an unlimited capacity for growth, but rather show only a restricted growth of from six to eight generations. They grow well during this time period, but then lose the capacity.

Are there any stigmata of the macromolecular alterations in the original cell population in this new hyperplastic population, and if so, can one use this to separate the relevant from irrelevant initial interactions? In the case of nodules induced by AAF, altered DNA has been found. (1) The nodule DNA shows absorption in the range of 300 to 340 mμ, very similar to that observed when double-stranded liver or thymus DNA is reacted in vitro with N-acetoxy-AAF. This is absent from the DNA from the surrounding liver. (2) The nodule DNA, but not that from the surrounding liver, has a small population (2 to 3%) with a greater buoyant density in CsCl than the bulk of liver DNA. (3) By electron microscopy, the nodule DNA shows many areas of strand separation and "puddles" not seen in DNA from normal liver, from surrounding liver, or from regenerating liver at two different times (17 and 23 hr) after partial hepatectomy.

Thus, a retrospective approach can uncover altered cellular macromolecules that may be used in the analysis of relevance, and could be used as a basis for a working hypothesis of liver carcinogenesis with AAF. For example, the hyperplastic cell population, having lost the ability to repair its altered DNA, may now show a progressive distortion of its DNA with each cycle of replication. Such a phenomenon could play a role in the slow but progressive changes in the premalignant cell leading to a stepwise appearance of discrete properties characteristic of cancer.

This formulation may not be unique to AAF. Dimethylaminoazobenzene or its active derivatives bind in a covalent-like manner to liver nucleic acids, the binding to DNA persists for months after termination of exposure to the carcinogen, and a noncarcinogenic derivative becomes carcinogenic when combined with partial hepatectomy. These findings, coupled with the observations concerning cell populations during azo dye carcinogenesis, suggest that the hypothesis outlined may be applicable, in principle, to carcinogenesis with chemicals other than AAF.

However, caution is again required. On examining another macromolecule, glycogen, clear-cut evidence for a bound AAF derivative is present. This could theoretically account for the observation of some alteration in glycogen in nodules made by many investigators of liver cancer, beginning with Sasaki and Yoshida in 1935 with o-aminoazotoluene and including recent studies with nitrosamines, ethionine, and virtually every hepatic carcinogen. Also, a similar type of bound AAF derivative is present in the small amount of glycogen in liver cancer induced by AAF, even though the animal has not had any exogenous carcinogen for months. Could such an altered macromolecule, by feedback or other mechanisms of information expression, play an important role in the genesis of malignant transformation by a non-DNA pathway?

In conclusion, it is evident that the assessment of the interaction of chemicals with cellular components at the tissue and cellular level will require us to focus on different cell populations during carcinogenesis, but in so doing we may uncover interesting and potentially important new properties of cells and cell constituents altered by carcinogens. Hopefully, such studies may aid in the ultimate analysis and synthesis of the molecular events that are responsible for and that accompany the sequence of cellular changes leading to malignant neoplasia.

2

Chemical Carcinogenesis In Vitro

"Spontaneous" Neoplastic Transformation In Vitro

KATHERINE K. SANFORD

Tissue Culture Section, Laboratory of Biology, National Cancer Institute,
National Institutes of Health, Bethesda, Maryland, USA

THE ONLY CONCLUSIVE TEST at present for the neoplastic transformation
of cells in vitro is to implant the cells in compatible hosts and obtain
from the implants invasive, progressively growing neoplasms. Almost
all cell lines that have been adequately tested by this method have
been found to undergo neoplastic transformation even in the absence
of any deliberately added carcinogen or carcinogenic agent. Such transformations have occurred repeatedly in cells from embryonic, neonatal, or adult tissues of several strains of mice, Syrian and Chinese
hamsters, different strains of rat, and man.[1] The cells converted after
various periods of culture. Mouse cells appear to be the most unstable, with transformations occurring as early as 56 days in vitro.[2]
However, in other rapidly proliferating mouse cell lines grown in the
same type of medium and subcultured on the same schedule, the cells
transformed after more than three years in culture. Syrian hamster
embryo cells have transformed by 90 days and after more than 300
days in vitro,[3, 4] Chinese hamster adult tissue cells by six months,[5]
and rat cells after more extended periods of nine to 30 months.[6] This
high incidence of "spontaneous" neoplastic transformation must be
considered in evaluating data from chemical carcinogenesis studies.

The etiology of these transformations attendant on serial culture in
vitro has not been identified to date. Their occurrence in chemically

76

defined medium would appear to eliminate chemical carcinogens as a cause.[7, 8] Chromosomal aberrations, which occur early in many normal and neoplastic cells in culture, and tumor viruses, especially leukemia virus, have been suggested as causative. Efforts to associate the time of chromosomal alterations with the onset of neoplastic conversion or to identify any specific chromosomal alteration in neoplastic as compared with nonneoplastic cell populations in vitro have not been successful to date.[6, 9] In collaborative studies with Dr. Hartley, more than 75 murine cell lines from 24 mouse cell pools were examined for complement-fixing mouse leukemia virus antigens and for recoverable virus.[5, 10] All lines were also assayed for neoplastic transformation. Of the cell pools, 42% gave rise to lines showing the presence of leukemia virus. Some of these lines also underwent neoplastic transformation; others have not in tests to date. The remaining 58% gave rise to lines with no evidence of leukemia virus, but most of these also underwent neoplastic transformation. These results, although not excluding the possibility of a viral etiology, suggest that spontaneous neoplastic transformation can occur in the absence of detectable mouse leukemia virus. Neoplastic transformations have also occurred in rat cells; no leukemia virus has as yet been isolated from the rat.

Another possible cause is the abnormal environment in vitro which lacks certain of the homeostatic controls operative in vivo. In our search for means of preventing neoplastic transformation, which is probably one of the most urgent problems for further use of long-term cells in cancer research and for vaccine production, certain more physiologic methods of culture should be explored.

The observation by Evans and Andresen[11] that neoplastic transformation is reproducible with respect to time of occurrence in C3H mouse embryo cells grown in chemically defined medium (CDM) supplemented with gelding horse serum (HS) provided an experimental baseline for studies on factors influencing this transformation. The type of serum supplement was found to be important. Cells grown in HS-supplemented CDM converted after approximately 90 to 180 days in vitro. Cells from the same pool grown in CDM with fetal calf serum (FCS) as supplement converted only after significantly longer periods, sometimes up to several years, even though proliferating at similar rates.[2] When cells were transferred from one serum to the other, the longer the time in HS before transfer to FCS, the shorter the time required for neoplastic conversion. Cells grown for only 15 days in HS before transfer converted sooner than cells initiated and maintained in FCS.[12]

In explanation of these observations, we have been considering the following possibilities: (1) The type of serum may have a direct effect on the cells or an indirect effect by supporting the proliferation of different cell types. Certain observations support the latter concept, but clonal studies are needed to resolve this point. (2) Some component (s) of HS may induce neoplastic transformation. (3) Some component (s) of FCS may inhibit conversion. If some component of FCS inhibits, it might also be inhibitory in a medium containing HS. We have found that cells grown in CDM with both FCS and HS show a greatly delayed conversion as compared with cells maintained continuously in HS medium. Further studies are in progress to identify the possible stabilizing fraction (s) in FCS.

The different effects of these two serums on cells in vitro have made it possible to compare properties of paired nonneoplastic and neoplastic cell lines derived from a common cell pool after equal periods of culture in vitro and when proliferating at approximately the same rate. Such comparisons should be useful in developing some reliable criteria of neoplastic state applicable to populations of cells or even individual cells in culture.

A change in growth pattern characterized by a random orientation and piling up of cells has been observed in response to certain tumor viruses and chemical carcinogens. This response, referred to as "transformation," appears in certain studies to be associated with neoplastic transformation, although this response may also be obtained in cells already neoplastic when treated.[13] Since neoplastic cells may exhibit confluent monolayer growth and nonneoplastic cells may grow in randomly oriented multilayers, as shown in Figure 2-1 (for review see reference 1; also 13, 14), additional criteria of neoplastic transformation are obviously needed.

In collaboration with Dr. Barker, we tested whether cytologic diagnoses of neoplastic transformation could be made accurately on cultured cells in vitro.[5, 14] Cytologic criteria of malignancy as applied to tissues or exfoliated cells in vivo served as guidelines for the diagnoses in vitro. Diagnosis was made on stained cover slip preparations sent coded to Dr. Barker. We determined the neoplastic state by animal assay. In two studies, several populations of mixed cell types from embryos of the C3Hf and germ-free ALB-M2 mouse, Syrian hamster, and ALB/N rat were followed during long-term culture. Of the 14 cell lines initiated, all but one underwent neoplastic transformation. Most lines undergoing such transformation showed a progression of cytologic changes in the following order: increase in cytoplasmic basophilia, increase in number and size of nucleoli, slight retraction of cytoplasm resulting in cell separation and apparent increase in nuclear:cytoplasmic ratio, further extensive retraction of cells from glass substrate frequently resulting in bipolar or rounded cell form, and finally, cohesion of cells in cords and clusters. This cohesion or sticking might conceivably be associated with the accumulation of specific mucopolysaccharides on the cell surface. In the first study, diagnoses of 93% of the 95 cultures were consistent with results of in vivo assays; in the second study, all 41 cultures were correctly diagnosed.

One of the earliest cytologic changes associated with neoplastic conversion was an increase in cytoplasmic basophilia. Usually the cells

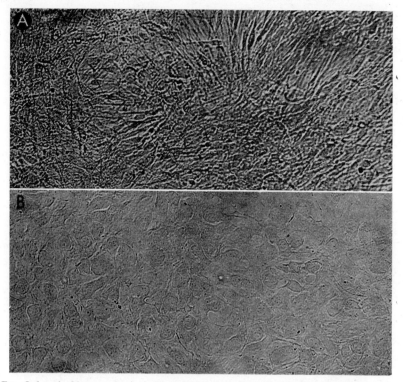

Fig. 2–1.—A—Nonneoplastic cells derived from Syrian hamster embryos after 42 days in vitro. Note criss-cross, multilayered growth pattern. B—Cells from mouse mammary carcinoma. Note lack of "piling up" and flattened monolayer growth pattern. Reduced from ×200.

showing this change retracted from each other and from the glass substrate to assume a more bipolar or rounded form. We did not know whether the increased cytoplasmic basophilia resulted from an actual increase in numbers of ribosomes and polysomes or whether this characteristic reflected the change in cell shape. If the cells assumed a more bipolar shape and retracted from the glass surface, their cytoplasmic basophilia on microscopic observation might appear to be increased.

Examination by electron microscopy of sectioned cells showed that the cytoplasmic basophilia of the neoplastic cells was associated with more numerous ribosomes occurring free or clumped as well as coating numerous surfaces of rough ER. In nonneoplastic cells proliferating at approximately the same rate in culture as the neoplastic cells, the rough ER had greatly dilated cisternae and the cytoplasm contained relatively fewer ribosomes scattered singly or in clumps. From these observations on the increase in cytoplasmic basophilia associated with increased densities of ribosomes and polysomes in the cytoplasm of the neoplastic cells, we might infer that protein synthesis is more active in the neoplastic as compared with the nonneoplastic cells even when growing at similar rates in vitro. However, further studies on protein synthesis and mitotic rates in clonal derivatives are needed to establish this point.

A conspicuous difference between many of the neoplastic and non-neoplastic cells was the loose attachment of the neoplastic cells to glass

FIG. 2–2.—Film sequence to show division of NCTC strain 2071 cell *(arrow)* completely surrounded by and in contact with neighboring cells. Cells are growing in unsupplemented chemically defined medium and under these conditions grow as a monolayer without piling up.[17] Although there appears to be a white space around each cell, cell membranes are actually in contact. Reduced from ×176.

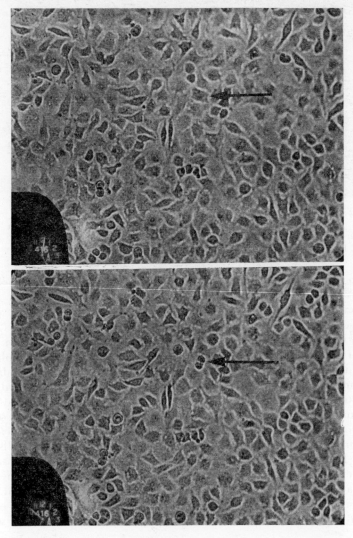

substrate, and their clumping, detachment, and sloughing in dense culture. While this characteristic was particularly noticeable in HS-supplemented CDM, it appeared also in FCS medium. These observations on the living cells confirmed those on the cytology of the fixed and stained cells. Whereas the nonneoplastic cells were well spread on the solid substrate, the neoplastic cells showed extensive retraction from each other and from the glass substrate, tending to grow on each other in cords and clusters rather than as a confluent sheet.

This growth pattern change has sometimes been attributed to a loss of contact inhibition of mitosis.[16] Cessation of division in confluent monolayer cultures particularly of nonneoplastic cells has been interpreted as resulting from cell contact. However, other interpretations are also possible. The cessation of division in such cultures might result from the lack of surface substrate for outgrowth. From microcinematographic studies[17] we have observed, as have others,[18] that certain cells that tend to grow as monolayers continue to divide when surrounded by and in contact with neighboring cells (Figure 2-2). Thus, contact alone appears not to be the inhibiting factor in such monolayer growth. As the cells continue to divide, they gradually change shape from a flattened to a more rounded form. Rates of mitosis ultimately decline with this change in shape and with the decrease in the substrate area occupied by the cell. These observations suggest that the rate of cell division may depend on the area of surface substrate available for cell spreading. Most cells derived from fixed tissues in vivo require a surface substrate which allows membrane spreading and serves as a stimulus for migration and division. The tendency of many neoplastic cells to retract from each other and from the substrate and also to acquire the capacity to grow in suspension suggests that they are less dependent on surface substrate. When a well-spread cell retracts, its surface exposed to the medium may be reduced manyfold. This reduced surface:volume ratio, in turn, could conceivably have profound effects on rates of exchange through the cell membrane and on membrane activity. This reduced substrate dependency, rather than loss of contact inhibition, may account for the growth pattern change observed in the neoplastic transformation of certain cell types in culture and may also have considerable biologic significance.

References

1. Sanford, K. K.: Malignant transformation of cells *in vitro*. Internat. Rev. Cytol., 18:249-311, 1965.
2. Evans, V. J., and W. F. Andresen: Effect of serum on spontaneous neoplastic transformation *in vitro*. J. Nat. Cancer Inst., 37:247-249, 1966.
3. Gotlieb-Stematsky, T., A. Yaniv, and A. Gazith: Spontaneous malignant transformation of hamster embryo cells *in vitro*. J. Nat. Cancer Inst., 36:477-482, 1966.
4. Sanford, K. K., and R. E. Hoemann: Neoplastic transformation of mouse and hamster cells *in vitro* with and without polyoma virus. J. Nat. Cancer Inst., 39:691-703, 1967.
5. Sanford, K. K., and associates: Unpublished data.

6. Jackson, J. L., K. K. Sanford, and T. B. Dunn: Neoplastic conversion and chromosomal characteristics of rat embryo cells *in vitro*. J. Nat Cancer Inst. In press.

7. Andresen, W. F., F. M. Price, J. L. Jackson, T. B. Dunn, and V. J. Evans: Characterization and spontaneous neoplastic transformation of mouse embryo cells isolated and continuously cultured *in vitro* in chemically defined medium NCTC 135. J. Nat. Cancer Inst., 38:169-183, 1967.

8. Waymouth, C.: The cultivation of cells in chemically defined media and the malignant transformation of cells *in vitro*. In: Tissue Culture Seminar, Baroda, India (C. V. Ramakrishnan, ed.), Dr. W. Junk, Hague, Netherlands, 1965, pp. 168-179.

9. Mitchell, J. T., W. F. Andresen, and V. J. Evans: Comparative effects of horse, calf, and fetal serums on chromosomal characteristics and neoplastic conversion of mouse embryo cells *in vitro*. J. Nat. Cancer Inst., 42:709-721, 1969.

10. Hall, W. T., W. F. Andresen, K. K. Sanford, V. J. Evans, and J. W. Hartley: Virus particles and murine leukemia virus complement-fixing antigen in neoplastic and nonneoplastic cell lines. Science, 156:85-88, 1967.

11. Andresen, W. F., V. J. Evans, F. M. Price, and T. B. Dunn: Neoplastic transformations in cells explanted from the kidneys of 3-day old C3H mice. J. Nat. Cancer Inst., 36:953-963, 1966.

12. Andresen, W. F., J. L. Jackson, J. T. Mitchell, and V. J. Evans: Effects of changing horse and fetal calf serum supplements on neoplastic conversion and chromosomal characteristics of mouse embryo cells *in vitro*. J. Nat. Cancer Inst., 43:377-383, 1969.

13. Sanford, K. K., B. E. Barker, M. W. Woods, R. Parshad, and L. W. Law: Search for "indicators" of neoplastic conversion *in vitro*. J. Nat. Cancer Inst., 39:705-733, 1967.

14. Kakunaga, T., and J. Kamahora: Properties of hamster embryonic cells transformed by 4-nitroquinoline-1-oxide *in vitro* and their correlations with the malignant properties of the cells. Biken J., 11:313-332, 1968.

15. Barker, B. E., and K. K. Sanford: Cytologic manifestations of neoplastic transformation *in vitro*. J. Nat. Cancer Inst., 44:39-63, 1970.

16. Todaro, G. J., G. K. Lazar, and H. Green: The initiation of cell division in a contact inhibited mammalian cell line. J. Cell. Comp. Physiol., 66:325-333, 1965.

17. McQuilkin, W. T., and W. R. Earle: Cinemicrographic analysis of cell populations *in vitro*. J. Nat. Cancer Inst., 28:763-799, 1962.

18. Castor, L. N.: Flattening, movement and control of division of epithelial-like cells. J. Cell Physiol., 75:57-64, 1970.

Hydrocarbon Carcinogenesis In Vitro

CHARLES HEIDELBERGER

American Cancer Society Professor of Oncology,
McArdle Laboratory for Cancer Research,
University of Wisconsin, Madison, Wisconsin, USA

I AM GLAD to have the opportunity to present to you some of the work that has been carried out in my laboratory on hydrocarbon carcinogenesis in vitro. Before doing so, I would like to point out that our system differs from those used by Professor Sachs and his group,[1, 2] by Kuroki and Sato,[3] and by DiPaolo[4] in the following ways: We are using C3H mouse cells, whereas they use hamster embryonic cells; we are using a permanent line of cells, whereas they use primary or secondary cultures for transformation; we use cells derived from an adult differentiated tissue, prostate, whereas their cells are mixed embryonic fibroblasts; and our cells are aneuploid, whereas theirs are probably euploid. Each system has its advantages. I will try to point out ours. We are well aware of the proclivity of mouse cells to undergo "spontaneous" malignant transformation, as Dr. Sanford has already pointed out.[5] However, as you shall see, our cells undergo spontaneous malignant transformation only rarely and after a very prolonged time of cultivation. Our cells, which I shall soon describe, resemble in some of their properties the 3T3 cells of Todaro and Green.[6]

Our work originated from the lead provided by Ilse Lasnitzki,[7] who found that organ cultures of mouse ventral prostate grown in the presence of methylcholanthrene (MC) underwent massive hyperplasia and squamous metaplasia. She kindly trained me in these methods in her laboratory, and upon my return to Madison, Röller and I adapted the method to liquid media and obtained with carcinogenic hydrocarbons morphologic changes that some pathologists read as malignant. However, when 872 such pieces, cultured from the prostates of C3H mice in the presence of hydrocarbons, were implanted into isologous mice under a variety of conditions, no tumors were obtained.[8] However, Iype and I dispersed the organ culture pieces so treated, and obtained permanent lines of cells that did give tumors on inoculation into C3H mice.[9] This was our first indication of carcinogenesis in vitro in our system, although Berwald and Sachs had already reported their success.[1]

When Chen joined my laboratory, he was able to culture pronase-dispersed organ cultures that had not been treated with carcinogens.

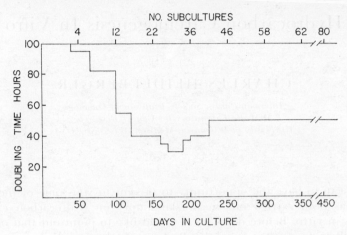

FIG. 2–3.—The life history of a line of cells derived from adult C3H mouse prostate.[10]

These cells grew very slowly at first, but upon patient cultivation their rate of cell division increased, as shown in Figure 2-3.[10] However, in spite of the fact that this became a permanent line, no spontaneous malignant transformation was found until 570 days in culture. On treatment with MC, these cells underwent malignant transformation.[11] The control cells grew to a monolayer, did not pile up, and reached a saturation density as shown in Figure 2-4. On the other hand, the transformed cells continued to grow after reaching a monolayer, piled up, and did not reach a saturation density, as shown in Figure 2-4.[11] The controls did not give tumors on inoculation of 10⁶ cells into irradiated C3H mice (Table 2-1), whereas, on subcutaneous injection, as few as

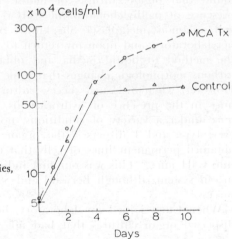

FIG. 2–4.—The saturation densities, under comparable conditions, of control and in vitro transformed prostate cells.[11]

TABLE 2–1.—TUMOR FORMATION IN ADULT C3H MALE MICE
AFTER INOCULATION SUBCUTANEOUSLY OF PROSTATE BY CELLS

TREATMENT	DAYS IN CULTURE AFTER ISOLATION OF COLONIES	NO. CELLS INOCULATED	DAYS AFTER INOCULATION	PALPABLE TUMORS
Control	3	1×10^4	150	0/4 X-ray
MCA	3	1×10^4	21	4/4
Control	7	1×10^6	146	0/4 X-ray
MCA	7	1×10^6	14	6/6
Control	11	1.3×10^6	142	0/4 X-ray
MCA	11	1×10^3	28	2/2
MCA	11	1×10^4	21	2/2
MCA	11	1×10^5	14	2/2
MCA	11	1×10^6	14	2/2

1,000 transformed cells gave 100% tumors in nonirradiated C3H mice.[11] These tumors were rapidly growing, lethal, transplantable, and metastasizing fibrosarcomas.[11]

The system was now ready to make quantitative. When 1,000 control prostate cells were plated in a dish and treated with 0.5% dimethyl sulfoxide (DMSO), they grew to a monolayer and did not pile up, as shown on the left of Figure 2-5. However, when 1,000 cells were treated with MC, a number of piled-up colonies were obtained, which could be easily seen and counted after fixing and staining, as shown on the right in Figure 2-5.[12] When six such colonies were picked and grown from a single MC-treated dish, every one, as shown in Table 2-2, gave rise to tumors on inoculation into the brains of C3H mice, whereas cells from the monolayer areas of the dish did not.[12] Thus, we are completely justified in scoring the individual piled-up colonies as malignant.

We then wished to test a series of carcinogenic and noncarcinogenic

FIG. 2–5.—Photograph of dishes containing fixed and stained control cells *(left)* and MCP-treated cells *(right)*.[12]

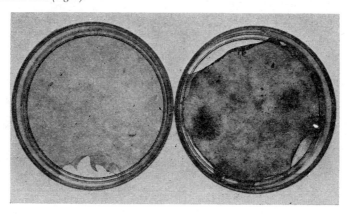

TABLE 2-2.—INOCULATION OF INDIVIDUAL PILED-UP COLONIES AND MONOLAYER AREAS INTO THE BRAINS OF C3H MICE

DISH No.	TYPE OF AREA ISOLATED	NO. CELLS INOCULATED/ MOUSE	NO. MICE	DURATION OF OBSERVATION DAYS	TIMES OF TUMOR APPEARANCE DAYS	NO. TUMORS
1	Monolayer	1,000	4	150	—	0
1	Piled-up	1,000	3	90	30-90	3
1	Piled-up	100	3	150	30-150	2
1	Piled-up	10	3	150	36	1
2	Monolayer	1,000	3	60	—	0
2	Piled-up Colony 1	500	3	60	30-60	3
2	Piled-up Colony 2	500	3	60	30	1
2	Piled-up Colony 3	500	3	60	30	1
2	Piled-up Colony 4	500	3	60	30	1
2	Piled-up Colony 5	500	3	60	30-60	2
2	Piled-up Colony 6	500	3	60	30-60	2

MCA at 1 μg/ml was added to each dish. Each experiment represents one 35 mm dish. For description, see text.

hydrocarbons in our system, where we could determine the transformation frequencies as well as the plating efficiencies, which are a measure of toxicity. When we treated our cells with the noncarcinogenic hydrocarbons, pyrene, 1,2,3,4-dibenzanthracene, and 3-fluoro-10-methyl-1,2-benzanthracene, no piled-up transformed colonies were observed. The results obtained with the powerful carcinogenic hydrocarbons, 9,10-dimethyl-1,2-benzanthracene (DMBA) and 4-fluoro-10-methyl-1,2-benzanthracene are shown in Figure 2-6.[12] It is evident that they produce a relatively high frequency of transformed colonies. Similarly,

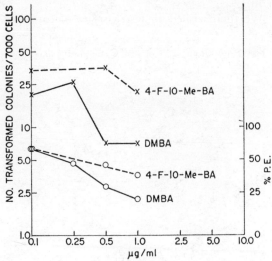

FIG. 2-6.—The transformation frequencies and toxicities produced on mouse prostate cells by DMBA and 4-fluoro-10-methyl-1,2-benzanthracene.[12]

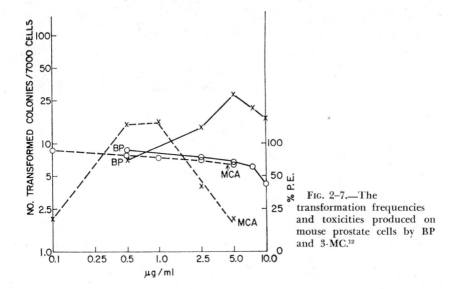

Fig. 2-7.—The transformation frequencies and toxicities produced on mouse prostate cells by BP and 3-MC.[12]

the carcinogenic MC and 3,4-benzpyrene (BP) produced many transformed colonies, although at different doses, as shown in Figure 2-7. It is also clear from these graphs that the shapes of the dose-response curves for toxicity and transformation are not the same, indicating that these are two different processes. Huberman and Sachs[2] found the same lack of a direct relationship between the toxicity of benzpyrene and the frequency of transformation it produced at different doses. The data we obtained with 1,2,5,6-dibenzanthracene, a moderately potent carcinogen, are shown in Figure 2-8.[12] Again, note the lack of correspondence between the curves for toxicity and transformation. It is clear from these experiments that there is a good correspondence be-

Fig. 2-8.—The transformation frequencies and toxicities produced on mouse prostate cells by 1,2,5,6-dibenzanthracene.[12]

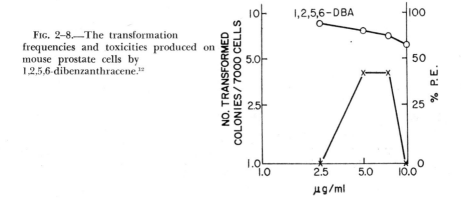

tween the carcinogenic activities of these hydrocarbons and the frequency of transformed colonies they produce in this in vitro system.

We were now ready to approach the unsettled question of the cellular mechanism of hydrocarbon carcinogenesis. Three such cellular mechanisms can be stated: (1) The carcinogen directly transforms normal cells into cancer cells (although I have used the word "transformation," this has so far been an operational term used with no implications about mechanism); (2) the carcinogen because of its toxicity selects for pre-existing malignant cells, as proposed by Prehn;[13] and (3) the hydrocarbon activates a latent oncogenic virus (this theory, although old, has recently been revived and propounded with great vigor by Huebner and Todaro).[14]

We thought that if we could clone our cells and grow individual single cells in separate dishes and transform them at the one-cell stage with MC, we could find out whether a selection of pre-existing malignant cells occurred. Dr. Sukdeb Mondal succeeded most beautifully in doing this in my laboratory, and although he will give the full details of the experiments elsewhere at the Main Congress[26] (see pages 269-273, this volume), and these experiments have been published very recently,[15] I cannot refrain from mentioning these experiments here. Dr. Mondal isolated individual single cells in separate dishes, and was able to grow them into clones with 72% efficiency, as shown in Table 2-3. Of the 18 clones that grew in the presence of 0.5% DMSO, one transformed spontaneously for a 5% incidence. In a subsequent similar experiment, spontaneous transformation was not seen.

When the individual single cells were treated with the proper concentration of MC, 100% of the clones became transformed with little or no toxicity,[15] as shown in Table 2-3. This experiment, because of the very high efficiencies, rules out the cellular mechanism involving selection of pre-existing transformed cells. We then asked whether all the progeny of the treated single cells were transformed. By means of a suitable recloning experiment, Dr. Mondal and I showed that this was so.[15] This is a remarkably efficient process.

Since we have shown that the transformation is direct, we are now

TABLE 2–3.—SINGLE CELL TRANSFORMATION EXPERIMENTS

TREATMENT	CLONING EFF.		TRANSFORMATION	
0.5% DMSO, 6 days	18/25	72%	1/18	5.5%
MCA, 0.25 μg/ml, 6 days	6/10	60%	2/6	33%
MCA, 0.50 μg/ml, 6 days	9/14	64%	8/9	88%
MCA, 1.0 μg/ml, 6 days	26/36	72%	26/26	100%
MCA, 1.0 mg/ml, 1 day	13/21	62%	13/13	100%
MCA, 2.5 μg/ml, 6 days	11/16	68%	11/11	100%
MCA, 5.0 μg/ml, 6 days	12/22	55%	8/12	67%
MCA, 10.0 μg/ml, 6 days	12/28	43%	8/12	67%
MCA, 10.0 μg/ml, 1 day	11/25	44%	8/11	72%

TABLE 2–4.—SUMMARY OF IMMUNOLOGY

17 Clones Tested for Immunogenicity.
    14 Antigenic, 1 Non-Antigenic, 2 Uncertain.
7 Pairs of antigenic clones from the same dish tested
    reciprocally for cross reactivity, 0 Cross-reactive.
3 Antigenic clones derived from 3 different dishes
    tested reciprocally for cross-reactive, 0 Cross-reactive.

fully justified in using that word, and we would like to know whether the hydrocarbon is carrying out this process by itself or with the intervention of an oncogenic virus. At present I can say only that we have tried many experiments designed to reveal such a virus if it existed, and all of them were negative. Moreover, Drs. Hartley and Huebner failed to detect the antigens of the murine leukemia-sarcoma virus complex either in our control or transformed cells. Although we have no evidence for a virus in our system, even if we did we would not know whether it was a passenger or causative. So this question must remain open.

It is well known from the work of Prehn,[16] Klein,[17] and Old[18] that hydrocarbon-induced sarcomas have individual transplantation antigens. In fact, Globerson and Feldman[19] found that two tumors induced by the same hydrocarbon in the same mouse had different antigens. As a check on the validity of our model, we investigated the antigenicity of the in vitro transformed clones. This work will be reported in this volume by Dr. Mondal,[26, 27] but the conclusions are summarized in Table 2-4. It is evident that pairs of clones derived from the same MC-treated dish are antigenic and not cross-reactive, in complete analogy with the situation in vivo. This gives us additional confidence in the validity of our model.

In the case of hamster cells transformed with polyoma and Simian 40 viruses, Rabinowitz and Sachs[20] and Pollack et al.[21] by different methods were able to select variants of less malignancy than that of the original transformed cells. We have preliminary data to indicate that in a thrice-cloned population of chemically transformed cells we have been able to select with FUdR a clone that requires 2.5 log more cells to produce a tumor in C3H mice than did the original clone. Thus, the permanence of the process of chemical carcinogenesis is in question.

It is clear that the development of systems for in vitro chemical carcinogenesis has opened up a Pandora's box of exciting possibilities for understanding the cellular and molecular mechanisms involved in this process. It now puts us in a situation as favorable as the virologists have had for some time. Hopefully, we may be able to catch up with them, since I believe it is correct to state that the virologists still do not fully understand the mechanisms of viral oncogenesis. It is perhaps of passing interest that I, who was trained as an organic chemist, have thus far reported only biologic experiments in our system. It appears self-evident that we must understand the biology of the system before we can proceed intelligently to biochemical studies.

What vistas have opened up in our laboratory? Mr. Corbett, under the supervision of Dr. Dove and myself, has studied the mutagenesis of a series of carcinogenic and noncarcinogenic compounds in bacteriophage T4. Although we have clarified the molecular mechanisms of mutagenesis of some of these compounds,[22] the fact that T4 phage does not get cancer represents a severe limitation to interpretation. The exciting possibility now exists that it may be possible to study carcinogenesis and mutagenesis in the same cells, which would lead to a considerably more valid correlation or lack of correlation between these two processes. Dr. Huberman, one of Professor Sachs' most able students, is currently investigating the feasibility of performing such a study in our system. Assuming that the hydrocarbon produces the transformation directly, then the molecular mechanism can be either a somatic mutation, which many favor, or a perpetuated epigenetic alteration of gene expression. Pitot and I,[23] based on Jacob and Monod ideology, have proposed how perpetuated derepression might be caused by a single pulse of a carcinogen.

In our work on the in vivo interactions of topically applied hydrocarbons to the skin of mice, we have studied intensively their covalent binding to proteins[24] and DNA.[25] I am very fortunate to have Dr. Kuroki visiting my laboratory, and he is now busily engaged in studying the binding of hydrocarbons to these macromolecules in our system; Dr. Huberman is studying their metabolism at the same time. We hope that this integrated biologic and biochemical study in cells that can undergo controlled in vitro hydrocarbon carcinogenesis will contribute toward a complete understanding of the cellular and molecular mechanisms of the process that Percival Pott discovered in 1775. It is about time!

References

1. Berwald, Y., and L. Sachs: J. Nat. Cancer Inst., 35:641, 1965.
2. Huberman, E., and L. Sachs: Proc. Nat. Acad. Sci., USA, 56:1123, 1966.
3. Kuroki, T., and H. Sato: J. Nat. Cancer Inst., 41:53, 1968.
4. DiPaolo, J. A., P. Donovan, and R. Nelson: J. Nat. Cancer Inst., 42:867, 1969.
5. Sanford, K. K.: Nat. Cancer Inst. Monogr., 26:387, 1968.
6. Todaro, G. J., and H. Green: J. Cell Biol., 17:299, 1963.
7. Lasnitzki, I.: Nat. Cancer Inst. Monogr., 12:381, 1963.
8. Röller, M.-R., and C. Heidelberger: Internat. J. Cancer, 2:509, 1967.
9. Heidelberger, C., and P. T. Iype: Science, 155:214, 1967.
10. Chen, T. T., and C. Heidelberger: J. Nat. Cancer Inst., 42:903, 1969.
11. Chen, T. T., and C. Heidelberger: J. Nat. Cancer Inst., 42:915, 1969.
12. Chen, T. T., and C. Heidelberger: Internat. J. Cancer, 4:166, 1969.
13. Prehn, R. T.: J. Nat. Cancer Inst., 32:1, 1964.
14. Huebner, R. J., and G. J. Todaro: Proc. Nat. Acad. Sci. USA, 64:1087, 1969.
15. Mondal, S., and C. Heidelberger: Proc. Nat. Acad. Sci. USA, 65:219, 1970.
16. Prehn, R. T.: Cancer Res., 28:1326, 1968.
17. Klein, G.: Cancer Res., 28:625, 1968.

18. Old, L. J., E. A. Boyse, E. Carswell, and D. A. Clarke: Ann. N. Y. Acad. Sci., 101:80, 1962.
19. Globerson, A., and M. Feldman: J. Nat. Cancer Inst., 32:1229, 1964.
20. Rabinowitz, Z., and L. Sachs: Virology, 38:343, 1969.
21. Pollack, R. E., H. Green, and G. J. Todaro: Proc. Nat. Acad. Sci. USA, 60:126, 1968.
22. Corbett, T. H., C. Heidelberger, and W. F. Dove: Molec. Pharmacol., 6:667, 1970.
23. Pitot, H. C., and C. Heidelberger: Cancer Res., 23:1694, 1963.
24. Abell, C. W., and C. Heidelberger: Cancer Res., 22:931, 1962.
25. Goshman, L. M., and C. Heidelberger: Cancer Res., 27:1678, 1967.
26. Mondal, S.: Hydrocarbon carcinogenesis in vitro. In: Oncology, 1970, Vol. I, A. Cellular and Molecular Mechanisms of Carcinogenesis; B. Regulation of Gene Expression. (Proceedings of the 10th International Cancer Congress). Year Book Medical Publishers, Inc., Chicago, Illinois, 1971, pp. 269-273.
27. Mondal, S., L. Griesbach, and C. Heidelberger: Noncross-reactivity of antigenic clones obtained by in vitro malignant transformation of mouse prostate cells by methylcholanthrene. (Abstract) Tenth International Cancer Congress, Abstracts, Houston, Texas, 1970, p. 33.

Carcinogenesis In Vitro with Nitroquinoline-N-Oxide Derivatives

TOSHIO KUROKI AND HARUO SATO

Cancer Research Laboratory, Tohoku University, Sendai, Japan

Introduction

IN THE PAST four years since the Ninth International Cancer Congress in Tokyo, several reports on chemical carcinogenesis in vitro have accumulated. The first success in transformation with chemical carcinogens was reported by Berwald and Sachs[1, 2] after the treatment of hamster embryonic (HE) cells with carcinogenic hydrocarbons. This work was confirmed later by DiPaolo,[3–5] Sivak,[6] and Goetz, Hill, and Kinoshita.[7] Heidelberger and his colleagues established a quantitative system of hydrocarbon carcinogenesis using aneuploid cell lines derived from organ-cultured mouse prostate tissue.[8–11] Transformations with water-soluble carcinogen nitrosamine derivatives were achieved by Huberman and Sachs with HE cells and dimethylnitrosamine,[12] by Sanders et al. with a Chinese hamster cell line and nitrosomethyl-

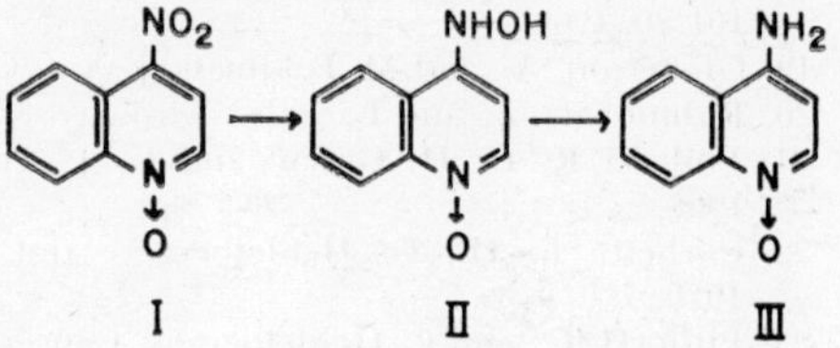

FIG. 2-9.—Chemical structures of 4 NQO and its derivatives.

urea[13, 14] and by Takaki et al. with rat thymus cells and N-methyl-N'-nitro-N-nitrosoguanidine.[15] Another type of carcinogen, 4-nitroquino-line-1-oxide (4 NQO) and its derivatives are also able to convert normal cells to cancer cells in tissue culture. We[16–18] and Kamahora and Kakunaga[19, 20] originally reported malignant transformation of HE cells after the exposure to this type of carcinogen. These studies were later confirmed by Kinoshita et al.[7, 21] and Moriyama and Yamada et al.[22] Recently, it has been shown by Katsuta et al. and Sato et al. that rat embryonic cells and liver parenchymal cells are also sensitive to transformation by 4 NQO.[23, 24]

Ochiai in 1947 first synthesized 4 NQO, and its carcinogenic activity was demonstrated by Nakahara in 1958.[25] The manifold carcinogenicity of 4 NQO and its derivatives rivals that of the most potent carcinogenic hydrocarbons. It was reported by Sugimura et al.[26] that 4 NQO (I in Figure 2-9) can be converted metabolically into noncarcinogenic 4-aminoquinoline-1-oxide (4 AQO; III in Figure 2-9) through a N-hydroxy metabolite 4-hydroxyaminoquinoline-1-oxide (4 HAQO; II in Figure 2-9) in mammalian cells. It is generally accepted that 4 HAQO is a more active carcinogenic form of 4 NQO.[27] The mode of action of 4 NQO and 4 HAQO has been extensively studied in various biologic materials. 4 NQO and 4 HAQO can bind covalently to DNA from calf thymus,[28] Euglena,[29] and rat ascites hepatoma cells.[30, 31] Treatment with these compounds results in single- and double-strand scission of DNA,[32, 33] inhibition of macromolecular synthesis,[34–38] inhibition of glycolysis,[39, 40] inactivation of DNA of bacteriophage T4,[41] and inactivation of transforming DNA from Bacillus subtilis.[42] They also induce chromosomal aberrations in Yoshida sarcoma cells,[43] uneven division of Tetrahymena pyriformis,[44] inhibition of division of sea urchin egg,[45] nuclear caps in tissue culture cells,[27, 37] and nontransplantable mutant clones from an ascites tumor.[46] They are carcinostatic,[39] and also mutagenic for viruses[47] and yeast.[48, 49] In the present paper, we will mainly discuss our studies on transformation of HE cells by 4 NQO and its derivatives. Based on the results obtained, an analysis will be made of the process of carcinogenesis.

General Pattern of Transformation

HE cells were prepared by digestion of near-term hamster embryos by 0.05% pronase and cultured with Eagle's minimum essential medium plus 1.0 mM pyruvate, 0.2 mM serine, 10% heated calf serum, and 60 mg/l of kanamycin. Preparation of solution of the carcinogens has been described previously.[18] The carcinogens were applied usually to a subconfluent, exponentially growing secondary culture of HE cells at a concentration of $10^{-5.5}$ to 10^{-6} M in 4 NQO or $10^{-5.0}$ in 4 HAQO. The effects of the carcinogens were apparent two or three days after the treatment and were characterized by cell necrosis and a criss-cross arrangement of fusiform cells in parts of the culture. In the subculture, these fusiform cells were not apparent, but three or four weeks later there was the appearance of cells that grew actively and formed a dense, piled-up layer. This we define as transformation. The transformed cells revealed stable and logarithmic increase in cell number, as clearly shown in cumulative growth curves (Figure 2-10). Within several passages after this transformation, the cells usually acquired the ability to produce fibrosarcomas in hamsters. The duration of the effective 4 HAQO treatment was successfully shortened to 15 min.[18]

The chromosomal constitution of the transformed cells varied among different transformed lines. Five of 11 lines had the modal number in the tetraploid range, four had diploid and near diploid chromosomes, and the remaining two showed a bimodal distribution of diploid and tetraploid. The details were reported elsewhere.[50]

Biochemically, the transformed cells exhibited an increased aerobic glycolysis and an inhibition of respiration by addition of glucose (Crabtree effect).[51]

FIG. 2–10.—Cumulative growth curves of the treated and untreated control cultures. The ordinate shows cumulative increase in cell number with the cell number at the first subculture referred to one. NQ-, Cl-NQ-, and HA- indicate the cells treated with 4 NQO, 6-chloro 4 NQO, and 4 HAQO respectively. Zen-12 shows the control cells transformed spontaneously.

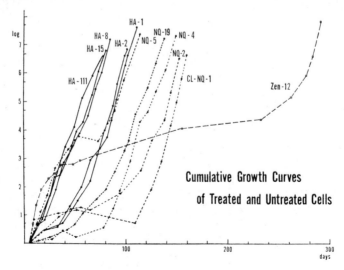

Cumulative Growth Curves
of Treated and Untreated Cells

Control cultures in which carcinogens were not applied showed a striking contrast with the treated cultures. During the first two or three weeks, the cells grew rapidly and exhibited generation times of 14.4 hr (S: 7.6 hr, G1: 4.2 hr, and G2: 2.6 hr).[38] However, the cells gradually lost their ability to proliferate and there was no or little increase in cell number after six or seven weeks in vitro. Ten of 12 control cultures died within 400 days, although the medium was changed regularly. In two cultures (Zen -4 and Zen -12), a focus of growing cells was found after about 260 days in vitro, and the cells continued to proliferate to form a dense layer. This could have been "spontaneous transformation." A typical growth history of the control cells in which spontaneous transformation took place is shown in Figure 2-10.

The cultures treated with the noncarcinogenic derivatives, 4 AQO and 3-methyl 4 NQO, followed essentially the same growth pattern as that of control cells, and failed to transform.

Quantitation of Transformation

The above-mentioned experiments were carried out in mass cultures and represent, therefore, a gross, rather than a quantitative, study of transformation. Commencing in 1963, papers published from Sachs' laboratory have mainly concerned the quantitation of the morphologically transformed colonies.[1, 2, 52] DiPaolo et al. later confirmed this technique,[4] and demonstrated that transformed clones eventually develop into malignant cells during further cultivation in vitro.[5] Chen and Heidelberger established a quantitative system by scoring the piled-up colonies, which they proved to be malignant.[11]

In 4 NQO carcinogenesis in vitro, we attempted to quantitate the transformed colony by the essentially same method as that of Sachs, i.e. HE cells were plated on a feeder layer, treated with 4 NQO or 4 HAQO, followed by incubation for two or three weeks, and then were fixed, stained, and scored. When the cells were treated with $10^{-5.0}$ M 4 HAQO, morphologically somewhat altered colonies were seen, although isolation and further cultivation of an altered colony failed to prove their significance in transformation. These colonies were different in appearance from those described by Sachs. It was also shown that 4 NQO was not adequate for such cloning experiments because of its enhanced cytotoxicity at low cell densities. We then attempted another system in which carcinogens were applied to a mass culture and then the cells were plated in a carcinogen-free medium. After two or three weeks of cultivation, it was found that morphologically distinct colonies of randomly oriented piled-up cells that stained deeply with Giemsa were formed (Figure 2-11A). No such colonies were found in the untreated controls so far examined (Table 2-5). These morphologically altered colonies are referred to as early transformed (ET) colonies. As shown in Table 2-5, the frequency (%) of ET colony per total colonies

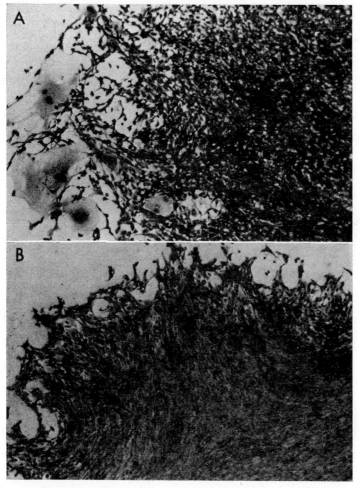

FIG. 2–11.—Early transformed colony *(A)* and late transformed colony *(B)* of the HA-8 culture. The former was obtained by plating on feeder cells just after the treatment with 4 HAQO for nine days and the latter on 64 days when the cells became fully malignant. Note that the cells in the former piled up in a criss-cross arrangement, but those in the latter in a parallel rather than a criss-cross arrangement.

was relatively constant in the different culture conditions (number of cells plated and presence or absence of feeder layer). However, the percentage of ET as a function of the number of cells plated varied greatly under the different conditions. This suggested that the plating efficiency of the ET cells might be the same as that of nontransformed cells, and the value percentage of ET colony/colonies formed may be preferable as a measure of the frequency of ET cells in the population. It is therefore conceivable that about 3.0% of the cells in the NQ-5 culture and

TABLE 2–5.—FREQUENCY OF EARLY TRANSFORMED COLONIES

CULTURE*	CULTURE CONDITIONS† Inoculum	Feeder Layer	PLATING EFFICIENCY (%)	EARLY TRANSFORMED COLONIES Total Colonies (%)	Total Cells
HA-8	10,000	(+)	0.89	6.0 (16/288)	0.053
	1,000	(+)	4.13	6.4 (8/128)	0.27
	10,000	(−)	0.46	6.5 (9/138)	0.03
NQ-5	1,000	(+)	6.66	2.5 (5/200)	0.017
	10,000	(−)	0.68	3.4 (7/205)	0.0023
Control	1,000	(+)	6.50	0 (0/130)	
	10,000	(−)	0.945	0 (0/189)	

* HA-8: treated with $10^{-5.0}$M 4 HAQO for 9 days. NQ-5: treated with $10^{-5.5}$M 4 NQO for 9 days. Control: untreated control culture. Cells were plated just after treatment for 9 days and cultured for 3 weeks.
† Inoculum: cells/60 mm Petri dish. Feeder layer: 4.000r irradiated mouse embryonic cells (100,000 cells/60 mm dish).

6.0% of the cells in the HA-8 culture were in the state of early transformation at the time of replating, i.e. just after the treatments for nine days. However, this does not describe the true rate of transformation. We have not yet established conditions to determine the accurate rate of transformation in 4 NQO carcinogenesis in vitro.

Some morphologic differences were noted between the early and the late transformed colony. In the HA-8 culture, for example, the early transformed colony showed piled-up growth in a cross-cross arrangement, while the colonies in the later passage where the cells became fully malignant revealed a piled-up growth in a parallel, rather than a random, orientation (Figure 2-11B). It seemed likely that late transformed colonies are not identical with the early one, although the latter may have been the ancestor of the former.

Early Events of 4 NQO Carcinogenesis In Vitro

Early events of carcinogenesis in this in vitro system were investigated with respect to the effect of carcinogens on macromolecular syn-

TABLE 2–6.—ACTION OF 4 NQO, 4 HAQO AND 4 AQO ON MACROMOLECULAR SYNTHESES AND CELL LIFE CYCLE[38]

	4 NQO	4 HAQO	4 AQO
Carcinogenicity	+	+	−
Inhibition of synthesis			
DNA	+	+	−
RNA	+	+	−
Protein	+	−	−
Block of cell life cycle			
G1 to S	+	−	−
S to G2	+	+	−
G2 to M	+	+	−

thesis and cell life cycle,[38] and the mode of incorporation of [14]C-4 NQO into the cells.[53, 54]

When 4 NQO or 4 HAQO was added at an effective concentration for transformation to exponentially growing HE cells, inhibitions of macromolecular synthesis and cell life cycle were observed. This is shown qualitatively in Table 2-6, which summarizes earlier work, i.e. 4 NQO inhibited synthesis of DNA, RNA, and protein and blocked the cycle from G1 to S and G2 to M, while the proximal carcinogen, 4 HAQO, acted selectively on nucleic acid syntheses and blocked the flow from S to G2; consequently the treated cells are left in the S-period for a longer time than the untreated cells. The noncarcinogenic 4 AQO had no effects on macromolecular syntheses and cell life cycle (Table 2-6). Recovery from the carcinogen-induced inhibition took place within 48 hr after the treatment. Still unanswered is the question of whether such a selective action of the proximal carcinogen 4 HAQO on nucleic acid syntheses is indeed involved in the trigger mechanism reaction of cancerization, or is merely a cytotoxic action of the compound.

The mode of incorporation of the carcinogen into the cells was investigated using 4 NQO [5,6,7,8,9,10-^{14}C] (7.76 mCi/mM, Daiichi Chemical, Tokyo). Within a short time 4 NQO was incorporated and bound to macromolecules of HE cells with a characteristic time course, i.e. the curve is characterized by a sharp peak of radioactivity in the acid-soluble pool of the cells at 30 min after the treatment. The bound carcinogen reached a maximum value at 30 to 60 min, then decreased gradually. After 72 hr, the bound radioactivity remained at about 50% of the two-hr value.

The physiologic state of the cells in which incorporation and binding of carcinogen takes place was investigated using specific inhibitors of macromolecular syntheses such as hydroxyurea, actinomycin D, and puromycin. However, 4 NQO was incorporated into the acid-insoluble fraction independently of the inhibition of macromolecular synthesis. This was more clearly indicated in an experiment in synchronous cultures of HE cells.[53, 55] These findings are in a good agreement with the reports on binding in vivo of hydrocarbons to DNA by Goshman and Heidelberger[56] and binding in vitro of DMBA to replicating and nonreplicating DNA by Yuspa et al.,[57] but are not consistent with the finding in vivo by Suss et al.[58] It is, however, still uncertain whether there is really a competent physiologic state of the cells for cancerization. Studies on the early events of carcinogenesis from the viewpoint of fixation of transformation would be necessary, and our preliminary study will be shown below.

Fixation and Expression of Transformation

When carcinogen is added to the target cells, it is incorporated and bound to macromolecules, although the real target (s) for cancerization is still unknown. It is probably this initial change that determines whether transformation occurs. However, the cells at this point are not yet in the transformed state. It is apparently necessary to culture the cells for more than 20 days to express their state of transformation. If the initiation change (s) induced by carcinogen is genetically unstable, a process to fix the change (s) in a form capable of being replicated may be required. A competitive process would be repair of the initiation change (s) and that fixation must take place before repair. It has been suggested by Berwald and Sachs[2] and Chen and Heidelberger[11] that transformation by hydrocarbons may require a process associated with cell replication. Borek and Sachs reported that two cell generations may be required for fixation of transformation by X-irradiation.[59] In viral carcinogenesis, it has been concluded that cellular DNA synthesis and/or one cell generation is sufficient to fix the transformed state.[60–64] The following experiments were undertaken to determine the cellular condition required for fixation and expression of transformation in 4 NQO carcinogenesis in vitro.

TABLE 2–7.—DAYS AND CELL GENERATIONS
REQUIRED FOR EXPRESSION OF TRANSFORMATION

CELLS*	DAYS†	CELL GENERATIONS‡
NQ-2	60	4.1
NQ-3	230	NE§
NQ-4	80	4.1
NQ-5	20	2.8
NQ-19	30	1.8
ClNQ-1	75	2.8
HA-1	20	1.8
HA-2	20	2.0
HA-4	80	NE
HA-6	50	NE
HA-7	50	NE
HA-8	15	2.6
HA-15	20	7.9
HA-108	48	3.3
HA-109	48	3.9
HA-110	20	3.4
HA-111	20	4.2
HA-151 A	20	6.4
Zen-4	260	NE
Zen-12	260	17.0

* NQ-, ClNQ- and HA- indicate cells treated with 4 NQO, 6-chloro 4 NQO and 4 HAQO, respectively. Zen- shows the cells transformed spontaneously.
† Days after the treatment.
‡ Cell generations were calculated from the cumulative growth curves (Fig. 2-10).
§ NE: not examined.

The requirement of DNA synthesis for fixation was studied using hydroxyurea which can inhibit DNA synthesis of HE cells 95% at 1 mM.[53] Secondary cultures of HE cells were exposed to 1 mM hydroxyurea for 12 or 24 hr immediately after or 12 hr after the treatment with $10^{-5.0}$ M 4 HAQO for 24 hr. There was no transformation in cultures when DNA synthesis was suppressed during 24 hr after the treatment with carcinogen, while in the cultures where hydroxyurea was not applied transformation was observed 20 days after the treatment. Thus, our preliminary experiment suggested that DNA synthesis within 24 hr after the treatment with the carcinogen is required to fix the transformed state. Of interest in this connection are the observations by Gelboin[65] and by Hennings and Boutwell[66] which demonstrated that skin carcinogenesis by 9,10-dimethyl-1,2-benzanthracene (DMBA) was greatly reduced when large doses of actinomycin D were applied. Quite recently, Chan et al. reported that two-stage skin carcinogenesis was significantly suppressed when hydroxyurea was injected at 24 and 48 hr after the first painting with croton oil.[67]

The number of cell generations required to express the transformation was calculated from the cumulative growth curves on the assumption that all the cells in culture have divided at the same rate. As shown in Table 2-7, it seemed likely that the transformation is usually expressed three or four cell generations after the treatment with the carcinogens, while spontaneous transformation occurred after 17 cell generations.

Progression of Malignancy

When transformed cells were transplanted into the cheek pouch or the subcutaneous tissue of adult hamsters, some differences were seen in the process of tumor formation, i.e. the stages of neoplastic development M1, M2, and M3.[18] At stage M1, the transplanted cells grew and formed histologically malignant (fibrosarcoma) nodules, but regressed. At stage M2, there was either a temporary regression of tumor nodules or a long latent period before the tumor began to grow progressively. At stage M3, the tumor grew progressively without regression or recognizable latent period. As shown in Table 2-8, the stage of neoplastic development M1, M2, and M3 was progressive with the time of cultivation. Thus, for example, neoplastic development of the HA-8 culture was in stage M1 at 28 and 35 days, in stage M2 at 54 days, and in stage M3 at 60 days. These correspond to the cell generations of 6.0, 13.3, and 14.8, respectively. Generally speaking, approximately 20 cell generations were required for neoplastic development. Such enhancement of malignancy with time should be interpreted as an example of "tumor progression" that was proposed by Foulds.[68] The cultures of NQ-4, HA-7, and HA-7F, in which neoplastic development was considerably delayed, were interesting. Although interpretation of such "delayed de-

TABLE 2–8.—DAYS AND CELL GENERATIONS REQUIRED FOR PROGRESSION OF MALIGNANCY (M1, M2 AND M3)

CELLS	DAY			CELL GENERATIONS		
	M1	M2	M3	M1	M2	M3
NQ-2	—	106	106	—	8.5	12.1
NQ-3	—	302	—		NE	
NQ-4	—	85	364	—	6.1	107.5
NQ-5	23	86	109	7.4	15.6	24.4
NQ-19	—	134	170	—	24.2	38.6
ClNQ-1	—	—	110	—	—	6.3
HA-1	49	49	70	6.6	6.6	11.5
HA-2	—	—	58	—	—	7.3
HA-4	—	—	121		NE	
HA-6	—	101	110		NE	
HA-7	—	139	279		NE	
HA-7F	—	—	286		NE	
HA-8	28	54	60	6.0	13.3	14.8
HA-15	30	74	NE	7.9	22.6	NE
Zen-4	—	—	319		NE	
Zen-12	—	342	NE	—	32.7	NE

velopment" remains speculative, it suggested that transformation and neoplastic development may be different biologic processes.

To investigate the mechanisms underlying a progressive increase in neoplastic potential, clonal analysis was carried out at various stages of neoplastic development of the newly established cell lines NQ-19 and HA-111. The results obtained are as follows:

1. Progressive change in neoplastic development as M1, M2, and M3 was seen in clonal populations (NQ-19/cl. 4, cl. 3, HA-111/cl. 9).

2. There was considerable variation in the progressive development among clonal populations; for example, NQ-19/cl. 3 and HA-111/cl. 7 became malignant much later than the parental lines and the other clones.

3. In the earlier passages in which the cells had not yet become malignant, the population was mixed with different types of clones such as clones growing fast, those growing slowly, those having limited life span, or those consisting of the highly contact-inhibited cells. However, in the later passage where the cells became fully malignant, almost all clones isolated were malignant. It is likely from these results that at least two mechanisms may operate in the progressive development of malignancy: (1) progressive change in neoplastic potential within a clone, and (2) selective overgrowth of the cells from highly malignant clones. The latter may be explained by the finding of Pollack et al.[69] that tumorigenic cells are less sensitive to density-dependent inhibition of growth. This result is in a good agreement with the investigation of Jarret et al. on BHK-21 cells[70] and of Enders et al. on Simian virus-40 transformed hamster heart cell line.[71]

Conclusions

Our studies on 4 NQO carcinogenesis in vitro permit us to distinguish the following cancerization process. First, the carcinogen is incorporated into the cells and bound to macromolecules DNA, RNA, and protein. This binding may result in the interruption of cellular functions, and killing and transformation of the cells. However, there is still no available evidence on the type and extent of binding that is responsible for these biologic reactions. Second, the initial change induced by carcinogen is fixed and expressed as the state of transformation. As suggested by our preliminary study, DNA synthesis within 24 hr after the treatment may play a role in the fixation of transformation. Expression of transformation is usually achieved after four cell divisions, while spontaneous transformation is apparent after 17 cell generations. This suggests that carcinogen-induced transformation may be a different process from spontaneous transformation. Finally, the cells acquire neoplastic potential through cell divisions. This process is a progressive change, recognized as tumor progression by Foulds.[68] Clonal analysis indicates that progression of neoplastic development may involve both the mechanism of progressive change in neoplastic potential within a clone and that of selective overgrowth by the malignant cells among clones.

Although it is still uncertain whether there is the intervention of oncogenic viruses as was proposed by Huebner and Todaro,[72] the cellular mechanisms underlying chemical carcinogenesis are being elucidated by these in vitro systems. For example, quite recently, Mondal and Heidelberger reported that carcinogen does not select for pre-existing malignant cells, but acts to convert nonmalignant control cells to malignant cells.[73] It is likely that these in vitro systems now provide an opportunity for biochemical studies to elucidate the molecular mechanisms of chemical carcinogenesis.

Acknowledgments

We are indebted to Professor Hajim Katsuta (University of Tokyo, Tokyo, Japan) for his criticism throughout this work, and to Professor Charles Heidelberger (The University of Wisconsin, Madison, Wisconsin, U.S.A.) for reading the manuscript.

References

1. Berwald, Y., and L. Sachs: Nature, 200:1182, 1963.
2. Berwald, Y., and L. Sachs: J. Nat. Cancer Inst., 35:641, 1965.
3. DiPaolo, J. A., and P. J. Donovan: Exp. Cell Res., 48:361, 1967.
4. DiPaolo, J. A., P. J. Donovan, and R. L. Nelson: J. Nat. Cancer Inst., 42:867, 1969.
5. DiPaolo, J. A., R. L. Nelson, and P. J. Donovan: Science, 165:917, 1969.
6. Sivak, A., and B. L. Van Duuren: Exp. Cell Res., 49:572, 1968.

102 / KUROKI AND SATO

7. Goetz, I. E., B. R. Hill, and R. Kinoshita: Proc. Amer. Ass. Cancer Res., 10:30, 1969.
8. Heidelberger, C., and P. T. Iype: Science, 155:214, 1967.
9. Chen, T. T., and C. Heidelberger: J. Nat. Cancer Inst., 42:903, 1969.
10. Chen, T. T., and C. Heidelberger: J. Nat. Cancer Inst., 42:915, 1969.
11. Chen, T. T., and C. Heidelberger: Internat. J. Cancer, 4:166, 1969.
12. Huberman, E., S. Salzberg, and L. Sachs: Proc. Nat. Acad. Sci. USA, 59:77, 1968.
13. Sanders, F. K., and B. O. Burford: Nature, 213:1171, 1967.
14. Sanders, F. K., and B. O. Burford: Nature, 220:448, 1968.
15. Takaki, R., M. Takii, and T. Ikegami: Gann, 60:661, 1969.
16. Sato, H., and T. Kuroki: Proc. Jap. Acad., 42:1211, 1966.
17. Kuroki, T., M. Goto, and H. Sato: Tohoku J. Exp. Med., 91:109, 1967.
18. Kuroki, T., and H. Sato: J. Nat. Cancer Inst., 41:53, 1968.
19. Kamahora, J., and T. Kakunaga: Proc. Jap. Acad., 42:1079, 1966.
20. Kamahora, J., and T. Kakunaga: Biken J., 10:219, 1967.
21. Kinoshita, R., I. E. Goetz, and J. Mori: Proc. Amer. Ass. Cancer Res., 9:37, 1968.
22. Moriyama, Y., and M. Yamada: Personal communication.
23. Katsuta, H., and T. Takaoka: Personal communication.
24. Sato, J., and M. Namba: Personal communication.
25. Nakahara, W., F. Fukuoka, and T. Sugimura: Gann, 48:129, 1957.
26. Sugimura, T., K. Okabe, and H. Endo: Gann, 56:489, 1965.
27. Endo, H., and F. Kume: Gann, 54:443, 1963.
28. Nagata, C., M. Kodama, Y. Tagashira, and A. Imamura: Biopolymer, 4:409, 1966.
29. Malkin, M. F., and A. C. Zahalsky: Science, 154:1665, 1966.
30. Matsushima, T., I. Kobuna, and T. Sugimura: Nature, 216:508, 1967.
31. Tada, M., M. Tada, and T. Takahashi: Biochem. Biophys. Res. Comm., 29:469, 1967.
32. Sugimura, T., H. Otake, and T. Matsushima: Nature, 218:392, 1968.
33. Ando, T., and H. Katsuta: Personal communication.
34. Amsterdam, D., J. Berek, A. C. Zahalsky, and S. S. Lazarus: Exp. Cell Res., 48:499, 1967.
35. Paul, J. S., R. C. Reynolds, and P. O'B. Montgomery: Cancer Res., 29:558, 1969.
36. Paul, J. S., R. C. Reynolds, and P. O'B. Montgomery: Nature, 215:749, 1967.
37. Floyd, L. R., T. Unuma, and H. Busch: Exp. Cell Res., 51:423, 1968.
38. Kuroki, T., J. Ishizawa, and H. Sato: Gann, 60:261, 1969.
39. Fukuoka, F., T. Sugimura, and S. Sakai: Gann, 48:65, 1957.
40. Ono, T., T. Tomaru, and F. Fukuoka: 50:189, 1959. [sic]
41. Ishizawa, M., and H. Endo: Biochem. Pharmacol., 16:637, 1967.
42. Ono, T.: Tanpakushitsu-Kakusan-Koso, 9:1122, 1964.
43. Yosida, T. H., Y. Kurita, and K. Moriwaki: Gann, 56:523, 1965.
44. Mita, T., R. Tokuzen, F. Fukuoka, and W. Nakahara: Gann, 56:293, 1965.
45. Kamahora, J., and T. Kakunaga: Biken J., 11:139, 1968.
46. Koyama, K., and K. Ishii: Gann, 60:367, 1969.
47. Endo, H., A. Wada, K. Miura, J. Hidaka, and C. Hiruki: Nature, 190:833, 1961.
48. Okabayashi, T.: Chem. Pharmacol. Bull., 10:1127, 1962.
49. Mifuchi, I., Y. Hosoi, Y. Yanagihara, and M. Otsubo: Gann, 54:1205, 1963.
50. Yosida, T. H., T. Kuroki, H. Masuji, and H. Sato: J. Nat. Cancer Inst. Submitted.
51. Sato, K., T. Kuroki, and H. Sato: Proc. Soc. Exp. Biol. Med. In press.
52. Huberman, E., and L. Sachs: Proc. Nat. Acad. Sci. USA, 56:1123, 1966.
53. Kuroki, T., R. Kanamura, and H. Sato: Gann. Submitted.
54. Kanamura, R., T. Kuroki, and H. Sato: In preparation.
55. Kuroki, T., and H. Sato: Exp. Cell Res. In press.
56. Goshman, L., and C. Heidelberger: Cancer Res., 27:1678, 1967.
57. Yuspa, S. H., S. Eaton, D. L. Morgan, and R. R. Bates: Chemico-Biol. Interac., 1:223, 1969/1970.
58. Suss, R., and H. Rainer-Maurer: Nature, 217:752, 1968.
59. Borek, C., and L. Sachs: Proc. Nat. Acad. Sci. USA, 57:1522, 1967.
60. Todaro, G. J., and H. Green: Proc. Nat. Acad. Sci. USA, 55:302, 1966.

61. Temin, H.: J. Cell. Physiol., 69:53, 1967.
62. Nakata, Y., and J. P. Bader: Virology, 36:401, 1968.
63. Nakata, Y., and J. P. Bader: J. Virology, 2:1255, 1968.
64. Yoshikura, H., Y. Hirokawa, Y. Ikawa, and H. Sugano: Internat. J. Cancer, 3:743, 1968.
65. Gelboin, H. V., M. Klein, and R. R. Bates: Proc. Nat. Acad. Sci. USA, 53:1353, 1965.
66. Hennings, H., H. C. Smith, N. H. Colburn, and R. K. Boutwell: Cancer Res., 28:543, 1968.
67. Chan, P. C., A. Goldman, and E. L. Wynder: Science, 168:131, 1970.
68. Foulds, L.: Cancer Res., 14:327, 1954.
69. Pollack, R. E., H. Green, and G. J. Todaro: Proc. Nat. Acad. Sci. USA, 59:1144, 1968.
70. Jarret, O., and I. McPherson: Internat. J. Cancer, 3:654, 1968.
71. Enders, J. F., and G. Th. Diamondopoulas: Proc. Roy. Soc. London, B, 171:431, 1969.
72. Huebner, R. J., and G. J. Todaro: Proc. Nat. Acad. Sci. USA, 64:1087, 1969.
73. Mondal, S., and C. Heidelberger: Proc. Nat. Acad. Sci. USA, 65:219, 1970.

Liver Carcinogenesis In Vitro

HAJIM KATSUTA

Department of Cancer Cell Research, Institute of Medical Science, University of Tokyo, Tokyo, Japan

LIVER CARCINOMA has a high incidence among Japanese. However, liver cells had not been employed in experimental chemical carcinogenesis in tissue culture, probably because of the difficulty in the cultivation of liver cells. Ten years ago a research team was organized in Japan and is still working to investigate chemical carcinogenesis in tissue culture. This team consists of tissue culturists working in different research institutions. Kuroki was also one of the members. These members, including myself, were interested in the cultivation of liver cells, and tried to transform liver cells of the rat, first, by treatment with azo dyes.

In the beginning, liver cells did not proliferate in the primary culture, but survived for a long time, several months or more.[2] However, when the culture was treated with 4-dimethylaminoazobenzene (DAB) in a final concentration of 1 γ/ml for the initial four days, proliferation of liver cells was abruptly and frequently induced about seven to 10 days after the treatment and has continued indefinitely. These proliferating cells, however, did not produce tumors on backtransplantation into animals of the same origin.[3]

Various second treatments were given to these cells, e.g., no renewal of culture fluid for a long period, and addition of hormones, DAB, or thalidomide into culture fluid. The cells, however, did not become malignant.[4]

Sato[12] of Okayama University, who is one of the members of our research team, confirmed this finding by the use of liver tissue from rats of another line and with 3'-methyl-4-dimethylaminoazobenzene (3'-methyl-DAB) as well.

Since then, we have found a way to grow liver parenchymal cells of the rat in culture. The clue was the age of rats: When the liver tissue of two- to three-week-old rats is used, we can grow liver cells with little difficulty. However, in rats more than one month old, proliferation is obtained with difficulty.

In relation to this finding, Sato and Yabe[15] got an interesting result. They gave a diet containing DAB to rats for periods of 44 to 312 days, and cultured the liver tissue of these animals following the course. In the early stage of this course, proliferation of liver cells was slight. However, when the rats were fed DAB for more than 57 days, at which stage degenerated and regenerating liver cells were observed histologically in liver tissue, proliferation was exhibited in the culture of these cells.

By using young suckling rats, we have established many cell strains of liver parenchymal cells from normal rats and utilized these cell strains for our experiments of chemical carcinogenesis.

Long-term addition of DAB or 3'-methyl-DAB into the cultures of rat liver cell strains was carried out by Sato and Yabe[14] in the concentration of 1 γ/ml continuously for about 300 days. Considerable changes were found in the morphology of cells. On backtransplantation, however, no tumors were produced.

Sato[13] also treated rat liver cell strains with 3'-methyl-DAB in high concentrations, such as 10 to 40 γ/ml, and repeatedly for various periods. On backtransplantation into rats, the treated cells gave rise to tumors. In this experiment, untreated control cells also produced tumors on backtransplantation. However, in terms of the backtransplantability rate of the cells and the survival days of the tumor-bearing rats, 3'-methyl-DAB was shown to accelerate the tumor-producing capacity and the malignancy of cells.

In our laboratory, we found the transformation of liver cells of normal rats without use of chemical carcinogens:[6] We inoculated liver cells showing a diploid number of chromosomes into the tubes with flattened surfaces and incubated the tubes in stationary culture keeping them slanted at an angle of 5°. When the culture fluid was renewed twice a week routinely, but the cells not subcultured for a long period such as 1 or 2 months, tremendous changes appeared in the morphology of the cells scattering on the zone nearest to the air-liquid interface, named "Nagisa." The changes consisted of marked pleomorphism and atypism of cells, abnormal and multipolar mitosis, and others. Eventually we obtained mutant cell lines in which cells grow piling up on each other. These cells, however, did not produce tumors when inoculated into rats.

After the Nagisa culture, we treated liver cells with high concentrations of DAB.[5] After a week of DAB treatment, marked changes were noticed in the cultures, e.g., loss of the activity of metabolizing DAB, changes in cell morphology and in the modal number of chromosomes, and others. Mutant cell lines were established from all the cultures. These cells closely resembled hepatoma cells in morphology. Some lines later recovered the capacity to metabolize DAB to an abnormally high extent. On backtransplantation, however, no tumors were formed by any of the lines.

Kuroki treated the cultures of hamster embryonic cells with a very active carcinogen, 4-nitroquinoline-1-oxide (4NQO), and its derivatives.[8, 9, 11] By means of these carcinogens, the cells became malignant, as confirmed by the tumor death of the animals inoculated with the treated cells.

Since then, most of the members of our research team have treated cultures with 4NQO and its derivatives.

Namba et al.[10] of Okayama University treated the cultures of rat liver cells repeatedly with 4NQO in various concentrations for a period of 25 days and obtained malignant transformation of these cells. On backtransplantation, the formation of tumors was detected an average of about six months after transplantation. Most of the tumors were diagnosed histologically as hepatomas.

In our laboratory, we employed one of the cell strains, RLC-10, derived from normal rat liver cells preserving a diploid number of chromosomes as a mode. 4NQO was given to these cultures in a final concentration of 3.3×10^{-6}M each time for 30 min. We tried to decrease the number of treatments as little as possible.

As illustrated in Figure 2-12, four lines of experiments, #CQ39 to #CQ42, were made. In all of the experiments, liver cells were transformed by treatment with 4NQO. It should be noticed that, in the experiment of #CQ40, malignant transformation was obtained by one treatment with 4NQO. In the control culture, the cells did not produce tumors on backtransplantation in the fourth month of experiment, i.e. around the time when the cells were transformed in all of the treated cultures. However, in the seventeenth month, it was found that they had undergone spontaneous transformation. This was the first case of spontaneous transformation in our laboratory during the past 20 years. After the transplantability of cells was confirmed, the cell lines were given the names of "RLT-". The tumors produced in animals have

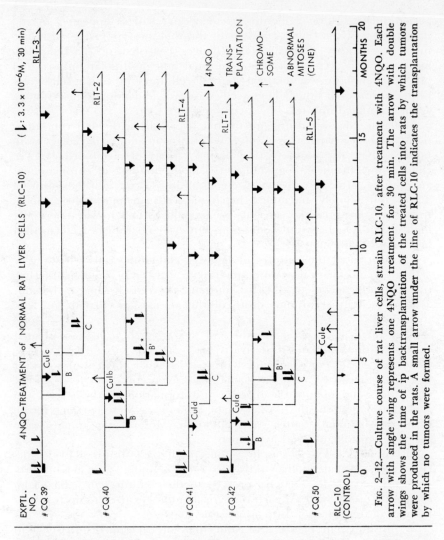

Fig. 2-12.—Culture course of rat liver cells, strain RLC-10, after treatment with 4NQO. Each arrow with single wing represents one 4NQO treatment for 30 min. The arrow with double wings shows the time of ip backtransplantation of the treated cells into rats by which tumors were produced in the rats. A small arrow under the line of RLC-10 indicates the transplantation by which no tumors were formed.

been passaged through rats, and these animal lines were given the names such as "Cula, Culb, Culc and so on."

More detailed results of backtransplantation in the experiment #CQ40 are given in Figure 2-13: The cultures were treated only once and, after 3.5 months, the cells were transplanted ip into two newborn rats. One of the two died of tumor 3.6 months after the transplantation. In other branch lines of experiment, the cultures were treated more times with 4NQO. The survival time of the rats transplanted appears to suggest that too frequent treatments do not necessarily accelerate malignancy. In other experiments, we have also employed single administration and obtained transformation. These findings indicate that one treatment for 30 min is sufficient to transform the cells under the conditions employed, at least, in rat cells.

In morphology, the 4NQO-transformed cells were little different from control cells when examined on fixed specimens. By cinemicrography, however, some changes were noticed, e.g. greatly decreased adhesiveness between cells. This finding suggests a change in cell membrane.

In the mode of chromosome numbers, the control culture showed the diploid number, 42, with high frequency. In all of the cultures treated with 4NQO, however, one or two chromosomes were reduced.

In the culture course after 4NQO treatment, changes in an electric mobility of the cells have been chased by means of cytoelectrophoresis by Yamada of the National Cancer Center Institute in Tokyo. The ascites hepatoma cells passaged through rats exhibited widely distributed, high values of mobility, on the average. When the cells were treated with neuraminidase at 37 C for 30 min, however, the values were found apparently to have been decreased. In contrast, untreated liver cells of the control culture showed low values, and the values were increased by the treatment with neuraminidase. The liver cells transformed by Nagisa culture scarcely changed the values by the same treatment. 4NQO-transformed liver cells behaved similarly to ascites hepatoma cells.

We have cell strains of rat liver cells transformed by Nagisa culture. These cells are capable of growing in protein- and lipid-free chemically

FIG. 2–13.—The results of backtransplantation of rat liver cells, RLC-10, treated with 4NQO into newborn rats (Expt. #CQ40). Each arrow indicates one 4NQO treatment for 30 min in the concentration of 3.3×10^{-6}M.

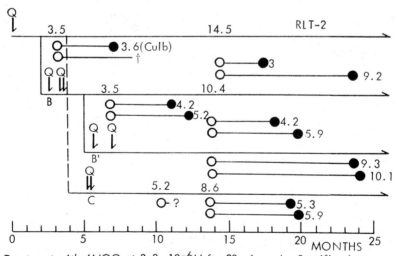

Q: Treatment with 4NQO at 3.3×10^{-6}M for 30 min.   †: Sacrificed.
?: **Accidental** death. O: No. of rats transplanted. ●: No. of rats died of tumor.

defined synthetic media. To exclude the possibility that the carcinogen may first interact with the proteins in the medium and the possibility of viral contamination, we have also employed these strains in our works. Biochemical analyses of these cells have been carried out by Andoh of our institute, especially of the interaction between the carcinogens and macromolecular substances in the cells.

After treatment of RLH-5·P3 cells with 4NQO, he analyzed DNA of the cells by sucrose density gradient centrifugation and found the break of DNA not only at the single strand level but also at the double strand level, the extent of break being dependent on the concentration of the carcinogen. When treated with 4NQO in the concentration of $10^{-5}M$, the double strands of one DNA molecule were fragmented into an average of 100 pieces. The molecular weight of each fragment corresponded to about 10^8 daltons. When the cells treated in this way were further incubated in the medium without carcinogen, rejoining of broken pieces was observed. This rejoining was confirmed also with L·P3 cells, one of substrain of L-929 which has been propagated in a protein- and lipid-free synthetic medium.[1, 7] By the use of ^{3}H-4NQO, he detected no binding of 4NQO to a special fraction of proteins such as slow h2 protein.

It has yet to be determined whether misrejoining of DNA might play a certain role in the production of tumor cells.

We hope the mechanism of carcinogenesis will be clarified in the near future.

References

1. Kagawa, Y., T. Takaoka, and H. Katsuta: Mitochondria of mouse fibroblasts, L-929, cultured in a lipid- and protein-free chemically defined medium. J. Biochem., 65:799-808, 1969.
2. Katsuta, H., and T. Takaoka: Carcinogenesis in tissue culture. I. Cultivation of normal rat liver cells. Jap. J. Exp. Med., 33:265-275, 1963.
3. Katsuta, H., and T. Takaoka: Carcinogenesis in tissue culture. II. Proliferation-inducing effect of 4-dimethylaminoazobenzene on normal rat liver cells in culture. Jap. J. Exp. Med., 35:209-230, 1965.
4. Katsuta, H., and T. Takaoka: Carcinogenesis in tissue culture. III. Effects of the second treatments on DNA-induced proliferating liver cells of normal rats in culture. Jap. J. Exp. Med., 35:231-248, 1965.
5. Katsuta, H., and T. Takaoka: Cytobiological transformation of normal rat liver cells by treatment with 4-dimethylaminoazobenzene after Nagisa culture. In: Cancer Cells in Culture (H. Katsuta, ed.), University of Tokyo Press, Tokyo, 1968, pp. 321-334.
6. Katsuta, H., T. Takaoka, Y. Doida, and T. Kuroki: Carcinogenesis in tissue culture. VII. Morphological transformation of rat liver cells in NAGISA culture. Jap. J. Exp. Med., 35:513-544, 1965.
7. Katsuta, H., T. Takaoka, and K. Kikuchi: Further studies on amino acid requirements of a subline of strain L cells (mouse fibroblasts) in synthetic media. Jap. J. Exp. Med., 31:125-136, 1961.
8. Kuroki, T., M. Goto, and H. Sato: Malignant transformation of hamster embryonic cells by 4-hydroxyaminoquinoline N-oxide in tissue culture. Tohoku J. Exp. Med., 91:109-118, 1967.
9. Kuroki, T., M. Goto, and H. Sato: Malignant transformation of hamster embry-

onic cells with 4-nitroquinoline-1-oxide and its derivatives in tissue culture. In: Cancer Cells in Culture (H. Katsuta, ed.), University of Tokyo Press, Tokyo, 1968, pp. 364-381.

10. Namba, M., H. Masuji, and J. Sato: Carcinogenesis in tissue culture. IX. Malignant transformation of cultured rat cells treated with 4-nitroquinoline-1-oxide. Jap. J. Exp. Med., 39:253-265, 1969.

11. Sato, H., and T. Kuroki: Malignization in vitro of hamster embryonic cells by chemical carcinogens. Proc. Jap. Acad., 42:1211-1216, 1966.

12. Sato, J.: Carcinogenesis in tissue culture. IV. Proliferation-inducing effect of 4-dimethylaminoazobenzene and 3'-methyl-4-dimethylaminoazobenzene on liver cells from normal Donryu rats in culture. Jap. J. Exp. Med., 35:433-444, 1965.

13. Sato, J.: Malignant transformation in culture of rat liver cells treated with and without 3'-methyl-4-dimethylaminoazobenzene. In: Cancer Cells in Culture (H. Katsuta, ed.), University of Tokyo Press, Tokyo, 1968, pp. 335-350.

14. Sato, J., and T. Yabe: Carcinogenesis in tissue culture. V. Effects of long-term addition of 4-dimethylaminoazobenzene and 3'-methyl-4-dimethylaminoazobenzene on liver cells in culture. Jap. J. Exp. Med., 35:445-462, 1965.

15. Sato, J., and T. Yabe: Carcinogenesis in tissue culture. VI. Tissue culture of liver cells from DAB-feeding rats. Jap. J. Exp. Med., 35:491-511, 1965.

3

Cell-Virus Interaction: Biological Aspects

Historical Review and Perspectives

HILARY KOPROWSKI

Wistar Institute of Anatomy and Biology, Philadelphia, Pennsylvania, USA

HISTORY BEING a subject dear to my heart, I have, over the years, developed definite likes and dislikes for historians. Toynbee, for instance, is not my cup of tea, whereas Trevor-Roper, Cecily Wedgewood, to mention a few, are among my favorites. The master of them all is, however, for me, the Dutch historian, Johan Huizinga. Thus, when confronted with the task of developing ideas on the "historical aspects" of the virus-host cell relationship in carcinogenesis, I turned to Huizinga for guidance as to the role of historical perspective in furthering the progress of ideas in a given field.

Huizinga expresses the opinion that "the discipline of history is suffering from the defect that the issues are insufficiently formulated." He describes the uncomfortable feeling, very familiar to us today, that is engendered by the "flood of countless monographs, articles and source publications that are being added to the material of history from month to month in every country." With Huizinga, we must ask ourselves, "Is the labor expended by the machinery of scholarship a hopeless waste of energy?" As he himself states, "only a very few of all these studies seem to point back to a central core of knowledge."[17]

Abetted by Huizinga's advice, as well as that of Hegel, that we learn from history only that men never learn anything from history, my presentation will not be based on the illusion that general historical concepts developed in the past form an "image" which today helps us to formulate principles on which the structures of our investigations are built. I suspect that my fellow scientists, in reporting their scientific discoveries, refer studiously and piously to the past, not because their discovery was engendered from past knowledge, but because it is considered proper for each of us to play the historian's role. So, rather than crediting present ideas to past accomplishments with "historical hindsight," I shall attempt to include in my presentation only that knowledge of the past which has proved conducive to new ideas, i.e. ideas of the past which are assimilated in one's conceptions of today.

Vertical Transmissions

For more than two decades, the term vertical transmission was used rather indiscriminately to represent the concept of hereditary transmission of oncogenicity engendered by tumor viruses. Except, however, for the fact that milk of certain strains of mice was shown to contain mammary tumor virus, the actual mechanism of "vertical transmission" remained obscure. Many questions awaited answers: If the infection occurs in utero, at what stage of embryonic development is the fetus susceptible? Is the virus blood-borne? Does it pass through the placenta? Could transmission of infection through the ovum by virus-carrying spermatozoa be considered?

During the last year, my associate, Dr. Baranska, directed her efforts toward the problem of susceptibility of mammalian eggs to infection with tumor viruses. Results of her investigations[1] revealed that oncogenic DNA viruses indigenous to mouse species, such as polyoma virus, exercised a marked degenerative effect on parthenogenetically stimulated mouse eggs deprived of their zona pellucida. When mouse eggs were exposed instead to Simian virus 40 (SV40), for which mouse somatic cells are nonpermissive, the eggs were stimulated to divide by the presence of the virus or its DNA, and virus could be recovered from the eggs up to 72 hr after exposure. This time limit was imposed by the inability to maintain the eggs in culture for a longer period.[1]

The ability of mouse eggs to support growth of Moloney sarcoma virus (MSV) is even more interesting, since the virus can be placed inside the eggs either by fusion with mouse fibroblasts carrying MSV or by direct exposure to a viral suspension. The presence of MSV in the ovum also seems to stimulate division of eggs, but to a lesser extent than does SV40. As shown in Table 3-1, the virus can easily be recovered from eggs 72 hr after infection by co-cultivation of the eggs with the XC line of rat cells transformed by Rous sarcoma virus.[2] Thus, it was possible to show that unfertilized eggs are capable of being infected with at least three tumor viruses, and that except for polyoma virus, the other two viruses did not adversely affect development of the eggs. What remains to be seen is whether the ovum, a cell which contains all of the information as well as the capacity for differentiation, will "overcome" the effect of tumor viruses and develop normally, fol-

TABLE 3–1.—EFFECT OF ONCOGENIC VIRUSES ON
PARTHENOGENETIC DEVELOPMENT OF MOUSE EGGS*

VIRUS	RATIO OF DIVIDING EGG CELLS	RATIO OF DIVIDING EGGS YIELDING INFECTIOUS VIRUS
SV40 DNA	231/416	38/48†
MSV	82/466	54/104†
None	4/60	NT

* Without zona pellucida.
† After co-cultivation with susceptible cells.
MSV: Moloney sarcoma virus.
NT: Not tested.

lowing either parthenogenetic stimulation or fertilization; or whether the cell will succumb to the effect of the tumor virus, and develop into an abnormal mouse.

It should be mentioned in passing that incorporation of SV40 DNA into the genome of the egg may serve as a useful marker for the timing of the turning-off point for certain host genes which regulate development.

Transmission of oncogenic viruses through spermatozoa presents an entirely different, but just as interesting, aspect of viral carcinogenesis. Spermatozoa have no ribosomes to speak of, and do not synthesize protein. Are such structures capable of incorporating a genome of an oncogenic virus and then transmitting it to the fertilized egg? The answer to the first question is affirmative. Although it is impossible for complete SV40 to penetrate rabbit spermatozoa, SV40 DNA can do so and can be recovered 72 hr later "integrated" into cellular DNA. Biologic activity of the viral DNA has been maintained, as indicated by the isolation of infectious SV40 from African green monkey kidney (AGMK) cells after their fusion with SV40 DNA-infected spermatozoa. The second question represents a more formidable problem. Until now, the presence of labeled SV40 DNA could be observed only in the spermatozoon found inside the fertilized egg.[3] It is still uncertain, however, whether, following digestion of the spermatozoon, biologically active DNA will be recovered from the fertilized egg at different stages of embryonic development. Equally uncertain is the fate of the fetus.

Early Events

It was, I think, in 1969, during a cancer meeting at the Abbaye de Royaumont in France, that Roger Weil posed a series of questions directed as much to himself as to the audience. Noticing the general feeling of futility prevailing at that meeting, Weil suggested that we all return to our laboratories and each, in domo sua, re-examine the effect of tumor viruses on the cell, paying particular attention to the early events following adsorption and penetration of the virus. Because there was already so much information available about the phase following replication of viral DNA, from which so little had been gained, new approaches might shed light on the eternal unanswered question: if and why cells infected with oncogenic virus become cancer cells.

Using SV40 and permissive AGMK cells, my associates, Hummeler and Sokol,[4] and Barbanti-Brodano and Swetly,[5] investigated the sequence of early events of virus uptake by the cell. Morphologic studies by Hummeler and Sokol[4] of the initiation of the infectious process revealed that following viral penetration by monopinocytosis and acquisition by the virus of an extra membrane, the virus then proceeded, possibly within 10 min after infection, to the nucleus, reaching maximum concentration at two hr after infection. During penetration of the nucleus, the newly acquired envelope is shed, and viral uncoating takes place in the nucleus.

Barbanti-Brodano and Swetly[5] confirmed and amplified these morphologic observations. They were able to show the presence of parental SV40 particles in the isolated nuclei of infected permissive cells as early as 20 min after infection. A ^{3}H-thymidine-labeled component isolated from the nuclei between one-half and two and one-half hr after infection bands after equilibrium density centrifugation at a buoyant density identical to that of SV40 virions (1.34 g/cm^3). From that point, a gradual conversion of the DNA to a component of 1.37 g/cm^3 buoyant density occurs. After labeling the protein of the virus with ^{3}H-leucine, a shift in the buoyant density of the preparation from 1.34 g/cm^3 toward a lighter component occurring at four hr after infection is indicative of the initiation of the uncoating process, which terminates at six hr. At six hr the protein coat is separated from the virus genome, and parental DNA probably becomes associated with either cellular or newly synthesized viral protein at a density of 1.30 g/cm^3. Vulnerability of SV40 DNA present in the nuclei to the action of nucleases, which does not become apparent before one to one and one-half hr after infection, adds further support to the hypothesis of early nuclear penetration of the SV40 particles and their uncoating within the nucleus.

"Virus Fiat Ubi Vult"

I have dwelt at length upon the early events of infection of a cell by an oncogenic virus because I suspect that what happens during the latter stages of the infectious process can best be expressed by the motto, "Let the virus appear where it will"; it may be of no consequence to the host cell.

I have no more experimental evidence to support this contention than you have to deny it. I would like, however, to drive a few stakes into the ground in order to mark my claim.

TABLE 3–2.—EFFECT OF GUINEA PIG ANTI-C57BL/6 EGG SERUM ON UNFERTILIZED EGGS OF SYNGENEIC, ALLOGENEIC, OR XENOGENEIC ORIGIN

ORIGIN OF EGGS	SERUM	RATIO OF EGGS DESTROYED IN PRESENCE OF SERUM DILUTIONS					
		und.	1:5	1:10	1:20	1:40	1:80
C57BL/6	I		14/14	14/14	8/8	12/17	0/16
	C	0/20		0/20			
BALB-C	I		10/10		10/10		
	C	0/7					
Rat	I	0/21					

I: Immune serum.
C: Prebleeding specimen of serum of guinea pig subsequently immunized with mouse eggs.
Numerator: Number of eggs observed.
Denominator: Number of eggs destroyed.

The nature of the antigens engendered in the host cell exposed to an oncogenic virus remains obscure. The contribution of viral components to the synthesis of either the T or transplantation antigen is essentially unknown. Recently, however, my associates, Drs. Baranska and Koldovsky, approached this problem in an oblique manner through the study of a serum containing antibodies against mouse eggs.[6] As shown in Table 3-2, this serum is cytotoxic in the presence of complement for any strain of mouse eggs, but not for either rat or hamster eggs. Table 3-3 shows that the anti-egg serum is not cytotoxic for normal cells obtained from adult C57BL/6 mice whose eggs were used to immunize a guinea pig. It shows also, however, that the serum is cytotoxic for PF-1 and 3T3-SV mouse cells transformed by SV40 but not for "normal" 3T3 cells. Finally, the close relationship between the antigen present in a parthenogenetically stimulated egg and the surface SV40 antigen is confirmed by the data presented in Table 3-4, which shows adsorption of anti-egg antibody following treatment of the serum with SV40-transformed mouse cells.

One may argue that the future of this study lies in determination of the possibility of immunizing against pregnancy by immunization

TABLE 3–3.—EFFECT OF GUINEA PIG ANTI-C57BL/6 EGG SERUM ON SOMATIC MOUSE CELLS OF SYNGENEIC AND ALLOGENEIC ORIGIN

STRAIN OF MICE	CELLS	SERUM	CYTOTOXICITY
	PF-1 (SV40-transformed embryonic cells)	I	65/112*
		C	16/100
C57BL/6	3T3-SV (SV40-transformed 3T3 cells)	I	50/98
		C	19/106
	3T3 ("normal" embryonic cells)	I	25/114
		C	26/116

* Numerator: Number of cells observed.
Denominator: Number of cells either destroyed in cytotoxicity test or showing membrane fluorescence in the immunofluorescence test.

TABLE 3–4.—Cytotoxicity Test on C57BL/6
Eggs with Anti-Egg Serum Adsorbed with
PF-1 and MC57G Cells

Anti-Egg Serum Diluted 1:10 Absorbed with Cells	Ratio of Eggs Destroyed
PF-1	2/30
None	26/29

against SV40 transplantation antigen, a problem which may be of much greater importance than prevention of death by cancer. Be that as it may, this study has shown that at least one of the antigens engendered by an oncogenic virus is very similar to the antigen detected at the earliest stage of embryonic development. A parallel can be drawn between these results and those pointing to the relationship between cancer cell antigens and embryonic antigens of the same species. These investigations did not, however, go as far back as ours did in relation to the earliest stages of embryonic development.

Additional support for the claims of lesser involvement of complete oncogenic viruses in the actual process of carcinogenesis comes from the discovery by Michel et al.,[7] Winocour,[8] and later of Trilling and Axelrod[9] and Levine and Teresky[10] of pseudovirions in cells infected either by polyoma or SV40. Levine's data[10] indicate that purified SV40 virions obtained from AGMK cells labeled before infection with ^{3}H-thymidine contained ^{3}H-labeled DNA obviously of cellular origin and that, following complexing with anti-SV40 rabbit antibody, the preparation can be precipitated by antirabbit serum, thus indicating the enclosure of DNA in a viral capsid. Additional data[10] indicate that pseudovirions contain cellular DNA made before infection of the cell with SV40 but also some synthesized after infection.

The removal and subsequent encapsulation of a portion of the cellular genome may be of greater importance in determining the fate of the host cell than synthesis of a complete oncogenic virus inside the cell. It is hoped that the role of "oncogenic pseudovirions" in transduction of cellular genetic markers and cell transformation will be elucidated in the near future.

One or Two Viruses

It is difficult even to hypothesize at present why Vero and AGMK cells produce pseudovirions, whereas BSC and CV-1 cells do not. Since the phrase "to speculate" is derived from "specula," which means a watchtower, I would like at the end of my talk to climb into the watchtower and speculate on the possibility that phenomena such as the formation of pseudovirions may be explained by the interaction of two or more viral agents not even closely related. The latter statement is made in view of the results presented by Choppin[11] on transcapsidation between such unrelated viruses as vesicular stomatitis virus and SV5.

Historically, Stenback et al.[12] demonstrated in adeno- or SV40-induced hamster tumors presence of C-type virions and R-type virions. The biologic activity of the R-type virions is still unknown; however, high concentrations of virions resembling the C-type particles were present in the blood of these animals but were found to be nononcogenic per se.[13] Conversely, Graffi et al.[14] observed that cell-free extracts of hamster papillomas containing large concentrations of papova-like virions, found in newborn hamsters, will produce leukemias. In the leukemic cells, however, they observed only the C-type virions and could not detect the papova virions. Jensen et al., working with 12 SV40-transformed hamster cell lines from which the SV40 genome could be rescued by co-cultivation with AGMK cells, recovered a syncytia-producing paramyxovirus hitherto unidentified.[15] There is good evidence that many hamster colonies are infected with this agent.

Finally, I would point out that the agents observed in and isolated from Burkitt lymphomas of man and from Marek neurolymphomatotic tumors of chickens are herpeslike viruses containing DNA, whereas viruses observed in murine, cat, dog and hamster leukemias and in other types of chicken lymphomatosis are of the RNA-C particle variety.

The multiple virus theory could not be presented even as a hypothesis unless we could speculate on the nature of the interaction between the viral agents present in the same cell. For example, in the cytoplasm of human brain cells, papovalike virions persist in the presence of nucleocapsids or of virus particles related to measles virus.[16]

The role of paramyxoviruses found in SV40-transformed hamster cells may be simply that of producing a factor which facilitates fusion between various types of cells, with the resulting rescue of the viral genome occurring during co-cultivation experiments. The relationship between two or more viral agents and their host cell, however, may go beyond a simple mechanical interaction. Some of the myxoviruses and paramyxoviruses are known to cause breakage and pulverization of chromosomes, and may thus directly cause breaks in host cell DNA. Whether this hypothesis explains the formation of pseudovirions is at present beyond the horizon which we observe from our watchtower. As easily as the multivirus theory is made into a hypothesis, as difficult will it be to prove or disprove it, particularly since it is more difficult to document the absence of a second virus than its presence. Ultimately, the hypothesis may succumb to the fate described by T. H. Huxley as "the great tragedy of science—the slaying of a beautiful hypothesis by an ugly fact." But so with other hypotheses.

Samuel Butler said, "If science tends to thicken the crust of ice on which, as it were, we are skating, it is all right. If it tries to find, or professes to have found, the solid ground at the bottom of the water, it is all wrong."[18] Let us, apprentices in research in the etiology of tumors, continue to skate safely rather than to drown while searching for the bottom of the water.

Acknowledgments

This investigation was supported in part by U. S. Public Health Service Research Grants No. P01-CA 10815 and No. R01-CA 04534 from the National Cancer Institute, No. S01-FR 05540 from the General Research Support Branch, and funds from The Lalor Foundation.

References

1. Baranska, W., and H. Koprowski: Fusion of unfertilized mouse eggs with somatic cells. J. Exp. Zool. In press.
2. Baranska, W., and H. Koprowski: In preparation.
3. Brackett, B. G., W. Sawicki, W. Baranska, and H. Koprowski: In preparation.
4. Hummeler, K., and F. Sokol: Morphological aspects of the uptake of simian virus 40 by permissive cells. J. Virol. In press.
5. Barbanti-Brodano, G., P. Swetly, and H. Koprowski: Early events in the infection of permissive cells with simian virus 40: Adsorption, penetration and uncoating. J. Virol. In press.
6. Baranska, W., P. Koldovsky, and H. Koprowski: Antigenic study of unfertilized mouse eggs cross reactivity with SV40-induced antigens. Proc. Nat. Acad. Sci. USA. In press.
7. Michel, M. R., B. Hirt, and R. Weil: Mouse cellular DNA enclosed in polyoma viral capsids (pseudovirions). Proc. Nat. Acad. Sci. USA, 58:1381-1388, 1967.
8. Winocour, E.: Some aspects of the interaction between polyoma virus and cell DNA. Adv. Vir. Res., 14:153-200, 1969.
9. Trilling, D. M., and D. Axelrod: Encapsidation of free host DNA by simian virus 40: A simian virus 40 pseudovirus. Science, 168:268-271, 1970.
10. Levine, A. J., and A. K. Teresky: Deoxyribonucleic acid replication in simian virus 40-infected cells. J. Virol., 5:451-457, 1970.
11. Choppin, P. W., and R. W. Compans: Phenotypic mixing of envelope proteins of the parainfluenza virus SV5 and vesicular stomatitis virus. J. Virol., 5:609-616, 1970.
12. Stenback, W. A., G. L. Van Hoosier, Jr., and J. J. Trentin; Virus particles in hamster tumors as revealed by electron microscopy. Proc. Soc. Exp. Biol. Med., 122:1219-1223, 1966.
13. Stenback, W. A., G. L. Van Hoosier, Jr., and J. J. Trentin: Biophysical, biological and cytochemical features of virus associated with transplantable hamster tumors. J. Virol., 2:1115-1121, 1968.
14. Graffi, A., T. Schramm, E. Bender, I. Graffi, K. H. Horn, and D. Bierwolf: Cell-free transmissible leukoses in syrian hamsters, probably of viral aetiology. Brit. J. Cancer, 22 (3):577-581, 1968.
15. Jensen, F. C., F. S. Lief, and K. Hummeler: Correlation between SV40 rescue and presence of a paramyxo-like virus in SV40-transformed hamster cells. (Abstract) Fed. Proc., 29 (2):372, 1970.
16. Koprowski, H., G. Barbanti-Brodano, and M. Katz: Interaction between papova-like virus and paramyxovirus in human brain cells: A hypothesis. Nature, 225: 1045-1047, 1970.
17. Huizinga, J.: Men and Ideas: History, the Middle Ages, the Renaissance. (J. S. Holmes, and H. Van Marle, trans.), Meridian Books, Inc., New York, 1959, pp. 19-20.
18. Auden, W. H., and L. Croninberger, eds.: The Viking Book of Aphorisms. Viking Press, New York, 1963, p. 259.

Virus-Induced Cell Transformation

MICHAEL G. P. STOKER

Imperial Cancer Research Fund Laboratories, Lincoln's Inn Fields, London, England

SINCE THE LAST CONGRESS, intensive studies on the action of DNA tumor viruses at the cellular level have been continued, particularly with polyoma viruses and Simian virus 40 (SV40). With their small genomes, polyoma and SV40 remain the simplest known tumor viruses and, therefore, the viruses most amenable to detailed investigation. As Huebner and Todaro[10] have suggested, the RNA tumor viruses may be of more general importance in naturally occurring cancers, but these are difficult to work with because of their large size and their ubiquity. In addition, many of the RNA tumor viruses are defective and can only be studied in mixed infections with helper viruses.

This paper is restricted to a discussion of the early events, particularly the altered physiology of transformed cells, during transformation by polyoma and SV40. It is possible, however, that many of the common features of polyoma and SV40-transformed cells are also shared by cells transformed by the large DNA viruses, by the RNA viruses, and even by chemical carcinogens.

Requirements for Transformation

There are probably three essential requirements if transformation is to follow infection with polyoma virus or SV40: first, continued cell survival and multiplication; second, expression of transforming viral gene (s) ; and third, stable perpetuation of the viral genome.

NONCYTOCIDAL INFECTION

While RNA tumor viruses can replicate and emerge from the host cell by budding without killing it, the production of progeny by DNA tumor viruses kills the host cell; by analogy with similar bacteriophage infections, this is known as the lytic cycle. The cytocidal action of DNA tumor viruses is associated with, but not necessarily caused by, synthesis of viral capsid proteins, specified by genes expressed late in the virus growth cycle.

Since transformation obviously depends on survival and continued growth of the cell, it must follow an incomplete virus infection in which the cytocidal genes are not expressed. It is now believed that non-lethal infection, sometimes leading to transformation, may occur in a cell, which supports lytic replication of wild-type virus, if it is infected by a mutant virus with a defect affecting the cytocidal genes. Transformation of mouse cells by polyoma virus and human cells by SV40 virus probably arises in this way. Although viral DNA can be detected by hybridization with viral RNA,[26] intact, nondefective viral genomes cannot be recovered by the cell fusion technique (except in the case of SV40-transformed cells, by special procedures which may allow complementation between different defective viruses).[11]

Other cell types do not even allow the expression of all the genes of wild-type virus. Because of this, they are called nonpermissive cells, in contrast to permissive cells which support the lytic cycle of wild-type virus. Certain hamster and rat cells are nonpermissive for polyoma virus and SV40, and mouse cells are nonpermissive for SV40. In such cells, the late genes responsible for the cytocidal effect and for specifying the viral capsid are not expressed, while other genes constituting at least a third of the virus genome, and including those responsible for transformation, are active.[1, 16] Transformed cells, arising after nonpermissive infection with SV40, may contain the complete viral genome, which can be recovered by hybridization with a permissive cell.[12, 24] Polyoma virus has not been recovered by this method, however, despite the presence of virus-specific DNA in the transformed cells. The difference between permissive and nonpermissive cells is of considerable interest and importance, but will be discussed more appropriately at the molecular level in another session.

Certain events which occur in the lytic cycle, notably induction of host DNA synthesis, may be important clues to the mechanism of transformation.[4, 8, 25] Transformation is, however, a rare event in permissive cells, so it is more convenient to use nonpermissive cells, infected with large doses of virus, to study the initial stages of transformation in a measurable number of cells. The two model systems extensively studied are the 3T3 mouse cell line infected with SV40[22] and the BHK21 hamster cell line infected with polyoma virus.[14] With these systems, it is possible to distinguish the physiologic from the hereditary aspects of transformation, and I shall deal now with our own work on BHK21 cells infected with polyoma virus.

PHYSIOLOGIC EXPRESSION AND STABILIZATION

Some 2 to 4% of BHK21 cells, exposed to high multiplicities of polyoma virus, give rise to transformed clones, which can be recognized by their randomly arranged, piled-up colonies on surfaces or their ability to grow in suspension in viscous medium containing agar or methyl cellulose.[13] Other alterations in transformed cells include increased transplantability, and the continued synthesis of virus-specific T antigen and transplantation antigen. Virus DNA is detectable in the cells by hybridization with virus-specific RNA.[26] Since these characters

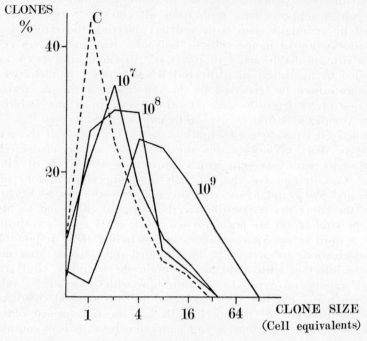

FIG. 3–1.—Frequency of clone sizes seven days after exposure of suspended BHK21 cells to polyoma virus, in doses indicated as plaque-forming units (for methods see Stoker[18]).

are normally inherited by all daughter cells, the phenomenon is called "stable transformation."

The remaining 96 to 98% of cells, despite virus uptake,[6] were originally thought to remain unaltered, but further examination has shown that a large number temporarily develop the ability to grow in suspension.[18] This continues for several days, giving rise to clones of as many as 32 cells. The cells then lose the ability to grow in suspension and regain their original character. This temporary change is called "abortive transformation." The cells which revert to normal contain no T antigen and are susceptible to reinfection, again leading to abortive and stable transformation.

Further studies in our laboratory with higher virus input have shown that virtually all cells can be transformed abortively. Figure 3-1 shows the distribution of clone sizes seven days after exposure of suspended BHK21 cells to the virus doses indicated. The whole population shows a shift in clone size after exposure to 10^9 plaque-forming units of virus, giving rise to clones varying from two to 64 cells. The few stable transformants are included in the larger clones of 32 to 64 cells, which continue to enlarge. Some arise after one or more divisions, giving rise to mixed clones containing both stably and abortively transformed cells. Lowering the virus dose reduces the number of cells dividing and the number of divisions by each cell. The relationship to virus dose is, therefore, complex and does not show the simple first order relationship given by stable transformation.

Initial transformation of all cells, even if only temporary, means that some initial stages of transformation can be investigated. Besides ability to grow in suspension, abortively transformed cells show other temporary changes.[27] They develop random orientation and, perhaps distinct from this, accelerated movement. BHK21 cells show density-dependent inhibition of growth in low serum concentrations (see below), and this inhibition is also overcome in abortive as well as stable transformation.

It is not known whether the expression of the transformed cell physiology requires synthesis of viral proteins. Full DNA-containing particles, and not empty shells, are required, but the full particles may contain "core" polypeptides[15, 17] besides DNA, which might conceivably cause the cell changes, particularly in view of the high virus dose required.

These results show that the virus can induce changes characteristic of transformation, which may be either transient or permanent. It suggests that the expression of the physiologic changes and their hereditary perpetuation are distinct processes, both of which are essential for transformation. If both are caused by the virus, more than one viral gene may be required for transformation. If so, it should be possible to obtain mutants affecting either the physiologic expression or the stable perpetuation of transformation. Until recently, only one type of mutant affecting transformation, the Tsa mutant, was available.[7] Though this mutation prevented the development of stable transformants, it did not affect abortive transformation.[19] This shows that a viral gene is involved in stabilization. We would now anticipate another type of mutant, which prevented the expression of the transformed cell physiology, but did not affect the stable perpetuation of the viral genome. Cells infected with such a mutant should not show abortive transformation, and the viral genome might be detected in clones with otherwise normal characteristics.

Figure 3-2 summarizes the three main consequences of the infection by polyoma virus and probably also SV40 in permissive and nonpermissive cells.

One plausible explanation of the findings would be as follows: the changed cell physiology would be the result of expression of an early viral gene or genes. This occurs whether the viral DNA is or is not free or attached to host cell DNA, and is expressed even in permissive infections for a brief period before cell lysis, where it may be de-

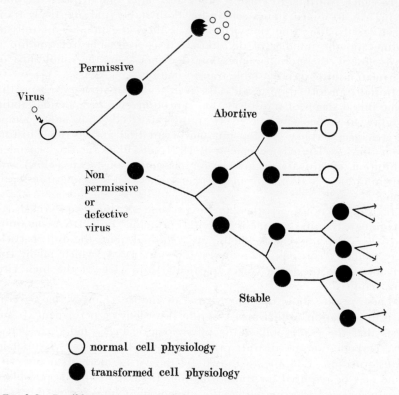

FIG. 3–2.—Possible consequences of infection by small DNA-containing tumor viruses.

tected, in resting cells as induction of host cell DNA synthesis. In non-permissive infection, the manifestations of this transforming gene would last longer and persist until the (free) viral DNA or viral gene products were lost by dilution or decay. In a few cells however, re-combination, requiring another viral gene, would occur between the viral and host cell DNA, leading to linear insertion. In such stably transformed cells, the viral genome would be perpetuated and the transforming gene expressed indefinitely.

This theory would imply that the integration of viral and host DNA is incidental to the expression of the transformed cell physiology but necessary for its hereditary stability. It must, however, be admitted that there are other possible explanations. For example, abortive trans-formation could be caused by unstable integration of viral DNA, or the integration might be stable, but at a site in a cell chromosome which prevented transcription of viral genes. Further studies are, therefore, needed on the fate of viral DNA during abortive transforma-tion, and in the cells which revert to normal.

Growth of Normal and Transformed Cells

We have now seen that the physiology can be distinguished from the genetics of transformation, and I should now like to discuss briefly one important aspect of the transformed cell physiology, namely the altered control of cell growth.

Transformed cells grow in environmental conditions which are restrictive for normal cells. This obviously applies in vivo and also to cells in culture. There are several ways of restricting the growth of normal fibroblastic cells, which are affected by transformation with tumor viruses, and which can be studied in detail. It is for example, well known that cell growth is inhibited under conditions of high density, while the transformed cells under the same conditions continue to grow. Growth of certain fibroblasts also depends on anchorage to a rigid surface,[20] and I have already mentioned that transformed cells are able to escape this restriction and grow in suspension. Finally, the growth of normal fibroblasts is dependent on naturally occurring factors present in serum, while transformed cells will grow in medium deprived of these factors.[2, 9, 21, 23]

Since all of these characteristics of normal growth can be affected concurrently by the introduction of perhaps one or two viral genes of average size, it seems possible that they are different aspects of one process. Accordingly, my colleagues and I have been studying the interrelationship of these growth controls to search for common features.[3] Following earlier studies on BHK21 cells by Burk[2] in our laboratories, we have examined the requirement of individual BHK21 cells for calf serum under differing conditions of density and anchorage. Serum contains many factors essential for cell integrity and growth, but since the inhibition of growth of cultured cells occurs in the G1 phase of the cell cycle, we have limited our investigations to the initiation of events leading to DNA synthesis, as shown by incorporation of thymidine detected by autoradiography.

When BHK21 cells were deprived of serum and were incubated in Eagle's medium alone, in a variety of conditions of density and suspension, a low proportion, usually less than 2%, showed evidence of DNA synthesis.

Resting cells deprived of serum, as surface cultures in various densities, and in suspension, were then exposed to increasing doses of serum. Figure 3-3 shows the percentage of cells which entered the first cycle of DNA synthesis. (The extrapolation for the absence of serum is taken from other experiments.) The following points may be noted:

1. The number of cells in which DNA synthesis is initiated is proportional to serum dose.

2. The probability of initiation of DNA synthesis in a given cell is affected by cell density. It is reduced about threefold for a given serum dose if there are 10 times more surrounding cells. Thus, even BHK21

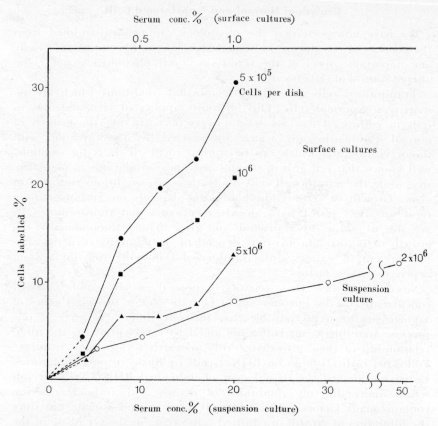

Serum conc.% (surface cultures)

FIG. 3–3.—Initiation of ³H-thymidine incorporation in resting (serum-deprived) BHK21 cells after addition of calf serum, showing percentage of radioactive nuclei after 20 hr exposure. (Data from Clarke et al.[3])

cells are subject to density-dependent inhibition if the serum concentration is low, though they are obviously less sensitive than, for example, 3T3 cells. This effect of density is not attributable to depletion of serum by the larger cell numbers, since the same change in sensitivity is seen as cells migrate to lower density in the same medium along the edge of a wound.[3, 5]

3. The proportion of suspended cells which enter DNA synthesis is also related to the amount of serum, but the cell sensitivity is low: at least 40 times less than anchored cells at an equivalent density. (It may also be noted that in high serum DNA synthesis is followed by cell division and appearance of clones in suspension.)

Although grains were not counted, the uptake of thymidine per cell does not vary greatly with serum dose, so DNA synthesis is an all-or-none phenomenon. This means that the probability of initiation of the early events in the cell cycle by a given dose of serum factor is altered by the cell topography, the interaction of cells with one another, or with a rigid surface, or by changes in cell shape. Density-dependent inhibition, for example, could be explained by the increased requirement by each cell for factor as crowding increased, in addition to depletion of available factor in the medium. Whether these changes in sensitivity are the result of variation in uptake or some other aspect of the interaction with serum factor is unknown.

Figure 3-4 shows the results of similar measurements on polyoma virus-transformed BHK21 cells derived from the same clone. In contrast to the data in Figure 3-1, this shows that: (1) At least one half of

Fig. 3–4.—Initiation of thymidine incorporation in serum-deprived polyoma-transformed BHK21 cells after addition of calf serum (see Figure 3-3: data from Clarke et al.[3]). Layer culture, 3×10^5 cells per dish. Suspension culture, 2×10^6 cells per dish.

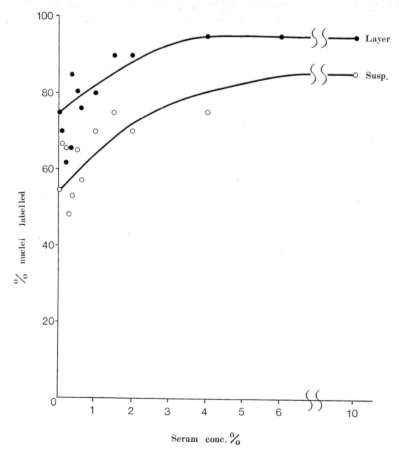

the cells are already synthesizing DNA without added serum; (2) the sensitivity to added serum of the remaining cells is very high; and, (3) suspended cells respond nearly as well as anchored cells.

As well as the stably transformed cells, abortively transformed cells tested up to 48 hr after addition of virus and before reversion occurred showed the same lack of serum requirement for initiation of DNA synthesis.[27]

These results and those obtained in other laboratories with other types of tumor virus and cell[9, 21, 23] suggest that an important feature of transformation is the removal or reduction of the requirement for an external factor to initiate the cell cycle. It follows that transformed cells have the greatest selective advantage in those conditions where the requirement of normal cells for such a factor is highest, for example, high density and suspension. It would be interesting to know if conditions in vivo also restrict the initiation of the cell cycle by an extracellular factor equivalent to serum factor.

There are several hypotheses which might explain the effect on the basis of a single virus gene. For example, a viral gene product inside the cell may act as an analog of serum factor, or a later product in the initiation chain, so that the external factor is not required. Alternatively, a viral gene product could activate cell genes which include an otherwise repressed gene for a serum factor equivalent.

Unfortunately, a simple replacement of serum factor activity may not account for other manifestations of the transformed cell physiology. It has recently been shown, for example, that both serum and virus will initiate cell movement in serum-deprived cultures.[27, 28] This could be explained if movement and growth were causally linked, but virus-induced movement is random and less subject to contact inhibition, so the replacement is probably not a simple one, and may involve distinct membrane changes.

Meanwhile, further knowledge about changes in the physiology of cell growth will probably depend on the purification and characterization of active growth factors, both as naturally occurring molecules in serum, and as viral specified products, and also on the isolation of viral mutants, and eventually cell mutants, affecting the different components of growth regulation.

References

1. Aloni, Y., E. Winocour, and L. Sachs: J. Molec. Biol., 31:145, 1968.
2. Bürk, R. R.: In: Growth Regulating Substances for Animal Cells in Culture (V. Defendi and M. G. P. Stoker, eds.), Wistar Symposium Monograph No. 7, 1967.
3. Clarke, G. D., M. G. P. Stoker, A. Ludlow, and M. Thornton: In press.
4. Dulbecco, R., L. H. Hartwell, and M. Vogt: Proc. Nat. Acad. Sci. USA, 53:403, 1965.
5. Dulbecco, R., and M. G. P. Stoker: Proc. Nat. Acad. Sci. USA. In press.
6. Fraser, K. B., and E. M. Crawford: Exp. Molec. Path., 4:51, 1965.
7. Fried, M.: Proc. Nat. Acad. Sci. USA, 53:486, 1965.

8. Gershon, D., P. Hausen, L. Sachs, and E. Winocour: Proc. Nat. Acad. Sci. USA, 54:1584, 1965.
9. Holley, R. W., and J. A. Kiernan: Proc. Nat. Acad. Sci. USA, 60:300, 1968.
10. Huebner, R. J., and G. J. Todaro: Proc. Nat. Acad. Sci. USA, 64:1087, 1969.
11. Knowles, B. B., F. C. Jensen, Z. Steplewski, and H. Koprowski: Proc. Nat. Acad. Sci. USA, 61:42, 1968.
12. Koprowski, H., F. C. Jensen, and Z. Steplewski: Proc. Nat. Acad. Sci. USA, 58:127, 1967.
13. Macpherson, I., and L. Montagnier: Virology, 23:291, 1964.
14. Macpherson, I., and M. G. P. Stoker: Virology, 16:147, 1962.
15. Murakami, W. T., R. Fine, M. R. Harrington, and Z. B. Susman: J. Molec. Biol., 36:153, 1968.
16. Oda, K., and R. Dulbecco: Proc. Nat. Acad. Sci. USA, 60:525, 1968.
17. Schlumberger, H. D., F. A. Andever, and M. A. Koch: Virology, 36:42, 1968.
18. Stoker, M.: Nature, 218:234, 1968.
19. Stoker, M., and R. Dulbecco: Nature, 223:397, 1969.
20. Stoker, M., C. O'Neill, S. Berryman, and V. Waxman: Internat. J. Cancer, 3:683, 1968.
21. Temin, H. M.: Internat. J. Cancer, 3:771, 1968.
22. Todaro, G. J., and H. Green: Virology, 23:117, 1964.
23. Todaro, G. J., Y. Mutsuya, S. Bloom, A. Robbins, and H. Green: In: Growth Regulating Substances for Animal Cells in Culture (V. Defendi and M. G. P. Stoker, eds.), Wistar Symposium No. 7, 1967.
24. Watkins, J. F., and R. Dulbecco: Proc. Nat. Acad. Sci. USA, 58:1396, 1967.
25. Weil, R., M. R. Michel, and G. K. Rushman: Proc. Nat. Acad. Sci. USA, 53:1468, 1965.
26. Westphal, H., and R. Dulbecco: Proc. Nat. Acad. Sci. USA, 59:1158, 1968.
27. Taylor-Papadimitriou, and M. G. P. Stoker: Unpublished data.
28. Dulbecco, R.: Personal communication.

Role of Herpesviruses in Neoplastic Diseases

WERNER HENLE, M.D.

The Children's Hospital of Philadelphia, Philadelphia, Pennsylvania, USA

To DISCUSS the herpes group of viruses at a cancer congress would have been startling some five years ago, but recent reports have linked members of this group to the etiology of Marek's disease (the neurolymphomatosis of chicken), the Lucké adenocarcinoma of the leopard frog kidney, and, at least experimentally, to lymphomas of certain

South American monkeys, marmosets, and rabbits. It therefore should no longer be surprising to find herpesviruses implicated in the etiology of certain human malignant diseases.

I shall not discuss the evidence for oncogenic activities of the animal herpesviruses, but shall concentrate on the Epstein-Barr (EB) virus and its possible relation to Burkitt's lymphoma (BL) and nasopharyngeal carcinoma (NPC). After all, we do not have to depend, for once, on animal models, but can turn with the available tools directly to the study of human neoplasms.

The fact that EB virus has a world-wide distribution and causes infectious mononucleosis (IM) in young adults, but mostly milder or inapparent infections in children, does not exclude that it possesses an oncogenic potential. Indeed, ubiquitousness might almost be considered a prerequisite for an oncogenic virus, since nearly all animal tumor viruses are widely disseminated among their respective host species, yet induce malignant change only rarely under natural conditions.

Study of virus-induced animal tumors has provided methodologic approaches to linking a virus, such as the EB virus, to tumors, such as BL or NPC. These are: (1) search for virus, or virus-related antigens, or virus-related nucleic acids in biopsy or cultured cells of the neoplasms; (2) induction of neoplasms by inoculation of virus into nonhuman primates or other animals; (3) malignant transformation of normal human cells by virus in vitro; and (4) detection of antibodies to virus-related antigens at higher frequency and at higher titers in sera of patients with the neoplasm, as compared to healthy controls and patients with other neoplasms.

Much of the pertinent information regarding the relation between EB virus and BL or NPC has been obtained in Dr. George Klein's laboratory in Stockholm or ours (my wife's and mine) in Philadelphia, often in close collaboration between the two, as well as with Drs. Peter Clifford, Nairobi, Richard Morrow and John Ziegler, Kampala, John C. Ho, Hong Kong, de Thé, Lyon, Lloyd Old and his group, New York, and many others too numerous to mention in this brief summary.

Before discussion of the current status of the four types of approaches, I shall present briefly the immunologic techniques which have been most useful in the detection of EB virus-related antigens and the corresponding antibodies. Three of these involve immunofluorescence. The first, employing acetone-fixed smears of lymphoblastoid cells from established continuous cultures, detects those cells which contain, among others, viral capsid antigens, i.e., cells which produce virus particles. Immunofluorescent cells from BL (or IM leukocyte) cultures were shown by electron microscopy to harbor numerous virus particles, and positive human sera or pooled human gamma globulin were shown to cause antibody coating and agglutination of EB viral capsids detectable by electron microscopic examination. Undoubtedly other, nonvirion antigens also participate in this reaction.

In the second test, acetone-fixed smears are prepared from cultures of EB virus antigen-free blastoid cell lines which had been exposed several days previously to graded doses of EB virus. Under appropriate conditions, only abortive cellular infections may result; that is, early EB virus-induced antigens are synthesized but not viral capsids. Antibodies to early antigens (EA) are absent in pooled human gamma globulin and many human sera, which have antibodies to viral capsid antigens (VCA). They are especially found in many but not all sera from patients with IM, BL or NPC.

The third test, developed by Dr. George Klein and his co-workers, employs live cells from BL biopsies or from cultures of BL cells or IM leukocytes. It detects cell membrane antigens (MA) which are distinct from EA and VCA. Antibodies to the MA are frequently found in IM, BL, or NPC patients' sera, but also in some other human sera with anti-VCA titers.

In addition, double diffusion precipitation tests with concentrated extracts of EB virus-positive cell lines have been described first by Old and his associates, which may yield up to five precipitation lines. Again, mainly sera from patients with BL or NPC were reactive, but the exact nature of the antigens remains to be elucidated. Also, complement fixation tests have been described by Armstrong, Gerber, Trentin, and Benyesh-Melnick, and their associates.

Turning to EB virus or EB virus-related antigens in Burkitt's tumors and early cultures, it was shown by Dr. George Klein and his group that live cells from biopsies often have cell surface antigens detectable by indirect immunofluorescence with the patient's own or other patients' sera, which are not present on bone marrow or other cells from the biopsy donors. When biopsy cells failed to give this reaction, they were usually already coated with IgG, the patient's antibodies.

The membrane antigens are found also on cells from continuous BL or IM cultures, provided they harbor EB virus in a sufficiently large proportion of the cells. In a collaborative study with Dr. Klein, the percentages of cells with MA and with viral antigens in recently established BL cultures were compared. Arranged in descending order of the frequency of MA-positive cells, the EB virus-positive cells showed a roughly parallel decline. It should be noted, though, that approximately 10 times more cells showed MA than VCA.

These and other data indicated that the membrane antigens are EB virus-induced. Yet, herpes-type virus particles have been found only very rarely in tumor biopsies. Likewise, EB viral antigens are rarely noted in biopsy cells. In collaboration with the Nadkarnies in Dr. Klein's laboratory, 79 BL biopsies were examined by immunofluorescence, but only yielded specifically stainable cells, which amounted to less than 1 in 100,000. Yet when biopsy cells were placed in culture, viral antigen-producing cells appeared in 68% within three to seven days, at times in substantial numbers, that is, up to 3% of the cell population. On further maintenance, ultimately all cultures which survived showed the presence of EB virus in a small proportion of the cells (0.1 to 10%).

EA are as rare as VCA in biopsy cells, which prevents us at this stage to consider them the equivalent of neo- or T antigens. In some continuous cultures, cells with EA may exceed those with VCA, or even be the only ones present to indicate a persistent EB virus infection.

These observations denote that the EB viral genome is present in the majority, if not all of the BL cells in vivo and in vitro, but that its messages are often only partially translated, or not at all. This conclusion is supported by additional evidence. Clones were raised by our associates, Drs. Zajac and Kohn, from singly picked cells of the EB-2 line of BL cells in the presence of antibodies to EB virus to exclude transfer of extracellular virus. All clones obtained at an efficiency of greater than 40% harbored EB virus, even though the parent EB-2 cultures contained no more than 0.5% virus-producing cells. Furthermore, our former co-worker, Dr. zur Hausen, now at Würzburg, Germany, found a noncellular DNA in biopsy cells and cultured BL cells, whether from lines with or without detectable EB virus-related antigens, which corresponded in its physical properties to EB viral DNA.

No doubt, EB virus is intimately associated with BL. As shown by Dr. de Thé, the lymphoblastoid cell lines derived from NPC biopsies also harbor regularly EB virus.

The second approach, the induction of tumors by EB virus or EB virus-containing cells in nonhuman primates (or other animals), has been totally unsuccessful in spite of intensive efforts by various investigators. Many primates have antibodies interacting with EB virus, as first shown by Gerber, and thus might be immune. However, if EB virus has an oncogenic potential, additional factors are likely required for expression of this potential which were absent in the transmission experiments.

As to transformation of normal cells by EB virus in vitro, three types of experiments have shown that the virus has at least a growth-stimulating effect on peripheral lymphocytes, which has been suggested also by the fact that leukocytes of patients in the acute stage of IM become more rapidly established in culture than leukocytes from other donors.

In the first procedure, lethally X-irradiated blastoid cells of lines from donors of one sex were co-cultivated with leukocytes from healthy donors of the opposite sex and without antibodies to EB virus. The X-irradiated cells and the leukocytes cultured separately usually died within three weeks. Co-cultivation of leukocytes with irradiated cells from EB virus antigen-negative lines likewise failed to yield growing cultures, but co-cultivation with irradiated cells from EB virus-positive lines yielded many continuous cultures, whether the blastoid cells were derived from Burkitt's tumors, IM leukocytes, or co-cultivation experiments. All growing cultures harbored EB virus and were composed of descendants of the leukocytes on the basis of their chromosomal sex.

In experiments reported by Dr. John C. Pope and co-workers, continuous lines of blastoid cells were established from leukocytes cultured in cell-free media of EB virus-positive lines. No growth was obtained when the virus was removed from the medium by Millipore filtration, inactivated by heat, or neutralized by antibodies to EBV.

Most recently, Dr. Paul Gerber as well as ourselves exposed leukocytes from anti-EB virus-negative donors to EB virus derived from the HRI-K line of BL cells. Several continuous cultures were obtained, but the results were erratic, possibly because many of the cells may rapidly succumb to potent virus preparations.

These results fulfill most of the criteria for transformation of cells by oncogenic viruses; that is the blastoid cell lines show: (1) a change in morphology from lymphocytes into lymphoblasts; (2) loss of contact inhibition, since the cells grow in large aggregates in suspension or in multilayered colonies when attached to fibroblasts; (3) they have a permanent growth potential, having been maintained for years; (4) they show chromosomal aberrations; and (5) they acquire new surface antigens but the equivalent of neo- or T antigens has not as yet been clearly demonstrated.

A transformed cell is not necessarily a malignant cell, however, and final proof would depend upon transplantation of transformed cells to syngeneic hosts, which for several reasons is impossible.

We have succeeded, though, in collaboration with Dr. Haff of the Smith, Kline and French laboratories, in establishing lines by the co-cultivation procedure from leukocytes of three gibbons. When 10^8 cells from these lines were transplanted to the autochthonous animals, they were rejected. The animals responded with antibodies to EB virus, having had none before.

Finally, in the fourth approach, the association of antibodies to EB virus-related antigens in patients with BL or NPC, all BL patients studied were found to have antibodies to EB viral antigens, usually at high titers (geometric mean 1:360). These persist also generally at high levels during prolonged remissions. In contrast, among age-, sex-, and tribe-matched control children, or siblings and other relatives of patients, an appreciable number had no antibodies and those who did had generally low titers (geometric mean 1:40).

If EB virus were merely a passenger in this tumor, with increased antigen production and correspondingly increased antibody responses, one should expect similar antibody levels in patients with related malignant diseases (chronic lymphocytic leukemia, Hodgkin's disease, LYS, MM, etc.). This is evidently not the case. Some patients had no antibodies, but the incidence of high titers in several of these groups was somewhat greater than that expected in appropriate controls.

A similar association of high anti-EB virus titers is seen in NPC. A series of NPC patients were compared with other patients having carcinomas of similar histologic descriptions but arising elsewhere in the head and neck. Carcinomas other than NPC did not show an association with high anti-EB virus titers but were comparable to controls.

The incidence of high anti-EB virus titers and their geometric means in NPC clearly depend on the stage of the disease according to Dr. Ho's classification. There is a steady increase in antibody titers from stage I to V, which probably reflects an increasing tumor mass.

Patients with BL or NPC generally also show high levels of antibodies to cell membrane antigens which tend to persist during long-term remissions. Of particular interest is one patient who has been followed for several years. Antibodies to MA and VCA persisted during remission at high levels for several years, but those to the MA fell to insignificant levels about six months before a recurrence was noted. Antibodies to MA reappeared as the recurrent tumor grew, and precipitating antibodies also became detectable. It is suggestive that the tumor recurred because of loss of membrane-reactive antibodies, but such an interpretation obviously requires confirmation by study of other, similar patients.

Most recently, tests for antibodies to EB virus-induced EA were applied to numerous BL patients. Sera from African control children generally were negative. There is a suggestion that there are more patients with low or no anti-EA levels among the one-year survivors than among the patients who died within one year. At the time of death, few patients had no antibodies to EA. In contrast, among the long-term survivors (two years) were many with no anti-EA. Sera were available which had been taken at the time of admission of several patients and which also were found to be negative. Among the long-term survivors with high anti-EA titers were several with histories of intermittent recurrences. It would seem that patients with few or no antibodies to EA have a better chance for long-term survival.

These findings, if confirmed in a larger series, would denote that the anti-EA titer may be of prognostic significance. If true, the passenger hypothesis would no longer remain tenable. It would be difficult to understand how an antibody induced by a passenger could reflect the prognosis of the patients.

Simian Virus 40 Specific "Repressor" in Infected and Transformed Cells

ROLAND CASSINGENA

Laboratoire de Virologie, Institut de Recherches sur le Cancer (CNRS), Villejuif, France

CELLS TRANSFORMED by simian virus 40 (SV40) do not produce virions although they contain functioning viral genes.[1, 2, 10, 21] In several lines of SV40-transformed cells, the production of virions can be induced by fusion of these cells with permissive cells and, in some cases, by chemical treatment.[4, 5, 13, 14, 20, 26]

In inducible as well as in noninducible transformed cells, autonomous replication of viral DNA and synthesis of viral capsid proteins are generally not detectable.[6, 13, 19, 20, 21, 25] Therefore, the expression of selected viral genes is blocked. One possible explanation for this phenomenon could be the presence of a specific repressor. We have attempted to verify this hypothesis by studying whether an extract of SV40-transformed cells, added to SV40-infected monkey cells, reduces plaque formation.[7]

An extract of SV40-transformed hamster, mouse, or cat cells inhibits plaque formation in SV40-infected monkey cells, provided it is added with a basic polymer (poly-L-lysine) known to stimulate pinocytosis,[22] and diluted in certain proportions (Table 3-5). Under these conditions, the inhibition rate averages 30%.

Plaque reduction is not observed either with extracts of normally or of "spontaneously" transformed cells, or with cells transformed by 20-methylcholanthrene, adenovirus 12, or polyoma virus. It also is not observed with an extract of monkey cells transformed by an irradiated adeno 7-SV40 hybrid virus, in which SV40 can replicate (Table 3-5).

An extract of SV40-transformed hamster cells does not inhibit plaque formation in monkey cells infected with vesicular stomatitis virus (VSV), poliovirus type 1, vaccinia, or herpesvirus (Table 3-6).

This extract is ineffective in preventing SV40 lytic infection when it is heated at 56 C for 30 min, or treated with trypsin; it is still effective when treated with DNAse or RNAse (Table 3-7).

It has been concluded that nonpermissive SV40-transformed cells contain a protein which specifically inhibits SV40 plaque formation in permissive cells. This protein has been tentatively called "repressor."

In a second series of experiments,[8] we first tried to enhance the rate of inhibition of SV40 plaque formation by using other basic polymers,

TABLE 3-5.—EFFECT OF VARIOUS CELLULAR EXTRACTS ON THE FORMATION OF SV40 PLAQUES IN MONKEY CELLS (BSC-1)

Cellular Species	Transforming Agent	Cells Utilized for Extracts (5 × 10⁷ Cells/ml)	Extract + Poly-L-lysine (10γ/ml)† Crude	½	¼	⅛	Extract without Poly-L-lysine Crude	½	¼	⅛	Poly-L-lysine (10γ/ml) Control
	0	Syrian hamster embryos in primary culture EHB³	None				None				None
	"Spont." transf.‡	T.20-MC XV³									
Syrian hamster	Adenovirus 12	T.Ad.12 III³	None				None				None
	Polyoma virus	T.Py. XV³									
	SV40 virus	TSV-11²⁵	2	31	16	2					
	SV40 virus	EHSVi²⁵	0	36,5	13,5	3					
	SV40 virus	Clone 2 TSV-5²⁵	2	36	17	6,5					
	0	Mouse embryos (C3H) in primary culture L¹²	None								
Mouse	"Spont." transf.	Cl.1.1.mKS-BU 100³¹	6	29	13	4,5	—				—
	0	BSC-1¹⁶									
	0	CV-1¹⁸									
Cercopithecus monkey	Irrad. hybrid Adeno 7-SV40 virus	CV-1LL "E-46"¹⁷	None				—				—
	0	CH²³	None								
Cat	SV40 virus	CHSV²³	2,5	29	18	6,5	—				—

* Compilation of 2 experiments (12 Petri dishes/point, with an average of 100 SV40 plaque/control plate).
† Basic polyaminoacid increasing the cellular permeability.²²
‡ Spontaneous transformation.

TABLE 3–6.—Assay of the Action of SV40-"Repressor" on
the Multiplication of Vesicular Stomatitis Virus (VSV) ,
Poliovirus Type 1, Vaccinia Virus and Herpesvirus
in Monkey Cells (BSC-1)

Virus	% Reduction of the Number of SV40 Plaques[*] EHSVi Cellular Extract[†] (5×10^7 cells/ml) + 10 γ Poly-L-lysine/ml			
	Crude	$\frac{1}{2}$	$\frac{1}{4}$	$\frac{1}{8}$
SV40 l.p.[‡]	5	29	14	2,5
SV40 s.p.[§]	0	30	12	3
VSV	0	0	0	0
Poliovirus, type 1	0	0	0	0
Vaccinia virus	0	0	0	0
Herpesvirus	0	0	0	0

* Average of 6 Petri dishes/point, with an average of 60 plaques/
control plate.
† Syrian hamster cells transformed by SV40.
‡ SV40 large plaque.
§ SV40 small plaque.

such as poly-D-lysine or poly-L-ornithine,[22] with the repressor extract.
We then tried to test, by the plaque reduction assay, if the repressor is
made in productive and abortive infections.

The number of SV40 plaques in infected monkey cells can be reduced
by approximately 40% when the extract is added with poly-D-lysine,
and by approximately 50% with poly-L-ornithine (Table 3-8). Because
of this, this polymer was adopted.

The repressor is detectable in both productive and abortive infections, but only in reduced amounts in the former case. The kinetics of
appearance of the repressor are different in these two cases: in abortive
infection, it appears earlier after infection and is detectable over a
longer period (Tables 3-9 and 3-10).

TABLE 3–7.—Sensitivity of the SV40-"Repressor" to
Trypsin, Temperature, RNAse, and DNAse

EHSVi Cellular Extract[*] (5×10^7 cells/ml) + 10 γ Poly-L-lysine/ml	% Reduction of the Number of SV40 Plaques[†]			
	Crude	$\frac{1}{2}$	$\frac{1}{4}$	$\frac{1}{8}$
Control	4	31	17	6
+ Trypsin[‡]	0	0	0	0
30 min. at 56°C	0	0	0	0
+ RNAse[§]	3,5	29	17	4,5
+ DNAse[#]	5	31	15	4

* Syrian hamster cells transformed by SV40.
† Compilation of two experiments (12 Petri dishes/point, with an
average of 100 SV40 plaques/control plate).
‡ 170 γ/ml; 30 min. at 37°C; trypsin inactivation by Iniprol
(170,000 U.I.P./ml).
§ 200 γ/ml; 30 min. at 37°C.
# 250 γ/ml (in the presence of 5×10^{-3}M MgSO$_4$); 30 min. at 37°C.

TABLE 3-8.—EFFECT OF DIFFERENT BASIC POLYMERS ON THE INHIBITION OF SV40 MULTIPLICATION IN BSC-1 CELLS BY EXTRACTS OF EHSVI* CELLS

POLYMER	γ OF POLYMER/ML	% REDUCTION OF THE NUMBER OF SV40 PLAQUES[†] EHSVi Extract (5×10^7 cells/ml) + Polymer								Polymer
		Crude	½	¼	⅛	$\frac{1}{16}$	$\frac{1}{32}$	$\frac{1}{64}$	$\frac{1}{128}$	mer
Poly-L-lysine	5	0	28	15	0	ND‡	ND	ND	ND	
(M.W. = 195.000)	10	0	36,5	13,5	0	ND	ND	ND	ND	
	20	0	15	30	13	0	ND	ND	ND	
Poly-D-lysine	10	0	10	29	45	31	14	0	0	None
(M.W. = 65.000)	20	0	14	31	39	24	0	0	0	
Poly-L-ornithine	5	0	19	28	36	25	18	0	ND	
(M.W. = 90.000)	10	0	22	35	53	27	23	15	0	
	20	0	33	44	56	40	21	ND	ND	

* Syrian hamster cells transformed by SV40.
† Average of 12 Petri dishes/point, with an average of 70 SV40 plaques/control plate.
‡ Not done.

These data have suggested that uninfected permissive cells contain a factor which is able to counteract the effect of the repressor.

In order to test this hypothesis, an extract of cells containing the repressor (EHSVi) was mixed in vitro with an extract of uninfected permissive or nonpermissive cells. The persistence of the action of the repressor in these mixed extracts was then measured by the usual technique.[7]

Extracts of uninfected permissive or nonpermissive cells have, by themselves, no effect on SV40 plaque formation in monkey cells (Tables 3-11 and 3-12).

An extract of EHSVi cells, mixed with an extract of uninfected permissive cells, can no longer inhibit plaque formation (Table 3-11). The mixture is capable, under conditions described in Table 3-11, even of enhancing the number of SV40 plaques.

An extract of EHSVi cells, mixed with an extract of uninfected nonpermissive cells, retains its inhibitory activity (Table 3-12).

The factor in uninfected permissive cells which is able to block the action of the repressor (FBR) is temperature- and trypsin-sensitive and insensitive to DNAse and RNAse (Table 3-13).

The existence of an FBR in uninfected permissive cells allows one to understand how the repressor can be present during productive infection. Furthermore, it may help to explain the phenomenon of induction of SV40 replication in transformed cells after their fusion with permissive cells.

That extracts of uninfected permissive cells containing FBR are ineffective on SV40 plaque formation in monkey cells could mean either that the FBR penetrates poorly, if at all, into the mammalian cells; or that once penetrated, it is rapidly degraded.

TABLE 3-9.—SYNTHESIS OF SV40-"REPRESSOR" AFTER INFECTION OF PERMISSIVE (BSC-1, MA-104) AND NONPERMISSIVE CELLS (ES, EH) WITH SV40

CELLS Perm. / Nonperm.	M.O.I. (PFU/CELL)	HOURS AFTER INFECTION	% REDUCTION OF THE NUMBER OF SV40 PLAQUES* + 10 γ Poly-L-ornithine/ml Cellular Extract (5×10^7 cells/ml)								
			Crude	$\frac{1}{2}$	$\frac{1}{4}$	$\frac{1}{8}$	$\frac{1}{16}$	$\frac{1}{32}$	$\frac{1}{64}$	$\frac{1}{128}$	$\frac{1}{256}$
Cercopithecus monkey kidney (BSC-1)	10		0	0	0	0	0	0	ND†	ND	ND
	20	18	0	0	17	30	14	0	0	0	ND
	40		ND	20	36	54	31	28	16	ND	ND
Rhesus monkey kidney (MA-104)	10		ND	ND	0	0	0	0	0	ND	ND
	20	18	ND	0	19	36	22	0	0	ND	ND
	40		ND	19	35	48	30	17	0	ND	ND
Mouse embryos (ES)	10		ND	ND	25	36	23	0	0	0	0
	20	18	ND	15	25	41	29	18	0	ND	ND
	40		ND	25	28	42	53	40	32	20	0
Hamster embryos (EH)	10		ND	0	18	32	15	0	0	ND	ND
	20	18	ND	26	39	47	42	21	14	ND	ND
	40		ND	ND	16	31	41	29	15	0	0

* Average of 6 Petri dishes/point, with an average of 70 SV40 plaques/control plate.
† Not done.

TABLE 3–10—KINETICS OF SYNTHESIS OF SV40 "REPRESSOR" IN PERMISSIVE (BSC-1) AND NONPERMISSIVE (ES) CELLS AFTER SV40 INFECTION

Cells Perm.	Cells Nonperm.	M.O.I. (PFU/ CELL)	HOURS AFTER INFECTION	% REDUCTION OF THE NUMBER OF SV40 PLAQUES* Cellular Extract (5×10^7 cells/ml) $+ 10\,\gamma$ Poly-L-ornithine/ml					
				$\frac{1}{2}$	$\frac{1}{4}$	$\frac{1}{8}$	$\frac{1}{16}$	$\frac{1}{32}$	$\frac{1}{64}$
Cercopithecus monkey kidney (BSC-1)		20	6	0	0	0	0	0	0
			12	0	0	0	0	0	0
			18	0	21	29	16	0	0
			24	0	12	20	15	0	0
	Mouse embryos (ES)	20	6	0	0	0	0	0	0
			12	0	0	12	0	0	0
			18	15	25	41	29	18	0
			24	23	38	46	42	26	10
		10	6	0	0	0	0	0	0
			12	0	0	10	0	0	0
			18	11	19	30	25	0	0
			24	13	27	35	21	10	0

* Average of 6 Petri dishes/point, with an average of 70 SV40 plaques/control plate.

We have observed that the blocking of the repressor in the extract of EHSVi cells reveals the presence of a substance, whose nature is unknown, capable of enhancing the number of SV40 plaques in monkey cells. This could explain why, in order to detect the repressor in an extract of this type, it is necessary to dilute the extract.

TABLE 3–11.—BLOCKAGE OF THE ACTION OF SV40-"REPRESSOR" BY EXTRACTS OF PERMISSIVE CELLS (BSC-1, CV-1, CV-1LL"E-46", MA-104)

CELLULAR EXTRACTS (5×10^7 CELLS/ML) $+ 10\,\gamma$ POLY-L-ORNITHINE/ML	% INCREASE (+) OR REDUCTION (−) OF THE NUMBER OF SV40 PLAQUES* Dilutions of Cellular Extract $+ 10\,\gamma$ Poly-L-ornithine/ml						
	Crude	$\frac{1}{2}$	$\frac{1}{4}$	$\frac{1}{8}$	$\frac{1}{16}$	$\frac{1}{32}$	$\frac{1}{64}$
EHSVi† ..... crude-1:64 in medium	0	−10	−24	−42	−26	−14	0
BSC-1 .... crude-1:64 in medium	0	0	0	0	0	0	0
EHSVi ...... 1:2-1:64 in crude BSC-1		+45	+27	+10	0	0	0
EHSVi ...... crude-1:64 in medium	0	−17	−29	−45	−32	−15	0
CV-1 .... crude-1:64 in medium	0	0	0	0	0	0	0
EHSVi ...... 1:2-1:64 in crude CV-1		+54	+35	+19	0	0	0
EHSVi ...... crude-1:64 in medium	0	−20	−41	−48	−34	−23	0
CV-1LL"E-46" crude-1:64 in medium	0	0	0	0	0	0	0
EHSVi ...... 1:2-1:64 in crude CV-1LL"E-46"		+43	+25	+19	0	0	0
EHSVi ...... crude-1:64 in medium	0	−22	−39	−52	−28	−23	0
MA-104 ..... crude-1:64 in medium	0	0	0	0	0	0	0
EHSVi ...... 1:2-1:64 in crude MA-104		+35	+21	0	0	0	0

* Average of 12 Petri dishes/point, with an average of 70 SV40 plaques/control plate.
† Syrian hamster cells transformed by SV40.

TABLE 3–12.—ABSENCE OF BLOCKAGE OF THE ACTION OF SV40-"REPRESSOR" BY EXTRACTS OF NONPERMISSIVE CELLS (ES, L, EH, EHB, T.Py XV, T.Ad. 7)

CELLULAR EXTRACTS (5 × 10⁷ CELLS/ML) + 10 γ POLY-L-ORNITHINE/ML		% INCREASE (+) OR REDUCTION (−) OF THE NUMBER OF SV40 PLAQUES* Dilutions of Cellular Extract + 10 γ Poly-L-ornithine/ml						
		Crude	½	¼	⅛	¹⁄₁₆	¹⁄₃₂	¹⁄₆₄
EHSVi†	crude-1:32 in medium	0	−26	−34,5	−47	−37	−26	
ES	crude-1:32 in medium	0	0	0	0	0	0	0
EHSVi	1:2-1:64 in crude ES		−22,5	−36	−45	−30,5	−23	−19
EHSVi	crude-1:32 in medium	0	−23	−32	−47	−41	−23	
L	crude-1:32 in medium	0	0	0	0	0	0	0
EHSVi	1:2-1:64 in crude L		−24	−37	−54	−35	−32	−20
EHSVi	crude-1:32 in medium	0	−22	−37	−43	−32	−29	
EH	crude-1:32 in medium	0	0	0	0	0	0	0
EHSVi	1:2-1:64 in crude EH		−16	−33,5	−41	−27	−24	−13
EHSVi	crude-1:32 in medium	0	−13	−25	−35	−22	0	
EHB	crude-1:32 in medium	0	0	0	0	0	0	0
EHSVi	1:2-1:64 in crude EHB		−14	−27	−39	−27	−15	0
EHSVi	crude-1:32 in medium	0	−28	−36	−51	−40	−28	
T.Py XV	crude-1:32 in medium	0	0	0	0	0	0	0
EHSVi	1:2-1:64 in crude T.Py XV		−20	−41	−45	−38	−26	0
EHSVi	crude-1:32 in medium	0	−14	−30	−42	−25	−11	
T.Ad. 7	crude-1:32 in medium	0	0	0	0	0	0	0
EHSVi	1:2-1:64 in crude T.Ad. 7		−21	−21	−38	−26	−13	0

* Average of 12 Petri dishes/point, with an average of 70 SV40 plaques/control plate.
† Syrian hamster cells transformed by SV40.

In summary: (1) Nonpermissive SV40-transformed cells contain a protein, named repressor, which specifically inhibits SV40 plaque formation in permissive cells by 30-50%; (2) the "repressor" is made in productive and abortive infections; and (3) its effect can be counteracted by a constitutive protein present only in permissive cells.

TABLE 3–13.—SENSITIVITY OF FBR* TO TEMPERATURE AND TRYPSIN

CELLULAR EXTRACTS (5 × 10⁷ CELLS/ML) + 10 γ POLY-L-ORNITHINE	% INCREASE (+) OR REDUCTION (−) OF THE NUMBER OF SV40 PLAQUES† Dilutions of Cellular Extract + 10 γ Poly-L-ornithine/ml						
	Crude	½	¼	⅛	¹⁄₁₆	¹⁄₃₂	¹⁄₆₄
EHSVi‡ crude-1:64 in medium	0	−21	−36	−48	−37	−23	−12
EHSVi 1:2-1:64 in crude BSC-1		+45	+31	+11	0	0	0
EHSVi 1:2-1:64 in crude BSC-1 heated 30 min. at 56°C		−25	−32	−47	−35	−20	−10
EHSVi 1:2-1:64 in crude BSC-1 trypsin-treated§		−20	−34	−47	−39	−22	−19

* Factor blocking the action of SV40-"repressor."
† Average of 12 Petri dishes/point, with an average of 70 SV40 plaques/control plate.
‡ Syrian hamster cells transformed by SV40.
§ 170 γ/ml; 30 min. at 37°C; trypsin inactivation by Iniprol (170,000 U.I.P./ml).

The mechanism by which an extract of SV40-transformed cells (EHSVi) inhibits plaque formation in SV40-infected monkey cells is presently under study.

Results to be published have already shown that in single growth experiments, the extract reduces the yield of virions by approximately 50% in monkey cells infected either with SV40 or with SV40 DNA.

References

1. Aloni, Y., E. Winocour, and L. Sachs: Characterization of the Simian virus 40-specific RNA in virus-yielding and transformed cells. J. Molec. Biol., 31:415-429, 1968.
2. Benjamin, T.: Virus-specific RNA in cells productively infected or transformed by polyoma virus. J. Molec. Biol., 16:359-373, 1966.
3. Bernhard, W., and P. Tournier: Modification persistante des mitochondries dans des cellules tumorales de hamster transformées par l'adénovirus 12. Internat. J. Cancer, 1:61-80, 1966.
4. Burns, W. H., and P. H. Black: Analysis of simian virus 40-induced transformation of hamster kidney tissue in vitro. V. Variability of virus recovery from cell clones inducible with mitomycin C and cell fusion. J. Gen. Virol., 2:606-609, 1968.
5. Burns, W. H., and P. H. Black: Analysis of SV40-induced transformation of hamster kidney tissue in vitro. VI. Characteristics of mitomycin C induction. Virology, 39:625-634, 1969.
6. Cassingena, R., and P. May: Etude du mécanisme de l'induction du développement du virus SV40 dans des cellules de hamster syrien transformées: Cinétique de l'apparition de l'ADN infectieux. Compt. Rend. Acad. Sci. (PARIS) Série D, 267:250-252, 1968.
7. Cassingena, R., and P. Tournier: Mise en évidence d'un "répresseur" spécifique dans des cellules d'espèces différentes transformées par le virus SV40. Compt. Rend. Acad. Sci. (PARIS) Série D, 267:2251-2254, 1968.
8. Cassingena, R., P. Tournier, E. May, S. Estrade, and M. F. Bourali: Synthèse du "répresseur" du virus SV40 dans l'infection productive et abortive. Compt. Rend. Acad. Sci. (PARIS) Série D, 268:2834-2837, 1969.
9. Cassingena, R., P. Tournier, S. Estrade, and M. F. Bourali: Blocage de l'action du "répresseur" du virus SV40 par un facteur constitutif des cellules permissives pour ce virus. Compt. Rend. Acad. Sci. (PARIS) Série D, 269:261-264, 1969.
10. Defendi, V.: Effect of SV40 virus immunization on growth of transplantable SV40 and polyoma virus tumors in hamsters. Proc. Soc. Exp. Biol. Med., 113:12-16, 1963.
11. Dubbs, D. R., S. Kit, R. A. De Torres, and M. Anken: Virogenic properties of bromodeoxyuridine-sensitive and bromodeoxyuridine-resistant simian virus SV40-transformed mouse kidney cells. J. Virol., 1:968-979, 1967.
12. Earle, W. R.: Production of malignancy in vitro. IV. The mouse fibroblast cultures and changes seen in the living cells. J. Nat. Cancer Inst., 4:165-212, 1943.
13. Gerber, P.: Virogenic hamster tumor cells: Induction of virus synthesis. Science, 145:833, 1964.
14. Gerber, P.: Studies on the transfer of subviral infectivity from SV40-induced hamster tumor cells to indicator cells. Virology, 28:501-509, 1966.
15. Gerber, P., and R. Kirschstein: SV40 induced ependymomas in newborn hamsters. I. Virus-tumor relationships. Virology, 18:582-588, 1962.
16. Hopps, H. E., B. C. Bernheim, A. Nisalak, and J. E. Smadel: Biological characteristics of a continuous kidney cell line derived from the African Green-Monkey. J. Immunol., 91:416-424, 1963.
17. Jensen, F., and V. Defendi: Transformation of African Green-Monkey kidney cells by irradiated adenovirus-7-simian virus 40-hybrid. J. Virol., 2:173-177, 1968.
18. Jensen, F., A. J. Girardi, R. V. Gilden, and H. Koprowski: Infection of human and

simian tissue cultures with Rous sarcoma virus. Proc. Nat. Acad. Sci. USA, 52:53-59, 1964.

19. Kit, S., T. Kurimura, M. L. Salvi, and D. R. Dubbs: Activation of infectious SV40-DNA synthesis in transformed cells. Proc. Nat. Acad. Sci. USA, 60:1239-1246, 1968.

20. Koprowski, H., F. C. Jensen, and Z. Steplewski: Activation of production of infectious tumor virus SV40 in heterocaryon cultures. Proc. Nat. Acad. Sci. USA, 58:127-133, 1967.

21. Pope, J. H., and W. P. Rowe: Detection of specific antigen in SV40-transformed cells by immunofluorescence. J. Exp. Med., 120:121-128, 1964.

22. Ryser, H. J. P.: A membrane effect of basic polymers dependent on molecular size. Nature, 215:934-936, 1967.

23. Samolyk, D.: Unpublished data.

24. Sabin, A. B., and M. A. Koch: Behaviour of non-infectious SV40 genome in hamster tumor cells: Induction of synthesis of infectious virus. Proc. Nat. Acad. Sci. USA, 50:407-417, 1963.

25. Tournier, P., R. Cassingena, R. Wicker, J. Coppey, and H. Suarez: Etude du mécanisme de l'induction chez des cellules de hamster syrien transformées par le virus SV40. I. Propriétés d'une lignée cellulaire clonale. Internat. J. Cancer, 2:117-132, 1967.

26. Watkins, J. F., and R. Dulbecco: Production of SV40 virus in heterocaryons of transformed and susceptible cells. Proc. Nat. Acad. Sci. USA, 58:1396-1403, 1967.

4

Cell-Virus Interaction: Molecular Aspects

The Transcription of the DNA Tumor Virus Genome

GERHARD SAUER

Institut für Virusforschung am Deutschen Krebsforschungszentrum, Heidelberg, Germany

THE INFECTION of a cell with a DNA tumor virus leads to either of two entirely different pathways. Either the cell is productively infected—virus multiplication occurs with ensuing cell death—or there is no virus multiplication but the infected cell is undergoing various alterations leading to the transformed state.

The elucidation of this particular dualism may help us greatly to understand the molecular mechanisms responsible for malignant transformation. The phenotypic differences between the productively infected and transformed cells may be characterized briefly as follows: Shortly after productive infection there is a stimulation of various enzyme activities related to DNA metabolism,[1] and new antigens, in particular, tumor antigen, are being synthesized. These so-called "early" functions are not dependent on viral DNA replication,[2] unlike the "late" viral functions which include viral coat protein synthesis and virus maturation. In contrast, in the case of the transformed cell, one can only detect the early viral functions. Thus, the expression of the viral genome is somehow restricted. The question therefore arises whether this curtailed gene activity in transformed cells is caused by incomplete transcription of the viral genome, by incomplete translation of viral messenger RNA (mRNA), or by a combination of both.

This report will deal mainly with the transcription of the simian

142

virus 40 (SV40) genome. I shall try to survey the state of our current knowledge concerning the transcription of the viral DNA in either the productively infected cell or in the transformed cell.

To study this problem, the technique of DNA-RNA hybridization[3] has been employed. This procedure takes advantage of the complementarity between the viral DNA nucleotide sequences and the base sequences of the viral mRNA. We shall consider first the amount of mRNA present during the various stages of the infectious cycle. The RNA transcribed early, that is, before viral DNA replication, comprises only about 0.06% of the total RNA present in the cell.[4] After the onset of SV40 DNA synthesis, late in infection, the amount of viral mRNA increases 25- to 40-fold.[4, 5, 6] The relative amount of SV40 mRNA which is detectable in SV40-transformed 3T3 cells is also very small. It corresponds to about the amount synthesized early in productive infection.[6] These quantitative aspects, however, do not allow any conclusions to be drawn concerning the actual species of mRNA present at these various times, and whether these species are transcribed sequentially during viral infection.

Using hybridization competition experiments, the events occurring during productive infection were studied first.[4, 6, 7] Radioactively labeled late SV40 mRNA has been added at saturation level to SV40 DNA. Unlabeled RNA obtained at various times during productive infection was then added in increasing amounts to the reaction mixture. Late mRNA is used as competitor because it most likely contains all the base sequences necessary for the production of viral progeny. The results of this experiment are as follows: At three hr postinfection there are no detectable mRNA sequences available to compete with late mRNA for homologous sites on the viral DNA. By six hr postinfection, however, a section of the SV40 genome is transcribed which effectively competes with 25% of late-labeled mRNA. RNA extracted 17 hr postinfection competes to the same extent. Thus, it appears that by six hr postinfection, most of the early mRNA sequences are being transcribed (Figure 4-1).

To determine precisely the onset of transcription of late mRNA sequences, arabinofuranosylcytosine (Ara-C), an inhibitor of DNA synthesis,[1] has been used. Ara-C allows the expression of early SV40 functions but effectively prevents the expression of late viral functions.[2] The RNA synthesized up to 19.5 hr postinfection in the presence of Ara-C competes with late RNA to the same extent as RNA extracted six hr postinfection, indicating that Ara-C prevented transcription of new sequences. In the absence of Ara-C, however, between 17 and 19.5 hr postinfection, new sections of the SV40 genome are being transcribed. A plateau has not been attained, which shows that only a few copies of the new mRNA species are present (Figure 4-1).

To summarize, the onset of transcription of SV40-specific RNA in productively infected cells occurs sequentially. Most of the early mRNA

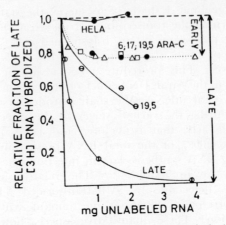

Fig. 4–1.—Transcription of the SV40 genome in productively infected monkey kidney cells. In hybridization competition experiments (³H), late SV40 RNA was added in saturating amounts to 0.05 μg of immobilized SV40 DNA. The late (³H) RNA was obtained 51 hr post-infection of CV-1 cells with 20 plaque-forming units of SV40/cell. The RNA had been labeled with 20 μc (³H) uridine/ml from 48 to 51 hr post-infection. Unlabeled RNA was extracted at the times indicated post-infection and added in increasing amounts to the reaction mixture. The hybridization reaction was performed as described previously.[4] The concentration of Ara-C was 5 μg/ml. The cultures were grown in the presence of the inhibitor from two to 19.5 hr post-infection. The level of hybridization of late (³H) RNA without any unlabeled RNA is indicated by the broken line.

sequences are synthesized by six hr postinfection. Late mRNA transcription begins shortly after 17 hr postinfection. At this later time, both early and late mRNA species are being copied.

I will now describe the SV40 gene activity in transformed cells. Using RNA extracted from SV40-transformed 3T3 cells, hybridization competition experiments were performed. The RNA from transformed cells displayed only 40% homology with late mRNA from productively infected cells. Thus, in this cell line, the viral functions are regulated at the level of transcription, although more SV40 mRNA sequences are present than are available early in a productive cycle of infection. These conclusions have been reached by Aloni, Winocour and Sachs, Oda and Dulbecco, and by our group.[4, 6, 7] It has also been shown by Oda and Dulbecco that most, but not all, of the early SV40 mRNA sequences are represented in SV40-transformed 3T3 cells.

Up to this point in the investigation, only 3T3 cells had been employed. This cell line is derived from mouse embryo cells that do not permit productive infection with SV40. It was of particular interest to determine whether the same mechanism of regulation of transcription applied in transformed cell lines of different origins, using, for example, SV40-transformed African green monkey kidney cells which were originally permissive for the multiplication of SV40. In such cells, considerably more SV40-specific mRNA nucleotide sequences are represented than in transformed 3T3 cells. A competitive experiment revealed 80% homology with late SV40 mRNA, and it also appeared that most, if not all, early mRNA sequences were present.[4] Thus, when investigating mRNA in transformed cells, one is confronted with a pattern of transcription that is extremely variable. The homology of the SV40 mRNA from transformed cells with late SV40 mRNA varies from 17% (in mouse embryo cultures six days postinfection) to 30,[8] 40,[4] and even 100%[8] in various transformed mouse cell lines. Considering adenovirus type 2 transformed cells, 4 to 10% homology with late lytic adenovirus type 2 mRNA has been reported.[9] In the case of polyoma virus, 40% homology was observed.

The only feature in common is that in all transformed cell lines, with one exception, fewer sections of the viral genome are copied than one detects late during productive infection. The presence in some of these cell lines of more RNA sequences than one finds early in lytic infection, and the absence of late viral functions in those cells that exhibit 80 to 100% homology between transformed and lytic mRNA suggest the existence of additional blocks subsequent to transcription, perhaps at the level of translation.

The restricted expression of the viral genes in most of the transformed cell lines could be accounted for by the presence of defective or mutant genomes. However, in both transformed 3T3 and monkey kidney cells, the formation of infectious SV40 can be induced upon fusion with permissive cells.[10, 11] Thus, all viral genes necessary for transformation and for virus multiplication are present. It must be concluded, therefore, that in transformed cells, a particular mechanism is controlling the transcription of the viral genes.

The nature of this mechanism remains unknown at present. It does seem to be different, however, from the control exerted on the transcription of the viral DNA during the lytic cycle of infection, where infectious viral DNA is present at any time. Late mRNA is copied only when DNA replication is permitted, as revealed by the experiments with Ara-C. In transformed cells, despite the absence of viral DNA in an infectious configuration, at least some late viral mRNA sequences could be demonstrated in several cell lines. Thus, the state of the viral DNA may play a role with regard to its transcription.

There is little doubt that cellular factors also have to be taken into account as possible control elements. In view of the recently discovered initiation and termination factors in *Escherichia coli* that exert a controlling influence on the DNA-dependent RNA polymerase,[12, 13] one would not be surprised if the presence or absence of such factors in mammalian cells might decide whether a cell is rendered permissive for viral infection, or whether, instead, the cell undergoes malignant transformation.

References

1. Kit, S., D. R. Dubbs, P. M. Frearson, and J. L. Melnick: Virology, 29:69, 1966.
2. Butel, J. S., and F. Rapp: Virology, 27:490, 1965.
3. Gillespie, D., and S. Spiegelman: J. Molec. Biol., 12:829, 1965.
4. Sauer, G., and J. R. Kidwai: Proc. Nat. Acad. Sci. USA, 61:1256, 1968.
5. Carp, R. I., G. Sauer, and F. Sokol: Virology, 37:214, 1969.
6. Aloni, Y., E. Winocour, and L. Sachs: J. Molec. Biol., 31:415, 1968.
7. Oda, K., and R. Dulbecco: Proc. Nat. Acad. Sci. USA, 60:525, 1968.
8. Martin, M. A., and D. Axelrod: Proc. Nat. Acad. Sci. USA, 64:1203, 1969.
9. Fujinaga, K., and M. Green: Proc. Nat. Acad. Sci. USA, 65:375, 1970.
10. Koprowski, H., F. C. Jensen, and Z. Steplewski: Proc. Nat. Acad. Sci. USA, 58:127, 1967.
11. Watkins, J. F., and R. Dulbecco: Proc. Nat. Acad. Sci. USA, 58:1396, 1967.
12. Burgess, R. R., A. A. Travers, J. J. Dunn, and E. K. F. Bautz: Nature, 221:43, 1969.
13. Travers, A. A.: Nature, 225:1009, 1970.

State of the Viral Genome in Simian Virus 40 Transformed Cells

SAUL KIT

*Division of Biochemical Virology, Baylor College of Medicine,
Houston, Texas, USA*

Introduction

THE ONCOGENICITY of Simian virus 40 (SV40) has been demonstrated only in hamsters and mastomys.[19, 42] SV40 has, however, a very broad transforming capacity for cells in culture. Transformation has been obtained in cell cultures of mouse, rat, rabbit, guinea pig, hamster, cow, pig, mongoose lemur (*Lemur mongoz*), monkey, man,[2, 7, 8, 13, 14, 18, 30, 38, 60] cat, and dog.[66] Mammalian species differ considerably in susceptibility to SV40 virions and in conditions required for transformation. SV40 DNA can be used advantageously in those species where adsorption, penetration, or uncoating of virions is inefficient. It has been found to be about 1,000 times more efficient than whole virus in transforming human cells.[2] It has also transformed bovine embryo cells, which were very resistant to transformation by intact virus.[14]

Are cell lines transformed in culture malignant? The answer is affirmative for SV40-transformed hamster cells. It has been more difficult, however, to demonstrate that transformed mouse cells are malignant. In part, this is because SV40-specific transplantation antigens give rise to rejection of inoculated cells. Recently, a transplantable sarcoma in mice was obtained by Kit et al.[28] after inoculation of SV40-transformed mouse kidney cells into adult untreated syngeneic mice. Prolonged growth in vitro and in vivo seemed to be important for the development of the progressively growing tumor. Highly malignant transplantable tumors have also been obtained in rats and mice by inoculation of transformed cells into irradiated hosts and passages of the tumor tissue in irradiated, and later, in nonirradiated hosts.[63]

Regardless of whether all SV40-transformed mouse cells are malignant, they grow rapidly and can be subcultured indefinitely. Capacity for continued growth in culture is achieved within, at most, a few days after primary cell cultures are infected by SV40. Hence, SV40 transformation in vitro provides an important model for study of the interaction between tumor viruses and their hosts.

Do tumors and transformed cells produce SV40 after the malignant transformation has taken place? In contrast to cells transformed by leukosis viruses, cells transformed by SV40 usually do not release infectious virus into the culture medium. Furthermore, infectious virus and virus particles are not detectable in cell lysates of most SV40-transformed cells. Some exceptions to this generalization will be noted later.

Despite the absence of detectable viral infectivity, the SV40-cell interaction does not appear to be of the "hit-and-run" variety. Several observations indicate that the SV40 genome is integrated in transformed cells:

1. Products of SV40 genes are present because transformed cells contain: (A) an SV40-specific intranuclear antigen demonstrable by complement fixation or immunofluorescence techniques;[43] (B) specific transplantation antigens, demonstrable by immunorejection experiments;[63] and (C) virus-specific RNA, detectable by DNA-RNA hybridization in cells.[3, 37, 47]

2. SV40 DNA sequences are demonstrable in transformed mouse and hamster cells. Nuclear DNA from cells transformed by SV40 is homologous to virus-specific RNA made in vitro.[54, 64] The viral DNA is localized in the chromosomal, and not the mitochondrial, fraction of the cell.[4, 45] It occurs in a high molecular weight form joined to cellular DNA by alkali-stable covalent linkages.[45]

3. Interferon studies suggest that SV40 mRNA is not recognized as a foreign nucleic acid in transformed mouse (3T3) cells. Continuous passage in the presence of interferon fails to reduce the content of SV40 T antigen in these cells. However, marked inhibition of SV40 T antigen formation and of transformation results when normal 3T3 cells are pretreated with interferon and subsequently infected with SV40 virus.[40, 56] Interferon acts by inducing the synthesis of an active intracellular protein that selectively inhibits the translation of viral mRNA.

However, there is no apparent alteration in the translation of host cell mRNA. The mRNA coding for the T antigen must, at least in part, be transcribed from the SV40 genome present in transformed cells since its product, the SV40 T antigen, is indistinguishable from that formed in cells acutely infected with SV40. An attractive hypothesis would be the presence of some host cell information, presumably host mRNA, in the molecule of mRNA coding for the T antigen in the transformed cells. The presence of such cellular mRNA in the RNA coding for T antigen could act to prevent its recognition as viral. If true, this also suggests that integration of SV40 DNA involves the physical linkage of viral and host DNA in a manner permitting uninterrupted transcription of mRNA across the point of junction.

4. Conclusive evidence that the entire SV40 genome is integrated in transformed cells has been obtained through rescue experiments. In the author's laboratory, following co-cultivation with, or UV-irradiated Sendai (UV-Sendai) virus-induced fusion with susceptible green monkey kidney cells, infectious SV40 has been rescued from over 70 lines of mouse cells independently transformed by nondefective virus. Furthermore, infectious virus has been recovered from mouse kidney lines that have been cloned twice in the presence of SV40 antisera. This shows that each transformed cell in the population, or its progeny, has the potential for SV40 production.[18]

The conclusion that SV40 nucleotide sequences are integrated does not signify that the state of the viral genome is uniform in all transformed cells. Whether the integration is stable or unstable, and the extent to which SV40 will replicate following release of the SV40 genome from the integrated state, depends upon the species of origin, the karotype of the transformed cell, and upon the number and types of SV40 genomes present.

Recovery of SV40 from Transformed Lines of Different Species

TRANSFORMATION OF MOUSE CELLS BY NONDEFECTIVE SV40

In contrast to African green monkey kidney (GMK) cells, which are highly susceptible, mouse cells are very nonpermissive for SV40 replication. Other species exhibit intermediate levels of permissiveness. It will be useful to describe first the state of the SV40 genome in transformed mouse cells. The SV40-mouse cell interaction seems less complicated than that of other species since replication of SV40 DNA does not occur. Following the presentation of experiments with mouse cells, studies involving other mammalian species such as hamster, human, and monkey will be described.

SV40 infection of mouse cells is abortive even when infection occurs at high input multiplicities—100 to 1,000 plaque-forming units (PFU) per cell.[30] Early SV40 functions are expressed: induction of T antigen, enhancement of enzymes of DNA metabolism, and stimulation of cellular DNA synthesis. However, few, if any, rounds of SV40 DNA replication take place, and neither virion proteins nor virus particles are made.[30, 34] Some abortively infected cells do undergo transformation. Superhelical SV40 DNA (Form I) and nicked-circular DNA (Form II) are infectious.[29] However, infectious DNA has not been detected in extracts of transformed mouse cells, indicating that neither Form I nor Form II SV40 DNA is present. Indeed, radioisotope experiments have shown that SV40 DNA does not exist in transformed mouse cells in a free form of any configuration of molecular weight comparable to the DNA of the virion.[45] These observations and the experiments discussed previously suggest that SV40 DNA is linked to cellular DNA at one or more chromosomal sites.

Rescue of SV40 entails the release of the genome from the integrated state, replication of the SV40 DNA, and maturation of infectious virus. Rescue is readily accomplished when mouse cells are transformed by nondefective SV40 virions.[17, 18] The probability of successful rescue does not depend on the input multiplicity of SV40 used in the initial transformation.[27] In a study of the relationship between input multiplicity during transformation and subsequent rescue, mouse kidney cultures were infected by nondefective SV40 virions at multiplicities varying from 0.06 to 200 PFU/cell. Clonal lines of all of the transformed cells yielded infectious SV40. Virus rescued from transformed cells can initiate transformation of new primary mouse kidney cultures, virus can once again be rescued from the second step transformation, and the virus rescued in the second step can initiate a third round of transformation. SV40 can again be rescued from the cells transformed in the third round.

Rescue of SV40 is accomplished by co-cultivating transformed mouse kidney cultures (MKS) with susceptible GMK cells, or by fusing cell mixtures in the presence of UV-Sendai virus.[15, 16] Primary African green monkey kidney (PGMK) or established monkey cell lines (CV-1, BSC-1, Vero) can be utilized for rescue experiments.[18, 59] UV-Sendai treatment of cell mixtures facilitates rescue by increasing the number of monkey-mouse heterokaryons. The total yield of SV40 is thereby enhanced and the time required to detect rescue is reduced.[15, 16] Infectious SV40 has been detected by 19 hr and infectious virus by 29 hr after UV-Sendai-induced fusion.[15, 32] These times are very similar to the times required to initiate SV40 replication in productively infected CV-1 cells, indicating that activation of SV40 synthesis occurs very shortly after fusion.

The initial site of virus synthesis during rescue of SV40 from heterokaryons of SV40-transformed hamster and susceptible monkey cells was studied by Wever et al.[65] Nuclei were isolated from fused cells at various times after fusion, separated on sucrose density gradients, and assayed for infectious center formation and virus content on CV-1 monolayers. Virus was first detected in the transformed nucleus (40 hr postfusion), and later associated with both transformed and susceptible nuclei (68 to 72 hr). Based upon these results, the following time table of events is suggested: SV40 DNA synthesis is activated in the transformed nucleus, and a pool of virus particles is formed. Virus particles are subsequently released into the cytoplasm 40 hr after cell fusion and secondarily infect other nuclei in the heterokaryon. A second cycle of SV40 replication then takes place in the monkey nucleus.

After UV-Sendai treatment of monkey and mouse cell mixtures, approximately 50 to 70% of the transformed mouse kidney (MKS) nuclei are found in heterokaryons.[16] However, only a fraction of the heterokaryons initiate SV40 formation. The number of cells activated to synthesize SV40 varies greatly with different MKS lines. Frequency of induction tests have shown that about 3×10^{-3} MKS-BU100 heterokaryons form infectious centers when plated with freshly trypsinized CV-1 cells. The frequency of induction is 10^{-2} to 10^{-4} for transformed MKS lines classified as "good" yielders, and about 10^{-4} to 10^{-5} for lines classified as "average" yielders. Heterokaryons formed with "poor" and "rare" yielder MKS lines produce even fewer infectious centers.[17] Thus, heterokaryon formation with monkey cells is necessary, but not sufficient for activation of SV40 replication in transformed mouse lines. The rate limiting step is not known, but it could perhaps be the release of the SV40 genome from the integrated state.

The finding that SV40 replication commences in some MKS cells after they form heterokaryons with susceptible monkey cells suggests that a substance essential for SV40 replication is missing in nonpermissive mouse cells and is supplied by monkey cells. The properties and precise function of SV40 essential replication factor (SERF) are not known. Some speculative possibilities are that SERF is an initiator of DNA replication or of DNA transcription (e.g., a sigma-type factor), or that SERF is required for translation of SV40 messenger RNA (e.g., a special tRNA). Another possibility is that SERF is an antirepressor.

In all probability, SERF activates SV40 replication after SV40 DNA has been released from integration. Swetly et al.[53] studied SV40 replication after non-transformed mouse fibroblasts, LM (TK⁻)Cl 1D, were infected with SV40 DNA. Replication did not occur in the nonpermissive mouse fibroblast cells. However, if LM (TK⁻)Cl 1D were fused with monkey kidney cells 24 hr after they were infected with SV40 DNA, then replication of SV40 did occur.

The following experiment suggests that a monkey chromosome controls the availability of SERF. Somatic hybrid monkey-mouse cells were isolated from survivors of mixed cultures of CV-1 (monkey kidney) and MKS-BU100 (SV40-transformed mouse kidney) cells by constantly culturing the cells in selective HAT (hypoxanthine-aminopterin-thymidine) medium.[33] The parental MKS-BU100 cells, a thymidine kinase-deficient cell line, perish when cultured in HAT medium. Parental CV-1 cells are destroyed by the presence of SV40 in some of the monkey-mouse heterokaryons. The hybrid monkey-mouse cells receive the determinant for thymidine kinase from the CV-1 cell, and grow in HAT medium. The SV40 genome remains integrated in the monkey-mouse hybrid cells, as has been shown by positive tests for the SV40 T and transplantation antigens.

The surviving monkey-mouse hybrid cells contain a substantial complement of mouse chromosomes, but gradually lose monkey chromosomes until only a few are left. The hybrid cells are resistant to superinfection with SV40 virions or SV40 DNA. Hence, the few monkey chromosomes that remain do not supply the SERF which permits SV40 replication. However, SV40 virus can be rescued from the hybrid cells by fusing them with additional CV-1 cells. Studies of chromosome reduction in monkey-mouse hybrids may, perhaps, lead to the identification of the chromosome which controls SERF.

In the preceding discussion, it has been emphasized that an SV40 genome is integrated during transformation. The total number of integration sites per cell and their location are not known. It would not be surprising if there were two or more integration sites. Nucleic acid hybridization experiments by Westphal and Dulbecco[64] have shown that the number of SV40 DNA equivalents per transformed cell varies from five to 60 in different lines. This could signify that there are many integration sites in each cell, or that long catenated molecules are integrated at a single site.

Dubbs and Kit[17] recently demonstrated that at least two different SV40 genomes can be integrated in a single cell. 3T3 mouse cells were transformed by simultaneously infecting them with SV40 (MKS-U4), a fuzzy plaque strain, and SV40 (MKS-U88), a small clear plaque strain. From one of the transformed lines, 3T3 (4-88) G, 14 tertiary clones were isolated. After fusion of each of the clonal lines with CV-1 cells, fuzzy and small clear plaque strains of SV40 were recovered. There are several possible ways in which the double lysogens could have been generated. In a diploid cell, it is reasonable to assume that there are at least two integration sites. Either integration of fuzzy and small clear genomes occurs independently at each of the sites, or sequential integration occurs at one of the sites. Another possibility is that double-length circular molecules generated by joining SV40 (MKS-U4) and SV40 (MKS-U88) DNAs are integrated in tandem with or without secondary integration of SV40 (MKS-U4) and SV40 (MKS-U88) DNAs. Multiple length rings of S13 and ϕx174 replicative forms have been demonstrated and suggested as possible intermediates in recombination. Multiple length rings of polyoma DNA have also been found after induction of polyoma ts⁻a mutants by temperature shift.

It is attractive to postulate that the site of integration contains nucleotide sequences homologous to SV40 DNA. If the cellular sequences were reiterative,[62] the probability of multiple SV40 integrations would be increased.

Cell lines can be transformed not only by two distinct SV40 genomes, but also by SV40 and an unrelated virus. Todaro et al.[57] found that polyoma virus-transformed mouse 3T3 cells, superinfected with SV40 virus, possess the T antigens induced by both SV40 and polyoma virus. In the "reverse" direction, SV40 hamster tumor cells were superinfected and transformed by polyoma virus; such doubly transformed cells had the T and the transplantation antigens specific for both tumor viruses.[55] Moreover, SV40-transformed mouse cells can be transformed by murine leukosis viruses. These doubly transformed cells continuously produce leukemia-sarcoma viruses, as do 3T3 cells transformed by leukosis viruses.[67]

TRANSFORMATION OF MOUSE CELLS BY DEFECTIVE SV40

Primary mouse kidney cultures transformed by UV-irradiated SV40 have been named MKS-U lines.[15] Eighty-three MKS-U lines were isolated in the author's laboratory. Forty-eight of these failed to yield virus when fused with CV-1 cells. In further experiments, it was shown that these nonyielder lines are frequently produced when mouse cells are transformed at very low input multiplicities of UV-irradiated SV-40.[27] Another way to produce nonyielder lines is by transforming 3T3 cells with defective SV40 "T particles."[59] SV40 T particles are "light" virions isolated by equilibrium centrifugation. They induce T antigen, but are defective in plaque-forming ability. The light defective virions have been demonstrated by velocity sedimentation and electron microscopy to contain heterogeneous circular DNA molecules slightly shorter than those from plaque-forming virions.

The failure to rescue SV40 from nonyielder MKS-U lines does not stem from the failure of these cells to fuse with CV-1. In fact, 12 of 14 nonyielder lines of MKS-U cells fused as well with CV-1 as did various good yielder lines. In further attempts to rescue SV40 from nonyielder MKS-U lines, PGMK and Vero monkey kidney cells were used for fusion. This procedure was based upon the possibility that PGMK or Vero cells might be more permissive for SV40 variants than CV-1. Vero cells were also chosen because they fail to produce interferon after infection with Newcastle disease, Sendai, Sindbis, or rubella viruses. The induction of interferon by UV-Sendai virus-treated cell mixtures would be expected to reduce the yield of rescued SV40. Hence, yielder and nonyielder lines were mixed with PGMK, CV-1, and/or Vero cells, then treated with UV-Sendai virus. The virus yields obtained after seven days incubation were measured on CV-1 monolayers (Table 4-1). No virus was recovered from fusion mixtures of poor, rare, or nonyielders with Vero or PGMK cells. Moreover, the virus yields obtained from fusion mixtures of good or average yielders with Vero or PGMK cells were usually lower than those obtained in fusion mixtures with CV-1 cells.

TABLE 4-1.—A COMPARISON OF CV-1, VERO, AND PRIMARY GMK FOR THE RESCUE OF SV40 FROM TRANSFORMED MOUSE KIDNEY LINES IN THE PRESENCE OF UV-SENDAI

| | | | VIRUS YIELD (PFU/CULTURE)[*] | | |
| | | PASSAGE | RESCUE AFTER FUSION WITH: | | |
CLASSIFICATION	CELL LINE	NUMBER	CV-1	Vero	GMK
Nonyielder	MKS-U5	116	0	0	0
		127	0	0	
	MKS-U7	116	0	0	0
		129	0	0	
Rare yielder	MKS-U16	119	0	0	0
		139	0	0	
	MKS-U18	127	0	0	0
		146	0	0	
Poor yielder	MKS-U1	120	0	0	0
		141	0	0	
	MKS-U3	118	0	0	0
Average yielder	MKS-A	54	4.0×10^4	4.8×10^3	
	MKS-U4	81	1.0×10^2	0	0
Good yielder	MKS-U13	118	2.0×10^5	3.3×10^3	1.9×10^3
		139	8.8×10^5	3.4×10^4	
	MKS-BU100	269	5.8×10^3	1.1×10^3	

[*] Virus yields were determined by assay on CV-1 monolayers. Samples from nonyielders, rare yielders and poor yielders after fusion with Vero cells were also assayed on Vero monolayers. No plaques were obtained.

The possibility was considered that defective SV40 might be rescued from the rare or nonyielder MKS-U cells after fusion with Vero, which, in turn, might plaque poorly on CV-1 monolayers. Therefore, all fusion mixtures of poor, rare, and nonyielders with Vero cells were also assayed on Vero monolayers. No plaques were produced.

Two additional procedures have been used in an attempt to rescue SV40 from nonyielder MKS-U lines: (1) Nonyielder lines were propagated in medium containing the mutagen 5-bromodeoxyuridine (BUdR) in an effort to induce pseudorevertants. (2) Transformed cell lines were pretreated with mitomycin C prior to fusion with CV-1 to induce the release of defective SV40 genomes from integration. The techniques employed did not permit rescue of SV40 from nonyielder MKS-U lines.

Taking into account the negative experiments that have been described, it seems probable that the integrated SV40 genomes of nonyielder MKS-U lines contain lesions in genes essential for release of SV40 from the integrated state, for replication of viral components, or for viral maturation. Another possibility not rigorously excluded, however, is that inhibitors present in MKS-U cells prevent activation or replication of SV40.

TRANSFORMATION OF RAT, GUINEA PIG, BOVINE, CAT, AND DOG CELLS

SV40 replicates to only a limited extent in rat, guinea pig, and bovine cells. Transformed cultures of rat and guinea pig kidney cells have been studied by Diderholm et al.[13] Virus was not detected in extracts of transformed rat cultures after the twentieth passage, nor in those of the transformed guinea pig cultures after the seventeenth passage. Rescue experiments by co-cultivation or fusion with GMK cells were not attempted. In the case of bovine embryonic lung cultures transformed by SV40 DNA, sporadic production of small amounts of infectious virus were observed through the twenty-fourth tissue culture passage.[14] Studies of clonal lines of transformed bovine or rat cells have not been reported.

SV40-transformed cat and dog cells have been studied in the author's laboratory. Cell-free extracts of transformed cat cells did not contain infectious virus, nor was virus rescued after fusion with CV-1 cells. Cell-free extracts of transformed dog cells were also virus free. However, small amounts of virus were recovered from transformed dog cells after fusion with CV-1 cells.

The replication of SV40 in primary cultures of porcine and rabbit kidney cells was studied by Black and Rowe.[8] Large amounts of virus were produced in primary cultures of pig cells and moderate amounts of virus were found in extracts of transformed pig cells. Replication of SV40 was also detected after infection of primary rabbit kidney cultures by either SV40 virions[8] or SV40 DNA.[21]

The response of rabbit kidney cells to SV40 infection varies with the passage level of the tissue culture cells.[49] Rabbit kidney cells of increasing passage levels passed through various stages of response to SV40 inoculation. Primary rabbit cells inoculated with high multiplicities of SV40 did not show lytic cytopathic effects and produced little infectious virus. Continued passage of rabbit kidney cells resulted in augmented susceptibility to SV40, as indicated by shortened incubation time, enhanced cytopathic effects, and augmented virus yield. A high passage rabbit embryo kidney line, MA-111, was studied by Schell and Maryak.[49, 50] SV40 elicited a fulminant cytolytic effect in MA-111 cells. Virus and complement fixing antigen yields in MA-111 cells approached those in GMK cells.

Because of their susceptibility to SV40, primary and established lines of rabbit kidney cells can be used for the rescue of SV40 from transformed cells. Gerber[21] first showed that SV40 was rescued from hamster tumor cells by seeding them onto rabbit kidney monolayers. Margalith et al.[39] recovered small amounts of infectious SV40 after fusion of transformed monkey cells with MA-111 rabbit kidney cells. In the author's laboratory, MA-111 cells have been utilized to rescue SV40 from transformed mouse cells.

In the early study of Black and Rowe,[8] SV40 was not detected either in culture fluids or in suspensions of transformed rabbit kidney cells. In contrast, another transformed cell line established from SV40-infected rabbit kidney cultures exhibited a steady state of virus production.[48, 49] Only a small proportion of transformed cells (1.4 to 1.7%) released virus into the supernatant medium at any given time. However, on prolonged contact with GMK cells, each transformed cell or its progeny was shown to release virus eventually.

HAMSTER TUMOR AND TRANSFORMED HAMSTER CELLS

Virus was readily recovered from culture fluids of weanling hamster kidney or embryonic hamster kidney primary cultures for prolonged periods.[9] These observations indicate that hamster cells are partly susceptible to SV40.

Following transformation of hamster cultures, a progressive decline in virus titer was observed.[9] Virus was recovered from culture fluids of the first three cell passages, but in distinctly lesser amounts than from primary cultures. Supernatant fluids from continuous cell lines were consistently negative. Virus was also recovered from cell lysates at the twenty-fourth passage, but not at the fifty-first or fifty-ninth passages.

The virogenic properties of SV40-induced hamster tumors have been studied by Sabin and Koch.[44] Extracts of primary tumors developing many months after injection of large amounts of SV40 virus in newborn hamsters usually yielded little or no infectious SV40. After transplantation of the tumors, only minute amounts of virus were detected during the course of 31 serial transplant passages in adult hamsters. Tumors without virus could give rise to tumors with virus, and vice versa. In primary cultures, large numbers of tumor cells either failed to release virus or did so in single bursts of minute amounts on rare occasions. Prolonged propagation and serial passage of the tumor cells in tissue cultures induced the release of larger, though still small, amounts of virus in cultures that were previously virus-free for a month or more. Nine of 12 tumors produced by transplantation of approximately two cells in adult hamsters yielded minute amounts of virus, indicating that most, and perhaps all, of the tumor cells carried the SV40 genome in a noninfectious state, and that maturation of the virus occurred only rarely in an occasional cell.

SV40 rescue experiments on cultured lines of hamster tumor cells and on hamster cell lines transformed in vitro have yielded interesting results.[6, 21-23, 58] Some of the hamster cultures resembled mouse cell lines transformed by defective SV40 virions. These hamster lines failed to yield SV40 even after co-cultivation or fusion with susceptible monkey cells.[6, 58] H-50 hamster tumor cells have been shown by nucleic acid hybridization experiments to contain about 60 equivalents of SV40 DNA,[64] and the SV40 tumor and transplantation antigens. Yet, after fusion with susceptible GMK cells, neither infectious virions nor infectious SV40 DNA was detected.[17, 32]

Several other hamster tumor and transformed cell lines exhibited the properties of mouse cells transformed by nondefective SV40 virions. Infectious SV40 was not detected in cell-free extracts of these cell lines. Nevertheless, SV40 was rescued following co-cultivation or UV-Sendai virus-induced fusion with either GMK or rabbit kidney cells.[6, 21-23, 58] Virus was also recovered from clonal lines of transformed hamster cells.[6] In the case of TSV-5 clone 2, another hamster line, from 4 to 13% of the cells released virus when plated on GMK cells.[17, 58]

A few of the yielder lines of hamster tumor cells had a unique property. These hamster lines produced small amounts of infectious SV40 after they were incubated overnight with mitomycin C.[10, 22] Furthermore, passage through hamsters of one SV40-transformed hamster kidney cell line not inducible by mitomycin C resulted in its becoming inducible.[11] Most transformed hamster cells and all transformed mouse cells so far tested were not inducible by mitomycin C.

The mitomycin C induction experiments are highly significant in that they show that fusion with monkey or rabbit cells is not always necessary for recovery of SV40. The number of cells yielding infectious virus has not yet been established. Fluorescent antibody staining for V antigen suggests that less than one out of 10^4 cells is activated by mitomycin C treatment.

The mechanism of induction by mitomycin C is not understood. One possibility is that mitomycin C promotes the "excision" of the integrated viral genome, perhaps through the production of an endonuclease. If SERF were present in hamster cells that released the SV40 genome, replication of viral DNA, expression of late viral gene functions, and formation of viral particles would take place.

Also not understood is the reason why in vivo passage of a hamster cell line not inducible by mitomycin results in its becoming inducible. Perhaps tumor cells fuse with normal hamster cells during in vivo passage. If the normal cells contributed a more permissive protoplasm to the hamster-hamster somatic hybrid, greater inducibility by mitomycin C might be expected.

SV40-TRANSFORMED HUMAN CELLS

Numerous studies have shown that human diploid cell lines are susceptible to infection by SV40 virions.[1, 2, 5, 12, 24, 41, 46, 52] Susceptibility varies with the metabolic condition of the cell, the number of passages in tissue culture, and the source of the human cells. Cells derived from persons with genetic diseases associated with a high risk of neoplasia, and cells at the end of their in vitro lifetime generally had an increased susceptibility to SV40. Nevertheless, the percentage of productively infected cells was low compared with GMK cells. Even when high input multiplicities were employed, only about 3 to 20% of the human cell lines developed the SV40 T antigen,[2, 5, 12, 46] whereas 80 to 100% of GMK cells did so. In human cultures infected with SV40, little virus production or cell destruction occurred. The cells could be maintained for extended periods with eventual transformation of growth, morphologic, and chromosomal characteristics. In contrast to human cells, SV40 replicated extensively in GMK cells. Furthermore, SV40 produced cytopathic effects in all cells, but usually did not morphologically transform the cells. Although few virion-infected human diploid cells initiate T antigen formation, the average virus yield per T antigen positive cell may be of the same order of magnitude as that found in monkey cells. Since limited SV40 replication occurs in human cells infected by SV40, the SERF is probably present, at least in low concentrations, in normal human cells. The production of SV40 virions in cells infected with SV40 DNA represents further evidence that SERF is either present or is produced in normal human cells.[2, 53]

In human cell lines transformed by SV40, all cells are positive for the SV40 T antigen. In contrast to transformed mouse cells, however, a small number of transformed human cells also sometimes contain the SV40 V antigen. For example, after twice cloning one subline of transformed human cells, Aaronson and Todaro[1] found that up to 1% of the cells cultivated with SV40 antiserum contained V antigen. Moreover, infectious SV40 was detected when transformed human cultures were cultivated without SV40 antiserum. In spite of two clonings, several sublines shed virus spontaneously.

In studies carried out in the author's laboratory, infectious SV40 was detected in cell-free extracts of transformed human buccal mucosa (W18 Va2-P363) and embryonic lung (WI38 Va13A) cells. Virus yield was not significantly increased by fusing either cell line with CV-1 cells. Infectious center studies indicated that about 10^{-2} W18 Va2-P363, and 10^{-5} to 10^{-6} WI38 Va13A cells produced virus. Twelve clonal lines of WI38 Va13A cells were isolated. Eight of these spontaneously shed small amounts of virus. Some transformed human lines may appear to be free of virus for several passages, but on further testing, they do produce infectious SV40.

In contrast to the WI38 Va13A cells, clonal lines isolated from W18 Va2-P363 cultures did not produce virus spontaneously. Moreover, no virus was detected after fusion of the clonal lines with CV-1. Similarly, two sublines of transformed human skin cells (W98 VaD and W98 VaH) did not produce virus spontaneously, or after fusion with CV-1 cells. Furthermore, attempts to induce virus formation by mitomycin C treatment, or by growth at sub- or supraoptimal temperatures were also unsuccessful.

To determine whether SV40 DNA could be detected in the non-yielder human lines, transformed human cells were grown in medium containing ³H-thymidine, and DNA extracts were prepared by the method of Hirt.[25] Neither infectious DNA nor labeled Form I SV40 DNA was found. The SV40 genomes integrated in these cell lines may be defective. An alternative possibility is that nondefective SV40 genomes were integrated in the nonyielder lines. However, release from integration may have been an extremely rare event.

Experiments by Koprowski and co-workers[26, 53] have shown that normal and transformed human cell cultures are capable of supporting at least some SV40 replication. Jensen and Koprowski[26] were able to rescue small amounts of SV40 from fusion mixtures of SV40-transformed human and SV40-transformed mouse (SV40-3T3-101) or SV40-transformed hamster (TSV-5) cells. Control cultures of fused SV40-3T3-101 cells alone did not yield virus, nor was virus recovered when TSV-5 cells were self-fused or fused with another transformed hamster line. It was not established, however, whether the progeny SV40 was derived from the viral genome in the transformed mouse cell, the transformed human cell, both cells, or whether the rescued virus was a recombinant. Swetly et al.[53] showed that normal and SV40-transformed human lines relatively resistant to infection by intact SV40 virions do produce infectious SV40 when infected with SV40 DNA. Again, it was not shown whether the virus progeny was derived from the superinfecting SV40 DNA, from the SV40 genome resident in the transformed human cells, or from both.

To determine the derivation of the virus progeny, rescue experiments were performed using mouse cells transformed by plaque morphology mutants of SV40.[31] The transformed mouse lines which were used yielded fuzzy, small clear, and large clear plaque strains of SV40 when fused with CV-1 cells. In addition, replication of SV40 was studied after human cells were infected with DNA isolated from the plaque morphology mutants of SV40.

The experiments in which transformed human cells were fused with transformed mouse cells demonstrated four significant facts: (1) The SV40 recovered from the fusion mixtures was always of the same plaque morphology as the SV40 resident in the transformed mouse cells. Either the SV40 genome resident in the transformed human cells was not activated, or defective particles were produced which were not detected in the plaque assay on CV-1 cells. (2) Virus yields were much lower when transformed mouse cells were fused with transformed human cells than when fused with CV-1 cells. (3) In many instances, fusion of transformed mouse cells with transformed human cells failed to yield SV40, although fusion with CV-1 cells always resulted in rescue of virus. (4) The rate of SV40 formation was greater from monkey-mouse than from human-mouse heterokaryons.

In experiments in which SV40 DNA was used to infect CV-1 and transformed human cells, the rate of virion formation and the final SV40 yields were much higher from monkey than from transformed human cells. Figure 4-2 shows an experiment in which cells were infected with DNA from SV40 (MKS-U4), a fuzzy plaque strain. Only virus of the fuzzy plaque type was found in extracts from the infected cells. Similarly, when SV40 DNA which gave small clear or large clear plaques on CV-1, respectively, were used to infect transformed human cells, only small clear or large clear plaques were found in extracts from the infected cells. Thus, only the replication of the superinfecting DNA was detected. The fate of the SV40 genome resident in the transformed human cells is unresolved; it may have been released from integration in cells superinfected by SV40 DNA. Either replication was minimal, however, or the particles produced were noninfectious for CV-1 cells.

The yields of SV40 in rescue experiments and after infection with SV40 DNA were lower from transformed human lines than from monkey cells. This suggests that the designation "semipermissive" or "semirestrictive" would be appropriate for the human cell lines used in our study. In contrast, primary and established lines of GMK cells are highly permissive for nondefective SV40 virion infection. Normal and transformed mouse cell lines are very nonpermissive. Semipermissiveness could mean that transformed human cell lines contain lower concentrations of SERF than GMK cells. Further studies are needed to elucidate the mechanisms underlying semipermissiveness or semirestriction.

With respect to the DNA superinfection experiments, fewer transformed human cells might have initiated replication of the superinfecting SV40 DNA, or the yield per cell may have been lower than from monkey cells. The induction of T antigen or synthesis of early SV40-messenger RNA cannot be used as a measure of initiation of infection, since all transformed cells contain T antigen and early SV40 mRNA.

The plaque-forming efficiency of SV40 DNA is very low—about 10^5 to 10^6 DNA molecules/PFU. Experiments with ^{3}H-SV40 DNA have shown that SV40 DNA molecules are converted to Form II (nicked) DNA shortly after infection of CV-1 or transformed human skin cells. Within 14 hr of infection, most of the parental input DNA was extensively nicked. We do not know the percentage of parental SV40 DNA molecules that ultimately reach replication sites. Perhaps few molecules do so, and the percentage of SV40 DNA molecules that reach the replication sites differs in CV-1 and in transformed human cells.

In order to determine the percentage of DNA-infected cells that initiate SV40 replication, infectious center experiments have been performed (Table 4-2). Approximately 1 to 5% of the CV-1 (monkey) and the KB (human) cells produced T antigen after SV40 DNA infection. Also, about 2% of the CV-1 and KB cells formed infectious centers. The virus yields were about 2,000 PFU/infectious center from CV-1 and about 430 for KB cells. With nonpermissive 3T3 mouse and HT-1 (MSV) hamster cells, no infectious centers were detected. Two trans-

FIG. 4–2.—Replication of SV40 after infection of monkey and human cell lines with SV40 (MKS-U4) DNA, a virus strain which produces fuzzy-type plaques. The input multiplicities (PFU/cell) were as follows: CV-1 (monkey), 0.2; HEK (human embryonic kidney), 0.5; W98 VaD and W98 VaH (transformed human skin), 0.4 and 0.2, respectively. Only fuzzy plaque type progeny SV40 were detected.

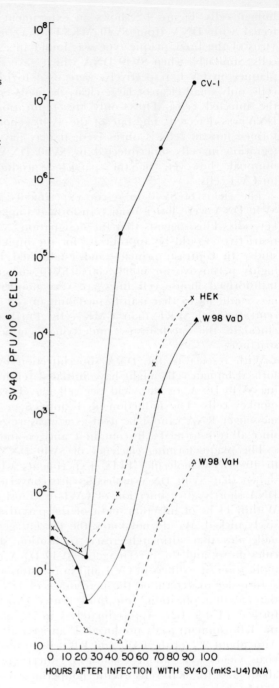

TABLE 4-2.—Properties of SV40-Transformed Cell Lines of Different Species

Species of Origin	Transformed Cell Line	Integrated SV40 Genome	Recovery of Infectious SV40*			SV40 DNA Infectious Centers per 10^5 Cells†	PFU per Infectious Center
			Cell Extracts	Mitomycin C Treated	Co-cultivation or Fusion with Monkey or Rabbit Cells		
Mouse	MKS-U5, 7, 25	Defective	−		−	0	0
	MKS-BU100	Nondefective (1c)‡	−	−	+		
	MKS-U13	Nondefective	−		+	0	0
	MKS-U4, 3T3 (U4)	Nondefective (f)	−		+		
	MKS-U88, 3T3 (4-88) J-3	Nondefective (sc)	−		+		
Golden hamster	H-50	Defective	−	−	−		
	TSV-5 C12	Nondefective (1c)	−	−	+		
	THK-1 (T-6)	Nondefective	−	+	+		
	Hamster tumor (Sabin & Koch)	Nondefective	+				
Human	W98 VaD (P124)	Defective	−	−	−	288	299
	W98 VaH (P117)	Defective	−	−	−	142	81
	W18 Va2 (P363)	Nondefective (r) plus defective	+				
	WI38 Va13A	Nondefective (1c) or leaky mutant	+				
Monkey	BSC/SV40 cl 1-1	Defective	−		−	25	86
	GMK-EVa-2-A-1	Defective	−		−		
	BSC/SV40 (NCM₄)	Nondefective or leaky mutant	−	+	+	216	1435
	GMK-EVa-5-1	Nondefective	−		+		

* "+" denotes that virus was recovered; "−" means rescue trials were negative.

† The values of infectious center formation for 10^5 cells was 2,200 for CV-1 (monkey), 1900 for KB (human), and 0 for 3T3 mouse and HT-1(MSV) hamster cells. The values for PFU/infectious center were 2,020 for CV-1 and 426 for KB cells.

‡ Rescued virus produces large clear (lc), small clear (sc), fuzzy (f), or large ragged (r) type plaques on CV-1 monolayers.

formed human lines, W98 VaD and W98 VaH, produced 10-fold fewer infectious centers than CV-1 cells. The average yield in PFU/infectious center was 299 for W98 VaD and 81 for W98 VaH cells. These results support the notion that the transformed human lines studied are semipermissive or semirestrictive as compared with CV-1 cells for SV40 DNA replication. Fewer transformed human cells were productively infected, and the average burst size per cell was reduced.

TRANSFORMATION OF GREEN MONKEY KIDNEY CELLS

SV40 may cause both cytolysis and transformation in the same cell system. GMK cells are highly permissive for SV40; the usual result of infection is cytopathic change and lysis of the cultures. Under special conditions, however, transformation can be obtained. Fernandes and Moorhead,[20] Koprowski et al.,[36] and Wallace[61] achieved transformation of primary GMK cultures by infecting at very low SV40 multiplicities. In contrast, Margalith et al.[38] employed a high multiplicity of SV40 and obtained a carrier BSC-1/SV40 culture. They suggested that autointerference may have played an important role in the establishment of the system. During passage of the chronically infected BSC-1/SV40 cultures, a cell line was selected in which all of the cells exhibited T antigen and only 0.2 to 1% of the cells produced infectious virus (transformed state).

The transformed monkey cells were resistant to superinfection by SV40 virions, although they were susceptible to SV40 DNA.[38, 53] The resistance to superinfection by SV40 virions permitted the small number of transformed cells to survive in monkey kidney cultures that were producing infectious virus.

Thirteen clonal lines of SV40-transformed BSC-1 cells were selected by Margalith et al.[38] Only two of the clonal lines were free of detectable V antigen and exhibited T antigen in all the cell nuclei. No virus was detected in cell-free extracts of the latter two clones. The efficiency of cloning of the transformed virus-free clones was tested in parallel with cells of the virus carrier state (BSC/SV40). The virus-free cloned cell line BSC/SV40 (NCM$_4$) had a 90% efficiency of cloning and its colonies were large, whereas the virus carrier cells had only 7% efficiency of cloning and formed small colonies.

Eight clones were established from an SV40-transformed culture (GMK-EVa) of PGMK cells.[36] During continuous passage for 12 months, the eight clones remained free of infectious virus. Four of the GMK-EVa clones yielded virus when fused with primary GMK cells, and four clones did not.[35]

Rescue experiments have been performed with the virus-free clonal line BSC/SV40 (NCM$_4$).[38, 39] Although virus was not recovered from fusion mixtures of NCM$_4$ with PGMK cells, occasional recovery of small amounts of virus were obtained after fusion with an established line of rabbit kidney, MA-111,[39] or with CV-1 cells.[68] Another clonal line of transformed monkey cells (BSC/SV40 cl 1-1) studied in the author's laboratory did not produce infectious virus spontaneously or after fusion with CV-1 or rabbit kidney cells.

Extracts of transformed monkey lines, BSC/SV40 (NCM$_4$) and BSC/SV40 cl 1-1, have been tested for the presence of infectious DNA. No infectivity was detected. However, when BSC/SV40 (NCM$_4$) cells were labeled with ^{3}H-thymidine, a radioactive DNA fraction which banded in cesium chloride-ethidium bromide density gradients in the position of Form I SV40 DNA was detected. Further studies are being done to determine whether this ^{3}H-thymidine-labeled fraction is noninfectious SV40 DNA.

Margalith et al.[39] have shown that heating to 45 C induced the synthesis of SV40 viral antigen in transformed monkey BSC/SV40 (NCM$_4$) cells. Up to 3.8% of the cells exhibited V antigen 72 hr after heating to 45 C for 30 min. Depletion of arginine from the medium of the heated cells enhanced and increased the percentage of cells synthesizing V antigen to 11%. No infectious virus was recovered from the cells in which synthesis of V antigen was induced. However, small amounts of infectious SV40 were rescued by treatment of the BSC/SV40 (NCM$_4$) cells with mitomycin C.

The recovery of small amounts of SV40 after mitomycin C treatment and occasionally after fusion with CV-1 monkey or MA-111 rabbit cells suggests (1) that at least a fraction of the cells contain a complete complement of SV40 genetic information, and (2) that some of the transformed monkey cells contain SERF. The latter hypothesis is supported by DNA superinfection experiments. Swetly et al.[53] showed that clonal lines of GMK-EVa cells infected with SV40 DNA produced infectious SV40. Dubbs and Kit[68] also found that clonal lines of transformed BSC-1 cells infected with SV40 DNA produced virus. The nonyielder BSC/SV40 cl 1-1 line produced 100 times fewer infectious centers, and the virus yield per infectious center was only about one tenth of that from SV40 DNA-infected CV-1 cells (Table 4-2). In contrast, the BSC/SV40 (NCM$_4$) clonal line, which occasionally yielded virus, produced about one tenth as many infectious centers, but the virus yield per infectious center was over one half of that obtained with CV-1 cells. It would appear that transformed monkey lines differ quantitatively in their ability to support replication of SV40 DNA. The BSC/SV40 (NCM$_4$) (transformed monkey) cells resemble KB human cells in being slightly less permissive than CV-1 for SV40 DNA replication. In contrast, the BSC/SV40 cl 1-1 cells were found to be much less permissive than CV-1 and resembled transformed human lines W98 VaD and W98 VaH.

Discussion

SV40-transformed cells contain the SV40 genome in an integrated state. The transformed cells are positive for SV40-specific T antigen, transplantation antigen, and SV40 mRNA. With few exceptions, however, SV40-transformed cells do not contain infectious virus, SV40 particles demonstrable by electron microscopy, V antigen, infectious DNA, or molecular forms of SV40 DNA corresponding to those extractable from SV40 virions. There are three general requirements for recovery of infectious SV40 from transformed cells: (1) A complete complement of the SV40 genetic information necessary for infectivity must be present, (2) the genome must be released from integration, and (3) SERF must be available.

The properties of SV40-transformed cell lines of different species are shown in Table 4-2. The requirements for recovery of SV40 from transformed cells will be discussed on the basis of the data summarized in this table.

SERF probably exists in SV40-infected and SV40-transformed monkey and human cells. SERF is also present in rabbit, pig, and hamster cells. The concentration of SERF may vary in different cell lines, in cells of a particular population, and with the metabolic condition of the cells. Primary and established lines of GMK and high passage rabbit kidney (MA-111) cells probably contain the highest concentrations of SERF. Normal and transformed mouse cells and certain transformed hamster cells contain little or none. Intermediate amounts of SERF may be present in cells from many other species.

The following lines of evidence suggest the existence of SERF: (1) SV40 is spontaneously released in small amounts by a few hamster tumor and SV40-transformed human cells; (2) production of small amounts of SV40 can be induced by treating THK-1 (T-6) hamster kidney and BSC/SV40 (NCM$_4$) monkey kidney cells with mitomycin C; (3) SV40 can be recovered from transformed mouse, hamster, dog, human, and monkey cells after co-cultivation or fusion with normal GMK or rabbit cells; (4) the genome resident in some transformed mouse cells can be recovered after the mouse cells are fused with normal or transformed monkey or human cells; (5) the virus that is produced after transformed human cells are superinfected with SV40 DNA has the same plaque morphology as the superinfecting SV40 DNA; and (6) transformed monkey cells superinfected by SV40 DNA, but not transformed mouse or hamster cells, produce infectious virus.

Availability of SERF may be necessary but not sufficient for recovery of SV40 from SV40-transformed cells. The release of the genome from integration may be the rate-limiting step even when SERF is present. This might explain the puzzling finding that transformed human and monkey cells contain enough SERF to activate virus production in transformed mouse cells, and yet the transformed human and monkey cells produce little or no virus spontaneously or after fusion with CV-1 cells. After fusion with CV-1 (monkey) cells, only a fraction of transformed mouse or transformed hamster cells in heterokaryons produce virus. The proportion of heterokaryons that produce virus varies considerably in different lines. Mitomycin C treatment probably enhances the release step.

The molecular events underlying the release mechanism are unknown. The release step could be under either positive or negative control, or it might be coupled to rare recombinational events. In transformed human or monkey cells, if release did not take place, the availability of SERF would be inconsequential. In transformed mouse cells, even if the release of the SV40 genome from integration did occur, there would be no virus production because SERF was unavailable.

Some transformed mouse and hamster lines do not produce infectious virus even after they are fused with permissive GMK cells. This is comprehensible if the transformed cells integrated SV40 mutants defective in SV40 DNA or capsid protein formation or defective in virus maturation. (The complex problems of complementation and recombination of mutant SV40 genomes will not be discussed in this article.) A number of transformed human and monkey lines also fail to produce SV40 spontaneously, after mitomycin C treatment, or even after fusion with susceptible monkey cells (Table 4-2). DNA superinfection experiments and fusion studies with transformed mouse cells indicate that at least some cells in the nonyielder cultures of transformed human and monkey cells contain SERF. The tentative conclusion, therefore, is that the nonyielder human and monkey lines have integrated mutant SV40 genomes. This conclusion should be accepted with caution, however, since the release mechanism may be faulty or the metabolic conditions may not be favorable for the expression of SERF.

A general picture of the state of the SV40 genome has emerged from recent studies. It appears now that the SV40-cell interaction does not differ in principle from the polyoma virus-cell interaction. However, with both viruses, many details have not yet been worked out. Among the most important of these are the enzymology of the integration and release mechanisms, the molecular mechanisms by which they are regulated, and the isolation and characterization of the postulated SERF substances.

Acknowledgments

This research was aided by grants from the Robert A. Welch Foundation (Q-163), and by U. S. Public Health Service Grants Ca-06656-08 and 1-K6-AI-2352.

References

1. Aaronson, S. A., and G. Todaro: SV40 antigen induction and transformation in human fibroblast cell strains. Virology, 36:254-261, 1968.
2. Aaronson, S. A., and G. J. Todaro: Human diploid cell transformation by DNA extracted from the tumor virus SV40. Science, 166:390-391, 1969.
3. Aloni, Y., E. Winocour, and L. Sachs: Characterization of the simian virus 40-specific RNA in virus-yielding and transformed cells. J. Molec. Biol., 31:414-429, 1968.
4. Benjamin, T. L.: Absence of homology between polyoma or SV40 viral DNA and mitochondrial DNA from virus-induced tumors. Virology, 36:685-687, 1968.

5. Bissett, M. L., and F. E. Payne: Development of antigens in human cells infected with simian virus 40. J. Bact., 91:743-749, 1966.
6. Black, P. H.: An analysis of SV40-induced transformation of hamster kidney tissue in vitro. III. Persistence of SV40 viral genome in clones of transformed hamster cells. J. Nat. Cancer Inst., 37:487-493, 1966.
7. Black, P. H., and W. P. Rowe: Transformation in hamster kidney monolayers by vacuolating virus, SV40. Virology, 19:107-108, 1962.
8. Black, P. H., and W. P. Rowe: SV40-induced proliferation of tissue culture cells of rabbit, mouse, and porcine origin. Proc. Soc. Exp. Biol. Med., 114:721-727, 1963.
9. Black, P. H., and W. P. Rowe: An analysis of SV40-induced transformation of hamster kidney tissue in vitro. I. General characteristics. Proc. Nat. Acad. Sci. USA, 50:606-613, 1963.
10. Burns, W. H., and P. H. Black: Analysis of simian virus 40-induced transformation of hamster kidney tissue in vitro. V. Variability of virus recovery from cell clones inducible with mitomycin C and cell fusion. J. Virol., 2:606-609, 1968.
11. Burns, W. H., and P. H. Black: Analysis of SV40-induced transformation of hamster kidney tissue in vitro. VI. Characteristics of mitomycin C induction. Virology, 39:625-634, 1969.
12. Carp, R. I., and R. V. Gilden: A comparison of the replication cycles of simian virus 40 in human diploid and African green monkey kidney cells. Virology, 28:150-162, 1966.
13. Diderholm, H., R. Berg, and T. Wesslen: Transformation of rat and guinea pig cells in vitro by SV40, and the transplantability of the transformed cells. Internat. J. Cancer, 1:139-148, 1966.
14. Diderholm, H., B. Stenkvist, J. Ponten, and T. Wesslen: Transformation of bovine cells in vitro after inoculation of simian virus 40 or its nucleic acid. Exp. Cell Res., 37:452-459, 1965.
15. Dubbs, D. R., and S. Kit: Isolation of defective lysogens from simian virus 40-transformed cells in the presence of ultraviolet-irradiated Sendai virus. J. Virol., 2:1272-1282, 1968.
16. Dubbs, D. R., and S. Kit: Heterokaryon formation of simian virus 40-transformed cells in the presence of ultraviolet-irradiated Sendai virus. J. Virol., 3:536-538, 1969.
17. Dubbs, D. R., and S. Kit: Isolation of double lysogens from 3T3 cells transformed by plaque morphology mutants of SV40. Proc. Nat. Acad. Sci. USA, 65:536-543, 1970.
18. Dubbs, D. R., S. Kit, R. A. de Torres, and M. Anken: Virogenic properties of bromodeoxyuridine-sensitive and bromodeoxyuridine-resistant simian virus 40-transformed mouse kidney cells. J. Virol., 1:968-979, 1967.
19. Eddy, B. E., G. S. Borman, G. E. Grubbs, and R. D. Young: Identification of the oncogenic substances in rhesus monkey kidney cell cultures as simian virus 40. Virology, 17:65-75, 1962.
20. Fernandes, M. V., and P. S. Moorhead: Transformation of African green monkey kidney cultures infected with simian vacuolating virus (SV40). Tex. Rep. Biol. Med. 23:242-258, 1965.
21. Gerber, P.: Tumors induced in hamsters by simian virus 40: Persistent subviral infection. Science, 140:889-890, 1963.
22. Gerber, P.: Virogenic hamster tumor cells: Induction of virus synthesis. Science, 145:833, 1964.
23. Gerber, P.: Studies on the transfer of subviral infectivity from SV40-induced hamster tumor cells to indicator cells. Virology, 28:501-509, 1966.
24. Girardi, A. J., F. C. Jensen, and H. Koprowski: SV40-induced transformation of human diploid cells: Crisis and recovery. J. Cell. Comp. Physiol., 65:69-84, 1965.
25. Hirt, B.: Selective extraction of polyoma DNA from infected mouse cell cultures. J. Molec. Biol., 26:365-369, 1967.
26. Jensen, F. C., and H. Koprowski: Absence of repressor in SV40-transformed cells. Virology, 37:687-690, 1969.

27. Kit, S., and M. Brown: Rescue of simian virus 40 from cell lines transformed at high and at low input multiplicities by unirradiated or ultraviolet-irradiated virus. J. Virol., 4:226-230, 1969.
28. Kit, S., T. Kurimura, and D. R. Dubbs: Transplantable mouse tumor line induced by injection of SV40-transformed mouse kidney cells. Internat. J. Cancer, 4:384-392, 1969.
29. Kit, S., T. Kurimura, and D. Trkula: The infectivity of molecular forms of simian virus 40 (SV40) DNA. Biophysical Society Abstracts, 1970, p. 156.
30. Kit, S., D. R. Dubbs, L. J. Piekarski, R. A. de Torres, and J. L. Melnick: Acquisition of enzyme function by mouse kidney cells abortively infected by papovavirus SV40. Proc. Nat. Acad. Sci. USA, 56:463-470, 1966.
31. Kit, S., T. Kurimura, M. Brown, and D. R. Dubbs: Identification of the SV40 which replicates when SV40-transformed human cells are fused with SV40-transformed mouse cells or superinfected with SV40 DNA. J. Virol. In press.
32. Kit, S., T. Kurimura, M. L. Salvi, and D. R. Dubbs: Activation of infectious SV40 DNA synthesis in transformed cells. Proc. Nat. Acad. Sci. USA, 60:1239-1246, 1968.
33. Kit, S., K. Nakajima, T. Kurimura, D. R. Dubbs, and R. Cassingena: Monkey-mouse hybrid cell lines containing the SV40 genome in a partially repressed state. Internat. J. Cancer, 5:1-14, 1970.
34. Kit, S., R. A. de Torres, D. R. Dubbs, and M. L. Salvi: Induction of cellular deoxyribonucleic acid synthesis by simian virus 40. J. Virol., 1:738-746, 1967.
35. Knowles, B. B., F. C. Jensen, Z. Steplewski, and H. Koprowski: Rescue of infectious SV40 after fusion between different SV40-transformed cells. Proc. Nat. Acad. Sci. USA, 61:42-45, 1968.
36. Koprowski, H., F. C. Jensen, and Z. Steplewski: Activation of production of infectious tumor virus 40 in heterokaryon cultures. Proc. Nat. Acad. Sci. USA, 58:127-133, 1967.
37. Levin, M. J., M. N. Oxman, G. T. Diamandopoulos, A. S. Levine, P. H. Henry, and J. F. Enders: Virus-specific nucleic acids in SV40-exposed hamster embryo cell lines: Correlation with S and T antigens. Proc. Nat. Acad. Sci. USA, 62:589-596, 1969.
38. Margalith, M., R. Volk-Fuchs, and N. Goldblum: Transformation of BSC-1 cells following chronic infection with SV40. J. Gen. Virol., 5:321-327, 1969.
39. Margalith, M., E. Margalith, T. Nasialski, and N. Goldblum: Induction of SV40 antigen in BSC_1 transformed cells. J. Virol., 5:305-308, 1970.
40. Oxman, M. N., S. Baron, P. H. Black, K. K. Takemoto, K. Habel, and W. P. Rowe: The effect of interferon on SV40 T antigen production in SV40-transformed cells. Virology, 32:122-127, 1967.
41. Pertursson, G., J. Fogh, E. de Harven, and D. Armstrong: Rapid cytopathic changes and transformation in human foreskin cell cultures infected with simian virus 40. Virology, 28:303-317, 1966.
42. Rabson, A. S., G. T. O'Conlor, R. L. Kirschstein, and W. J. Branigan: Papillary ependymomas produced in Rattus (mastomys) natalensis inoculated with vacuolating virus (SV40). J. Nat. Cancer Inst., 29:765-787, 1962.
43. Rapp, F., J. S. Butel, and J. L. Melnick: Virus-induced intranuclear antigen in cells transformed by papovavirus SV40. Proc. Soc. Exp. Biol. Med., 116:1131-1135, 1969.
44. Sabin, A. B., and M. A. Koch: Evidence of continuous transmission of noninfectious SV40 viral genome in most or all SV40 hamster tumor cells. Proc. Nat. Acad. Sci. USA, 49:304-311, 1963.
45. Sambrook, J., H. Westphal, P. R. Srinivasan, and R. Dulbecco: The integrated state of viral DNA in SV40-transformed cells. Proc. Nat. Acad. Sci. USA, 60:1288-1295, 1968.
46. Sauer, G., and V. Defendi: Stimulation of DNA synthesis and complement-fixing antigen production by SV40 in human diploid cell cultures: Evidence for "abortive" infection. Proc. Nat. Acad. Sci. USA, 56:452-457, 1966.
47. Sauer, G., and J. R. Kidwai: The transcription of the SV40 genome in productively infected and transformed cells. Proc. Nat. Acad. Sci. USA, 61:1256-1263, 1968.

48. Schell, K.: Persistence of SV40 virus in transformed rabbit kidney cells. Proc. Soc. Exp. Biol. Med., 128:1145-1148, 1968.
49. Schell, K., and J. Maryak: Susceptibility of rabbit kidney cells of various passage levels to infection with SV40 virus. Archiv Virusforsch., 19:403-414, 1966.
50. Schell, K., and J. Maryak: SV40 virus growth and cytopathogenicity in a serial rabbit kidney cell line. Proc. Soc. Exp. Biol. Med., 124:1099-1102, 1967.
51. Shein, H. M., and J. F. Enders: Transformation induced by simian virus 40 in human renal cell cultures. I. Morphology and growth characteristics. Proc. Nat. Acad. Sci. USA, 48:1164-1172, 1962.
52. Shein, H. M., and J. F. Enders: Multiplication and cytopathogenicity of simian vacuolating virus 40 in cultures of human cells. Proc. Soc. Exp. Biol. Med., 109: 495-500, 1962.
53. Swetly, P., G. B. Brodano, B. Knowles, and H. Koprowski: Response of simian virus 40-transformed cell lines and cell hybrids to superinfection with simian virus 40 and its deoxyribonucleic acid. J. Virol., 4:348-355, 1969.
54. Tai, H. T., and R. L. O'Brien: Multiplicity of viral genomes in an SV40 transformed hamster cell line. Virology, 38:698-701, 1969.
55. Takemoto, K. K., and K. Habel: Hamster tumor cells doubly transformed by SV40 and polyoma viruses. Virology, 30:20-28, 1966.
56. Todaro, G. J., and S. Baron: The role of interferon in the inhibition of SV40 transformation of mouse cell line 3T3. Proc. Nat. Acad. Sci. USA, 54:752-756, 1965.
57. Todaro, G. J., K. Habel, and H. Green: Antigenic and cultural properties of cells doubly transformed by polyoma virus and SV40. Virology, 27:179-185, 1965.
58. Tournier, P., R. Cassingena, R. Wicker, J. Coppey, and H. Suarez: Etude du mechanisme de l'induction chez des cellules de hamster syrien transformee par le virus SV40. I. Properties d'une lignee cellulaire clonale. Internat. J. Cancer, 2:117-132, 1967.
59. Uchida, S., and S. Watanabe: Transformation of 3T3 cells by T antigen forming defective SV40 virions (T particles). Virology, 39:721-728, 1969.
60. Ushijima, R. N., C. E. Gardner, and E. Cate: Transformation of renal cells from a prosimian by simian virus 40 (SV40). Proc. Soc. Exp. Biol. Med., 122:676-679, 1966.
61. Wallace, R.: Viral transformation of monkey kidney cell cultures. Nature, 213: 768-770, 1967.
62. Waring, M., and R. J. Britten: Nucleotide sequence repetition: A rapidly reassociating fraction of mouse DNA. Science, 154:791-794, 1966.
63. Wesslen, T., H. Diderholm, and R. Berg: Studies on the malignancy of SV40 transformed cells from animals resistant to the oncogenic action of SV40 in vitro. Acta path. microbiol. scand., Suppl., 187:114, 1967.
64. Westphal, H., and R. Dulbecco: Viral DNA in polyoma- and SV40-transformed cell lines. Proc. Nat. Acad. Sci. USA, 59:1158-1165, 1968.
65. Wever, G. H., S. Kit, and D. R. Dubbs: Initial site of synthesis of virus during rescue of SV40 from heterokaryons of SV40-transformed and susceptible cells. J. Virol. In press.
66. Cassingena, R.: Unpublished data.
67. Somers, K., and S. Kit: Unpublished data.
68. Dubbs, D. R., and S. Kit: Unpublished data.

Protein Compositions of DNA Tumor Viruses

WILLIAM T. MURAKAMI

Graduate Department of Biochemistry, Brandeis University, Waltham, Massachusetts

THE DNA TUMOR viruses, SV40, polyoma virus, and the adenoviruses, are icosahedral in shape and are composed of only protein and DNA. The morphologic characteristics and the chemical compositions of these viruses are summarized in Table 4-3.

SV40 and polyoma virus particles are about 45 mμ in diameter. The adenoviruses are larger, having diameters of about 72 mμ. The symmetry of the icosahedral surface lattice of SV40 and polyoma virus has been established to be T = 7 by Klug.[5] The capsids are made up of 72 capsomeres: 60 hexagonal and 12 pentagonal capsomeres located at the vertices of the icosahedron. The adenovirus capsid (T = 25) is made up of 252 capsomeres: 240 hexagonal (hexons) and 12 pentagonal capsomeres, each with a knobbed fiber projecting from it (pentons).

The DNA contents of the three viruses have been determined to represent 12 to 13% of the particle weight. The DNA of SV40 and polyoma virions has been shown to be a twisted closed circular duplex molecule with a molecular weight of 3×10^6 daltons.[15] The adenovirus DNA appears to be a linear duplex with a molecular weight of 23×10^6 daltons.[9] Particle weights of 24×10^6 daltons for SV40 and polyoma virus and 177×10^6 daltons for adenovirus can be calculated from the

TABLE 4-3.—MORPHOLOGICAL CHARACTERISTICS AND CHEMICAL COMPOSITIONS OF SV40, POLYOMA VIRUS AND ADENOVIRUS

	SV40	POLYOMA VIRUS	ADENOVIRUS
Size (diameter)	45 mμ	45 mμ	720 mμ
Symmetry of icosahedral surface lattice	T = 7	T = 7	T = 25
Number of capsomeres	72	72	252
pentagonal clusters	12	12	12 (pentons)
hexagonal clusters	60	60	240 (hexons)
DNA content	12.5%	12.3%	13%
DNA (molecular weight)	3×10^6	3×10^6	23×10^6
Particle weight (calculated)	24×10^6	24×10^6	177×10^6
Particle weight (measured)	17.3×10^6	23.6×10^6	—
Protein content (calculated)	$14.3 - 20.6 \times 10^6$	20.6×10^6	154×10^6

DNA contents and molecular weights of the viral DNAs. The molecular weight of the SV40 virion has been determined to be 17.3 × 10⁶ from sedimentation velocity and diffusion measurements.[6] The particle weight of polyoma virions has been estimated to be 23.6 × 10⁶ daltons by sedimentation equilibrium measurements.[16] It can be calculated that SV40 and polyoma virus contain 14 to 21 × 10⁶ daltons of protein and adenovirus, 154 × 10⁶ daltons.

The protein of SV40 virions and empty capsids (Table 4-4) has been separated into three components (polypeptides A, B, and C) by electrophoresis.[2] The relative amounts of the three polypeptides were determined by densitometry of the stained electropherograms, and similar results were obtained with virion and empty capsid preparations (polypeptide A = 45%, polypeptide B = 45%, polypeptide C = 10%). Molecular weights of 16,400, 16,900, and 16,800 daltons were obtained for purified polypeptides A, B, and C, respectively, by sedimentation equilibrium centrifugation.[12]

Evidence for the internal localization of the minor C polypeptide was obtained by trypsin digestion of full and empty particles.[2] The proteins of both particle types are completely digested by extended trypsin treatment. Partial tryptic digests showed that polypeptides A and B were more rapidly degraded than polypeptide C. This conclusion has been further substantiated by the isolation of an alkali-stable DNA-polypeptide C complex from pH 10.5-dissociation products of virions.[1] The amino acid compositions of the separated polypeptides show that the C peptide contains more basic residues (about 20% of the total residues) than either polypeptides A or B. It has been concluded that polypeptides A and B together constitute the protein shell of the virus, and that polypeptide C is an internal component which might play a role in orienting the DNA within the virus particle.

Polyoma virus protein, dissociated with sodium dodecyl sulfate (SDS), was first analyzed by polyacrylamide gel electrophoresis by Thorne and Warden.[14] They observed one major peak with several

TABLE 4-4.—PROTEIN COMPOSITIONS OF SV40 AND POLYOMA VIRUS

VIRUS	PROTEIN	MOLECULAR WEIGHT	PERCENT OF VIRION PROTEIN
SV40			
Capsid	Polypeptide A	16,400	45
	Polypeptide B	16,900	45
Internal	Polypeptide C	16,800	10
Polyoma virus			
Capsid	Capsid protein	42,000	80
Internal	IP-1	30,000	3–7
	IP-2	23,000	3–7
	IP-3	20,000	3–7
	IP-4	17,000	3–7

minor peaks. The minor peaks were thought to represent, at least in part, contaminants of cellular origin, and it was concluded that the polyoma virus is composed of one type of structural polypeptide. A single protein band was obtained also by Fine et al.[4] when SDS-dissociated viral protein was electrophoresed in SDS-containing polyacrylamide gels by a discontinuous buffer system. However, virions dissociated by acid-urea treatment and electrophoresed in polyacrylamide gels in the presence of 10 M urea revealed the presence of two protein components. Subsequent investigation of SDS-dissociated proteins, using a continuous buffer system,[13] has revealed the presence of a total of five different polypeptides in virion preparations.[16] The proteins have been designated capsid protein and internal proteins (IP) 1, 2, 3, and 4 (Table 4-4). The molecular weights of the polypeptides have been estimated to be: capsid protein, 42,000; IP-1, 30,000; IP-2, 23,000; IP-3, 20,000; and IP-4, 17,000 daltons.

The relative proportions of the different proteins in the gel have been approximated by measuring the distribution of radioactivity of lysine-labeled virus proteins among the protein bands. The major band (capsid protein) represents about 80% of the total radioactivity, and each of the minor components 3 to 7%. Distinct amino acid compositions have been found for each of the purified proteins. The minor components contain more basic amino acid residues than the capsid protein. Proteins from the two bands obtained by polyacrylamide gel electrophoresis of acid-urea treated particles have been re-electrophoresed in the SDS gels. The major component has been shown to migrate as capsid protein and the minor component as IP-1 in the SDS system. The absence of internal proteins 2, 3, and 4 from the acid-urea gels has been found to be caused by incomplete dissociation of the virus by the urea treatment utilized. Sucrose gradient centrifugation of the dissociation products has shown that although 40 to 60% of the protein is dissociated, the remainder is still complexed to DNA. The dissociated protein consists largely of capsid protein and internal protein-1, indicating that about 50% of the capsid protein and all of the internal proteins 2, 3, and 4 are in the DNA-protein complex.

Among the 31 serotypes of the human adenovirus group, antigenic types 12, 18, and 31 have been designated to be highly oncogenic and types 3, 7, 11, 14, 16, and 21, weakly oncogenic. The protein composition of adenovirus type 2 has been analyzed by Maizel, White and Scharff.[7, 8] The SDS-dissociated virion has been shown to contain at least nine different polypeptides by acrylamide gel electrophoresis (Table 4-5). The electrophoretic patterns obtained with the weakly oncogenic type 7 and the highly oncogenic type 12 adenovirions were broadly similar to that of adenovirus type 2.

About 50% of the total protein of adenovirus type 2 is made up of polypeptide II. It has a molecular weight of 120,000 daltons and has been identified to be the structural peptide of the hexons. Polypeptides

TABLE 4–5.—PROTEIN COMPOSITION OF ADENOVIRUS

PEPTIDE	PERCENT OF VIRION PROTEIN	MOLECULAR WEIGHT	MORPHOLOGICAL UNIT
II	50.9	120,000	hexon
III	4.6	70,000	penton base
IV	4.0	62,000	fiber
V	5.4	44,000	core
VI, VII	14.2	24,000	core
VIII, IX	3.5	13,000	hexon aggregates
		7,500	—

III and IV make up the pentons. Peptide III, 70,000 daltons, is the structural peptide of the penton base and peptide IV, 62,000 daltons, makes up the fiber projections of the pentons.

Polypeptides V, VI, and VII, with molecular weights 44,000, 24,000, and 24,000 daltons, respectively, have been isolated from the nucleoprotein core of the adenovirus. The proteins are basic, somewhat arginine-rich, and represent about 20% of the total virion protein.[3, 7, 8, 10, 11] They are not histonelike, since they have been shown to contain tryptophan.[3, 7]

Polypeptides VIII and IX have been shown to be associated with aggregates of nine hexons but not with single hexons. It has been suggested that these peptides might have the role of stabilizing the hexon aggregates.

The location and role of peptide X is unknown.

The three DNA viruses exhibit some diversity in protein composition. The capsid of SV40 appears to be composed of a single structure unit which is made up of two different polypeptides. The structure unit of the polyoma capsid is a single polypeptide. The adenoviruses, which are larger and structurally more complex, utilize three different proteins to form the hexons and pentons. All of the viruses contain basic internal components which are complexed to the DNA. The function of these minor components remains to be elucidated. They may play a structural role in stabilizing and/or orienting the DNA in the virion. Conversely, their histonelike properties suggest a possible role in the regulation of macromolecular synthesis in the infected cell.

No information is available as to the genetic specification of the minor components. The genetic capacity of SV40 and polyoma virus is limited. The DNA can specify, at most, about 2×10^5 daltons of protein. In the extreme case that all of the polypeptides found in virions are structural, nonfunctional proteins, and are specified by the viral DNA, about one third of the SV40 and about two thirds of the polyoma virus genome would be required for structural protein synthesis. In either case, very little residual information would be available for the synthesis of functional and/or regulatory proteins. About one third of the adenovirus genome would be required to specify all of the proteins found in adenovirions.

References

1. Anderer, F. A., M. A. Koch, and H. D. Schlumberger: Virology, 34:452, 1968.
2. Anderer, F. A., H. D. Schlumberger, M. A. Koch, H. Frank, and H. J. Eggers: Virology, 32:511, 1967.
3. Boulanger, P. A., F. Jaume, P. Flamencourt, and G. Biserte: J. Virol., 5:109, 1970.
4. Fine, R., M. Mass, and W. T. Murakami: J. Molec. Biol., 36:167, 1968.
5. Klug, A.: J. Molec. Biol., 11:424, 1965.
6. Koch, M. A., H. J. Eggers, F. A. Anderer, H. D. Schlumberger, and H. Frank: Virology, 32:503, 1967.
7. Maizel, J. V., Jr., D. O. White, and M. D. Scharff: Virology, 36:115, 1968.
8. Maizel, J. V., Jr., D. O. White, and M. D. Scharff: Virology, 36:126, 1968.
9. Piña, M., and M. Green: Proc. Nat. Acad. Sci. USA, 54:547, 1965.
10. Prage, L., U. Pettersson, and L. Philipson: Virology, 36:508, 1968.
11. Russell, W. C., W. G. Laver, and P. J. Sanderson: Nature, 219:1127, 1968.
12. Schlumberger, H. D., F. A. Anderer, and M. A. Koch: Virology, 36:42, 1968.
13. Shapiro, A. L., E. Viñuela, and J. V. Maizel, Jr.: Biochem. Biophys. Res. Comm., 28:815, 1967.
14. Thorne, H. V., and D. Warden: J. Gen. Virol., 1:135, 1967.
15. Weil, R., and J. Vinograd: Proc. Nat. Acad. Sci. USA, 50:730, 1963.
16. Fine, R., Bancroft [sic], and W. T. Murakami: In preparation.

The Nucleic Acid and Protein of the Avian Tumor Viruses

WILLIAM S. ROBINSON, PAUL HUNG,

HARRIET L. ROBINSON, AND DAVID RALPH

Department of Medicine, Stanford University School of Medicine, Stanford, California, USA

ULTRASTRUCTURAL AND chemical studies indicate that the avian tumor viruses have a complex structure. An outer membrane or envelope, an intermediate membrane, and an electron-dense "nucleoid" have been described in electron micrographs of negatively stained virions.[1, 57, 58] Lipid has been shown to make up 30-35% of the dry weight of avian myeloblastosis virus (AMV),[2] and it consists of a mixture of cholesterol, neutral lipids and phospholipids similar but not identical to cellular lipid.[3] The lipid of the virion is probably derived from host cells, as is the lipid of influenza virus.[4] The sensitivity of the viruses to disruption by various detergents and organic solvents suggests that lipid is near the surface of the virion or in the viral envelope.

Viral RNA

The RNA recovered from purified avian tumor viruses (ATVs) after disruption with a detergent such as sodium dodecyl sulfate (SDS), followed by phenol extraction, sediments in two major components[5-7] (Figure 4-3A). The more quickly sedimenting component has a sedimentation coefficient around 70S in 0.1 m salt, it has properties of single-stranded RNA, and its sedimentation boundary indicates significant heterogeneity.[8] The RNAs recovered from several different ATVs are indistinguishable in rate of sedimentation and base composition.[9]

Recently the 70S RNA has been shown to dissociate into a more slowly sedimenting form after denaturation with dimethyl sulfoxide (DMSO) or heat.[10, 11] Two components around 35S and 25S are commonly observed after incubating the 70S RNA in 90% DMSO (Figure 4-3). The sedimentation of the 57S ^{32}P RNA from Sendai virus is not altered by DMSO treatment (Figure 4-3). The change in sedimentation of Rous sarcoma virus (RSV) RNA probably represents dissociation of a large noncovalently bonded complex into smaller RNA components, but it has not been completely excluded that the change in sedimentation behavior is attributable to a conformational change in a single RNA molecule. The transition from 70S to 35S has not been shown to be reversible.

The studies of AMV[12] and RSV (Rous associated virus 1 [RAV-1])[13] RNA by electron microscopy have demonstrated multiple lengths of single-stranded RNA with some molecules around 8 to 11 μm in length. Whether these are single covalently bonded molecules is not certain because of the presence of "curled regions" of unknown structure.[13] The RNAs of other RNA tumor viruses have been shown to have structures similar to ATV RNA.[9, 13-20]

The more slowly sedimenting RNA component from ATVs has a sedimentation coefficient around 4S.[8] The pattern of ^{3}H-uridine incorporation into the 4S RNA component of AMV suggests that it is derived at least in part from host cell RNA,[7] although some of the RNA in the 4S component may have a different origin, such as from degradation of 70S RNA by RNase within the virion or during RNA isolation.[5, 21] Degradation of 70S RNA in the virion is suggested by the observation that 70S RNA-^{3}H from RSV (RAV-1) and Schmidt-Ruppin Rous sarcoma virus (SR-RSV) is converted to 4S RNA-^{3}H by freezing and thawing virus and during incubation of virus at 37°.[5, 21] That the 4S RNA from virus contains cellular RNA is also suggested by the observation that growth of AMV[11] and RSV (RAV-1)[21] in the presence

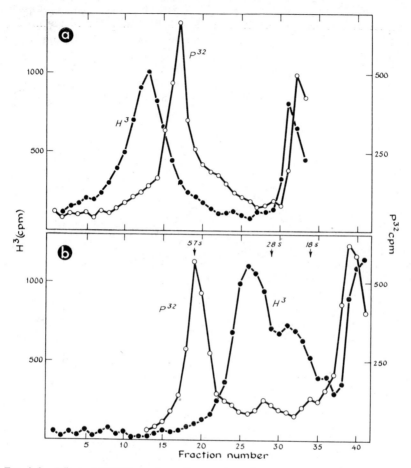

FIG. 4–3.—Effect of DMSO on the sedimentation of RSV RNA. RSV (RAV-1) RNA labeled with ^{3}H-uridine was prepared as previously described.[5] *A*—To one aliquot of ^{3}H-RNA plus ^{32}P RNA from Sendai virus and unlabeled chick cell RNA carrier, 9 vol of buffer containing 0.10 m NaCl, 0.01 m Tris HCl pH 7.5 and 0.001 m EDTA was added; *B*—to a second aliquot in the same buffer, 9 vol of DMSO was added. Both were then incubated at room temperature for 10 min and the RNA in each was precipitated with 6 vol of ethanol. The RNA was collected and redissolved in the same buffer for sedimentation as previously described.[5]

of ^{3}H-methymethionine results in methylation of the 4S RNA of virus to the same extent as 4S cell RNA, and almost no methylation of viral 70S RNA results.

The 4S RNA component recovered from partially purified preparations of AMV[22] has been shown to bind amino acids when incubated in a reaction mixture with amino acid-activating enzymes and adenosine triphosphate. This has also been shown with the 4S RNA from purified RSV (RAV-1).[21] More recently, Travnicek[23] has found amino acid acceptor activity for the 4S RNA from AMV with 14 of 15 amino acids tested. With the exception of two amino acids tested, the specific acceptor activity for the viral 4S RNAs was lower than for cellular 4S RNAs, although the relative order of individual amino acids based on specific activity was generally similar for viral and cellular 4S RNAs. Thus it appears likely that the ATVs contain cellular tRNAs, although the mixture of tRNAs in virus and in host cells is not identical. The individual transfer RNAs from virus and cell have not been compared to determine whether they are identical or whether the virus contains a unique tRNA.

The significance of the tRNA in virus preparations is not clear, and no biologic role of the tRNA for virus has been shown. It has not been directly proved that the tRNA is part of the virion, although it is clearly associated with a particle of similar size, buoyant density, and isoelectric point, because it follows virus during purification.[5, 21–23] It also is not digested by RNAse[21, 22] or venom phosphodiesterase[23] prior to disruption of virus. Cellular tRNA could be enclosed by chance within the viral envelope during virus formation and serve no specific role in virus replication, as may be the case for the adenosine triphosphatase reported to be present in AMV.[24]

A number of interesting problems arise from the observations on ATV RNAs. Since the RNAs from these viruses have not been shown to be infectious, and only 1 in 750 to 1,200 physical particles in virus preparations may be infectious,[25] it is not certain that any of the RNAs described above actually represent intact viral RNA rather than inactivated or degraded RNA. If more than one RNA molecule in the virus (e.g., the 70S or 35S and 4S RNA) is essential for virus infection, the probability of obtaining infection with free RNA molecules would be low. If the viral genome consisted of more than one piece of RNA, the high UV resistance of ATVs[26] might be explained by individual molecules complementing each other in cells infected with more than one virus. Similarly, the findings of Hanafusa and Hanafusa[27] suggesting high rates of genetic recombination by ATVs could result by random assortment and packaging of RNA pieces in cells infected by more than one virus, a mechanism proposed by Hirst[28] for influenza virus. A recent report of the formation in cells of one viral antigen but not infectious virus after treatment of cells with large amounts of RNA extracted from AMV[29] suggests that some but not all viral genes may function after exposure of cells to viral RNA. Finally, if another virion component besides the RNA was required for successful infection after RNA uncoating, the free viral RNA would not be infectious. The RNA polymerase in vaccinia,[30, 59] reovirus[31] and vesicular stomatitis virus[32] appears to be such a virion component. However, no RNA polymerase activity has so far been found in preparations of ATVs[21,33] (see Addendum).

Virus Coat Properties and Proteins

The type-specific antigen of the ATVs is considered to be on the virion surface because it reacts with virus-neutralizing antiserum.[34] The antigen appears to mediate specific viral interference among ATVs and to determine virus host range.[35, 37, 63] The ATVs have been placed in subgroups on the basis of their host range in genetically different types of chicken cells and in other avian cells.[36] The type-specific antigens of viruses in different subgroups generally do not cross-react,[38] and no specific interference is observed between viruses of different subgroups.[35, 37] Viruses with different type-specific antigens not only differ in host range but apparently differ in the efficiency with which they infect cells. Bryan high titer strain of Rous sarcoma virus (BH-RSV[RAV-1]) appears to infect cells with greatest efficiency. SR-RSV, BH-RSV(RAV-2), and BH-RSV(O) β[39, 40] probably infect susceptible cells with an intermediate efficiency, and the infectivity of these viruses is enhanced by DEAE dextran[41] and by extracts of RAV-1 infected cells.[40, 42] RSV(O) α[40] has not been shown to be infectious on any cell type tested.

A second antigen in the ATVs, the group-specific (GS) antigen, was first described by Huebner et al.,[43] and was detected with serum from hamsters with SR-RSV induced tumors. Hamster tumors produce no infectious virus and contain no type-specific viral antigen,[43, 63] and hamster cells are considered to be nonpermissive cells for replication of most strains of ATVs. Such hamster serum reacts in complement fixation and fluorescent antibody staining with all cells infected by and tumors induced by all known ATVs, hence the name GS antigen. The antigen is also part of the virion of all ATVs and is thought to be an internal antigen because antiserum reacts only with disrupted virus and not with intact virus.[44, 62] The GS antigen has been isolated from detergent disrupted ATVs and characterized.[44–47, 60, 61] Some evidence indicates that it consists of at least two proteins.[47]

Little work has been done to characterize the ATV type-specific antigens. There is a recent report of the detection of a component in between 20 disrupted ATVs which reacted with homologous virus-neutralizing antiserum in agar gel diffusion, absorbed homologous virus neutralizing antiserum, induced neutralizing antibody for homologous viruses in rabbits, and induced early interference for homologous viruses.[48] The component was sensitive to proteolytic enzyme digestion, indicating its protein nature. No further chemical characterization of this antigen was done.

There are no known chemical or physical differences in ATVs which might account for differences in coat properties. It has been shown that viruses with different type-specific antigens are very similar, if not indistinguishable, in physical properties such as buoyant density.[49]

We have recently compared several ATVs with different coat proper-

TABLE 4-6.—VIRUS PROPERTIES

| Virus | Focus Morphology | Host Range | | | Neutralized by Antibody | | | | Virus Focus Titer | | |
| | | C/O | C/B | Quail | Chicken Serum against | | | Serum from Hamster with SR Tumor | −DEAE Dextran | +DEAE Dextran | Enhanced by RAV-1 Cell Extract |
					RAV-1	RAV-2	SR				
BH-RSV (RAV-1)	BH	+	+	+	+	+	−	−	8.5×10^6	7.0×10^6	−
BH-RSV (RAV-2)	BH	+	+	−	−	+	−	−	7.5×10^2	5×10^4	+
SR-RSV	SR	+	+	−	−	−	+	−	4.2×10^4	1×10^6	+
BH-RSV-β	BH	−	−	+	−	−	−				+
BH-RSV-α	BH	−	−	−	−	−	−				+

Tissue culture methods for growing cells and viruses[54] and isolating RSV(O)[40] have been described. RSVα(O) and RSVβ(O) were distinguished by their ability to make foci on Japanese quail cells.[40] Neutralizing antibody was produced in chickens,[49, 54] and antiserum against gs antigen from hamsters with Schmidt-Ruppin RSV induced tumors was a gift of Flow Laboratories.

ties (Table 4-6) by electrofocusing. Figure 4-4A, B, and C shows that RSV (RAV-1) does not differ significantly in isoelectric point from SR-RSV, RSV (RAV-2), and RSVα (O) respectively; Figure 4-4D shows that RSV (RAV-2) is indistinguishable from RSVβ (O), indicating that if viruses with distinct type-specific antigens differ in over-all charge, the differences must be too small to be detected by this method. The isoelectric point of these viruses is about pH 3.9 to 4.0, indicating the presence of acidic groups on the virus surface. Phospholipid in the viral envelope could contribute such acidic groups.

Electrofocusing represents a method for further virus purification after sedimentation in sucrose density gradients.[5] Unfortunately, ATVs lose infectivity at pH 4.0 so that infectious virus cannot be recovered. Prolonged incubation in the electrofocusing column beyond 36 to 48 hr results in gradual breakdown of virus. The first protein components to be released are proteins with isoelectric points around pH 9 and pH 7 (e.g. Figure 4-4B and C), and the 70S viral RNA is degraded to 4S pieces.

We have also compared the dissociated protein components of two viruses with distinct type-specific antigens, RAV-1 and RSVβ (O) labeled with ^{14}C or ^{3}H amino acid mixtures and with ^{3}H-glucosamine. It is known that ATVs contain carbohydrate,[50] and radioactive glucosamine has been shown to be readily incorporated into AMV grown in tissue culture.[51]

Figure 4-5B shows the results of co-electrophoresis of amino acid-^{14}C-RSVβ (O) and amino acid-^{3}H-RAV-1 in a polyacrylamide gel containing 0.1% SDS after dissociation of the viruses in 1% SDS, 4 M urea, and 1% 2-mercaptoethanol at 37° for 30 min. Under these conditions, all of the radioactivity penetrated the gel. At least eight protein components can be identified in these viruses, and they are numbered P-1 to P-8. P-5 and 6 and P-7 and 8 were not completely separated in this experiment, but the two proteins of each pair have clearly distinct isoelectric points in electrofocusing.[52] Of the slowly moving amino acid-labeled proteins, P-1 was the major protein in RSVβ (O) (peak in fraction 23) and P-2 the major protein in RAV-1 (peak in fraction 30). In addition, the protein component from RAV-1 in the region of P-3 (peak in fraction 55) migrated slightly faster than the closely migrating protein from RSVβ (O) (peak in fractions 58 and 59). The electrophoretic profiles of ^{14}C amino acid RAV-1 and ^{3}H amino acid-labeled RAV-1 were shown to be indistinguishable, as were the profiles of RSVβ (O) labeled with each isotope. Components P-4, P-5 + 6, and P-7 + 8 correspond respectively to components RSV-3, RSV-2, and RSV-1 described previously and, as previously shown, no difference in electrophoretic mobility was observed for these proteins isolated from viruses with different type-specific antigens.[47]

Figure 4-5A shows the results of co-electrophoresis of amino acid-^{14}C-RSVβ (O) and ^{3}H-glucosamine RSVβ (O). It is clear that there are three major components labeled with ^{3}H-glucosamine designated

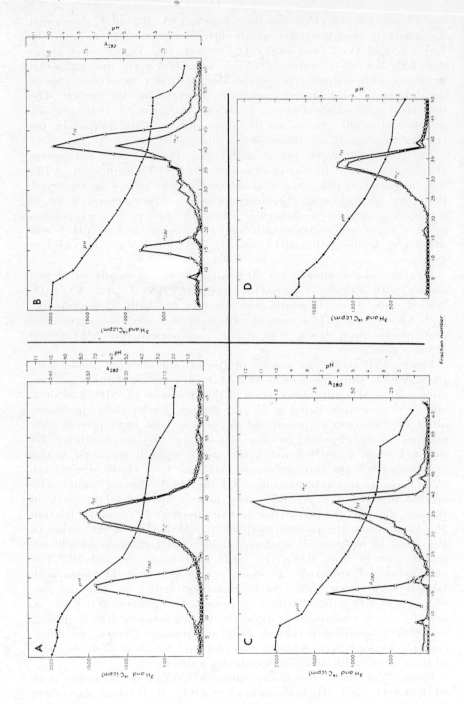

Fig. 4–4.—Isoelectric focusing of purified viruses with different type-specific antigens. Viruses were labeled in tissue culture with similar mixtures of 15 ^{3}H (1 to 10Ci/mM) or ^{14}C (10-100 mCi/mM) L-amino acids (New England Nuclear) added to 199 based growth medium I[54] containing one-tenth the regular amino acid concentration (^{14}C 1-2.5 μc per ml and ^{3}H 10 to 20 μCi per ml). Six ml of radioactive medium per 100 mm culture dish was changed at 12-hr intervals four times. Viruses were purified from culture medium,[5] and isoelectric focusing[55] with 2 mg human hemoglobin carrier was done in a 110 ml LKB column using 1% ampholine (LKB) in a 5 to 20% sucrose density gradient at 600 v 2 C for 48 hr. Fractions were collected and pH (-●-), A_{290} (-□-), trichloroacetic acid precipitable ^{14}C (-○-) and ^{3}H (-△-) were determined. A—shows ^{14}C-RSV (RAV-1) and ^{3}H-SR-RSV; B—^{14}C-RSV (RAV-1) and ^{3}H-RSV (RAV-2); C—^{14}C-RSV (RAV-1) and ^{3}H-BH-RSVα (○); and D—^{14}C-BH-RSVβ (○) and ^{3}H-RSV (RAV-2).

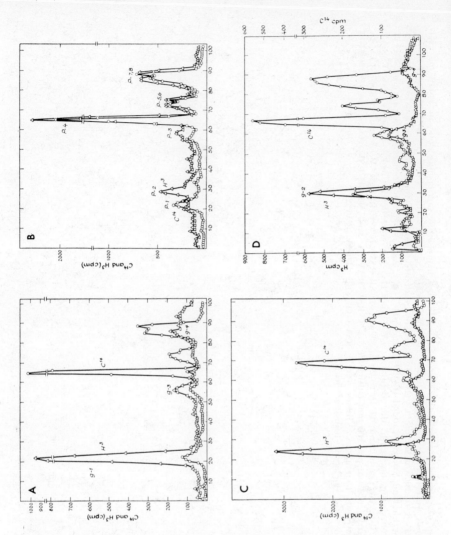

G-1, 3, and 4. G-1 had the same mobility as P-1 and G-3 the same as P-3. G-4 was more heterogeneous and in part migrated with P-7 and 8 and some ³H-labeled material moved more rapidly.

Figure 4-5D shows the results of co-electrophoresis of ³H-glucosamine RAV-1 and ¹⁴C amino acid RAV-1. It is clear that the two major ³H-glucosamine-labeled components G-2 and G-3 had the same mobilities as ¹⁴C amino acid-labeled components P-2 (peak in fraction 30) and P-3 (peak in fraction 59), respectively. As with RSVβ (O), some fast-moving ³H-glucosamine-labeled material (G-4) was more heterogeneous (fractions 85 to 105). Glucosamine-³H-labeled components G-1, G-2, and G-3 migrated with P-1, P-2, and P-3, respectively, in electrofocusing as well as in SDS gel electrophoresis, indicating that P-1,

FIG. 4-5.—Polyacrylamide gel SDS electrophoresis of dissociated RAV-1 and RSVβ (O). RAV-1 and RSV-β (O) were labeled with a mixture of ^{14}C or [3]H L-amino acids and purified as described in Figure 4-3. In a similar fashion, virus was labeled with ^{3}H-glucosamine (10 Ci per mM) 10 μCi per ml in growth medium 1.[54] Viruses were dissociated with 1% SDS, 4 m urea and 1% 2-mercaptoethanol at 37° for 30 min. Electrophoresis was done in 7% bisacrylamide gels 11 cm long and containing 0.1% SDS and 0.01 m sodium phosphate pH 7.2 at 10 ma per gel column.[56] Gel slices were shaken in 0.7 ml H_2O for two hr and then 10 ml Aquasol (New England Nuclear) was added for scintillation counting. A—[3]H-glucosamine-RSVβ (O) (-△-) and ^{14}C amino acid RSVβ (O) (-O-); B—[14]C amino acid RSVβ (O) (-O-) and ^{3}H amino acid RAV-1 (-△-); C—[3]H-glucosamine RSVβ (O) (-△-) and ^{14}C amino acid RAV-1, and D—[3]H-glucosamine RAV-1 (-△-) and ^{14}C amino acid RAV-1 (-O-).

P-2, and P-3 are glycoproteins. They contain about 5% of the radioactive amino acid in the total virion protein. ^{3}H-labeled G-3 did not follow P-7 or P-8 in electrofocusing and this glucosamine-containing component may not be a glycoprotein.[52] The radioactive peaks in fractions 2 and 12 (Figure 4-5D) did not appear in other experiments with these viruses, and may represent aggregated material.

Figure 4-5C shows the results of co-electrophoresis of ^{3}H-glucosamine RSVβ (O) and amino acid-^{14}C-RAV-1. In agreement with the results in Figure 4-4A and B the major ^{3}H-glucosamine-labeled component of RSVβ (O) with a peak in fraction 24 (G-1) moved more slowly than the ^{14}C amino acid-labeled RAV-1 component P-2 (peak in fraction 30). Similarly, glucosamine component G-3 (peak in fraction 58) moved more slowly than amino acid-labeled P-3 (peak in fraction 60 and 61).

We have also found significant differences in the electrophoretic mobilities of glycoproteins in RSV (RAV-1), RSV (RAV-2), and SR-RSV.[52]

These experiments indicate that viruses with different type-specific surface antigens have glycoproteins that are related to the type-specific antigen.

Separation of ^{14}C amino acid-labeled BH-RSV (RAV-1) proteins by electrofocusing after disruption of the virus with 1% Brij 58 and 4 M-urea is shown in Figure 4-6. Seven distinct components are apparent. Table 4-7 summarizes the characteristics of the virion proteins. The isoelectric point of six of the seven virion proteins isolated in this way is greater than the isoelectric point of whole virus. The individual components separated by electrofocusing were recovered and electrophoresed in SDS polyacrylamide gels to establish their identity in that system. SDS gel components 5 and 6 and components 7 and 8 corresponding to isoelectric focus components IV and I and components VI and III, respectively, are seen to have distinct isoelectric points.

Fig. 4–6.—Dissociated ^{14}C amino acid-labeled RSV (RAV-1) components separated by isoelectrofocusing. RSV (RAV-1) labeled and purified as described for Figure 4-4 was dissociated with 1% Brij 58, 4 m urea and 1% mercaptoethanol at 37° for 30 min. Isoelectric focusing was done as described in Figure 4-4 (pH- ●-, [14]C-○-) .

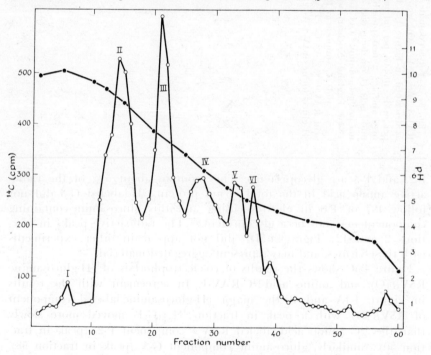

TABLE 4–7.—BH-RSV (RAV-1) PROTEINS

PROTEIN COMPONENT SDS GEL ELECTROPHORESIS	ELECTROFOCUS	% TOTAL ^{14}C	GLUCOSAMINE	pI	MOL. WT. $\times 10^{-3}$ BY SDS GEL ELECTROPHORESIS	PROTEIN µG. PER ML. REACTING IN MICRO CF WITH HAMSTER ANTISERUM
1	VII	2	+++	3.5	96.	>100.
2	V	9	+++	5.3	75.	25.3
3	IV	5	++	6.3	35.	18.5
4	II	31	– –	8.9	27.5	0.105
5	IV	14	– –	6.3	21.	18.5
6	I	2	– –	9.9	19.	>100.
7	VI	8	– –	4.9	16.5	10.2
8	III	27	– –	7.4	14.	0.715

Table 4-7 gives the tests of each protein from the electrofocus column for reaction by complement fixation with hamster group-specific antiserum. It can be seen that components II and III corresponding to SDS gel proteins 4 and 8 react at the lowest protein concentration in microcomplement fixation with antiserum to GS antigen. The poor reaction of the other proteins may represent cross-contamination with small amounts of components II and III. Positive reactions with components II and III are in agreement with the previous finding[47] that two components, prepared by preparative polyacrylamide electrophoresis, react with antiserum to GS antigen, although we now know that the previously described protein component RSV-1 can be separated into two components (P-7 and P-8) and only P-8 reacts in complement fixation. The components P-4 and P-8 represent the proteins present in greatest amount in the virion, indicating that nonpermissive cells transformed by RSV synthesize the major proteins present in the virion.

These results suggest a number of questions about the virion proteins. One is the chemical nature of the glycoproteins in the virion and differences in these proteins in viruses with different type-specific antigens. Our results[52] suggest that different viruses may contain either component P-1 or P-2 or both. The significance of glycoprotein P-3, which appears to have a slightly different mobility when isolated from viruses with different coat antigens, is also not clear. Two questions about the carbohydrate portion of the glycoproteins are obvious. First is the mechanism of its synthesis and whether it is cell or virus directed. Second is the functional role of the carbohydrate in the virion. It is known that sialic acid residues on cell surfaces are involved in myxovirus attachment to cells and, similarly, carbohydrate on the virion surface could play a role in virus attachment to cells. Finally, the origin and function of most of the eight virion proteins are not clear. Certain virion proteins are very likely viral coded (e.g. those reacting with antibody to group-specific antigen and those related to the type-specific antigen). However, enzymes have been found to be associated with ATVs,[24, 53] and these may be cellular enzymes incorporated into the virion. Similarly, some of the virion proteins we describe could have a cellular origin.

Acknowledgments

This work was supported by U. S. Public Health Service Research Grant CA 10467.

We wish to thank Miss Virginia Rimer and Miss Nona Stone for excellent technical assistance.

David Ralph was supported by U. S. Public Health Service Training Grant AI 0185 from the Institute of Allergy and Infectious Diseases.

Addendum

Since the delivery of this manuscript, Temin and Mizutani (Nature, 226:1211, 1970) and Baltimore (Nature 226:1209, 1970) have reported enzyme activities in preparations of RSV and Rauscher mouse leukemia virus, respectively, which incorporate deoxynucleoside triphosphates into TCA-insoluble products. These enzymes may represent RNA-dependent DNA polymerases in the virions which are essential for virus infectivity and explain the apparent dependence of replication of these RNA viruses on DNA synthesis.

References

1. Bonar, R. A., U. Heine, D. Beard, and J. W. Beard: J. Nat. Cancer Inst., 30:949-997, 1963.
2. Bonar, R. A., and J. W. Beard: J. Nat. Cancer Inst., 23:183-197, 1959.
3. Roa, P. R., and J. W. Beard: Nat. Cancer Inst. Monogr., 17:673-675, 1964.
4. Kates, M., A. C. Allison, D. A. J. Tyrrell, and A. T. James: Biochim. Biophys. Acta, 52:455-466, 1961.
5. Robinson, W. S., A. Pitkanen, and H. Rubin: Proc. Nat. Acad. Sci. USA, 54:219, 1965.
6. Harel, J., J. Huppert, F. Lacour, and L. Harel: Compt. Rend. Acad. Sci. Paris, 261:2266, 1965.
7. Baur, H.: Zeitschr. Naturforsch., 21b:453-460, 1966.
8. Robinson, W. S., and M. A. Baluda: Proc. Nat. Acad. Sci. USA, 54:1686, 1965.
9. Robinson, W. S., H. L. Robinson, and P. H. Duesberg: Proc. Nat. Acad. Sci. USA, 58:825-834, 1967.
10. Duesberg, P. H.: Proc. Nat. Acad. Sci. USA, 60:1511-1518, 1968.
11. Erikson, R. L.: Virology, 37:124-131, 1969.
12. Granboulan, N., J. Huppert, and F. Lacour: J. Molec. Biol., 16:571-575, 1966.
13. Kakefuda, T., and J. P. Bader: J. Virol., 4:460-474, 1969.
14. Galibert, R., C. Bernard, P. Chenaille, and M. Boiron: Compt. Rend. Acad. Sci. Paris, 261:1771, 1965.
15. Mora, P. T., V. W. McFarland, and S. W. Luborsky: Proc. Nat. Acad. Sci. USA, 55:438, 1966.
16. Blair, C. D., and P. H. Duesberg: Nature, 220:396-399, 1968.
17. Duesberg, P. H., and Cardiff [sic]: Virology, 36:696-700, 1968.
18. Montagneir, L. A., A. Goldé, and P. Vigier: J. Gen. Virol., 4:449-452, 1969.

19. Bader, J. P., and T. L. Steck: J. Virol., 4:454-459, 1969.
20. Sarkar, N. H., and D. H. Moore: J. Virol., 5:230-236, 1970.
21. Robinson, W. S.: Unpublished data.
22. Bonar, R. A., L. Sverak, D. P. Bologuesi, A. J. Langlois, D. Beard, and J. W. Beard: J. Nat. Cancer Inst., 27:1138, 1967.
23. Travnicek, M.: Biochim. Biophys. Acta, 182:427-439, 1969.
24. Thé, G. de: Nat. Cancer Inst. Monogr., 17:651-671, 1964.
25. Crawford, L. V., and E. M. Crawford: Virology, 13:227-232, 1961.
26. Rubin, H., and H. Temin: Virology, 7:75-91, 1959.
27. Hanafusa, H., and T. Hanafusa: Virology, 34:630-636, 1968.
28. Hirst, G. K.: Cold Spring Harbor Symp. Quant. Biol., 27:303-309, 1962.
29. Hlozanek, I., V. Sovova, J. Riman, and L. Veprek: J. Gen. Virol., 6:163-168, 1970.
30. Kates, J. R., and B. R. McAuslan: Proc. Nat. Acad. Sci. USA, 58:134, 1967.
31. Shatkin, A. J., and J. D. Sipe: Proc. Nat. Acad. Sci. USA, 61:1462-1469, 1968.
32. Baltimore, D.: Personal communication.
33. McAuslan, B. R., W. Levinson, and M. J. Bishop: Personal communication.
34. Hanafusa, H., T. Hanafusa, and H. Rubin: Virology, 51:41-48, 1964.
35. Hanafusa, H.: Virology, 25:248-255, 1965.
36. Vogt, P. K., and R. Ishizaki: Virology, 26:664-672, 1965.
37. Vogt, P. K., and R. Ishizaki: Virology, 30:368-374, 1966.
38. Ishizaki, R., and P. K. Vogt: Virology, 30:375-387, 1966.
39. Vogt, P. K.: Proc. Nat. Acad. Sci. USA, 58:801-807, 1967.
40. Hanafusa, H., and T. Hanafusa: Virology, 34:630-636, 1968
41. Vogt, P. K.: Virology, 33:175-177, 1967.
42. Hanafusa, H., and T. Hanafusa: Proc. Nat. Acad. Sci. USA, 58:818-825, 1967.
43. Huebner, R. J., D. Armstrong, M. Okuyan, P. S. Sarma, and H. C. Turner: Proc. Nat. Acad. Sci. USA, 51:742-749, 1964.
44. Bauer, H., and W. Schafer: Virology, 29:494-496, 1966
45. Eckert, E. A., R. Rott, and W. Schafer: Virology, 24:426-433, 1964.
46. Allen, D. W.: Biochim. Biophys. Acta, 133:180-183, 1967
47. Duesberg, P. H., H. L. Robinson, W. S. Robinson, R. J. Huebner, and H. C. Turner: Virology, 36:73-86, 1968.
48. Tozawa, H., H. Bauer, T. Graf, and H. Gelderblom: Virology, 40:530-539, 1970.
49. Robinson, H. L.: Proc. Nat. Acad. Sci. USA, 57:1655-1662, 1967.
50. Bonar, R. A., and J. W. Beard: J. Nat. Cancer Inst., 23:183-197, 1959.
51. Baluda, M. A., and D. P. Nayak: J. Virol., 4:554-566, 1969.
52. Hung, P., H. L. Robinson, and W. S. Robinson: In preparation.
53. Bauer, H., and W. Schafer: In: Subviral Carcinogenesis (Y. Ito, ed.), 1967, pp. 337-352.
54. Hobom-Schnegg, B., H. L. Robinson, and W. S. Robinson: J. Gen. Virol., 7:85-93, 1970.
55. Svensson, H.: Arch. Biochem. Biophys., Suppl. 1:132-138, 1962.
56. Summers, D. F., J. V. Maizel, and J. E. Darnell: Proc. Nat. Acad. Sci. USA, 54: 505-513, 1965.
57. Eckert, E. A., R. Rott, and W. Schafer: Zeitschr. Naturforsch., 18b:339-340, 1963.
58. Thé, G. de: In: Experimental Leukemia (M. Rich, ed.), 1968, p. 277.
59. Munyon, W., E. Paoletti, and J. T. Grace: Proc. Nat. Acad. Sci. USA, 58:2280, 1967.
60. Allen, D. W.: Biochim. Biophys. Acta, 154:388-396, 1968.
61. Allen, D. W.: Virology, 38:32-41, 1969.
62. Kelloff, G., and P. K. Vogt: Virology, 29:377-384, 1966.
63. Hanafusa, H., and T. Hanafusa: Proc. Nat. Acad. Sci. USA, 55:532-538, 1966.

5

Tumor-Specific Antigens

Historical Review and Perspectives

RICHMOND T. PREHN

Institute of Cancer Research, Philadelphia, Pennsylvania, USA

ENTHUSIASM FOR the prospects of tumor immunology, like so much of medical research, has followed a typical sine curve. At about the turn of the century, following the tremendous success of vaccination against certain infectious diseases, enthusiasm reached a high point. It was demonstrated that immunization could prevent the growth of transplantable animal tumors and, consequently the immunologic prevention of cancer seemed almost at hand.

Doubts began to occur when it was demonstrated that immunization with embryonic or, in some cases, normal adult tissues could inhibit cancer growth. Confidence in immunology as an answer to the cancer problem began to decline rapidly. It reached a low point with the apparent demonstration, as the result of the development of inbred mice, that immunity to transplanted tumors was not tumor-specific, but rather a form of homograft reaction. A number of studies showed that immunity could not be produced within an inbred strain against tumors arising in that strain. (In retrospect, these negative results were probably attributable to an unfortunate selection of tumor systems, and perhaps also to the firm notion that immunity was philosophically not possible because of the principle of "horror autotoxicus"—a notion which may have prevented notice of subtle effects.)

In 1957, the curve of expectations again started upward with the demonstration of the existence of true tumor-specific antigenicity in 3-methylcholanthrene-induced mouse sarcomas. This observation, followed by the almost simultaneous discovery that a viral-induced tumor system also exhibited tumor antigens, precipitated a new rise in the curve of immunologic expectations. This rise has accelerated to the present day. Indeed, so much has the climate of opinion now altered that it is seriously suggested by some that cellular immunity has as its raison d'etre the suppression of neoplasia. It is argued that cancer may be largely a vertebrate disease and that cellular acquired immunity may have evolved in the early vertebrates specifically to cope with this new problem! According to these enthusiasts, neoplasia probably occurs frequently in all vertebrate animals, but is usually promptly suppressed by an immunologic surveillance mechanism. Only the rare exceptional neoplasm may, for a variety of reasons, escape this surveillance mechanism and give rise to a clinically manifest lesion. Recently the enthusiasm for the immunologic approach to cancer has begun to spill over into the clinic, and there are increasing reports of the demonstration of tumor antigens in human neoplasia and even attempts at immunotherapy in man.

There can be no question that much of the present enthusiasm is well justified. Tumor antigens are, this time, here to stay! However, I think it probable that the enthusiasm for the immunologic approach to cancer prevention, diagnosis, and therapy may again decline—certainly not to its former abysmal level, but to levels considerably below those currently existing. Some disquieting notes are already beginning to appear, suggesting that enthusiasm for the immunologic approach may eventually again be somewhat dampened. Although no one can foresee the future with clarity, I predict, and I hope I am proved wrong, that limitations of the immunologic approach will become increasingly evident. In particular, the importance of immunity as a surveillance mechanism may be found to be much less than many investigators currently believe.

If classical acquired immunity is to serve as an efficacious surveillance mechanism, a number of prerequisites must be largely met. First among these is the prerequisite that the cells of most neoplasms must have sufficiently abnormal surfaces to serve as antigens in the animal in which the neoplasm arises. It is currently believed that most and perhaps all neoplasms are antigenic in the animal of origin. However, in our enthusiasm for the immunologic approach, we may be overstating the case. The trouble lies in the fact that it is theoretically impossible to prove the absolute absence of antigenicity; therefore we tend to discount those cases in which it is not demonstrable. Perhaps antigenicity is really there but too slight to be detected by current means or is masked by some unknown process. This belief is supported by the fact that there is no known class of neoplasms of which all members fail to exhibit antigenicity. Thus, tumors arising by the spontaneous transformation of mouse cells in tissue culture usually have little or no antigenicity, but occasionally such a neoplasm is clearly immunogenic. Lung adenomas induced by urethan are seldom antigenic, but are in certain instances. Similar results have been obtained with rat mammary carcinomas induced by 2-acetylaminofluorene. Many but not all "spontaneous" neoplasms have little or no antigenicity. Perhaps rather than emphasizing, as was necessary 10 years ago, that most tumors are probably antigenic, we would be better advised to say that most spontaneous and some experimentally-induced tumors have little or no measurable immunogenicity. If one assumes a priori the efficacy of immunologic surveillance, the lack of antigenicity of spontaneous tumors is to be expected; these would represent the small minority of neoplasms that are able to survive such surveillance. However, immunoselection cannot account for the lack of antigenicity in the spontaneously transformed tissue cultures. Thus, the basic premise upon which the hypothesis of effective immunologic surveillance depends, namely the nearly universal existence of effective levels of immunogenicity in tumor cells, remains questionable.

Effective immunosurveillance demands not only nearly universal antigenic potential in the neoplastic cells; it also demands that this potential be realized while the neoplasm is still small and in situ. The larger and more widespread the neoplasm at the time when the immune reaction is first aroused, the less likely that mechanism is to succeed. Direct experimental evidence from chemically induced mouse skin carcinogenesis and chemically induced mouse breast carcinogenesis suggests that the immune mechanism may often not be activated until relatively late in the course of the disease. Furthermore, the "sneaking through" phenomenon, first described by Humphreys et al., suggests that a very small incipient neoplasm may not stimulate host immunity until after the neoplasm is too large and well established to be overtaken by the immune reaction.

One of the best arguments in favor of the effective role of immunosurveillance is the alleged increase in tumor incidence in experimental or clinical situations in which immunocompetence is reduced. The experimental situations include the very young or newborn animal's susceptibility to induced oncogenesis; the fact that most oncogenic agents interfere with immune responses; and that in most systems, depression of immune reactivity by newborn thymectomy or antilymphocyte serum increases tumor incidence. However, the effects in newborn animals could well be caused by differences in newborn physiology having nothing to do with lack of immunocompetence. At least one potent oncogen does not appear to interfere with immune capacity, and the increase in tumor incidence as a result of immunodepression by newborn thymectomy has proved to be usually a rather weak and subtle effect. In fact, in the viral-induced mouse breast cancer system, both newborn thymectomy and treatment with ALS delay tumor appearance.

The clinical situations in which lack of normal immunocompetence is associated with an increased risk of neoplasia include patients being treated with immunosuppressive drugs, congenital disorders of the immune system, various cytogenetic defects, and last but not least, aging. However, the most prevalent neoplasm accompanying each of these states, with the exception of aging, is some form of leukemia or lymphoma. A grossly deranged immune mechanism might well result in leukemia or lymphoma for reasons not directly related to a relative lack of immunosurveillance. In aging, there are so many abnormalities other than a decrease in immunocompetence that too much significance cannot be attached to that one parameter.

In sum, it seems to me that the effects of immunodepression on oncogenesis, both in the experimental and clinical situations, are not as great as one might expect if immunosurveillance were a really important tumor-suppressive mechanism. However, the apparent effectiveness in several systems, both in man and mouse, of nonspecific stimulation of the immune mechanism, as by BCG or specific immunization, suggests that the effectiveness of immunosurveillance can be artificially increased. Perhaps these approaches hold clinical promise.

Although I have cast some doubt upon the probable importance of the immune mechanism as a surveillance device against incipient neoplasms, there is no doubt that in some systems an immunologic defense against tumor cells is demonstrable. However, it seems to me that this defense, even when demonstrable, is usually a rather late and ineffective phenomenon. It therefore seems doubtful that cellular acquired immunity evolved specifically as an antitumor mechanism.

It is not necessary a priori to postulate an effective immunosurveillance mechanism to account for the low incidence (considering the numbers of cells at risk) of neoplasia. Other control mechanisms have been demonstrated and more will undoubtedly be found. It appears to be a general rule that early neoplasms are inhibited by surrounding normal tissues of the same type. Thus, in the mouse breast, the premalignant hyperplastic alveolar nodule is inhibited by the presence in the fat pad of normal mammary gland. Stoker has shown inhibition of tumor cells by normal cells in tissue culture. Lewis has observed that malignant melanomas of the soles of African negroes never invade or metastasize to pigmented areas of skin. Thus, it is evident that effective homeostatic mechanisms exist to control early neoplasia without invoking effective immunosurveillance.

I hope that with increased realization of the limitations of the immune mechanism, the present enthusiasm is not followed by a repetition of the past period of discouragement. Such a reaction would be even less justified than is the present possible over-enthusiasm.

Detection of Murine Leukemia Virus Antigens

JANET W. HARTLEY, Ph.D.,

WALLACE P. ROWE, M.D., AND

ROGER E. WILSNACK, D.V.M.

Laboratory of Viral Diseases, National Institute of Allergy and Infectious Diseases, National Institutes of Health, Bethesda, Maryland, and Huntingdon Research Center, Inc., Baltimore, Maryland, USA

THE MURINE LEUKEMIA viruses have presented unusual problems for virologists because of the great difficulty in demonstrating infectivity. In contrast, highly reactive antigens were relatively easy to detect and immunologic markers have, therefore, been widely exploited to approach the basic problems of virus infection and oncogenicity.

Utilizing the antigens found in disrupted virus preparations, it has been possible to establish the many murine type-C virus isolates as members of one large group, and attempts have been made to distinguish individual envelope specificities by virus neutralization tests. Tests which detect naturally occurring virus and virus growth in mice and tissue culture followed the discovery of the type-specific Gross soluble antigen (GSA) and the group-reactive internal antigens. Searches for virus-specific cell surface antigens were required in order to study transplantation immunity and tumor prevention, and the detection of GSA and of the natural Gross (G) antibody which occurs in some antigen-negative mouse strains[1] has permitted the study of immune tolerance mechanisms in murine leukemia virus infection.

Unfortunately, the variety of questions studied by immunologic methods has led to the revelation of an almost bewildering variety of antigens. Based on the method of demonstration, there are four broad classes of virus-induced antigens, which may or may not have overlapping identities (Table 5-1).

By use of transplantation rejection,[2,3] in vitro cytotoxicity,[4,5,6] and immunofluorescence[3] techniques, two serologic classes of virus-specific cell surface antigens have been recognized,[7] which probably reflect protein of the viral envelope incorporated in the cell membrane. The G antigen is found in leukemic cells induced by Gross passage A virus and in spontaneous leukemias or normal lymphoid tissue of mice of strains with a high incidence of spontaneous leukemia ("G+" strains), as well as in many leukemias in lower-incidence strains. The second class, designated FMR, includes the cross-reacting cellular antigens found in leukemias induced by the Friend, Moloney, and Rauscher viruses.[8]

TABLE 5–1.—Major Antigens of the Murine Leukemia Virus Group

Source		Designation	Speci-ficity	Method of Detection	Presumed Origin in Virus
Infected cells	Tumor and lymphoid cells	Cell surface (G, FMR)	Type	Transplant rejection Cytotoxicity and absorption of cytotox. Immunofluorescence	Envelope protein
	Plasma and tissue extracts	Soluble (GSA, FMR sol.)	Type	Absorption on indicator cells— —cytotox. (FMR) —immunofl. (G)	Envelope protein
	Plasma and tissue extracts, tissue culture harvests	Soluble (gs)	Group	Immunodiffusion Complement fixation Immunofluorescence	Internal protein
Virion		Virion surface	Group and type	Neutralization (Immunofluorescence)	Envelope protein
		Soluble (gs)	Group	Immunodiffusion Complement fixation Passive HA	Internal protein

Second, there are type-specific soluble antigens found in plasma or tissue extracts of G+ mice and mice with leukemias induced by naturally occurring virus,[9] and in mice with FMR leukemias,[10] which have the serologic specificity of the G and FMR cellular antigens and which may be components of the viral envelope. These antigens are detected, after absorption to viable indicator cells, by indirect immunofluorescence (for GSA) and by cytotoxicity (for FMR soluble antigen). Testing for the G and FMR cellular and soluble antigens in uninoculated mouse populations showed that only the G antigens occur in naturally infected animals. FMR antigen has never been detected in nature.

Third, antigens demonstrable in the envelope of the infective virus (i.e., the reactive sites in virus neutralization tests) have also indicated two broad antigenic subgroups, referred to here as Gross-AKR and FMR. Depending on the type and potency of the antiserum used, both shared and distinct antigens, between and within subgroups, can be demonstrated.[11-17] Typing of viruses isolated from naturally infected animals has confirmed the observation that only Gross-AKR subgroup strains are found in nature.[18]

Finally, there is the nonsedimentable antigen common to all murine leukemia viruses, found in plasma and tissue extracts of naturally and experimentally infected animals and in tissue culture harvests. It is demonstrable by complement fixation (CF),[19] immunodiffusion,[12] and immunofluorescence[20] tests with sera from rats immunized with isolo-

TABLE 5–2.—COMPARISON OF MOUSE AND RAT ANTISERA
FOR USE IN DETECTING MuLV ANTIGENS

	SERUM	
USEFULNESS OF ANTIBODY INDUCED	MOUSE	RAT
Detection of G and FMR cellular antigen	+	+
Detection of GSA and FMR soluble antigen	+	Not tested
Neutralization	FMR only	+
Immunodiffusion	−	+
Complement fixation	−	+
Immunofluorescence in tissue culture cells	Not tested	+

gous tumors induced by viruses of the murine leukemia-sarcoma complex, and by passive hemagglutination inhibition procedures.[21] This group-specific (gs) antigen or complex of antigens is an internal component of the virion; it is found free in tissue and virus-infected tissue cultures, and can be released from intact virus by treatment with ether.[14, 18, 19, 21–23] The group-reactive specificity of this antigen allowed the development of tests for isolation and quantitation of virus in tissue culture systems, increasing the sensitivity of infectivity assays manyfold.[18, 19, 24]

To avoid the complications of histocompatibility reactions, the most widely used tests for murine leukemia viruses are based on antisera prepared by immunization of mice or rats with isogenic tumors, either by transplantation or hyperimmunization with viable cells. The usefulness of these sera for detecting murine leukemia virus antigens is shown in Table 5-2. Mouse sera have the advantage of being type-specific, but their use is limited by the poor antigenicity in mice of naturally occurring Gross-AKR subgroup viruses and the failure of mice to respond to the gs antigen.[12, 25] Most studies in our laboratory have been based on tests which utilize rat antisera for detection of group-specific antigen by complement fixation and immunofluorescence and for serologic classification by virus neutralization.

Sera are obtained from inbred Fischer rats three to four weeks after a single subcutaneous implantation as weanlings with tumor cells derived from rat tumor cell lines induced by the Moloney strain of murine sarcoma virus (M-MSV) or by an isolate from a naturally infected AKR mouse. Sera are selected for having high titer to several murine leukemia virus antigen preparations (animal tissue as well as infected mouse embryo tissue culture) and for lack of reaction with control tissue culture and rat lymphoid tissue antigens. Such sera may or may not have precipitating or virus neutralizing capacity. Representative CF antigen titers obtained with such sera are shown in Table 5-3.

The M-MSV tumor cell line induces the highest frequency of group-reactive antibody; however, only a relatively small proportion of rats develop broadly reactive CF antibody. The antibody developed after immunization with the AKR rat tumor cell line is more type-specific, de-

TABLE 5-3.—REPRESENTATIVE MuLV* COMPLEMENT-FIXING ANTIGEN TITERS AS DETECTED BY RAT ANTISERA

					ANTIGEN METC†			
RAT SERUM POOL (4-8 UNITS)	M-MSV RAT TUMOR	MLV	RLV	GrLV	AKR L_1	Ether Treated AKR L_1	Control	RAT THYMUS
M-MSV #R22560	8‡	32	64	64	64		0	0
" #16	16	64	16	32	32	32		
AKR #3	0	0	0	0	16	0	0	0
" #5	2	8	32	16	32		0	0
" #8	2	8		32	32	8		

* Murine leukemia virus.
† Mouse embryo tissue culture antigens: MLV: Moloney virus; RLV: Rauscher virus; GrLV: Gross passage A virus; AKRL1: AKR virus, strain L_1.
‡ Reciprocal of dilution; 0: <2.

tecting higher antigen titers with Gross-AKR subgroup viruses than with FMR, although group reactivity can also be demonstrated.

In susceptible animals and tissue cultures inoculated with murine leukemia viruses, the development of gs antigen demonstrable by CF is always associated with the appearance of infectious virus. Similarly, the presence of gs antigen in spontaneous leukemias and solid tumors and in normal lymphoid tissues of mice from high and intermediate incidence strains is usually indicative of virus isolatable in an appropriate tissue culture system.

However, a third class of antigen preparations is encountered—those which fix complement but have no detectable infectious virus. Such cases occur rarely, if ever, in high spontaneous leukemia strains, occasionally among spontaneous or carcinogen-induced tumors in BALB/c, DBA, and C_3H mice, and relatively frequently in carcinogen-induced tumors of very low incidence strains, such as NIH Swiss.[25] In some cases, such as NIH Swiss, virus has never been isolated from any specimen; that the lack of correlation of antigen with virus recovery is attributable to failure to find a suitable host cell system must still be considered.[24] In other cases, where techniques are well established, it must be presumed that gs and possibly viral envelope antigens are made but not assembled into infectious virus particles.

Using the most reactive rat sera available, MSV antiserum with high CF and neutralizing titers and with precipitating activity, Huebner et al.[26] have recently detected antigen in tissue extracts generally negative with previously used rat serum pools. Antigen has been found in adult, young, and embryo mice of strains with extremely low spontaneous leukemia rates. These antigens generally have the properties of gs antigen, i.e. they are nonsedimentable and ether-resistant. However, the special properties of the antisera used to detect these reactions have not yet been clearly defined. Rats exposed to the antigenic stimulus of tumor cells which release infectious virus as well as gs antigen may be expected to respond with antibodies against a variety of virus-specific antigens. The complete antibody spectrum of these rat sera has by no means been fully explored.

For studying growth of virus in tissue culture, another application of detection of group specific antigen by rat serum is available. Indirect immunofluorescence (FA) techniques can be used to demonstrate diffuse cytoplasmic staining in acetone-fixed cells or particulate antigen on the membrane of unfixed cells. As shown in Table 5-4, when FMR and Gross-AKR subgroup reagents are tested reciprocally, clear cross-reactivity is seen, with homologous titers being slightly higher. Less significant cross-reactivity has been found with sera which are more type-specific by complement fixation, and sera which are broadly CF reactive but negative for homologous neutralizing antibody. In contrast to the avian leukosis virus system, where membrane antigens are type-specific,[27] the staining of unfixed murine leukemia virus infected cells gives essentially the same pattern as in fixed cells. However, it is probable that the rat sera are detecting some virus envelope antigens in addition to gs antigen.

In tests with the broadly reactive M-MSV rat antiserum on acetone-fixed cultures, typical FA staining has been obtained with every tissue culture isolate of murine leukemia virus tested, including laboratory strains of both the FMR and Gross-AKR subgroups (Gross passage A, Moloney, Rauscher, Friend, WM1-B, Graffi, Kirsten, and FBJ) and more than 20 field strains isolated from AKR, C58, C_3H, BALB/c, CF-1, CFW, C57B1, and SJL mice.

The formation of discrete foci of FA-stainable cells in the infected cultures has provided the basis for a quantitative assay system. Dose response studies (Fig. 5-1) have shown one-hit kinetics, but with a tendency for the number of foci to decline somewhat less than the dilution factor. The reasons for this phenomenon are not clear. In secondary mouse embryo cultures, where the phenomenon is most marked, this may be attributable to the diffuseness of the foci; closely spaced foci at lower virus dilutions cannot be resolved, resulting in falsely low counts. However, the same pattern occurred in the cultures with agar overlay, where the foci are small and sharply circumscribed.

Because of this aberrant dose-response relation, calculation of virus titers is done only with virus dilutions giving less than 20 foci. Within this limitation, determination of virus titers by FA focus counts has proved to be sensitive and reproducible.

It has been shown by a number of investigators that both type and group neutralization can be demonstrated,[11-18] the results depending on the nature and potency of the antiserum used. The broadness of antibody response in rats, although of great advantage in detecting any member of the murine leukemia virus group, limits its usefulness for the detection of antigens. However, some serologic classification is possible using selected rat antisera; the results obtained using tissue

TABLE 5–4.—SERUM ANTIBODY TITERS OF BROADLY REACTIVE M-MSV AND AKR RAT ANTISERA TO MOLONEY (MLV) AND AKR-L1 VIRUS ANTIGENS IN DIFFERENT SEROLOGICAL TESTS

| | FLUORESCENT ANTIBODY* | | | | | | NEUTRALIZATION† | | CF (Tissue Culture Antigen) | | |
| | Unfixed Cells | | | Acetone-fixed Cells | | | | | | | |
RAT SERUM	MLV	AKR-L1	Control	MLV	AKR-L1	Control	MLV	AKR-L1	MLV	AKR-L1	Control
MSV #22560	1000	300	0‡	300	100	0	640	40-80	160	160	< 20
AKR #6	30	300	0	10	100	0	20	80	20	160	< 20
Normal	0	0	0	0	0	0					

* Tested on chronically infected NIH-3T3 cell cultures.
† Tested by focus reduction method using pseudotypes of M-MSV.
‡ 0: < 10.

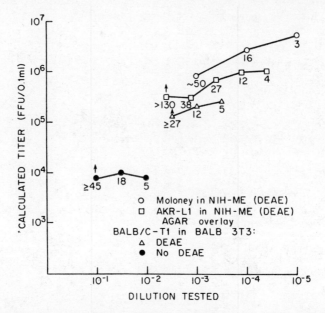

FIG. 5–1.—Dose-response relations of murine leukemia viruses titrated by fluorescent focus assay. The numbers under each point are the number of foci per half cover slip. Titrations were done by inoculating serial dilutions of virus on NIH Swiss mouse embryo (NIH-ME) or BALB 3T3 cell cultures (60 mm plastic dishes containing 1 or more 11 × 22 mm glass cover slips, plated 24 hr previously with 3.5 × 10⁵ cells), untreated or treated with DEAE-dextran.[24] Cover slips were fixed in cold acetone at five or six days after inoculation and tested by indirect immunofluorescence (FA) with M-MSV rat antiserum and fluorescein isothiocyanate-labelled goat anti-rat globulin, using a lissamine rhodamine bovine serum albumin counterstain. The number of FA-stainable foci per half cover slip were counted; titers were calculated by multiplying the number of foci by the dilution factor by 16 (the ratio of the area of the culture dish to that of the half cover slip) and were expressed as focus forming units (FFU) per 0.1 ml.

culture infectivity end-points are in general agreement with tests done by others, including those using in vivo assays. Antisera were obtained from rats immunized with M-MSV, AKR, and Gross Passage A transplanted rat tumors, and in a few cases from rats hyperimmunized with tissue culture-grown virus. The most reproducible and accurate assays measure inhibition of focus induction by MSV pseudo-types prepared with various strains of murine leukemia virus,[13] or plaque reduction using a recently developed assay based on formation of syncytia by the XC Rous rat tumor cell line when in contact with cells infected with murine leukemia viruses.[28, 29]

Separation of murine leukemia viruses into subgroups is based on high ratios of homologous to heterologous neutralization (Table 5-5). Moloney-MSV antiserum neutralizes Friend, Moloney, and Rauscher viruses to essentially the same titer; using homologous antiserum to each strain, Moloney virus can be distinguished from the Friend and Rauscher strains. These FMR strains, however, are neutralized only by high concentrations of Gross Passage A and AKR antisera, or the anti-Gross (C58 virus) rat serum of Geering et al.[12]

A second well-defined subgroup includes Gross Passage A and all naturally occurring strains thus far tested, including one or more isolates from AKR, C58, C3H (substrains Fg, He, and Bi), CF$_1$, DBA, BALB/c, RF, and SJL mice. These virus strains are all neutralized by rat antiserum to Gross Passage A virus, but not by FMR neutralizing antibody except in high concentration.

Within this subgroup a further subdivision is possible, based on neutralization by antiserum against the AKR virus isolate (Table 5-6). The majority of AKR rat antisera with high homologous titer to AKR virus do not efficiently neutralize Gross Passage A virus. Similar patterns are seen with the Kirsten leukemia virus and Kirsten sarcoma virus and with some strains isolated from BALB/c mice; other BALB/c isolates are neutralized like AKR virus. It is possible that the Gross Passage A-induced rat tumor used for immunization contained a mixture of viruses, one being like AKR virus, another being like the variant isolates. Clarification of these cross-reactivities is dependent on preparation of homologous antisera, ideally with plaque-purified viruses.

A number of laboratory passage strains have not been studied as to serotype, or have not been clearly defined. One of the latter is the Graffi leukemia virus. Although leukemic cells of Graffi virus-infected mice possess a surface antigen (the "FMRGi" surface antigen) which cross-reacts with FMR leukemia cellular antigen,[30, 31] by neutralization tests with mouse antisera it has been shown that Graffi virus is distinct from FMR subgroup viruses.[16, 17] Preliminary tests in our laboratory indicate that Graffi virus is not neutralized by typing dilutions of Moloney-MSV, Gross Passage A, or AKR rat antisera. The virus may represent a third subgroup, as suggested by Levy et al.[17]

TABLE 5-5.—NEUTRALIZATION PATTERNS OF MuLV PSEUDOTYPES
WITH RAT ANTISERUM

RAT SERUM	MLV	RLV	SERUM TITER* AGAINST FLV	Gross Pass. A.	AKR-L1	C58 E1
M-MSV R22560	640			40	40	
R18996	80	80	40	0	0	0
Moloney	40	0	0	0	0	
Rauscher	0	40	20	0	0	
Friend	0	20	40	0	0	
Gross Pass. A	0	0	0	40	80	> 40
AKR	0	0	0	0	160	> 80
C58 (L.J.O.)	20	20	20	320	320	>160
Normal	0	0	0	0	0	0

* Titers expressed as reciprocals of dilution giving 67% or greater reduction in number of foci when tested against approximately 30 focus-forming units of M-MSV pseudotype (13). 0 = < 20.

TABLE 5–6.—SPECIFICITIES WITHIN GROSS-AKR
SUBGROUP AS INDICATED BY PLAQUE REDUCTION
NEUTRALIZATION TESTS

| VIRUS | RAT ANTISERUM | |
	AKR	Gross Passage A
AKR-L$_t$	320*	160
B/C S3-B	320	80†
B/C S3-N	320	NT‡
B/C S2-N	320	80
Gross Pass. A	20	40-80
Kirsten	< 40	> 40
B/C S2-B	40	80
B/C T1	40	80
C57 B1 MC-1	40	40

* Reciprocal of highest dilution giving 67% or greater reduction in number of plaques when tested against approximately 50 plaque-forming units of leukemia virus.[29]
† Titer determined by reduction in number of focal areas detected by immunofluorescence.
‡ Not tested.

There are many unresolved questions raised by efforts to detect virus-specific antigens in murine leukemia virus infection, whether induced or naturally acquired. The relationship between antigens detected by different techniques is not yet clear and the results given by some procedures may reflect the reactivity of one or several minor antigens as well as that of the major antigen. Distinctions between qualitative and quantitative measurements must be made, particularly where antisera of varying breadths of reactivity are used. Control mechanisms governing the expression of antigens in different host systems are not fully defined. For example, in the high leukemia-incidence AKR mouse, infectious virus and all Gross-type antigens are detectable throughout life. In contrast, no murine leukemia virus antigens are found in MSV nonproducer tumors and transformed cells, although the sarcoma genome is rescuable. The function of antigens found in low leukemia-incidence strains of mice with undetectable infectious viruses, and the implications of these antigens in understanding the natural history of murine leukemia virus infection have yet to be established.

References

1. Aoki, T., E. A. Boyse, and L. J. Old: Occurrence of natural antibody to the G (Gross) leukemia antigen in mice. Cancer Res., 26:1415-1419, 1966.
2. Klein, G., H. O. Sjögren, and E. Klein: Demonstration of host resistance against isotransplantation of lymphomas induced by the Gross agent. Cancer Res., 22:955-961, 1962.
3. Klein, E., and G. Klein: Antigenic properties of lymphomas induced by the Moloney agent. J. Nat. Cancer Inst., 32:547-568, 1964.
4. Slettenmark-Wahren, B., and E. Klein: Cytotoxic and neutralization tests with

serum and lymph node cells of isologous mice with induced resistance against Gross lymphomas. Cancer Res., 22:947-954, 1962.

5. Old, L. J., E. A. Boyse, and F. Lilly: Formation of cytotoxic antibody against leukemias induced by Friend virus. Cancer Res., 23:1063-1068, 1963.

6. Old, L. J., E. A. Boyse, and E. Stockert: The G (Gross) leukemia antigen. Cancer Res., 25:813-819, 1965.

7. Aoki, T., L. J. Old, and E. A. Boyse: Serological analysis of the leukemia antigens of the mouse. Nat. Cancer Inst. Monogr., 22:449-457, 1966.

8. Old, L. J., E. A. Boyse, and E. Stockert: Typing of mouse leukemias by serological methods. Nature, 201:777-779, 1964.

9. Aoki, T., E. A. Boyse, and L. J. Old: Wild-type Gross leukemia virus. I. Soluble antigen (GSA) in the plasma and tissues of infected mice. J. Nat. Cancer Inst., 41:89-96, 1968.

10. Stück, B., L. J. Old, and E. A. Boyse: Occurrence of soluble antigen in the plasma of mice with virus-induced leukemia. Proc. Nat. Acad. Sci. USA, 52:950-958, 1964.

11. Fink, M. A., and F. J. Rauscher: Immune reactions to a murine leukemia virus. I. Induction of immunity to infection with virus in the natural host. J. Nat. Cancer Inst., 32:1075-1082, 1964.

12. Geering, G., L. J. Old, and E. A. Boyse: Antigens of leukemias induced by naturally occurring murine leukemia virus: Their relation to the antigens of Gross virus and other murine leukemia viruses. J. Exp. Med., 124:753-772, 1966.

13. Huebner, R. J., J. W. Hartley, W. P. Rowe, W. T. Lane, and W. I. Capps: Rescue of the defective genome of Moloney sarcoma virus from a noninfectious hamster tumor and the production of pseudotype sarcoma viruses with various murine leukemia viruses. Proc. Nat. Acad. Sci. USA, 56:1164-1169, 1966.

14. Huebner, R. J.: The murine leukemia-sarcoma virus complex. Proc. Nat. Acad. Sci. USA, 58:835-842, 1967.

15. Fefer, A., J. L. McCoy, and J. P. Glynn: Neutralization of the oncogenicity of Moloney sarcoma virus and Moloney leukemia virus by anti-Gross serum. Internat. J. Cancer, 2:647-650, 1967.

16. Steeves, R. A., and A. A. Axelrad: Neutralization kinetics of Friend and Rauscher leukemia viruses studied with the spleen focus assay method. Internat. J. Cancer, 2:235-244, 1967.

17. Levy, J. P., B. Varet, E. Oppenheim, and J. C. Leclerc: Neutralization of Graffi leukemia virus. Nature, 224:606-608, 1969.

18. Hartley, J. W., W. P. Rowe, W. I. Capps, and R. J. Huebner: Isolation of naturally occurring viruses of the murine leukemia virus group in tissue culture. J. Virol., 3:126-132, 1969.

19. Hartley, J. W., W. P. Rowe, W. I. Capps, and R. J. Huebner: Complement fixation and tissue culture assays for mouse leukemia viruses. Proc. Nat. Acad. Sci. USA, 53:931-938, 1965.

20. Rowe, W. P., J. W. Hartley, and R. E. Wilsnack: Unpublished data.

21. Fink, M. A., L. R. Sibal, N. A. Wivel, C. A. Cowles, and T. E. O'Connor: Some characteristics of an isolated group antigen common to most strains of murine leukemia virus. Virology, 37:605-614, 1969.

22. Gregoriades, A., and L. J. Old: Isolation and some characteristics of a group-specific antigen of the murine leukemia viruses. Virology, 37:189-202, 1969.

23. Schäfer, W., F. A. Anderer, H. Bauer, and L. Pister: Studies on mouse leukemia viruses. I. Isolation and characterization of a group-specific antigen. Virology, 38:387-394, 1969.

24. Hartley, J. W., W. P. Rowe, and R. J. Huebner: Host-range restrictions of murine leukemia viruses in mouse embryo cell cultures. J. Virol., 5:221-225, 1970.

25. Huebner, R. J.: Identification of leukemogenic viruses: Specifications for vertically transmitted, mostly "switched off" RNA tumor viruses as determinants of the generality of cancer. Proceedings of the IVth International Symposium on Comparative Leukemia Research. In press.

26. Huebner, R. J., R. V. Gilden, G. Kelloff, H. Meier, D. D. Myers, R. L. Peters,

C. E. Whitmire, P. S. Sarma, W. T. Lane, and H. C. Turner: Group specific (gs) expression of the C-type RNA tumor virus genome during embryogenesis: Implications for a possible role in ontogenesis as well as in oncogenesis. Proc. Nat. Acad. Sci. USA. In press.

27. Vogt, P. K.: Phenotypic mixing in the avian tumor virus group. Virology, 32:708-717, 1967.
28. Klement, V., W. P. Rowe, J. W. Hartley, and W. E. Pugh: Mixed culture cytopathogenicity: A new test for growth of murine leukemia viruses in tissue culture. Proc. Nat. Acad. Sci. USA, 63:753-758, 1969.
29. Rowe, W. P., W. E. Pugh, and J. W. Hartley: Plaque assay techniques for murine leukemia viruses. Submitted for publication.
30. Pasternak, G.: Serologic studies on cells of Graffi virus-induced myeloid leukemia in mice. J. Nat. Cancer Inst., 34:71-83, 1965.
31. Levy, J. P., J. C. Leclerc, B. Varet, and E. Oppenheim: Studies of the antigenic specificity of Graffi leukemic cells. J. Nat. Cancer Inst., 41:743-750, 1968.

Antigens of Chemically Induced Tumors

CHARLES F. McKHANN, M.D., AND
GERALD W. HAYWOOD, PH.D.

*Departments of Surgery and Microbiology, University of Minnesota,
Minneapolis, Minnesota, USA*

TUMORS INDUCED by chemical carcinogens are characterized by alterations in their normal transplantation antigens and the acquisition of new tumor-specific antigens. A wealth of evidence, going back to the initial studies of Prehn, indicate that the new tumor antigens are specific for each individual tumor, even though they are induced by the same agent in identical animals of an inbred strain. A graphic demon-

TABLE 5–7.—COMMON ANTIGENS OF MCA TUMORS DETECTED BY ANTIBODY

McKHANN—I^{125} ANTI-MOUSE GLOBULIN

	Target Cells			
Antiserum A	E	G	H	M
2.0	1.0	1.7	1.0	1.0

Antibody absorption is recorded as an "absorption ratio," relative to the absorption of normal serum. (1.0 indicates no absorption in excess of normal.) Antiserum directed against Tumor A also reacted with Tumor G.

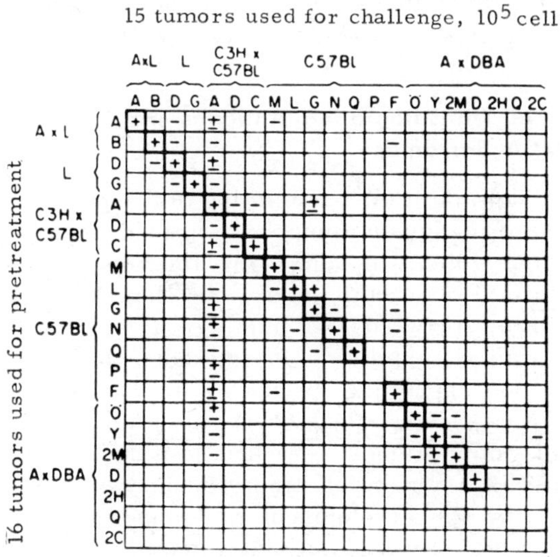

15 tumors used for challenge, 10^5 cells

FIG. 5–2.—Fifteen tumors indicating no tumor immunized any animal against any other tumor of the series.

stration of this was provided by Klein et al., in which 15 different tumors were matched against each other with the finding that no tumor consistently immunized animals against any other tumor of the series (Figure 5-2).

Three studies have raised the possibility that some methylcholanthrene-induced sarcomas may share common antigens. Using an indirect isotope-labeled antiglobulin technique, it was found in our laboratory that antisera recovered after amputation of a methylcholanthrene sarcoma was strongly positive for that sarcoma (Table 5-7). It failed to show any absorption to cells of two other similar sarcomas, but reacted strongly with a fourth tumor. Also using immune serum, Hellstrom found evidence of cross-reactions when immune serum and complement were used to inhibit colony formation of tumor cells in tissue culture (Table 5-8). Finally, Reiner and Southam show that in vivo immunization of mice simultaneously with several MCA tu-

TABLE 5–8.—COMMON ANTIGENS OF MCA TUMORS DETECTED BY ANTIBODY

HELLSTROM—COLONY INHIBITION

Target Cell						Antisera					
$\frac{49}{}$	$\frac{49}{80}$	$\frac{35}{}$	$\frac{44}{}$	$\frac{45}{}$	$\frac{61}{}$	$\frac{74}{46}$	$\frac{81}{}$				% Inhibition
$\frac{81}{}$	$\frac{81}{51}$	$\frac{32}{}$	$\frac{33}{45}$	$\frac{44}{41}$	$\frac{47}{}$	$\frac{49}{}$	$\frac{51}{}$	$\frac{53}{}$	$\frac{61}{}$	$\frac{71}{}$	% Inhibition

Inhibition of colony growth of tumor cells exposed to antibody and C^1 is recorded as per cent inhibition, compared to cells exposed to normal sera. Tumor 49 reacted with serum 49 and 46. Tumor 81 reacted with sera 81, 33, and 44.

mors caused immunity against a different tumor that was not included in the immunization group.

Alterations of Normal Transplantation Antigens in MCA Sarcomas

The concept of "antigenic simplification" accounting for increased host range of transplantability of malignant tumors was provided with an experimental foundation by Moller. In comparing the concentration of antigen sites on the surface of several tumors, she showed that there was an inverse relationship between the number of antigenic sites and the host range for transplantability of the tumors. Tumors that retained a narrow host range, remaining specific for the strain in which the tumor originated, usually showed a higher concentration of surface H-2 antigens than did similar tumors that had lost their host specificity and grew successfully in a variety of strains. A more refined study has been made possible by the development of "monospecific" H-2 antisera by Snell and others. Utilizing antisera directed against seven specificities of C3H mice, a study was undertaken in our lab-

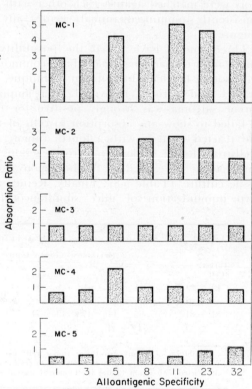

Fig. 5-3.—Absorbing capacity of different MCA tumors relative to Tumor MC-1.

oratory of the surface antigenic properties of five different methyl-cholanthrene-induced tumors of that strain. Quantitative absorption of the antisera by various numbers of cells of each tumor was followed by a cytotoxic assay for residual antibody activity against C3H lymphocytes. Using numbers of cells adjusted to compensate for minor differences in surface area, the five tumors were compared for their capacity to absorb each of the H-2 specificities. It can be seen in Figure 5-3 that the surface representation of the different H-2 specificities on the five tumors was not randomized. Instead, each tumor could be characterized as having a large, intermediate, or small amount of each of the antigenic specificities for which it was tested. For convenience, these were standardized against one tumor, MC3. It can be seen that no single antigenic moiety was found to be completely absent from any tumor studied, and there was a definite quantitative pattern of the different antigens with respect to each other. No tumor had high levels of one antigen with low levels of others or vice versa. These studies suggest that control is influenced over the entire complex locus to the same degree, influencing all of the antigens uniformly. The level at which this control is exerted and the mechanism of its alteration are not known.

Reciprocal Relationship Between Tumor and Normal Antigens

Each tumor of the preceding study was also evaluated with respect to its tumor-specific immunogenicity. Immunization was standardized by injecting all mice in the leg with the same dose of tumor cell and amputating the leg at seven days. Five days later, groups of mice were challenged with different numbers of cells of the appropriate tumors, and the development and growth rate of tumors were noted. The results of this study, shown in Table 5-9, indicated that tumor-specific immunogenicity had an inverse relationship to the H-2 antigenicity previously found. Tumor 1, which was strongly H-2 antigenic, showed the least capacity to immunize against its tumor-specific antigens in isologous mice. Tumor 5, which had little H-2 antigenicity, was strongly tumor immunogenic. Finally, the same tumors were also compared with respect to one other property, their capacity to metastasize to the

TABLE 5–9.—SUMMARY

| | H-2 | | TUMOR ANTIGEN | |
	Absorption	Cytotoxicity	LD$_{50}$	Metastasis
MC-1	+++++	+++++	+	++++
MC-2	++++	++++	+	++++
MC-3	++	++	++	++
MC-4	++	+	+++	+
MC-5	+	+	+++	+

lung. This was measured by excising the lungs at 1, 2, or 3 weeks following a standard injection of tumor cells subcutaneously. The lungs were minced and transferred subcutaneously to freshly irradiated isologous mice. The development of subcutaneous tumor nodules was considered indicative of pulmonary metastases in the original animal. This function correlated positively with H-2 antigenicity and negatively with tumor-specific immunogenicity, as might be expected. Tumors that were highly tumor-immunogenic gave fewer and later metastases than those that were weakly immunogenic.

Models of Cell Surface

Recent studies indicate that cellular antigens may not be distributed randomly over the surface of the cell, but may be present in clusters separated by large or small areas of surface that are antigenically barren. The reciprocal relationship between normal transplantation antigens and tumor-specific antigen in MCA tumors suggests two alternative configurations (Figure 5-4): 1. The tumor-specific antigens may be independent entities, separate from clusters of normal antigens. If great in number, the tumor-specific antigens may encroach upon the normal clusters and crowd them out, resulting in fewer such clusters. The implication here is that the clusters are of normal size and characteristics, but that their number is inversely related to the number of

Fig. 5-4.—The reciprocal relationship between normal transplantation antigens and tumor-specific antigen in MCA tumors.

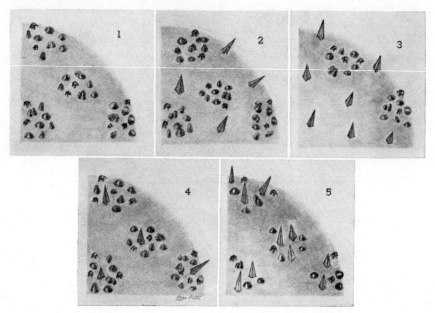

FIG. 5–5.—Topographical rearrangements of existing normal antigens. The deletion of varying numbers of normal antigenic specificities from the clusters with a spatial rearrangement of the remaining antigens.

tumor-specific antigenic sites on the cell. 2. The tumor-specific antigens may be intimately related to the H-2 clusters, rendering the individual no longer normal in composition. The new antigens would be at the expense of normal antigens in the same cluster. An alternative to this that bears consideration is that there are no new tumor-specific antigens, but only topographical rearrangements of existing normal antigens (Figure 5-5). The above findings could all be explained by the deletion of varying numbers of normal antigenic specificities from the clusters with a spatial rearrangement of those remaining. The implication here is that the total antigenic picture reflects not only the individual specificities but also their spatial relationship to each other.

Mechanisms of Antigenic Alteration

Chemical carcinogens are probably able to combine with many different components of the cell. It is still premature to indicate that any one of the several target materials is more important than the others. From a functional point of view, however, some of the possible mechanisms of chemical carcinogenesis are more accountable for the observed cell properties than are others.

INTERACTION WITH DNA RESULTING IN MUTATIONS OF STRUCTURAL GENES

Unless it is postulated that a single mutation can affect much of the cell function, such as a general disruption of membrane architecture, one must assume that many mutations would be required to accommodate the diverse properties of malignancy. These would have to be precise enough that substitution of amino acids was the usual result. Randomized losses or additions of nucleotide bases would all too frequently result in lethal mutants resulting in death of the cell. The mutation of structural genes would account well for the diversity of the new tumor-specific antigens seen in MCA sarcomas. However, it does not account for the reciprocal modulation of normal antigens unless they are passively crowded out by the new antigens.

DNA-SPONTANEOUS MUTATION

Burnet has postulated that a high level of spontaneous mutation may take place in cells other than those accounting for the immune response and that such mutations may result in new antigens. In this way, every somatic cell may have built in the possibility of being antigenically different from most or all other cells. Chemical carcinogenesis would then provide a selective advantage to one cell whose antigenicity was already established but which was "lost in the crowd" until augmented in number by malignant growth. Again, the modulation of normal antigens is not easily accounted for by this theory.

ELIMINATION OF GENETIC DUPLICATION

The studies of Brittan and Kohne indicate that mammalian cells may have an enormous amount of genetic duplication. The elimination of multiple identical messages in a tumor cell could very well reduce the amount of antigenic material produced and presented on the cell surface. With few exceptions, it is not known how direct is the genetic dose effect in mammalian cells, particularly in areas of large-scale genetic duplication. If new antigens are truly new and not secondary to rearrangement of existing specificities, the quantitative reduction of genetic duplication would not account for the appearance of new specificities.

GENETIC CONTROL LEVEL (REPRESSOR, INDUCER, OPERATOR)

Operations at the genetic control level are usually thought to be capable of switching on or off entire sets of structural genes. The appearance of new antigens would require that the genetic information be predetermined in the cell and available for derepression. This raises the very important question of whether the new antigens are actually new.

DNA-HISTONE

The uncovering or derepression of genetic information already existing in the cell, resulting in the formation of new antigens, can also be accomplished by alterations of the DNA-histone relationship. This particular mechanism lends itself well to speculation, because so little is actually known of this relationship and its control over genetic expression.

mRNA and Protein Synthesis

Selective transcription and selective translation both imply that the necessary information for new antigens is available in the cell and has been processed up to that level. Both of these mechanisms could easily accommodate alterations in the surface concentration of normal antigens or tumor antigens, but do not help much in determining why a new tumor antigen should be present at all.

Membrane Properties—Spatial Arrangement

The surface membrane of the cell is a complicated structure that can be viewed from several vantage points. In cross-section it is undoubtedly composed of several layers, the removal of any one of which may uncover material that may be antigenic in the next deeper layer. These materials may be perfectly normal to the cell but not previously exposed to the immune systems, so that their antigenicity went "unrecognized." Similarly, viewed from the top, the surface of the cell may actually be an intricate mosaic of materials, some of which are easily recognized as antigens. As previously implied, the rearrangement of these materials may result in entirely new configurations and new antigens. Finally, a generalized disruption or alteration of the cell surface, or even all of the cell membranes, could result in both vertical and horizontal structural changes eventuating in the production of new antigens and the revealing of hidden specificities.

The alternative mechanisms for antigenic alterations in chemical carcinogenesis may yield to further study. A major question is to determine whether the tumor-specific antigens are truly new primary entities, or whether they represent phenomena secondary to rearrangements of existing cellular components. Much of this question can be answered by determining the localization of tumor and normal antigens with respect to each other. If they are remote from each other and not intimately associated, it will be unlikely that the new antigens are merely the result of rearrangements. Similarly, chemical isolation and characterization of both tumor-specific and normal antigens should demonstrate whether they are identical, similar, or unrelated materials. The cloning of several cells from a single MCA tumor will help to determine how many different antigenic specificities may be present in one tumor, and prolonged passage of the tumor will determine the genetic stability of the antigen(s). It can be anticipated that more detailed study of cellular antigens, both tumor-specific and normal, in malignant cells may contribute to our understanding of the mechanisms of chemical carcinogenesis.

Acknowledgments

Work reported from the authors' laboratory was supported in part by American Cancer Society Grant T428, and U. S. Public Health Service Grants CA-08832-03, AI-0090, CA 39382-02, and CA-10910.

Altered Surface Properties of
Neoplastic Cells

PAUL H. BLACK, JEFFREY J. COLLINS,
AND LLOYD A. CULP

*Department of Medicine, Massachusetts General Hospital, and
Harvard Medical School, Boston, Massachusetts, USA*

THIS PRESENTATION will be concerned with the changes, both antigenic and biochemical, which have been found on the surface membranes of cancer cells, principally virus-transformed cells. This subject is of much importance, since immunologic mechanisms are primarily involved in the elimination of cancer cells and the principal immunity seems to be mediated by immunocompetent cells sensitized to new surface antigens. Changes in the composition of the surface membrane are also of importance since several properties of cancer cells may be causally related to such changes. Some of these properties include the loss of contact inhibition, the increased electronegative surface charge, and the diminished adhesiveness which characterize the cancer cell.

In this report, the new antigens which appear in cancer cells will be classified as specific or nonspecific. The former antigens are the viral transplantation antigens which appear to be coded for by viral genetic information. The nonspecific antigens are coded for by host genetic information, which may normally be repressed. The fetal antigens which have been found in some cancers may be an example of new antigens which are derived from derepressed genetic information. A major portion of the changes in the surface membrane of tumor cells seems to occur by exposure of cryptic membrane sites. These sites may be exposed either by failure to synthesize membrane constituents distal to these sites, by uncovering or unmasking surface sites caused by the elimination of surface material, or by a restructuring or conformational change of the membrane surface. Immunologic and biochemical studies on which of these mechanisms may be operative in causing changes in the surface membrane of tumor cells will be presented. Last, the significance of the presence of these changes will be briefly assessed, both with respect to the altered growth potential of the transformed cell and the host response to the cancer cell.

Specific Antigens

VIRAL

The viral transplantation rejection antigens are coded for by viral genes contained within the transformed cell.[1] The main evidence for this is derived from the specificity of the viral transplantation rejection antigens. This has been most thoroughly investigated with cells transformed by the oncogenic DNA viruses in which each transplantation antigen is virus-specific and not cell-specific. The viral transplantation antigens are presumably located on the plasma membrane, although direct demonstration of these antigens by techniques other than transplantation rejection tests has not been achieved. Several studies have suggested that an antigen detected by surface immunofluorescence (S antigen) is virus-specific.[2-5] The evidence for this, however, is not conclusive. Studies have shown that the S antigen is not directly related to the presence of the transplantation resistance antigen.[6] Moreover, S antigen may be present in a cell line in which no transcription of viral genetic information has been demonstrated by nucleic acid hybridization techniques.[7] Recent evidence, in addition, suggests that the S antigen may be a fetal antigen (see below).

In addition to the virus-specific transplantation antigens which appear in virus-transformed cells, results obtained in our laboratory indicate that antigenic changes characteristic for each transformation event may be present as well.[8] Using the indirect membrane immunofluorescence technique, in both an autochthonous and homologous system, we have demonstrated that cells of the same species, hamster, transformed by a given pool of purified SV40 virus, contain new S antigens unique for each individual cell line. This is reminiscent of the antigenic conversion with chemical carcinogens; it implies that oncogenic viruses may code for specific transplantation antigens as well as induce the appearance of nonspecific antigenic moieties which apparently differ with each transformation event. Whether the specific or nonspecific antigen (s) will be detected depends, of course, upon the nature of the assay procedure utilized.

Nonspecific Antigens

DEREPRESSED HOST GENETIC INFORMATION

The nonspecific antigens are coded for by host genetic information. They may arise either from a derepression of host cell genetic information or exposure of membrane sites (in the case of S antigens) attributable to either a failure to synthesize membrane component (s) or a restructuring of the membrane. The former mechanism has been invoked to explain the growing number of instances in which tumor tissues have been found to contain or produce materials normally associated with fetal tissues.

Several laboratories have reported the synthesis and secretion into the blood of a specific component of the embryonal serum α_1 fetoprotein, by a variety of human (and other mammalian) tumors, although primarily those of liver origin. Abelev et al.[9] demonstrated that synthesis of this globulin occurs in approximately 70% of adult patients with primary carcinoma of the liver (thereby suggesting possible diagnostic value in such cases), as well as in the sera of some adult patients with testicular teratoblastomas. From their study of a series of malignant diseases of children, Mawar et al.[10] detected fetoprotein only in the sera of those patients with testicular or ovarian embryonal carcinomas, and suggested a rough correlation between the tumor mass (including metastases) and the amount of serum fetoprotein. In a much more extensive study, Masopust et al.[11] found that fetoprotein usually appears in two types of tumors only, hepatocellular carcinoma and malignant undifferentiated teratoma, although many other tumors of widely varying differentiation, including those of an embryonal nature, were negative. The diagnostic value of this test for patients of less than one year of age is suspect, as fetoprotein was also found in the sera of some patients of this age suffering from hepatitis or other liver diseases. The precise mechanism of the reappearance of this material is not known, nor why teratomas should be capable of synthesizing fetoprotein, which in human fetuses is considered to be produced only in the liver under normal developmental conditions.[12] All of the above investigators favor an explanation based on derepression of genetic information normally expressed at some stage of fetal development.

In addition to monitoring the synthesis of proteins of undefined function, such as α-fetoprotein, functional proteins have been demonstrated to revert to a more primitive nature in certain malignant conditions. For one, serum alkaline phosphatase isozyme (Regan isozyme), which is indistinguishable from the placental isozyme, has been shown to appear in a number of adult human cancer patients with tumors at a variety of primary organ sites.[13, 14] Again, this phenomenon is postulated to represent an example of genomic derepression leading to the synthesis of embryonic protein in a series of human cancers, thus far not including hepatomas.

Of potentially greater significance in the growth or rejection of a neoplasm is the appearance of new cellular antigens on or in the tumor cells. Work by Ivanov et al.[15] has demonstrated that the appearance of normal embryo-specific antigens in Zagdela ascitic rat hepatoma cells is accompanied by a sharp increase in the concentration of heteroorganic antigens (nonliver) and the complete loss of normal organospecific liver antigens. In this regard, the elegant studies of Gold and his colleagues over the past five years have clearly demonstrated the identity of a tumor-specific antigen with that of a normal fetal antigen.[16-22]

By working with adenocarcinoma of the human colon, these workers had the advantage of a highly localized neoplasm, which enabled them to obtain control tissue and tumor material from the same patients, thereby eliminating the complication of isoantigens in their search for a tumor-specific antigen.[16] Heterologous rabbit sera were made specific for tumor antigens both by adsorption with control colon tissue and by preparing some sera in rabbits previously made tolerant to control tissue. Using these sera in a variety of immunologic procedures, they demonstrated the presence of new antigens identical in all colon adenocarcinomas studied from unrelated individuals, and absent in control colonic tissue from these same patients.[16] In a subsequent study,[17] the distribution of this antigen was examined; it was found that this antigenic moiety could be detected in all malignant tumors of the adult digestive system (with a gradient of decreasing concentration proportional to the higher levels of the gastrointestinal tract), yet it was absent in the corresponding normal tissue. It was also found to be present in normal human fetal gut, liver, and pancreas between two and six months' gestation. However, in the third trimester of pregnancy, it was absent from these fetal tissues. The antigen has thus been denoted the carcinoembryonic antigen (CEA) of the human digestive system. Analysis of its distribution revealed that CEA can be found only in tissues derived from (or part of) the embryonic entoderm. With respect to the mechanism of the appearance of CEA in digestive system tumors, the authors state, ". . . the carcinoembryonic antigens represent cellular constituents which are repressed during the course of differentiation of the normal digestive system epithelium and reappear in the corresponding malignant cells by a process of derepressive-dedifferentiation."[17] It should be noted that the presence of CEA is a function of the site of tumor origin and not tumor growth, in that metastases from the digestive system contain CEA while metastases to the digestive system from organs outside of it lack CEA. Also, the degree of tissue disorganization appears to be involved, since benign tumors of the gastrointestinal tract lack CEA.

What is the relevance of CEA to the fate of a digestive system tumor? As might be expected of a potential transplantation antigen, CEA has been localized to the tumor cell surface.[18] Purification and biochemical characterization of CEA reveal it to be a glycoprotein containing no abnormal sugars;[19] the antigenic specificity resides in the carbohydrate portion. Studies of the sera of patients with digestive system tumors have detected anti-CEA antibody activity in 70% of patients with nonmetastatic cancer, but no activity in normal subjects of those with tumors of other organs.[20] Furthermore, anti-CEA antibodies were also found in the majority of pregnant and postpartum women studied. The ability of a primary tumor to grow in the presence of high anti-

CEA antibody titers suggests that this antibody may have little relevance to tumor rejection, and it may, in fact, represent enhancing antibody. The inability to detect anti-CEA antibody activity after tumor metastasis led to the hypothesis that the increased tumor mass is acting as an "antigenic sponge" to remove specific circulating antibody.[20] However, more recent studies have demonstrated the presence of CEA-anti-CEA antibody complexes in the serum; it now appears that CEA is readily solubilized from the surface of the tumor cell and proceeds to bind to circulating antibody, thereby lowering the titer of free antibody.[21, 22] Thus, instead of the increased tumor mass after metastasis removing antibody by "antigenic sponging," it appears that increased amounts of CEA are solubilized, which then bind greater amounts of antibody. The potential diagnostic use of this situation has been suggested in preliminary experiments, where, by monitoring the level of these complexes in the serum after surgical removal of primary colon and rectum tumors, an early indication of tumor regrowth or undiscovered metastases has been provided by a rise in their level.

As stated earlier, Gold and coworkers,[16–22] in agreement with the other studies mentioned above, proposed a genetic mechanism to explain the disappearance of CEA during embryogenesis and its reappearance in neoplastic tissues. Preliminary studies suggest that some of the new antigens induced by oncogenic DNA viruses may represent antigens normally expressed in fetal tissue. Such cross-reactions have recently been obtained between polyoma-transformed hamster cells and normal hamster embryonic cells.[23] Furthermore, sera from gravid hamsters never having experienced infection with SV40 virus or exposure to transformed cells behave similarly in membrane immunofluorescent staining to sera from hamsters immunized against the SV40 S antigen.[2, 25] Last, initial studies suggest that the SV40 cytostatic antibody in hamsters can be induced both by hamster and mouse embryonic cells, but not by adult cells of either species.[26]

EXPOSURE OF CRYPTIC MEMBRANE SITES

As stated, the appearance of new surface antigens may be attributable to the failure to synthesize membrane materials. This same result can be achieved experimentally by treating normal cells with various enzymes which can be shown to expose underlying antigenic sites. We shall review the immunologic as well as biochemical data which may provide insights into the mechanism of exposure of cryptic antigenic sites.

FAILURE TO SYNTHESIZE MEMBRANE SUBSTANCE.—The loss of organospecific antigens in tumor tissue has been mentioned. Although the precise biochemical delineation of such loss is not available, several studies have provided biochemical explanations for the loss of blood group antigens in neoplastic tissue. Loss of blood group antigens has been reported in several human cancers, including bladder carcinoma[27] and carcinoma of the lung.[28] In the latter study, antigenic analysis revealed a loss of isoantigens A, B, and H in the tumor tissue. A thorough biochemical analysis has been made of a human adenocarcinoma derived from a patient with Blood Group A.[29] It was found that a fucose-containing glycolipid isolated from this tumor lacked Blood Group A reactivity. Instead, it had weak H reactivity, moderate Lewis[a] activity, and was precipitated by Type 14 pneumococcal antiserum after mild acid hydrolysis. Since the chemical groups for these antigenic reactivities appear as the substructure within the glycolipid core of Blood Group A, it was postulated that the tumor glycolipid arose from aberrations in the synthesis of glycolipids possessing Blood Group A reactivity. Such aberrations in this instance would correspond to the loss of N-acetylgalactosaminyl, galactosyl, and $\alpha(1,2)$-L-fucosyl residues from the glycolipids and/or the glycoproteins of the carcinoma. According to this hypothesis, the precursors which are the core structures of the blood groups would accumulate at the cell surface.

Other studies have revealed the presence of a new heterophile antigenic reactivity in certain virus-transformed cells. Such Forssman reactivity has been found on the surfaces of SV40- and polyoma-transformed hamster cells.[30, 31] The chemical structure of horse Forssman glycolipid has been described;[32] it is believed that the antigenic reactivity of Forssman glycolipid resides in the terminal disaccharide portion of the molecule. This disaccharide portion of the molecule is similar to that of Blood Group A, but differs from Blood Group A in that a fucose moiety is attached to the galactosyl portion of the latter compound by an $\alpha(1\rightarrow2)$ linkage. Thus, it was postulated that Forssman reactivity may be covered normally by the presence of a blocking sugar, in this case fucose.[30] Inability to add this fucose moiety to the glycolipid substructure of the blood groups might then result in the appearance of Forssman reactivity. It is of interest that hamster cells cultivated in vitro become Forssman-reactive after several days in tissue culture.[33, 34] This would suggest that the Forssman reactivity becomes uncovered as cells are propagated in vitro, which may be similar to the uncovering which occurs with viral transformation.

Hakomori and Murakami[35] have shown that the major glycolipid of a continuous line of hamster fibroblasts (BHK-21) was hematoside (N-acetylneuraminyllactosylceramide), while the main glycolipid of polyoma virus-transformed BHK-21 cells was lactosyl ceramide (cytolipin H).[35] Thus, it appears that the transformed cell glycolipid lacks a sialic acid residue. These authors have correlated the degree of contact inhibition with the amount of hematoside present in normal and transformed cells; cells which are most contact-inhibited contain the most hematoside. Antisera were prepared against the gangliosides of the malignant cell; these cause cytoagglutination of the transformed cell. Gangliosides from normal cells would not inhibit this cytoagglutination. However, normal gangliosides could be converted to a material capable of inhibiting the malignant cytoagglutination by the Smith degradation (oxidation of normal ganglioside fraction in aqueous solution with 0.01 M sodium metaperiodate for 1 hour, followed by sodium borohydride treatment and weak acid hydrolysis). This suggests that a reactive group is masked in the normal ganglioside by a periodate-susceptible group, either galactose or fucose. In a recent study, it was found that further exposure of hematoside in the normal cell could be achieved by treatment with the proteolytic enzyme trypsin.[36] This suggests that the normal cell has a proteinaceous or glycoprotein cover on the surface. In the cancer cell, the cryptic hematoside component is further uncovered. Although the total amount of hematoside in transformed cells was significantly lower than in normal cells, the reactivity of surface hematoside to antihematoside serum was found to be higher in the transformed cells; trypsin-treated normal cells, however, had the highest reactivity. Thus, these studies indicate that in the polyoma-transformed BHK-21 cell there seems to be a failure to add sugars such as galactose or fucose, as determined by the Smith degradation studies; amino sugars such as sialic acid, as determined by the ganglioside analyses; and glycoprotein or protein material, as determined by the trypsin treatment of normal cells, as compared to the cell membrane of the transformed cells.

In still other studies, Mora et al. reported a decrease in the higher ganglioside homologues disialo-ceramidetetrahexoside and monosialo-ceramidetetrahexoside in SV40-transformed mouse cells.[37] The absence of these higher gangliosides corresponded with increased saturation density and increased transplantability of these transformed mouse cell lines. The higher gangliosides were not found to be diminished in spontaneously transformed cells which had saturation densities which were intermediate between that of normal and virus-transformed cells.

The studies enumerated, namely the glycolipid analyses of a human colon cancer, the ganglioside studies of polyoma-transformed BHK-21 and SV40-transformed mouse cells, and the Forssman studies, all suggest that there is a failure to complete synthesis of ganglioside or glycolipid portions of the cell membrane of tumor cells. It had previously been found that lactosyl ceramide (cytolipin H) is a tumor-specific hapten which is found in many human tumors.[38] We have seen that cytolipin H is the predominant sphingoglycolipid in polyoma-transformed hamster cells. The presence of this tumor-specific hapten in tumors evokes the formation of an agglutination factor which may be found in sera of cancer patients and normal pregnant females,[39] which again suggests a relationship between tumor and fetal components. This factor is specifically inhibited by cytolipin H, but not by similar glycosphingolipids. In HeLa cells and other cancer cells, the cell surface receptor for this factor was found to be identical to cytolipin H.[39] This phenomenon, whereby new agglutinable sites appear on the surface of cancer cells, will now be considered.

AGGLUTINABLE SITES.—In 1963, Aub and coworkers reported that an agglutinin, present as a contaminant in a wheat germ lipase extract, produced clumping in mouse tumor cells.[40] In general, malignant cells agglutinated more strongly than their nonmalignant counterparts. Burger and Goldberg purified the active component and found it to be a glycoprotein with a mol wt of approximately 26,000.[41] They also demonstrated that the specific surface site that interacts with the agglutinin contains N-acetyl-glucosamine. Agglutination could be inhibited by N-acetyl-glucosamine, di-N-acetyl-chitobiose, and ovomucoid; these compounds all contain N-acetyl-glucosamine.

Burger further isolated the receptor complex from the surface of neoplastic cells.[42] This agglutination site had strong hapten-inhibition properties. The agglutination site could be uncovered in normal cells after trypsin or other protease treatments.[43] The same inhibitors, in the same concentrations, prevented agglutination of enzyme-treated normal cells and the dissociation kinetics with inhibitors were similar. It was further found that this cytoagglutinin, which had been purified from wheat germ lipase, agglutinated various transformed lines in direct proportion to their saturation densities, i.e. the most agglutinable lines were the least contact-inhibited and grew to highest saturation densities.[44] Preincubation of the tumor lines with trypsin enhanced their agglutinability. Thus, it appears that this receptor site, present in tumor cells, is covered in normal cells; its presence seems to be correlated with the loss of contact inhibition.

It is not known at this time whether the N-acetyl-glucosamine or di-N-acetyl-chitobiose in the membrane is linked to glycolipids or glycoproteins; actually, the major portion of these amino sugars is found in the glycoprotein and mucopolysaccharide fractions of the cell membrane. Thus, these may be the agglutination receptors. A recent study pointed out a lack of correlation between agglutinability of tumor and nontumor cells by wheat germ agglutinin and their transplantability.[45] In these studies, there did seem to be a direct relationship between saturation density and agglutinability. However, the cell lines utilized were maintained in different types of media and in some cases without serum; thus limited conclusions from this study seem warranted.

Another agglutinin, Concanavalin A, is a protein isolated from crystalline jack bean meal. This protein agglutinates cells transformed by viruses, chemicals and x rays.[46] The specific agglutinable site has been found to be alpha-methyl-D-glucopyranoside, and the agglutination reaction can be specifically inhibited by adsorption with this substance. Normal cells treated with trypsin agglutinate with Concanavalin A.

The studies with various agglutinins indicate that agglutinin-specific sites are unmasked in cancer cells. Treatment of normal cells with various enzymes can expose these specific sites. Additional enzymatic studies in which surface components are hydrolized to reveal antigenic sites will now be considered.

ENZYME TREATMENT OF TUMOR CELLS.—We have seen that tumor cells have exposed antigenic or agglutinable sites caused by failure to synthesize membrane material. We have also considered several instances in which similar sites have been revealed after treatment of normal cells with proteolytic enzymes. We shall briefly consider some studies in which tumor-specific transplantation antigens are unmasked in tumor as well as normal cells by enzymatic treatment.

Many of these studies have been directed at the cell wall sialomucins, and have been made with the enzyme neuraminidase. They have revealed that tumor cell antigens are exposed after treatment of tumor cells with neuraminidase. Thus, use of this enzyme has unmasked the antigenicity of several experimental tumors, including the TA_3 ascites mouse tumor,[47] L 1210 murine leukemia cells,[48] and the Landschultz ascites tumor.[49] After exposure to neuraminidase, inoculation of the treated cells resulted in enhanced tumor immunity and an increase in circulating antitumor agglutinins. In addition to uncovering tumor-specific transplantation antigens, it has been found that normal transplantation-resistant antigens can be unmasked by neuraminidase. Thus, treatment of mouse trophoblast cells with neuraminidase resulted in the appearance of H2 antigenic reactivity which is normally masked.[50] These results suggest that further uncovering of cryptic antigenic sites results in an enhanced antigenicity.

Biochemical Studies of Sugars and Glycoproteins

The finding of lower amounts of sialic acid in polyoma-transformed BHK-21 cells by Hakamori and Murakami has been mentioned.[35] Other reports of lower amounts of sialic acid in polyoma virus- and SV40-transformed cells have appeared.[51, 52] Thus, data from three laboratories indicate that there is a diminished amount of sialic acid in transformed cells; this is in contrast to previous studies which indicated increased amounts of sialic acid in polyoma-transformed cells.[53, 54] Comparative biochemical studies have been done with normal and SV40-transformed mouse fibroblasts. These studies have indicated a lower amount of neutral and amino sugars in transformed cell surface membranes.[51] The sugars analyzed were N-acetyl-neuraminic acid, N-acetyl-galactosamine, N-acetyl-glucosamine, fucose, mannose, galactose, and glucose. It is of interest that a spontaneously transformed mouse cell line, derived from the normal cell line, contained levels of neutral and amino sugars which were intermediate between those of normal and virus-transformed lines. The spontaneously transformed cells also grew to a saturation density which was intermediate between the normal and transformed lines. The neutral and amino sugar levels were the same in all particulate fractions of a given cell line; however, levels of these sugars were comparable in the nucleotide sugar fraction. Thus, the changes in membrane carbohydrate composition in virus-transformed cells could not be attributed to a lack of particular nucleotide sugar precursors. It was postulated that the defect in transformed cells was attributable either to the absence or diminished concentration of transferase enzymes, which transfer sugars from the nucleotide pool to the membrane, or to a defect in the membrane attachment site.[51, 55] Recent studies have revealed diminished levels of sialyl transferase enzyme, which transfers sialic acid from the nucleotide sugar pool to the cell surface, in transformed cell lines.[56] The levels of sialyl transferase, in general, are proportional to the amounts of sialic acid present in the cell membrane. Thus, they are lowest in transformed cell lines, intermediate in spontaneously transformed cells, and highest in untransformed cells. These studies suggest that the sialyl transferase enzyme may be rate-limiting with respect to the amount of sialic acid on the various cellular membranes. It is of interest that another transferase enzyme, the collagen-glucosyl transferase, has been found to be lower in SV40-transformed mouse cells.[57] However, one report provides data that SV40-transformed fibroblasts contained greater activities of membrane glycoprotein:glycosyl transferases per cell or unit protein than untransformed cells; the increases were approximately twice the levels of enzyme in nontransformed cells.[58] In these studies, transferase enzymes were extracted with 0.1% Triton X-100; however, the differential solubilities of these enzymes, whether from normal or transformed cells, were not established. Additional studies, therefore, will be needed in order to establish, definitively, the role of the transferase enzymes in determining the altered sugar composition of the transformed cell membranes.

Other enzymes participating in carbohydrate metabolism may, of course, be responsible for the observed changes in the composition of transformed cell membranes. The galactose-epimerase "choke" which has been investigated by Kalckar should be mentioned.[59, 60] Very low levels of Gal-1-P uridyl transferase and UDP-galactose 4-epimerase were found in several lines of tumor cells; it was postulated that the latter enzyme may be rate-limiting in determining the availability of galactose to the tumor cell.[61] It should be mentioned, however, that membrane galactose levels of transformed cells in the studies described above were the least depressed.[51]

To examine the change in the composition of membrane glycoproteins in greater detail, labeled membrane fractions derived from normal and SV40-transformed mouse cells were fractionated and chromatographed on Sephadex G-150 columns in the presence of sodium dodecyl sulfate.[55] In another series of experiments, membrane glycoproteins were digested with the proteolytic enzyme, pronase, followed by fractionation of the glycopeptide mixture on Sephadex G-50.[55] The pattern of glycopeptides seen with one membrane fraction were reflected in all the membranes of a given cell line. Several differences between normal and transformed cell glycoprotein and glycopeptide fractions were revealed. In particular, a glycoprotein (s) appearing in a fraction corresponding to a mol wt of approximately 20,000 was found to be present in greater amounts in normal mouse cells than in SV40-transformed mouse cells. A similar diminution of this glycopeptide (s) was seen when normal mouse cells were analyzed while in the logarithmic phase of cell growth. These studies suggest that certain components of the membrane may be altered rather drastically, not only as a result of transformation but even as a result of the shift from the growing state to confluence, and provide evidence that there may be a physiologic control of membrane structure. The findings reaffirm the existence of structural changes in the cellular membranes accompanying viral transformation.

The biochemical studies described provide an explanation for the failure to complete glycolipid and/or glycoprotein synthesis of the surface membrane. They further indicate that the changes observed in the plasma membrane are reflected in other membranes of the cell. Thus, if the transferase enzymes are rate-limiting, it might be postulated that an individual transferase enzyme transfers a sugar or amino sugar from the nucleotide pool to all membranes of the cell. This finding is of interest, since it indicates that changes observed in the plasma membrane may be accompanied by changes in the nuclear membrane, for example. Since DNA synthesis in bacteria,[62] and mammalian cells as well,[63] may be dependent on binding of DNA to the nuclear membrane, changes in this membrane could, conceivably, result in abnormal DNA biosynthesis. Such a hypothesis would provide the long-sought connection between the plasma membrane and DNA replication in the cancer cell. The biochemical findings described supplement immunologic data which indicate that similar antigenic groupings may be present on the various membranes of the cell. For example, an immunologic cross-reactivity has been demonstrated between the plasma membrane and the endoplasmic reticulum in Ehrlich ascites carcinoma cells.[64] In addition, tumor-specific antigens have been found in various membranes of an amino azo-dye induced rat hepatoma.[65]

Reversion

To determine the relationship between the viral genome and the phenotypic changes observed in the transformed cells, revertant cells have been isolated from transformed cells in several laboratories. Using the FUdR method of Pollack et al.,[66] revertant cells which are contact-inhibited have been recovered. These cells have a diminished plating efficiency, do not grow in agar, and are less transplantable to animals.[67] However, the tumors that did arise were similar to wild-type tumors in morphology and pattern of tumor growth. When cell lines were established from these tumors, the cells were as contact-inhibited as the inoculated cells; this indicates that passage through the animal did not lead to selection of a common transplantable cell type. All revertants isolated by this FUdR method contained the complete SV40 viral genome[66, 71] and did not agglutinate with wheat germ agglutinin.[44]

Revertants have also been isolated in vivo[68] and in vitro[69] by other techniques; the latter revertants have been recovered when plated on glutaraldehyde-fixed cells. As with the FUdR revertants, these show diminished cloning efficiency in fluid or agar and grow to saturation densities similar to the untransformed cells. These revertants agglutinate with Concanavalin A to a variable degree.[70] Restoration of the ability to be agglutinated by Concanavalin A can be effected by treatment of the cells with trypsin. Unlike the FUdR revertants, these transplant to animals with a higher degree of tumorigenicity.[70]

The isolation of revertant cells which contain the viral genome offers an opportunity to answer two important questions: (1) Does the viral genome specify the changes in neutral and amino sugars present in transformed cell membranes? (2) Are the sugar changes responsible for the altered growth pattern and neoplastic potential of the transformed cell?

Answers to these questions were sought by investigating the chemical properties of a revertant isolated by the FUdR technique.[71] It was found that the sialic acid content of the plasma membrane of the revertant cell was approximately that of the nontransformed cell.[72] These studies indicate that the viral genome does not specify the sugar changes which have been described. They suggest, furthermore, that these changes may be related to the growth characteristics of these cells in vitro; transplantation of this revertant cell line has not been attempted.

Significance

One may question the significance of the changes described in transformed cells. Do they contribute in any way to the loss of growth restraint of or offer any growth advantage to the transformed cell? In this respect it is noteworthy that various growth-promoting substances isolated from the medium bathing transformed cells have the ability to promote growth and increase plating efficiency. Thus, the factor described by Rubin which promotes growth can be mimicked by treatment with the proteolytic enzyme, trypsin.[73] Moreover, other growth factors, such as the nerve growth factor[74] and a growth factor isolated from submaxillary glands,[75] also have proteolytic activity. These studies suggest that proteolytic cleavage of a portion of the cell membrane might be related to the enhanced growth potential. The observations that transformed cells have incomplete glycolipids and/or glycoproteins in the plasma membrane would be compatible with this hypothesis.

Increasing evidence is accumulating that glycoproteins and sialic acid may be important mediators of normal cell-to-cell contact. The studies of Crandall and Brock have indicated that complementary macromolecules, which are glycoproteins of low molecular weight, are present in yeasts of opposite mating types.[76] The strong adhesion between cells during sexual agglutination, therefore, is dependent on the presence of these complementary glycoproteins.

Sialic acid may be an important factor regulating cell-to-cell relationships since it is a terminal amino sugar and has an electronegative charge at physiologic pH. Studies of embryonic chick muscle in tissue culture have indicated that aggregation can be prevented by treatment of these cultures with neuraminidase.[77] This implies that normal aggregation is dependent on the presence of sialic acid. We have mentioned that sialic acid concentrations are lower in transformed cell membranes. Furthermore, the revertant cells which contain normal levels of sialic acid have growth properties similar to those of untransformed cells.[71] It is possible that the absence of this amino sugar may be a factor in the loss of normal cell-to-cell interaction which characterizes the cancer cell.

In view of the studies presented, it seems unlikely, as has been postulated in the past,[78] that the sialic acid in transformed cells is responsible for the increase in the electronegative surface charge which characterizes tumor cells in general. The increased net negative charge could be caused by a loss of positively charged amino sugars and, indeed, may be responsible for the lack of adherence between tumor cells because of mutual repulsion.[79] What the relationship of this negative charge is to the asocial behavior of the tumor cell, if any, is not known. Several interesting experiments are being carried out at present to determine the importance of the increased electronegative surface charge. Organ cultures of fetal mouse heart have been exposed to the cationic polyelectrolyte poly-l-lysine and toluidine blue dye in an effort to neutralize the negative charge.[80] It was found that poly-l-lysine adsorbed to the cell and diminished the ability of the cell to move and therefore invade. Toluidine blue produced polarization of polyoma-transformed BHK-21 cells and also seemed to diminish their invasive powers. It cannot be concluded, however, from these studies that the effects were attributable to a neutralization of the negative charge. These same authors attempted to remove sialic acid enzymatically from tumor cells and to determine the effect of such removal on the invasive properties of the cell.[81] Some suggestion that the invasive properties of polyoma-transformed BHK-21 cells were lessened was obtained, but there was no evidence that this was followed by an enhanced mutual adhesion or any return of mutual contact inhibition.

The role that the surface glycoproteins and/or glycolipids play in the electrical coupling of cells is unknown. It would be of immense importance to relate any changes in sugar and/or glycoprotein composition of the surface membrane with the inability to form tight junctions or nexus or to be electrically coupled with an adjacent cell.[82-83]

Perhaps the most important aspect of the appearance of new antigenic reactivity on the surface of transformed cells has to do with the host response. The viral transplantation antigens are foreign to the cell and evoke a cell-mediated immune response. That the new non-specific antigens derived from host information, whether derepressed or uncovered, are antigenic is apparent from the antibody response of the host. Thus, for example, humoral immunity is evoked by the carcinoembryonal antigens. The role of this circulating antibody in the rejection or enhancement of tumor formation is unknown, as has been mentioned earlier. It is most probable that cellular immune mechanisms are the prime defense against the elimination of tumor cells. Whether cell-mediated immune mechanisms are directed against derepressed or uncovered antigenic sites is not readily apparent at the present time. If a "split-tolerance" exists, in which the host fails to respond with a cellular immunity, an explanation of persistent tumor growth will be available. Moreover, a rational approach for the therapy of such cancers might involve attempts to break such tolerance. It should be noted, however, that the presence of enhancing antibodies might also account for progressive tumor growth, despite the presence of an active cellular immune response.

Acknowledgments

This investigation was supported by Grant CA-10126-04 from the National Cancer Institute, U. S. Public Health Service.

References

1. Habel, K.: Cancer Research, 28:1825, 1968.
2. Tevethia, S. S., M. Katz, and F. Rapp: Proc. Soc. Exp. Biol. Med., 119:896, 1965.
3. Kluchareva, T. E., K. L. Shachanina, S. Belova, V. Chibisova, and G. I. Deichman: J. Nat. Cancer Inst., 39:825, 1967.
4. Irlin, I.: Virology, 32:725, 1967.
5. Malmgrem, R. A., K. K. Takemoto, and P. G. Carney: J. Nat. Cancer Inst., 40:263, 1968.
6. Tevethia, S. S., G. T. Diamandopoulos, F. Rapp, and J. F. Enders: J. Immunol., 101:1192, 1968.
7. Levin, M. J., M. N. Oxman, G. T. Diamandopoulos, A. S. Levine, P. H. Henry, and J. F. Enders: Proc. Nat. Acad. Sci. USA, 62:589, 1969.
8. Collins, J., and P. H. Black: Unpublished data.
9. Abelev, G. I., I. V. Assecritova, N. A. Kraevsky, S. D. Perova, and N. I. Perevodchikova: Internat. J. Cancer, 2:551, 1967.
10. Mawas, C., M. Kohen, J. Lemerle, D. Buffe, O. Schwersguth, and P. Burtin: Internat. J. Cancer, 4:76, 1969.
11. Masopust, J., K. Kithier, J. Radl, J. Koutecky, and L. Kotal: Internat. J. Cancer, 3:364, 1968.
12. Gitlin, D., and M. Boesman: J. Clin. Invest., 45:1826, 1966.

13. Fishman, W. H., N. R. Inglis, L. L. Stolbach, and M. J. Krant: Cancer Res., 28:150, 1968.
14. Fishman, W. H., N. R. Inglis, S. Green, C. L. Anstiss, N. K. Gosh, A. E. Reif, R. Rustigian, M. J. Krant, and L. L. Stolbach: Nature, 219:697, 1968.
15. Ivanov, V. A., V. Ja. Fel, and J. M. Olenov: Cancer Res., 28:1524, 1968.
16. Gold, P., and S. O. Freedman: J. Exp. Med., 121:430, 1965.
17. Gold, P., and S. O. Freedman: J. Exp. Med., 122:467, 1965.
18. Gold, P., M. Gold, and S. O. Freedman: Cancer Res., 28:1331, 1968.
19. Krupey, J., P. Gold, and S. O. Freedman: Nature, 215:67, 1967.
20. Gold, P.: Cancer, 20:1663, 1967.
21. Thomson, D. M. P., J. Krupey, S. O. Freedman, and P. Gold: Proc. Nat. Acad. Sci. USA, 64:161, 1969.
22. Gold, P.: Personal communication.
23. Pearson, G., and G. Freeman: Cancer Res., 28:1665, 1968.
24. Tevethia, S. S., L. A. Corivillion, and F. Rapp: J. Immunol., 100:358, 1968.
25. Duff, R., and F. Rapp: Bacteriol. Proc., p. 172, 1970.
26. Ambrose, K. A., and J. H. Coggin, Jr.: Bacteriol. Proc., p. 187, 1970.
27. Kay, H. E. M., and D. M. Wallace: J. Nat. Cancer Inst., 26:1349, 1961.
28. Davidsohn, I., and Y. N. Louisa: Amer. J. Path., 57:307, 1969.
29. Hakomori, S., J. Koscielak, K. J. Bloch, and R. W. Jeanloz: J. Immunol., 98:31, 1967.
30. Robertson, H. T., and P. H. Black: Proc. Soc. Exp. Biol. Med., 130:363, 1969.
31. O'Neill, C. H.: J. Cell Sci., 3:405, 1968.
32. Makita, A., C. Suzuki, and Z. Yosizawa: J. Biochem., 60:502, 1966.
33. Fogel, M., and L. Sachs: Exp. Cell Res., 34:448, 1964.
34. Fogel, M., and L. Sachs: Dev. Biol., 10:411, 1964.
35. Hakomori, S., and W. T. Murakami: Proc. Nat. Acad. Sci. USA, 59:254, 1968.
36. Hakomori, S., C. Teather, and H. Andrews: Biochem. Biophys. Res. Comm., 33:563, 1968.
37. Mora, P. T., R. O. Brady, R. M. Bradley, and V. W. McFarland: Proc. Nat. Acad. Sci. USA, 63:1290, 1969.
38. Rapport, M. M., L. Graf, V. P. Skipski, and N. F. Alonzo: Nature, 181:1803, 1958.
39. Tal, C.: Proc. Nat. Acad. Sci. USA, 54:1318, 1965.
40. Aub, J. C., C. Tieslan, and A. Lankester: Proc. Nat. Acad. Sci. USA, 50:613, 1963.
41. Burger, M. M., and A. R. Goldberg: Proc. Nat. Acad. Sci. USA, 57:359, 1967.
42. Burger, M. M.: Nature, 219:499, 1968.
43. Burger, M. M.: Proc. Nat. Acad. Sci. USA, 62:994, 1969.
44. Pollack, R. E., and M. M. Burger: Proc. Nat. Acad. Sci. USA, 62:1074, 1969.
45. Gantt, R. R., J. R. Martin, and V. J. Evans: J. Nat. Cancer Inst., 42:369, 1969.
46. Inbar, M., and L. Sachs: Proc. Nat. Acad. Sci. USA, 63:1418, 1969.
47. Gasic, G., T. Gasic, and C. C. Stewart: Proc. Nat. Acad. Sci. USA, 61:46, 1968.
48. Bagshawe, K. D., and G. A. Currie: Nature, 218:1254, 1968.
49. Currie, G. A., and K. D. Bagshawe: Brit. J. Cancer, 22:588, 1968.
50. Currie, G. A., W. van Doorninck, and K. D. Bagshawe: Nature, 219:191, 1968.
51. Wu, H. C., E. Meezan, P. H. Black, and P. W. Robbins: Biochemistry, 8:2509, 1969.
52. Ohta, N., A. B. Pardee, B. R. McAuslan, and M. M. Burger: Biochim. Biophys. Acta, 158:98, 1968.
53. Forrester, J. A., E. J. Ambrose, and I. A. MacPherson: Nature, 196:1068, 1962.
54. Forrester, J. A., E. J. Ambrose, and M. Stoker: Nature, 221:945, 1964.
55. Meezan, E., H. C. Wu, P. H. Black, and P. W. Robbins: Biochemistry, 8:2518, 1969.
56. Grimes, W., and P. W. Robbins: Unpublished data.
57. Bosmann, H. B., and E. H. Eylar: Nature, 218:582, 1968.
58. Bosmann, H. B., A. Hagopian, and E. H. Eylar: J. Cell. Physiol., 72:81, 1968.
59. Kalckar, H. M.: Nat. Cancer Inst. Monogr., 14:21, 1964.
60. Kalckar, H. M.: Science, 150:305, 1965.

61. Robinson, E. A., H. M. Kalckar, and H. Troedsson: J. Biol. Chem., 241:2737, 1966.
62. Svedka, N., and W. G. Quinn: Cold Spring Harbor Symp. Quant. Biol., 33:695, 1968.
63. Comings, D. E., and T. Kakefuda: J. Molec. Biol., 33:215, 1968.
64. Wallach, D. F. H., and V. Vlahovic: Nature, 216:182, 1967.
65. Baldwin, R. W., and M. Moore: Internat. J. Cancer, 4:753, 1969.
66. Pollack, R. E., H. Green, and G. Todaro: Proc. Nat. Acad. Sci. USA, 60:126, 1968.
67. Pollack, R. E., and G. W. Teebor: Cancer Res., 29:1770, 1969.
68. Rabinowitz, Z., and L. Sachs: Virology, 38:336, 1969.
69. Rabinowitz, Z., and L. Sachs: Virology, 38:343, 1969.
70. Inbar, M., Z. Rabinowitz, and L. Sachs: Internat. J. Cancer, 4:690, 1969.
71. Culp, L., and P. H. Black: Unpublished data.
72. Culp, L., W. Grimes, and P. H. Black: Unpublished data.
73. Rubin, H.: Science, 167:1271, 1970.
74. Greene, L. A., E. M. Shooter, and S. Varon: Proc. Nat. Acad. Sci. USA, 60:1383, 1968.
75. Attardi, D. G., M. J. Schlesinger, and S. Schlesinger: Science, 156:1253, 1967.
76. Crandall, M. A., and T. D. Brock: Science, 161:473, 1968.
77. Kemp, R. B.: Nature, 218:1255, 1968.
78. Ambrose, E. J.: Progr. Biophys. Molec. Biol., 16:243, 1966.
79. Curtis, A. S. G.: Amer. Nature, 94:37, 1960.
80. Yarnell, M. M., and E. J. Ambrose: Europ. J. Cancer, 5:255, 1969.
81. Yarnell, M. M., and E. J. Ambrose: Europ. J. Cancer, 5:265, 1969.
82. Loewenstein, W. R.: Ann. N. Y. Acad. Sci., 137:441, 1966.
83. Loewenstein, W. R., and Y. Kanno: Nature, 209:1248, 1966.

6

Tumor Antigens:
Clinical and Experimental

Historical Perspective

EVA KLEIN

Department of Tumor Biology, Karolinska Institute,
Stockholm, Sweden

THE DEVELOPMENT of tumor immunology has proceeded in three phases. During the first phase, the so-called "transplantable" tumors were used which grew also in allogeneic recipients. Their progressive growth was frequently taken as evidence for host-tumor compatibility (which it is not), and the high levels of resistance that could be attained by various forms of immunization generated the belief that tumor cells carry specific and strong antigens and that an immunologic solution of the cancer problem was near. This belief was badly shaken when inbred mouse strains were developed in the 1930's and 1940's, and it was shown that the antigenicity of tumors which arose in and were propagated in members of inbred strains could not be demonstrated in the same simple immunization procedures. The immunogenetic laws of tissue transplantation were, in fact, first discovered by experimenting with such systems.[1] These experiments led to the realization that the Mendelian segregation of histocompatibility genes governed the transplantability of neoplastic as well as of normal tissues. These "transplantable" tumors, which grew freely across genetic barriers, did so not because they lacked the relevant histocompatibility antigens, but because they somehow avoided the host response, and preimmunization against the relevant histocompatibility antigens caused their rejection. This evidence led to the opinion that all tumor rejection responses were probably transplantation artifacts and to gloomy conclusions about the role of immunology in cancer research.

A new era started around 1950 after the experiments by Gross[2] and Foley.[3] Foley ligated isografted, methylcholanthrene-induced sarcomas in C3H mice, inducing tumor necrosis. Subsequent challenge of the hosts with the same sarcoma frequently led to rejection, whereas previously uninoculated controls readily accepted identical grafts. It was unlikely that this was caused by residual heterozygosis within the strain, because mammary carcinomas of spontaneous origin, derived from and carried in the same strain, failed to show a similar difference between "ligated" and control groups. Prehn and Main[4] confirmed Foley's findings and showed that skin grafts could be readily exchanged between different members of their inbred strain, while MC sarcoma isografts were frequently rejected by hosts which had previously had a similar tumor ligated. Final proof of the existence of tumor-associated antigens was obtained when the capacity to reject methylcholanthrene-induced sarcomas was demonstrated in the autochthonous host.[5] These findings were rapidly followed by other reports on rejection responses by syngeneic or autochthonous hosts against indigenous tumors.

The reasons for the success of the experiments of the 1950's, particularly by contrast with the lack of success of similar experiments in the 1930's and '40's, is to be found in the attitudes and the level of expectations. Since it was possible to immunize against large numbers of cells from genetically foreign transplanted tumors, experiments to search for tumor-specific reactions in inbred strains were first designed in a similar manner. However, we know now that, with rare exceptions, tumor-specific antigens seldom induce more than relative resistance. The host response may, in fact, be indicated only by a prolongation of the latent period. When expectations became more realistic and the methodology was refined by using graded cell doses to compare growth in syngeneic preimmunized and control hosts, it became clear that most tumors can evoke at least a weak rejection response.

Studies on tumor-specific surface antigens in animals soon revealed a very important rule. Tumors induced by chemical carcinogens have individual antigens; cross immunization thus is rarely possible, even with tumors of similar morphology induced in members of an inbred strain by an identical carcinogen.[5, 6] This is true even for independently induced primary tumors in the same host.[7] In contrast, virus-induced tumors carry a virus-determined surface antigen which is common to all the tumors induced by the same virus, even if they are different in morphology. This fact makes cross-immunization feasible.[8-15]

We know more about the relation of tumor-specific transplantation antigen to the oncogenic stimulus in virus-induced tumors than in chemically induced ones. Cell surface antigens in tumors induced by DNA viruses are not identical to the antigens of the mature virion, and cellular antigens are present even when infectious virus production by the transformed cells cannot be demonstrated.[16] As the antigen is specific for the inducing virus, its presence and permanence provided the first evidence that viruses leave part of their genetic information in a cell after neoplastic transformation. In view of the cross-reactivity between cells of many different types and also between tumors induced in different species, it appears likely that the new transplantation antigens appearing on the surface of tumor cells induced by oncogenic DNA viruses are determined by the viral rather than the cellular genome. In leukemias induced by RNA viruses, the cell surface antigens may be shared with those of the virion.[17] These viruses mature at the cell membrane by budding, and during this process, the virus particles, which are continuously shed by the leukemia cells, receive an outer coat derived from the cell membrane.

The individually distinct antigenicity of chemically induced tumors is of considerable interest. Although it is often suggested that chemical carcinogens may act by the activation of latent oncogenic viruses, it is difficult to see how this explanation can be reconciled with known antigenic patterns. If altered antigenicity reflects a basic change in the neoplastic cell clone, occurring in relation to the transformation process, it follows that the exact details of the cellular change involved are likely to be at least slightly different in different interaction events between the same carcinogen and target cell type. The antigenic uniformity of virus-induced tumors may indicate that the cell changes in tumors arising in this way are identical. Recent results indicate that some viral tumors which carry a common group-specific transplantation antigen have, in addition, individually distinct rejection-inducing antigens as well.[18, 19] In the ordinary graft rejection test, as it usually is carried out with virus-induced tumors, i.e. by immunizing previously unexposed adult syngeneic recipients with irradiated cells or allogeneic tumor cells induced by the same virus, the existence of minor individual differences between tumors is masked by the group-specific cross-reacting antigen. The weaker individual antigens can be detected in conditions where tolerance prevails against the group-specific component.

The strength of antigenicity is usually determined in transplantation tests by assessing the maximum number of tumor cells which are rejected by preimmunized but accepted by untreated syngeneic hosts. While preimmunization either completely inhibits tumor takes or increases the threshold dose necessary for successful tumor transplantation, experimental manipulations known to inhibit immune response, such as total body irradiation,[20] neonatal thymectomy,[21] or treatment with antilymphocytic serum,[22] reduce the threshold dose.

That it is necessary to transplant a large number of tumor cells to ensure outgrowth is of itself suggestive of the presence of tumor-specific antigens. This initial transplant can evoke an immune response without any further manipulation; consequently, the minimum dose for a successful take depends at least in part on the antigenic strength of the tumor cells. The introduction of a small number of cells during the latent period can induce efficient immunization and lead to the rejection of subsequent tumor challenges; a larger number of cells, though it can evoke an immune response, may reach a large and unmanageable population size before significant immunity develops. One can often observe that small and large inocula grow, while medium-sized populations do not. The ability of a small primary inoculum to avoid rejection, to "sneak through" a self-induced immune response, is most probably caused by a discrepancy in timing which happens to favor the tumor rather than the host. Small numbers of tumor cells apparently present an inadequate antigenic stimulus to the host. The host is unable to respond with a sufficiently strong immune reaction before tumor growth has passed a threshold beyond which it is no longer possible to influence it by immunologic mechanisms acting alone. This phenomenon may partly explain why antigenic tumors can arise. It is known, too, that small numbers of tumor cells may grow relatively undisturbed within the shelter of a compact, differentiated tissue until they reach irreversible size. It follows from these observations that reinforcement of the host response during the latent period should reduce the frequency of tumor occurrence. This has, indeed, been found to occur in several systems.

Immunization against an antigenic tumor graft can be achieved by: (1) pretreatment with cells rendered incapable of multiplication; (2) pretreatment with living allogeneic tumor cells (obviously only in virus-induced, cross-reacting systems); (3) pretreatment with subthreshold doses of tumor cells; (4) pretreatment with subcellular fractions derived from tumor cells; (5) surgical removal or ligation of an existing tumor; and (6) contact with the inducing virus. (Viral tumors can usually be induced only after neonatal injection. If adult animals are infected with a virus, immunity develops against the virus and against isografts of tumors induced by that virus.)

The classic experiments demonstrating tumor-specific cell surface antigens were all done with transplantation tests. Later, attention turned to the analysis of different parameters of the immune response and the development of in vitro test systems. (This was most important since in the studies of human tumors, transplantation tests can be used to only a limited extent.) The role of cellular and humoral immunity was therefore studied by selecting animal host-tumor systems in which antigenicity was proved by transplantation. Techniques for these studies were provided by work on the immune response to histocompatibility antigens in which tumor cells were often used. Specific humoral antibodies and cell-mediated responses have been demonstrated. Humoral antibodies can be demonstrated by membrane immunofluorescence,[23-26] mixed hemadsorption,[27, 28] and immune adherence.[29, 30] Cytotoxicity tests work in some systems but not in others,[31, 32] but this is also true for the genetically determined transplantation antigens. Lymphoma and leukemia cells generally are more often sensitive in short-term cytotoxicity tests than are sarcoma or carcinoma cells.

Delayed cytotoxicity, measured by the reduction of cellular efficiency in tissue culture ("colony inhibition test"), is often successful in systems where short-term cytotoxicity experiments do not work.[33] It may be questioned, however, whether colony inhibition by antibodies in vitro necessarily means that the same antibodies will exert an inhibitory effect in vivo. The paradoxic phenomenon of immunologic enhancement[34] has been found to occur with tumor-specific antigens.[35, 36] A blocking action of humoral antibodies and the protection of antibody-coated target cells from the killing action of sensitized host lymphoid cells is illustrative of what may happen in vivo, at least in the case of relatively immunoresistant target cells.[37]

Sensitized lymphoid cells exert a more consistent inhibitory effect against target cells than do humoral antibodies. Their action can be demonstrated by mixing lymphoid cells and target cells before inoculation to syngeneic hosts,[38] or by studying the effect of lymphoid cells in tissue culture systems on target cell survival, growth, or plating efficiency.[33, 39]

The transplantation systems in which tumor-specific antigens are studied and in which healthy recipients are suddenly confronted with tumor cells differ in many ways from the host in which a tumor arises spontaneously. Differences in the relationship of the tumor cell to the host tissue, its growth pattern, and degree and timing of antigen release are factors which have to be considered. The successful outgrowth of a primary tumor may be facilitated by depressed immune reactivity of the primary host. It is therefore important to distinguish between immunologic host-tumor relationships in syngeneic and autochthonous hosts. The evidence that rejection-inducing potential in the experimental autochthonous host exists is provided by spontaneous regression of the Shope papilloma in the rabbit[40] and the murine sarcoma virus (MSV) induced sarcoma in mice.[41] Also, surgical removal of primary MC sarcomas followed by three inoculations of X-irradiated autochthonous sarcoma cells led to resistance to subsequent challenge of viable cells.[5] As a rule, the autochthonous resistance was weaker than the resistance of similarly preimmunized syngeneic controls. Similar results were obtained by Takeda et al. with rat MC tumors.[42] In these studies, a relationship also was found between antigenic strength and recurrence tendency, with strongly antigenic tumors showing fewer recurrences than weakly antigenic ones.

There is increasing evidence from in vitro studies of host antitumor activity in a variety of human tumors. However, in many cases antibodies and active lymphoid cells are detectable in patients with growing tumors, suggesting that the immune response, though active, had no significant tumor-limiting effect. In a number of cases this may be attributable to the interaction of effector components, in that instead of rejection, its opposite, enhancement dominates the eventual outcome.

In others, it may be attributable to the relative quantitative aspects discussed before, which also indicate important practical consequences. An immune response which might be inefficient when a large number of tumor cells are present may achieve decisive importance when the population size is brought down by some form of therapy.

Since tumors induced by the same virus possess common cell surface antigens, it is appropriate to consider whether the identification of such membrane-associated antigens in tumor groups could be interpreted as favoring the possibility of a viral etiology. In principle, this interpretation is feasible, but the situation is complicated by the occurrence of the phenomenon known as "antigenic conversion."[43-45] Virus-determined, group-specific transplantation or membrane-associated antigens can appear in established tumors because of the fortuitous acquisition of oncogenic or nononcogenic agents as passengers. For instance, the polyoma antigen can be introduced into methylcholanthrene-induced sarcomas or Moloney virus-induced lymphomas by superinfection with polyoma virus.[43,45] Antigens characteristic of murine leukemia agents can appear on the surface of carcinoma or sarcoma cells of other, independent origin and even on normal skin cells, by infection with the appropriate leukemia viruses.[46] This makes it obvious that the presence of a group-specific membrane antigen cannot of itself be regarded as conclusive evidence of viral etiology of a group of tumors. Collateral evidence will have to be sought, often on indirect lines, in order to distinguish between passenger viruses and oncogenic agents. The dilemma may be illustrated by findings in Burkitt's lymphoma and nasopharyngeal cancer.

It has been suggested that Burkitt's lymphoma has a viral etiology[47] and, indeed, in the majority of culture lines derived from Burkitt's lymphoma, a new herpeslike virus, Epstein-Barr (EB) virus, was detected by electron microscopy.[48-50] Later the EB virus was found to be involved most probably in the etiology of one form of infectious mononucleosis.[51, 52]

Antibodies reacting with the surface of Burkitt's cells have been detected by the immunofluorescence technique in the sera of most patients with Burkitt's lymphoma.[53] It was found that cells of culture lines which harbor the EB virus showed surface reactivity, but when virus was no longer present in the cell line, the membrane antigen disappeared.[54] It is thus considered that the cell membrane antigen is closely associated with the presence of EB virus in the culture.

In addition to the sera of Burkitt's lymphoma and infectious mononucleosis patients (the latter with comparatively lower titers), sera from patients with nasopharyngeal carcinoma regularly have high titers of EB virus-associated antibodies.[55] Based on analogy with findings in experimental systems, these findings would suggest that the EB virus is involved in the etiology of Burkitt's lymphoma and nasopharyngeal cancer also. If the virus were present in lymphoid cells merely as a passenger (nasopharyngeal cancer is usually heavily infiltrated with lymphoid cells), the same serologic pattern could also be obtained. However, no high titers of EB virus-associated antibodies occur regularly in other lymphoid malignant conditions.

After the demonstration of tumor-specific immunity, it is necessary to consider the various routes by which tumor cells can evade known forms of immune inhibition. Experimental evidence suggests that the mechanism of evasion may be: (1) inherent to the tumor cell, (2) related to host responses, and (3) active at the level of the host-tumor interaction.

1. The development of immunoresistance may be as important in tumor biology as drug resistance. The mechanisms underlying the development of immunoresistance on the cellular level are poorly understood, but in some instances this phenomenon is associated with decrease in surface antigen concentration.[56]

2. At the level of the host, immunologic tolerance is of considerable importance. So far, this has been demonstrated only when an essentially noncytopathogenic virus is transmitted vertically, i.e. from parent to offspring, within the natural host species.[57–60] This includes murine leukemia viruses, such as the Gross agent, carried in AKR mice and transmitted by both males and females,[57] or the mammary tumor agent, transmitted via the milk.[60] Horizontal transmission of the same agents to susceptible strains which have not received them by vertical transmission can induce tumors proved to be antigenic in syngeneic, agent-free recipients or in recipients infected with the agent as adults. Tolerance can also be brought about by the neonatal inoculation of other leukemogenic viruses, not known to be carried and vertically transmitted in the mouse strain studied.[58, 59] Such animals are unable to develop virus-neutralizing antibodies or antibodies directed against new cellular antigens determined by the same virus.

The radiation-induced leukemia virus of Kaplan represents an interesting situation. This virus is transmitted vertically in C57BL mice in a proviral or "switched off" form. Radiation activates the virus, which becomes extractable and capable of inducing leukemia. Although they carry the proviral agent, C57BL mice are not tolerant to the antigens which characterize the activated virus and the leukemias induced by it.[61] This suggests that the characteristic antigens for this virus system do not appear until and unless the virus is "switched on."

Immunosuppression, brought about by X-radiation, immunosuppressive drugs, antilymphocyte serum, or the natural decline in immune reactivity with old age, may be another important factor at the level of host responsiveness. A remarkable illustration was the demonstration that neonatal thymectomy renders adult mice liable to develop tumors after exposure to low doses of polyoma virus (e.g. room infection),[62] which are quite harmless to intact mice.

3. At the level of the host-tumor interaction, we have already dealt with the phenomenon of insufficient antigen release. An inadequate

supply of effector cells is also conceivable, particularly if the immune system is preoccupied with other immune reactions directed against antigens of different kinds. In addition to the inefficiency of the "numbers game" related to the race between tumor cell growth and rejector cell recruitment, the site of tumor proliferation may be inaccessible, e.g. tumor cells in the central nervous system. Neonatal thymectomy, known to increase the incidence of Rous sarcomas in virus-inoculated mice, had no effect when the virus was inoculated into the brain. This suggests that in an immunologically privileged site, surveillance plays no role in antagonizing tumor development. It is also of interest that the ultimately fatal course of Burkitt's lymphoma, a tumor in which host defenses are believed to play a relatively important role in inhibiting localized tumor growth, is frequently caused by the involvement of the central nervous system.[63]

The main immunotherapeutic dilemma is what the proper stimuli are, specific or nonspecific, and how they are best administered in order to achieve the objective, rejection, and avoid its opposite, enhancement. The rationale of introducing immune stimuli at a time when the tumor load confronting the host is minimal, i.e. after regression has been induced by chemotherapy, is obvious,[64] but the optimal form of stimulus and the best mode and timing of its administration is not. No a priori guidance can be given from experimental studies, because the same mode of administration, dosage, vehicle, etc. of the same preparation may favor rejection in one system and enhancement in another, depending on host species, tumor type, and individual characteristics of the tumor line.[65–67] Ideally, it would be desirable to develop methods that allow the quantitative assessment of cell-bound immunity and the synergistic or antagonistic action of humoral antibodies in relation to it in each untreated patient, and follow it subsequently during treatment. While this should be feasible, its practical application is still in the future. Meanwhile, an empirical approach, based on as much rational reasoning as the experimental models will allow, may yield important information, as the work of Mathé and his group clearly indicates.[68]

Acknowledgments

This work has been supported by grants from the Swedish Cancer Society, Contract No. 69.2005, within the Special Virus-Cancer Program of the National Cancer Institute, NIH, PHS, and the Medical Research Council.

References

1. Snell, G. D.: Biology of the Laboratory Mouse, McGraw-Hill, New York, 1966, p. 457.
2. Gross, L.: Cancer Res., 3:326, 1943.
3. Foley, E. J.: Cancer Res., 13:835, 1953.
4. Prehn, R. T., and J. M. Main: J. Nat. Cancer Inst., 18:769, 1967.
5. Klein, G., H. O. Sjögren, E. Klein, and K. E. Hellström: Cancer Res., 20:1561, 1960.

6. Sjögren, H. O., I. Hellström, and G. Klein: Cancer Res., 21:329, 1961.
7. Glöberson, A., and M. Feldman: J. Nat. Cancer Inst., 32:1229, 1964.
8. Sjögren, H. O., I. Hellström, and G. Klein: Cancer Res., 21:329, 1961.
9. Habel, K.: Proc. Soc. Exp. Biol. Med., 106:722, 1961.
10. Klein, G., H. O. Sjögren, and E. Klein: Cancer Res., 22:955, 1962.
11. Old, L. J., E. A. Boyse, and E. Stockert: J. Nat. Cancer Inst., 31:977, 1963.
12. Klein, E., and G. Klein: J. Nat. Cancer Inst., 32:547, 1964.
13. Goldner, H., A. J. Girardi, V. M. Larson, and M. R. Hilleman: Proc. Soc. Exp. Biol. Med., 117:851, 1964.
14. Pasternak, G.: J. Nat. Cancer Inst., 34:71, 1965.
15. Rich, M. A., J. Geldner, and P. Meyers: J. Nat. Cancer Inst., 35:523, 1965.
16. Sjögren, H. O.: Progr. Exp. Tumor Res., 6:289, 1965.
17. Klein, E., and G. Klein: Nature, 209:163, 1966.
18. Morton, D. L., G. F. Miller, and D. A. Wood: J. Nat. Cancer Inst., 42:289, 1969.
19. Vaage, J.: Nature, 218:101, 1968.
20. Klein, G., and E. Klein: Cold Spring Harbor Symp. Quant. Biol., 27:463, 1967.
21. Law, L. W.: Cancer Res., 26:551, 1966.
22. Bremberg, S., E. Klein, and J. Stjernswärd: Cancer Res., 27:2113, 1967.
23. Irlin, I. S.: Virology, 32:725, 1967.
24. Klein, E., and G. Klein: J. Nat. Cancer Inst., 32:547, 1964.
25. Pasternak, G.: J. Nat. Cancer Inst., 34:71, 1965.
26. Tevethia, S. S., L. A. Couvillion, and F. Rapp: J. Immunol., 100:358, 1968.
27. Barth, R. F., J. Å. Espmark, and A. Fagraeus: Biological Properties of the Mammalian Surface Membrane (L. P. Manson, ed.), Wistar Institute Symposium Monograph No. 8, 1968, p. 105.
28. Metzgar, R. S., and S. R. Eoltenisk: Cancer Res., 28:1366, 1968.
29. Nishioka, R., I. R. Furuse, T. Kawana, and S. Takeuchi: Internat. J. Cancer, 41:139, 1969.
30. Nishioka, K., T. Tachibana, G. Klein, and P. Clifford: Gann Monogr., 7:49, 1968.
31. Old, L. J., E. A. Boyse, D. A. Clarke, and E. A. Carswell: Ann. N. Y. Acad. Sci., 101:80, 1962.
32. Slettenmark, B., and E. Klein: Cancer Res., 22:947, 1962.
33. Hellström, I., and K. E. Hellström: Internat. J. Cancer, 5:195, 1970.
34. Kaliss, N.: Cancer Res., 18:992, 1958.
35. Batchelor, J. R.: Cancer Res., 28:1410, 1968.
36. Weiss, D. W., D. H. Lavrin, M. Dezfulian, J. Wager, and P. B. Blair: Viruses Inducing Cancer, Implications for Therapy (W. J. Burdette, ed.), University of Utah Press, Salt Lake City, 1966, p. 138.
37. Hellström, I., K. E. Hellström, C. A. Evans, G. H. Heppner, G. E. Pierce, and J. P. S. Yang: Proc. Nat. Acad. Sci. USA, 62:362, 1969.
38. Klein, E., and H. O. Sjögren: Cancer Res., 20:452, 1960.
39. Rosenau, W., and D. L. Morton: J. Nat. Cancer Inst., 36:825, 1966.
40. Evans, C. A., R. S. Weiser, and Y. Ito: Cold Spring Harbor Symp. Quant. Biol., 27:453, 1962.
41. Fefer, A., J. L. McCoy, K. Perk, and J. P. Glynn: Cancer Res., 28:1577, 1968.
42. Takeda, K., M. Aizawa, Y. Kikuchi, S. Yamawaki, and K. Nakamura: Gann, 57: 221, 1966.
43. Stück, B., L. J. Old, and E. A. Boyse: Nature, 202:1016, 1964.
44. Svet-Moldavsky, G. J., D. M. Mkheidze, and A. L. Liozner: J. Nat. Cancer Inst., 38:933, 1967.
45. Sjögren, H. O., and I. Hellström: Exp. Cell Res., 40:208, 1965.
46. Breyere, E. J., and L. B. Williams: Science, 146:1055, 1964.
47. Burkitt, D.: Internat. Rev. Exp. Path., 2:69, 1963.
48. Epstein, M. A., Y. M. Barr, and B. G. Achong: In: Methodological Approaches to the Study of Leukemia. Wistar Institute Symposium Monograph No. 4, 1965, p. 69.
49. Dalton, A. J., and V. H. Zeve: Cancer Res., 27:2465, 1967.
50. Epstein, M. A., and B. G. Achong: Cancer Res., 27:2489, 1967.

51. Niederman, J. C., R. W. McCollum, G. Henle, and W. Henle: J. Amer. Med. Ass., 203:205, 1968.
52. Henle, G., W. Henle, and W. Diehl: Proc. Nat. Acad. Sci. USA, 59:94, 1968.
53. Klein, G., P. Clifford, E. Klein, and J. Stjernswärd: Proc. Nat. Acad. Sci. USA, 55:1628, 1966.
54. Klein, G., G. Pearson, J. S. Nadkarni, J. J. Nadkarni, E. Klein, G. Henle, W. Henle, and P. Clifford: J. Exp. Med., 128:1011, 1968.
55. De Schryver, A., S. Friberg, G. Klein, W. Henle, G. Henle, G. De Thé, P. Clifford, and H. C. Ho: Clin. Exp. Immunol., 5:443, 1969.
56. Fenyö, E. M., P. Biberfeld, and E. Klein: J. Nat. Cancer Inst., 42:837, 1969.
57. Axelrad, A. A.: Nature, 199:80, 1963.
58. Chieco-Bianchi, L., L. Fiore-Donati, G. Tirdente, and N. Panelli: Nature, 214: 1227, 1967.
59. Klein, E., and G. Klein: Cancer Res., 25:851, 1965.
60. Morton, D. L.: J. Nat. Cancer Inst., 42:311, 1969.
61. Haran-Ghera, N.: Nature, 222:992, 1969.
62. Law, L. W., and C. J. Dawe: Proc. Soc. Exp. Biol. Med., 104:414, 1960.
63. Clifford, P., S. Singh, J. Stjernswärd, and G. Klein: Cancer Res., 27:2578, 1967.
64. Skipper, H. E.: Cancer Res., 27:263, 1967.
65. Klein, E., and H. O. Sjögren: Transpl. Bull., 26:442, 1960.
66. Batchelor, J. R., E. A. Boyse, and P. A. Gorer: Transpl. Bull., 26:449, 1960.
67. Brondz, B. D.: Transplantation, 3:356, 1965.
68. Mathé, G.: Brit. Med. J., 4:7, 1969.

Human Fetal Antigens: Liver

JOSÉ URIEL

Institut de Recherches Scientifiques sur le Cancer, Villejuif, France

IN THE COURSE of the developmental history of multicellular organisms, the expression of some biosynthetic products seems to be restricted to a limited period of the over-all process of cell diversification and maturation. Such products are normally absent in fully differentiated cells.

These particular cell substances, which we have proposed to designate by the general term of "transitory cell antigens,"[1] can reappear in adult animals under different pathologic situations, including cancer. I will outline recent data on the association of primary liver cancer with these antigens, and discuss briefly their possible relevance to the general mechanism of carcinogenesis.

The transitory cell antigens associated with primary hepatoma are all synthesized by the liver, and for this reason can be considered as molecular markers of hepatocyte differentiation. Another property is that of being secreted into blood, where they are known as "feto-specific serum proteins."

The first of these circulating transitory cell antigens in mammals was described under the name of "fetuin" by Pederson in 1944. The experimental work on mouse and rat hepatomas[2, 3] has focused attention on other serum constituents belonging to the same group and particularly the α-fetoprotein (α-FP). (Recommendations for a uniform terminology of fetospecific serum proteins have been proposed in the course of the "Meeting of Investigators for Evaluation of a Serological Test for Liver Cancer" IARC, Lyon [France] July, 1969. The proposed terminology is used in this paper. See also reference 1.) This protein is the first α-globulin to appear in mammalian sera during ontogenic development, and is the dominant serum protein in early embryonic life.

Traces of the protein are detectable in human and rat newborns up to one month of postnatal life. The α-FP can be characterized and quantified by immunodiffusion techniques using specific antisera.

As far as the association of transitory cell antigens with clinical disorders in man is concerned, the occurrence of α-FP in patients with primary liver cancer was first reported by Tatarinov.[4] An extensive survey of the incidence of fetospecific serum proteins in liver diseases and other clinical disorders in man has been undertaken since 1966 by Abelev and his co-workers in Moscow[5] and by our group at Villejuif.[6, 7] Additional studies relevant to the same problem have also been made by other groups of investigators. The information gained during the last four years in the search for α-FP in thousands of serum samples can be summarized as follows:

The α-FP has never been found in the sera of: (1) healthy adults and children; (2) adults with various forms of nonneoplastic diseases, including hepatopathies; (3) adults with tumors of nonhepatic origin, even when these tumors metastasize to the liver; and (4) patients with liver tumors other than those of the parenchymal cells.

In contrast, the α-FP has been demonstrated in the sera of (1) infants, up to 12 months of age, when suffering from hepatitis or other nonneoplastic hepatopathies; (2) patients with malignant teratoblastomas; and (3) patients with hepatoblastomas and hepatocellular carcinomas. The frequency of positive tests in the different pathologic situations where the presence of α-FP has been demonstrated is variable.

Table 6-1 shows the incidence of α-FP associated with primary liver cancer in seven geographic areas. Whether genetic, etiologic, nutritional or ecologic factors might be implicated in such differences is unknown. What I believe is important to point out is that histologically confirmed hepatocellular carcinomas can develop without secretion of α-FP.

TABLE 6–1.—INCIDENCE OF SERUM α-FETOPROTEIN IN CASES OF
PRIMARY LIVER CANCER

	COUNTRY OF ORIGIN	NUMBER OF PATIENTS	% OF POSITIVE REACTIONS	REF.
	Great Britain	17*	29	14
Primary	U.S.A.	39	38	15
	Uganda	40	50	16
Liver	France	22†	55	7, 9
Cancer	USSR	28	60	5
	South Africa	130	75	17
	Senegal	102	80	7

* All patients of British origin.
† All patients of French origin.

Conversely, no correlation has been found between the absence or presence of serum α-FP in patients with hepatocellular carcinoma and any of the clinical and biochemical parameters investigated, nor is there any correlation with the size, histologic type, or degree of differentiation of the neoplastic livers. The serum titer of α-FP in patients with primary liver cancer varies over an extremely broad range when different individuals are compared. In the same patient, the titer can also change from nondetectable traces of α-FP to significant values; it can increase in the course of the disease or decrease under the action of chemotherapeutic agents.

A survey of the incidence of α-FP in childhood neoplasms (hepatomas and teratoblastomas) made in France during the past two years by Mawas and co-workers[8] gives consistently higher values than in adults, as shown in Table 6-2.

At present, there is general agreement about the specificity of the association between serum α-FP and hepatocellular carcinoma as well as malignant teratoblastoma. Hence, the serologic test which allows the demonstration of α-FP is of great value for the diagnosis of these diseases. In addition, the simplicity of the immunodiffusion technique makes the test available for routine purposes and particularly useful in epidemiologic studies.

Another human transitory cell antigen appears frequently in the

TABLE 6–2.—SERUM α FETOPROTEIN AND CHILDHOOD NEOPLASMS*

DIAGNOSIS	No. OF CASES	AGE RANGE	% OF POSITIVE TESTS
Hepatomas	23	6 months to 9 years	93
Malignant teratoblastomas	21	2 months to 16 years	71

* From C. Mawas et al. (personal communication).

sera of patients with neoplasms of nonhepatic origin or with primary liver cancer and also with other nonneoplastic liver disorders such as hepatitis and some forms of cirrhosis.[9] The nature and physiocochemical properties of this antigen, which after immunoelectrophoresis in agarose has the mobility of a β-globulin, are poorly known. This protein is, apparently, the equivalent in man of the rat α_M-FP also known as α_2-acute phase globulin.[1, 10]

As to the association with pathologic states, a striking parallelism is observed between rat serum α-FP and α_M-FP and their assumed counterparts in human serum, α-FP and β-fetoproteins (β-FP). Thus: (1) both rat and human α-FP are specifically induced in primary hepatoma; (2) both rat α_M-FP and human β-FP are associated with liver regeneration concomitant with neoplastic or nonneoplastic situations, and (3) the secretion into blood of both α-FPs follows in time that of rat α_M-FP or human β-FP.

Transitory Liver Antigens and Retrodifferentiation

The reappearance of transitory liver antigens in adult animals under several pathologic situations brings us to the problem of cell differentiation. The two following questions arise from the specific association of α-FP with adult individuals bearing hepatocellular carcinoma: (1) Is the synthesis of α-FP due to: (a) the activation by growth of incompletely differentiated cell clones, or (b) the true derepression of a silent gene? (2) Is the reappearance of α-FP: (a) a unique property of neoplastic hepatocytes, or (b) one of the multiple biologic transitions which occur in reverting cells?

Fig. 6–1.—Reappearance of α-FP in newborn rats subjected to intraperitoneal injections of CCl$_4$.

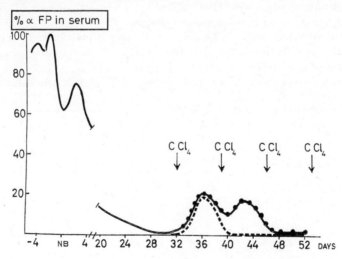

TABLE 6–3.—QUANTITATIVE CHANGES IN ENZYME LEVELS

ENZYME	ADULT LIVER	IMMATURE LIVER	REGENERATING LIVER	HEPATOMA	REF.
Deoxycytidylate deaminase	100*	(18-day embryo) increased 40-fold	(48 hours) increased 20-fold	(Morris 5123) † increased 6-fold	27
Thymidylate synthetase	undetectable	(18-day embryo) increased 1,850-fold	(48 hours) increased 1,000-fold	(Morris 5123) † increased 960-fold	27
Thymidine kinase	100*	(21-day embryo) increased 23-fold	(23 hours) increased 25-fold	(Morris 5123)† increased 24-fold	28 29 30
LDH$_4$ LDH$_5$	0.025‡	(15-day embryo to 6-day neonates) 0.40	(36 hours) 0.40	(3′-Me-DAB) § 0.30-0.45	10
G-6-PDH	adult pattern	(ib.) immature pattern	(24 hours) immature pattern	(3′-Me-DAB) § immature pattern	
Aldolase	adult pattern	immature pattern		(3′-Me-DAB) § immature pattern	10 31
G-6-Phosphatase	100*	(15-day embryo to 6-day neonates) <1 to 50		(3′-Me-DAB) § 10 to 60	10

* Enzymatic activity of normal adult liver taken as 100 per cent.
† Slow-growing hepatoma.
‡ Ratio estimated from electrophoretic patterns.
§ Primary hepatomas induced by oral ingestion of carcinogen.

The experiments described below were designed to approach the first question.

Serum α-FP becomes undetectable in rats around the thirtieth day of postnatal life. When newborn rats, up to one month old, are subjected to a series of injections of CCl_4, the disappearance of the fetoprotein takes place one to two weeks later than the normal period of 30 days. If the same treatment is applied to rats aged between 32 and 44 days, one or several waves of α-FP synthesis can be observed (Figure 6-1). The fetoprotein appears in serum 24 hr after CCl_4 injections, reaches a maximum between 48 and 72 hr, and then declines, disappearing two days later. The number of waves varies according to individuals, although rarely exceeding three.[11] A transient reappearance of α-FP in the sera of newborn rats subjected to partial hepatectomy has been reported by Perova and Abelev.[12] α-FP induction cannot be provoked by CCl_4 or by partial hepatectomy in rats older than five weeks. These results parallel the observation reported above that α-FP can be demonstrated in infants up to one year old who have hepatitis or other nonneoplastic hepatopathies.[13] These facts suggest that the resurgence of α-FP after hepatic injury in neonates is a consequence of the enhanced activity of some incompletely differentiated cell clones. Such clones probably exist in all individuals undergoing the terminal stages of liver maturation, but their production of α-FP ranges below the sensitivity of the immunologic methods which allow the characterization of the fetoprotein.

In contrast, the same facts strongly support the alternative hypothesis that the association of α-FP with primary hepatoma in adults is a true derepression phenomenon, since liver tissue repair subsequent to nonneoplastic situations never induces α-FP synthesis in adult animals.

As far as the second question, the possible coexistence of other biologic transitions with the derepression of fetoproteins, is concerned, we have undertaken comparative studies on several biochemical patterns in embryonic, regenerating, and neoplastic rat liver.[1]

Table 6-3 groups our results together with literature data relative to the same subject. The data refer to quantitative changes in enzyme levels and changes in the molecular forms of several enzymes. The analogies encountered relative to these biochemical transitions suggest that the reappearance of α-FP and other serum feto-specific proteins is not a unique event.

In order to explain some of the clinical and experimental facts already available, I have drawn the hypothesis that the resumed synthesis of transitory liver antigens could reflect a sequential process of retrodifferentiation.[1] The hypothesis, schematically represented in Figure 6-2, assumes that differentiation and retrodifferentiation represent alternatives between the convergent directions of a unique chain of events. Thus, when a mature liver cell enters retrodifferentiation, the synthesis of certain fetoprotein and/or the transition to a given pattern of enzymatic activity may depend on how far the reversion proceeds and how it modulated between the stages of the sequence.

On the left of Figure 6-2 is represented the period of synthesis of rat human transitory liver antigens within the developmental sequence

Fig. 6-2.—Diagram suggesting the dynamics of the synthesis of transitory liver antigens in man and rat, and their association with different liver states. See explanations in the text.

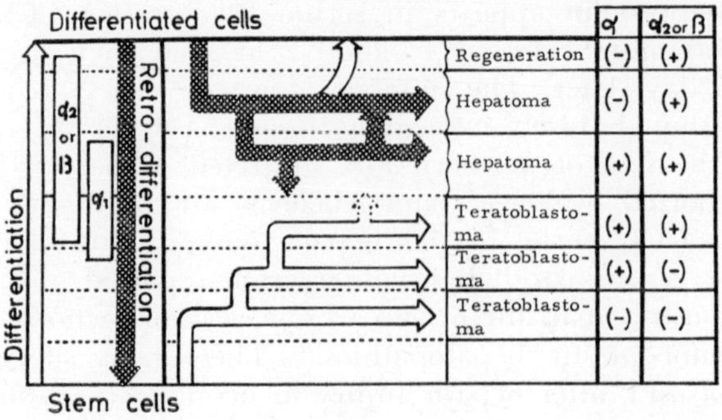

	α	α_2 or β
Regeneration	(-)	(+)
Hepatoma	(-)	(+)
Hepatoma	(+)	(+)
Teratoblastoma	(+)	(+)
Teratoblastoma	(+)	(-)
Teratoblastoma	(-)	(-)

of the hepatocyte lineage. On the right side are indicated the association patterns of these antigens in relation with liver regeneration, hepatocellular carcinoma, and malignant teratoblastomas.

It appears that the synthesis of transitory liver antigens from fully differentiated cells can be explained as being the consequence of retrodifferentiation. Therefore, no causal relationship need account for the association between human or rat α-FP and primary hepatoma. What probably happens is that in some hepatomas, but not in other hepatic lesions, retrodifferentiation proceeds to the stage where the synthesis of α-FP takes place. The situation is different in the case of rat α_M-FP and β-FP, because the genes coding for them are still operative in the terminal stages of hepatocyte differentiation or because they are easily derepressible.

The presence of transitory liver antigens in some cases of malignant teratoblastomas can be explained on the same basis. The synthesis of such antigens should logically occur when precursors of liver parenchymal cells progress far enough in their developmental differentiation.

While retrodifferentiation is probably the underlying cause for the similarities encountered in regenerating liver and hepatocellular carcinoma, the dynamics of the process are clearly distinct. In regeneration, the whole change is a cyclic one: the cell retrodifferentiates to some degree and, after a period of active growth, differentiates again until complete maturity. In hepatoma, there is also retrodifferentiation, and the cell can either progress far in this way or modulate through several stages of the sequence but, once stabilized, it does not undergo full compensatory differentiation. Thus, unbalanced retrodifferentiation apparently characterizes hepatocellular carcinoma.

Is this a peculiarity of liver cancer, or is retrodifferentiation a general mechanism for the neoplastic transformation of adult cells? Obviously, no reply can be given today. Nevertheless, the idea that analogous mechanisms are probably implicated in both differentiation and neoplastic transformation is now gaining general acceptance. Therefore, the developmental history of cells, as well as the reverse process, retrodifferentiation, may become one of the key references for further understanding of the intricate mechanism of carcinogenesis.

References

1. Uriel, J.: Path. Biol., 17:877, 1969.
2. Abelev, G., S. Perova, S. Kramkova, Z. Postnikova, and I. Irlin: Biokhimiya, 28: 625, 1963.
3. Stanislawski-Birencwajg, M.: Compt. Rend. Acad. Sci. (Paris), 260:364, 1965.
4. Tatarinov, Y. S.: Vop. med. Khim., 11:20, 1965.
5. Abelev, G., I. Assecritova, N. Kraevski, S. Perova, and N. Perevodchikova: Internat. J. Cancer, 2:551, 1967.
6. Uriel, J., B. de Nechaud, M. Stanislawski-Birencwajg, R. Masseyeff, L. LeBlanc, C. Quenum, F. Loisillier, and P. Grabar: Compt. Rend. Acad. Sci. (Paris), 265: 75, 1967.
7. Uriel, J., B. de Nechaud, M. Stanislawski-Birencwajg, R. Masseyeff, L. LeBlanc, C. Quenum, F. Loisillier, and P. Grabar: Presse méd., 76:1416, 1968.

8. Mawas, C., D. Buffe, O. Sweissguth, and P. Burtin: In: Coll. Prot. Biol. Fluids, Brugge. In press.
9. de Nechaud, B., P. Economopoulos, and J. Uriel: Presse méd., 52:1945, 1969.
10. Weimer, H. E., and D. C. Benjamin: Amer. J. Physiol., 209:736, 1965.
11. de Nechaud, B., and J. Uriel: In: Coll. Prot. Biol. Fluids, Brugge. In press.
12. Perova, S. D., and G. I. Abelev: Voprossi meditsinskoi chimii (Moscow), 13:369, 1967.
13. Masopust, J., K. Kithier, J. Radl, J. Houstek, and L. Kotal: Internat. J. Cancer, 3:364, 1968.
14. Foli, A. K., S. Sherlock, and M. Adinolfi: Lancet, 2:1267, 1969.
15. Hull, et al.: Lancet, 1:779, 1970.
16. Alpert, M. E., J. Uriel, and B. de Nechaud: New Eng. J. Med., 278:984, 1968.
17. Purves, L. S., E. W. Geddes, M. MacNab, and I. Bersohn: Lancet, 1:921, 1968.

Immunologic Factors in Malignant Melanomas, Skeletal and Soft Tissue Sarcomas of Man

DONALD L. MORTON, M.D.,

FREDERICK R. EILBER, M.D., AND

RICHARD A. MALMGREN, M.D.

Tumor Immunology Section, Surgery Branch, and Laboratory of Pathology, National Cancer Institute, National Institutes of Health, Bethesda, Maryland, USA

DURING THE PAST DECADE it has become increasingly apparent that cells acquire new antigens in the process of neoplastic transformation. Tumor-specific antigens capable of inducing a host immune response which specifically retards the growth of neoplastic cells have been demonstrated in a wide variety of viral[24] and carcinogen-induced neoplasms,[13] as well as in certain spontaneous animal neoplasms.[9] It is logical to assume that neoplasms in man contain cancer-specific antigens similar to those found in animal tumors; but until recently, there was little evidence for the existence of such antigens. Since the tumor transplantation techniques used to demonstrate tumor-specific antigens in animal neoplasms were not applicable to man, it was necessary to study these antigens by other methods. Recently, the application of sensitive serologic techniques, including immunofluorescence, colony inhibition, immunodiffusion, and complement fixation, have revealed the presence of tumor-associated antigens in a variety of neoplasms in man, including Burkitt's lymphoma,[12, 14, 25] malignant melanoma,[15, 16, 19, 21, 23] neuroblastoma,[10] skeletal and soft tissue sarcomas,[4, 17, 18] colonic neoplasms,[8, 11] and other tumors.[1, 7, 11] Thus, there is increasing evidence that human cancers, like animal neoplasms, contain tumor-specific antigens which are immunogenic in the autologous host.

Some of our immunologic studies with human melanomas and sarcomas will be reviewed.

Immunologic Studies with Human Malignant Melanoma

We have previously suggested that certain clinical features of malignant melanoma may indicate the importance of immunologic factors in this disease.[19, 20] Examples of host immunity in malignant melanoma include the unexpectedly high rate of spontaneous regressions,[5] observations of induced regressions of malignant melanoma in recipients of transfusions,[27, 28] reports that therapeutic cross-transplantation of tumors and sensitized leukocytes is sometimes successful,[22] and the demonstration of cytotoxic effects of autologous sera against melanoma cells in short-term tissue culture.[15] Additional experimental evidence to support the presence of immunologic factors in malignant melanoma was provided by our demonstration of a common tumor antigen in malignant melanoma which was immunogenic in patients with this disease.[23] Since then, additional reports have appeared which confirm and extend our earlier immunofluorescence studies.[16, 23, 26] In addition, the existence of cellular immunity is suggested by the demonstration of delayed cutaneous hypersensitivity reactions to autologous extracts of malignant melanoma.[6]

Additional studies which indicate the presence of an immunologic response to malignant melanoma in man will be reviewed.

Immunofluorescence Studies

The immunofluorescence technique and method of preparing tumor imprints on glass slides for these studies have been described.[19] Tumor imprints from 16 melanoma specimens were tested for reactivity against serial dilutions of autologous serum by the indirect immunofluorescence technique. In addition, sera from 38 patients with malignant melanoma and 25 control sera from normal blood bank donors have been tested against tumor imprints of eight different malignant melanomas.

Prominent cytoplasmic and perinuclear fluorescence were seen when each patient's serum was tested against his own melanoma imprints. As previously described,[19] intranuclear fluorescence was also observed

TABLE 6–4.—CORRELATIONS BETWEEN STAGE OF DISEASE AND IMMUNO-
FLUORESCENCE REACTIONS OF AUTOLOGOUS SERUM WITH ACETONE-FIXED
IMPRINTS OF MALIGNANT MELANOMA

| | DISEASE LOCALIZED TO SKIN AND NODES | | | ADVANCED DISEASE WITH VISCERAL METASTASES | | |
| | Antibody | Immunoglobulin | | | Antibody | Immunoglobulin |
Patient	Titer*	Type	Patient		Titer*	Type
H P	1:64	IGG	R L		1:2	
H M	1:64		B C		1:16	
J M	1:64	IGM	R G H		1:16	
H B	1:128		N I		1:32	IGM
H R	1:128		M W		1:32	
F D	1:128	IGM, IGG	R H		1:32	
			R S		1:32	IGM, IGG
			H R		1:32	IGM, IGG
			H O		1:32	
			F A		1:128	
Mean						
Titer	1:96				1:35	

* Titers are significantly different by Mann Whitney Test (p < .05).

with some melanomas, but with progressive serum dilutions, the nuclear fluorescence disappeared and only the cytoplasmic fluorescence
persisted.[19] Table 6-4 gives the titers of antibody to the intracytoplasmic
antigen found when autologous sera from 16 different patients were
tested in serial dilutions against each patient's own melanoma. All patients were found to have autoantibody to their own melanomas.
However, patients with localized melanoma were found to have significantly higher titers of antibody than did patients with widespread
disease.

The results of testing undiluted melanoma sera against eight different homologous melanomas are summarized in Table 6-5. Again it

TABLE 6–5.—CORRELATIONS BETWEEN THE CLINICAL STATUS OF MELANOMA
PATIENTS AND THE REACTIVITY OF THEIR SERA BY IMMUNOFLUORESCENCE
AGAINST EIGHT DIFFERENT HOMOLOGOUS MALIGNANT MELANOMAS

SERA OBTAINED FROM	No. PATIENTS	No. POSITIVE TESTS Total No. Tests	POSITIVE TESTS %
Patients with melanoma localized to the primary site and regional nodes	17	64/86†	75
Patients with widespread metastatic disease	16	33/66†	50
Patients exhibiting unusual host resistance*	5	24/35†	69
Normal blood bank donors	25	32/178	18

* Sera from four patients with spontaneous remissions and one with remission
following chemotherapy.
† Values differ significantly by X² (p < .01) from normal blood bank donors.

will be noted that patients with localized melanoma or those exhibiting unusual host resistance had a significantly higher incidence of antibody (75%) than did patients with advanced disease (50%). Both of these groups, however, had a higher incidence of antibody than was found in the sera of normal blood bank donors (18%). The possible explanations for the presence of antimelanoma antibody in the sera of apparently healthy donors has been previously discussed.[19]

The observation that 100% of sera reacted with autologous melanomas regardless of the extent of disease, whereas only 75% of sera from patients with localized melanoma and 50% of sera from patients with advanced disease had antibody to homologous melanomas suggests the presence of an antigen which is individually specific for each melanoma in addition to the common antigen which is found in most or all melanomas. Thus, some sera had antibody to only the individual specific antigen since they possessed antibody to their own melanoma but no cross-reacting antibody, whereas other sera have antibody to both antigens. In this respect, it is interesting that Lewis[16] has reported that the cell surface antigens demonstrated by the membrane immunofluorescent technique are individually distinct for each melanoma, whereas the intracytoplasmic antigens are shared by most or all melanomas. These observations are contrary to our earlier studies[19] and the more recent work of Rhomsdahl,[26] who found common cell surface as well as intracytoplasmic antigens.

Fluorescein-labeled antisera specific for the heavy chains of human immunoglobulins (Hyland Laboratories) were used to determine the immunoglobulin type of these antimelanoma antibodies from six patients. The results are given in Table 6-4. None of the sera contained IgA antibody, two of the sera contained only IgM, three contained both IgM and IgG, and one serum had only IgG. The patient with pure IgG antibody was somewhat unusual in that she had a metastatic melanoma to lymph nodes in the left groin which had gradually increased in size over a period of seven years before it was excised. This patient had evidence of in vivo fixation of antibody of the IgG class to cell surface antigens by both the membrane immunofluorescent reaction and the antiglobulin consumption technique.

Complement-Fixation Studies

Recently, we have been able to demonstrate antisarcoma antibodies in the sera of sarcoma patients to a sarcoma-specific antigen derived from tissue cultures of human sarcomas by a sensitive and quantitative complement-fixation technique.[4] The applicability of this technique to our studies with human melanomas was tested after we had initiated tissue cultures from three different malignant melanomas.

The complement-fixation techniques, the technique for preparation of antigens, and complement source have been previously described.[4]

TABLE 6-6.—DISTRIBUTION OF ANTIBODY TO HuMEL-1 MELANOMA
ANTIGENS DETECTED BY COMPLEMENT FIXATION IN PATIENTS
WITH MALIGNANT NEOPLASMS

TYPE OF SERUM	No. Pos./No. TESTED*	% Pos.
Normal blood donors	11/50	22
Epidermoid CA—head & neck	1/10	10
Epidermoid CA—cervix	3/10	30
Epidermoid CA—lung	2/10	20
Adenocarcinoma—breast	2/10	20
Adenocarcinoma—colon	1/10	10
All melanoma patients	42/63†	67
Patients with localized disease	31/35†	89
Patients with unusual host resistance	5/5	100
Patients with metastatic disease	6/23	26

* Antigen was HuMel-1 diluted ⅛, positive sera had titer ⅛ or >.
† Values differ significantly (p < .01) by X^2 from normal blood donors.

The HuMel-1 melanoma cell line used for most of these studies was derived from an amelanotic melanoma and did not form melanin in the tissue culture.

The distribution of antibody in sera from patients with various types of malignant disease to the HuMel-1 melanoma antigen is shown in Table 6-6. Using four units of antigen (determined by box titration with autologous serum), 67% of patients with malignant melanoma had detectable antibody which was significantly higher than the 22% incidence of antibody in normal blood bank donors. Patients with epidermoid carcinoma of the head and neck, cervix, and lung or those with adenocarcinoma of the breast and colon did not have a higher incidence of antibody than did normal blood bank donors. Also, the incidence of antimelanoma antibody in patients with different stages of disease may be compared in Table 6-6. It will be noted that patients with localized melanoma (89%) or those undergoing spontaneous regression of their melanomas (100%) had a significantly higher incidence of antimelanoma antibody than did those with advanced metastatic disease. The incidence of antibody in the latter group did not differ significantly from the incidence of antibody in normal sera.

The specificity of this antigen for melanoma cells was demonstrated by the following studies: Three sera previously found to have a high titer of antibody against the HuMel-1 antigen were diluted 1/10 and used to assay various tissue culture cell lines for the presence of sarcoma-specific antigens. Serial dilutions of antigenic preparations of tissue cultures derived from three different melanomas had antigenic titers of 1/16 to 1/64. However, no antigen was detected in tissue culture fibroblasts derived from muscle of the same melanoma patient from which one of the melanoma cell lines originated (HuMel-3). Similarly, cells derived from other malignant tumors, normal adult organs, and fetal organs had no detectable reaction with the same test sera. Therefore, it appears that tissue culture cell lines derived from human melanomas possess a common melanoma antigen that is specific for melanomas. This antigen is not an artifact of the tissue culture process, as test sera do not react with tissue culture cell lines derived from normal tissues or from other malignant conditions. The melanoma antigen in these cell lines is not melanin, since only one of the three melanoma cell lines contained melanin. The antimelanoma antibody found in the sera of melanoma patients is not an isoantibody directed against histocompatibility antigens, since sera of patients from which the melanoma cultures were derived reacted with their own melanoma cells but not with normal cells from the same patient.

Delayed Cutaneous Hypersensitivity in Malignant Melanoma

We have recently reported that cancer patients who have normal immunologic competence, as indicated by their ability to manifest delayed cutaneous hypersensitivity, usually have a good prognosis after surgical therapy, whereas those exhibiting cutaneous anergy developed early recurrence or were inoperable because of metastatic disease.[2, 3] Since some melanoma patients with widespread metastatic disease exhibited normal immunologic reactivity, it was of interest to test a larger series of melanoma patients for delayed cutaneous hypersensitivity to dinitrochlorobenzene (DNCB) and a battery of common skin test antigens (blastomycin, coccidioidin, histoplasmin, mumps, mixed trees, dermatophytin, and tuberculin). The methods of sensitization and testing have been previously described.[2, 3]

The results of skin tests in 24 melanoma patients are summarized in Table 6-7. Patients with localized melanoma and those undergoing spontaneous regression of their melanomas were found to have normal delayed cutaneous hypersensitivity, whereas most patients with wide-

TABLE 6–7.—INCIDENCE OF DELAYED CUTANEOUS HYPERSENSITIVITY TO
DINITROCHLOROBENZENE AND COMMON SKIN TEST ANTIGENS
IN MELANOMA PATIENTS

TYPE OF PATIENTS	DNCB No Pos./ No. Tested	Pos. %	SKIN TEST ANTIGENS No. Pos. to One or More Antigens No. Tested	Pos. %
Control	19/20	95	18/20	90
Spontaneous regression of melanoma	2/2	100	2/2	100
Melanoma patients with localized disease	10/10*	100	6/10	60
Melanoma patients with metastatic disease	3/12*	25	3/10	30

* Values differ significantly by Fisher's exact probability test (p < .05).

spread metastatic disease exhibited impaired immunologic reactivity. It is not certain at the present time whether the cutaneous anergy exhibited by these patients is the cause or the result of the metastatic disease. Whatever the explanation, it is quite evident that patients who exhibit cutaneous anergy are likely to have metastatic disease, whereas those who have localized disease maintain their immunologic competence.

Immunologic Studies with Human Sarcomas

Recently, with immunofluorescent techniques, specific antibody to a common antigen in human osteosarcomas was demonstrated in 100% of the sera from patients with this disease.[17] Because specific antibody was also detectable in 29% of the normal blood donors and in 85% of healthy family members of these patients, an associated infectious agent capable of producing unrecognized infections in healthy contacts of sarcoma patients was suspected. Subsequently, a tissue culture cell line (SA-1) has been established from a human liposarcoma which was found by electron microscopy to contain viral particles morphologically similar to the avian and murine sarcoma viruses.[18]

Additional immunologic studies have revealed a high incidence of antibody to sarcoma-specific antigens prepared from this human liposarcoma in the serum of patients with various types of skeletal and soft tissue sarcomas.[4, 18] The sarcoma-specific antigen was found in tissue culture cells derived from different histologic types of sarcomas, but not in normal fibroblasts obtained from sarcoma patients nor in cells from nonsarcomatous malignant disease.

Since the antigen (s) appeared to be specific for sarcoma cells and common to different histologic types of sarcomas, the next phase of this study was to determine if specific antibody to the sarcoma antigen (SA-1) could be detected in sera of a larger number of patients with sarcomas; and whether this antibody was present in normal sera, or in sera of patients with other nonsarcomatous malignant disease. The distribution of antisarcoma antibody in the sera of various patients using four units of the SA-1 (liposarcoma) antigen is given in Table 6-6. Of the sera from patients with skeletal and soft tissue sarcomas, 92% (72/78) had detectable antibody to this sarcoma antigen to a titer of $1/8$ or greater, whereas only 21% of normal blood donors had antibody activity. Both incidence and range antibody titer in sarcoma patients were significantly higher than those of the normal blood donors. However, patients with nonsarcomatous malignant disease of various histologic types did not have significantly higher incidence or titers of antibody than did the normal donors.

We then investigated the relationship between the antisarcoma antibody titer and the course of the patient's disease. For these studies, serum samples were obtained preoperatively and at various intervals during the postoperative period in patients with skeletal and soft tissue

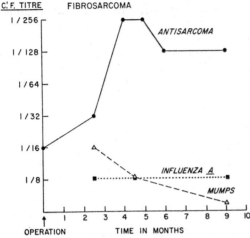

Fig. 6–3.—Antisarcoma antibody titers determined by complement fixation against the HuSA-1 liposarcoma antigen. Serial serum samples obtained following resection of the primary sarcoma in a patient who remained free of disease.

sarcomas undergoing definitive resection of their neoplasms. A total of 21 patients have been studied to the present time, but the results are typical of those illustrated in Figures 6-3 and 6-4. Note that the anti-body titer usually increases following surgical resection of the tumor mass, and remains elevated in patients who remain free of disease (Figure 6-3). However, all patients who developed recurrent disease with pulmonary metastases almost simultaneously were noted to have a de-clining level of antisarcoma antibody, which dropped to 0 with pro-gressive disease (Figure 6-4). Thus, there is an extremely good correla-tion between recurrent disease and declining antisarcoma antibody

Fig. 6–4.—Antisarcoma antibody titers determined by complement fixation against the HuSA-1 liposarcoma antigen. Serial serum samples obtained following resection of the primary sarcoma in a patient who developed recurrent disease with pulmonary metastases.

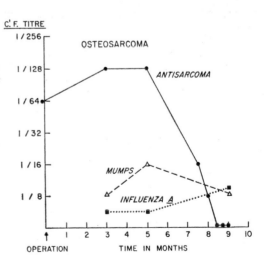

titer. Furthermore, patients who have remained tumor-free for several years postoperatively have been found to maintain their antisarcoma antibody at relatively stable levels.

Because of the similarity of these results with the immunofluorescent data of a cross-reacting antigen among sarcomas of the same histologic type and findings that sarcoma of other histologic types contained a similar antigen, the possibility of an associated viral agent was investigated.

Attempts were made to determine if the antigenic activity of the sarcomas was transmissible to normal human tissue culture cells (Table 6-8). Extracts prepared from a human chondrosarcoma and an osteosarcoma tumor by the Moloney technique, placed on normal human embryonic tissue culture cells, resulted in antigenic transformation after seven to 14 days. Additionally, supernatants from tissue cultures of one osteosarcoma, one fibrosarcoma, and one liposarcoma after passage through a .45 micron Millipore filter induced antigenic transformation of normal target cells. Uninfected control cells never developed antigens recognized by the test sera. The new antigen was usually not detectable seven days following infection, but by day 14 the antigenic titer usually had risen to 1/32 and sometimes as high as 1/64 by 28 days after infection. One transformed cell line has retained its antigenic activity now for 18 months. Evidence that the new antigen these sera detected is the same sarcoma antigen as was in the original cell line comes from the observation that absorption of these sera with the SA-1 antigen removed all reactivity to the antigenically transformed cells, whereas absorption with Wi-38 or HeLa in an identical fashion removed no activity. Therefore, the filterable transferred antigen is the same as that detected in the original sarcoma cells.

TABLE 6–8.—Distribution of Antibody to SA_1 Sarcoma Antigen*
in Patients with Malignant Neoplasms

Serum Source	No. Pos./ No. Tested	% Pos.	Range of Antibody	Mean Titer of Pos. Sera
Sarcoma patients	72/78†	92	1/8-1/256‡	1/98
Adenocarcinoma of breast	8/35	22	1/8-1/16	1/10
Adenocarcinoma of colon	6/36	16	1/8-1/32	1/13
Carcinoma of liver and bile ducts	1/5	20	1/8	1/8
Carcinoma of thyroid	2/8	25	1/8-1/32	1/16
Hodgkin's disease	2/19	10	1/8	1/8
Leukemia (ALL & AML)	8/30	26	1/8-1/32	1/16
Malignant melanoma	9/51	17	1/8-1/16	1/9
Epidermoid carcinoma cervix	7/36	19	1/8-1/32	1/17
Epidermoid carcinoma head & neck	8/42	19	1/8-1/16	1/11
Epidermoid carcinoma lung	5/42	11	1/8-1/16	1/11
Normal blood donors	38/176†	21	1/8-1/32‡	1/19

* Antigen was SA_1 (liposarcoma) diluted 1/16, positive sera had a titer 1/8 or >.
† Values differ significantly (p < .005) by X^2.
‡ Distributions of antibody titers are significantly different (p < .005) by Mann-Whitney Test.

TABLE 6–9.—ANTIGENIC TRANSFORMATION OF NORMAL CELL LINES BY
EXTRACTS FROM HUMAN SARCOMA TISSUES AND CELL LINES

| | | | | ANTIGEN TITER BY C. F. | | | |
| | | TARGET | UNINFECTED | Days Following Infection | | | |
TYPE OF SARCOMA	EXTRACT	CELL	CONTROL CELL	7	14	21	28
SA$_6$-Chondro-tissue	Moloney	Wi-38	0	1/4	1/8		
SA$_5$-Osteo-tissue	Moloney	Monkey embryo				1/16	1/32-1/64
SA$_2$-Osteo-culture	100:1*	Wi-38	0	0	1/8		
SA$_4$-Osteo-culture	100:1*	Wi-38	0				1/8
SA$_1$-Lipo-culture	1000:1†	Monkey embryo	0	0	1/32		
SA$_2$-Osteo-culture	1000:1†	Monkey embryo	0	0	1/32		

* 1000 × 6 supernatant fluids from tissue culture frozen-thawed × 2 and concentrated 100:1.
† Supernatant fluids from tissue culture concentrated 1000:1 and passed through .45 μ Millipore filter.

The demonstration that a filterable agent is associated with the sarcoma tumors and tissue culture cell lines, which is capable of antigenically transforming normal cells, provides additional evidence of an associated virus with these sarcomas. Furthermore, when sera from relatives of patients with sarcoma were examined using the SA-1 antigen, it was found that 79% had detectable antisarcoma antibody (Table 6-9). The incidence of antibody was significantly higher than in the normal blood donors and significantly lower than the 92% incidence of all the sarcoma patients tested. Also, the range of antibody titers of the relatives was significantly higher than the normal donors, but not as high as the antibody titers of the sarcoma patients. None of the relatives of these patients or the normal blood donors had a history of clinically detectable sarcomas.

Discussion

These studies have revealed a remarkable correlation between the incidence and titer of antitumor antibodies detectable by complement fixation and immunofluorescence and the extent of disease in patients with malignant melanoma and skeletal and soft tissue sarcomas. Patients with localized disease were more likely to have antitumor antibodies than those with advanced disease. A rising titer of antisarcoma antibody was consistently observed following tumor resection in patients with skeletal and soft tissue sarcomas. Furthermore, study of serial serum specimens in patients with melanomas and sarcomas who developed recurrent disease have revealed a progressive decline in their titers of antitumor antibody with advancing disease.

There are several possible explanations for this correlation between the incidence and titer of antitumor antibody and stage of malignant disease. It is possible that the antitumor antibody is produced at a relatively constant rate but is constantly being absorbed from the circulation by a growing tumor mass. Therefore, one would expect removal of the tumor to result in an increase in the titer of antitumor antibody and regrowth of tumor to lower the titer of antibody. Since antibody cannot penetrate into the interior of a living cell, this would suggest that the effective antigens reactive with the antitumor antibody are located on the cell surface. Some support for this hypothesis comes from the observation that low titers of antisarcoma antibody have been eluted from the sarcoma tissues of two patients, thus suggesting that in vivo absorption of antibody to tumor cells had occurred.

However, another explanation for these findings is that the growing tumor mass produces specific immunosuppression because of the induction of high dose tolerance, and therefore the dropping antibody titer in patients with recurrent disease is caused by decreased production of antibody. Removal of the tumor would then remove the large antigenic mass and permit a return of immunologic competence to the sarcoma-specific antigens. There is no evidence to support this hypothesis and, in fact, the observation that antibody production can be stimulated in patients with advanced disease by immunization with autologous tumor suggests that high dose tolerance may not be a suitable explanation for these findings.

These studies demonstrate that human skeletal and soft tissue sarcomas contain a common tumor-associated antigen (s). The antigen is detectable in sarcomas of the same histologic type from different patients as well as in sarcomas of different histologic types. The antigenic activity is not attributable to histocompatibility antigens or blood group antigens, as skin and muscle fibroblasts from the same patient from whom the sarcoma cells were derived did not contain detectable antigenic activity and each patient's serum reacted with antigens derived from his own sarcoma in tissue culture. The antigen is specific for the sarcoma cell lines, as it was not found in tissue cultures of normal human and nonhuman primate cells or in cells derived from nonsarcomatous malignancies.

The sarcoma-specific antigen (s) may be recognized in tumor-bearing patients who develop specific antisarcoma antibody. The specificity of these antibodies was shown by the high incidence in patients who have skeletal and soft tissue sarcomas, the low incidence in patients with nonsarcomatous malignant disease, and by the correlation of the change in antisarcoma antibody titer with progression of the malignant disease. That the antibodies do not react with tissue culture cells derived from normal organs or other nonsarcomatous malignant disease and that the antibody activity can only be removed with antigens derived from sarcoma cells provide further evidence that they are directed specifically against antigens associated with skeletal and soft tissue sarcomas.

These data also suggest that a viral agent is associated with these antigenic tumors. From what is known of the antigens of tumors caused by oncogenic viruses in experimental animals, the existence of a common cross-reacting antigen in different histologic types of sarcomas would indicate a common viral etiology. The demonstration of a high incidence of antisarcoma antibody in the relatives of the sarcoma patients suggests the association of an infectious agent capable of producing unrecognized infection in healthy contacts of these patients. Also, we have shown that it is possible to antigenically transform normal tissue culture cells with cell-free extracts derived both from sarcomatous tumors and from the media of sarcoma tissue culture cells. Furthermore, this transformation has the capacity for replication and persistence through numerous subcultures. Whether the "C" particles observed in the SA-1 cell line are responsible for the antigenic activity or whether an additional helper agent is necessary remains to be established.

To determine whether the associated infectious agent could be a contaminant or antigenically related to a common, known virus, the high-titer sera used to assay the various cell lines for the presence of antigen have been screened against 15 known viral group antigens without any consistent positive reactions. Additionally, to date the SA-1 (liposarcoma) antigen has been assayed with 138 known viral antisera without any positive reactions.

If the infectious agent associated with these tumors is common enough to give a 20% incidence of antibody in normal sera and a 79% incidence of reactivity in healthy relatives of these patients, the question of why sarcomas are not seen more frequently and in more families is appropriate. However, similar seroepidemiologic studies of normal animals have frequently revealed antibodies to naturally occurring oncogenic viruses in the chicken and the mouse. Furthermore, in most infectious processes, both humoral antibody and cellular immunity are important for prevention of establishment and progression of an infectious agent. Infection of adult mice with Moloney sarcoma virus or chickens with the Rous sarcoma virus results in the temporary growth of a sarcomatous tumor which almost always regresses without treatment. However, in neonatal mice or in adult mice rendered immunodeficient by X-irradiation, the virus can be shown to produce progressive and lethal sarcomas.

Whether these filterable agents and observed viral particles in human sarcomas are incidental passengers or directly related to their etiology remains to be determined. Hopefully, with isolation of these particles and further immunologic studies, a more definitive relationship can be established.

Summary

Antimelanoma antibodies previously demonstrated in the sera of melanoma patients by immunofluorescence have now been detected by a sensitive and quantitative complement-fixation technique. The melanoma-specific antibodies detected by both of these techniques show a remarkable correlation with the stage of disease. Study of sera from 63 melanoma patients showed that both the incidence and titer of antibodies to the tumor antigens of malignant melanoma were higher in patients with localized melanoma than in those with widespread metastatic disease. Furthermore, study of serial serum specimens on melanoma patients revealed a drop in antibody titer to undetectable levels with advancing metastatic disease.

Additional evidence for the importance of immunologic factors in this disease came from studies of delayed cutaneous hypersensitivity in melanoma patients. All patients with localized melanoma were capable of being sensitized to DNCB, whereas all patients who could not manifest delayed cutaneous hypersensitivity to this chemical had widespread metastatic disease.

Immunologic studies have revealed a high incidence of antibodies to sarcoma-specific antigen (s) prepared from tissue culture cells derived from a human liposarcoma in the sera of patients with various types of skeletal and soft tissue sarcomas. A close correlation has been found between the antisarcoma antibody titers and the progression of the malignant disease in these patients. A rising titer of antisarcoma antibody was consistently observed following surgical removal of the tumor mass in patients with sarcomas. All patients with recurrent disease were found to have a progressive decline in their titers of antisarcoma antibody with advancing disease.

The discovery of a common antigen in different histologic types of human sarcomas, the demonstration of the presence of a filterable agent in these sarcomas capable of antigenically transforming normal tissue culture cells, and the presence of a high incidence of antisarcoma antibodies in close family members of the sarcoma patients support the hypothesis of an associated viral agent in skeletal and soft tissue sarcomas.

References

1. Dore, J. F.: New antigens in human leukemia cells and antibody in the serum of leukemic patients. Lancet, 2:1396, 1967.
2. Eilber, F. R., and D. L. Morton: Cutaneous anergy and prognosis following cancer surgery. Surg. Forum, 10:116-117, 1969.
3. Eilber, F. R., and D. L. Morton: Impaired immunologic reactivity and recurrence following cancer surgery. Cancer, 25:362-367, 1970.
4. Eilber, F. R., and D. L. Morton: Sarcoma specific antigens: Detection by complement fixation with serum from sarcoma patients. J. Nat. Cancer Inst., 44:651-656, 1970.
5. Everson, T. C.: Spontaneous regression of cancer. Ann. New York Acad. Sci., 114: 721, 1964.
6. Fass, L., R. B. Herberman, J. L. Ziegler, and J .W. M. Kiryabwire: Cutaneous hypersensitivity reactions to autologous extracts of malignant melanoma cells. Lancet, 1:116-118, 1970.
7. Fink, M. A., M. Karon, F. J. Rauscher, R. A. Malmgren, and H. C. Orr: Further observations on the immunofluorescence of cells in human leukemia. Cancer, 18: 1317-1321, 1965.

8. Gold, P.: Circulating antibodies against carcinoembryonic antigens of the human digestive system. Cancer, 20:1663-1667, 1967.
9. Hammond, W. G., J. C. Fisher, and R. T. Rolley: Tumor specific transplantation immunity to spontaneous mouse tumors. Surgery, 62:124-133, 1967.
10. Hellström, I., K. E. Hellström, G. E. Pierce, and A. H. Bill: Demonstration of cell-bound and humoral immunity against neuroblastoma cells. Proc. Nat. Acad. Sci. USA, 60:1231-1238, 1968.
11. Hellström, I., K. E. Hellström, G. E. Pierce, and J. P. S. Yang: Cellular and humoral immunity to different types of human neoplasms. Nature, 220:1352-1354, 1968.
12. Henle, G., and W. Henle: Immunofluorescence in cells derived from Burkitt's lymphoma. J. Bacteriol., 91:1248-1256, 1966.
13. Klein, G.: Tumor antigens. Ann. Rev. Microbiol., 20:223, 1966.
14. Klein, G., P. Clifford, E. Klein, R. T. Smith, J. Minowada, F. M. Kourilsky, and J. H. Burchenal: Membrane immunofluorescence reactions of Burkitt lymphoma cells from biopsy specimens and tissue cultures. J. Nat. Cancer Inst., 39:1027-1044, 1967.
15. Lewis, M. G.: Possible immunological factors in human malignant melanoma in Uganda. Lancet, 2:921, 1967.
16. Lewis, M. G., R. L. Idonopisov, R. C. Nairn, T. M. Phillips, H. G. Fairley, D. C. Bodenham, and P. Alexander: Tumour-specific antibodies in human malignant melanoma and their relationship to the extent of the disease. Brit. Med. J., 1:547-562, 1969.
17. Morton, D. L., and R. A. Malmgren: Human osteosarcomas: Immunologic evidence suggesting an associated infectious agent. Science, 162:1278, 1968.
18. Morton, D. L., R. A. Malmgren, W. T. Hall, and G. Schidlovsky: Immunologic and virus studies with human sarcomas. Surgery, 66:152, 1969.
19. Morton, D. L., R. A. Malmgren, E. C. Holmes, and A. S. Ketcham: Demonstration of antibodies against human malignant melanoma by immunofluorescence. Surgery, 65:233, 1968.
20. Morton, D. L., F. R. Eilber, R. A. Malmgren, and W. C. Wood: Immunologic factors which influence response to immunotherapy in malignant melanoma. Surgery. In press.
21. Muna, N. M., S. Marcus, and C. Smart: Detection by immunofluorescence of antibodies specific for human malignant melanoma cells. Cancer, 23:88-93, 1969.
22. Nadler, S. H., and G. E. Moore: Clinical immunologic study of malignant disease. Response to tumor transplants and transfer of leukocytes. Ann. Surg., 164:482-490, 1966.
23. Oettgen, H. F., T. Aoki, L. J. Old, E. A. Boyse, E. deHarven, and G. M. Mills: Suspension culture of a pigment-producing cell line derived from a human malignant melanoma. J. Nat. Cancer Inst., 41:827-831, 1968.
24. Old, L. J., and E. A. Boyse: Antigens of tumors and leukemias induced by virus. Fed. Proc., 24:1009, 1965.
25. Old, L. J., E. A. Boyse, H. C. Oettgen, E. deHarven, G. Geering, B. Williamson, and P. Clifford: Precipitating antibody in human sera to an antigen present in culture Burkitt's lymphoma cells. Proc. Nat. Acad. Sci. USA, 56:1699, 1966.
26. Rhomsdahl, M. D., and I. S. Cox: Immunofluorescent studies of antibodies against human malignant melanoma. Surg. Forum, 10:126-128, 1969.
27. Summer, W. C., and A. C. Foraker: Spontaneous regression of human melanoma, clinical and experimental study. Cancer, 13:79, 1960.
28. Teimourion, B., and W. S. McCune: Surgical management of malignant melanoma. Amer. Surg., 29:515, 1963.

Immunity to Neuroblastomas

INGEGERD HELLSTRÖM AND
KARL ERIK HELLSTRÖM

*Departments of Microbiology and Pathology, University of Washington
Medical School, Seattle, Washington, USA*

IT HAS BEEN well established that the majority of experimentally induced animal neoplasms possess tumor-specific transplantation antigens (TSTA) [8, 9, 10] and that immune reactions against such antigens can be demonstrated by in vitro techniques such as the colony inhibition (CI) assay.[5]

We have employed the CI technique to search for immunologic reactions against antigens specific for neoplasms in man and to analyze these reactions to some extent. The tumors first subjected to these studies were neuroblastomas. They were chosen for several reasons: the tumors occasionally regress,[1] indicating that an immunologic reaction against tumor-associated antigens might occur in vivo, their cells grow well in vitro and can be morphologically distinguished from contaminating stroma cells, and Dr. Alexander Bill at the Children's Orthopedic Hospital in Seattle offered excellent possibilities for a collaborative study, since he had a large number of neuroblastoma patients, some of whom he had followed clinically for years, and some of whom were symptom-free (cured?).

The data obtained have been described in two recent publications;[2, 4] we will therefore confine ourselves to summarizing the main findings, and will refer interested readers to the two original papers, as well as to three more general discussions of the field[5-7] which present our points of view.

The CI technique was used in all our studies in an attempt to demonstrate immune reactions mediated by peripheral blood lymphocytes against tumor-associated (specific?) antigens of human neuroblastomas. Lymphocytes from all of 11 patients carrying actively growing neuroblastomas as well as lymphocytes from all of 11 patients who were clinically symptom-free after therapy for neuroblastomas inhibited colony formation of plated neuroblastoma cells. They did not inhibit colony formation in normal skin fibroblasts derived from the same patients as the tumor cells. A specific colony inhibition of neuroblastoma cells was also seen with lymphocytes from 12 of 16 mothers of children with neuroblastomas and with lymphocytes from some fathers and siblings of such patients. No specific inhibition of neuroblastoma cell colony formation was seen with lymphocytes from patients not having neuroblastomas or from healthy subjects.

Sera from seven of seven patients with progressively growing neuroblastomas, but not from any of five patients who were clinically symptom-free after treatment for such tumors, could block lymphocyte-mediated colony inhibition of plated neuroblastoma cells. Most likely, the sera from patients with actively growing tumors contained antibodies which could mediate an efferent form of immunologic enhancement.

We have concluded from these studies that neuroblastomas of man possess antigens absent from normal adult human cells, that lymphocytes from patients carrying growing neuroblastomas can react against these antigens in vitro, and that progressive growth of neuroblastomas in vivo is at least partially made possible by the demonstrated blocking effect of sera from patients with growing neuroblastomas. It is so far uncertain whether the information obtained can be utilized therapeutically. Attempts in this direction might best be carried out in animal model systems.

Findings very similar to those obtained with neuroblastomas have been obtained with other neoplasms as well,[3] indicating that the neuroblastoma results have a general applicability.

Acknowledgments

The authors' studies on neuroblastomas have been supported by grants CA-10188 and CA-10189 from the National Institutes of Health, by grant T-453 from the American Cancer Society, and by contract NIH-69-2061 from the National Institutes of Health to Dr. Charles McKhann, University of Minnesota, subcontracted to us.

References

1. Everson, T. C., and W. H. Cole: Spontaneous Regression of Cancer. Saunders, Philadelphia, 1966, 560 pp.
2. Hellström, I., K. E. Hellström, G. E. Pierce, and A. H. Bill: Demonstration of cell-bound and humoral immunity against neuroblastoma cells. Proc. Nat. Acad. Sci. USA, 60:1231-1238, 1968.
3. Hellström, I., K. E. Hellström, G. E. Pierce, and J. P. S. Yang: Cellular and humoral immunity to different types of human neoplasms. Nature, 220:1352-1354, 1968.
4. Hellström, I., K. E. Hellström, A. H. Bill, G. E. Pierce, and J. P. S. Yang: Studies on cellular immunity to human neuroblastoma cells. Internat. J. Cancer. In press.
5. Hellström, K. E., and I. Hellström: Cellular immunity against tumor antigens. Adv. Cancer Res., 12:167-223, 1969.
6. Hellström, K. E., and I. Hellström: Immunological defenses against cancer. Hosp. Prac., 5:45-61, 1970.
7. Hellström, K. E., and I. Hellström: Immunological enhancement as studied by cell culture techniques. Ann. Rev. Microbiol. In press.
8. Klein, G.: Tumor antigens. Ann. Rev. Microbiol., 20:223-252, 1966.
9. Old, L. J., and E. A. Boyse: Immunology of experimental tumors. Ann. Rev. Med., 15:167-186, 1964.
10. Sjögren, H. O.: Transplantation methods as a tool for detection of tumor specific antigens. Progr. Exp. Tumor Res., 6:289-322, 1965.

7

Tests for Carcinogenic Activity in Cell or Organ Culture

A Specific Common Chromosomal Pathway for the Origin of Human Malignancy. III. Extended Observations

JOHN W. GOFMAN, JASON L. MINKLER, ROBERT K. TANDY, DOLORES PILUSO, MARGARET SODERBERG, FRANK FICKEL, ERMA KOVICH, STUART P. STONE, AND JAMES L. LITTLEPAGE

Bio-Medical Division, Lawrence Radiation Laboratory, University of California, Livermore, California, USA

ADVANCES IN THE STUDY of human chromosomes in the past decade have produced a startling body of evidence that derangements in cellular chromosomal complement are responsible for several important human disease entities, such as Down's disease, Turner's disease, and others. In 1960, Nowell and Hungerford demonstrated a specific chromosomal abnormality characteristic of most cases of chronic granulocytic leukemia.

Over 60 years ago, Boveri originally proposed the hypothesis that an imbalance in cellular chromosome content, no matter what physical, chemical, or biologic mechanism was responsible for achieving it, might destine such cells to malignant behavior. In essence, this was a proposed explanation of all forms of human cancer. Recently we presented evidence supporting Boveri's hypothesis of a possible specific chromosomal origin of human cancer. An excess of E16 chromosomes was found in all of seven human cell lines and in two human cancers studied directly.

One major purpose of this communication is to provide the data from extensive further tests, in material from man, of the relationship of excess E16 chromosomes and cancer in man.

For the study of human chromosomes and cancer, the ideal material is fresh cancer tissue directly obtained from surgical specimens. The data for 11 such specimens will be presented. However, for reasons not clear at present, investigators throughout the world, ourselves included, have found that only 10 to 20% of human cancers lend themselves to such direct study. The difficulties have been of two types: (1) an adequate number of mitoses is not present in some of the fresh cancers obtained surgically, and/or (2) the quality of chromosome preparations from some cancers is poor. It is certainly to be hoped that future technologic improvements will solve these two problems. At the moment they plague all such investigations. It might appear, superficially, that this problem is obviated through the simple expedient of studying a larger number of cancer cases. This, however, is not a satisfactory solution, for, when 80% of the material does not lend itself to study, the possibility of bias is ever present.

Pending the ultimate technical solution of the problem of preparing fresh cancers for chromosome analysis, there exists a supply of very pertinent material of great relevance for the human cancer problem. This is in the form of the spontaneous human cell lines now available. Cell lines of human origin have arisen from explanted material of either nonmalignant or malignant origin. Once these lines have become established, they are characterized by essential immortality, in contrast with the limited life span of normal human cells in similar culture. Further, where tested, such immortal cell lines have been proved to show malignant properties, either by homotransplantation into man or by heterotransplantation into hamsters. Indeed, some investigators believe that cell lines in vitro are the malignancy equivalent to cancer in the living subject. Whether this analogy is as thorough going as this is subject to debate, and we shall by no means insist upon it here. It does appear clear, however, that such human cell lines have many properties of malignancy, and, hence, represent suitable material for evaluation of clues concerning human cancer. With this proviso in mind, the results of the study of the chromosomal constitution of 17 human cell lines will be presented.

The method we have developed for these studies utilizes electronic scanning of carefully traced chromosomes, and subsequent arm measurement and centromeric index determination by computer. Using this method, we have been able to circumvent many of the problems associated with automatic chromosome analysis. As a result, the data presented here are based upon the karyotypes of more than 6,000 cells, rather than the one or few often reported in the literature.

Measurements obtained from the karyotypes of some 1,800 normal cells are used to establish a cutting line diagram with boundary limits, both for length and for centromeric index, which is consistent with the Denver karyotype classification method. Normalization of measurements made on cell lines and cancers, to be consistent with measurements made on normal cells, is based upon the following postulate: In a cancer or cell line, chromosomes of any particular class, e.g., B chromosomes, have the same average length as do B chromosomes in a large group of normals. Indeed, unless this is broadly true, it is impossible to speak meaningfully of chromosome classes at all. So we can start using the same average length of each chromosome class in an unknown cancer as in normals. The chromosomes are then normalized with this arbitrary sum of lengths and classified. If we have overestimated the sum of lengths, then each of our classified chromosome groups will show too long a length. In such a case, a second iteration is made, and normalization again carried through. We have found that three or four iterative calculations lead to convergence, and the normalization correction is then completed.

The Experimental Results—Human Cell Lines

The human cell lines investigated are of three origins: (1) spontaneously occurring cell lines originating from nonmalignant explanted human tissue, (2) spontaneously occurring cell lines originating from malignant tissue or effusions from patients with known malignant growth, and (3) cell lines obtained from group (1) by selection for resistance to chemical antimetabolites.

For the 17 cell lines studied, we found that the mean number of E16 classified chromosomes was 6.36, as compared to 2.05 E16 mean number in the normals, or an increase of over three to one in the occurrence of E16 chromosomes in the cell lines.

We should digress for a moment to discuss the nonintegral chromosome numbers reported. Clearly, in any one cell the number of chromosomes in a particular classification must be integral. However, in a series of 50 cells, biologic plus technical variation can make the integral number of chromosomes in a particular cell different from the integral number in other cells. As a result, the final mean number of chromosomes per class is nonintegral. Thus for any chromosome class such as A1, A2, etc., we generally end up with a nonintegral mean number of chromosomes per cell, together with a standard error of that mean number which is the result of variability. All other factors being equal, the standard error of each mean varies inversely as the square root of the number of cells studied.

Returning to the results again, we next consider the effect of the increased number of chromosomes per cell in the cell lines on the E16 ratio. Consider, for example, the HeLa cell line. We find that the mean total chromosomes per cell is 69.72. For normal female cells, the E16 level is 2.05 chromosomes per cell. Therefore, simply on the basis of the ratio of 69.72 to 46, we would expect to find 3.11 E16 chromosomes per HeLa cell. But we observe 8.23 E16 chromosomes per HeLa cell. Therefore, there is an excess of 5.12 E16 chromosomes per cell, even after correcting for total number of chromosomes. If we carry through such an analysis for every chromosome class in every cell line studied, we find that only for E16 chromosomes is consistent behavior observed —namely, an elevation of E16 mean chromosome number above the corrected expectation. For the 17 cell lines studied, the mean E16 level is 2.03 times the corrected E16 expectation.

Experimental Results—Freshly Obtained Human Cancers

All the data presented to this point confirm our previous hypothesis that an E16 chromosome level elevation, absolute or relative to other chromosome classes, characterizes human cell lines—cell lines regarded by many as malignant—in vitro. How well does this hypothesis obtain when applied to freshly obtained human cancers? The latter represent the ultimately desirable test material, for with such material the argument cannot be raised that long-continued cell culture accounts for the chromosome findings, rather than a relationship of chromosome constitution with malignancy per se. Eleven fresh cancers have now been studied, in every case with chromosome preparations made from two to 20 hours after excision of the malignant tissue or withdrawal of the malignant effusion. The material included specimens of carcinomas of the breast, colon, bladder, ovary, and lung.

Ten of the 11 fresh cancers show appreciable and highly significant elevations in absolute E16 chromosome level; in the eleventh specimen, we were unable to demonstrate a significant absolute elevation in E16 level. This one cancer is extremely unusual in that it has only 37.13 total chromosomes per cell. Such cancers with total chromosome numbers this low have been reported before, but they are extremely rare. Although this cancer does not demonstrate an absolute elevation, it does show a significant elevation in E16 chromosomes after correction for total number of chromosomes per cell. The mean number of E16 chromosomes per cell for all 11 cancers is 3.72 or a ratio of 1.81 to 1 over normal cells on an absolute basis.

After including corrections for the number of chromosomes per cell, we find that 10 of the 11 cancers have a significant E16 chromosome elevation above the corrected expectation. The eleventh, with a demonstrable E16 level elevation on an absolute basis, fails to meet the more rigorous criterion of elevation above corrected expectation. The mean E16 chromosome levels corrected for total number of chromosomes per cell for all 11 cancers is 2.69 E16 chromosomes per cell. This is a ratio of observed E16 to corrected expected E16 of 1.38 to 1.

Possible Exceptions to the E16 Hypothesis

Nowell and Hungerford's discovery of the Philadelphia chromosome in chronic granulocytic leukemia was the first specific chromosome abnormality identified in a malignant disease. This chromosome is considered to represent a G chromosome from which approximately 40% of the DNA content has been deleted. An E16 chromosome excess was not reported. We have now had an opportunity to examine a specimen from a patient with chronic granulocytic leukemia by quantitative chromosome analysis. The data clearly demonstrate that no absolute excess of E16 chromosome exists.

The deletion of some G chromosomal material means that the G + Y level is lower than normal in chronic granulocytic leukemia. Therefore, even with a normal absolute E16 level, the ratio of E16 to G + Y may well be higher, in effect, than normal. It is to be noted that this ratio, E16 to G + Y, is high in every human cell line and every one of the 11 fresh cancers studied. It is, therefore, possible that chronic granulocytic leukemia may not represent an exception to the E16 hypothesis. Final decision must await determination of whether the E16 to G + Y imbalance is a necessary or sufficient condition for malignancy.

Burkitt's lymphoma is a special case among malignant diseases in two major respects. First, virus or viruslike particles are commonly demonstrable in involved tissues. Second, cell lines derived from Burkitt's lymphoma grow only in suspension culture, in contrast to those previously described, which all grow as monolayers, but which may also grow in suspension culture. We have subjected one such cell line to quantitative chromosome analysis, and found that the E16 level was 1.67 chromosomes per cell, which is within normal limits in the Burkitt's lymphoma cells with 46 and 47 chromosomes. Every cell, however, shows a specific marker chromosome, the content of which is unknown. If E16 genetic material is present in this marker chromosome, Burkitt's lymphoma would be consistent with all the cell lines and cancers. If not, this will represent a distinct exception to the E16 hypothesis.

Conclusions

There does exist a consistent chromosome abnormality in 17 human cell lines and in 11 fresh cancers, a finding strongly supportive of our original support of Boveri's concept of a chromosomal imbalance origin of human cancer. This abnormality is in the form of an excess of E16 chromosomes per cell, either absolute or in relationship to other chromosome classes. If the ratio of E16 chromosomes to those of other classes be the crucial parameter, several ratios involving E16 chromosomes must be considered as candidates. We believe the choice between such possible ratios might be better made when 100 or more human cancers have been studied, rather than now. It may be that imbalance in E16 chromosomes relative to certain other classes represents a necessary condition for malignant cell behavior, but that more than one such E16 imbalance may be a sufficient condition.

Acknowledgment

This work was performed under the auspices of the United States Atomic Energy Commission.

Effects of Carcinogenic Agents on Organ Cultures

ILSE LASNITZKI

Strangeways Research Laboratory, Cambridge, England

ORGAN CULTURES OFFER a convenient system for investigating the direct effects of carcinogenic agents under strictly controlled and easily reproducible experimental conditions. The anatomic relationships of the various tissue components and their functional activities are, with suitable techniques, preserved for long periods in vitro, and organ cultures are, therefore, more closely like their parent tissue than cell cultures. Although the system is more complex, it is, at the same time, more physiologic and allows study of the action of carcinogens on several parameters of tissue growth, such as cell proliferation, changes in the direction of/or loss of differentiation, and normal functional activity. The effects on the epithelium can be separated from those on the connective tissue, and alterations in their relationships determined. In hormone-dependent organs, the interaction of target-specific hormones with the carcinogens can be investigated.

In this paper is described the effect of carcinogenic hydrocarbons and cigarette smoke condensates on organ cultures of embryonic human lung, of embryonic and suckling mouse trachea, of embryonic mouse and rat skin, and of adult rat and mouse prostate glands.

Methods

Portions of the organs were grown in the presence of carcinogenic hydrocarbons in doses of 1 to 6 μg/ml medium or cigarette smoke condensate in concentrations of 100 to 300 μg/ml. Human and mouse lung were exposed continuously for periods of up to 28 days; and mouse trachea and rat and mouse epidermis for up to 14 days. Mouse and rat prostate glands were treated for 10 to 11 days and then transferred to normal control medium.

Various media were used. In earlier work, a mixture of cock plasma with horse serum and chick embryo extract was employed;[1, 2, 6] in recent experiments this was superseded by fluid media consisting of Morton and Parker's 199 with 3% chick embryo extract and/or varying concentrations of horse serum.[4, 7, 8]

Effects on Lung and Trachea

EMBRYONIC LUNG

HUMAN.—Most experimental data relating to effects of cigarette condensate have been obtained on rodents, and the organ culture method is a convenient way to compare the response of human and rodent lung. The condensates contain small amounts of noncarcinogenic and carcinogenic hydrocarbons, including benzpyrene, and the activity of this compound was tested on human embryonic lung.[1]

The lung consists of primitive bronchi lined with one row of secretory cells and embedded in cellular connective tissue. In benzpyrene-treated explants, the bronchial epithelium multiplies to form several layers projecting into the lumen. The original epithelium is shed and not replaced. The newly formed cells remain undifferentiated, show prominent nuclei and vary greatly in size. Occasionally, they undergo squamous metaplasia.

With increasing dose, the hyperplasia appeared earlier, but the final incidence was similar after all concentrations: 85% of treated explants.

The neutral fraction of cigarette smoke condensate has been widely tested in animal experiments. The effects of two of its subfractions, one containing the normal amount of hydrocarbons and another one that was enriched in them, were tested.[2, 3] Both compounds induced epithelial hyperplasia in bronchi and bronchial glands (Figure 7-1). In contrast to the benzpyrene effect, the secretory activity in some bronchi was initially increased or preserved for longer periods, and the hyperplastic epithelium was less pleomorphic and remained of the basal cell type or underwent squamous metaplasia. The "enriched"

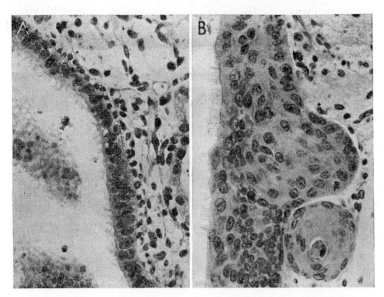

Fig. 7–1.—Bronchi of human lung after two weeks' growth in organ culture. *A*— Control bronchus showing one row of ciliated epithelium. *B*—Bronchus exposed to "enriched" hydrocarbon fraction of cigarette smoke condensate, showing hyperplastic epithelium and squamous metaplasia in bronchial gland. Periodic acid-Schiff stain after diastase digestion. Reduced from × 400.

fraction induced more extensive hyperplasia than the ordinary hydrocarbon fraction. Both benzpyrene and the two smoke condensates depressed stromal growth and severely damaged the cells and matrix of the bronchial cartilage.

MOUSE.—In organ cultures of embryonic mouse, neither benzpyrene nor the "enriched" hydrocarbon fractions were active. Conversely, methylcholanthrene and 1.2.3.5.6 dibenzanthracene induced considerable basal cell hyperplasia in the epithelium of the main bronchi. The secretory activity of the cells lining the bronchi was maintained for longer periods than in the human lung, but the newly formed cells underneath the secretory elements frequently became pleomorphic and in some explants broke through the basement membrane into the underlying connective tissue.

MOUSE TRACHEAS

In contrast to embryonic mouse lung, tracheas from late embryonic or suckling mice were susceptible to the "enriched" hydrocarbon fraction. The compound induced considerable hyperplasia of the tracheal epithelium.[4] Early effects seen were cell enlargement and increased secretory activity of the superficial cells combined with basal cell multiplication. As the exposure was extended, basal cell proliferation continued and many layers of irregularly enlarged cells were formed. As they moved up toward the lumen, secretory activity ceased, and the superficial cells became pyknotic and were shed into the lumen. Cells and matrix of the tracheal cartilage were severely damaged by the condensate.

Effects on Epidermis

The effect of carcinogenic hydrocarbons was also studied in non-secretory tissues. Epidermis of late embryonic mice and rats was exposed to dimethylbenzanthracene.[5] The carcinogen induced considerable basal cell hyperplasia in many explants and promoted the growth of the hair follicles. In some cultures, papilloma-like structures appeared, in others the hyperplastic epithelium broke through the basement membrane into the dermis, which was not visibly affected by the carcinogen.

Effects on Adult Mouse and Rat Prostate Glands

Carcinogens act not only on embryonic or postnatal tissues, but affect fully differentiated organs with a very low rate of cell division.

In prostate glands from adult mice and rats, epithelial cell proliferation was promoted by methylcholanthrene (Figure 7-2) and persisted after withdrawal of the carcinogen. The cells lost their secretory character, became pleomorphic, or underwent squamous metaplasia.[6, 7]

In both mouse and rat prostates, methylcholanthrene increased epithelial cell division to about four times the control value during a 10-day exposure. After withdrawal of methylcholanthrene, it fell to almost the control level, but then rose again to the previous high level.

The early effects of methylcholanthrene on RNA and protein synthesis were examined by autoradiography in rat prostate glands labeled with uridine T5 and leucine 4-5T, and assessed as the percentage of labeled epithelial cells. After two days, the incorporation of uridine was unchanged, but after six days' treatment, it was significantly increased in the experimental cultures. In contrast, the uptake of leucine was temporarily raised after two days' exposure and returned to the control level at six days.[8]

Prostate glands depend for their maintenance on androgenic hormones; the influence of such hormones and of estrogens on the induction of prostatic tumors by methylcholanthrene had been studied in animal experiments,[9, 10] without clear-cut results. The influence of testosterone, hydrocortisone, and estradiol on the methylcholanthrene effect in organ cultures of the rat prostate was investigated.[11] The hormones were added simultaneously with the carcinogen or after its withdrawal. It was found that (1) testosterone inhibited the hyperplasia normally seen after methylcholanthrene alone, whether added

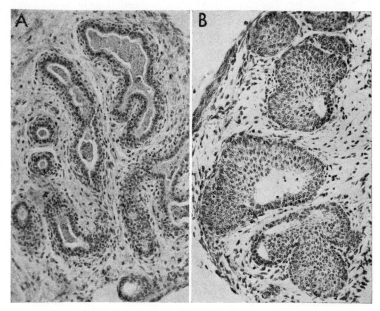

FIG. 7–2.—Organ cultures of rat ventral prostate gland after 11 days' growth. *A*—Control explant showing alveoli lined with one row of epithelium, embedded in cellular connective tissue. *B*—Explant exposed to 20-methylcholanthrene showing epithelial hyperplasia. Periodic acid-Schiff stain after diastase digestion. Reduced from × 130.

with or after the carcinogen; (2) hydrocortisone suppressed the hyperplasia if added simultaneously but only partially, if administered following the carcinogen; and (3) estradiol increased the hyperplasia and induced squamous metaplasia under both conditions.

In the mouse prostate gland, methylcholanthrene induced similar changes as in the rat, but the hyperplastic epithelium showed more dedifferentiation. In some explants, foci of disorganized, irregularly enlarged cells with polyploid divisions and multinucleate cells appeared, in others the hyperplastic epithelium underwent squamous metaplasia and became stratified into layers of basal, transitional, and precornifying cells. Vitamin A modified these changes. If added with the carcinogen, it prevented the squamous transformation but did not influence the hyperplasia; if added after the carcinogen, it inhibited both the hyperplasia and the squamous metaplasia.[12]

Conclusions

In all treated tissues, the carcinogens stimulated epithelial cell proliferation and, except for the epidermis, inhibited connective tissue growth.

The hyperplasia was associated with anaplasia or metaplasia of the newly formed cells. The term anaplasia is defined here as loss of differentiation accompanied by pleomorphic changes. The cells showed irregular increase of cell and nuclear size, prominent nucleoli, multipolar divisions, and multinucleate cells. Occasionally, they lost their organization, as in the mouse prostate, or acquired invasive properties, as in mouse lung and epidermis. Metaplasia, defined as a change in the direction of differentiation from the secretory to the squamous type, occurred in the mouse prostate and in human lung.

In all treated tissues, the extent of hyperplasia varied considerably in individual epithelial structures independently of the compound used or the duration of exposure. It is unlikely that this was caused by a difference in the concentration of the carcinogens in different areas of the explants, since "normal" bronchi or alveoli lined with one row of epithelium were often adjacent to others with a high degree of cell multiplication. But it might reflect a difference in susceptibility of the epithelial stem cells to the carcinogens.

The effects of the cigarette smoke condensates on human lung suggest that the hydrocarbons present in it play a role in the causation of human lung cancer. Mouse lung was, under the conditions of the experiment, not affected by them, and one should be cautious to extrapolate from mouse to man. Conversely, mouse trachea responded similarly to human lung; this organ could, therefore, be used as a substitute for human lung.

References

1. Lasnitzki, I.: The effect of 3-4 benzpyrene on human foetal lung grown in vitro. Brit. J. Cancer, 10:510, 1956.
2. Lasnitzki, I.: Observations on the effects of condensates from cigarette smoke on human foetal lung in vitro. Brit. J. Cancer, 12:547, 1958.
3. Lasnitzki, I.: The effect of a hydrocarbon enriched fraction of cigarette smoke condensate on human fetal lung grown in vitro. Cancer Res., 28:510, 1968.
4. Lasnitzki, I.: The effect of a hydrocarbon enriched fraction from cigarette smoke condensate on mouse tracheas grown in vitro. Brit. J. Cancer, 22:105, 1968.
5. Lasnitzki, I.: Tissue Culture of Skin. Progress in the Biological Sciences in Relation to Dermatology. Cambridge University Press, 1965.
6. Lasnitzki, I.: Precancerous changes induced by 20-methylcholanthrene in mouse prostates grown in vitro. Brit. J. Cancer, 5:345, 1951.
7. Lasnitzki, I.: The effect of methylcholanthrene on rat prostate glands grown in natural and semi defined medium. Cancer Res., 24:973, 1964.
8. Lasnitzki, I.: The effects of actinomycin D and methylcholanthrene on the cytology, RNA and protein synthesis in prostatic epithelium grown in vitro. Cancer Res., 29:318, 1969.
9. Allen, J. M.: Responses of the rat prostate gland to methylcholanthrene. J. Exp. Zool., 123:289, 1953.
10. Mirand, E. A., and W. J. Staubitz: Prostatic neoplasms of the Wistar rat induced with methylcholanthrene. Proc. Soc. Exp. Biol. Med., 93:457, 1956.
11. Lasnitzki, I.: Interaction of steroid hormones and methylcholanthrene in the rat prostate gland grown in organ culture. Europ. J. Cancer, 1:289, 1965.
12. Lasnitzki, I.: Influence of a hypervitaminosis on the effect of 20-methylcholanthrene on mouse prostate glands grown in vitro. Brit. J. Cancer, 9:434, 1955.

Hydrocarbon Carcinogenesis In Vitro

SUKDEB MONDAL

Department of Oncology, McArdle Laboratory for Cancer Research,
University of Wisconsin, Madison, Wisconsin, USA

THE MECHANISM of chemical carcinogenesis is at present an important problem to many investigators in the field of cancer research. There are at least three biologic theories of chemical carcinogenesis: (1) The carcinogen directly transforms normal cells into cancer cells; (2) the carcinogen selects for pre-existing cancer cells; and (3) the carcinogen activates a latent oncogenic virus in the cells.[12] Another important question is whether the process of carcinogenesis can be reversed.

In the laboratory of Professor Charles Heidelberger in the McArdle Laboratory for Cancer Research, University of Wisconsin, the problem of the mechanism of chemical carcinogenesis has been studied for a long time.[7, 8] Toward this end, a quantitative system for hydrocarbon carcinogenesis in vitro has been developed.[2-4, 9] Aneuploid lines of cells derived from C3H mouse ventral prostate can be cultured indefinitely. The cells grow to a monolayer and reach a saturation density without piling up in the dishes. They do not give rise to tumors on subcutaneous inoculation of 10^6 to 10^7 cells into irradiated C3H mice. When such cells were treated for one day in culture with 3-methylcholanthrene (3-MC), they piled up after reaching a monolayer (see Figure 2-5). The cells from these piled-up areas, when inoculated into non-irradiated C3H mice, gave rise to progressively growing, transplantable and metastasizing fibrosarcomas with only 10^3 cells.

Other workers in chemical carcinogenesis[1, 5, 15] use mouse and hamster embryonic cells at the early passage for their studies. Those cells are probably diploid and they do not form a permanent line.

The question of direct transformation of normal cells to malignant cells or selection for pre-existing clones of malignant cells from the parent line by the carcinogen was investigated by us.[16] In that experiment, individual single cells were isolated by using very small bits of cover slips (1 to 2 mm^2), and the bits containing only one cell by inspection were treated either with 0.5% dimethyl sulfoxide (DMSO) or with various concentrations of 3-MC for 24 hr or six days. The results (see Table 2-3) showed that under optimal conditions, treatment of individual single cells with 3-MC led to the development of piled-up transformed colonies in 100% of the clones, whereas with 18 DMSO-treated individual single cells, only one (about 5%) gave rise to a transformed clone. This 5% transformation in the control series may be considered as a spontaneous transformation, and did not recur in comparable subsequent experiments. However, the 100% transformation of the 3-MC-treated single cells was definitely attributable to the carcinogen. This result also indicated that the dose range of 1 to 2.5 μg/ml of 3-MC had a low toxicity (as expressed by cloning efficiency), but the highest carcinogenicity in comparison to the dose of 10 μg/ml where the toxicity was higher but the carcinogenicity was lower. Thus, there was no direct relationship between the toxicity of the carcinogenic hydrocarbon and its ability to produce transformation. This is in agreement with the previous findings in our laboratory[4] and those of Huberman and Sachs.[13] From a recloning experiment (Figure 7-3) it was demonstrated that all the progeny of the 3-MC-treated single cells were potentially transformed, but the time taken for the expression of transformed state as piled-up colonies was variable. We do not know the reason for this. These experiments completely rule out the mechanism that 3-MC acts by the selection of pre-existing malignant cells in our system.

It is now well known that sarcomas and carcinomas induced in mice and rats by carcinogenic hydrocarbons exhibit tumor-specific trans-

FIG. 7–3.—Outline of the recloning experiments.

Individual single cell

MCA 1 μg/ml, treatment for 1 day

↓

cultured in normal media for 36 days

↓

No piled up colonies

↓

400 of these cells plated in 10 dishes

↓

cultured for 8 days

↓

36 clones isolated

↓

33 clones grew successfully

↓

All clones developed piled up colonies

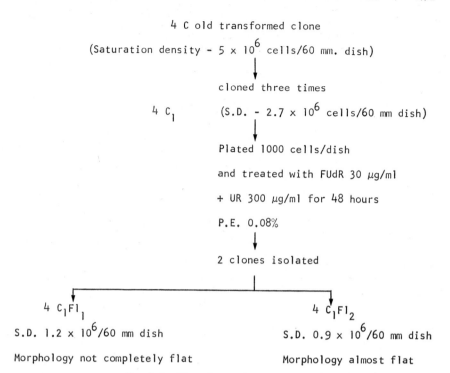

4 C old transformed clone

(Saturation density - 5×10^6 cells/60 mm. dish)

cloned three times

$4 C_1$ (S.D. - 2.7×10^6 cells/60 mm dish)

Plated 1000 cells/dish

and treated with FUdR 30 μg/ml

+ UR 300 μg/ml for 48 hours

P.E. 0.08%

2 clones isolated

$4 C_1Fl_1$ $4 C_1Fl_2$

S.D. 1.2×10^6/60 mm dish   S.D. 0.9×10^6/60 mm dish

Morphology not completely flat   Morphology almost flat

FIG. 7–4.—Plan of reversion experiment.

plantation antigens.[6, 11, 17, 18, 20] We wanted to see whether the cells transformed in vitro by chemical carcinogens also exhibited transplantation antigens and, if so, whether those antigens were cross-reactive. Seventeen clones of transformed cells were tested for their immunogenicity in C3H mice (the details of this experiment will be described elsewhere at this Congress[22]). Eleven of these clones were definitely antigenic and only one was nonantigenic. No cross-reactivity was found within seven pairs of clones isolated from the same dish or within three clones derived from three different dishes. Thus our in vitro experiments are in good accord with the in vivo experience. This agreement lends support to the validity of our system as a model of carcinogenesis.

The question of the activation of a latent oncogenic virus by the chemical carcinogen is also under intensive study in our laboratory. Some experiments done in our laboratory have failed to provide any evidence in favor of the activation or "switching on" of a latent virus by carcinogens, as follows:

1. Cell-free extract of transformed cells were not cytopathic to various other cell lines.[9]

2. Cell-free extracts of transformed cells did not induce any tumor

TABLE 7-1.—TUMOR PRODUCTION OF CLONE 4 C_1
AND ITS VARIANTS

No. of Cells Injected	4 C_1	Clone 4 C_1FL_1	Clone 4 C_1FL_2
10^6	4/4	4/4	1/4
5×10^5	4/4	—	0/4
10^5	4/4	4/4	0/4
5×10^4	3/4	0/4	0/4
10^4	1/4	0/4	0/4

or neoplastic disease after inoculation into newborn C3H mice, observed throughout their lifetime.[10]

3. Few viruslike particles have been observed in electron micrographs of both control and transformed cells.

4. Drs. Hartley and Huebner of the National Cancer Institute have failed to detect the group-specific antigens of the murine leukemia-sarcoma complex of viruses in our control or transformed cells either by direct complement fixation test or by their Comul test.[11, 23] Although negative experiments cannot constitute proof, there is no evidence at present in favor of the activation or "switching on" of a latent oncogenic virus in our system for chemical carcinogenesis in vitro.

Last, we are interested in the question of whether chemical carcinogenesis is a reversible process. Both Drs. Howard Green[19] and Leo Sachs[21] with their collaborators have isolated from clones of cells transformed by polyoma and Simian 40 (SV40) viruses some less malignant variants. For this Green treated the transformed cells with FUdR while Sachs plated the transformed cells over a glutaraldehyde-fixed normal cell layer. We wanted to see whether less malignant chemically transformed cells could also be obtained by the use of both the techniques. The preliminary results showed that it was possible to obtain with FUdR from a thrice-cloned transformed cell line a clone that required 2·5 logs more cells to induce a tumor (Figure 7-4 and Table 7-1). Thus it is possible that the process of chemical carcinogenesis may not be absolutely irreversible.

Summary

Single cells were isolated and treated individually with 3-MC and DMSO. All the cells treated with 3-MC developed into malignant clones, whereas only one cell out of 18 DMSO-treated cells gave rise to a malignant clone. This proved that the carcinogen produced a direct transformation, rather than selecting a pre-existing malignant clone in our system. It has been shown that the cells transformed in vitro by chemical agents exhibit transplantation antigens that are not cross-reactive. This agrees with the fact that many of the chemically induced tumors in animals exhibit tumor-specific transplantation antigens. Efforts to substantiate the theory of activation or "switching on" of some latent oncogenic virus by the carcinogen have so far failed. The possibility of reversion of the process of carcinogenesis has also been studied. Less malignant variant clones were isolated from a chemically transformed thrice cloned cell line by treating it with FUdR or plating it over gluteraldehyde-fixed normal cells, as had been shown with the cells transformed by viruses.

References

1. Berwald, Y., and L. Sachs: J. Nat. Cancer Inst., 35:641, 1965.
2. Chen, T. T., and C. Heidelberger: J. Nat. Cancer Inst., 42:903, 1969.
3. Chen, T. T., and C. Heidelberger: J. Nat. Cancer Inst., 42:915, 1969.
4. Chen, T. T., and C. Heidelberger: Int. J. Cancer, 4:166, 1969.
5. DiPaolo, J. A., P. Donovan, and R. Nelson: J. Nat. Cancer Inst., 41:53, 1968.
6. Foley, E. J.: Cancer Research, 13:835, 1953.
7. Heidelberger, C.: J. Cell Comp. Physiol., 64 (Suppl. 1) :129, 1964.
8. Heidelberger, C.: Canadian Cancer Conference, 7:323, 1967.
9. Heidelberger, C., and P. T. Iype: Science, 155:214, 1967.
10. Heidelberger, C., P. T. Iype, M.-R. Röller, and T. T. Chen: Studies of hydrocarbon carcinogenesis in organ and cell culture. In: The Proliferation and Spread of Neoplastic Cells (The University of Texas M. D. Anderson Hospital and Tumor Institute at Houston, 21st Annual Symposium on Fundamental Cancer Research) . The Williams and Wilkins Company, Baltimore, 1968, pp. 137-154.
11. Hartley, J. W., W. P. Rowe, W. I. Capps, and R. J. Huebner: J. Virol., 3:126, 1969.
12. Huebner, R. J., and G. J. Todaro: Proc. Nat. Acad. Sci. USA, 64:1087, 1969.
13. Huberman, E., and L. Sachs: Proc. Nat. Acad. Sci. USA, 56:1123, 1966.
14. Klein, G., H. O. Sjögren, E. Klein, and K. E. Hellström: Cancer Res., 20:1561, 1960.
15. Kuroki, T., and H. Sato: J. Nat. Cancer Inst., 41:53, 1968.
16. Mondal, S., and C. Heidelberger: Proc. Nat. Acad. Sci. USA, 65:219, 1970.
17. Old, L. J., E. A. Boyse, E. Carswall, and D. A. Clarke: Ann. N. Y. Acad. Sci., 101:80, 1962.
18. Prehn, R. T., and J. M. Main: J. Nat. Cancer Inst., 18:769, 1957.
19. Pollack, R. E., H. Green, and G. Todaro: Proc. Nat. Acad. Sci. USA, 60:126, 1968.
20. Revesz, L.: Cancer Res., 20:443, 1960.
21. Rabinowitz, Z., and L. Sachs: Nature, 220:1203, 1968.
22. Mondal, S., L. Griesbach, and C. Heidelberger: Noncross-reactivity of antigenic clones obtained by in vitro malignant transformation of mouse prostate cells by methylcholanthrene. (Abstract) Tenth International Cancer Congress Abstracts, Houston, Texas, 1970, p. 33.
23. Huebner, R. J.: Personal communication.

Chemical Carcinogenesis In Vitro

JOSEPH A. DiPAOLO

Cytogenetics and Cytology Section, Biology Branch, Etiology,
National Cancer Institute, National Institutes of Health,
Bethesda, Maryland, USA

INVESTIGATION OF chemical carcinogenesis in vitro dates from the time of Earle[1] and Gey,[2] who showed that cells cultured serially over a long period of time in heterologous media underwent malignant transformation in the presence or absence of known carcinogenic agents. These studies, which were performed with cell lines derived from mice or rats, have two major disadvantages. It now appears that in vitro spontaneous transformation occurs most often with fibroblasts such as from inbred mouse material, particularly when medium is supplemented with horse serum. The other drawback is that the recognition of transformation in mass populations is difficult because recognition depends on the original change as well as upon conditions in the population which allow for selection of transformed and untransformed cells.

Nevertheless, because carcinogenesis studies in vivo frequently utilize mice, we thought that it would be desirous to use mouse material for in vitro assay. To produce a normal cell line with properties of "normal" cells, the heart was the organ of choice since it is rarely associated with malignancy. Cell strains derived from mammalian heart tissue are rare, and even the cells thought at first to have been derived from cynomolgus monkey heart and reported by Salk[3] to produce fatal tumors when injected into pretreated Wistar rats were later thought to be a line of human heteroploid cells similar to HeLa cells that had contaminated the culture and overgrown the monkey heart cells.

In our study, within four months the cultures derived by mechanical dispersion of polyoma-free strain A mouse hearts and grown in Eagle's basal medium plus 15% fetal bovine serum were growing steadily and rapidly and extended up the sides of the 8-oz "gem oval" bottles. Growth became so heavy after three weeks that several layers of cells peeled off in sheets. Cells would survive mechanical or enzyme removal from the glass surface.

Strain A male mice given 1.25 mg of cortisone acetate 24 hr previously were injected with cultures four to five months old (15 subcultures). All 10 animals injected subcutaneously with at least 3×10^6 viable cells developed tumors. Tumors appeared approximately three weeks after inoculation and grew at a steady rate; the tumors later grew in unconditioned mice.[4]

The tumor masses that developed consisted of mesenchymal tissue. The cultures were made up of fibroblasts. Cells exhibited dispersion of chromosome numbers with at first no mode in the distribution curve. Thus with the culture conditions cytologic and neoplastic transformation had occurred, proving again that mouse connective tissue, regardless of source, can be expected to produce fibroblasts that may undergo spontaneous transformation.

In order to have a standardized, easily reproducible bioassay, we next considered the use of permanent lines such as the 3T3, WI-38, and more recently the Al/N line. Carcinogenic polycyclic hydrocarbons had no effect. We concluded that contact-inhibited cell lines do not yet represent the ideal system for chemical carcinogenesis. Special situations, however, do exist: the pseudodiploid Chinese hamster "Don" line adapted to grow in agar produced more tumors after carcinogen treatment than before;[5] aneuploid fibroblast cell lines derived from C3H mouse prostate tissue used during a finite period produce a low frequency of tumors which is augmented by carcinogenic hydrocarbons.[6]

Because of the successful viral studies with Syrian hamsters, we shifted our attention to this species. Probably the most successful studies reported in chemical carcinogenesis in vitro have been with the treatment of mass cultures of Syrian hamster embryo cells.[7-11] The exposure of these cells either as primaries, secondaries, or tertiaries to chemical carcinogens belonging to the polycyclic hydrocarbon or to the 4-nitroquinoline-N-oxide class have resulted in transformed cells which, when implanted into animals, produced tumors, while control cells failed to produce tumors. Our studies in this area were first reported at the International Cancer Congress held in Tokyo in 1966.[12] The transformed cells had a number of properties known to be common indices of neoplastic transformation. The cytopathic effect was determined by the carcinogen used, 3-methylcholanthrene being more toxic than benzo[a]pyrene, and dimethylbenz[a]anthracene being the most toxic compound of the polycyclics, and by the concentration of the suspension which varied from 0.01 μg to 10 μg/ml of medium. Cells originally exposed to 3-methylcholanthrene or benzo[a]pyrene were re-exposed to 3-methylcholanthrene, benzo[a]pyrene, or pyrene, and results obtained were compared to secondary hamster embryo cultures exposed to the same compounds in the same manner. Both transformed lines are resistant to the carcinogen to which they were originally exposed as well as to a second carcinogen. Suspension of benzo[a]pyrene and methylcholanthrene as high as 100 μg/ml did not inhibit the multiplication of cells which had been exposed originally to carcinogen 90 days previously; in fact, these cells were approximately 20 times more dense than at the start. These were also unaffected by the noncarcinogen. In contrast, the normal cells were extremely sensitive to the two carcinogens used, but insensitive to the noncarcinogen. The doubling rate of transformed lines was 15 to 17 hr, while the optimal division time of the secondary hamster embryo cells was 24 hr. With repeated change of tissue culture medium, a progressive increase in cell numbers occurred which eventually reached a saturation level. For a 50-mm petri dish, the total number was 4×10^6 cells for the normal secondary, while the benzo[a]pyrene-transformed line had 3×10^7 cells and the methylcholanthrene-exposed cells had 9×10^7 cells. Another property of some cell lines transformed by chemical carcinogens was the ability of the transformed lines to produce colonies in agar medium. No such colonies were found when normal control cells were plated at 10^4 to 10^6 cells per dish. Chromosome analysis of transformed lines indicated that the populations were at first near diploid, and eventually that the lines developed hypotetraploid elements. The control cultures, however, remained diploid for at least the first 10 passages. Further transformation was obtained by exposing chemically transformed cells to Simian virus 40 (SV40) or LLE 46 strain of adenovirus.[13] It has been routine in our laboratory to test all transformed cell lines for viruses known to transform hamster cells in vitro or in vivo. These have included polyoma, the adenoviruses, and SV complex. Complement fixation tests have been negative. In addition, viruses found as contaminants by the MAP test have also been examined, and the cultures have been negative for a number of viruses such as Sendai, K, MBM, LCM, LDH, M. *hepatitis*, Rheo3 and PBM.

On the basis of the foregoing studies, we decided that early subcultures of hamster cells were prime candidates for developing an in vitro system for carcinogenesis. Subsequently, we were fortunate in having Doctors Sachs and Huberman demonstrate their system for in vitro transformation by chemical carcinogens.[14] Our published procedure used as a standard transformation assay incorporates some modifications of their basic technique.[15] We reported the establishment of clonal transformation from cultures derived from random and inbred Syrian hamsters. The results obtained with in vivo polycyclic hydrocarbons which are noncarcinogens, weak carcinogens, or potent carcinogens, as well as the degree of decrease in cloning efficiency, may be taken as an indication that the transformed colonies were induced by the carcinogen used.

By carrying out experiments in which cells were grown on cover slips, it was possible to propagate the transformed clones and to produce cell lines which were homogeneous.[16] We then reported that lines developed from chemically altered clones produced serially transplantable fibrosarcomatous tumors, whereas cell lines derived from normal-appearing clones did not produce tumors. Thus we showed the quantitation of clonal alterations and the correlation of the morphologically altered colonies with tumor production.

Our next interest was in determining some of the factors which can affect transformation.[17] Our assay method has the advantage that it uses freshly isolated diploid cells from animals known to be sensitive to the polycyclic hydrocarbons. However, the disadvantage lies in the low cloning efficiency and transformation rate and in the fact that growth or expression of transformed clones is suppressed at high cell densities. If one treats varying numbers of cells with 10 μg of benzo[a]-pyrene/ml medium and scores for t/cell per cent, there is very little variation between 300 and 1,000 cells/petri dish; furthermore, if one expresses these results as percentages (number of transformed clones divided by total clones $\times$ 100), the results fluctuate between 8 and 9%. This is again evidence that induction rather than selection is occurring. Once one gets beyond 1,000 cells, all scoring methods become less reliable because there are too many colonies to count accurately. Also, the large number of growing cells approach the situation in mono-layer cultures, and it becomes difficult to recognize the transformed areas. Thus we conclude that it is not possible to increase the number of countable transformed colonies per culture by increasing the total cells plated.

A feeder layer of irradiated rat cells may increase the cloning efficiency and the number of transformations, or it may actually be responsible for inhibiting the growth of hamster clones. The cloning efficiency of untreated cells was increased by a factor from four to 10 when they were grown in the presence of irradiated feeder cells. The proportional increase in the number of transformed colonies was lower and more variable than that in the control colonies on feeders. The interdependence of the transformation rate and the over-all cloning efficiency was investigated by adding feeder cells at different times before and after plating the hamster cells to be treated. The hamster cells were added to the various parts of the experiment at the same time. The cloning efficiency was highest when the feeders had been added 48 hr prior to the addition of hamster cells and decreased to a minimum if they were added 24 or 48 hr subsequent to the addition of the hamster cells. The transformation rate generally followed the over-all plating efficiency. If varying numbers of feeder cells are added at 0 time, they will also influence the transformation rate. For example, 30,000 irradiated rat cells have a very poor feeder effect, while 60 to 100,000 cells produce the optimal feeder effect; as the number of feeder cells increases beyond this, it becomes increasingly difficult to recognize the transformed colonies. The addition of one million feeder cells practically suppresses the recognition of transformed colonies. Therefore, it is likely that feeder cells can also check the formation of hamster colonies and consequently inhibit the growth of these transformed colonies. The sensitivity of the system was checked by using concentrations of 0.1 to 20 μg benzo[a]pyrene/ml medium. No threshold response was noted with these concentrations. Furthermore, once 10 μg/ml was exceeded, there was only further slight increase in the toxicity while there was still increase in the transformation rate. This probably indicates that all the cells sensitive to the cytotoxic action of the carcinogen have been eliminated, and that only those cells which are genetically and physiologically capable of being transformed or not are remaining.

In another series of experiments using a conditioned feeder layer, it was noted that there was an increase in proportionality of transformation between 0.1 and 10 µg of benzo[a]pyrene/ml of medium. The increase in number of transformations was Poissonian in distribution, and the transformation frequency was fitted to the curve by Dr. Gart. The results were consistent with a "one hit" hypothesis. When these data were plotted again, expressing the transformation as t/cell per cent vs. carcinogen concentration on a semilog scale, it was noted that the transformation increase fitted the concept that transformation is caused by induction. If this had not been increasing on a t/cell per cent basis, the line would have been static rather than increasing.

In conclusion, these observations on the quantitation of transformation, transformation following a linear relationship with dose, and the previous observations that transformed colonies can produce lines with the attributes of neoplastic cells, including the production of tumors, provide evidence that chemically induced oncogenesis can be studied in vitro by using diploid hamster cells as an in vitro model.

Acknowledgment

I wish to thank Mr. P. J. Donovan and Mr. R. L. Nelson for their capable assistance.

References

1. Earle, W. R.: Production of malignancy in vitro. IV. The mouse fibroblast cultures and changes in the living cells. J. Nat. Cancer Inst., 4:165-212, 1943.
2. Gey, G. O.: Cytological and cultural observations on transplantable rat sarcomata produced by inoculation of altered normal cells maintained in continuous culture. Cancer Res., 1:737, 1941.
3. Salk, J. E., and E. N. Ward: Some characteristics of a continuously propagating cell derived from monkey heart tissue. Science, 126:1338-1339, 1957.
4. DiPaolo, J. A.: In vitro spontaneous neoplastic transformation of mouse heart tissue. Nature, 213:932-933, 1967.
5. Borenfreund, E., M. Krim, F. K. Sanders, S. S. Sternberg, and A. Bendich: Malignant conversion of cells in vitro by carcinogens and viruses. Proc. Nat. Acad. Sci. USA, 56:672-679, 1966.
6. Chen, T. T., and C. Heidelberger: In vitro malignant transformation of cells derived from mouse prostate in the presence of 3-methylcholanthrene. J. Nat. Cancer Inst., 42:915-925, 1969.
7. Berwald, Y., and L. Sachs: In vitro transformation of normal cells to tumor cells by carcinogenic hydrocarbons. J. Nat. Cancer Inst., 35:641-661, 1965.
8. DiPaolo, J. A., and P. J. Donovan: Properties of Syrian hamster cells transformed in the presence of carcinogenic hydrocarbons. Exp. Cell Res., 48:361-377, 1967.
9. Kuroki, T., and H. Sato: Transformation and neoplastic development in vitro of hamster embryonic cells by 4-nitroquinoline-1-oxide and its derivatives. J. Nat. Cancer Inst., 41:53-71, 1968.
10. Sivak, A., and B. L. Van Duuren: Studies with carcinogens and tumor-promoting agents in cell culture. Exp. Cell Res., 49:572-583, 1968.
11. Goetz, I. E., B. R. Hill, and R. Kinosita: Evaluation of neoplastic transformation in vitro. Proc. Amer. Ass. Cancer Res., 10:30, 1969.

12. DiPaolo, J. A.: Morphological and growth response of hamster cells to carcinogenic hydrocarbons in vitro. IX International Cancer Congress, Abstracts of Papers, 1966, Tokyo, Japan, p. 100.
13. DiPaolo, J. A., A. S. Rabson, and R. A. Malmgren: In vitro viral transformation of chemically transformed cells. J. Nat. Cancer Inst., 40:757-770, 1968.
14. DiPaolo, J. A., P. J. Donovan, and R. L. Nelson: Quantitative studies of in vitro transformation by chemical carcinogens. J. Nat. Cancer Inst., 42:867-874, 1969.
15. Huberman, E., and L. Sachs: Cell susceptibility to transformation and cytotoxicity by the carcinogenic hydrocarbon benzo[a]pyrene. Proc. Nat. Acad. Sci. USA, 56:1123-1129, 1966.
16. DiPaolo, J. A., R. L. Nelson, and P. J. Donovan: Sarcoma producing cell lines derived from clones transformed in vitro by benzo[a]pyrene. Science, 165:917-918, 1969.
17. DiPaolo, J. A., P. J. Donovan, and R. L. Nelson: Conditions influencing in vitro transformation by chemical carcinogens. Proc. Amer. Ass. Cancer Res., 11:21, 1970.

Detection of Oncogenic Adenoviruses by the Use of Cell Transformation In Vitro

ROBERT M. McALLISTER

Children's Hospital of Los Angeles, Los Angeles, California, USA

By 1966, the 31 serotypes of human adenoviruses had been divided into three subgroups on the basis of their capacity to induce tumors in hamsters: the highly oncogenic (types 12, 18, and 31), the weakly oncogenic (types 3, 7, 14, 16, and 21), and the nononcogenic group composed of all other serotypes.[1-5] The highly oncogenic viruses induced tumors in a higher percentage of hamsters and after a shorter incubation period than the weakly oncogenic viruses. Of interest, the highly oncogenic subgroup corresponded to hemagglutination group 4 and the weakly oncogenic subgroup to hemagglutination group 1.[6] An interesting biologic feature of the adenovirus hamster tumor system was that the tumor cells contained no infectious virus but produced antigens, so-called tumor antigens, which resulted in complement-fixing antibody responses in the animals bearing the tumor. These antibodies reacted not only with the antigens in the tumor cell but also with early nonvirion antigens, designated T antigens, synthesized in tissue culture cells infected with the same adenovirus. The tumor and T antigens were found to be subgroup-specific, that is, shared by members of the two oncogenic subgroups.[4, 5] The finding of these subgroup-specific nonvirion tumor antigens in the tumor cells served as a marker in adenovirus-induced tumors.

In 1964 McBride and Wiener reported that adenovirus type (Ad) 12, in addition to inducing tumors in vivo, could transform newborn hamster kidney cells in vitro.[7] The transformed cells were epithelioid, piled on each other, did not contain detectable virus, but did produce Ad 12 tumor antigen. This finding was followed by reports of in vitro transformation of hamster, rat, and rabbit cells by Ad 12.[8-11] The cells used in these studies were in primary or early tissue culture passage, and therefore consisted of heterogeneous populations of cell types. The low rates of transformation observed (0.01 to 0.001%) may have been caused by a scarcity of susceptible cells, as suggested by Yamane and Kusano.[10] Also, Reed reported that batches of hamster embryo cells varied in their susceptibility to transformation.[11]

Since previous studies had shown that in vitro transformation by polyoma viruses and Simian 40 viruses (SV40) were most amenable to detailed studies in established cell lines with a high degree of autonomy in vitro, McAllister and Macpherson attempted to transform four clones of the NIL-2 hamster cell line[12] with Ad 12 virus to compare the transformation with that of primary rat embryo cells by the same virus.[13] Two methods were described for the in vitro transformation by Ad 12 of the hamster cell line NIL-2[14] (Figure 7-5). One method was similar to that developed by Temin and Rubin for the assay of Rous sarcoma virus-transformed chick cells[15] and the other was the same as that described by Macpherson and Montagnier for the assay of polyoma-transformed cells.[16]

For these studies a liquid medium described by Freeman et al. was used.[13] It consisted of Eagle's medium without calcium and with twice the normal concentration of amino acids and vitamins supplemented with 0.1 MM calcium chloride, 5% dialyzed calf serum, and 2% fetal calf serum. Agar overlay medium contained the same components and 0.5% agar. Media for agar suspension cultures consisted of Eagle's medium supplemented with 20% fetal calf serum and either 0.33% or 0.5% agar.[16]

In the first assay method, semiconfluent monolayers of NIL-2 cells (about 1.5×10^6 cells per culture) in 5-cm plastic petri dishes were rinsed with tris buffer solution, exposed to 0.1 ml of virus suspension for three hr at 37°, and overlaid with 2.5 ml of 0.5% agar medium. The plates were incubated at 37° in humidified atmosphere constantly gassed with approximately 10% CO_2 in air. After two days, 2.5 ml of liquid Freeman's medium were pipetted on top of the agar and replaced every two to three days for 25-50 days. Foci of transformed cells appeared after 17 days in the monolayer culture, and were as-

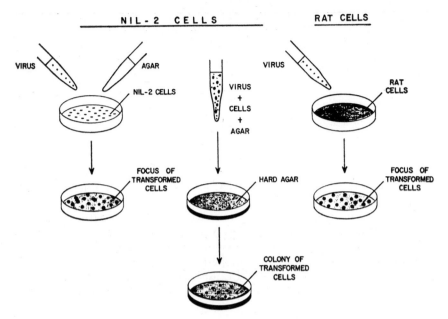

FIG. 7–5.—Adenovirus transformation assay systems.

sayed after pouring off the agar and staining the culture with Giemsa stain.

In the second method, centrifuged pellets of trypsin-dispersed NIL-2 cells were suspended in 1 ml of virus suspension, agitated for one hr at room temperature, and 5×10^5 cells in 1.5 ml of 0.33% agar medium were added to 5-cm petri dishes containing a preset base of 0.5% agar medium. After one week, 2 ml of Eagle's medium containing 10% fetal calf serum were pipetted on top of the agar and replaced weekly. Colonies 0.1 to 0.2 ml in diameter were present in the agar suspension culture after 21 days' incubation, and were counted with the aid of a low-power microscope after 25 days. These colonies, when transplanted to liquid medium, yielded transformed cells. The highest transformation rate, 0.002% of cells, was obtained by both methods using clone 3.

In addition, the NIL-2 cell assay methods were compared with the rat embryo cell transformation method described by Freeman et al.[13] This was identical to that described for monolayers of NIL-2 cells, except that a confluent sheet (about 4×10^6 cells) was exposed to virus and no agar overlay was used. The results obtained were approximately the same as those with NIL-2 cells. The rat cells did not form colonies when infected and suspended in agar; however, rat cells transformed in using Freeman's method under liquid medium did form colonies when suspended in agar medium.

TABLE 7–2.—TRANSFORMATION OF NIL-2 CELLS AND RAT EMBRYO
CELLS BY ADENOVIRUS 12*

	NIL-2 CELLS	RAT EMBRYO CELLS
Focus forming units (FFU) /ml virus stock	2.8×10^2	1×10^3
VP/FFU	1.7×10^7	5×10^6
PFU/FFU	3.9×10^6	1.1×10^6
Percent cells transformed (50-80 PFU/cell)	0.002	0.001

* Contain 5×10^9 total virus particle (VP)/ml and 1.1×10^9 PFU/ml.
(From McAllister and Macpherson.[14])

In summary, it was found in these studies that a virus stock containing 5×10^9 virus particles and 1.1×10^9 PFU/ml contained 2.8×10^2 focus-forming units per ml in NIL-2 cells (Table 7-2). The number of cell foci and of colonies induced by serial dilutions of virus were consistent with a linear dose response. Approximately 2×10^7 total virus particles or 4×10^6 infectious units were required to induce one focus of transformed NIL-2 cells. The highest transformation rate was 0.002% for cells exposed to about 80 PFU of virus per cell. The results obtained in the rat embryo cell transformation assay method were approximately the same as those with NIL-2 cells. Our results indicate that several clones of hamster fibroblasts were transformed by Ad 12 with about the same low efficiency as a heterogeneous population of rat embryo tissues. This suggests that the efficiency of transformation is primarily a function of virus and not attributable to a dearth of susceptible cells in these cultures.

With this background and because Freeman observed that the weakly oncogenic Ad 3 could transform rat cells in vitro,[17] our group decided to study the hitherto nononcogenic adenoviruses for their transforming capacity using the NIL-2 cell and rat embryo cell adenovirus transformation assay systems. During our studies of Ad 1, Freeman and associates reported transformation of rat cells by types 2 and 5.[18] All three of these viruses, types 1, 2 and 5, were in hemagglutination group 3. The results of our studies with type 1 indicated that the virus could transform rat cells in vitro but that it was cytopathic for

TABLE 7–3.—SPECIFICITY OF ADENOVIRUS TUMOR ANTIGEN AS DETERMINED
BY COMPLEMENT FIXATION

ANTIGEN	HAMSTER TUMOR ANTISERA					Schmidt-Ruppin
	Ad-1-SV40	Ad-2-SV40	Ad-5-SV40	Ad-12	SV40	
Ad-1 transformed rat cells	32-64*	16-32	16-32	0+	0	0
Ad-2 transformed rat cells	4-8	4-8	ND	0	0	0
Ad-12 transformed rat cells	0	0	ND	32-64	0	0

* Reciprocal of complement fixing antigen titer (20% cell extracts.)
+ 0: < 4
ND: Not done
(From McAllister et al.[19])

TABLE 7–4.—NUCLEIC ACID HOMOLOGY

DNA	AD-1 TRANSFORMED WHOLE-CELL RNA INPUT (counts/min.)	RNA BOUND (counts/min.)*	INPUT BOUND (%)
Adenovirus-1, 3 μg	26,900	200	0.74
	269,000	746	0.28
Escherichia coli K 996, 3 μg	26,900	24	0.08
	269,000	3	0.001

* Blank value: filter incubated in [^{32}P]RNA in absence of DNA was subtracted from each sample.
(From McAllister et al.[19])

hamster cells.[19] Approximately 6.5×10^5 PFU of virus were required to induce one focus of transformed cells. The transformed rat cells formed colonies in agar medium which had the cytologic characteristics of adenovirus-induced hamster tumors. Antigenic analysis of Ad 1 transformed cells by immunofluorescent and complement-fixing reactions indicated that the cells contained adenovirus-specific tumor antigens (Table 7-3). In addition, in agreement with the findings of Green et al., with cells transformed by the strongly oncogenic and the weakly oncogenic adenoviruses[20] and those of Freeman et al. with Ad 2 transformed rat cells,[18] the rat cells transformed by Ad 1 synthesized Ad 1 specific RNA which formed RNase-resistant hybrids with Ad 1 DNA (Table 7-4). These results, along with those of Freeman et al.,[18] suggested that in addition to the highly oncogenic viruses, now called subgroup A, and the weakly oncogenic viruses, subgroup B, a third group, subgroup C, composed of types 1, 2 and 5, have demonstrated transforming potential in vitro. Further studies by Green et al.[20] and Gilden et al.[21] indicated that members of subgroup C included types 1, 2, 5, and 6 and produced a common T antigen and a subgroup-specific messenger RNA.

As noted, these subgroups correspond to hemagglutination subgroups. Since HA group 2 had not induced tumors in vivo and had

TABLE 7–5.—TRANSFORMATION OF RAT EMBRYO CELLS BY ADENOVIRUS 19*

VIRUS INPUT PFU/CELL	NUMBER OF FOCI PER MONOLAYER CULTURE (1.4×10^6 cells per culture exposed to virus)
14.3	57, 46, 40
2.8	139, 130, 127, 118, 95, 89
1.4	97, 92, 76, 65, 65, 59
0.7	65, 57, 55, 54, 35, 30
0.35	23, 19, 18, 14, 11, 9
Control	0, 0, 0, 0, 0, 0

* 2×10^8 PFU/ml.
(From McAllister et al.[22])

not been tested for transforming activity in vitro, a number of these were tested by our group in the NIL-2 and rat embryo cell assay systems. The results of these studies indicated that primary rat embryo cells and NIL-2 hamster cells were transformed by Ad 9, 10, 13, 15, 17, 19 and 26[22] (Table 7-5). The transformed cells formed multilayered foci in monolayer cultures (Figure 7-6). Approximately 2.7×10^4 PFU of Ad 19 were required to induce one focus of transformed rat cells. Cell lines derived from such foci formed colonies when suspended in soft agar medium. In hamsters, Ad 19 and Ad 26 transformed NIL cells formed tumors with the morphologic characteristics of adenovirus tumors. In addition, the histology of cell colonies of Ad 19 transformed cells also resembled that of adenovirus tumors.

Antigens prepared from Ad 19 transformed NIL-2 cells or hamster tumors induced by these cells reacted with sera from hamsters bearing tumors induced by Ad 19 or Ad 26 transformed cells but not with sera from hamsters with tumors induced by Ad 12, Ad 7, Ad 2/SV40, or SV40 viruses (Table 7-6). The sera from hamsters with Ad 19 tumors or Ad 26 tumors reacted with cell pack antigens of Ad 13 and Ad 15 transformed NIL-2 cells, with 20% suspensions of KB cells infected with all members of hemagglutination group 2, and also with types 20, 25, and 28. These sera did not react with T antigens of human adenovirus groups A, B, or C, simian adenovirus subgroups 1-3, canine adenoviruses, bovine adenovirus type 3, polyoma, or SV40 (Table 7-7).

Unlike groups A, B, and C, no virus-specific RNA could be detected in adenovirus transformed rat or NIL-2 cells or in hamster tumors induced by Ad 19 cells.

The results of these studies suggest that all members of hemag-

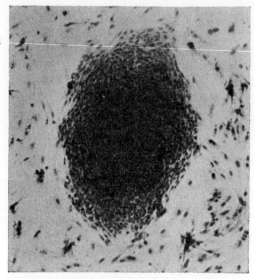

FIG. 7–6.—Focus of transformed rat embryo cells 60 days after infection. Giemsa stain. Reduced from × 42.5. (From McAllister et al.[22])

TABLE 7–6.—Specificity of Adenovirus Tumor Antigens as
Determined by Complement Fixation

	Hamster Tumor Antisera					
Source of Antigen	Ad-19	Ad-26	Ad-2-SV40	Ad-7	Ad-12	SV40
Ad-19 transformed NIL cells	80*	80	< 10	< 10	< 10	< 10
Ad-19 tumor extract	320	160	< 10	< 10	< 10	< 10
Ad-2-SV40 tumor extract	< 10	< 10	160	< 10	< 10	160
Ad-7 tumor extract	< 10	< 10	< 10	80	< 10	< 10
Ad-12 tumor extract	< 10	< 10	< 10	< 10	320	< 10
SV40 tumor extract	< 10	< 10	160	< 10	< 10	160

* Reciprocal of serum dilution reacting with 4 U of tumor antigen based on homologous tests. Representative results of multiple tests.
(From McAllister et al.[22])

glutination group 2 can be considered subgroup D of the human adenoviruses. All the members tested transformed rat and hamster cells in vitro, and the complete subgroup was readily defined by studies of T antigen using sera from hamsters bearing tumors induced by Ad 19 or Ad 26 transformed NIL cells.

Subgroup C as well as subgroup D viruses can transform rat cells in vitro, but have not been reported to cause tumors in rats, although, admittedly, extensive tests have not been made. In addition, rat cells transformed by these viruses do not induce tumors in rats unless, as in the present study, rats are treated with cortisone or Freund adjuvant. Possibly these viruses produced strong transplantation antigens in the cells they transform, thus minimizing their chances of initiating a focus of tumor cells.

As demonstrated by the results of transformation assays of subgroup C and subgroup D, Ad 1 and Ad 19 are approximately equally efficient to Ad 12 in inducing the neoplastic transformation in rat cells. Such data show that the classification of human adenoviruses

TABLE 7–7.—Specificity of Adenovirus Subgroup D-T Antigens

Source of Antigen Subgroup (Virus Type)*	Tumor Antiserum			
	Ad-19	Ad-7	Ad-12	Ad-2-SV40
A—Ad-12	< 8†	< 8	16	< 8
B—Ad-7	< 8	32	< 8	< 8
C—Ad-2	< 8	< 8	< 8	64
D—Ad-8, 9, 10, 13, 15, 17, 19, 22, 23 24, 26, 27, 29, 30; also 20, 25, 28	8-64	< 8	< 8	< 8
KB cell control	< 8	< 8	< 8	< 8

* Twenty per cent cell suspensions of infected KB cells collected 48 hours post-infection. Adenovirus group antigen titers were in the range 32-128. Representative types given for the A, B, and C subgroups.
† CF titer reciprocals with 4-8 U of indicated tumor antiserum. Of the viruses listed under subgroup D, all except types 8 and 27 have given titers of 16 or greater. Titers of 8 were obtained for 8 and 27 which, based on relatively low group antigen titers, could refer to low virus input.
(From McAllister et al.[22])

TABLE 7–8.—CHARACTERISTICS OF ADENOVIRUS-TRANSFORMED CELLS

Morphologic:	Epithelioid, piled
Physiologic:	High saturation density
	Form colonies in agar medium*
Transplantation:	Induce tumors in hamsters or rats*†
Serologic:	Contain subgroup specific tumor antigens
Biochemical:	Contain subgroup specific adenovirus RNA‡

* With morphologic characteristics of adenovirus-induced tumors.
† Except rat cells transformed by subgroup C.
‡ Except hamster or rat cells transformed by subgroup D (tentative).

into highly, moderately, or weakly oncogenic subgroups depends on the assay system.

In summary, it appears that all serotypes of human adenoviruses have the potential to induce tumors in hamsters (subgroups A and B) or to transform hamster or rat cells in vitro (subgroups A, B, C, and D). That subgroups C and D have oncogenic potential is suggested by their capacity to transform rodent cells in vitro and the fact that the transformed cells share morphologic, physiologic, transplantation, serologic, and biochemical similarities to hamster tumors induced in vivo by subgroups A and B (Table 7-8).

References

1. Trentin, J. J., Y. Yabe, and G. Taylor: The quest for human cancer viruses. Science, 137:835, 1962.
2. Huebner, R. J., W. P. Rowe, and W. T. Lane: Oncogenic effects in hamsters of human adenovirus types 12 and 18. Proc. Nat. Acad. Sci. USA, 48:2051, 1962.
3. Pereira, M. S., H. G. Pereira, and S. K. R. Clarke: Human adenovirus type 31. A new serotype with oncogenic properties. Lancet, 1:21, 1965.
4. Huebner, R. J., M. J. Casey, R. M. Chanock, and K. Schell: Tumors induced in hamsters by a strain of adenovirus type 3: Sharing of tumor antigens and "neoantigens" with those produced by adenovirus type 7 tumors. Proc. Nat. Acad. Sci. USA, 54:381, 1965.
5. Huebner, R. J.: Adenovirus-directed tumor and T antigens. In: Perspectives in Virology (M. Pollard, ed.), Academic Press, Inc., New York, Vol. 5, 1967, pp. 147-166.
6. Rosen, L.: A hemagglutination-inhibition technique for typing adenoviruses. Amer. J. Hygiene, 71:120, 1960.
7. McBride, W. D., and A. Wiener: In vitro transformation of hamster kidney cells by human adenovirus type 12. Proc. Soc. Exp. Biol. Med., 115:870, 1964.
8. Pope, J. H., and W. P. Rowe: Immunofluorescent studies of adenovirus 12 tumors and of cells transformed or infected by adenoviruses. J. Exp. Med., 120:577, 1964.
9. Leventhal, J. D., and W. Petersen: In vitro transformation and immunofluorescence with human adenovirus type 12 in rat and rabbit kidney cells. Fed. Proc., 24:74, 1965.
10. Yamane, I., and T. Kusano: In vitro transformation of cells of hamster brain by adenovirus type 12. Nature, 213:187, 1967.
11. Reed, S.: Transformation of hamster cells in vitro by adenovirus type 12. J. Gen. Virol., 1:405, 1967.

12. Diamond, L.: Two spontaneously transformed cell lines derived from the same hamster embryo culture. Int. J. Cancer, 2:143, 1967.
13. Freeman, A. E., P. H. Black, R. Wolford, and R. J. Huebner: The adenovirus type 12-rat embryo transformation system. J. Virol., 1:362, 1967.
14. McAllister, R. M., and I. Macpherson: Transformation of a hamster cell line by adenovirus type 12. J. Gen. Virol., 2:99, 1968.
15. Temin, H. M., and H. Rubin: Characteristics of an assay for Rous sarcoma virus and Rous sarcoma cells in tissue culture. Virology, 6:669, 1958.
16. Macpherson, I., and L. Montagnier: Agar suspension culture for the selective assay of cells transformed by polyoma virus. Virology, 23:291, 1964.
17. Freeman, A. E., E. A. Vanderpool, P. H. Black, H. C. Turner, and R. J. Huebner: Transformation of primary rat embryo cells by weakly oncogenic adenovirus type 3. Nature, 216:171, 1967.
18. Freeman, A. E., P. H. Black, E. A. Vanderpool, P. H. Henry, J. B. Austin, and R. J. Huebner: Transformation of primary rat embryo cells by adenovirus type 2. Proc. Nat. Acad. Sci. USA, 58:1205, 1967.
19. McAllister, R. M., M. O. Nicolson, A. M. Lewis, Jr., I. Macpherson, and R. J. Huebner: Transformation of rat embryo cells by adenovirus type 1. J. Gen. Virol., 4:29, 1969.
20. Green, M., M. Piña, K. Fujinaga, S. Mak, and D. Thomas: Transcription of viral genes in adenovirus-infected and transformed cells. In: Perspectives in Virology (M. Pollard, ed.), Academic Press, Inc., New York, Vol. 6, 1968, pp. 15-36.
21. Gilden, R. V., J. Kern, A. E. Freeman, C. E. Martin, R. M. McAllister, H. C. Turner, and R. J. Huebner: T and tumour antigens of adenovirus group C-infected and transformed cells. Nature, 219:517, 1968.
22. McAllister, R. M., M. O. Nicolson, G. Reed, J. Kern, R. V. Gilden, and R. J. Huebner: Transformation of rodent cells by adenovirus 19 and other group D adenoviruses. J. Nat. Cancer Inst., 43:917, 1969.

8

Hormones and Cancer: Clinical and Experimental

Historical Perspective

JACOB FURTH

*Institute of Cancer Research and Department of Pathology,
Columbia University, New York, New York, USA*

A Unified Concept of Neoplasia

ALL NEOPLASMS are caused by derangement of the highly ordered communication system (homeostasis) which limits the number of each cell type.[2, 8, 26] The fluid regulators of normal tissues are hormones; the basic alteration is attributable either to a change in the cell's code or in the regulatory system itself (see Figure 8-1). This concept evolved from several basic discoveries. Beatson introduced the concept of hormonal control of human breast cancer when he recommended ovariectomy. The research which followed led to recognition of the role of hormones in formation and growth of many neoplasms. Kennaway, with his colleagues, discovered that cancer is not caused by chronic irritation but by carcinogenic chemicals which, as we know, either change the genetic code (DNA) of cells or induce an abnormal differentiation or derepression of the code. Independent investigations have shown that the two other classes of carcinogenic agents, radiations and viruses, share with chemical carcinogens the induction of this basic change in cells.

Carcinogens are best conceived as modifiers of the cell's genetic code, creating cells that either fail to recognize their hormonal regulators (stimulators or inhibitors) or if they do, respond to them inadequately. Cancer cells are transformed cells which have a preferential proliferative advantage over their normal ancestors. In contrast, hormones are homeostatic (short- or long-acting) regulators but not code changers (see Figure 8-2). By stimulating DNA synthesis, hor-

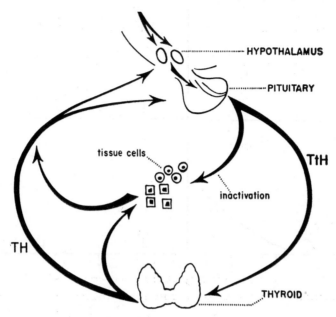

FIG. 8–1—Scheme of homeostatic regulation. Feedback regulation of the thyroid-thyrotrope system. Tumors can be produced in the thyroid by sustained stimulation with thyrotropic hormones (inducible by blocking thyroid hormone synthesis) or in the pituitary thyrotropic cells by inhibition of their physiologic inhibitors T3 or T4 (best done by thyroidectomy).

mones enhance the action of carcinogens. They can also stimulate or retard proliferation of neoplastic cells as long as the altered cells still recognize the hormones. Whichever direction cancer research takes, comprehension of the role of hormones is essential, as I hope will be evident from this review.

I have chosen to limit this presentation to breast cancer. For a comprehensive review of basic and practical aspects of hormones and neoplasia, I refer to the many recent monographs to which our Chairmen were major contributors.[9, 21]

Breast Cancer

HISTORICAL

Following Beatson's idea, research on breast cancer was done in mice by Leo Loeb, Lacassagne, and Little et al. of the Jackson Memorial Laboratory, and others (see Gardner et al.[9]). A high mark was Bittner's formulation of the three cooperative factors in causation of breast cancer: ovarian hormone, a specific "milk factor" (virus), and genes.

The multifactorial concept of Bittner was amplified and modified

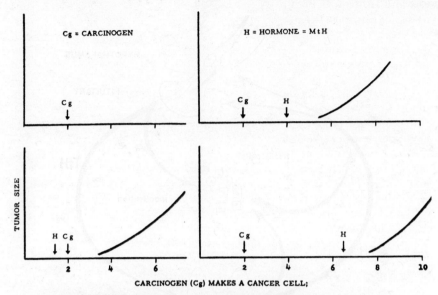

CARCINOGEN (Cg) MAKES A CANCER CELL;

HORMONE (MtH) PROMOTES GROWTH OF MAMMARY EPITHELIUM AND ITS TUMORS

FIG. 8-2.—Simplified scheme of the two-stage (inducer and promoter) concept of carcinogenesis as applied to the mammary gland. Carcinogens change the cytogenetic code demonstrable by delayed application of the promoter MtH to animals that were given a subcarcinogenic dose or are resistant to the carcinogen. In contrast, the action of the promoters (as hormones) is readily reversible.

by Rous, Berenblum, and others, leading to the concept of initiation and promotion and to the existence of latent cancer cells. Woolley et al. discovered that the adrenal compensates for lack of ovarian hormones. Huggins introduced adrenalectomy in the treatment for human breast cancer, and the rat as the experimental animal for studies on the role of hormones in breast cancer. Similarly, recognition of the physiology of the pituitary led Luft and Ray to introduce hypophysectomy for breast cancer control.

For several decades, steroids were the focal point of induction, progression, and treatment for neoplasia. Even today, investigators and editorial writers, ignoring that estrogens act indirectly by stimulating mammotropic hormone (MTH) production, consider as the cardinal question the determination of whether a breast cancer cell is estrogen-sensitive, rather than MTH-responsive, and what the blood level of MTH is.

Recognition of the effects of hypophysectomy and isolation of pituitary units and their hormones shifted the emphasis to protein hormones, with steroids still remaining a vital link in the chain of events. Presently we look upon the pituitary MTH as the centrum in the gen-

esis and control of breast cancer and on the hypothalamus as the mod-
ulator of pituitary function.[8, 18, 19, 27]

Huggins,[11] by introduction of breast cancers of the rat as a model,
gave a strong stimulus to research on mammary tumors. Rat tumors are
highly hormone-responsive and do not seem to contain a causative virus.

Clinicians are alternately elated and disappointed with discoveries
made in laboratories. So it was with the discovery of Bittner, because
until this year, no virus was found in breast cancer of species other
than the mouse, and because the usual mouse cancers are highly autonomous even though estrogens are essential for their induction.
Presently, cancer research is being successfully pursued in many specific areas. However, the generalizations to which they lead are often
shaky because of extreme specialization. In the area of endocrines, the
hypothalamus is a major target. As concerns neoplasia in general, research on intercellular communication of cells not under the influence of conventional hormones (e.g. liver, skin, and kidney) is still
in its infancy.[17, 26]

In rats, mammary tumors can be readily induced by chemical carcinogens and by ionizing radiation, but not by virus. Ovariectomy
causes regression of breast tumors. These regressed tumors remain
silent in estrogen-free and hypophysectomized rats; estrogens fail to reverse them. However, administration of MTH, not estrogens, can re-
suscitate these latent tumors in ovariectomized as well as in hypophysectomized hosts several months after regression (Figures 8-3 and

FIG. 8–3.—Scheme showing repression of mammary tumors induced by methylcholanthrene following hypophysectomy or ovariectomy (but not after adrenalectomy)
and reappearance of the tumors, with heightened growth, following administration
of pituitary hormones of mammotropic cells (done by grafts of the latter).

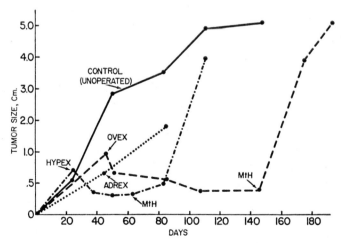

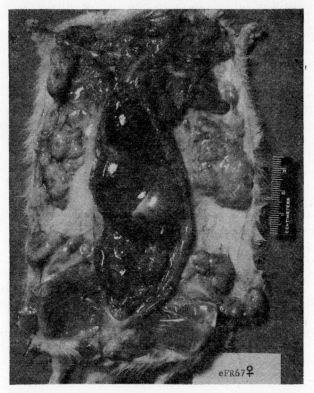

Fig. 8-4.—Rat in which the hormones of mammotropic cells not only caused reappearance of the tumor that was induced by methylcholanthrene and regressed following ovariectomy, but also "activated" latent cancers induced by this carcinogen.

8-4).[6, 13, 23] Whether, in time, these latent cells degenerate and die and actual cures of cancers can thereby be achieved remains to be demonstrated.

ESTROGENS VS. MTH

Estradiol and stilbestrol have several target organs. Jensen et al.[12] have demonstrated the receptor sites for free estradiol. With respect to the mammary gland in adult rats, the action of estrogens is indirect by way of the pituitary and the hypothalamus.[7, 10, 13, 27] The major direct target cells are the acidophilic cells of the pituitary. The present tendency to accept estrogens as the direct specific stimulant of the mammary gland is a roadblock to progress.

The role of MTH in carcinogenesis is further indicated by experiments showing that subcarcinogenic doses of the three classes of carcinogens produce breast cancer only if the MTH level of the host is highly elevated (Table 8-1). The simplest way to attain high levels of

TABLE 8–1.—Breast Cancer Induction with Subcarcinogenic
Doses of Carcinogens

Carcinogen:	Radiation	Chemical*	Virus
Dose:	50 r	10 mg	0.1 ml milk
Species:	Rat	Rat	Mouse
Carcinogen alone	0	0	0
MTH† alone	0	0	0
Carcinogen + MTH	58%	85%	40%

* 3-Methylcholanthrene
† Mammotropic hormone, used synonymously for prolactin.
This table is a schematic summary of a series of experiments (8) indicating that resistance to subcarcinogenic doses of either of the three classes of carcinogens can be overcome by hormones. These hormones can be the determinant factors in carcinogenesis even though they are not direct inducers of cancers.

MTH is by administration of estrogen pellets or by extrasellar pituitary grafts. In experiments performed with K. H. Clifton, very high levels of MTH alone attained by grafts of mammotropic isologous tumors failed to produce a neoplastic change. It did so in experiments on mice which carry a latent MTV (Haran-Ghera).

Homeostasis of the Mammary Gland and Neoplasia

Returning to hormonal regulation of the mammary gland, presently three levels have to be considered: hypothalamic, hypophyseal, and peripheral (see Figure 8-5). (This holds for most target endocrine organs.) Derangement at any point can lead to either increase or decrease of target cell tumors, depending on the kind of interference. It follows that better understanding of homeostasis of the endocrine systems is needed to advance knowledge of the related cancers.

There are several gray and black areas in the understanding of the normal communication systems, and consequently of the derangements which lead to neoplasia.

That a hypothalamic hormone inhibits MTH release is well known. Lesions in a hypothalamic area, cutting the pituitary stalk, or extrasellar grafts of the pituitary will increase MTH blood levels and secondarily raise the incidence of mammary and mammotropic tumors (MTT) (Figure 8-6).[18, 19, 27] Knowledge of the physiologic inhibitors of MTH and the postulated hypothalamic hormone which stimulates MTH production is deficient.

In principle, the findings in rodents seem applicable to man, but none of the known endocrine manipulations which can actually control the highly hormone-responsive rat cancer give better palliation to cancer patients than that attainable by nonendocrine treatment. Further, most if not all human breast cancers seem to be fully autonomous even though about 30 to 40% are somewhat hormone-responsive, and androgens proved to be no more effective in causing remissions than large doses of estrogens. Recent developments now to be discussed point to avenues of investigations with promise of better control of human breast cancer.

The excellent animal model systems for the study of breast cancer in rats and mice supplement each other. If the rat exaggerates hormone responsiveness, it also yields a wide variety of hormone-responsive and autonomous mammary cancers. Further, the rat MTH is readily separable from growth hormone and immunologically does not cross-react with it. Inability to separate human mammotropic from somatotropic hormone (STH) blocks the development of an assay for detection of hormone sensitivity of human breast tumors. In the rat, MTH and STH are readily separable and can be quantitated in a few drops of normal serum. Radioimmunoassays indicate that these two hormones are closely linked (Ito et al., to be published). Estrogen stimulates production of both, but under certain physiologic conditions, and the two activities appear to move independently.

"Prolactin" refers to a stimulator of milk secretion. This term is used synonymously with mammotropin, and most assays for mammotropic hormone are based on assaying secretion. Human breast can-

FIG. 8–5.—Scheme of relationships between the mammary gland, pituitary, and hypothalamus. Note that the mammary gland does not "feed back." The number, character, and intimate interrelationship of hormones involved in growth and function of the mammary gland are still not well known.

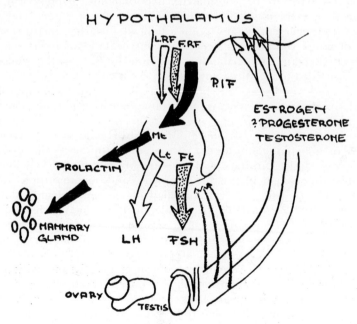

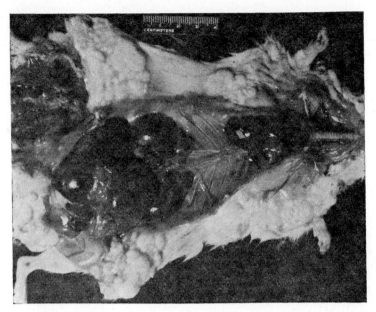

FIG. 8–6.—Illustration of extraordinary mammary gland hyperplasia which hormones of the mammotropic cells can induce in virgin female and in male rats. The level of mammotropic hormones in these rats exceeded 10,000 ng/ml; that of somatotropic hormones was also elevated.

cers rarely, if ever, are secretory, and studies with experimental MTT indicate that extensive mammary gland stimulation can occur without secretion. Milk secretion is under strong influence of glucocorticoids. A technique is needed to distinguish and quantitate these two activities.

VIRAL GENES AND ANTIGENS

For about three decades the mouse tumor virus was the only known breast cancer virus. To this DeOme et al.[4] added the mammary nodule-inducing virus. Technologic developments led to the isolation of more and more tumor viruses in diverse species. One, found recently, is associated with breast cancer of the rhesus monkey; this can be grown in human cells.[3]

Latent viral genes can now be detected by immunologic or physicochemical analyses of their nucleic acids or by the products of viral nucleic acids. Analysis of viral and virus-induced host cell antigens (Huebner, Old, and many others)[14] led to detection of latent, defective noninfectious, but potentially pathogenic tumor viruses. These developments revived interest in mouse-limited Bittner virus, the study of which has been kept alive in the United States by the team of DeOme at Berkeley and of our Chairman, Dr. Muhlbock of Amsterdam, and a few others.

Advances in viral neoplasia have many milestones. Currently research has been accelerated in several directions; some are based on discoveries of isolation and synthesis of infectious viral RNA, developments of methods of their physical characterization and homology; some on immunology of viruses and of antigenic changes in host cells coded by them; and some on developments in high resolution electron microscopy. The applicability of basic research on bacterial to mammalian viruses has been solidly proved. The cell's nuclear code (DNA) is now looked upon as "polluted" with viral genes (RNA or DNA).

In Vitro Test for Hormone Responsiveness

The first clinical problem is how to recognize in vitro the hormone responsiveness of a tumor. Jensen's[12] technique can identify the receptor sites of estradiol which are ubiquitous;[24] thus far the various types of pituitary cells have not been distinguished. It seems to bind nuclei of 80% of pituitary cells which could include mammotropes or gonadotropes. A technique is needed to identify the specific receptor sites of MTH. Such a technique might be developed by following the procedure of Lefkowitz,[15] who identified the receptor sites of ACTH on the plasma membrane of cells of the adrenal cortex. Radioactive MTH might pinpoint specific receptor sites on cells of the mammary gland, distinguish between hormone-responsive and fully autonomous mammary tumors, and quantitate responsiveness; it may also be used for detection of tumor-inhibiting analogs. A simpler procedure may be an adaptation of the technique of Graham and Karnovsky, who labeled antibodies with oxidases. This was applied by Nakane and Pierce[20] for identification of pituitary hormones.

Hormone-responsive tumor cells recognize and probably combine with their regulatory hormones. Fully autonomous tumor cells will probably fail to translate the hormonal message. We have been attempting to test this supposition by incubating in organ cultures known hormone-responsive and autonomous rat tumors in media rich or poor in MTH and observing the rate of synthesis of DNA, quantitating it chemically, and checking the events in radioautographs. MTH enhances DNA synthesis of the responsive but not of the autonomous tumors.[25] To have some such reliable technique for human breast cancers seems to require only patient developmental work.

Human Cancers—The Three Questions

Once a specific human MTH assay is available, the physician facing treatment of a patient with breast cancer will have to answer three questions: The first question will remain as before, whether the tumor is operable; the second, whether the tumor is hormone-responsive (this question need not delay operation); and the third question should be whether the cancer is autoantigenic.

Early diagnosis of hormone responsiveness is essential because of the tendency of tumor cells to give rise to new and more independent variants. The host selects the more autonomous and more aggressive variants.

IMMUNOTHERAPY

The relationship of immunotherapy to hormonal therapy remains to be established.[14] Presently we consider immunotherapy only for fully autonomous tumors, but it is possible that hormone-responsive tumors also possess tumor antigens. If so, the use of combinations of hormonal therapy with immunotherapy will have to be worked out. A step in this direction is the observation that the steroidal alkylating agent Phenesterine has antitumor as well as immunosuppressive effect. An extract of *Mycobacterium butyricum* can counteract the immunosuppressive effect.[1, 5]

Should breast cancers possess specific fetal antigens, as do cancers of some other organs, immunodiagnosis of latent breast cancer is feasible.

NUTRITIONAL INFLUENCE

There are indications that underfeeding or certain nutritional deficiencies inhibit MTH production and, secondarily, mammary tumor development.[22] The half-life of MTH is a matter of minutes, that of normal large polypeptides as globulins and albumins is two to three weeks. This may explain how deficiencies may exert their effect via the hypothalamus.

Knowledge of the complete amino acid composition and sequence in MTH may enable synthesis of MTH analogs which may block MTH receptors and thereby inhibit mammary tumors. It should be emphasized that hormonal therapy can be applied soon after surgical therapy whenever it is suspected that operation failed to remove all tumor cells.

HORMONE THERAPY

Isolation of human MTH, free from growth hormone, would open new diagnostic and therapeutic possibilities, such as attaching to the hormone cytocidal agents (chemicals or radionuclides) without destroying their receptor sites. In utilizing hormones combined with radiation or chemicals, proper timing of administration of these agents is needed. Transient hyperstimulation with hormones (i.e. bringing tumor cells in the sensitive phase), well timed with administration of cytotoxic agents or radiations, may result in "lethal stimulation." Development of RIA for blood levels of human MTH will simplify the search for inhibitors of synthesis or release of MTH. Androgens are commonly conceived to act as MTH inhibitors, but in treatment for human breast cancers, androgens proved to be no improvement over treatment with large doses of estrogens. This puzzle remains to be solved.

It has been suggested that inadequate conversion of E2 to E3 is a risk to development of human breast cancer. Estriol (E3) may be the physiologic inhibitor of estradiol (E2). Unlike E2, E3 is not carcinogenic. It has been reported that E3 prevented mammary tumor induction by DMBA (Lemon[16]). This is thought to be caused by competitive attachment of E2 to receptors of cells of the mammary gland, but it is also possible that E2 operates competitively via pituitary mammotropes and blocks MTH production.[16]

Summary

This sketchy historic review of problems of breast cancer demonstrates how experimental and clinical observations (basic and practical) are intertwined. The specific recent advances, made in the study of mammary cancer of experimental animals of different species, justify intensification of efforts, broadly based, cooperative and individualistic, in both the laboratory and the clinic.

Acknowledgments

I am grateful to Dr. William Gardner for reading this manuscript for me and for his editorial corrections. Also to my past and present associates from whom I learned so much in this area.

The investigations in our laboratories have been supported by United States Public Health Service Grants Ca-06215 and CA-02332.

References

For references prior to 1959, see Gardner et al.[9]

1. Bogden, A. E., D. J. Taylor, and F. F. Menninger, Jr.: Immunosuppressive activity of phenesterin, a steroidal alkylating agent. Proc. Amer. Ass. Cancer Res., 61st Abstract, No. 35, 1970.
2. Burch, P. R. J.: New approach to cancer. Nature, 225:512-516, 1970.
3. Chopra, H. C.: Electron microscopic detection of an oncogenic-type virus in a monkey breast tumor. Proc. Amer. Ass. Cancer Res., 61st Abstract, No. 60, 1970.
4. DeOme, K. B., and S. Nandi: The mammary-tumor system in mice, a brief review. In: Viruses Inducing Cancer (W. J. Burdette, ed.), University of Utah Press, 1966.
5. Esber, H. J., A. E. Bogden, and D. J. Taylor: Counteraction of the immunosuppressive effect of tumor growth by methanol soluble fraction of mycobacterium butyricum. Proc. Amer. Ass. Cancer Res., 61st Abstract, No. 90, 1970.
6. Furth, J.: The role of mammosomatotropin in tumorigenesis of the mammary gland. In: Endogenous Factors Influencing Host-Tumor Balance (R. W. Wissler, T. L. Dao, and S. Wood, eds.), University of Chicago, 1967, pp. 49-62.
7. Furth, J.: Hormones and neoplasia. In: Thule International Symposia, Cancer and Aging (A. Engeland, and T. Lasson, eds.), Nordiska Bokhandelns Forlag, Stockholm, 1968, pp. 131-151.

8. Furth, J.: Pituitary cybernetics and neoplasia. In: The Harvey Lectures, Series 63. Academic Press, Inc., New York, 1969, pp. 47-71.
9. Gardner, W. U., C. A. Pfeiffer, and J. J. Trentin: Hormonal factors in experimental carcinogenesis. In: The Physiopathology of Cancer (F. Homburger, ed.), Harper (Hoeber), New York, 1959, pp. 152-237.
10. Guillemin, R.: The adenohypophysis and its hypothalamic control. Ann. Rev. Physiol., 29:313-348, 1967.
11. Huggins, C., L. Grand, and R. Fukunishi: Aromatic influences on the yields of mammary cancers following administration of 7,12-dimethylbenz (a) anthracene. Proc. Nat. Acad. Sci. USA, 51:737-742, 1964.
12. Jensen, E. V., E. R. DeSombre, and P. W. Jungblut: Estrogen receptors in hormone responsive tissue and tumors. In: Endogenous Factors Influencing Host-Tumor Balance (R. W. Wissler, T. L. Dao, and S. Wood, Jr., eds.), The University of Chicago, 1967, pp. 15-30.
13. Kim, U.: Pituitary function and hormonal therapy of experimental breast cancer. Cancer Res., 25:1146-1161, 1965.
14. Klein, G.: Experimental studies in tumor immunology. Fed. Proc., 28:1739-1753, 1969.
15. Lefkowitz, R. L., J. Roth, W. Pricer, and I. Pastan: ACTH receptors in the adrenal: Specific binding of ACTH-^{125}I and its relation to adenyl cyclase. Proc. Nat. Acad. Sci. USA, 65:745-752, 1970.
16. Lemon, H. M.: Inhibition of rat mammary carcinogenesis by an impeded estrogen, estriol. Proc. Amer. Ass. Cancer Res., 61st Abstract, No. 188, 1970.
17. Loewenstein, W. R.: Communication through cell junctions. Implications in growth and differentiation. Devel. Biol. 19 (Suppl. 2):151-183, 1968.
18. Lu, K. H., Y. Koch, Y. Amenomori, C. L. Chen, and J. Meites: In vivo and in vitro effects of drugs on prolactin release by the rat pituitary. Fed. Proc., 54th Abstract, No. 1868, 1970.
19. MacLeod, R. M., and E. H. Fontham: Influence of hormone-secreting pituitary tumors and catecholamics on pituitary hormone synthesis. Proc. Amer. Ass. Cancer Res., 61st Abstract, No. 200, 1970.
20. Nakane, P. K., and G. B. Pierce, Jr.: Enzyme-labeled antibodies for the light and electron microscopic localization. J. Cell Biol., 33:307-318, 1967.
21. Segaloff, A., K. K. Meyer, S. DuBakey, eds.: Current Concepts in Breast Cancer. The Williams and Wilkins Co., Baltimore, 1967.
22. Srebnik, H. H., and R. E. Grindeland: Reduced luteotropic activity in the anterior pituitary gland and plasma of protein-deficient rats. Fed. Proc., 54th Abstract, No. 1096, 1970.
23. Sterental, A., J. M. Dominguez, C. Weissman, and O. H. Pearson: Pituitary role in the estrogen dependency of experimental mammary cancer. Cancer Res., 23:481-484, 1964.
24. Stumpf, W. E.: Nuclear concentration of ^{3}H-estradiol tissues. Dry-mount autoradiography of vagina, oviduct, testis, mammary tumor, liver and adrenal. Endocrinology, 85:31-37, 1969.
25. Takizawa, S., J. J. Furth, and J. Furth: DNA synthesis in autonomous and hormone-responsive mammary tumors. Cancer Res., 30:206-210, 1970.
26. Teir, H., and T. Rytomma, eds.: Control of Cellular Growth in Adult Organisms. Academic Press, New York, 1967.
27. Welsch, C. W., H. Nagasawa, and J. Meites: Increased incidence of spontaneous mammary tumors in female rats bearing hypothalamic lesions. Proc. Amer. Ass. Cancer Res., 61st Abstract, No. 326, 1970.

Transplantable Endocrine Tumors

RIGOBERTO IGLESIAS

Instituto de Medicina Experimental of the National Health Service, Santiago, Chile

Introduction

AFTER Dr. Furth's "Historical Perspective," I feel free to begin immediately speaking on our transplantable endocrine tumors, without referring to the important bibliography on the subject. Notwithstanding, the following references are mentioned: van Nie,[41] Furth and Clifton,[7] Gardner et al.,[10] and Kirschbaum.[28]

All of our work has been done with AxC rats, an inbred strain of brown rats started more than 40 years ago by Wilhelmina F. Dunning in the United States, and which we received from Albert Segaloff in 1949. They are maintained by strict brother-sister matings. The animals receive food prepared by a local mill (Benedicto Aguado y Cía.) according to a formula provided by the National Institute for Medical Research from England.

In Table 8-2 are summarized autopsy data on all of the AxC rats examined in our Institute from 1950 to December 31, 1969.

Some tumors, most probably spontaneous, have been found in the 32,969 animals belonging to experiments and in the 750 castrated rats, but we will refer to tumors found in the 4,059 normal intact rats only. The tumors have been found in routine careful autopsy examination; systematic microscopic studies in search of tumors have not been made. Many tumors have been found, many have been grafted with success, and many have been lost. Maybe now we are prepared to find tumors. As neoplasia appears in aged rats, it is not difficult to find tumors if it is possible to maintain animals for their life-span. It must be kept in mind that a three-year-old rat may be compared to a 90-year-old hu-

TABLE 8-2.—AxC RATS NECROPSIED AT THE INSTITUTE FROM 1950 TO DECEMBER 31, 1969

GROUPS	Intact	NORMAL Castrated	Totals	EXPERIMENTAL Intact and Castrated
Males	1777	444	2221	17389
Females	2282	306	2588	15580
Totals	4059	750	4809	32969

man being. I think it is necessary to insist that in the genesis of our tumors, "spontaneous" or experimentally produced, exogenous factors do not play any role. They appear as the result of the distortion of the physiologic process.

In my presentation, which will be sketchy because of the large amount of material, I will emphasize our established transplantable tumors and how they are now.

Spontaneous Transplantable Endocrine Tumors

Of 533 tumors of endocrine glands found, 73 have been grafted; 54 of these grew progressively, killing the host. As many as 22 of these were lost or discarded. There are 17 tumors maintained as established transplantable tumors. Another 15 tumors are still in the first and second transplant generations, and they may become established transplantable tumors or may be lost or discarded (Table 8-3).

FUNCTIONAL OVARIAN TUMORS

Our first ovarian tumor (TOF) was found in New Orleans May 3, 1949.[15, 25] Now, in the one hundred and eighth transplant generation, it still shows the morphology of a granulosa cell tumor and still shows estrogenic activity (Table 8-4). I think the preservation of the capacity to produce hormones for more than 20 years is an interesting biologic fact. The tumor still produces metastases. It does not produce bone. We do not know whether the tumor is sensitive to gonadal hormones as it was years ago.

The second ovarian tumor (TR.DXCI) was found in August 1963, in a 702-day-old rat, with congenital sterility. It is of complex histologic structure and shows estrogenic activity. It grows very irregularly. In experiments with the fourth transplant generation, it grew in the eight intact males with latent periods of 30 days. In castrated males,

---

TABLE 8–3.—SPONTANEOUS TUMORS OF ENDOCRINE GLANDS FOUND IN 4059 NORMAL INTACT AxC RATS NECROPSIED FROM 1950 TO DECEMBER 1969

				NUMBER OF TUMORS TRANSPLANTED No. of Generations December 31, 1969		Lost or
TUMORS	Found	Total	"Positive"	3 or More	1 and 2	Discarded
Ovary	9	4	4	2*	—	2
Testis	154	33	27	8	8	11
Adrenals	84	8	4	4	—	0
Pituitary	286	28	19	3	7	9
Totals	533	73	54	17	15	22

* The first ovarian tumor we found in USA at Segaloff's laboratory in 1949.

TABLE 8–4.—TOF II. The Spontaneous Ovarian Tumor of the AxC
Rat Found May 3, 1949, Is Still Functional: Estrogenic

No. Gener.	Date Inoc. 1969	Hosts	Survival Days	Mam. Gland*	Testis[†] (Ovaries)[‡] mg	Sem. ves.[§] (Uterus)[#] mg
103rd	9.26	4 ♂	61-94	10-15	174-198	42-69
104th	12.5	4 ♂	52-88	n-5	127-251	39-80
107th	10.28	3 ♀	56-118	n-5	(5-7)	(291)
108th	12.23	4 ♀	44-77	n-5	(4-4)	(228)

* Development equivalent days pregnancy.
Normal weights: † 1128 ± 69 mg; ‡ 29 ± 5 mg; § 478 ± 58 mg; # 374 ± 77 mg.

it grew only in four of eight, with latent periods of 146 to 629 days. Testosterone propionate and estradiol, but not progesterone, stimulate the growth of this tumor. It may produce bone, sometimes in a remarkable way, as it was with TOF 15 to 20 years ago.

FUNCTIONAL ADRENAL TUMORS

Of the four transplantable tumors of the adrenal cortex which we have established, one never has shown hormonal activity and will not be included in this paper.

The first functional adrenal tumor (TD) was found July 6, 1953, in an intact 550-day-old rat.[16] It was a tumor of 20 mm, which gave metastasis to the lungs, liver, adrenals, and spleen, but never to the kidneys (Table 8-5). The other adrenal gland weighed 9 mg, i.e. half the normal size. The tumor is in the ninety-third transplant generation, with a survival of 53 to 68 days, and still must produce corticoids, with the weight of one adrenal gland 6 mg. It still gives metastases.

The second adrenocortical (TR.LXVII) was found March 14, 1956, in a 623-day-old virgin female rat.[18] It was a tumor with a diameter of 18 mm; the weight of the other adrenal was 12 mg; there were no metastases. The grafts of the tumor gave metastases to the lungs, liver, adrenals, and kidneys, but never to the spleen. It was very similar to our first adrenal tumor. Since the twenty-second transplant generation, February 1965, it is no longer functional. This tumor should be discarded, but we keep it because it has been useful in experiments on

TABLE 8–5.—TD-IV. The Spontaneous Adrenal Tumor of the
AxC Rat Found July 6, 1953, Is Still Functional

No. Gener.	Date Inoc. 1969	Hosts	Survival Days	Adr.* mg	Metastases
92nd	11.3	4 ♀	39-78	5-8	Spl. Liv. Lung
93rd	12.23	4 ♀	53-68	6-6	Adr. Spl.

* Normal weight: 21 ± 2 mg.

TABLE 8–6.—TR.CMVIII. The Spontaneous Transplantable Adrenal Tumor of the AxC Rat Found August 19, 1965, Is Still Functional; It Produces Corticoids, Estrogens and Androgens

No. Gen.	Date Inoc. 1969	Hosts	Corticoids		Estrogens			Androgens		
			Adrenals[a] mg.	Mam. gl.*	Ovaries[b] mg.	Uterus[c] mg.	Clit.[e] mm.	Clit. gl.[d] mg.	Para- uretr. gl.[e] mg.
15th	7.30	4 ♀	7- 8	10-15	9-11	274-750	3	69-103	71-85
16th	10.27	4 ♀	11-12	10-15	11-15	470-600	+	77-92	65-82

* Development equivalent to days pregnancy.
Normal weights: [a] 21 ± 2 mg; [b] 29 ± 5 mg; [c] 374 ± 77 mg; [d] 32 ± 8 mg. [e] Clitoris and paraurethral glands are not visible in normal AxC rats.
The survival in these 2 last generations was from 80 to 118 days.

metastasis. It is now in the sixtieth transplant generation, with survivals of 38 to 43 days.

The third adrenocortical tumor is the most interesting. It was found August 19, 1965, in an 864-day-old AxC rat, which had been a normal breeder. The tumor measured 20 × 14 × 14 mm; the other adrenal weighed 6 mg. The mammary gland was developed as in a 10 days' pregnant rat and there was a mammary fibroadenoma. The ovaries, uterus, pituitary gland and thyroids were of normal weight. Young adult intact and castrated male and female rats, four in each group, were subcutaneously inoculated with a suspension of the original tumor. Another group of eight female rats was inoculated, to be adrenalectomized after the tumor had grown. The tumor grew progressively in all of the animals; the latent period was 50 to 83 days in males and 42 to 58 days in females; the survival was 96 to 184 days, and 86 to 134 days, respectively. The gonads did not affect the growth of the tumor. In the animals adrenalectomized when the tumor was palpable, 67 days after the inoculation, the survival was from 96 to 179 days.

We call this tumor trifunctional because it must produce corticosteroids, estrogens, and androgens, as can be appreciated by its biologic effects: (1) corticosteroids: atrophy of the adrenals, which

TABLE 8–7.—TR.CMVIII. The Spontaneous Transplantable Adrenal Tumor of the AxC Rat Found August 19, 1965, Is Still Functional

No. Gener.	Date Inoc. 1969	Hosts	Corticoids	Androgens	
			Adrenals[a] mg.	Sem. Ves.[b] mg.	Ventr. Prost.[c] mg.
16th	8.26	1 ♂	21-24	980	—
		3 ♂	8-12	1000	970
17th	11.27	1 ♂	11-12	1060	850
		3 ♂	8-9	1520	1090

Normal weights: [a] 21 ± 2 mg; [b] 478 ± 58 mg; [c] 587 ± 84 mg.
Survival in these 2 last generations was from 88 to 130 days.

weighed 7, 6, 5, 3, and even 2 mg (normal 20 mg) ; edema, hydrothorax, and survival after adrenalectomy; (2) estrogens: atrophy of the ovaries with well-developed uterus; this last in spayed rats also; testicular atrophy and well-developed mammary glands in females and males; and (3) androgens: well-developed seminal glands and prostate in castrated males, as well as in intact ones with atrophic testes. The seminal vesicles in castrated males with tumor may reach a weight of 1,520 mg, as compared with 15 to 25 mg in castrated males without tumor. Hypertrophy of the clitoris, of the clitoridean glands, and development of the vestigial prostate in females occurred.

This tumor is in the seventeenth transplant generation and is still functional (Tables 8-6 and 8-7).

FUNCTIONAL TESTICULAR TUMORS

Of 154 testicular tumors found, 33 were transplanted. Of these, 27 grew, but 11 were lost or discarded. Eight are established transplantable tumors; another eight are in the first or the second transplant generation. All are interstitial cell tumors. One of the established tumors is not functional now, others are estrogenic only, and the majority are androgenic and estrogenic. Some of these produce mammary tumors. So we have two groups of testicular tumors:

TESTICULAR TUMORS WHICH DO NOT PRODUCE MAMMARY TUMORS.— Four belong to this group. Three (TR.X, TR.XVIII, and TR.LIV) were found in 1955.[19] Two of these, TR.X and TR.XVIII, are still functional and they are estrogenic as they were since the beginning (Tables 8-8 and 8-9).

TR.LIV, which was androgenic, also is no longer functional; or perhaps a little estrogenic, and is growing very fast. It is now in the one hundred and twenty-eighth transplant generation, with a survival of 23 to 25 days (Table 8-10). As it gives precocious, not visible, metastases to the lungs, one subline of this tumor is maintained by subcutaneous inoculation of suspension of apparently healthy lungs. The first tumor, TR.X, which was found 11 months before the third, TR.LIV, is now in the nineteenth transplant generation only, with a survival of six to 11 months.

TABLE 8–8.—TR.X. THE SPONTANEOUS TRANSPLANTABLE TESTICULAR TUMOR OF THE AxC RAT, WHICH WAS FOUND JANUARY 11, 1955, IS STILL FUNCTIONAL: ESTROGENIC

No. GENER.	DATE INOC.	HOSTS	SURVIVAL DAYS	MAM. GLAND[a]	OVARIES[b] mg	UTERUS[c] mg	HYPOPH.[d] mg
18th	9.23.68	4 ♀	140-168	0->N	6-10	231-408	8-10
19th	3.8.69	4 ♀	191-343	0-n	7-11	497-890	—

[a] n = normal.
Normal weights: [b] 29 ± 5 mg; [c] 374 ± 77 mg; [d] 10 ± 1.5 mg.

TABLE 8–9.—TR.XVIII. The Spontaneous Transplantable Testicular Tumor of the AxC Rat Found February 2, 1955, Is Still Functional: Estrogenic

No. Gener.	Date Inoc. 1969	Hosts	Mam. Gland[a]	Testes[b] mg	Sem. Ves.[c] mg	Hypophysis[d] mg
56th	7.25	4 ♂	5-15	108-323	27-67	14-20
57th	10.13	4 ♂	5-15	125-213	30-55	12-21

[a] Development equivalent days pregnancy.
Normal weights: [b] 1128 ± 69 mg; [c] 478 ± 58 mg; [d] 10 ± 1.5 mg.
Survival in these 2 last generations was 73 to 115 days.

The fourth tumor of this group, found July 7, 1964, is in the seventh transplant generation and is androgenic and estrogenic.

Testicular Tumors Which Produce Mammary Tumors.—Three of these tumors were found, one in 1962, TR.CDLXXXI, and two in 1964, TR.DCLXIII and TR.DCLXXXIX. Mammary and pituitary tumors develop in animals grafted with these tumors. I will describe TR.CDLXXXI.[14, 22] It was found February 5, 1962, in a congenitally blind, fertile male, 749 days old. The right testis was occupied almost completely by a tumor and weighed 2.40 g; the left testis was of normal appearance and weighed 1.16 g. The weights of other organs were: seminal vesicles, 143 mg with secretion and 86 mg without secretion; adrenal glands, 27 and 30 mg; and hypophysis, 12 mg. The mammary gland was not visible. This testicular tumor is of interstitial cells, as are the others already studied. The original tumor did not show hormonal activity, but when transplanted it became functional and produced androgens: there is great development of the seminal vesicles and of the prostate in castrated males, and hypertrophy of the clitoris in females. It produces estrogens also: there is atrophy of the ovaries and great development of the uterus with pyometra in intact and spayed females and great development of the mammary gland (see Tables 8-11 and 8-12). Pasqualini et al.[34] in France have studied in vitro the biosynthesis of testosterone by this tumor and have established some biogenetic pathways and suggested others. Surprisingly, with the tumor so

TABLE 8–10.—TR.LIV. The Spontaneous Transplantable Testicular Tumor of the AxC Rat, Found November 23, 1955, Is No Longer Functional

No. Gener.	Date Inoc. 1969	Hosts	Survival Days	Mam. Gland[a]	Testis[b] mg	Sem. Vesic.[c] mg	Hypophysis[d] mg
127th	1.26	1 ♂	28	—	—	282	—
		3 ♀	27-28	n->n	—	72-97	n-13
128th	2.23	1 ♂	24	>n	148-850	128	—
		3 ♀	23-25	n->n	—	158-270	11-13

[a] n = normal.
Normal weights: [b] 1128 ± 69 mg; [c] 478 ± 58 mg; [d] 10 ± 1.5 mg.
Maintained with inoculation of suspension of lungs.

TABLE 8–11.—INTACT AND CASTRATED AxC MALE RATS WITH SPONTANEOUS
TRANSPLANTABLE FUNCTIONAL TESTICULAR TUMOR, TR.CDLXXXI—ANIMALS
WITHOUT TUMORS FOR COMPARISON

GROUPS		TESTES, MG.		SEMINAL VESICLES mg. Full	WITH SCROTAL HERNIA
		Right	Left		
With tumor	8 ♂	115-129[a]	117-142[a]	650-1450[a]	8
	8 ♂̸	—	—	700-1250[a]	8
Without tumor	8 ♂	1128 ± 69	1127 ± 42	478 ± 58	0
	8 ♂̸	—	—	20 ± 3	0

[a] Only 4 or 5 were weighed, the others destroyed by cannibalism.

estrogenic, very little estradiol-17β or estrone was detected using different labeled precursors.

Another sign of estrogenic action is the development of scrotal hernia in intact and castrated males. This was previously observed in mice by Burrows[2] and subsequently studied in the same species by Miller and Gardner.[32] Inguinal hernia are seen in females grafted with the tumor.

The most impressive feature of this tumor is the production of mammary and pituitary tumors. The incidence of pituitary tumors is 6.7% and of mammary tumors 1.8% in our group of 4,809 normal adult and aged AxC rats, including 444 castrated males and 306 spayed females. In Table 8-13 they are compared with animals grafted with the testicular tumor. In these, the frequency of pituitary tumors was 43.7% and of mammary tumors, 46.8%.

The pituitary tumors may be found in animals autopsied six months after the inoculation of the testicular tumor. They are dark red, soft, and macroscopically very similar to the majority of spontaneous tumors and to those experimentally produced by continuous and prolonged action of estrogens. Their weights range from 23 to 324 mg. We have not studied the transplantability of these tumors.

The mammary tumors[14, 23] appear later than those of the pituitary,

TABLE 8–12.—INTACT AND SPAYED FEMALE AxC RATS WITH SPONTANEOUS
TRANSPLANTABLE FUNCTIONAL TESTICULAR TUMOR, TR.CDLXXXI—ANIMALS
WITHOUT TUMORS FOR COMPARISON

GROUPS		OVARIES, MG.		UTERUS MG.	WITH MASCULINI-ZATION
		Right	Left		
With tumor	8 ♀	4.5 ± 1.6	7.0 ± 3.5	710-1400[a]	5
	8 ♀̸	—	—	284-800[a]	8
Without tumor	10 ♀	28.8 ± 5.4	37.6 ± 10.2	374 ± 77	0
	8 ♀̸	—	—	78 ± 25	0

[a] Majority with pyometra; weighed empty, but 4 and 5 only.

TABLE 8–13.—FREQUENCY OF PITUITARY AND MAMMARY TUMORS OF NORMAL AxC RATS AND OF RATS WITH THE TRANSPLANTABLE TESTICULAR TUMOR

| | NORMAL | | | WITH TESTIC. TUMOR | |
| | | Tumors | | | Tumors | |
Groups	Pituit.	Mamm.	Groups	Pituit.	Mamm.
1777 ♂	68	5	8 ♂	3	3
444 ♂	16	1	8 ♂	4	3
2282 ♀	223	83	8 ♀	3	5
306 ♀	19	1	8 ♀	4	4
4809	326	90	32	14	15
%	6.7	1.8		43.7	46.8

10 to 12 months after the inoculation of the testicular tumor. They may be small, of 2 to 3 mm, or may reach a diameter of 40 mm and a weight of 24 g. They are soft, dark brown with white pinkish zones, and are multiple; they are mammary adenocarcinoma. In one case there was an associated mammary fibroadenoma. The mammary glands are always well developed and contain milk.

The original mammary tumor appears after the grafted testicular tumor has reached some size. The following is a typical case: On August 10, 1965 one intact female rat, 85 days old, was subcutaneously inoculated with the third transplant generation of the testicular tumor, TR.CDLXXXI. One hundred days after the inoculation there was a tumor of 5 mm. At 326 days, when the testicular tumor measured 36 × 23 × 23 mm, one mammary tumor of 5 mm was discovered. The animal was killed 422 days after the inoculation. Then the dimensions of the testicular tumor were 37 × 30 × 30 mm, and there was another of 14 mm. In all the mammary groups there were mammary tumors, varying in size from 3 to 55 mm. The mammary gland itself was well developed. The pituitary gland was tumoral and measured 8 × 5.5 × 4 mm. The ovaries were atrophic, and there was a big uterus with pyometra.

Knowing that continuous and prolonged treatment with estrogens produces pituitary and mammary tumors in the rat, 100% and 85%, respectively, in the AxC strain, we may accept that the pituitary and mammary tumors developed in our animals are the final result of the action of the estrogens produced by the grafted testicular tumor. The chain of events seems to be as follows: testicular tumor = estrogens→pituitary gland = pituitary tumor = prolactin→mammary gland = mammary cancer. This would be the confirmation of the experimental concept of Furth, co-workers and followers. He has long postulated that estrogens are the "specific and main stimulants of the mammotropes," and 13 years ago he showed a picture of a mammary adenocarcinoma developed in a rat grafted with a mammotropic tumor.[8] At the same occasion he said, "Future research should be designed to explain more

TABLE 8–14.—SPONTANEOUS TRANSPLANTABLE TESTICULAR TUMORS OF AxC RATS
WHICH PRODUCE MAMMARY TUMORS

| TESTIC. TUMOR | TRANSPLANT GENERATIONS | | | ANIMALS WITH | | GENER. WITH |
	First	Last	Total[a]	Test. T.	Mam. T.[b]	MAM. T.
TR.CDLXXXI	2.5.62	7.15.69	11	102	24	2, 3, 4, 5, 7, 8
TR.DCLXIII	7.10.64	8.4.69	7	50	8	3, 4, 7
TR.DCLXXXIX	11.10.64	5.28.69	9	35	9	2, 3, 4, 7, 8

[a] The 3 testicular tumors continue growing in new transplant generations in 1970.
[b] Appear in intact and castrated male and female rats grafted with testicular tumor.

completely the role of mammotropic hormone in mammary tumorigenesis and should attempt to control mammary tumors by specific inhibition of the mammotropes." Meites and Sinha[30] have seen mammary adenocarcinoma in Wistar rats implanted with the W15 "mammosomatotropic tumor" of Furth, which releases large amounts of prolactin and growth hormone. Kim[27] says that "changes in the mammary tumor size are directly related to the changes in the prolactin levels." And finally, Boot[5] has been able to produce mammary carcinoma in mice with exogenous prolactin.

The mammary cancer produced by the testicular tumor is transplantable, but grows only in animals grafted with the testicular tumor or treated with estrogens. I will show some experiments with the mammary tumor later on.

In Table 8-14 there is some information on the three testicular tumors which produce mammary tumors. As may be seen, no mammary tumors appear in the first transplant generation, nor in any generation afterwards. The second tumor, TR.DCLXIII, and the third, TR. DCLXXXIX, resemble the first and will not be described. There is a fourth transplantable testicular tumor, TR.MCV, which belongs to this group, but which has not been included in Table 8-14 because it has given mammary tumor in only one transplant generation, in this case in the first. The tumor appeared in a spayed female rat and histologically is a true cancer. TR.MCV is now in the fifth transplant generation.

FUNCTIONAL SPONTANEOUS TRANSPLANTABLE PITUITARY TUMORS

Pituitary tumors are frequent in aged rats. We have found 286 in our group of 4,059 intact normal rats. Of the 28 which were grafted, 19 grew; nine of these have been lost or discarded. There are now three established tumors and seven which are in the first or the second transplant generation.

Pituitary tumors have been so well studied by Furth and co-workers that I will speak but very briefly on our findings and observations.

Among our transplantable pituitary tumors we may distinguish four types: (1) mammosomatoadrenocorticotropic; (2) mammotropic which produces mammary tumors; (3) co-existent mammary and pituitary tumors; and (4) co-existent pituitary and testicular tumors.

MAMMOSOMATOCORTICOTROPIC TUMORS.—There are two of these tumors. They were found in 1962 and 1964, both in aged intact males. We will describe only the first, TR.DXXXVI. It grew very slowly during the first transplant generation, the survival being five to eight months. It showed great mammotropic effect: the mammary glands contained abundant milk and reached a weight of 50 g. In a lactating rat, the weight is 7 to 8 g. Big mammary glands have been observed also in males and in spayed females. This was, for me, unexpected before knowing the work of Furth with mammotropic tumor and the endocrinologic studies of Lyon et al. In the first transplant generation, the tumor showed somatotropic activity only after adrenalectomy; great increase in body weight, with big thymus (1,200 mg) has been observed. With new transplant generations, somatotropic effects were produced in nonadrenalectomized animals with atrophic thymus and with big adrenals. Polydipsia, polyuria, glucosuria, edema, and atrophy of the thymus with enormous adrenals of 200 and 300 mg (20 mg normal) had to be attributed to ACTH. Enlargement of the liver, kidney, and heart, with sclerotic lesions in the two last organs, have been observed. Similar changes have been produced in rats by Selye[38] and by Ingle[26] with corticoids. These tumors are not interesting now. But as may be seen in Table 8-15, they are still functional in the last transplant generations.

MAMMOTROPIC PITUITARY TUMOR PRODUCING MAMMARY TUMORS WHEN GRAFTED.—More interesting is our third transplantable pituitary tumor, TR.MIX, which was found January 4, 1966, in an 838-day-old female rat, nonbreeder, weighing 143 g. The weight of other organs was: ovaries, 44 and 26 mg; uterus, with one horn only, 235 mg; and adrenal glands, 37 and 39 mg. The mammary gland was developed as in pregnancy of 20 days, and contained very little secretion. The pi-

TABLE 8–15.—ESTABLISHED SPONTANEOUS TRANSPLANTABLE PITUITARY TUMORS OF THE AxC RAT*

| NUMBER OF TUMORS | DATE OF FINDING | No. GENER. | Last Gener. | HORMONAL ACTIVITY | | |
				LTH Mam. Gl.[a] mg.	STH Length[b] cm.	ACTH Adrenals[c] mg.
TR.DXXXVI	12.19.62	22	4 ♂[d]	1320	38-42	65-108
TR.DCXXV	2.4.64	5	4 ♀[e]	2450	43.5-49.5	82-118

* They are still functional in the last transplant generation.
[a] Weight of one inguinal group.
[b] Normal length of adult ♀ AxC rat 38 to 40 cm.
[c] Normal weights, group of 8 animals: 21 ± 2 mg.
Survival days: [d] 67-71; [e] 266-279.

tuitary tumor measured $8 \times 6 \times 6$ mm, and was of irregular surface, pinkish with a white anterior zone. It was grafted in four intact males, but grew in two only. Subsequently it grew in 100% of animals inoculated. This tumor shows very weak hormonal activity. In Table 8-16 are summarized data on the fourth transplant generation of this tumor. Apparently it does not produce growth hormone, nor ACTH. Adrenal glands are larger than normal, but as Furth has pointed out, increased adrenal size does not always mean adrenal hyperfunction. Its mammotropic effect was weak also: the mammary gland was normal sometimes; the weight of one inguinal group was 1.90 g in the animal with the largest mammary glands. With the first tumor, the mammary gland reached a weight of 50 g. The small size of the testes is, conversely, in favor of prolactin.[6] We have insufficient information on prostatic and preputial glands and on seminal vesicles, which are effectors of prolactin.[1, 37]

In the fourth transplant generation of this tumor, in a total of 16 animals, including males and females, intact and castrated, mammary tumors appeared in two intact females. One of these cases was as follows: The pituitary tumor was subcutaneously inoculated in an intact female 173 days old, on March 19, 1968. After 199 days a small nodule of 3 mm was palpated, which, after 60 days, grew to a size of $15 \times 10 \times 10$ mm, and to a size of $37 \times 25 \times 17$ mm after 106 days more. At this time, i.e. one year after the inoculation of the pituitary tumor, one mammary tumor 10 mm in diameter was palpated. Next day the animal was killed; the pituitary tumor (TR.MIX) weighed 13.5 g, and the mammary tumor 980 mg. The weights of other organs were: ovaries, 36 and 28 mg; uterus, 598 mg; adrenals, 24 and 39 mg; and hypophysis, 9 mg. The mammary glands were well developed but did not contain secretion; the weight of one inguinal group was 1.9 g. It seems as if estrogens would have played no role in the production of this mammary tumor. The development of the mammary gland and the mammary tumor would be the result of direct stimulation by the mammotropic factor, prolactin, or maybe some other factor produced by the inoculated tumor.

With the mammary tumor, 14 intact female rats were inoculated; of these, four received pituitary tumor at the same time. This grew in three animals, in which the inoculated mammary tumor developed also. In the 10 animals grafted with the mammary tumor only, this has not grown, and more than a year has passed since the inoculation. Now the mammary tumor is in the second transplant generation and grows only in animals inoculated with the pituitary tumor. It is apparently hormone-dependent. We have not yet studied its responsivity or sensitivity to some hormones. I am almost certain that estrogens and prolactin will stimulate the growth of this mammary tumor.

This pituitary tumor, TR.MIX, became more and more dark and now is as black as a melanoma. I think we will lose this tumor soon. But we have to save the mammary tumor.

TABLE 8-16.—TR.MIX. Spontaneous Transplantable Pituitary Tumor of the AxC Rat, Which Apparently Produces Prolactin Only and Not Somatotropin and Adrenocorticotropin

No. GENER.	DATE INOC.	ANIMALS Inoc.	With T.	SURVIVAL DAYS	TUMOR G.	MAMM. GLAND[a]	TESTES[b] (OVARIES)[c] MG.	SEM. VES.[d] (UTERUS)[e] MG.	ADRENALS[f] MG.	HY- POPHYSIS[g] MG.	TOTAL LENGTH[h] CM.
1st	1.4.66	4♂	2	318	0.14-6.0	5,s-550,s	130-1250	100-570	30-55	8-9	—
2nd	11.18.66	4♂	4	222-432	10.0-20.0	120-156,s	179-950	51-134	31-66	6-8	40-43
3rd	6.28.67	4♂	4	224-264	13.0-16.0	>n-278,s	416-474	58-52	37-44	6	—
4th	3.19.68	4♂	4	268-581	29.0-37.0	5,s-600,s	163-1350	45-700	32-57	8-12	40-41
		4♀	4	302-510	29.0-34.0	n-> n,s	—	25-44	47-68	11-13	43
		4¹♀	4	283-460	5.0-14.0	0.7-1.90	(14-34)	(367-720)	24-57	9-12	40.5
		4♂	4	456-581	39.0-45.0	10,s-150	—	(84-103)	35-56	9-11	36.5-40

[a] Weight of one inguinal group; n: normal; s: secretion. Normal weights, mg, groups of 8 animals: [b] 1128 ± 69; [c] 29 ± 5; [d] 478 ± 58; [e] 374 ± 77; [f] 21 ± 2; [g] 10 ± 1.5. [h] Normal length, cm, groups of 8 animals: ♂ 40-43; ♀ 41-42; ♂ 35,5-38,5; ♀ 37,5-40. [1] 2 with mammary tumor.

SPONTANEOUS CO-EXISTENT PITUITARY AND MAMMARY TUMORS.—In this group are included animals which have original pituitary and mammary tumors at the same time (Table 8-17). Evidently it is not mere co-existence. Some kind of causal relationship must exist; it is not unreasonable to think that the pituitary tumor is the cause of the mammary tumor. The three tumors were found, one (TR.DCCCXLIV) in 1965 and the other two (TR.MCCCXLI and TR.MCDXVI) in 1967, in intact female rats aged 962, 818, and 866 days, respectively. They resemble, functionally, TR.MIX, especially the first and the third. They have shown mammotropic activity only and not very greatly; this increased when the tumor was grafted. The first pituitary tumor of this group was not weighed; the other two weighed 340 and 250 mg, respectively. The mammary tumors measured 12 mm, 9 mm, and 50 × 44 × 19 mm. The last was as hard as fibroadenoma; the others were as soft as mammary cancer.

The three pituitary tumors were grafted in groups of six, seven and four intact female rats. They grew in all of the animals of the first group, and in three of the second and of the third groups. But more important was the fact that original mammary tumors developed in some of the animals of the first and of the third group in which the pituitary tumor grew. And with the first tumor, this was observed in the second transplant generation also. The pituitary glands of the animals grafted with the pituitary tumor and which developed original mammary tumors were of normal weight. So we may think that it is the grafted pituitary tumor which produces directly the mammotumorigenic factor.

The mammary tumors of the second and of the third pituitary tumor were grafted. That of the second grew in one of the animals in which the pituitary tumor grew and in one treated with estradiol. The mammary tumor of the third pituitary tumor is autonomous.

CO-EXISTENT PITUITARY AND TESTICULAR TUMORS.—These were found in a 984-day-old AxC rat, a nonbreeder. The pituitary tumor weighed

TABLE 8–17.—CO-EXISTENT PITUITARY AND MAMMARY TUMORS OF THE AxC RAT—FEMALES 27 TO 32 MONTHS OLD

Co-existent Tumors		Weight Dimensions		Ovaries mg.		Mamm.	Grafted		Orig. M. T. in Grafted with
Pituitary	Mammary	mg.	mm.	r.	l.	Gland[a]	s.c.	Posit.	Pit. T.
TR.DCCCXLIV		TUM		20	22	20,m	Yes	Yes	Yes
	TR.MCCCXLV		12				Not		—
TR.MCCCXLI		250		22	30	10,m	Yes	Yes	Not
	TR.MCCCLX		9				Yes	Yes	
TR.MCDXVI		340		15	21	5,m	Yes	Yes	Yes
	TR.MCDXV		50				Yes	Yes	—

[a] Equivalent to days pregnancy.
m: milk.

100 mg and the testicular tumor 3,550 mg. The other testis weighed 600 mg. The seminal vesicles and the prostate weighed 85 and 252 mg, the adrenals 27 and 30 mg. The mammary gland was a little bigger than normal and did not contain milk. Both tumors were grafted. The testicular tumor only grew. Now it is in the second transplant generation. As we have seen, testicular and pituitary tumors independently may produce mammary tumors. This did not happen in this case, as both tumors were in the same animal.

Transplantable Tumors Experimentally Produced

Our experience with spontaneous transplantable tumors of the gonads compelled us to study experimentally produced transplantable tumors of the ovary and testes. As has been known since the classic work of the Biskinds,[3] one ovary autografted into the spleen of a castrated rat becomes a tumor, if enough time elapses. To obtain testicular tumors, they grafted into the spleen one testis of a very young rat. The transplantability of these tumors has been studied[4, 40] but not extensively, as has been the experimental transplantable ovarian tumors of mice.[41]

The experimental transplantable pituitary tumors we owe to chance.

EXPERIMENTAL OVARIAN TUMORS

We call these experimentally produced transplantable tumors TOB. We maintain five of them (Table 8-18). They have been produced by autograft of one ovary in young adult spayed females, TOB.II, TOB. VIII, and TOB.XVI; or by grafting one ovary of a newborn rat in young adult castrated males, TOB.XIV and TOB.XV. Subcutaneous grafts were made of the intrasplenic tumors 14 to 24 months later. Some grew immediately in intact animals, others in castrated only. In the last transplant generations, they may grow more rapidly in intact animals. TOB.II and TOB.XVI are of interest. TOB.II is a granulosa cell tumor, macroscopically, microscopically and in general biologically

TABLE 8–18.—TOB. TRANSPLANTABLE EXPERIMENTAL OVARIAN TUMORS—STILL FUNCTIONAL

| TUMOR No. | DATE FIRST s.c. GRAFT | LAST GENERATIONS | | LAST GEN. SURVIVAL DAYS | HORMONAL ACTIVITY LAST GENER. |
		No.	Date Inoculation		
TOB.II	3.3.56	102	1. 9.70	38-56	Estrogenic
TOB.VIII	6.4.57	69	12.17.69	56-78	Estrogenic
TOB.XIV	3.3.64	4	12.12.68	264-424	Estrogenic
TOB.XV	3.19.64	8	5.19.69	80-109	Estrogenic
TOB.XVI	6.16.64	4	9.13.68	398-496	Estrogenic Androgenic

similar to our spontaneous functional transplantable ovarian tumor. All of our TOB are still hormonally active; they are estrogenic. TOB. XVI is androgenic also, although very weakly in the last transplant generation.

EXPERIMENTAL TESTICULAR TUMORS

As already explained, a testis of a newborn rat grafted into the spleen of castrated adults becomes a tumor. Thirty male and 16 female young adult AxC rats received an intrasplenic graft of one testis of a newborn rat. In 28 males and in 15 females, testicular tumors were found when the autopsies were made 11 to 28½ months afterwards. The largest tumor weighed 1.90 g, i.e. more than a normal testis of an adult rat, and almost a thousand times more than the testis of a newborn rat. Macroscopically these tumors resemble the spontaneous testicular tumors, being white or pink to yellowish in color and of soft consistency; they may be cystic. They are interstitial cell tumors and may contain vestigial seminal tubules.

Of 13 intrasplenic testicular tumors, 10 of males and three of females, grafts were made in intact and castrated males and females. They grew in all the groups, but better in castrated animals. They grow very slowly, surviving two years or more. In one case, considered unsuccessful, the tumor was found 32 months after the inoculation. Three tumors are maintained by subcutaneous grafts (see Table 8-19) and are now in the eleventh, fifth, and seventh transplant generations. The three are estrogenic; one is androgenic also.

EXPERIMENTAL PITUITARY TUMORS

Pituitary tumors are produced with radiation, antithyroid drugs, thyroidectomy, or continuous and prolonged estrogenic treatment. Such tumors are functional and transplantable, and have been one of the subjects of the pioneer work of Furth.

The pituitary tumors appearing in mice and rats castrated when young or newborn have been attributed to the action of estrogens produced by tumors of the adrenal cortex developing in such animals. Griesbach and Purves in 1960 observed pituitary tumors in female and

TABLE 8–19.—TTB. TRANSPLANTABLE TESTICULAR TUMORS OF THE AxC RAT EXPERIMENTALLY PRODUCED BY BISKIND'S METHOD, AND FIRST S.C. GRAFTED IN 1964—STILL FUNCTIONAL

No.	DATE FIRST S.C. INOC.	No. TRANSPL. GENER.	DATE LAST TRANSPL. GENER.	SURVIVAL LAST TRANSPL. GENER.	HORMONAL ACTIVITY	
TTB.II	2.18.64	11	11.25.69	56-58	Androgenic	Estrogenic
TTB.III	2.19.64	5	9.27.68	191-290	—	Estrogenic
TTB.V	2.19.64	7	8. 8.69	189-213	—	Estrogenic

TABLE 8–20.—AxC Female Rats Spayed between 24 hr. and 6 Days after Birth Compared with Female Rats Spayed at 2 Months and Intact Females

With Tumor (10-30 mg)	Hypophysis Large (15-27)	Normal Weight (8-12)	Survival or Age (Days)	Uterus (mg)
7			755-1128	31; 35; 40; 47; 64; 81; 115
	3		979-1120	21; 27; 58
		25[a]	362-1102	16-86
6 females spayed at 2 mos. (Hypophysis: 10-14 mg)			370-749	50; 60; 63; 84; 94; 117
10 intact females (Hypophysis: 10-12 mg)			428-627	288-513

[a] In one animal the weight of the hypophysis was 5 mg.

male rats castrated at the age of one and one-half, three, and nine months and autopsied when 14½ to 36 months old; there were no adrenal tumors and no signs of estrogenic action in these animals. These investigators concluded that the continuous and prolonged deficiency of gonadal hormones was the cause of these pituitary tumors, all of which were microscopic. In experiments with newborn and very young rats, we have obtained macroscopic pituitary tumors. One of these has been successfully transplanted.

Pituitary Tumors Produced by Deficiency of Gonadal Hormones. —Fifty male and 35 female AxC rats of less than 24 hr to six days of age were castrated under light ether anesthesia. The majority of autopsies were made one to three years later. In males as well as in females, pituitary tumors were found in animals without adrenocortical tumors and without signs of estrogenic action. In Table 8-20 are summarized the results obtained in females. Among the 35 females, there were seven with visible tumors of the pituitary gland, although their weight, except in one, did not surpass 30 mg, and some of the tumor-bearing pituitary glands had normal weight. In these cases without visible tumors, the weight of the hypophysis was from 15 to 27 mg, and in the other 25 the weight was normal and even subnormal. In all these animals, the uterus was smaller than normal. In the seven animals with a pituitary tumor, the weight of the uterus was 31 to 115 mg, as in spayed females without pituitary tumor. In intact females, the weight of the uterus was 288 to 512 mg and that of the hypophysis from 10 to 12 mg.

One of the pituitary tumors, found in a female which was spayed 24 hr after birth and killed at 26 months of age, was grafted. It was a big tumor with a calculated weight of about 100 mg, pink and soft. The uterus weighed 64 mg, the adrenals 18 and 21 mg, the thymus 24 mg, and the thyroids 8 and 4 mg. The mammary gland was developed as in a female pregnant 10 days. Since atrophy of the uterus is a certain sign of estrogen deficiency, there seems to be no doubt that the pituitary tumor was developed in the absence of estrogens. In the six animals inoculated, two intact and three spayed females and one intact male, the tumor grew after a latent period of 200 to 550 days. The survivals were of 633 to 680 days. This tumor is now in the eighth transplant generation, and the survivals are from 119 to 132 days. It does not show any hormonal activity. On March 20, 1970, a pituitary tumor weighing 300 mg was found in an 874-day-old female which was spayed at the age of 87 days; the uterus in this animal weighed 90 mg and the adrenals 26 and 29 mg; the mammary gland was not visible. This is another case of pituitary tumor developed in absence of estrogens. The tumor has been grafted.

PITUITARY TUMORS IN UNILATERAL OOPHORECTOMY.—We will describe now a pituitary tumor found in a female rat 677 days old, which was hemicastrated at 78 days of age. The tumor measured 9 mm. The mammary gland was developed as in a rat 20 days pregnant. The other organs were apparently normal. Three intact and three spayed females were inoculated with a suspension of the tumor. It grew in all the animals and showed weak mammotropic and adrenocorticotropic activity. Mammary tumors appeared in two spayed females in the first transplant generation. In the second transplant generation there were mammary tumors in two intact females. The pituitary glands were of normal weight, 8.8, 9, and 10 mg, in the four animals with mammary tumors. This would mean that there are no estrogens in action in the production of these mammary tumors. If we compare our hypermammotropic pituitary tumors which do not produce mammary tumors with this weak mammotropic tumor which produces mammary tumors, it would appear that it is not normal prolactin or prolactin alone that produces the mammary tumors. In any case, there is no direct relationship between mammary development and development of mammary tumors.

In the group of six animals with unilateral oophorectomy, there were four with pituitary tumors. But as all were animals aged 599 to 942 days, we are not sure whether the tumors were really caused by the experimental manipulation or whether they were spontaneous.

THE GONADOTROPIC PITUITARY TUMOR.—More interesting is the transplantable gonadotropic pituitary tumor.[24] The tumor, measuring 9 × 7 × 6 mm, was found in a 30-month-old castrated male AxC rat, which at the age of five months received an intrasplenic graft of a testis of a newborn rat of the same strain. A testicular tumor developed in the spleen as expected. The mammary gland was well developed and contained cysts with milk. The adrenals weighed 16 and 15 mg, i.e. a little less than normal. The tumor grew in four of five animals inoculated (see Table 8-21). The only female in the group died after 18 months (August 14, 1966) with a tumor of 31 g. The nipples and the mammary glands were large, and the ovaries weighed 908 and 1,040 mg (normally 29 mg). The uterus, with abundant fluid, weighed 2.5 g

TABLE 8–21.—TR.DCCXLIII. Transplantable Gonadotropic Pituitary Tumor
of the AxC Rat Found February 12, 1965
(1st transplant generation, s.c.)

Sex Hosts ♂	Survival Days	Tumor G.	Mamm. Gl.[a] G.	Testes[b], mg. Right	Testes[b], mg. Left	Sem. Ves.,[c] mg. R. Full	Sem. Ves.,[c] mg. L. Wide	Prostate[d] mg.	Adrenals[e] R.	Adrenals[e] L.	Hypophysis[f] mg.
♂	302	3	5	1200	288	800	192	600	14	16	9
	573	36	5	1450	1420	1150	350	1000	26	30	8
♂	551	T	n	—	—	6	6	4	20	24	n

				Ovaries[g] mg.	Uterus[h]						
♀	548	31	(1.3) s.	1040	908	2500			64	63	127

[a] Development equivalent days pregnancy; n: normal; ( ) weight one inguinal group. s: milk secretion.
Normal weights, mg: [b] 1128 ± 69; [c] 478 ± 58; [d] 369 ± 76; [e] 21 ± 2; [f] 10 ± 1.5; [g] 29 ± 5; [h] 374 ± 77.

(normally 374 mg) and the pituitary gland 127 mg (normal 10 mg). In males the testes weighed up to 1,650 mg (normal 1,200 mg), the seminal vesicles up to 1,150 mg (normal 400 mg) and the ventral prostate up to 1,000 mg (normal 350 mg). The hypophyses in males were of normal weight, 8 and 9 mg. In the castrated male the seminal vesicles weighed 6 mg and the prostate 4 mg.

In the third transplant generation, in three intact females there were three enormous ovaries weighing 820 to 2,800 mg, each ovary containing an ovarian tumor (Table 8-22). In one animal with big ovaries with ovarian tumor, and with pituitary tumor, there was a mammary fibroadenoma. A similar case was observed in the fifth transplant

TABLE 8–22.—TR.DCCXLIII. Transplantable Gonadotropic Pituitary Tumor
of the AxC Rat
(3rd transplant generation, s.c. inoc. 7.12.66)

Group	Survival Days	Tumor G.	Mamm. Gl.[a]	Testes[b] (Ovaries)[e] mg.	Sem. Ves.[d] (Uterus)[e] mg.	Prostate[f] mg.	Hypophysis[g] mg.
4 ♂	265-353	30-53	n- (142)	1400-1650	428-1050	230-350	8.5; 8; 6; 14
4 ♂	225-388	13-49	n-n	— —	17-28	4-13	12; 10; 12; 10
3 ♀	192-360	2-25	n,-10,S,MT[h]	(24-2800) [i]	(4600)	—	13; T; 95
3 ♀	254-374	12-58	0- (82)	— —	(53-75)	—	14; 11; 10

[a] n: normal; S: secretion; equivalent days pregnancy; ( ) weight of one inguinal group.
Normal weights, mg., groups of 8 animals: [b] 1128 ± 69; [c] 29 ± 5; [d] 478 ± 58; [e] 374 ± 77; [f] 369 ± 76; [g] 10 ± 1.5.
[h] Mammary tumor.
[i] Weight of the other ovaries: 25, 64, 820 and 860 mg; in the 3 big ovaries there were ovarian tumors.

TABLE 8–23.—TR.DCCXLIII. Transplantable Gonadotropic Pituitary Tumor of the AxC Rat Found February 12, 1965—Still Functional in Last Transplant Generations

No. Gener.	Date Inocu- lation	Hosts	Survival Days	Tumor g.	Mamm. Gland[a]	Ovaries[b] mg.	Uterus[c] mg.	Hypophysis[d] mg.
5th	3.27.68	4 ♀	235-303	12-64	15-1.30	28-1800	281-850	24; 10; 25; 39
6th	11.28.68	4 ♀	127-204	21-39	0.75-1.10	40-257	494-750	16; n; 30; 24
7th	6.17.69	4 ♀	217-267	49-56	15-1.45	115-375	600	35; 40; 38; 30

[a] Development equivalent to days pregnancy or weight, g, of one inguinal group.
Normal weights, mg, group of 8 animals: [b] 29 ± 5; [c] 374 ± 77; [d] 10 ± 1.5.

generation: intact female, survival 303 days, ovaries 154 and 1,800 mg, this last with tumor, uterus 1,800 mg with fluid, pituitary gland 39 mg, mammary gland well developed (one inguinal group 0.9 g), and mammary tumor of 900 mg. One may suggest the following chain of events in the production of the mammary tumor: grafted pituitary tumor=follicle-stimulating hormone→ovary=ovarian tumor=estrogens→ pituitary=pituitary hyperplasia or tumor=prolactin→mammary gland= mammary tumor.

The mammary fibroadenoma was grafted and grew in two transplant generations in animals grafted with the pituitary tumor or treated with estradiol. In the third transplant generation, leukemia appeared and the tumor was lost. The other mammary tumor was exclusively epithelial, but was found in a dead animal and was not grafted.

The pituitary tumor is still functional in the last transplant generations, as may be seen in Table 8-23.

Probably it is not difficult to produce gonadotropic tumors. It would be enough to implant one testis, or maybe an ovary (or maybe nothing) in the spleen of young adult castrated rats and wait two or three years.

Some Curious Observations

Scrotal Hernia

I have already mentioned the scrotal hernia developed in animals grafted with androgenic and estrogenic testicular tumors.

Catalepsy

Catalepsy has been observed occasionally in animals grafted with our first adrenal tumor, TD. The animals seem dead; after minutes or hours they recover completely. This may repeat two or three times in a period of several days. This phenomenon resembles that described by Selye[39] as steroid hormone anesthesia.

Myocardial Sclerosis

The splanchnomegaly or the kidney's and liver's pathology described by Furth in animals with grafted mammosomatocorticotropic pituitary tumors has been confirmed in our experiments with the corresponding tumors. Cardiomegaly and myocardial sclerosis have been observed also. All of these lesions must be the result of corticosteroids produced in excess by the action of ACTH. Splanchnomegaly must be produced by somatotropic hormone. Selye[38] and Ingle[26] have observed nephrosclerosis and myocardial necrosis in uninephrectomized salt-loaded rats treated with large doses of corticosteroids.

Precocious Invisible Metastasis

One of the testicular tumors (TR.LIV) with survival of 23 to 25 days is maintained by inoculating a suspension of an apparently normal lung. The neoplastic cells invade the lungs very early, but the animal does not live long enough to develop visible metastases. Based on this observation, one could say that if metastasis means malignancy, absence of metastasis may mean a greater degree of malignancy.

Some Experiments

Tumor-Stimulating Action of Subphysiologic Quantities of Testosterone

Large, masculinizing quantities of testosterone propionate stimulate the growth of the spontaneous ovarian tumor (TOF) and of one experimental ovarian tumor (TOB.II). In new experiments, it was demonstrated that very small quantities of the androgen, quantities not sufficient to maintain the weight of the seminal vesicles in castrated males, are able to stimulate the growth of these tumors.[13]

Change of Responsiveness

The spontaneous ovarian tumor (TOF) grows better in intact males or in castrated males treated with testosterone propionate than in castrated nontreated males. Since 1949 it has been maintained in intact males. In 1956, a subline of the tumor was started in castrated males. In 1961,[12] experiments were made with the tumor maintained in intact males and with the tumor maintained in castrated males. As expected, in the first, the tumor grew more rapidly in intact males and in castrated treated with testosterone propionate than in castrated nontreated. The contrary happened in the second: the tumor grew more rapidly in castrated males nontreated than in intact or castrated males treated with the androgen. Mercier and Furth[31] have

TABLE 8–24.—ANTITUMORAL ACTION OF ESTRADIOL ON ONE SPONTANEOUS
TRANSPLANTABLE TESTICULAR TUMOR, TR.CDLXXXI, 4TH TRANSPLANT GENERATION

| | | | ANIMALS WITH TUMOR | | | ANIMALS WITHOUT TUMOR | |
GROUPS	TREATMENT (SUBCUT. PELLET)	No.	Latent Period Days	Survival Days	Tumor Weight g.	No.	Survival Days
8 ♀	0	8	86-122	253-445	3-55	0	—
8 ♀̸	0	8	31-38	223-351	6-20	0	—
8 ♀̸ [a]	Estradiol 10%	2	276-432	287-502	0.056-0.505	6	384-827

[a] Treated for 9½ months; treatment withdrawn for 8 months.

studied this phenomenon experimentally with a thyrogonadotropic pituitary tumor in mice. Minesita and Yamaguchi[33] have described an autonomous mammary adenocarcinoma of the mouse which became androgen-dependent.

ANTITUMORAL ACTION OF ESTRADIOL

The testicular tumor (TR.CDLXXXI), which we have described in some detail, grows in 100% of males and females, intact and castrated; the latent period is longer in intact females.[14] Progesterone, testosterone propionate, or methyltestosterone had no action on the growth of the tumor, and all of the inoculated animals died with as big tumors as the non-treated. The results were thus impressive with estradiol (1 subcutaneous pellet, 10%, 25 mg); in a group of eight spayed females, only two developed tumors after a long latent period of 276 to 452 days and survival of 287 to 502 days, compared with a group of eight nontreated spayed females with a latent period of 31 to 38 days and a survival of 223 to 351 days, respectively (Table 8-24). The weight of tumors in these was 6 to 20 g, and in those treated with estradiol, 56 and 505 mg. In six animals of the group which have been treated with estradiol for nine and one-half months, the tumor did not grow after the estradiol was withdrawn, during a period of observation of eight months. This we call the antitumoral action of estradiol, which we must differentiate from the antitumorigenic action of a compound. All of these experiments were made with the third transplant generation of the tumor. In new experiments made with other generations, the results were somewhat different, which is expected when working with endocrine transplantable tumors; their responsiveness may change.

TUMOR-STIMULATING ACTION OF ESTRADIOL
AND CO-TUMOR-STIMULATING ACTION OF
TESTOSTERONE PROPIONATE

The mammary carcinoma (TR.MCII) produced by the testicular tumor (TR.CDLXXXI) already described did not grow in intact and castrated males and females, not treated or treated with testosterone propionate or progesterone, but grew in those treated with estradiol and faster in those treated simultaneously with estradiol and testosterone propionate. This we call the co-tumor-stimulating action of testosterone propionate.[23] In simple experiments, we have demonstrated that the stimulating action of estradiol is not direct on the tumor. This grows only in animals treated with estradiol subcutaneously. It does not grow in nontreated animals or in animals with estradiol implanted into the spleen; the steroid, in this case inactivated in the liver, does not reach the subcutaneous tumor. But the tumor does not grow when implanted into the spleen together with the estradiol. In this case, the estradiol is in direct contact with the inoculated tumor and this does not grow. So estradiol must go beyond the liver to stimulate the growth of the tumor. It is reasonable to think that the pituitary gland is the site where estradiol must go to produce the tumor-stimulating factor. And prolactin must be this factor. We have not observed inhibitory effects of estradiol on the growth of any of our transplantable mammary tumors, as has been established for other transplantable mammary tumors of the rat.[11, 27]

We give estradiol and testosterone in pellet form, 10% and 40%, repectively, weighing about 25 mg, which produces almost physiologic effects.

The Dormant Neoplastic Cell

We have seen that the mammary cancer grows only in animals treated with estradiol. What happens with the cancer cells inoculated in nontreated animals? Some of these animals were killed two years and more after the inoculation, and the interscapular tissue, where the tumor had been inoculated, was removed and inoculated in young rats; in these, which received estradiol, the tumor developed in about two months. The longest "sleeping" period was two years, two months, and 23 days. This is more than two thirds of the life-span of a rat, and equivalent to more than 60 years in a human being. Gardner[9] was the first to observe this phenomenon; he could awake with estrogen a testicular tumor of mice six and one-half months after the inoculation.

References

1. Apostolakis, M.: In: Vitamins and Hormones. Vol. 26, 1968, p. 197.
2. Burrows, H.: Brit. J. Surg., 21:507, 1934.
3. Biskind, M. S., and G. R. Biskind: Proc. Soc. Exp. Biol. (N.Y.), 55:176, 1944.
4. Biskind, M. S., and G. R. Biskind: Proc. Soc. Exp. Biol. (N.Y.), 59:4, 1945.
5. Boot, L. M.: Induction by Prolactin of Mammary Tumors in Mice. N. V. North Holland Publishing Co., Amsterdam, 1969, p. 77.
6. Coujard, R., and C. Coujard-Champy: Ann. d'Endocrinologie, 2:25, 1941.
7. Furth, J., and K. H. Clifton: In: Hormonal Production in Endocrine Tumors. Ciba Foundation Colloquia on Endocrinology, J. & A. Churchill, Ltd., London, Vol. 12, 1958, p. 3.
8. Furth, J., and K. H. Clifton: In: Endocrine Aspects of Breast Cancer. Livingstone, Ltd., Edinburgh, 1958, p. 276.

9. Gardner, W. U.: Cancer Res., 5:497, 1945.
10. Gardner, W. U., C. A. Pfeiffer, and J. J. Trentin: In: The Physiopathology of Cancer (Homburger, ed.), Hoeber, New York, 1959, p. 152.
11. Hilf, R., I. Michel, and C. Bell: Recent Progr. Hormone Res., 23:229, 1967.
12. Iglesias, R.: Proc. Amer. Ass. Cancer Res., 3:331, 1962.
13. Iglesias, R.: In: Hormonal Steroids. Proceedings of the First International Congress on Hormonal Steroids, Milan, 1962. Academic Press, New York, Vol. 2, 1965, p. 391.
14. Iglesias, R.: In: Proceedings of the Eighth International Conference of the International Planned Parenthood Federation, Santiago, Chile, 1967. Stephen Austin and Sons, Hertford, England, 1967, p. 468.
15. Iglesias, R., and E. Mardones: Cancer, 9:740, 1956.
16. Iglesias, R., and E. Mardones: Brit. J. Cancer, 12:20, 1958.
17. Iglesias, R., and E. Mardones: Brit. J. Cancer, 12:28, 1958.
18. Iglesias, R., and S. Salinas: In: Fifth Panam. Congress Endocrinology (Abstracts), Lima, Peru, 1961, p. 93.
19. Iglesias, R., and S. Salinas: Proc. Amer. Ass. Cancer Res., 5:30, 1964.
20. Iglesias, R., and S. Salinas: Proc. Amer. Ass. Cancer Res., 8:35, 1967.
21. Iglesias, R., S. Salinas, and A. Alvarez: In: Sixth Panam. Congress Endocrinology, Mexico, 1965. Excerpta Medica, Intern. Congress Series 99, p. E 120.
22. Iglesias, R., S. Salinas, A. Alvarez, and P. Vukusic: Acta Physiol. Lat. Amer., 16 (Suppl. 1) :63, 1966.
23. Iglesias, R., S. Salinas, A. Alvarez, P. Vukusic, and V. Panasevich: Proc. Amer. Ass. Cancer Res., 9:34, 1968.
24. Iglesias, R., S. Salinas, P. Vukusic, and V. Panasevich: Proc. Amer. Ass. Cancer Res., 10:43, 1969.
25. Iglesias, R., W. H. Sternberg, and A. Segaloff: Cancer Res., 10:668, 1960.
26. Ingle, D. J.: On Cancer and Hormones. University of Chicago Press, Chicago, 1962, p. 213.
27. Kim, U.: Cancer Res., 25:1146, 1965.
28. Kirschbaum, A.: In: Fundamental Aspects of Normal and Malignant Growth (Nowinski, ed.), Elsevier, Amsterdam, 1960, p. 823.
29. Lyon, W. R., C. H. Li, and R. E. Johanson: Recent Progr. Hormone Res., 14: 219, 1958.
30. Meites, J., and D. Sinha: Ninth International Cancer Congress. Abstract of Papers, 1966, p. 82.
31. Messier, B. [sic], and J. Furth: Cancer Res., 22:804, 1962.
32. Miller, O. J., and W. U. Gardner: Cancer Res., 14:20, 1954.
33. Minesita, T., and K. Yamaguchi: Cancer Res., 25:1168, 1965.
34. Pasqualini, J. R., R. Iglesias, and B. L. Nguyen: Testosterone. Proceedings of the Workshop Conference on Testosterone, Hamburg, 1967, p. 62.
35. Pasqualini, J. R., R. Iglesias, B. L. Nguyen, and S. Salinas: Research on Steroids. Vol. III, 1967, p. 108.
36. Russfield, A. B.: Tumors of Endocrine Glands and Secondary Sex Organs. Public Health Service Publication No. 1332. Washington, D. C., 1966.
37. Segaloff, A., S. L. Steelman, and A. Flores: Endocrinology, 59:233, 1956.
38. Selye, H.: J. Clin. Endocrinol., 6:117, 1946.
39. Selye, H.: Textbook of Endocrinology. Acta Endocr., Montreal, Canada, 1948, p. 59.
40. Twombly, G. H., D. Meisel, and A. P. Stout: Cancer, 2:884, 1949.
41. Van Nie, R.: Hormone Dependence of Transplanted Ovarian Tumors in Mice. Thesis. University of Utrecht, 1957.
(For references not listed above see Iglesias: Proceedings of the Second International Congress on Endocrinology, London, 1964, Part 2, p. 1072.)

Hormone-Producing Tumors from Nonendocrine Tissues

GRIFF T. ROSS, M.D., Ph.D.

*Endocrinology Branch, National Cancer Institute,
National Institutes of Health, Bethesda, Maryland, USA*

Introduction

TROPHIC HORMONES which stimulate endocrine target glands are sometimes secreted by tumors of nonendocrine tissues; this "ectopic hormone production" results in signs and symptoms of endocrine hyperfunction among patients with these tumors.[1, 2] Hormones identified include adrenocorticotropic hormone, antidiuretic hormone, erythropoietin, gastrin, glucagon, gonadotropins, melanocyte-stimulating hormone, parathormone, serotonin, substances producing hyperglycemia, and thyroid-stimulating hormone. Tumors of most organ systems have been implicated and, on occasion, more than one of these substances may be secreted by a single tumor.[3]

Recently these phenomena have been the subject of excellent comprehensive reviews.[1-6] To avoid needless repetition in the following discussion, basic principles documented in these reviews will be summarized briefly. Then, recent observations which provide additional insights will be presented in more detail.

Several generalizations can be made on the basis of information in the reviews mentioned:

1. Restricting use of the term "ectopic hormone production" to secretion of hormones by tumors of nonendocrine tissues "semantically" excludes from consideration some equally interesting tumors of endocrine glands.[2] Some of these tumors secrete hormones not characteristically produced by the nonneoplastic gland, such as secretion of gonadotropins by tumors of testis, ovary, or adrenal cortex, for example.[1, 3, 7]

2. Where studies have been possible, hormones produced by neoplasms of nonendocrine tissues have been found to be biologically, immunologically, and chemically similar to those produced by the tissues of which they are characteristic secretory products.[2, 8-11]

3. In some instances, evidence that tumor tissue is the source of hormone has consisted in biologic or immunologic identification of appropriate hormonal activity in extracts of tumor tissue. In other instances, evidence for hormonal secretion by tumor has been based upon decreased severity of signs and symptoms of hormone excess or re-

duced hormone concentrations in plasma or urine following reduction of tumor mass.[1, 3]

4. Endocrine hyperfunction in these syndromes is autonomous and not subject to methods of regulation which normally maintain a steady state in the endocrine milieu.[1-3] However, autonomous hyperfunction may also result from nonneoplastic diseases of the endocrine glands themselves, and at times it may be difficult to differentiate hyperfunction caused by ectopic hormone production by a tumor from hyperfunction of an endocrine gland unrelated to neoplasia. This is particularly true when a neoplasm of extra-endocrine tissues is not readily apparent; in such instances treatment may be misdirected.[12]

Methods

From these last two generalizations, it follows that sensitive methods for measurement of trophic hormones are needed to fully understand this fascinating area of tumor biology in man. Ideally, to establish secretion of hormone by tumor, one should be able to measure arteriovenous differences in hormonal concentrations across localized masses of tumor tissue.[2] In addition, methods should permit precise measurement of both target organ and trophic hormonal concentrations in the basal state in normal subjects. Then response to agents which either stimulate or suppress hormonal secretion in normal subjects could be evaluated among patients with tumors.

Tests with many of the requisite characteristics have been developed for some hormones, e.g. adrenocorticotropic hormone (ACTH) and adrenal cortical steroid hormones.[11-15] The frequency with which tumors producing ACTH have been identified may reflect both the quality of methods available and the comparative ease with which characteristic syndromes of target organ hormone excess can be diagnosed.

Recently, sensitive radioimmunoassays have been developed for measuring pituitary gonadotropins in plasma.[16-19] Pituitary gonadotropins and gonadotropins produced by tumors have common antigenic determinants so that whether the source of gonadotropin activity is pituitary or extrapituitary may be difficult to determine. This decision is particularly difficult in those instances where concentrations do not exceed those expected from pituitary secretion alone (Case 4 in reference 20, for example).

In addition to radioimmunoassays for gonadotropins, sensitive methods have been developed for measuring gonadal steroid hormones in plasma.[25-31] Ability to measure gonadotropins and steroids in aliquots of the same sample of plasma makes it possible to evaluate interactions of pituitary and gonads in normal human subjects.[32-34]

Results

Arteriovenous differences in hormone concentrations across localized masses of tumor tissue have been reported twice for tumors producing gonadotropins.[21, 22] Increased concentrations of a substance with antigenic determinants similar to those in human follicle-stimulating hormone were found in venous effluent from a bronchogenic carcinoma by Faiman and others.[21] Similarly, concentrations of immunoreactive gonadotropin were higher in spermatic vein blood than in mixed venous blood from a patient with a testicular tumor.[22] The long plasma half-life of chorionic gonadotropin[23, 24] may limit the usefulness of this type of study in some instances.

Gonadal steroid hormones, estrogens and progestins, given in appropriate doses singly or together to normal women suppress pituitary gonadotropin secretion, whether measured in urine[35–37] or in plasma.[38, 39] Suppression tests of this type are useful in ruling out an extrapituitary source of gonadotropin in women at risk for gestational trophoblastic neoplasms or other tumors producing gonadotropins.

In normal men, synthesis and secretion of testosterone (T) by Leydig cells is stimulated by luteinizing hormone (LH) secreted by the pituitary.[25, 32, 33] This stimulatory effect can be reproduced by administration of human chorionic gonadotropin (HCG) extracted from the urine of pregnant women.[25, 32, 33] Evidence exists for a negative feedback control operating between the Leydig cell and the pituitary by way of the hypothalamus. Thus, plasma concentrations of T decline when potent androgens (testosterone analogs such as fluoxymesterone) are given to normal men.[25, 32]

Plasma T concentrations can be restored to normal when HCG is

Fig. 8–7.—Plasma testosterone concentrations before and after 40 mg of fluoxymesterone have been given daily for three days to seven normal men, left panel, and seven men with testicular tumors containing trophoblast, right panel. (Courtesy of Kirschner, M. A., J. Clin. Endocrinol., in press.)

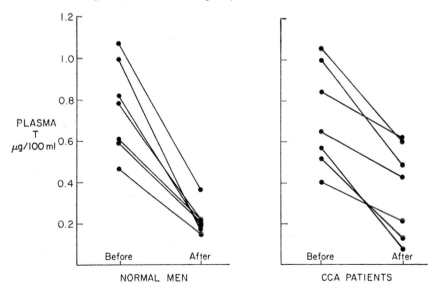

given concomitantly with the androgen,[25] indicating that the suppressive effect of the androgen is mediated indirectly by way of suppression of pituitary secretion of LH. Indeed, plasma LH concentrations, measured by radioimmunoassay, can be shown to decline in response to androgens.[32]

Kirschner and his associates, using these methods, have studied Leydig cell function in a series of men with testicular tumors producing gonadotropin.[40] Chemically and immunologically, this gonadotropin is very similar to HCG excreted in the urine of women during pregnancy.[41]

During control periods and periods when fluoxymesterone was given orally to men with tumors, plasma testosterone concentrations were indistinguishable from those in normal men (Figure 8-7), despite high levels of circulating tumor gonadotropins which varied over a thousandfold range in men with tumors. Measurements of immunoreactive gonadotropin concentrations in plasma showed no change while plasma testosterone concentrations were falling in response to fluoxymesterone (Figure 8-8). These results suggested that Leydig cell function was being stimulated by pituitary rather than tumor gonadotropin in these men with tumors.

To test biologic activity of the tumor gonadotropin in men, gonadotropin was extracted from the urine of one man with a tumor and given to other men with testicular tumors not producing gonadotropin. In these latter persons, tumor gonadotropin injections were followed by an increase in plasma testosterone concentrations. Under these conditions, then, biologic effects of tumor gonadotropin were similar to those of HCG in normal men. Thus, despite secretion of large

FIG 8-8.—Plasma LH and testosterone concentrations measured during a period when six men with testicular tumors containing trophoblast received 40 mg of fluoxymesterone per day. While plasma testosterone decreased, plasma gonadotrophin remained relatively constant. (Courtesy of Kirschner, M. A., J. Clin. Endocrinol., in press.)

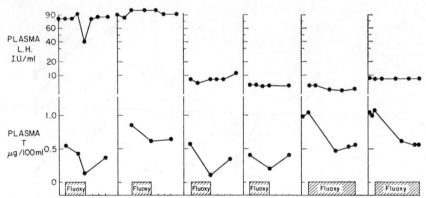

amounts of biologically active gonadotropin by testicular tumor tissue, no evidence for a steroidogenic effect of the hormone on Leydig cells of the host was observed. These data indicate that production of large amounts of trophic hormone by tumors may not always result in either stimulation of appropriate target organs or in a syndrome of endocrine hyperfunction in the host.

Target organ function may fail to be stimulated when tumor hormone production is minimal because of small masses of tumor tissue early in the course of disease or inefficient synthesis and secretion by larger masses of tumor. In these instances, too, ectopic hormone secretion may escape detection unless testing includes measurements of response to agents which stimulate or suppress hormone secretion in normal subjects. Rosen and others have reported failure of gonadal steroid hormones to suppress gonadotropin secretion in a patient with a bronchogenic carcinoma producing small amounts of gonadotropin.[42] In this patient, autonomous production of gonadotropin was apparent approximately one year before bronchogenic carcinoma was diagnosed.

For a variety of reasons, then, target organ stimulation may fail to occur despite ectopic hormone production. It follows that estimates of frequency of hormone production by tumors may be spuriously low if based exclusively upon the frequency with which symptoms and signs of hyperfunction occur. More accurate estimates of frequency of the phenomenon of hormone production by tumors will require wider use of methods which are sufficiently sensitive, precise, and specific to measure responses to suppressive and stimulatory tests in normal subjects.

It has been suggested that some neoplasms may produce imperfect replicates of a trophic hormone molecule: substances which are immunologically active but biologically inactive.[3] Evidence consistent with this hypothesis for tumors producing gonadotropins has been reported by Hobson and Wide, who examined immunologic and biologic activities of concentrates prepared by acetone precipitation of gonadotropins from urine of women with trophoblastic neoplasms.[43] They reported that the mean ratio of immunologic to biologic activity was greater in urine from women with chorioadenoma than in urine from women with choriocarcinoma. These results suggest that with increasing anaplasia of trophoblastic tissue, the immunologic to biologic ratio increases; this would make it seem logical to suppose that some highly anaplastic tumors might produce substances with only immunologic activity. However, evidence suggesting that Hobson and Wide's findings might relate to changes occurring in the molecule after secretion, has been obtained by Bridson et al., who studied immunologic and biologic activities of gonadotropin produced by clonal strains of human choriocarcinoma in tissue culture.[44] Surprisingly, in the light of Hobson and Wide's findings, Bridson found that biologic activity was greater than immunologic activity for gonadotropin secreted into tissue culture medium by some strains of these anaplastic cells.

It is possible to rationalize these apparent discrepancies between immunologic and biologic activities of gonadotropins in urine from women with choriocarcinoma and in media from choriocarcinoma cells in tissue culture. Chorionic gonadotropins contain sialic acid and desialation does not significantly alter immunologic activity.[45, 46] Conversely, increase in sialic acid content of chorionic gonadotropin during purification results in enhancement of biologic activity without proportionate increases in immunologic activity.[45, 46] If it is supposed that desialation of chorionic gonadotropin occurs in vivo after secretion by tumor, but either prior to or during excretion in urine, then these apparent discrepancies can be resolved. The question of whether tumors secrete hormone which is deficient in sialic acid cannot be resolved entirely from available data. The observations of Bridson et al. serve to emphasize Liddle's comment concerning the potential value of tissue cultures of tumors in studying properties of hormones they secrete.[2]

In addition to gonadotropins, some testicular tumors and some bronchogenic carcinomas produce chorionic somatomammotropin, a hormone which is usually produced only by normal trophoblast during pregnancy.[47] Since chorionic somatomammotropin normally is produced uniquely during pregnancy, demonstrating the hormone in plasma of nonpregnant subjects is likely to be indicative of the presence of a neoplasm. In contrast, then, to most other hormones, detection of chorionic somatomammotropin becomes a more specific test for malignancy.

Sensitive specific immunoassays have been developed for this hormone in plasma.[48] Using affinity chromatography, Weintraub has shown the feasibility of extracting and concentrating chorionic somatomammotropin from plasma prior to assay.[49] Measurement of concentrates from large volumes of plasma increases the sensitivity of detection by orders of magnitude and, hopefully, will permit application of the test to diagnosis of neoplasia early in the course of disease when tumor tissue may not be apparent by other methods of testing.

Summary and Conclusions

Recent studies of patients with tumors producing gonadotropins indicate that signs and symptoms of hormone excess need not always accompany ectopic hormone production. Consequently, ectopic hormone production may be more common than has usually been supposed on the basis of incidence of symptoms of hormone excess. All of these observations serve to emphasize the importance of appropriate methods of testing for recognition and study of these phenomena. Sensitive, automated methods for measurement coupled with practical methods for extraction and concentration of hormones prior to assay should provide a basis for wider evaluation of the significance of ectopic hormone production in tumor biology.

Finally, wide application of these tests for hormonal substances and other substances produced by neoplastic cells in high risk groups might conceivably result in earlier detection of neoplasms, thus allowing for any therapeutic benefits which may accrue by early treatment.

References

1. Lipsett, M. B.: Hormonal syndrome associated with neoplasia. Advance Metabol. Disorders, 3:111-152, 1968.
2. Liddle, G. W.: Preliminary characterization of some ectopic hormones. Vitamins and Hormones, 26:293-310, 1968.
3. Odell, W. D.: Humoral manifestation of non-endocrine neoplasms. In: Textbook of Endocrinology (R. H. Williams, ed.) , W. B. Saunders, Philadelphia, 4th Ed., pp. 1211-1222.
4. Sachs, B. A.: Endocrine disorders produced by non-endocrine malignant tumors. Bull. of N. Y. Acad. Med., 41:1069-1086, 1965.
5. Lipsett, M. B.: Humoral syndromes associated with cancer. Cancer Res., 25:1068-1073, 1965.
6. Bower, B. F., and G. S. Gordon: Hormonal effects of nonendocrine tumors. Ann. Rev. Med., 16:83-119, 1965.
7. Rose, L. I., G. H. Williams, P. I. Jagger, and D. P. Lauler: Feminizing tumor of the adrenal gland with positive "chorionic-like" gonadotrophin test. J. Clin. Endocrinol., 28:903-908, 1968.
8. Utiger, R. D.: Inappropriate antidiuresis and carcinoma of the lung: Detection of arginine vasopressin in tumor extracts by immunoassay. J. Clin. Endocrinol., 26:970-974, 1966.
9. Sawyer, W. H.: Pharmacological characteristics of the antidiuretic principle in a bronchogenic carcinoma from a patient with hypoproteinemia. J. Clin. Endocrinol., 27:1497-1499, 1967.
10. Sherwood, L. M., J. L. O'Riordan, G. D. Aurbach, and J. T. Potts: Production of parathyroid hormone by nonparathyroid tumors. J. Clin. Endocrinol., 27:140-146, 1967.
11. Orth, D. N., D. P. Island, W. E. Nicholson, K. Abe, and J. P. Woodham: ACTH radioimmunoassay: Interpolation, comparison with bioassay, and clinical application. In: Radioisotopes in Medicine: In Vitro Studies. U. S. Atomic Energy Comm., 1968, pp. 251-272.
12. Strott, C. A., C. A. Nugent, and F. H. Tyler: Cushing's syndrome caused by bronchial adenomas. Amer. J. Med., 44:97-104, 1968.
13. Liddle, G. W., D. P. Island, and C. K. Meador: Normal and abnormal regulation of corticotropin secretion in man. Rec. Prog. Hormone Res., 18:125-166, 1962.
14. Strott, C. A., K. Nakagawa, H. Nankin, and C. A. Nugent: A phenylalanine-lysine-vasopressin test for ACTH release. J. Clin. Endocrinol., 27:448-451, 1967.
15. Webb-Peploe, M. M., G. S. Spathis, and P. I. Reed: Cushing's syndrome: Use of lysine vasopressin to distinguish overproduction of corticotrophin by pituitary from other causes of adrenal cortisol hyperfunction. Lancet, 1:195-197, 1967.
16. Midgley, A. R., and J. S. Ram: Radioimmunoassay of human chorionic gonadotrophin (HCG) and human pituitary luteinizing hormone (LH). Fed. Proc., 24:162, 1965.
17. Odell, W. D., G. T. Ross, and P. L. Rayford: Radioimmunoassay for human luteinizing hormone. Metabolism, 15:287-288, 1965.
18. Bagshawe, K. D., C. E. Wilde, and A. H. Orr: Radioimmunoassay for human chorionic gonadotrophin and luteinizing hormone. Lancet, 1:1118-1121, 1966.
19. Faiman, C., and R. J. Ryan: Serum follicle stimulating hormone and luteinizing hormone concentrations during the menstrual cycle as determined by radioimmunoassay. J. Clin. Endocrinol., 27:1711-1716, 1967.
20. Fusco, F. D., and S. W. Rosen: Gonadotropin-producing anaplastic large-cell carcinomas of the lung. New Eng. J. Med., 275:507-515, 1966.

21. Faiman, C., J. A. Colwell, R. J. Ryan, J. M. Hershman, and T. W. Shields: Gonadotrophin secretion from a bronchogenic carcinoma: Demonstration by radioimmunoassay. New Eng. J. Med., 277:1395-1399, 1967.
22. Wieland, R. G., A. Guevara, M. C. Hallberg, E. M. Zorn, and C. Pohlman: Spermatic and peripheral venous levels of gonadotrophin and testosterone in a teratoma with embryonal cell carcinoma. J. Clin. Endocrinol., 29:398-400, 1969.
23. Rizkallah, T., E. Gurpide, and R. L. Vande Wiele: Metabolism of HCG in man. J. Clin. Endocrinol., 29:92-100, 1969.
24. Midgley, A. R., and R. B. Jaffe: Regulation of human gonadotropin. II. Disappearance of human chorionic gonadotropin following delivery. J. Clin. Endocrinol., 28:1712-1718, 1968.
25. Davis, T. E., M. B. Lipsett, and S. G. Korenman: Suppression of testosterone production by physiologic doses of 2α-methyldihydrotestosterone propionate. J. Clin. Endocrinol., 25:476-479, 1965.
26. Yoshimi, T., and M. B. Lipsett: The measurement of plasma progesterone. Steroids, 11:527-540, 1968.
27. Strott, C. A., and M. B. Lipsett: Measurement of 17-hydroxyprogesterone in human plasma. J. Clin. Endocrinol., 28:1426-1430, 1968.
28. Baird, D. T., and A. Guevara: Concentration of unconjugated estrone and estradiol in peripheral plasma in nonpregnant women throughout the menstrual cycle, castrate and postmenopausal women and in men. J. Clin. Endocrinol., 29:149-156, 1969.
29. Abraham, G. E.: Solid-phase radioimmunoassay of estradiol-17β. J. Clin. Endocrinol., 29:866-870, 1969.
30. Korenman, S. G., L. E. Perrin, and T. P. McCollem: A radioligand binding assay system for estradiol measurement in human plasma. J. Clin. Endocrinol., 29:879-883, 1969.
31. August, G. P., M. Tkachuk, and M. M. Grumbach: Plasma testosterone-binding affinity and testosterone in umbilical cord plasma, late pregnancy, prepubertal children and adults. J. Clin. Endocrinol., 29:891-899, 1969.
32. Bardin, C. W., G. T. Ross, and M. B. Lipsett: Site of action of clomiphene citrate in men: A study of the pituitary Leydig cell axis. J. Clin. Endocrinol., 27:1558-1564, 1967.
33. Bardin, C. W., G. T. Ross, A. B. Rifkind, C. M. Cargille, and M. B. Lipsett: Studies of the pituitary-Leydig cell axis in young men with hypogonadotropic hypogonadism and hyposmia: Comparison with normal men, prepubertal boys, and hypopituitary patients. J. Clin. Endocrinol., 48:2046-2056, 1969.
34. Ross, G. T., C. M. Cargille, M. B. Lipsett, P. L. Rayford, J. R. Marshall, C. A. Strott, and D. Rodbard: Pituitary and gonadal hormones in women during spontaneous and induced ovulatory cycles. Rec. Prog. Hormone Res., Vol. 26. In press.
35. Rosemberg, E., and I. Engel: Effect of methyltestosterone and estrogens on HPG excretion levels. In: Human Pituitary Gonadotropins: A Workshop Conference (A. Albert, ed.), Charles C Thomas, Springfield, Ill., 1961, pp. 215-222.
36. Stevens, V. C., and N. Vorys: The regulation of pituitary function by sex steroids. Obstet. Gynec. Survey, 22:781-811, 1967.
37. Rifkind, A. B., H. E. Kulin, C. M. Cargille, P. L. Rayford, and G. T. Ross: Suppression of urinary excretion of luteinizing hormone (LH) and follicle-stimulating hormone (FSH) by medroxyprogesterone acetate. J. Clin. Endocrinol., 29:506-513, 1969.
38. Ross, G. T., W. D. Odell, and P. L. Rayford: Oral contraceptives and luteinizing hormone. Lancet, 1:1255-1256, 1966.
39. Cargille, C. M., G. T. Ross, and P. L. Rayford: Effect of oral contraceptives on plasma follicle stimulating hormone. In: Gonadotropins 1968 (E. Rosemberg, ed.), Geron-X, Los Altos, 1968, pp. 355-360.
40. Kirschner, M. A., J. A. Wider, and G. T. Ross: Leydig cell function in men with gonadotropin-producing testicular tumors. J. Clin. Endocrinol. In press.
41. Canfield, R. E., G. A. Agosta, and J. J. Bell: Studies of the chemistry of human

chorionic gonadotropin. In: Workshop on the Study of Gonadotropins, Birmingham, England, Sept. 1969. In press.

42. Rosen, S. W., C. E. Becker, S. Schlaff, J. Easton, and M. S. Gluck: Ectopic gonadotropin production before clinical recognition of bronchogenic carcinoma. New Eng. J. Med., 279:640-641, 1968.

43. Hobson, B., and L. Wide: Human chorionic gonadotrophin excretion in men and women with invasive trophoblast assayed by an immunological and a biological method. Acta Endocrinol. (Kobenhavn), 58:473-480, July 1968.

44. Bridson, W. E., P. O. Kohler, and G. T. Ross: Immunologic and biologic activity of chorionic gonadotropin synthesized by cloned choriocarcinoma cells in tissue culture. Proc. Amer. Fed. Clin. Res., 18:356, 1970.

45. Goverde, B. C., F. J. N. Veenkamp, and J. D. H. Homan: Studies on human chorionic gonadotrophin. II. Chemical composition and its relationship to biological activity. Acta Endocrinol., 59:105-119, 1968.

46. Schuurs, A. H. W. M., E. de Jager, and J. D. H. Homan: Studies on human chorionic gonadotropin. III. Immunochemical characterization. Acta Endocrinol., 59:120-138, 1968.

47. Josimovich, J. B., and J. A. MacLaren: Presence in the human placenta and term serum of a highly lactogenic substance immunologically related to pituitary growth hormone. Endocrinology, 71:209-220, 1962.

48. Kaplan, S. L., and M. M. Grumbach: Immunoassay for human chorionic "growth hormone-prolactin" in serum and urine. Science, 147:751-753, 1965.

49. Weintraub, B. D.: Concentration and purification of human chorionic somatomammotropin (HCS) by affinity chromatography: Application to radioimmunoassay. Biochem. Biophys. Res. Comm. In press.

Hormonal Influences in Human Tumorigenesis

V. M. DILMAN

Prof. Petrov Research Institute of Oncology, Leningrad, USSR

EXPERIMENTALLY, disturbance of the feedback mechanism, produced by any means, stimulates tumorigenesis. This report substantiates the existence of a physiologic phenomenon—the age-associated increase of the sensitivity threshold of the hypothalamus to regulatory influences in the system of energetic and reproductive homeostasis, which gradually and regularly leads to disturbance of the feedback mechanism and the appearance of age pathology. Primarily, this includes age gain of body weight, prediabetes and adult onset of diabetes mellitus, atherosclerosis, cancer, and decreased resistance to infection. Such regular development of the definite pathologic processes is an important argument in favor of the existence of a specific mechanism that forms regular age pathology.

In any organism there are two basic homeostatic systems—the system of regulation of reproduction and the system of regulation of metabolism and energy. In this connection, biologists frequently define life as a "macromolecular system which is characterized by specific hierarchic organization and the ability for reproduction, metabolism and adequately regulated stream of energy."[23]

A proposed brief description of the concept of the nature of the mechanism of aging shows, in all the mentioned disturbances, the presence of one primary process. This process can be defined as the age-associated increase of the sensitivity threshold of the hypothalamus to the regulatory homeostatic influences in the system of energetic and reproductive homeostasis. The existence of this phenomenon alone

FIG. 8–9.—Effect of glucose load on the level of STH and NEFA in serum. *Note:* STH was determined radioimmunologically with the use of amino cellulose as immunosorbent. The absolute value of STH was somewhat higher than with the ordinary radioimmunologic methods. At the same time, after glucose load (100 g per os) in young persons (solid line) physiologic decrease of STH level was found at one hr. But this effect was not observed in typical age pathology: endometrial carcinoma (dotted line), breast carcinoma (double lines), coronary heart disease (dashed line).

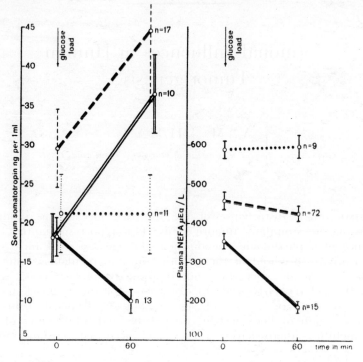

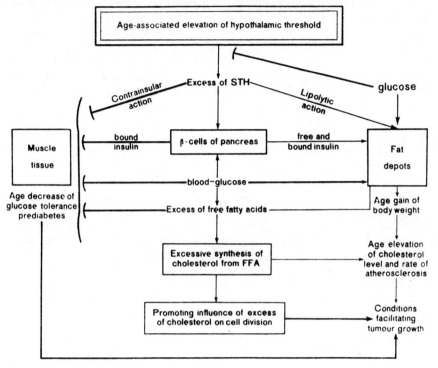

FIG. 8–10.—Schematic illustration of the relationship of age-associated hormonal and metabolic disturbances.

is sufficient for the age switching on and switching off of the reproductive cycle; for realization of the relationships between energetic and reproductive homeostasis in ontogenesis; the possibility of their interaction with stressor and environmental factors regulating the volume of population, as well as for regular development of those disturbances of homeostasis, which are manifested as the diseases of aging, lead to the termination of the individual existence of the organism.[14, 16]

Let us discuss the original data and some arguments in respect to the character of the mechanism of aging and related pathology.

One of the main processes in the energetic homeostasis is the effect of inhibition of somatotropic hormone (STH) secretion by glucose which affects the corresponding hypothalamic area.[20] On the contrary, starvation increases the secretion of STH which provides, through the mobilization of nonesterified fatty acids (NEFA), the supply of energy required for the organism. This homeostatic system is disturbed with aging and aging pathology. As can be seen from Figure 8-9, the standard glucose load fails to inhibit the levels of STH and NEFA in middle-aged persons and patients with endometrial and breast cancer.

The presence of this primary disturbance of regulatory mechanism is sufficient to bring into action a series of subsequent alterations, which facilitate or cause the conditions for age gain of body weight, development of prediabetes, atherosclerosis, and conditions promoting tumorigenesis. Figure 8-10 schematically shows the relationship of the mentioned metabolic disturbances. In this process, the excess of STH inhibits glucose utilization in the muscle tissue by direct contrainsular influence, excessive mobilization and utilization of NEFA,[39] and possibly by intensification of the binding of insulin with protein.[48] The age decrease of sensitivity to insulin is one of the early signs of these alterations. The stream of glucose is directed to utilization in the fatty tissue. All of these disturbances lead to the well-known age decrease in glucose tolerance. Simultaneously, a compensatory increase of the secretion of insulin develops, as is evident from the data on the increase of the blood level of insulin with aging.[8, 46] Bound insulin stimulates metabolism of glucose into fat in adipose tissue, but does not affect glucose uptake by muscle tissue.[2] In such a way the age gain of body weight develops. This results in fatty deposits from which STH obtains NEFA, which, in turn, provides the energy supply. Carbohydrates do not burn in the flame of lipids, and "circulus vitiosus" appears in which metabolic disturbances are constantly maintained. Excessive oxidation of NEFA leads to the excessive accumulation of acetylcoenzyme A and ultimately to increased synthesis of cholesterol. This order of disturbances explains why with aging the level of cholesterol in blood rises. The age hypercholesterolemia not only facilitates the development of atherosclerosis, but also creates conditions for intensive division of tumor cells, since cholesterol is necessary for the formation of the membranes of mitochondria. In this respect, it is of interest to note that many antitumorous preparations exert the ability to inhibit the synthesis of cholesterol,[30] and a hypocholesterolic diet inhibits tumor induction.[43] Moreover, a potent natural carcinogen —aflatoxin—considerably increases the synthesis of cholesterol many months before the appearance of hepatomas.[4] The changes described above involve a number of other systems of energetic homeostasis in the process of aging. Age increase of the appetite despite the relatively high level of glycemia after food intake and Cushingoid signs in aging persons reflect the resistance to inhibition of related centers of the hypothalamus.

Thus, the existence of one cause only, of one primary disturbance, namely, the increase of the threshold of the hypothalamus to homeostatic inhibition in energetic homeostasis, may result in a series of subsequent changes in the form of reduced sensitivity to insulin, compensatory hyperinsulinemia, fat storage, increased utilization of NEFA and reduced glucose tolerance, and age hypercholesterolemia, that is, the summation of metabolic abnormalities characterized by the loss of stability of internal environment and at the same time aging pathology. Undoubtedly, the details of the pathologic process are more complicated than can be analyzed in this paper. However, the described concept provides a uniform mechanism which covers different data and which gives evidence for the existence of the phenomenon of age-associated elevation of the hypothalamic threshold.

The presence of similar processes in the closed circuit of reproductive homeostasis allows an explanation of the physiologic nature of the above described disturbances in energetic homeostasis. In this respect, it is of interest to note that for suppression of gonadotropic function in immature rats, the required amount of estrogens is 100 times less than that for adult animals.[25] Therefore, at birth of the organism the hypothalamic regulator is within its initial stages of development and offers a high initial sensitivity to homeostatic inhibition. Because of this, a small amount of sexual hormones, produced by the immature organism, is sufficient for inhibition of the sexual center of the hypothalamus, and thus sexual maturity is retarded until the development of the organism is accomplished. A gradual age-associated increase of the threshold of the hypothalamus to inhibition releases the sexual center from suppression. As a result, the regular activity of the reproductive mechanism develops, which is necessary for reproduction.[13] The analogous mechanism of the switching on of the function of sexual glands takes place also in the male organism.[32] However, after the switching on of the reproductive system, the elevation of the hypothalamic threshold continues. This is evidenced by the age increase of the secretion of total gonadotropins and follicle-stimulating hormones (FSH) which starts long before the menopause (Figure 8-11). The results presented in Figure 8-11 are the distinct although indirect evidences of the age increase of the hypothalamic activity. That is identical in the physiologic sense to the increase of the hypothalamic resistance to homeostatic influences of estrogens. At the same time, induction of ovulation requires such a level of estrogens that could inhibit the hypothalamic center stimulating FSH secretion. This peculiarity of the mechanism of ovulation is manifested by the decrease of FSH level in blood before the "ovulation peak."[44] After FSH suppression, estrogens induce an additional output of luteinizing hormone (and FSH) that causes, as is known, the rupture of the follicle and ovulation. Therefore, if the hypothalamic threshold is significantly increased, then compensatory acceleration of ovarian function is required for the realization of the reproductive cycle, without which the mechanism inducing ovulation cannot manifest itself. Because of increased hypothalamic activity, the ovaries are actually subjected to progressively intensifying stimulation by the excess of gonadotropins, and acceleration of the function of the ovaries occurs. However, under the conditions of gonadotropic hyperstimulation, the ovaries start secreting, instead of standard estrogens, preferably their isohormones, nonclassic estrogens (so-called nonclassic phenolsteroids) (Figures 8-11 and 8-12).[16] This leads to the wrong impression that the activity of the ovaries decreases with aging, and in the postmenopausal period is completely ceased. Nonclassic phenolsteroids are also secreted by adrenals, especially intensively in the menopausal period. However, the compensatory ability of the ovaries is limited, and ultimately the switching off of the reproductive cycle is produced because the disturbance of feedback mechanism occurs as a result of the extremely high hypothalamic threshold. This, in particular, explains why the ovaries of old rats, when transplanted to young ones, restore their cyclic activity, showing that primary abnormalities lie in the range of the disturbances of the central regulation.[29] Therefore, both the switching on and the switching off of the reproductive cycle are realized by the uniform mechanism—age-associated elevation of the hypothalamic threshold to homeostatic influences.

FIG. 8–11.—Age-associated elevation of the excretion of total gonadotropins, FSH, and total phenolsteroids. *Note:* The hormone determinations were performed on the sixth to eighth day from the beginning of the menstrual flow. Total gonadotropins were tested by the modified method of Albert (1956), and expressed in mg of second IRP-HNG standard (dashed line). The FSH is determined by the method of Steelman and Pohley (1953), and the value is expressed per one hr equivalent of 24 hours' urine output in i.u. of second IRP-HMG standard (solid line). Total phenolsteroids (dashed-dotted line), which include both classic and nonclassic estrogens, were determined by the method of Dikun and Pavlova.[17]

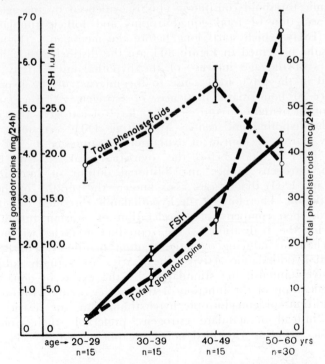

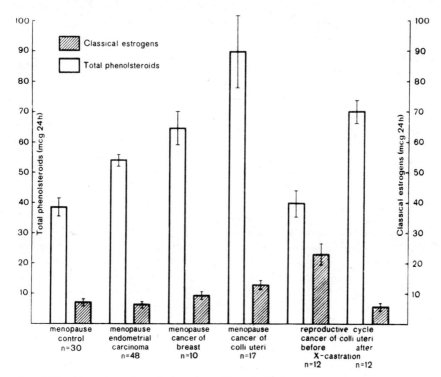

FIG. 8–12.—Excretion of total phenolsteroids and classic estrogens in normal menopausal women and in patients with cancer of breast, corpus and collum uteri. *Note:* Classic estrogens were determined by the method of Brown (1955); total phenolsteroids by the method of Dikun and Pavlova. The difference between values obtained at determination of total phenolsteroids and classic estrogens express the value for nonclassic phenolsteroids, though the determination of the latter is still insufficiently specific.[17]

Thus, in reproductive as well as in energetic homeostasis, physiologic compensation itself, which is necessary for the maintenance of the stability in the developing organism, forms at the same time a specific group of pathologic processes. A typical manifestation of this process is the increased secretion of nonclassic phenolsteroids with aging that allows the preservation, during a number of years, of the reproductive cycle under conditions of ever-intensifying hypothalamic activity. The more intensive is the compensation (namely, the higher is the production of nonclassic phenolsteroids) the longer the mechanism of ovulation can be manifested, despite the presence of the increased hypothalamic threshold. Late occurrence of menopause in patients with endometrial and breast carcinoma may be considered as the result of this phenomenon. In these patients, the excretion of total phenolsteroids during climacteric amenorrhea was 63.3 ± 6.7 mcg/24 hr as compared with 42.5 ± 4.5 mcg/24 hr in noncancerous women

with age amenorrhea. Excretion of nonclassic phenolsteroids is significantly increasing when hyperplasia of theca tissue develops in the
ovaries, for example, in the case of cancer of the corpus and collum
uteri, breast cancer, and after radiation castration (Figure 8-12). This
increase may be connected with synthesis of ovarian androgens in
theca tissue, while for their metabolism into classic estrogens, enzymatic
systems of follicles are required. Therefore, with their damage, for
example, after ovarian irradiation, metabolism of androgens is
changed, thus leading to the increase of secretion of nonclassic phenolsteroids. The increase of excretion of gonadotropins despite the unchanged excretion of classic estrogens in postmenopausal women after
ovariectomy may be explained by the decrease of the level of nonclassic phenolsteroids.[7, 19, 38]

Thus, with aging, target tissues are affected by the excess of both
central (gonadotropins) and peripheral (phenolsteroids) hormones
that facilitate tumor formation as observed experimentally, for example, in conditions of subtotal ovariectomy. This gives some explanation of the age-increased rate of tumors of the reproductive system
after the menopause when, according to classic estrogen criteria, the
activity of the ovaries ceases. It should be emphasized that the synthesis of nonclassic phenolsteroids instead of classic estrogens may be considered as a particular pattern of a more general process of qualitative
alterations of the spectrum of secreted hormones when the endocrine
gland is subjected to intensive stimulation, as is evident from the appearance of abnormal thyrotropin in thyrotoxicosis,[28] and the abnormal characteristics of gonadotropins in cancer.[27, 33, 34, 36] The compensatory increase of the level of bound insulin in aged persons is the
most demonstrative manifestation in respect to the process of age compensation in the system of energetic homeostasis.

Thus, the diseases, developing according to the discussed pattern,
can be designated as the diseases of compensation, because the intensifying compensation which is necessary for the maintenance of
homeostasis induces pathologic processes. During life there exists interaction between reproductive and energetic homeostasis that exerts
influence on the age peculiarities in the development of diseases of
compensation. This interaction can be briefly regarded in the example
shown in Figure 8-13. The continuous line shows the age changes in
energetic homeostasis (according to NEFA concentration). It can be
seen that in early childhood (up to the age of eight) when the reproductive homeostasis is not switched on, and in older ages when it
is switched off, a high NEFA level is observed.[24] Accordingly, before
sexual maturity[11, 37] and in aging, the tolerance to carbohydrates is
decreased. It allows the conclusion that in childhood and aging, similar changes occur in energetic homeostasis which might be connected
with the action of the excess of STH and insulin. In respect to the
early stage of diabetes, such condition was defined as prediabetes.[10]

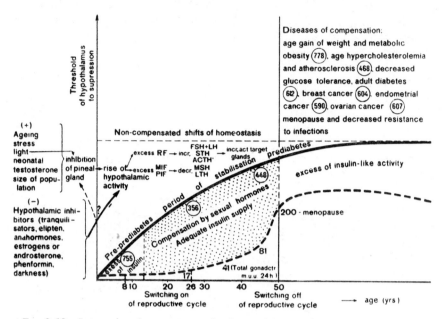

FIG. 8–13.—Interaction between reproductive and energetic homeostasis in onto-genesis and aging pathology.

Therefore, similar changes in childhood can be defined as pre-prediabetes. The switching on of the sexual cycle eliminates the symptoms of pre-prediabetes because of the action of estrogens, which in particular inhibit the lipolytic effect of STH.[26] This effect of estrogens is connected with the fact that they provide a rhythmic activity of the reproductive homeostasis in the female organism, and estrogens, therefore, exert pronounced action on the hypothalamus. This property facilitates the establishment of the phase of stabilization needed for reproduction. This role of estrogens can explain their ability to reduce age hypercholesterolemia, to increase the sensitivity to insulin, etc. The switching on of the reproductive cycle also suppresses the immunity by inhibiting the activity of the thymus with sex hormones. This influence of sex hormones is necessary for overcoming immunologic intolerance of the fetus and mother.

In the male organism, the reproductive homeostasis has a nonrhythmic pattern that biologically promotes overcoming of the limitations in reproduction connected with cyclic functions of the female sexual system. With nonrhythmic function of homeostasis, testosterone may fail to exert considerable inhibitory effect on the hypothalamus. Therefore, sexual maturity in the male organism does not eliminate compensatory excess of insulin as is observed with estrogens. This consideration explains why the rise of the level of plasma insulin in men in the age group of 20-49 is three times higher than that in women. The insulin increment during this interval constitutes 0.067 log serum insulin for men and only 0.021 log serum insulin for women.[46]

But the more intensive the elevation of the level of insulin, the more intensively aging develops and diseases of compensation are produced. This can explain the increased level of cholesterol at an earlier age and the earlier mortality in men from coronary atherosclerosis, and the temporary arrest of aging in females during the phase of stabilization. By the age of 70, a total age excess of insulin is of similar increment in men and women, reflecting the uniformity of the mechanism of the development and aging in both sexes. Thus, similar age dynamics in the energetic and reproductive homeostasis—the age elevation of the threshold of the hypothalamus to inhibition—determines three different periods in human ontogenesis: period of growth and maturation (pre-prediabetes); period of stabilization; and period of the loss of stability of internal environment (prediabetes), when changes nontolerable with life gradually develop in the form of specific age pathology—diseases of compensation.

The stated data on the mechanism of aging allow one to postulate the elevating nature of the mechanism of aging and related pathology, since the age increase of the threshold of the sensitivity of the hypothalamus should be regarded as the principal altering element in the mechanisms of development and aging.

The interaction may exist between diseases of compensation and diseases of adaptation, because the activation of the hypothalamus in stressor situations provides the mechanism of adaptation. But simultaneously, the resistance of the hypothalamus to homeostatic influence occurs, resulting in the disturbances of the stability of internal environment, that is, diseases. Thus, under the influence of the stressors, the same process develops which is characteristic of normal aging. Only the succession of the disturbances is different: the elevation of the resistance of the hypothalamus and then the increase of its activity with aging and controversial order of alterations in a stressor situation. External and internal causes of aging pathology and death ultimately are involved in the uniform mechanism. But in contrast to diseases of adaptation, the diseases of compensation gradually develop independently from the presense or absence of stressor factors. Regulation of the size of population, depending on the volume of population, is also performed through the increased activity in the system of the hypothalamus glucocorticoids that suppress the reproductive cycle and increase the mortality because of the reduced resistance to infections.[9] Such reduction is also characteristic for human aging. It should be emphasized, however, that any of the diseases of compensation may certainly develop at any age if the elevation of the hypothalamic threshold is caused by pathologic, but not age-associated, process. Moreover, disorders occurring at any other level of many-staged homeostatic systems can produce diseases clinically analogous to the diseases of compensation. An example of this kind of disturbance caused by the break of the feedback mechanism at the level of peripheral tissue is the finding that with plastic materials many more tumors are observed with plain than with perforated film.[35] In respect to diseases of compensation, these conditions of tumor formation represent a symptomatic variation of tumorigenesis similar to the relation of age atherosclerosis and symptomatic atherosclerosis, for example in hypothyroidism. However, the cancer process is less regular than atherosclerosis, because the latter is the direct manifestation of diseases of compensation, while for cancer appearance the age-associated disturbances of homeostasis is the main factor stimulating tumorigenesis; but ultimately development depends on whether the changes will or will not occur on the cellular level. The concept of special compensatory processes as the condition stimulating carcinogenesis explains why, in tumor patients, an increased body weight, decreased sensitivity to insulin, prediabetes, increased level of cholesterol and NEFA in blood, and late menopause are often observed, particularly in endometrial and breast carcinoma. These disturbances occur more frequently in persons in whom cancer developed in the postmenopausal period. That is one of the arguments for the differentiation of breast cancer in two forms: breast cancer in young patients (ovarian type), and maturity-onset breast cancer, in the pathogenesis of which the increase of the hypothalamic-pituitary activity is prevalent, as is observed with both juvenile and maturity-onset diabetes. In other words, we observe in persons in whom cancer develops the intensification of general metabolic disorders which are characteristic for regular physiologic loss of homeostasis regulation with aging.

Thus, the scope of diseases of compensation requires further specification. In this respect, it is of interest to note that, in rats, with the increase of the pituitary function the signs of premature aging have been observed, as well as the development of arteriosclerosis, hypertension, decreased tolerance to glucose, hyperplasia of the adrenals, and involution of the thymus. These disturbances, together with decreased level of Porter-Zilber chromogens, resemble the qualitative changes in hormone production observed in the climacteric.[47] ACTH suppresses the reproductive cycle also and causes lesions of renal vessels,[9] but restricted food intake considerably decreases the frequency of kidney diseases.[3] This effect may be connected with the so-called functional hypophysectomy produced by restricted food intake.

The group of diseases of compensation may involve an age gain of body weight, decreased glucose tolerance, age hypercholesterolemia and atherosclerosis, climacteric and climacteric neurosis, and some forms of cancer which can be represented by endometrial, breast and prostate carcinomas, although it is apparent that metabolic processes of aging (obesity, hypercholesterolemia, prediabetes) provide conditions for clinical manifestations of many other oncologic processes.

Hypertension is not a regular consequence of aging, however. The increase of the hypothalamic activity pertinent to aging promotes the development of hypertension with aging which explains its frequent association with obesity, hypercholesterolemia, decreased glucose tolerance, high level of plasma insulin, etc. A number of other characteristics of aging are also probably connected with the compensatory processes, although these relationships are not clearly obvious.[45] It should be mentioned that the function of some peripheral endocrine glands, primarily the thyroid gland, is decreased with advancing years, and production of classic sex hormones—estrogens and androgens —is reduced. However, in respect to estrogens, such decrease is the result of hypothalamic hyperactivity; age-increased rate of prostatic cancer may serve as a base for the studies of possible rearrangement of iso-hormones of androgenic type.

On the basis of the concept of the diseases of compensation, it is impossible to establish a clear distinction between the mechanism of aging and aging pathology. Moreover, the assumption of the presence of different normal limits for different age groups should be rejected, particularly in respect to the level of blood cholesterol or carbohydrate tolerance. It should be considered that the "normal value" is a constant pattern and should be within the limits characteristic for hypothalamic activity at the age of 20-25 when the phase of stabilization in the organism develops. At this period, such diseases as adult-onset diabetes, atherosclerosis, and cancer are of lower incidence. But prolonged stabilization in the developing organism can be obtained only by means of external influences. This conclusion is evident from the logical analysis of the cause which leads to alteration of the sensitivity of the hypothalamic threshold with advancing years. The existence of this phenomenon may be connected with self-development of the basic homeostatic systems, since the stability of internal environment can be provided if the mechanisms, maintaining the stability in the course of development, are developing themselves in time. Age dynamics of the hypothalamic threshold are the leading process in this mechanism of self-development of homeostatic systems. However, this internal process gradually results in the disturbance of homeostasis and diseases of compensation when the development of the organism is accomplished. Death from internal cause in the form of diseases of compensation appears with the transition of the unicellular organism into a multicellular specialized organization. This transition provides the appearance of specialized systems for the maintenance of an internal environment which decreases the influence of external factors on the organism. However, the transition itself introduces into animated nature the conflict leading to death from internal cause. Just for this reason, that the internal mechanisms of aging and death occur in the process of evolution as the response of nature to the damaging influence of the factors of external environment, these internal mechanisms will always obtain the ability to react with external factors. Therefore, the influence on the mechanism of aging and related pathology may be performed only by means of specific external influences. Ideally, the necessary means should obtain the ability to renew the rhythmic work of homeostatic systems by reducing the hypothalamic threshold to inhibition, i.e. counteract with the very process of self-development of homeostatic systems. It may be supposed that the pineal gland exerts such influence, but not so direct an inhibitory action on the hypothalamus and, therefore, other related means might be found. But at the present time, until this problem has been solved, the possibility should be investigated of prophylactic and therapeutic effects of estrogens, Sigetin,[16] androsterone, Atromide, α and l-thyroxine, rational diet, Elipten with the ability to suppress not only adrenal steroidogenesis but gonadotropin secretion also;[18] Dilantin in respect to inhibition of adrenal function and possibly influence on the synthesis of RNA;[22] and phenobarbital and other antiepileptic and neurotropic preparations. (Such preparations as chlorpromazine inhibit the secretion of gonadotropins but stimulate the secretion of prolactin and melanotropin (MSH). Continuous lighting is of similar action. These effects are connected with the peculiarities in the regulation of the latter hormones by PIF and MIF. Therefore, if with aging the activity of the hypothalamus is totally increased, similar to the reaction to lighting, it should be expected that in the course of aging secretion of MSH and prolactin will not increase but will decrease. This is of interest in respect to understanding the low incidence of melanoma after the age of 49 and peculiarities of adult-onset breast cancer, and also in respect to the possible role of the pineal gland in the mechanism of aging, similar to its transforming the influence of light in dual reaction of the hypothalamus. These observations are correspondent to the considerable incidence of atherosclerosis and cancer in progeria and the absence of skin cancer and melanoma in such patients.) [31] More attention should be directed to the study of phenformin, eliminating reactive hyperinsulinism and thereby age-gain of body weight and elevated levels of cholesterol and triglycerides.[40] For this reason, phenformin should be investigated in respect to its ability to suppress the development not only of atherosclerosis but also of tumor formation.

In a broad sense, anahormones, with their ability to induce antibodies, suppress the secretion or counteract the effect of protein hormones, and are of special interest as a tool for studies of age and pathologic processes.[6, 15, 16, 21]

More emphasis should be directed to the study of isohormones of the etiocholanolone type,[5] as well as to any other ways and means which, by affecting the threshold of the hypothalamus to inhibition or reducing the compensatory reactions, might facilitate the deceleration of the realization of the genetic program of development as well as aging and related pathology.

It seems to me that this way is more perspective in respect to prophylaxis of increased age-incidence of many tumors or prevention of cancer development when the elevation of the threshold of the hypothalamic activity occurs not only as a regular age-associated process, but also as a pathologic process independently of the mechanism of aging.

References

1. Albert, A.: Recent Progr. Hormone Res., 12:227, 1956.
2. Antoniades, H. V.: Lancet, 2:159-160, 1965.
3. Berg, B. N., and H. S. Simms: In: Biological Aspects of Aging (N. E. Shock, ed.) , New York, 1962.
4. Brown, J. B.: Biochem. J., 60:185-200, 1955.
5. Bulbrook, R. D., J. L. Hayward, and B. S. Thomas: Lancet, 1:945-947, 1964.
6. Bulovskaya, L. N., E. A. Prokhudina, V. L. Konstantinov, S. S. Tugunov, and V. M. Dilman: Acta Endocrinol., 61:193-197, 1969.
7. Charles, D., E. Bell, J. Lorain, and R. Harkness: Am. J. Obstet. Gynecol., 91: 1050, 1965.
8. Chlouverakis, C., R. J. Jarrett, and H. Keen: Lancet, 1:806-808, 1967.
9. Christian, J. J.: Coll. Int. Centre Nat. Recherche Sci., 173:289-322, 1968.
10. Conn, J. W.: Diabetes, 7:347-353, 1958.
11. Donowski, T. S.: Diabetes Mellitus with Emphasis on Children and Young Adults, Baltimore, 1957.
12. Dole, V. P.: J. Clin. Invest., 35:150-155, 1956.
13. Donovan, B. T., and J. J. van der Werff Ten Bosch: J. Physiol., 147:78-92, 1959.
14. Dilman, V. M.: Transact. Inst. Physiol. AMS USSR, Leningrad, 7:326-336, 1958.
15. Dilman, V. M.: Int. J. Cancer, 1:239-247, 1966.
16. Dilman, V. M.: Aging, Climacteric and Cancer. Leningrad, 1968.
17. Dilman, V. M., L. M. Berstein, Y. F. Bobrov, Y. V. Bohman, I. Kovaleva, and N. V. Krylova: Amer. J. Obst. Gynecol., 102:880-889, 1968.
18. Dilman, V. M., N. V. Krylova, E. V. Tsyrlina, and A. S. Vishnevsky: Vopr. Onkol., 3:94-95, 1969.
19. Dilman, V. M., and M. V. Pavlova: Vopr. Onkol., 9:75-79, 1963.
20. Glick, S. M., J. Roth, R. S. Valow, and S. A. Berson: Recent Progr. Hormone Res., 21:241-270, 1965.
21. Golubev, V. N., V. M. Dilman, I. G. Kovaleva, M. V. Pavlova, A. L. Remizov, and B. N. Sofronov: Reports AS USSR, 184:966-968, 1969.
22. Gordon, P.: In: Abstracts of the 8th International Congress of Gerontology, Washington, 1969, pp. 171-174.
23. Grobstein, C.: The Strategy of Life, San Francisco, 1965.
24. Heald, F. P., J. Arnold, W. Seabold, and D. Morrison: Amer. J. Clin. Nutr., 20:1010-1014, 1967.
25. Hohlweg, W., and M. Dohrn: Klin. Wochensch., 1:233-235, 1932.
26. Kovaleva, I. G., A. S. Vishnevsky, and V. M. Dilman: Fed. Proc. (Trans. Suppl.) , 24:863-864, 1965.
27. Krylova, N. V., V. N. Golubev, L. N. Simanovsky, and V. M. Dilman: Vopr. Onkol., 12:14-16, 1967.
28. Kumahara, J., H. Iwatsubo, K. Miyai, H. Masui, M. Fukuchi, and H. Abe: J. Clin. Endocrinol., 27:333-340, 1967.
29. Kushima, K., O. Kamio, and J. Okuda: Tohoku J. Exper. Med., 72:113-117, 1961.
30. Littman, M. L., T. Taguchi, and E. H. Mosbach: Cancer Chemother. Rep., 50:25-45, 1966.
31. Lynch, H. T.: Cancer, 24:277-288, 1969.
32. McCann, S. M.: In: Physiological Control and Regulations (W. S. Jamamoto and J. A. Brobeck, eds.) , W. B. Saunders Co., Philadelphia, 1965.
33. Marmorston, J.: Ann. N. Y. Acad. Sci., 125:959-973, 1966.
34. Mochizuki, M., V. Tokura, T. Tokura, J. Voshioka, V. Aschitaka, M. Tane, and S. Tojo: Acta Obst. Gynecol. Jap., 16:180-191, 1969.
35. Oppenheimer, B. S., E. T. Oppenheimer, J. Danishefsky, A. P. Stout, and F. B. Errich: Cancer Res., 15:334-340, 1955.

36. Ostroumova, M. N.: Vopr. Onkol., 4:76-80, 1970.
37. Pickens, J. M., J. N. Burkeholder, and W. N. Wamack: Diabetes, 16:11-14, 1967.
38. Procopé, B. J.: Acta Endocrinol., Suppl. 135:60, 1969.
39. Randle, P. J.: In: On the Nature and Treatment of Diabetes (B. S. Leibel and G. A. Wrenshall, eds.), Amsterdam, 1965.
40. Schwartz, M. J., S. Mirsky, and L. E. Schaefer: Metabolism, 15:808-815, 1966.
41. Siperstein, M. D.: Canad. Cancer Conf., 7:152-162, 1967.
42. Steelman, S. L., and F. M. Pohley: Endocrinology, 53:604-609, 1953.
43. Szepsenwol, J.: Proc. Soc. Exper. Biol. Med., 121:168-171, 1966.
44. Taymor, M. L., T. Aono, C. Pheteplace, and G. Page: Acta Endocrinol., 59:298-306, 1968.
45. Verzar, F.: Lectures on Experimental Gerontology, Charles C Thomas, Springfield, Illinois, 1963.
46. Welborn, T. A., N. S. Stenhouse, and C. G. Johnstone: Diabetologia, pp. 263-266, 1969.
47. Wexler, B. C., and G. W. Kittinger: J. Atheroscler. Res., 5:317-329, 1965.
48. Young, J. B.: Nature, 207:1199, 1965.

Alteration of Malignant Processes by Hormonal Manipulation

RENZO GRATTAROLA, M.D.

Istituto Nazionale dei Tumori-Milano, Italy

VOLUMES HAVE BEEN DEVOTED to the hormonal treatment of patients with hormone-dependent tumors, such as breast and endometrial carcinoma, but the subject is still controversial. It is accepted as possible that an abnormal hormonal secretion may exert a profound influence on the growth of neoplastic breast and endometrial cells, but which hormonal deviation is responsible for the pathogenesis of these diseases is still unknown. Until we know which hormonal factor acts as a carcinogen, our treatment can only be empirical, as it is today.

The reason why we have not changed our empirical approach to hormonal treatment for years is that we still think of breast or endometrial carcinoma as the outcome of an overproduction of estrogens. This assumption is based mainly on the observation that ovariectomy induces remissions in 30 to 50% of women with breast cancer, and it is presumed that this procedure exerts its favorable effect through a reduction of estrogen synthesis. Although this is a simplified view which equates ovarian activity with increased estrogen alone and does not take into account the numerous other endocrine features of the ovary, there is no evidence that estrogens are responsible for breast or endometrial neoplasia.

A number of investigators have demonstrated normal urinary estrogen levels in women with breast cancer, and none have shown a fall in urinary estrogens after castration.[1-3] Anyone reading the current literature gains the impression that there is a proved relationship between hyperplasia and carcinoma of the endometrium and prolonged estrogen stimulation. The "relationship" has been given most emphasis[4-6] in patients with ovarian abnormality, like cortical stromal (interstitial tissue) hyperplasia, thecomas, ovarian Leydig cell hyperplasia, and ovarian hilar rest resembling Sertoli and Leydig cells, in spite of the fact that androgenic hyperactivity is the major functional manifestation in such cases.

In our previous studies,[7-9] we pointed out that the hyperplastic pattern of the endometrium was present in premenopausal women with a significant increase in androgens, as revealed by the urinary levels of etiocholanolone and androsterone; no significant increase of urinary estrogens (estrone and estradiol-17β) was found in these patients.[10] This information led us to wonder whether it was not androgenic activity that was the cause of the hyperplastic pattern of the endometrium. We saw that when gonadotropic treatment induces ovulation in women with endometrial hyperplasia, the androgenic activity decreases to normal values; when the treatment does not induce ovulation, the endometrium shows a higher degree of proliferation and the urinary level of androgen metabolites increases.[9, 10]

Control Subjects

A wrong choice of controls is often made. Patients with endometrial hyperplasia frequently show no sign of irregular menstrual bleeding, except ovulation. This endometrial pattern may be found in women with polycystic ovaries, having regular menses and without sign of virilization. Such patients are often taken as controls, when obviously they are not. Such an error could not occur if a histologic examination of the endometrium were always made and excretion values of androgens always estimated. This error vitiates all the statistical analysis of such series. When these examinations are done, we discover that many patients who would otherwise have been considered normal show a hyperplastic endometrial pattern together with increased androgenic activity. We regard these women as an "at risk" group, because the hormonal situation closely resembles the one found in women with breast cancer.

It is well known, since the studies of Hertig and Sommers,[11] Gusberg and Kaplan,[12] and Speert,[13] that endometrial cancer may require many years to develop fully. Probably breast cancer has the same long silent phase before the disease manifests itself. The identification of the "at risk" group having the same abnormal hormonal activity of women with breast cancer can give us an opportunity to correct the hormonal abnormality, at the same time perhaps preventing the onset of breast cancer.

We take as controls premenopausal women with a premenstrual endometrium which has a progestational pattern, and postmenopausal women with a hypotrophic endometrial pattern. Both have a low urinary level of androgen metabolites or of testosterone.

Material and Methods

In all women examined, 24-hr specimens of urine were collected (at the twenty-second and twenty-third day of menstrual cycle, for premenopausal women). At the end of urine collection, endometrial tissue for histologic examination was obtained.

Ten premenopausal subjects (aged 39 to 46 years) with progestational premenstrual endometrium and 10 postmenopausal subjects (aged 51 to 62 years) with hypotrophic endometrium were considered as normal controls. Eleven premenopausal subjects with atypical endometrial hyperplasia (adenomatous hyperplasia) aged 38 to 48 years, four premenopausal patients with ovarian polycystic disease (aged 25 to 32 years) (Table 8-25), and six postmenopausal subjects with atypical endometrial hyperplasia (Table 8-28) served as "at risk" controls. None of these patients showed any sign of menstrual disorder or of irregular bleeding or any other relevant symptom. Of the 28 premenopausal patients with breast cancer (aged 40 to 47 years), 17 had a progestational endometrium and 11 atypical hyperplasia of the endometrium (Table 8-26). Of the 13 postmenopausal patients with

---

TABLE 8–25.—URINARY EXCRETION OF 11-DEOXY-17-KETOSTEROIDS— [DEHYDROEPIANDROSTERONE (D), ETIOCHOLANOLONE (E), ANDROSTERONE (A)], OF ESTRONE (EO), ESTRADIOL-17BETA (EOH) AND OF TESTOSTERONE OF NORMAL-CONTROLS AND OF WOMEN WITH ATYPICAL PREMENSTRUAL ENDOMETRIUM OR WITH POLYCYSTIC OVARIAN DISEASE (GROUP AT RISK)—PREMENOPAUSAL AGE

PATIENTS (NO. OF CASES)	D	E mg./24 hr.	A	EO mcg./24 hr.	EOH	TESTOSTERONE mcg./24 hr.
						(5 patients)
Normal-controls (5)	0.88	0.72	0.72	2.90	1.90	20.0-12.4-12.5
	(±0.14)	(±0.19)	(±0.09)	(±1.30)	(±0.87)	15.0-25.5
Women with atypical						(4 patients)
endometrium (7)	0.96	1.36	1.13	0.95	3.37	32.5-35.0-56.0
	(±0.25)	(±0.16)	(±0.11)	(±1.50)	(±0.86)	85.3
Women with polycystic						(4 patients)
ovaries						78.0-104.0-43.0
						32.0

TABLE 8–26.—URINARY EXCRETION OF 11-DEOXY-17-KETOSTEROIDS—
[DEHYDROEPIANDROSTERONE (D), ETIOCHOLANOLONE (E), ANDROSTERONE (A)], OF
ESTRONE (EO), ESTRADIOL-17BETA (EOH) AND OF TESTOSTERONE OF PATIENTS WITH
BREAST CANCER WITH OVULATORY CYCLE (PROGESTATIONAL ENDOMETRIUM) OR
WITHOUT OVULATORY CYCLE (ATYPICAL PREMENSTRUAL ENDOMETRIUM)

PATIENTS (No. OF CASES)	D	E mg./24 hr.	A	EO mcg./24 hr.	EOH	TESTOSTERONE mcg./24 hr.
Normal controls	0.88	0.72	0.72	2.90	1.90	aver. value: 17.0
Breast cancer patients						(8 patients)
with ovulatory cycle	0.53	0.69	0.48	6.26	5.26	26.0-32.0-10.6-24.5
(9 patients)	(±0.13)	(±0.08)	(±0.13)	(±2.10)	(±1.21)	29.6-37.0-35.0-21.7
Breast cancer patients						(5 patients)
with atypical	1.63	2.53	1.46	2.31	5.90	61.3-88.0-113.0
endometrium (6)	(±0.27)	(±0.20)	(±0.37)	(±0.82)	(±1.64)	153.0-71.5

breast cancer (aged 51 to 64 years) five had an atypical endometrial pattern, and eight a simple proliferative endometrium (Table 8-27). Finally, seven postmenopausal patients (aged 55 to 65 years) with endometrial carcinoma were examined (Table 8-28).

11-Deoxy-17-ketosteroids (i.e. dehydroepiandrosterone (Δ^5-androstene-3β-ol-17-one), etiocholanolone (5β-androstane-3α-ol-17-one), androsterone (5α-androstane-3α-ol-17-one) were determined according to Bush.[14] Estrone (3-hydroxy-1,3,5 (10)-trien-17-one) and estradiol-17β (estra-1,3,5 (10) triene-3, 17β-diol) were determined according to the method previously described.[15] Urinary testosterone was determined after enzymatic hydrolysis. The chromatographic purification of the ether extracts was done by Sephadex chromatography,[16] followed by thin-layer chromatography on silica gel as described by McRoberts et al.[17] The final quantitation was done by gas-liquid chromatography of trimethylsilyl ether derivative.

TABLE 8–27.—URINARY EXCRETION OF 11-DEOXY-17-KETOSTEROIDS—
DEHYDROEPIANDROSTERONE (D), ETIOCHOLANOLONE (E), ANDROSTERONE (A), OF
ESTRONE (EO), ESTRADIOL-17BETA (EOH) AND OF TESTOSTERONE OF WOMEN AT
POSTMENOPAUSAL AGE—NORMAL CONTROLS AND PATIENTS WITH BREAST CANCER
HAVING SIMPLE PROLIFERATIVE ENDOMETRIUM OR ATYPICAL ENDOMETRIUM

PATIENTS (No. OF CASES)	D	E mg./24 hr.	A	EO mcg./24 hr.	EOH	TESTOSTERONE mcg./24 hr.
Normal-controls (5)						(5 cases)
	0.19	0.34	0.32	2.78	0.82	15.0-12.5-10.0
	(±0.09)	(±0.10)	(±0.09)	(±1.31)	(±0.51)	8.6-12.0
Patients with breast cancer						(3 cases)
having simple prolifer-	0.37	0.61	0.60	5.58	7.66	22.5-20.0-7.0
ative endometrium (5)	(±0.09)	(±0.17)	(±0.09)	(±3.04)	(±2.09)	
Patients with breast						(5 cases)
cancer having atypical						60.0-56.2-36.0
endometrium						40.0-37.0

TABLE 8–28.—THE URINARY EXCRETION OF 11-DEOXY-17-KETOSTEROIDS—
DEHYDROEPIANDROSTERONE (D), ETIOCHOLANOLONE (E), ANDROSTERONE (A), AND OF
ESTRONE (EO), ESTRADIOL-17BETA (EOH) OF NORMAL-CONTROLS, OF WOMEN WITH
ATYPICAL ENDOMETRIUM (GROUP AT RISK), AND OF PATIENTS WITH
ENDOMETRIAL CARCINOMA

PATIENTS (NO. OF CASES)	D	E	A	EO	EOH
		mg./24 hr.		mcg./24 hr.	
Normal-controls (5)	0.19	0.34	0.32	2.78	0.82
Women with atypical endometrium	0.49	1.59	1.21	2.21	4.01
(group at risk) (6)	(±0.25)	(±0.35)	(±0.20)	(±0.85)	(±1.92)
Patients with endometrial	0.47	0.64	0.48	1.44	5.97
carcinoma (7)	(±0.14)	(±0.09)	(±0.15)	(±0.81)	(±1.87)

Results

Table 8-25 shows the excretion levels of 11-deoxy-17-ketosteroids (dehydroepiandrosterone, etiocholanolone and androsterone), of estrone, estradiol-17β and of testosterone observed in premenopausal normal controls (subjects with progestational endometrial pattern) and in our "at risk" group i.e. with atypical endometrial hyperplasia. Analysis of the variance of the values for estrogens (estrone and estradiol-17β) shows no significant difference between the groups examined (normal controls and "at risk" group), whereas a significant difference was found between the normal control and the "at risk" group when urinary excretion levels of androgen metabolites (etiocholanolone and androsterone) were considered ($P<0.05$). The urinary level of testosterone was significantly ($P<0.01$) higher in the "at risk" group than in the normal control.

Table 8-26 shows the excretion level of steroid hormones in the premenopausal breast cancer patients having a progestational or an atypical endometrium. In the group of patients with an atypical endometrial pattern, the androgenic activity was greatly increased. The excretion values of dehydroepiandrosterone and of etiocholanolone ($P<0.01$) and of androsterone ($P<0.05$) were significantly higher than in the normal controls, whereas in the group of patients with breast cancer having the ovulatory menstrual cycle (progestational endometrium), the androgen excretion values did not differ significantly from those in the normal controls. Moreover, the value of etiocholanolone of patients with breast cancer and with atypical endometrial pattern was found to be even higher than the etiocholanolone excretion value of the subjects in the "at risk" group ($P<0.01$).

Table 8-27 shows the excretion values of 11-deoxy-17-ketosteroids, estrone, estradiol-17β, and testosterone of postmenopausal women with hypotrophic endometrium (normal control), and of postmenopausal patients with breast cancer who have a simple proliferative endometrial pattern or an atypical endometrial pattern. No significant increase in androgenic activity was found between the normal control and the group of patients with breast cancer having a simple proliferative endometrium; in this group the excretion level of estradiol-17β was shown to be significantly higher ($P<0.05$) than in normal controls. On the contrary, the androgenic activity, as shown by the urinary levels of testosterone, was significantly higher ($P<0.01$) in the patients with breast cancer showing an atypical endometrial pattern than in the normal controls.

Table 8-28 shows the excretion level of 11-deoxy-17-ketosteroids, of estrone, estradiol-17β of postmenopausal women with atypical endometrial pattern and with endometrial carcinoma. In the group of patients with endometrial carcinoma, only a small and not significant increase of androgenic activity was observed; in this group of patients the excretion value of estradiol-17β was found to be significantly ($P<0.05$) higher than the normal controls. Even in these postmenopausal women, when the atypical endometrial hyperplasia was present, the androgen activity was shown to be significantly higher than in the normal controls, as shown by the urinary level of dehydroepiandrosterone ($P<0.05$) and of etiocholanolone and androsterone ($P<0.01$).

Discussion

The data given in this study confirm the impression gained in our previous studies, i.e. that it is an increased androgenic and not estrogenic activity that is responsible for the onset of the endometrial atypical hyperplasia.

In some premenopausal or postmenopausal patients, when the androgenic activity was greatly increased, the endometrial proliferation was so atypical that it was difficult to differentiate from carcinoma. We have shown in the present report that in patients with breast carcinoma having an atypical endometrial pattern, the androgenic activity is even more pronounced than in women not having breast cancer but only the atypical endometrial pattern. This proves that in these patients, androgens must play an important role in the development of breast cancer. We saw in our previous study[18] that atypical endometrial hyperplasia is present in a high proportion of breast cancer patients.

When the menstrual cycle is ovulatory in premenopausal breast cancer patients, or the endometrium does not show any proliferative activity (hypotrophic endometrium) in postmenopausal patients, androgenic activity is found to be normal. We suspect that breast cancer in such patients is not hormone-dependent.

In patients with endometrial carcinoma, the androgenic activity is close to normal; in these patients it was seen that the estradiol-17β excretion level was significantly higher than in the normal controls. We are still studying this group of patients and have as yet no conclusive proof that the androgenic activity does not play any role in the pathogenesis of this disease. The urinary level of testosterone was not de-

TABLE 8–29.—URINARY EXCRETION OF 11-DEOXY-17-KETOSTEROIDS—
[ETIOCHOLANOLONE (E) AND ANDROSTERONE (A)], OF ESTRONE (EO), AND
ESTRADIOL-17BETA (EOH) OF PATIENTS AT POSTMENOPAUSAL AGE WITH ATYPICAL
ENDOMETRIAL HYPERPLASIA AND OF PATIENTS WITH ENDOMETRIAL CARCINOMA,
AFTER TREATMENT WITH HCG (20,000 IU) AND DEXAMETHASONE

PATIENTS (NO. OF CASES)	E + A mg./24 hr.	EO + EOH mcg./24 hr.	ENDOMETRIUM AFTER TREATMENT
Patients with atypical endometrium (3)	2.80	6.80	
After treatment	0.50	10.60	proliferative (simple)
Patients with atypical endometrium (2)	2.20	8.00	atypical (adenomatous
After treatment	2.55	2.60	hyperplasia)
Patients with endometrial carcinoma (7)	1.13	5.80	
After treatment	0.85	2.79	adenocarcinoma

termined in this group. The determination of 11-deoxy-17-ketosteroids alone might not be sufficiently indicative of androgenic activity; in fact, testosterone can be metabolized not only as 17-ketosteroids but even as androstenediols, and the yield of androstenediols formed from testosterone might increase at the expense of 17-ketosteroids.[19] We have further seen that in the patients with endometrial carcinoma, human chorionic gonadotropin (HCG) stimulation given together with dexamethasone did not influence the androgenic activity of patients with endometrial carcinoma, whereas this combined treatment normalized the endometrial pattern in three of five postmenopausal patients with atypical endometrial pattern, together with greatly decreasing androgenic activity. We would point out that in two of these three patients the pattern was so atypical that adenocarcinoma was diagnosed. We tend to think that endometrial carcinomas which respond to hormonal treatments are not really carcinomas, but striking atypical endometrial hyperplasia misdiagnosed as adenocarcinoma.

HORMONAL TREATMENT OF BREAST CARCINOMA

In our previous study,[18] we saw that premenopausal breast cancer patients have a high incidence of atypical endometrial hyperplasia. We surmised at the time that the absence of progestational activity, with consequent hyperestrogenism, might be the hormonal factor responsible either for endometrial hyperplasia or breast carcinoma. Later[7-9] we found that in the absence of progestational activity (anovulatory menstrual cycle), an atypical proliferative pattern of the endometrium (adenomatous hyperplasia) was associated with the increased androgens; conversely, if the urinary output of androgen metabolites was not increased, the endometrium showed a simple proliferative pattern.[10] Our conclusion is that it is not the absence of progestational activity that is responsible for the atypical endometrial pattern but the high level of androgens. We think that the increased androgenic activity has an ovarian origin, first because the androgenic activity reverted to normal after ovarian resection, and second, because the androgen activity increased after the HCG stimulation, when this treatment failed to induce ovulation.[10] HCG treatment did not influence the urinary level of androgen metabolites in ovariectomized women.[10]

We concluded that when the atypical endometrial hyperplasia coexisted with breast carcinoma, the androgenic activity should be considered responsible for the breast cancer. As we showed in our previous paper[9, 10] that HCG alone can induce ovulation in women with adenomatous hyperplasia, depressing the androgenic activity, we gave this treatment to breast cancer patients with an atypical endometrial pattern for 10 days at the daily dose of 2,000 IU, starting on day 5 of the cycle, for a total dose of 20,000 IU. After this treatment, we observed that premenopausal patients with breast carcinoma may show two different responses: (1) ovulation followed by decreased androgenic activity, or (2) non-ovulation and an increase of androgenic activity, the endometrium maintaining its atypical pattern. Recently we began to treat this group of patients with a combination of HCG and dexamethasone (1.50 mg daily, given from day 3 to day 20 of the cycle). When the treatment with HCG alone or in combination with dexamethasone failed to reduce the androgenic activity, we performed ovarian resection. We have always found, at histologic examination of the resected ovaries, a high degree of interstitial tissue hyperplasia. Premenopausal breast carcinoma patients having an ovulatory cycle and low androgenic activity were not treated while this hormonal situation was present.

One patient (6R-32) was followed for two years after breast irradiation for carcinoma. During this period she was never given hormonal treatment because progestational activity was present and urinary testosterone low. After this period, the urinary testosterone increased and fibrocystic disease appeared in the untreated breast, while the endometrium was still showing progestational activity. Combined HCG and dexamethasone treatment was started. The urinary level of testosterone sharply increased after the treatment, and the endometrial

TABLE 8–30.—URINARY TESTOSTERONE LEVEL OF
PATIENT (6R-32) —44-YEARS-OLD

	URINARY TESTOSTERONE (mcg./24 hr.)	ENDOMETRIUM
Average value during 2 years	18.0	Progestational
Before treatment	35.0	Progestational
After combined treatment with HCG plus dexamethasone	102.0	Atypical hyperplasia
After ovarian resection	40.0	Progestational

TABLE 8–31.—URINARY TESTOSTERONE LEVEL OF WOMEN AT POSTMENOPAUSAL
AGE WITH BREAST CANCER AND ATYPICAL ENDOMETRIAL PATTERN,
AFTER TREATMENT WITH 20,000 IU HCG

PATIENTS (AGE)	TESTOSTERONE mcg./24 hr.	ENDOMETRIUM	TESTOSTERONE mcg./24 hr. (After Treatment)	ENDOMETRIUM
(7R-15) (53)	36.0	Atypical	16.0	Proliferative
(8R-4) (48)	60.0	Atypical	31.5	Proliferative
(7R-17) (57)	40.0	Atypical	120.0	Atypical
(7R-37) (53)	37.0	Atypical	198.0	Atypical

histologic pattern showed signs of hyperplasia. The patient was subjected to ovarian wedge resection. At histologic examination, large islets of interstitial luteinized cells were seen. Four months after ovarian resection, the fibrocystic disease of the breast disappeared, the urinary testosterone level decreased, and the endometrium showed a progestational pattern (Table 8-30).

The same HCG treatment was given to the postmenopausal patients with breast carcinoma having an atypical endometrial pattern and high androgenic activity. It was seen that gonadotropic treatment in this condition induced either a decrease of androgenic activity, as in the case of premenopausal patients with normalization of the endometrium, or an increase of androgenic activity with no change in the atypical endometrium (Table 8-31).

PROGESTATIONAL TREATMENT

On the strength of our earlier findings,[7] viz. that progestagen can depress androgenic activity, we treated 17 premenopausal breast carcinoma patients with 17α-acetoxyprogesterone cyclopentylenol ether for a total dose of 200 mg (20 mg each day) during the second half of the menstrual cycle. In this group, in which the patients had an atypical or a simple proliferative pattern of the endometrium, the

TABLE 8–32.—URINARY EXCRETION OF 11-DEOXY-17-KETOSTEROIDS—
[ETIOCHOLANOLONE (E) AND ANDROSTERONE (A)] AFTER
TREATMENT OF PATIENTS WITH BREAST CARCINOMA WITH
17ALPHA-ACETOXYPROGESTERONE CYCLOPENTYLENOL
ETHER (200 MG TOTAL DOSE)

PATIENTS (No. OF CASES)	E + A mg./24 hr.	E + A mg./24 hr. (After Treatment)
Patients with atypical endometrium (6)	3.61	1.92
Patients with proliferative endometrium (6)	3.01	1.13
Patients with progestational endometrium (5)	2.21	2.87

androgenic activity decreased. In the patients having an ovulatory pattern (progestational endometrium), progestagen treatment tended to increase the androgenic activity (Table 8-32).

In this study, we regard progestagen treatment as effective in breast carcinoma patients having an atypical or proliferative endometrium together with an increased androgenic activity. Sometimes we gave this treatment after a chorionic gonadotropic treatment, to obtain a further reduction of androgenic activity, as is reported for patient (8R-4) in Table 8-33. We should suggest that progestagens should not be given to patients with ovulatory cycle and that doses should be low; we administer up to 200 to 220 mg each month. One premenopausal patient with breast cancer and atypical endometrial pattern was given a total dose of 2,600 mg of 17alpha-acetoxyprogesterone cyclopentylenol ether (40 mg daily for 65 days). The urinary level of testosterone before treatment was 153.0 mcg/24 hr; after the high dosage of progestagen, the urinary testosterone increased to an extremely high level (525.0 mcg/24 hr), supporting the idea that at too high doses progestagen can be converted to androgens. When should we start hormonal treatment in breast carcinoma patients? We suggest immediately after diagnosis. As irradiation or operation may result in a temporary (two to four months) normalization of androgenic activity, if the hormone is not assayed before, a misleading impression is gained of the patients' real hormonal status. So ideally the hormonal examination should be made on diagnosis.

Figure 8-14 shows the urinary testosterone levels in premenopausal normal controls, in the "at risk" group and in breast carcinoma patients having an atypical endometrial pattern, examined shortly after mastectomy and not given hormonal treatment. The same figure shows a group of breast carcinoma patients who had been subjected to mastectomy or to irradiation of the breast some years before; they were treated with human chorionic gonadotropin with resulting ovulation. In all of these patients, breast cancer had been diagnosed five to seven years before and they are so far free from local recurrence or distant metastases. One of these patients was subjected to ovarian wedge resection; almost all had intermittently a course of treatment with pro-

TABLE 8-33.—URINARY TESTOSTERONE LEVELS OF BREAST CANCER PATIENT (8R-4), 48-YEAR-OLD—POSTMENOPAUSAL AGE, AFTER TREATMENT WITH 20,000 IU HCG AND AFTER TREATMENT WITH 800 MG. OF 17ALPHA-ACETOXYPROGESTERONE CYCLOPENTYLENOL ETHER

	TESTOSTERONE MCG./24 HR.
Before treatment	60.0
After 20,000 IU HCG	31.5
After progestagen	15.0

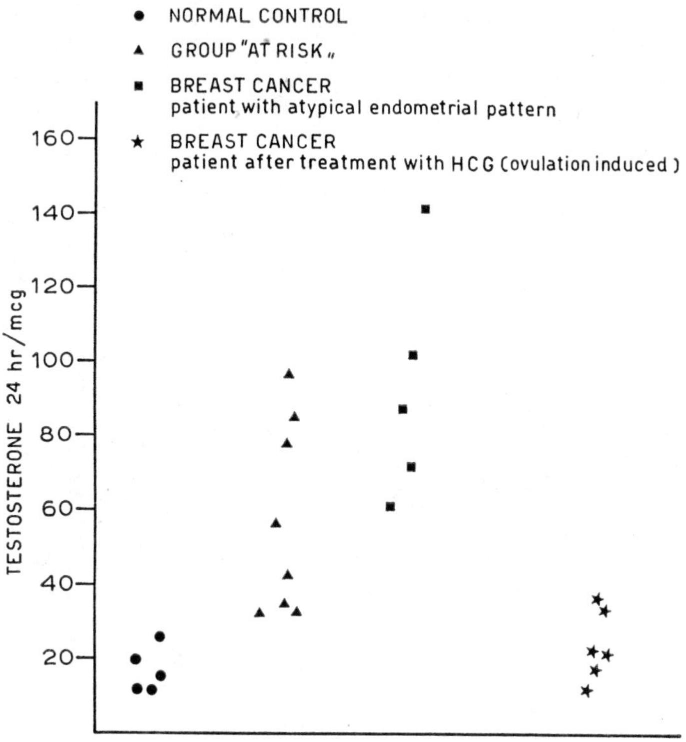

FIG. 8–14.—Testosterone levels in breast cancer patients at premenopausal age.

gestagen (17α-acetoxyprogesterone). Of the five patients with breast cancer and atypical endometrium who were not given hormonal treatment, two had a local recurrence three to four months after hormonal examination. All of these patients had been mastectomized five to six months before.

Figure 8-15 presents the urinary testosterone in postmenopausal women with breast cancer and a simple proliferative endometrium, breast cancer and atypical endometrium, and in normal controls. Patient (8R-4) had the left breast removed six years before, and the right a year later. She was subjected to hormonal examination five years ago. At that time the urinary testosterone level was above 50.0 mcg/24 hr; this excretion value was decreased to the level of 30.0 mcg/24 hr by HCG and kept at that level. A few months ago, this level fell to 15 mcg/24 hr as result of progestagen treatment. She is free from local or distant recurrences. Patient (7R-15) underwent mastectomy one year before (urinary testosterone level 36.0 mcg/24 hr). The patient was kept under treatment with HCG, and the urinary testosterone level after treatment was found to be 16.0 mcg/24 hr. The pa-

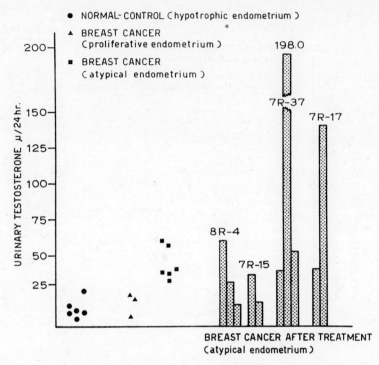

FIG. 8–15.—Testosterone levels in breast cancer patients at postmenopausal age.

tient is still well. Patient (7R-37) was recently subjected to irradiation of the breast; in this patient the HCG treatment induced a marked increase in androgenic activity. After this treatment, progestagen was given for a total dose of 800 mg. The urinary testosterone level remained above 50.0 mcg/24 hr. Ovariectomy was performed. At histologic examination of the ovary, a high degree of interstitial tissue hyperplasia was found. Patient (7R-17) was subjected to mastectomy six months before; after the HCG treatment, the testosterone urinary level increased greatly. The patient was lost sight of; when she was seen again five months later she had a local recurrence.

Conclusion

The results of this study indicate that overproduction of androgenic hormones rather than of estrogens is the most important etiologic factor in the development of breast cancer and of atypical endometrial hyperplasia, which is sometimes so atypical as to simulate adenocarcinoma histologically. We consider the ovary to be the site of the increased androgen biosynthesis. This abnormal ovarian activity is frequently observed in women suffering from sterility. As the incidence of infertility is increased in married women with breast cancer,[20] we must include these women in our "at risk" group. We recommend the determination of androgenic activity and examination of the premenstrual endometrium in these women; by inducing ovulation we could perhaps delay or inhibit the onset of breast carcinoma. When gonadotropic treatment is used to cure sterility by inducing ovulation, only the estrogens and pregnanediol excretion values are determined as a test of efficiency of the treatment.

In our view, the excretion of androgens should be evaluated too; when we observe that the androgenic activity is increased and the endometrium fails to revert to normal, even when dexamethasone is given together with gonadotropins, we perform ovarian resection, because the ovaries have consistently been found to be polycystic with a high degree of interstitial tissue hyperplasia. And we know that it is this interstitial tissue that produces androgens.[9, 21]

References

1. MacBride, J. M.: J. Clin. Endocrinol., 17:1440, 1957.
2. Bulbrook, R. D., and F. C. Greenwood: Brit. Med. J., 2:7, 1958.
3. Crowley, L. G., J. A. Demetrion, P. Kotin, A. J. Donovan, and S. Kushinsky: Cancer Res., 25:371, 1965.
4. Plotz, E. J., M. Wiener, A. A. Stein, and B. D. Hahn: Am. J. Obst. Gynec., 99:182, 1967.
5. Rivarola, M. A., J. H. Saez, H. W. Jones, J. G. Seegar, and C. J. Migeon: Johns Hopkins Med. J., 121:82, 1967.
6. Taylor, H. B., and H. J. Norris: Cancer, 20:1953, 1967.
7. Grattarola, R.: Advances in Exp. Med. Biol., 2:239, 1968.
8. Grattarola, R.: J. Endocrinol., 38:77, 1967.
9. Grattarola, R.: Excerpta Int. Congr., 161:234, 1968.
10. Grattarola, R.: Int. J. Gynec. Obst. Submitted for publication.
11. Hertig, A. T., and S. C. Sommers: Cancer, 2:946, 1949.
12. Gusberg, S. B., and A. L. Kaplan: Am. J. Obst. Gynec., 86:662, 1963.
13. Speert, H.: Surg. Gynec. Obst., 88:332, 1949.
14. Bush, I. E.: The Chromatography of Steroids. Pergamon Press, 1961, p. 336.
15. Grattarola, R.: Am. J. Obst. Gynec., 105:498, 1969.
16. Moxham, A., and J. D. Nabarro: Clin. Chim. Acta, 22:385, 1968.
17. McRoberts, J. R., A. O. Olson, and W. L. Herrmann: Clin. Chem., 14:565, 1968.
18. Grattarola, R.: Cancer, 17:1119, 1964.
19. Mauvais-Jarvis, P., H. H. Floch, and J. P. Bercovici: J. Clin. Endocrinol., 28:460, 1968.
20. Shimkin, M. B.: J. Amer. Med. Ass., 183:358, 1963.
21. Savard, K., J. M. March, and B. F. Rica: Recent Prog. Hormone Res., 31:285, 1965.

9

Cytogenetics and Cell Hybridization

Historical Perspectives in Cytogenetics and Cell Hybridization as Applied to Neoplasia

PETER C. NOWELL

Department of Pathology, School of Medicine, University of Pennsylvania, Philadelphia, Pennsylvania, USA

MAMMALIAN CYTOGENETICS and mammalian cell hybridization both represent relatively new fields, at least as related to the cancer problem. The significance of chromosome abnormalities in tumor cells has been debated since the 1890's, but it has only been within the last 15 years that modern cytogenetic techniques have made detailed study of this question possible. Mammalian somatic cell hybridization is an even newer field, dating back to the initial studies of Barski et al. in 1960.[1]

Despite this short history, however, research in these two areas during the past decade has been so vigorous that any attempt at a comprehensive review in this brief presentation is not possible. Therefore, these remarks will be largely limited to those topics with which I have had some personal experience, chiefly tumor chromosomes, although an attempt will also be made to provide some background on the application of cell hybridization studies to problems of neoplasia.

Cytogenetics of Neoplasia

From Von Hansemann in 1890 and Boveri in 1914 came suggestions that abnormalities of the mitotic apparatus and of chromosome constitution might play an essential role in the neoplastic process, but it was not until the development of modern techniques for mammalian chromosome study in the 1950's that these concepts were extensively investigated. These studies have now provided sufficient information to permit a number of generalizations to be made concerning the frequency, extent, and possible significance of chromosome alterations in mammalian neoplasms.[2-7]

The first generalization is that the neoplastic cells of most, but not all, mammalian tumors contain demonstrable chromosome changes. Nearly every human solid tumor reported to date, as well as most lymphomas and chronic leukemias, have been cytogenetically abnormal; this has also been true of most neoplasms investigated in animals. The human acute leukemias are exceptional in that approximately half of the cases have not had visible chromosome alterations,[8, 9] and changes have also been absent or minimal in some neoplasms induced in experimental animals by RNA viruses.[4, 10] Thus, there is no absolute requirement for chromosome alterations in malignant processes, but in most instances they have been present, varying from minor rearrangements to extensive aneuploidy.

A second generalization is that when present, the chromosome changes in a tumor are frequently clonal in nature. The neoplastic cells in a given case may all show the same abnormality or there may be a small number of stemlines with related chromosome changes, in both instances suggesting that the cells in a particular tumor all descended from a common ancestor. This clonal phenomenon has been particularly well documented in the human leukemias, where nearly all of the leukemic cells in an individual will commonly show the same chromosome alteration, and it has also been true in many solid neoplasms.[2-7] In either case, progression of a tumor to a more malignant stage is frequently associated with the appearance of a new predominant cell clone with additional chromosome changes superimposed on those originally observed.[2, 11]

The third generalization is that although cytogenetic abnormalities in mammalian neoplasms are clonal in nature, they generally differ from case to case.[2-7] Thus, the chromosome alteration characterizing one case of breast cancer may be quite different from the abnormality observed in the next case, even though the diseases are clinically identical. It is true that in some types of neoplasia, certain specific chromosome alterations have been observed with greater than random frequency, but only in human chronic granulocytic leukemia has it been possible to demonstrate a specific chromosome change associated with nearly every case of a particular neoplastic disorder. In this disease, the Philadelphia chromosome (Ph¹) is present in the neoplastic cells in approximately 90% of the typical cases.[5-9, 11, 12]

These three generalizations represent both the summation and the frustration of the recent history of chromosome studies in tumors. The demonstrated frequency and clonal nature of cytogenetic alterations have supported the suggestion that they play a significant role in the progression of the neoplastic process, conferring selective advantages on the cells bearing them, but their variability from case to case has made it difficult to assign them an etiologic role.

CHROMOSOME CHANGES AND THE ETIOLOGY OF CANCER

It is now known, from work done in recent years, that most agents which are carcinogenic are also capable of producing chromosome damage in human and other mammalian cells. Not only ionizing radiation, but also carcinogenic chemicals and oncogenic viruses have been shown to produce chromosome breakage both in vivo and in vitro.[10] Furthermore, an increased incidence of reticular tumors has been shown in those rare human diseases such as Bloom's syndrome and Fanconi's syndrome in which spontaneous chromosome breakage is excessive.[12] Unfortunately, it is not possible to assign quantitative risk estimates to the effects of various agents, and there may, in fact, be qualitative differences between the chromosome breakage produced by radiation and the lesions induced by certain viruses;[13] but the net effect of these studies has been to suggest that for a wide variety of agents there is a clear relationship between the capacity to damage chromosomes and the capacity to produce tumors. However, this does not imply that the visible chromosome changes ultimately seen in the resultant tumor are themselves the initiating events in the neoplastic process, but only that genetic damage may be a common mechanism by which many diverse carcinogenic agents act.

CLINICAL APPLICATIONS

The lack of precise quantitative relationships as well as the general lack of specificity of chromosome abnormalities for particular tumors has made it difficult to apply these concepts to the development of useful clinical applications. Physicians have occasionally found chromosome studies of diagnostic value (e.g. the Philadelphia chromosome in chronic granulocytic leukemia), and there have also been a few attempts to prognosticate the clinical course or response to therapy of certain types of neoplasms on the basis of chromosome findings. These efforts, to date, have proved of little practical value, although more work is needed, particularly with early neoplasms.[4-7] It has proved difficult to obtain adequate numbers of mitoses for study from such lesions as carcinoma in situ of the cervix and polyps of the bowel, but further investigation of such material might demonstrate useful correlations between chromosome changes and subsequent neoplastic progression.[14, 15] Attempts have also been made to use chromosome studies of the bone marrow for prognostic purposes in "preleukemic" states. Recent data suggest that if a clonal chromosome abnormality is found in the bone marrow, there is a significantly increased probability of overt leukemia developing within a few months; once beyond this critical period, however, those with an abnormality appear to carry little additional risk.[9]

It appears clear that before the role of chromosome changes in the initiation and progression of neoplasia can be more clearly elucidated, at least two additional kinds of information are needed. First, better data on what specific chromosome changes, if any, are associated with the earliest stages of various types of neoplasms must be obtained. Work along these lines is in progress, not only with early tumors in vivo, both in man and experimental animals, but also on the early chromosome changes in cultured mammalian cells transformed by oncogenic viruses.[10] Even more important than this knowledge, however, and also more difficult to obtain, is a clearer understanding of those metabolic changes critically involved in the initiation of neoplasia and the chromosomal location of the responsible genes. Attempts to develop such information in vivo through such systems as the transplantable "minimal deviation" rat hepatomas developed by Morris have not yielded consistent results,[16] and in vitro another approach is just beginning to be exploited: the cell hybridization phenomenon which is our second topic. Preliminary attempts at the mapping of mammalian, including human, chromosomes and investigation of the relationship of various chromosomal sites to neoplasia have been undertaken in hybrid cell systems, and some recent developments in this field will be briefly considered.

Cell Hybridization as Applied to Neoplasia

The pioneering studies of Barski et al., Ephrussi et al., and others in the early 1960's[1, 17] demonstrated that under the influence of certain viruses, in cultures containing a mixture of two different mammalian cell lines, single cells from each line would occasionally fuse, forming a hybrid element. Further work showed that these hybrids were capable of mitosis and clonal growth, and subsequently techniques were developed, both with and without the use of viral inducers, for producing combinations involving different species (e.g. rat-mouse, human-mouse).[18]

These hybrid elements provided potentially powerful tools for mammalian cell genetics. Many lines of investigation have been initiated relating to the control of cell differentiation and neoplastic growth, as well as to the chromosomal localization of genes responsible for metabolic products and other cellular characteristics such as permissiveness for infection by oncogenic viruses.

One particularly interesting aspect of this work has been the demonstration in several laboratories of the unusual propensity for human-mouse somatic cell hybrids to preferentially lose human chromosomes. Under circumstances in which the original mouse cell line was deficient and unable to grow in a given selective medium, it has been possible to develop, by continued propagation of the hybrid line in the selective medium, a population of cells containing a single human chromosome, presumably bearing the essential gene locus missing from the mouse cells. A number of such lines have now been developed, and although there are serious problems involved in the proper identification of the single human chromosome in the hybrid, this does represent one experimental approach which may ultimately contribute significantly to the mapping of the human genome.[18, 19] Any human products or characteristics identified in such a cell line can be assigned to the one remaining human chromosome, and by such means, a number of genes controlling specific enzymes have already been tentatively identified as grouped on the same human autosome. If and when specific metabolic alterations are shown to be critical in the initiation and progression of neoplasia, obviously such information on gene location will be of major importance in assessing the significance of specific chromosome anomalies in human tumors.

Another approach of particular relevance to the cancer problem has been the study of hybrid cells formed by the fusion of "malignant" cells with those from a relatively "nonmalignant" line, although results to date have been somewhat conflicting. Several early studies suggested that the introduction of a "normal" genome into a malignant cell did not result in suppression of the neoplastic state, whether the resultant hybrid does or does not retain all of the chromosomes of both parent cells.[20, 21] At least one recent study, however, has indicated that certain nonmalignant cell lines may be able to suppress the capacity to form tumors when fused with a number of different highly malignant cell types. It has even been suggested that the capacity of one particular cell line (clone A9) to do this might be related to its prolonged selection for azaguanine resistance.[22] Such conclusions would appear to be premature as yet, but they do indicate that further investigation is in order. It would be surprising if the introduction of a single altered metabolic characteristic into a series of highly aneuploid tumor cell lines consistently resulted in their loss of malignancy, but if similar studies could be carried out in malignant lines more nearly diploid, it is possible that more precise definition of both specific chromosome sites and specific metabolic pathways critically involved in the determination of neoplastic growth might be forthcoming.

Although its history is still very short, somatic cell hybridization does appear to offer one means by which the cytogenetic changes in neoplasia may be more precisely related to biochemical alterations, aiding in the long and frustrating process of eventually defining malignancy in molecular terms.

Acknowledgment

Original investigations by the author included in this review were supported by Research Grant CA-10320 from the National Cancer Institute, U. S. Public Health Service.

References

1. Barski, G., S. Sorieul, and Fr. Cornefert: Compt. Rend. Acad. Sci., 251:1825, 1960.
2. Hauschka, T. S.: Cancer Res., 21:957, 1961.
3. Stich, H. F.: Canad. Cancer Conf., 5:99, 1963.
4. Nowell, P. C.: Progr. Exp. Tumor Res., 7:83, 1965.
5. Sandberg, A. A.: Cancer Res., 26:2064, 1966.
6. Lejeune, J.: Science, 48:9, 1967.
7. de Grouchy, J.: Proceedings of the Third International Congress on Human Genetics. Johns Hopkins Press, Baltimore, 1967.
8. Conen, P. E.: Canad. Med. Ass. J., 96:1599, 1967.
9. Nowell, P. C.: Proceedings of the International Conference on Leukemia-Lymphoma (C. Zarafonetis, ed.), Lea and Febiger, Philadelphia, 1968, p. 47.
10. Aula, P., W. W. Nichols, and A. Levan: Ann. N. Y. Acad. Sci., 155:737, 1968.
11. de Grouchy, J., C. de Nava, and J. M. Cantu: Amer. J. Human Genet., 18:485, 1966.
12. Baikie, A. G.: Proceedings of the Eleventh Congress of the International Society of Hematology, Sidney, 1966, p. 198.
13. Nowell, P. C.: Fed. Proc., 28:1797, 1969.
14. Auersperg, N., M. J. Corey, and A. Worth: Cancer Res., 27:1394, 1967.
15. Enterline, H. T., and D. A. Arvan: Cancer, 20:1746, 1967.
16. Potter, V. R., M. Watanabe, H. C. Pitot, and H. P. Morris: Cancer Res., 29:55, 1969.
17. Ephrussi, B., L. J. Scaletta, M. A. Stenchever, and M. C. Yoshida: In: Cytogenetics of Cells in Culture. Academic Press, New York, 1964, p. 13.
18. Matsuya, Y., H. Green, and C. Basilica: Nature, 220:1199, 1968.
19. Heterospecific Genome Interaction (V. Defendi, ed.), Wistar Institute Symposium Monograph #9, The Wistar Institute Press, Philadelphia, 1969.
20. Barski, G., and Fr. Cornefert: J. Nat. Cancer Inst., 28:801, 1962.
21. Silagi, S.: Cancer Res., 27:1953, 1967.
22. Harris, H., O. J. Miller, G. Klein, P. Worst, and T. Tachibana: Nature, 223:363, 1969.

Chromosome Breakage by Oncogenic Viruses

H. F. STICH

Cancer Research Centre, University of British Columbia,
Vancouver, Canada

NUMERICAL AND STRUCTURAL chromosome alterations are implicated in a great variety of biologic phenomena involving evolution of animal and plant species, formation of cell strains and lines in vitro, induction of developmental anomalies, and transformation or progression of neoplastic cell populations. Concerning the latter problem, a certain disenchantment prevails. With the exception of one or two cases, no particular chromosome anomaly can be associated with the neoplastic behavior of a cell. Nevertheless, abnormal karyotypes comprise probably one of the few features present in a great variety of "spontaneous" or experimentally-induced neoplasms of several mammalian species. Chromosome anomalies were considered to provide a genetically heterogenous cell population and thus the raw material for the selection of neoplastic cells, to be involved in the fixation of neoplastic properties, to contribute to tumor progression, or to represent events superimposed on the transformation process. It now appears likely that the clue to the role of chromosome aberration is not to be found in any specific karyotypic changes, but rather must be sought in the randomly appearing additions, subtractions, and reshuffling of the chromosome complement.

Although the frequency and type of chromosome aberrations are widely used for measuring the effect of physical, chemical, or viral mutagens, they comprise a relatively insensitive tool to estimate genetic alterations. For example, the effect of the oncogenic[1] 4-nitroquinolin 1-oxide (4NQO) on the genome of mammalian cells can be estimated by measuring DNA-repair synthesis or by counting the frequency of chromatid breaks and exchanges. With the first procedure, it is possible to identify DNA lesions induced by a $1 \times 10^{-8}M$ 4NQO dose, whereas it needs at least a 4NQO concentration of $2 \times 10^{-6}M$ to raise significantly the incidence of visible chromosome breaks or exchange.[2] Nevertheless, the latter can be easily enumerated and represents at least an indicator for genetic changes occurring in a cell population. Unfortunately, the ratio between microscopically detectable and nondectable chromosome lesions is unknown. Thus it is not possible to assess whether chromosome anomalies represent a large or small part of the total genetic damage in a cell population.

Over the last decade, a considerable number of DNA and RNA viruses have been screened and found capable of inducing various chromosome and mitotic irregularities:[3-7, 10] herpes simplex; herpes zoster; human adenovirus type 2, 4, 7, 12, 16, 18; simian adenovirus SA7, SV11, SV15, SV40; measles, Sendai, mumps and Newcastle disease virus; poliovirus; vaccinia virus; and various strains of the Rous sarcoma virus. Aberrations of chromosomes and/or the mitotic apparatus were induced by viruses in cells of their natural host or in those of a phylogenic foreign species. In spite of these numerous studies, no particular pattern emerged. Apparently not all viruses capable of inducing chromosome anomalies are oncogenic, and not all oncogenic viruses (e.g. Friend and Rauscher leukemia virus) seem to interfere with the chromosome complement of the infected cell.

To distinguish cell responses which are directly involved in oncogenesis from unrelated events is a Herculean task; similarly, the role of chromosome aberration can only be guessed. Any interpretation is aggravated by the scarcity of karylogic data which are restricted to the very early stages following infection and to the end product, the rapidly proliferating neoplastic cell population. For example, one is tempted to link the high frequency of chromosome aberrations in Syrian hamster cells exposed to adenovirus 12 (AD12) with the abnormal karyotypes which prevail in AD12-transformed cells.[8] However it is difficult to prove or disprove such an idea. Chromosome aberrations are not limited to a preneoplastic period. They occur at a relatively high frequency in many adenovirus-induced neoplasms grown in vitro or in vivo, and continuously provide new abnormal karyotypes and increase the genetic heterogeneity of a neoplastic cell population.[9, 10] The viral genome, whether only temporarily present or integrated into the cell, seems to convey an instability to the chromosome complement. Thus abnormal karyotypes can become an integral part of a cell at almost any stage of the neoplastic transformation.

Many cytogenetic studies of viral oncogenesis emphasize experiments on the cellular rather than the viral level, e.g., responses of permissive and nonpermissive cells,[11] in vitro and in vivo systems, young and old cells at the "crisis,"[12] and infection at various stages of the cell cycle may be compared. Karyologic examinations combined with immunofluorescence procedures have revealed a wide spectrum of various cell types which evolve in a nonpermissive cell population (Syrian hamster cells) infected with AD12.[13] These cell variants include: (1) normal cells which have not been infected, (2) karyotypically normal cells which were infected but apparently lost the viral genome, (3) karyotypically normal cells with a functional viral genome as judged by the formation of neoantigen, (4) karyotypically abnormal cells with a viral genome, and (5) karyotypically abnormal cells which have either lost the viral genome or lack viral genomes capable of neoantigen formation. Considering that only two features were measured, karyotypes and neoantigens, the heterogeneity which is observed comprises only a fraction of the total. Cells of particular interest are those which survive an abortive viral infection or contain an altered chromosome complement and lack any detectable virus particles or genomes. When such genetically abnormal cells are encountered in vivo, it would be exceedingly difficult, if not impossible, to implicate a virus in their formation.

Another approach to the virus-chromosome interaction in early oncogenesis consists in varying the virus preparation. A few examples may suffice to exemplify these studies:

1. Virus types. All of the examined adenoviruses, including AD4, 7, 12, 16, 18, SA7, and SV11, are capable of inducing chromosome aberrations in Syrian hamster cells which comprise a nonpermissive system,[14] but the damage to chromosomes and/or mitotic apparatus in cells infected by the various virus types differs. For example, the chromosome lesions induced by AD12 or AD18 seem to copy those found in cells

exposed to ionizing irradiation, whereas the effect of AD4 resembles that resulting from x-irradiation followed by an extended colchicine treatment.

2. Viral dose. As was to be expected, there is a strict relationship between viral dose and the incidence of cells with chromosome anomalies and the incidence of chromosome breaks per metaphase plate.[15] The overwhelming majority of cells with severe chromosome aberrations lose their proliferative capacity.

3. Duration of virus-chromosome interaction. Nondividing Syrian hamster cells, blocked by arginine-deficient medium, were infected with AD12 and triggered into division one, two, three, or four days after infection. The chromosome damage persisted, but the incidence of breaks did not increase with time.

4. Impaired viruses. AD12 or 2 preparations exposed to UV retain their capacity to induce chromosome aberrations or anomalies of the mitotic apparatus in nonpermissive hosts, although they cannot complete an entire replicative cycle when tested in human cells. These impaired viruses can elicit chromosome aberrations in permissive host cells, although they have lost their mitosis-inhibiting and cytocidal effect.[8, 11] The experimentally impaired AD12 appears to exemplify the manner in which defective DNA viruses could be mutagenic for their own host.

Recently, attention has been given to the suitability of virus mutants as a tool to analyze the gene functions required for cell transformation or the maintenance of neoplastic properties.[16–19] Several AD12 mutants[18, 19] with greatly reduced oncogenic property (cyt 2, cyt 4, cyt 6, cyt 129, kb+; cyt 129, kb-; cyt 133, cyt 135) were examined for their capacity to induce chromosome aberrations in cultured Syrian hamster cells. The extent of chromosome damage induced by the nononcogenic mutants is equal to or even exceeds that elicited by the oncogenic mutant.[20] This result suggests an indirect rather than a direct involvement of visible chromosome aberration in neoplastic transformation. Furthermore, transformation comprises a rare event as compared to the frequency of chromosome aberration which occurs in most, if not all, AD12-infected cells. It is obvious that neither adenovirus infection nor genetic aberrations at the chromosome level are, by themselves, sufficient for neoplastic transformation.

Starting with the experiments of Hamper[21] with herpes simplex virus, evidence has accumulated that a great variety of viruses are potent radiomimetic or mutagenic agents for mammalian cells. Considering their ubiquitous distribution, viruses may represent the most common mutagen. So far, the emphasis has been placed mainly on virus-induced cell alterations which are caused by a complete or partially functional viral genome in the host cell. The presence of viruses, viral products, and viral genomes has been used as an indicator for the viral etiology of the morphologically or neoplastically transformed cell. Less consideration has been given to those genetically changed cells which result from an abortive infection and have lost the viral genome. The majority of nonpermissive cells following an adeno-virus infection may belong to this category. If one cannot follow the history of these genetically abnormal cells, their viral etiology would escape detection.

References

1. Nakahara, W., F. Fukuoka, and T. Sugimura: Gann, 48:128, 1953.
2. Stich, H. F., and R. H. C. San: Mutation Res. In press.
3. Stich, H. F., and D. S. Yohn: In: Progress in Medical Virology, 1970.
4. Nichols, W. W.: Hereditas, 55:1, 1966.
5. Black, P. H.: Ann. Rev. Microbiol., 22:391, 1968.
6. Nowell, P. C.: Progr. Exp. Tumor Res., 7:83, 1965.
7. Kato, R.: Hereditas, 59:120, 1968.
8. Stich, H. F., and D. S. Yohn: Nature, 216:1292, 1967.
9. Stich, H. F.: In: Radiation-induced Cancer, I.A.E.A., 1969, pp. 21-25.
10. Defendi, V.: Progr. Exp. Tumor Res., 8:125, 1966.
11. Stich, H. F., L. R. Avia, and D. S. Yohn: Exp. Cell Res., 53:44, 1968.
12. Moorhead, P. S., and D. Weinstein: Recent Results Cancer Res., 6:104, 1966.
13. Stich, H. F.: Jap. J. Genetics, 44 (Suppl. 1):65, 1969.
14. Cooper, J. E. K., D. S. Yohn, and H. F. Stich: Exp. Cell Res., 53:225, 1968.
15. Cooper, J. E. K., H. F. Stich, and D. S. Yohn: Virology, 33:533, 1967.
16. Eckhart, W.: Virology, 38:120, 1969.
17. di Mayorca, G., J. Callender, G. Marin, and R. Giordano: Virology, 38:126, 1969.
18. Takemori, N., J. L. Riggs, and C. D. Aldrich: Virology, 36:575, 1968.
19. Takemori, N., J. L. Riggs, and C. D. Aldrich: Virology, 38:8, 1969.
20. Stich, H. F., and N. Takemori: Nature. In press.
21. Hamper, B., and S. A. Ellison: Nature, 192:145, 1961.

Cell Hybridization and DNA Tumor Viruses

GUGLIELMO MARIN

Laboratorio di Embriologie Molecolere, Consiglio Nazionale delle Ricerche, Napoli, Italy

As a consequence of cell fusion, an event which is known to occur in vitro, nuclei of different mammalian cells are brought together in a common cytoplasm. The interaction of widely different somatic cell genomes can thus be studied, since effective fusion is not restricted to homologous cells, and viable hybrid lines have been derived from a number of heterospecific crosses.[1] Following fusion, two types of interactions are expected to take place: functional interactions between gene products already present or actively synthesized by the parental cells at the time of fusion, and physical interactions between the genetic determinants, i.e. chromosomes, contributed by each parent, and which may lead to the segregation of variants in the progeny of the hybrid. Functional interactions are expected to take place soon after fusion, and may be detected only when a significant proportion of the cell population takes part in it. For this reason, the frequency of fusion is usually increased artificially by exposing the cells to inactivated Sendai virus, one of a series of viruses which are known to induce polykaryocytosis. The reactivation of chicken erythrocyte nuclei fused into HeLa cells[2] is a typical example of this type of interaction. Furthermore, the very fact that viable hybrid lines can be established and sometimes display a generation time which is different from that of either parent[1] proves that early functional interactions do take place between fused cells. The proportion of fused cells that will give rise to viable hybrid lines is, however, low. A method based on complementation between cells deficient in different metabolic requirements has proved very effective in selecting for hybrid clones[3] but is dependent on the availability of the appropriate deficient variants of the lines to be crossed. In the absence of these, methods based on differential growth patterns or adhesiveness to the substrates can be useful.[4, 5] However, hybrid lines resulting from fusion and complementation of deficient cells have the additional advantage of providing a system which allows for the potential selection of genetic segregants.[6] Indeed, variants which had resumed parental characters as a consequence of chromosome loss have been selected from the progeny of intraspecific[7] as well as interspecific[8] hybrids of this category.

A number of questions related to cell transformation by DNA tumor viruses have been approached by making use of cell hybridization techniques, in the way of causing either short-term, functional, or long-term genetic interactions to take place between the appropriate cells. One question was whether neoplastic transformation might occur as the consequence of a loss of genetic information (deletion) caused by the infecting virus. The answer is that it does not. Tumorigenicity,[9] virus-specific tumor (T) antigens,[9, 10] and typical morphologic changes and growth properties acquired upon virus-mediated transformation[11] are usually preserved in hybrids of normal and virus-transformed cells. Although recent evidence indicates that this conclusion may not be extended to all cases of malignant development,[12] it supports the idea that oncogenic DNA viruses produce a hereditary dominant change in competent cells. It has been suspected for a long time that such a dominant change was the actual integration of viral genetic material in the cell's genome. This hypothesis has received strong support from the demonstration that DNA from SV40- and polyoma-transformed cells binds specifically RNA transcribed in vitro from the homologous viral DNA template.[13] But the actual proof that intact virus genomes can persist indefinitely in nonpermissive transformed cells was obtained by showing that SV40-transformed, virus-free mouse, human, or hamster cells release SV40 virus when artificially fused to susceptible African green monkey cells.[14, 15]

The third contribution of cell hybridization to the field of viral oncogenesis was the demonstration that the transformed phenotype may be lost by cells concurrently with the loss of chromosomes. T antigen-positive hybrid lines between SV40-transformed human and mouse cells were shown to give rise to T antigen-negative cells, and the disappearance of T antigen was shown to occur only in cells which had lost most, though not necessarily all, human chromosomes.[16] Loss of transformation traits was also observed in a polyoma-transformed hybrid cell line derived from BHK 21 variants by the selective method of Littlefield. This line gave rise to occasional clones of normal morphology (parallel orientation) which had lost the ability to grow in agar suspension[17] and the polyoma-specific complement-fixing antigen. Their tumorigenicity was reduced, and the amount of polyoma-specific transplantation antigen had also decreased.[18] The revertant cells were obtained by selecting for resistance to thioguanine (one of the markers of the parental cells used in the cross), and had lost about 20% of the chromosomes present in the hybrid. Two revertant clones were carried on for several months (over 100 generations), and their morphology appeared to be stable. When reinfected with polyoma virus, a small proportion of the cells were retransformed, regaining the ability to grow in agar suspension and to synthesize the polyoma-specific complement-fixing antigen. It thus appeared that the revertant cells were not simply variants incapable of expressing the transformed phenotype.

These results, when considered along with the demonstration that the DNA of polyoma- and SV40-transformed cells contains virus-specific base sequences,[13] suggest that it may become possible to map on the genome of somatic cells genes (viral or cellular) responsible for traits related to transformation, if the appropriate systems will be developed. The systems used so far are not entirely satisfactory. Homospecific hybrids between Syrian hamster cells have the advantage of retaining some of the growth properties which differentiate normal from transformed cells (parallel orientation in monolayers, inability to grow in suspension, low transplantability in vivo). However, the total number of chromosomes is too high and variable to allow for an easy identification of individual chromosomes, the absence of which could be correlated with the loss of phenotypic traits. Heterospecific hybrids between species with numerically low karyotypes and/or morphologically characteristic chromosomes would be potentially more valuable. It is to be expected, however, that the relevant changes in cell morphology, growth properties and transplantability may be difficult to detect in heterospecific hybrids. As for the virus of choice, SV40 seems at present more advantageous than polyoma because it can be rescued easily from transformed cells,[14, 15] and the demonstration of T antigen by immunofluorescence is easier in SV40-transformed than in polyoma-transformed cells.

Apart from being karyotypically suitable, the ideal hybrid should contain a number of independent markers that would allow selection for loss or retention of specific chromosomes. Resistance to purine or pyrimidine base analogs seems at present the best marker, since it usually involves a deficiency in the enzymes that normally account for their uptake from external sources. In a karyotypically unstable, genetically redundant cell, it is likely that resistance will be acquired by loss of the relevant chromosome(s), rather than by deletion or point mutation of the corresponding gene(s).

In testing the predictions that can be derived from the "lysogenic" model of transformation, one of the main questions to be asked is whether integration of viral genetic material takes place at a specific locus (or loci). If this were the case, it could be inferred that the mechanism of integration was similar to the one described for phage λ in E. coli, i.e. one involving base-pairing and crossing over in homologous regions of the viral and cellular genomes.[19] Consistent evidence for linkage of virus inducibility and/or transformation traits with cellular markers would support specific localization. To obtain this evidence, even a limited number of markers may be adequate, because it seems that chromosomes tend to be lost in "functional" groups rather than singly. When bromodeoxyuridine-resistant and thioguanine-resistant segregants were isolated from the hybrid cell line described by Marin and Littlefield,[17] there appeared to be little overlap between the groups of chromosomes lost in each case.[7] Nonrandom loss of specific groups of chromosomes would give rise to apparent linkage between markers located on different chromosomes. Evidence for specific localization of genes related to transformation could thus be obtained with a small number of markers, if they all shared these properties.

Most somatic cell hybrids are karyotypically unstable. With one exception,[8] however, the spontaneous loss of chromosomes in the hybrids tested so far occurs too slowly to be useful. In addition to producing appropriate markers that would allow the selection of specific chromosomal segregants, methods should be devised for inducing the controlled loss of chromosomes of either partner of a hybrid. For example, the induction of chromosomal aberrations in one of the partners before fusion may favor the loss of its chromosomes from the hybrids in which it participates. Preliminary observations on Chinese hamster-mouse cell hybrids seem, in fact, to show that x irradiation of one of the partners before fusion widens the distribution of chromosome numbers in the hybrids, and increases the frequency of hybrids with very few chromosomes of the irradiated partner.[20]

Another characteristic feature of the lysogenic state in bacteria is its dependence on the synthesis of a diffusible repressor. It has been suggested that transformation of animal cells may also involve the repression of some viral functions, the repressor in this case being synthesized by the cell. However, a strong argument against the existence of a diffusible repressor is the absence of immunity to superinfection with SV40 DNA in SV40-transformed, originally permissive cells, which could be shown to contain an inducible viral genome.[21] In general, failure of a cell to support the multiplication of SV40 or polyoma virus cannot be easily attributed to the action of a repressor because permissiveness appears to be strongly dominant. Sendai-induced heterokaryons of SV40-permissive and -nonpermissive cells always support the synthesis of SV40 T antigen and viral coat proteins, regardless of the ratio of permissive to nonpermissive nuclei in the cell.[22, 23] Stable hybrid lines between mouse (permissive) and Syrian hamster (nonpermissive) cells seem to support some multiplication of polyoma virus as long as an approximately full mouse chromosome complement is present, even when the number of hamster chromosomes far exceeds the diploid value.[24] This work probably is the first attempt at studying the genetic control of somatic cells by their ability to support the multiplication of a given virus. In the lines studied by Basilico et al.,[24] it would appear that the control of permissiveness is exerted at a specific stage of the viral cycle, preceding the synthesis of viral DNA. It may be inferred that the genetic basis of this control is a relatively simple one, and its mapping thus may be feasible. As in the case of the control of transformation traits, allocation of the relevant genes on individual chromosomes may have to await the production of cells with a sufficient number of genetically or morphologically marked chromosomes.

References

1. Ephrussi, B., and M. C. Weiss: Regulation of the cell cycle in mammalian cells: Inferences and speculations based on observations of interspecific somatic hybrids. Twenty-Sixth Symposium of the Society for Developmental Biology, Suppl. 1:136-169, 1967.
2. Harris, H., E. Sidebottom, D. M. Grace, and M. E. Bramwell: The expression of genetic information: A study with hybrid animal cells. J. Cell. Sci., 4:499-525, 1969.
3. Littlefield, J. W.: The selection of hybrid mouse fibroblasts. Cold Spring Harbor Symp. Quant. Biol., 29:161-166, 1964.
4. Davidson, R. L., and B. Ephrussi: A selective system for the isolation of hybrids between L cells and normal cells. Nature, 205:1170-1171, 1965.
5. Miggiano, V., M. Nabholz, and W. Bodmer: Hybrids between human leukocytes and a mouse cell line: Production and characterization. Wistar Institute Symposium Monograph No. 9, 1969, pp. 61-76.
6. Littlefield, J. W.: Selection of hybrids from matings of fibroblasts in vitro and their presumed recombinants. Science, 145:709-710, 1964.
7. Marin, G.: Selection of chromosomal segregants in a 'hybrid' line of Syrian hamster fibroblasts. Exp. Cell Res., 57:29-36, 1969.
8. Weiss, M. C., and H. Green: Human-mouse hybrid cell lines containing partial

complements of human chromosomes and functioning human genes. Proc. Nat. Acad. Sci. USA, 58:1104-1111, 1967.

9. Defendi, V., B. Ephrussi, H. Koprowski, and M. C. Yoshida: Properties of hybrids between polyoma-transformed and normal mouse cells. Proc. Nat. Acad. Sci. USA, 57:299-305, 1967.

10. Defendi, V., B. Ephrussi, and H. Koprowski: Expression of polyoma-induced cellular antigen(s) in hybrid cells. Nature, 203:495-496, 1964.

11. Marin, G.: Somatic cell hybridization and problems of viral oncogenesis. In Vitro, Vol. 5. In press.

12. Harris, H., O. J. Miller, G. Klein, P. Worst, and T. Tachibana: Suppression of malignancy by cell fusion. Nature, 223:363-368, 1969.

13. Westphal, H., and R. Dulbecco: Viral DNA in polyoma and SV40-transformed cell lines. Proc. Nat. Acad. Sci. USA, 59:1158-1165, 1968.

14. Watkins, J. F., and R. Dulbecco: Production of SV40 virlus in heterokaryons of transformed and susceptible cells. Proc. Nat. Acad. Sci. USA, 58:1396-1403, 1967.

15. Koprowski, H., F. C. Jensen, and Z. Steplewski: Activation of production of infectious tumor virus SV40 in heterokaryon cultures. Proc. Nat. Acad. Sci. USA, 58:127-133, 1967.

16. Weiss, M. C., B. Ephrussi, and L. J. Scaletta: Loss of T-antigen from somatic hybrids between mouse cells and SV40-transformed human cells. Proc. Nat. Acad. Sci. USA, 59:1132, 1968.

17. Marin, G., and J. W. Littlefield: Selection of morphologically normal cell lines from polyoma-transformed BHK21/13 hamster fibroblasts. J. Virol., 2:69-77, 1968.

18. Marin, G., and I. Macpherson: Reversion in polyoma-transformed cells: Studies on retransformation, induced antigens and tumorigenicity. J. Virol., 3:146-149, 1969.

19. Campbell, A.: Episomes. Adv. Genet., 11:101, 1962.

20. Pontecorvo, G.: Personal communication.

21. Jensen, F. C., and H. Koprowski: Absence of repressor in SV40-transformed cells. Virology, 37:687-689, 1969.

22. Steplewski, Z., B. B. Knowles, and H. Koprowski: The mechanism of internuclear transmission of SV40-induced complement fixation antigen in heterokaryocytes. Proc. Nat. Acad. Sci. USA, 59:769-776, 1968.

23. Knowles, R., Z. Steplewski, P. Swetly, G. Barbanti-Brodano, and H. Koprowski: Cell hybridization and tumour viruses. Wistar Institute Symposium Monograph No. 9, 1969, pp. 37-49.

24. Basilico, C., Y. Matsuia, and H. Green: The interaction of polyoma virus with mouse-hamster hybrid cells. Virology. In press.

10

Tumor Growth and Cell Kinetics

La Croissance Tumorale et la Cinetique Cellulaire: Perspectives Historiques

M. TUBIANA

Institut Gustave-Roussy, Villejuif, France

LA CINÉTIQUE CELLULAIRE est une discipline relativement jeune qui est née le jour où il a été possible de marquer les cellules et de suivre leur devenir, en utilisant pour cela un précurseur radioactif de l'acide désoxyribonucléique (DNA) qui est incorporée par la cellule au moment où celle-ci synthétise le DNA. Cette méthode marque parmi les cellules d'une population celles qui se trouvent en phase de synthèse de DNA. En suivant l'arrivée en mitose de la cohorte de cellules marquées on peut mesurer la durée des phases du cycle cellulaire. En associant ces techniques à la mesure du contenu en DNA des cellules, on obtient plusieurs informations sur les paramètres de la prolifération cellulaire des cellules: la durée des phases du cycle, la proportion de cellules se trouvant dans chacune de ces phases, la proportion de cellules se trouvant engagées dans un cycle cellulaire ou qui sont quiescentes en dehors du cycle (coefficient de prolifération ou growth fraction). A partir de ces données on peut calculer le taux de perte cellulaire.[41]

L'intérêt de ces méthodes en cancérologie est double: d'une part elles permettent de mieux comprendre les caractéristiques de la croissance d'une tumeur, d'autre part, elles peuvent en aidant à comprendre ce qui se passe pendant et après un traitement, donner des bases plus scientifiques à celui-ci et peut être accroître son efficacité.

Le but du traitement du cancer est de tuer le plus grand nombre de cellules tumorales, en épargnant autant que possible les tissus normaux. La recherche des différences entre les tissus sains et les tissus tumoraux est donc l'un de ses objectifs les plus importants. Reiskin[38] étudie le pourcentage de mitoses marquées dans l'épithélium de la poche du hamster. Quand l'animal vieillit, la durée de la phase S et celle du cycle augmente. Dans le cancer induit dans cet épithélium, la durée de la phase S est plus courte que dans le tissu adulte, mais plus longue que chez l'animal jeune; de plus on observe une seconde vague de mitoses marquées ce qui démontre qu'il y a dans ce cas, moins de variation de la durée du cycle et tout particulièrement de la phase G_1. C'est là d'ailleurs une constatation souvent faite dans les cancers induits ou transplantés.

Le Tableau 10-1 résume les résultats de quelques comparaisons entre les tissus normaux et cancéreux de même origine. Dans la plupart des cas, la phase S a une durée voisine, mais le cycle cellulaire a une durée plus longue dans les tissus normaux et ceci est essentiellement dû à une phase G_1 plus longue. Toutefois, dans les tissus normaux en régénération rapide, le cycle cellulaire peut devenir plus court que dans les cellules cancéreuses.

On peut se demander si ces conclusions obtenues généralement sur des tumeurs provoquées ou transplantées demeurent valables pour des tumeurs spontanées. Alors que dans les tumeurs transplantées, il existe en générale une seconde vague de mitoses marquées bien identifiée, ce qui indique qu'il y a relativement peu de variations dans la durée du cycle cellulaire d'une cellule à l'autre, on observe dans les tumeurs induites des rongeurs une tendance vers une durée plus longue du cycle cellulaire, de plus le second pic est moins marqué, ce qui indique une plus grande variabilité de la durée du cycle et notamment de G_1. Ceci est encore plus net dans les tumeurs spontanées du chien étudiées par Owen et Steel[33] la durée de S est relativement courte mais le cycle est beaucoup plus long.

Avec Frindel et Malaise[19] nous avons étudié 5 cancers de la peau

TABLE 10–1

		T_s(hrs)	T_c(hrs)	Réf.
Liver (rat)	Normal	8	21	34
	Hepatoma	17	31	35
Skin (mouse)	Normal	6-7	150	11
	Epithelioma	8	32	11
Mammary (C^3H)	Normal	21	64	
	Carcinoma	11	33	5
Cheek epithelium	Normal	8.6	130	
(hamster)	Carcinoma	5.8	11	6
Stomach (mouse)	Normal	7	28-55	14
	Sq. Cell carcinoma	3.6-5	8-12	15
Bone marrow (man)	Normal	13-14	24	25
	Ac. Leukemia	10-20	20-80	

TABLE 10-2.—HUMAN CANCERS—CELL KINETICS

TYPE	No. CASES	Ts	Tc	G.F.	CELL LOSS FACTOR
Skin (Basal cell carc.)	2 Frindel[19]	19 Hr.	3 d.	30%	95%
Skin (Ep. Ep.)	2 Frindel[19]	12 Hr.	38 Hr.	40%	90%
Cervix (Sq. cell. carc.)	2 Benington[3]	10 Hr.	15 Hr.	50%	
Melanoma	2 Shirakawa Tannock[43]	25 Hr.	3-4 d.	25%	
Ascitic Neop.	6 Clarkson[9]	15-35 Hr.	3-5 d.	20-90%	

chez l'homme, en faisant après injection de thymidine tritiée des biopsies répétées. De telles études ne peuvent être effectuées que chez les sujets dont l'espérance de vie est telle, que l'injection intra-veineuse de thymidine tritiée ne soulève pas de problème éthique. Il faut d'autre part que la tumeur soit volumineuse et peu sensible, afin que des biopsies répétées puissent être effectuées. Parmi près de 3000 malades atteints de tumeurs superficielles seules 5 ont paru pouvoir être retenues pour une telle étude.

Les durées des phases G_2 et S paraissent plus longues que dans les tumeurs animales mais la différence n'est pas importante, la seconde vague de mitoses marquées est généralement mal définies, ce qui indique là encore, une variation considérable de la durée du cycle cellulaire.[19, 30]

Une comparaison entre ces quatre groupes de tumeurs montre que les différences d'un type de tumeur à l'autre ne sont pas très importantes et souligne la tendance déjà notée, vers un cycle cellulaire plus long et présentant une plus grande variabilité d'une cellule à l'autre quand on passe d'une tumeur transplantée à un cancer humain. En tenant compte des caractéristiques des tumeurs spontanées, la différence entre les tissus sains et cancéreux est encore réduite. La durée de la phase S est voisine dans les deux types de tissus et il n'y a guère de différence dans la durée du cycle cellulaire, sauf peut être dans la durée de G_1.

Le Tableau 10-2 suivant résume les données de la littérature sur les quelques tumeurs humaines pour lesquelles on possède des informations complètes; il semble d'après ces résultats encore très peu nombreux que des tumeurs de même type histologique aient des paramètres de la prolifération cellulaire voisins, ou tout au moins comparables. Cette observation, si elle était confirmée, soulignerait l'intérêt de la cinétique cellulaire pour la caractérisation d'un type de tumeur et encouragerait à rassembler des données sur les différents types de tumeurs humaines. Malheureusement les méthodes actuellement utilisées soulèvent des problèmes techniques et éthiques tels, que seul un petit nombre de cancers peut être étudié: mais on peut espérer qu'avec le développement des nouvelles techniques, telles que les injections in situ[47] ou les études in vitro[13, 36] il sera possible de multiplier ces observations, aussi le développement de ces nouvelles techniques devrait être un objectif important.

Alors que la durée du cycle varie relativement peu d'une tumeur à l'autre, le temps de doublement d'une tumeur humaine présente de grandes variations et s'étale entre 4 jours et un an. Pour 522 cancers primitifs ou métastiques dont le temps de doublement a été rapporté dans la littérature, la durée médiane est de 58 jours. Parmi eux, il y avait 128 sarcomes avec une durée médiane de temps de doublement de 36 jours et 318 épithéliomas avec une durée médiane de 84 jours, la différence entre les deux temps de doublement est hautement significative.[7] Si la durée du cycle cellulaire n'a pas de corrélation avec le temps de doublement, deux autres facteurs peuvent expliquer les différences de vitesses de croissance.

1. Le coefficient de prolifération cellulaire, ou "growth fraction."

Chez l'animal on trouve une tendance vers un growth fraction plus petit dans les tumeurs à croissance lente.

2. La perte cellulaire.

Celle-ci peut être importante dans certaines tumeurs et en particulier nous l'avons trouvée notable dans trois tumeurs humaines. Il semble de plus qu'il existe dans les tumeurs animales une tendance vers une perte plus grande dans les tumeurs à croissance lente[41] et il est possible que le temps de doublement plus court des sarcomes soit lié à une moindre perte cellulaire.[10] Il faut d'ailleurs souligner que ce terme de perte cellulaire est assez vague et recouvre en fait, plusieurs phénomènes très différents sur le plan biologique; les uns tels la desquamation et la mort de cellules différenciées sont des phénomènes normaux survenant dans les tissus sains et qui peuvent exister aussi dans les tumeurs, en particulier les tumeurs différenciées. Les autres types sont plus spécifiques des tissues cancéreux, tels que la mort pendant la mitose, la nécrose dûe à des défauts d'apport nutritif ou à des réactions immunologiques. Il existe d'autre part des phénomènes de migration dont l'importance quantitative est difficile à évaluer mais qui ne doivent pas être négligés. Dans de nombreuses tumeurs, la production cellulaire n'est que de peu supérieure à la perte cellulaire, dans ce cas une petite augmentation du taux de perte cellulaire aurait pour effet de stabiliser la taille de la tumeur, voire même de la faire régresser.

Un problème essentiel est de savoir quels sont les facteurs qui influencent les différents paramètres de la prolifération cellulaire: la durée du cycle, le "growth fraction" et la perte cellulaire. Pour analyser ce problème, nous avons étudié une tumeur expérimentale à différentes phases de sa croissance et nous avons constaté que lorsqu'elle pousse sous forme solide, la durée du cycle cellulaire demeure identique cependant qu'on observe une diminution du coefficient de prolifération lié au fait que dans les grosses tumeurs, il y a des zones où les cellules sont au repos et des zones proches où elles sont en prolifération active. Au fur et à mesure que la tumeur grossit, d'une part les régions de la tumeur dans lesquelles les cellules sont au repos augmentent, d'autre part la perte cellulaire devient de plus en plus importante.[18]

Tannock[42] a étudié un tumeur dans laquelle les cellules poussent en boyaux autour des vaisseaux. Entre ces boyaux existent des régions de nécrose et il a mesuré les paramètres de la prolifération dans trois zones: au contact des vaisseaux, à mi-chemin entre ceux-ci et la région nécrotique, au contact de la région nécrotique. L'index mitotique et l'index de marquage diminuent au fur et à mesure qu'on s'éloigne des vaisseaux, ce qui traduit une diminution du coefficient de prolifération car la durée du cycle cellulaire est la même en ces trois régions. Tannock a pu par ailleurs mettre en évidence un mouvement des cellules de la zone des vaisseaux vers les zones de nécrose, où elles meurent (Tableau 10-3).

D'autres résultats expérimentaux ont confirmé ces données. Ils montrent que la durée du cycle cellulaire est relativement constante dans les tumeurs solides où les variations des conditions locales influencent surtout le taux de mortalité cellulaire et le coefficient de prolifération, qui dépend lui-même de ce qui se passe pendant la première phase du cycle, entre la mitose et le début de la phase de synthèse de l'ADN. Cependant la durée du cycle n'est pas une caractéristique de la cellule puisque si celle-ci pousse sous une autre forme, et en particulier sous forme de tumeur ascitique, on a pu mettre en évidence tant pour les cellules de l'ascite d'Erhlich[27] que pour les cellules NCTC,[16, 20] un allongement de la durée de toutes les phases du cycle au fur et à mesure que le nombre de cellules tumorales augmentent. Cet allongement est d'ailleurs réversible ce qui montre l'existence en milieu ascitique de facteurs allongeant la durée du cycle.[20, 27, 46]

Cette différence entre les caractéristiques de la prolifération selon que les mêmes cellules poussent soit sous forme solide, soit sous forme ascitique, est malheureusement difficile à utiliser pour l'identification des facteurs responsables. En effet les conditions in vivo sont si complexes qu'il est difficile de les analyser; cependant en testant in vitro l'influence de certaines des modifications observées in vivo, telles que l'augmentation de la concentration de l'acide lactique ou l'abaissement du pH, on a pu montrer que ce dernier facteur avait une importance primordiale.[31]

TABLE 10–3.—CELL LOSS IN 3 HUMAN SKIN TUMORS[44]

	BASAL CELL C.	BASAL CELL C.	EP. EP.
Clinical doubling time T_D	10 mo	4-6 mo	1 mo
Potential doubling time $T_p = T_c/G.F.$	10 days	5-12 d	2-5 d
Cell loss	97%	90-97%	92%

Hahn[22] a apporté une contribution importante en montrant que dans une culture où le milieu est changé fréquemment, le cycle cellulaire s'allonge au fur et à mesure que le nombre de cellules augmente, alors que dans une culture où le milieu n'est pas changé, le cycle cellulaire garde la même durée cependant que le coefficient de prolifération s'abaisse. Ces résultats suggèrent des rapprochements intéressants avec ce qui a été observé dans les tumeurs ascitiques ou solides. Au total au moins quatre types différents de facteurs semblent pouvoir influencer le taux de croissance des populations de cellules:

1. l'encombrement cellulaire, qui joue peut être par des mécanismes de contact entre les cellules.

2. les facteurs immunologiques.

3. les conditions métaboliques, telles que la concentration en oxygène ou la quantité de matériaux nutritifs disponible; le pH.

4. la présence de substances inhibitrices ou stimulantes.

Il est probable que chacun de ces facteurs peut jouer non seulement sur les caractéristiques du cycle cellulaire, mais aussi sur le fait qu'une cellule est ou non engagée dans un cycle. La quiescence d'une cellule peut être la conséquence de conditions différentes qu'il serait intéressant de distinguer les unes des autres car les caractéristiques des cellules quiescentes varient vraisemblablement avec la cause de cette quiescence comme le montre l'expérience de Hahn.[22] Certaines d'entre elles sont des cellules terminales incapables de se diviser, d'autres quoique capables de proliférer ne le font pas, soit du fait de l'absence de facteurs de stimulation ou de facteurs nutritifs, soit au contraire à cause de la présence d'inhibiteurs. Le fait que certaines cellules tumorales humaines puissent être quiescentes pendant de longs mois ou de longues années, montre l'importance de ce problème, il montre aussi que le concept apparement simple de coefficient de prolifération[32] (ou "growth fraction") mériterait maintenant d'être approfondi de façon à distinguer ces différentes catégories de cellules.

Une meilleure connaissance des traits serait utile non seulement pour une meilleure compréhension de la croissance tumorale, mais aussi parce qu'elle aidait à prédire le devenir d'une tumeur exposée à une perturbation telle qu'une radiothérapie ou chimiothérapie.

En radiothérapie ou en chimiothérapie, le traitement est fractionné et les modifications de la cinétique de prolifération provoquées par chaque traitement ont une importance capitale puisqu'elles influencent la façon dont la population va répondre au traitement ultérieur.

Plusieurs phénomènes doivent être considérés:

1. Considérons une population cellulaire dans laquelle les cellules sont distribuées uniformément dans toutes les phases du cycle. Comme la radiosensibilité ou la chimiosensibilité d'une cellule varie à travers le cycle, après un premier traitement seules survivront les cellules les plus résistantes; elles se trouveront donc groupées dans certaines phases du cycle. Leur progression ultérieure à travers le cycle, entraînera des

variations cycliques de sensibilité, donc de réactions aux agents thérapeutiques.[17, 48]

2. La prolifération cellulaire entre les traitements peut contribuer
à expliquer l'effet du fractionnement, et elle dépend de deux facteurs:
le nombre de cellules engagées dans le cycle et la durée du cycle. La
durée du cycle des cellules survivantes paraît peu modifiée après traitement chimiothérapique ou radiothérapique; dans une tumeur solide
après une dose de 600 R nous n'avons pas trouvé de modification du
cycle. Hermens et Barendsen[1, 24] ont trouvé un petit raccourcissement
après une dose de 1000 ou 2000 R. Nous avons fait la même observation
dans deux tumeurs ascitique, nous avons trouvé un allongement de la
durée du cycle: celui-ci est d'autant plus durable que la tumeur est plus
âgée, qui souligne encore l'importance des facteurs d'environnement.[21]

L'interprétation de ces expériences soulève cependant des problèmes.
En effet les méthodes autoradiographiques ne peuvent pas distinguer
les cellules viables survivantes de celles lésées mais néanmoins capables
d'encore une ou deux divisions, leur emploi pour de telles études a
paru à certains criticables.

Ce problème est d'ailleurs plus général, car dans toutes les tumeurs,
traitées ou non, seules sont intéressantes les cellules capables de donner
naissance à un clone c'est-à-dire possédant une capacité de prolifération
infinie. Or la proportion de cellules clonogènes peut varier d'un type de
tumeur à l'autre et est généralement inconnue. Lorsque cette proportion
est faible; les techniques autoradiographiques sont alors incapables, que
la tumeur ait ou non été traitée, d'étudier leurs caractéristiques. C'est
pourquoi il peut être utile d'utiliser d'autres méthodes qui étudient
uniquement les cellules clonogènes[4] techniques qui sont malheureusement difficiles à utiliser par tumeur dans lesquelles de fortes proportions
de cellules sont quiescentes.

En 1966, utilisant une technique indirecte, basée sur l'analyse de la
courbe de croissance des tumeurs après irradiation, nous avons montré
une accélération de la vitesse de croissance des cellules survivantes.[29]
L'analyse de tumeurs humaines irradiées aboutissait à la même conclusion.[37] Ces constatations avaient été accueillies avec quelques scepti-
cisme, elles viennent d'être confirmées et étendues par des expériences
directes de Barendsen,[1] dans lesquelles après irradiation, la variation du
nombre de cellules clonogènes est suivie dans une tumeur ayant reçue
une dose de 1000 ou 2000 rads. Après une période de latence d'environ
deux jours, la vitesse de prolifération des cellules survivantes est con-
sidérablement augmentée, par rapport aux tumeurs témoins. Quand la
tumeur est presque repeuplée la vitesse de croissance des cellules survivantes diminue et peut devenir plus lente que dans les tumeurs témoins.

Après administration d'une drogue cytotoxique, Skipper[39] a également
observé un raux élevé de repopulation de la tumeur par les cellules
clonogènes. On peut donc en conclure que la cinétique de prolifération
cellulaire des tumeurs survivantes est modifiée par le traitement et il

semble que cette accélération soit en partie due à un raccourcissement du cycle cellulaire et soit essentiellement causée par une augmentation du coefficient de prolifération.

Quant aux mécanismes en cause, ils sont encore discutés et peuvent être liés soit à la dépopulation qui augmente la quantité de matériaux nutritifs disponibles apporté par le système vasculaire, soit à libération de substances stimulantes par des cellules lésées.

Ainsi contrairement à ce que l'on pensait il y a quelques années, les cellules d'une tumeur ne restent pas indifférentes à l'action du traitement et réagissent en modifiant leurs caractéristiques de prolifération. Il y a là un phénomène voisin de celui constaté dans les tissus normaux où des mécanismes d'homéostasie stimulent la prolifération des cellules survivantes.

Tout l'art du traitement du cancer est d'utiliser les méthodes tuant sélectivement les cellules cancéreuses. Pour améliorer nos techniques de traitement, il faut donc choisir non seulement celles qui ont un maximum d'efficacité sur les tissus malins, mais encore les rythmes d'irradiation ou d'administration de drogues qui épargnent au maximum les tissus sains critiques. Ceux-ci sont dans le cas d'une irradiation ceux qui se trouvent dans la zone irradiée ou pendant une chimiothérapie ceux qui sont les plus sensibles, généralement la moelle osseuse et l'intestin.

Chaque tissu sain a sa propre façon de réagir à des agressions[28] tantôt en augmentant la proportion de cellules engagées dans un cycle tantôt en augmentant le nombre d'assises cellulaires au niveau desquelles les cellules peuvent se multiplier, tantôt enfin en raccourcissant la durée du cycle. De plus les mécanismes qui déclenchent ces réactions et le moment où celles-ci surviennent diffèrent d'un tissu à l'autre[28] il est donc nécessaire d'apprendre à les connaître puisqu'il faut en tenir compte, au même titre que celle des tissus cancéreux, dans la conduite du traitement.

Dans le cas d'une radiothérapie, comme le champ d'irradiation est limité, il faut également tenir compte des phénomènes de migration cellulaire qui déterminent un repeuplement des zones irradiées. L'accroissement de l'efficacité des méthodes thérapeutiques nécessite donc un important effort en recherche fondamentale et appliquée. Celui-ci doit être l'object d'une collaboration étroite entre cliniciens et chercheurs scientifiques. Les cliniciens doivent se familiariser avec la rigueur des méthodes scientifiques et avoir recours aux techniques statistiques pour établir un protocole thérapeutique et en exploiter les résultats. Les chercheurs doivent orienter leurs expériences en fonction des problèmes pratiques que pose la thérapeutique.

References

1. Barendsen, G. W., and J. J. Broerse: Experimental radiotherapy of a rat rhabdomyosarcoma with 15 MeV neutrons and 300 kV x-rays. I. Effects of single exposure. Europ. J. Cancer, 5:373-391, 1969.

2. Barrett, J. C.: A mathematical model of the mitotic cycle and its application to the interpretation of percentage labeled mitoses data. J. Nat. Cancer Inst., 37: 443-450, 1966.
3. Bennington, J. L.: Cellular kinetics of invasive squamous carcinoma of the human cervix. Cancer Res., 29:1082-1088, 1969.
4. Bergsagel, D. E., and F. A. Valeriote: Growth characteristics of a mouse plasma cell tumor. Cancer Res., 28:2187-2196, 1968.
5. Bresciani, F.: Cell proliferation in cancer. Europ. J. Cancer, 4:343-366, 1968.
6. Brown, J. M., and R. J. Berry: Effects of x-irradiation on cell proliferation in normal epithelium and in tumours of the hamster cheek pouch. In: Effects of Radiation on Cellular Proliferation and Differentiation, I.A.E.A., 1968, pp. 475-491.
7. Charbit, A., E. Malaise, and M. Tubiana: Europ. J. Cancer. Submitted for publication.
8. Choquet, C., N. Chavaudra, and N. Malaise: The influence of allogenic inhibition and tumour age on the kinetics of L 1210 leukemia in vivo. Europ. J. Cancer. In press.
9. Clarkson, B., K. Ota, T. Okhita, and A. O'Connor: Kinetics of proliferation of cancer cells in neoplastic effusions in man. Cancer, 18:1189-1213, 1965.
10. Denekamp, J.: Personal communication.
11. Dormer, P., H. Tulinius, and W. Oehlert: Untersuchungen über die Generationszeit, DNS-Synthesezeit und Mitosedauer von Zellen der hyperplastischen Emidermis und des Plattenepithelial Carcinoms der Maus nach Methylcholanthrenpinselung. Z. Krebsforsch., 66:11-28, 1964.
12. Ellis, F.: Dose-time and fractionation: A clinical hypothesis. Clin. Radiol., 20:1-7, 1969.
13. Fabrikant, J. I., C. L. Wisseman, and Vitak: The kinetics of cellular proliferation in normal and malignant tissues. II. An in vitro method for incorporation of tritiated thymidine in human tissues. Radiology, 92:1309-1321, 1969.
14. Frankfurt, O. S.: Cell proliferation and differentiation in the squamous epithelium of the forestomach of the mouse. Exp. Cell Res., 46:603-606, 1967.
15. Frankfurt, O. S.: Mitotic cycle and cell differentiation in squamous cell carcinomas. Int. J. Cancer, 2:304-310, 1967.
16. Frindel, E., and M. Tubiana: Durée du cycle cellulaire au cours de la croissance d'une ascite expérimentale de la souris C3H. Compt. Rend. Acad. Sci. (Paris), 265D:829, 1967.
17. Frindel, E., F. Charruyer, M. Tubiana, H. S. Kaplan, and E. L. Alpen: Radiation effects on DNA synthesis and cell division in the bone marrow of the mouse. Int. J. Rad. Biol., 11:435-443, 1966.
18. Frindel, E., E. Malaise, E. Alpen, and M. Tubiana: Kinetics of cell proliferation of an experimental tumor. Cancer Res., 27:1122, 1967.
19. Frindel, E., E. Malaise, and M. Tubiana: Cell proliferation kinetics in five human solid tumors. Cancer, 22:611-620, 1968.
20. Frindel, E., A. J. Valleron, F. Vassort, and M. Tubiana: Proliferation kinetics of an experimental ascites tumour of the mouse. Cell Tissue Kinet., 2:51-65, 1969.
21. Frindel, E., F. Vassort, and M. Tubiana: Effects of irradiation on the cell cycle of an experimental ascites tumor of the mouse. Int. J. Rad. Biol., 17:329, 1970.
22. Hahn, G. M., J. R. Stewart, S. J. Yang, and V. Parker: Chinese hamster cell monolayer cultures. I. Changes in cell dynamics and modifications of the cell cycle with the period of growth. Exp. Cell Res., 49:285-292, 1968.
23. Hermens, A. F., and G. W. Barendsen: Cellular proliferation patterns in an experimental rhabdomyosarcoma in the rat. Europ. J. Cancer, 3:361, 1967.
24. Hermens, A. F., and G. W. Barendsen: Changes of cell proliferation characteristics in a rat rhabdomyosarcoma before and after the x-irradiation. Europ. J. Cancer, 5:173-191, 1969.
25. Killman, S. A.: The kinetics of leukemic blast cells in man. Ser. Haematol., 1:38-102, 1968.

26. Lala, P. K., and H. M. Patt: Cytokinetic analysis of tumor growth. Proc. Nat. Acad. Sci. USA, 56:1735-1742, 1966.
27. Lala, P. K., and H. M. Patt: A characterization of the boundary between the cycling and resting states in ascites tumor cells. Cell Tissue Kinet., 1:137-146, 1968.
28. Lamerton, L. F., and G. G. Steel: Cell population kinetics in normal and malignant tissues. Progr. Biophys. Molec. Biol., 18:247-283, 1968.
29. Malaise, E., and M. Tubiana: Croissance des cellules d'un fibrosarcome expérimental irradié chez la souris C3H. Compt. Rend. Acad. Sci. (Paris), 263D:292-295, 1966.
30. Malaise, E., E. Frindel, and M. Tubiana: Cinétique de la prolifération cellulaire de deux tumeurs humaines étudiée grâce à l'injection de thymidine tritiée. Compt. Rend. Acad. Sci. (Paris), 264D:1104, 1967.
31. Malaise, E., and M. Tubiana: Etude in vitro de certains facteurs susceptibles d'influencer la croissance d'une ascite expérimentale. Compt. Rend. Acad. Sci. (Paris), 270D:539-542, 1970.
32. Mendelsohn, M. L.: Autoradiographic analysis of cell proliferation in spontaneous breast cancer of C3H mouse. III. The growth fraction. J. Nat. Cancer Inst., 28:1015-1030, 1962.
33. Owen, L. N., and G. G. Steel: The growth and cell population kinetics of spontaneous tumours in domestic animals. Brit. J. Cancer, 23:493-509, 1969.
34. Post, J., and J. Hoffman: The replication time and pattern of carcinogen induced hepatoma cells. J. Cell Biol., 22:341-350, 1964.
35. Post, J., and J. Hoffman: Further studies on the replication of rat liver cells in vivo. Exp. Cell Res., 40:333-339, 1965.
36. Rajewski, M. F.: Zell Proliferation in normalen und malignen Geweben: ³H Thymidine Einbau in vitro unter Standardbedingungen. Biophysik., 3:65, 1966.
37. Rambert, P., E. Malaise, A. Laugier, M. Schlienger, and M. Tubiana: Données sur la vitesse de croissance des tumeurs humaines. Bull. Cancer, 55:323-342, 1968.
38. Reiskin, A. B., and R. J. Berry: Cell proliferation and carcinogenesis in the hamster cheek pouch. Cancer Res., 28:898-905, 1968.
39. Skipper, H. E.: Biochemical, biological, pharmacologic, toxicologic, kinetic and clinical (subhuman and human) relationship. Cancer, 21:600-610, 1968.
40. Steel, G. G.: Cell loss as a factor in the growth rate of human tumours. Europ. J. Cancer, 3:381-387, 1967.
41. Steel, G. G.: Cell loss from experimental tumours. Cell Tissue Kinet., 2:193-207, 1968.
42. Tannock, I. F.: The relation between cell proliferation and the vascular system in a transplanted mouse mammary tumour. Brit. J. Cancer, 22:258-273, 1968.
43. Tannock, I. F.: A comparison of cell proliferation parameters in solid and ascites Ehrlich tumors. Cancer Res., 29:1527-1534, 1969.
44. Tubiana, M., E. Frindel, and E. Malaise: In vitro cell kinetics of human cancer. In: Recent Results in Cancer Research, Vol. 17, Normal and Malignant Cell Growth (R. J. N. Fry, M. L. Griem, and W. H. Kirsten, eds.), Springer Verlag, New York, 1969, pp. 202-217.
45. Tubiana, M., E. Frindel, and E. Malaise: The application of radiobiologic knowledge and cellular kinetics to radiation therapy. Amer. J. Roentgenol., 102:822-831, 1968.
46. Wiebel, F., and R. Baserga: Cell proliferation in newly transplanted Ehrlich ascites tumour cells. Cell Tissue Kinet., 1:273-289, 1968.
47. Young, R. C., and V. T. De Vita: Cell cycle characteristics of human solid tumors in vivo. Nature. In press.
48. Young, J. M., and J. F. Fowler: The effect of x-ray induced synchrony on two-dose cell survival experiments. Cell Tissue Kinet., 2:95-111, 1969.

Basic Problems of Cell Growth and Its Control

RENATO BASERGA

Department of Pathology and Fels Research Institute, Temple University School of Medicine, Philadelphia, Pennsylvania, USA

THE ULTIMATE GOAL of cancer research in general, and of research on tumor growth in particular, is to arrest tumor growth, that is, to control the proliferation of tumor cells. Therefore, a study of the basic problems of cell growth and its control is of fundamental importance if we are to understand the natural history of cancer and to design a rational therapeutic approach to it. The purpose of this paper is to discuss and identify the possible targets or target areas for the inhibition of tumor growth.

It is generally agreed that cells of the adult animal can be divided, as far as DNA synthesis and cell division are concerned, into three populations, namely: (1) continuously dividing cells that move around the cell cycle, (2) cells that leave the cycle and are destined to die without dividing again, and (3) quiescent cells that usually do not synthesize DNA or divide but can be stimulated to do so by an appropriate stimulus.[1] Cells representing these three types of populations are well known, and I can only add here that the same types of populations can be found in growing tumors. In tumors, too, we have continuously dividing cells, cells that leave the cell cycle but may re-enter it under favorable circumstances, and cells that die. It is upon the length of the cell cycle and the variable admixture of these three types of cells that the growth of a tumor depends. The question I would like to ask in this brief discussion is: What are the factors that control the length of the cell cycle and the shifting of tumor cells from one kind of population to the other, i.e., that control the growth of a tumor? The purpose, as mentioned above, is to identify some target areas where one can apply restrictive controls on the growth of tumors.

I must immediately confess that I will completely omit from this discussion the causes of cell loss, since, apart from cell death attributable to gross vascular abnormalities, we know very little about the causative factors leading to the death of a tumor cell. I will, instead, consider the biochemical events that control the onset of DNA synthesis and, therefore, cell division. I said: therefore, cell division, because although cell division and DNA synthesis can be dissociated and sometimes are dissociated, in the great majority of cases a cell that is synthesizing DNA is a cell that has taken the decision to divide. In fact, in bacteria, K. G. Lark[20] has formally demonstrated that cell division is controlled by DNA replication and that termination of DNA replication automatically triggers a cycle of division. Similarly, in bacteria, it has been shown that the initiation of DNA synthesis is controlled by specific genes. For instance, Mendelsohn and Gross[23] have found several lethal mutants of *Bacillus subtilis* in which the mutation affects the initiation of DNA synthesis although DNA polymerase activity is at normal levels and the concentration of the deoxynucleotide precursors necessary for DNA synthesis is also at normal levels. It is not unreasonable to extrapolate these results to mammalian cells in which, at any rate, there is already overwhelming evidence that the genome itself is involved in the control of DNA replication. The evidence has been discussed in detail in a recently published book (Baserga[1]), and I will not go into further detail in this paper.

I will, instead, discuss some of the biochemical events that have already been reported in the literature and are known to precede and regulate the onset of DNA synthesis in mammalian cells either in continuously dividing cells or in quiescent cells that can be stimulated to synthesize DNA by an appropriate stimulus. The first biochemical event in G_1 that could be related to the onset of DNA synthesis was the finding by Baserga et al.[3] in 1965 that in the G_1 of Ehrlich ascites tumor cells there was a step sensitive to very small doses of actinomycin D. If this step, presumably RNA synthesis, was inhibited, the onset of DNA synthesis was prevented. A similar actinomycin D-sensitive step was identified by Baserga et al.[4] in the G_1 phase of epithelial cells of the crypt of the mouse jejunum. Several reports since have shown that in mammalian cells the synthesis of some kind of RNA is necessary a few hours before the entrance of cells into the S phase. Protein synthesis was also found to be necessary during several steps in the G_1 period for the ordinate flow of cells into the S phase. The first demonstration goes back to the findings of Terasima and Yasukawa[28] in synchronized L cells, where they found that two-hr periods of exposure to either puromycin or cycloheximide produced a two-hr delay in the onset of DNA synthesis. Of particular significance were the findings of Borun et al.[6] that one hr before the onset of DNA synthesis an RNA messenger for histone synthesis was made in synchronized HeLa cells. The RNA messenger for histones appears on cytoplasmic ribosomes one hr before the onset of DNA synthesis, and since inhibition of histone synthesis promptly leads to inhibition of DNA synthesis, the lack of the appropriate mRNA also leads to failure of cells to initiate DNA synthesis.

Two enzymes are missing from G_1 cells that are present in cells in the S phase, namely, thymidine kinase, as demonstrated by Brent et al.,[7] and deoxycytidylate deaminase, as demonstrated in HeLa cells by Gelbard et al.[13] The synthesis of these two enzymes has also been demonstrated to be necessary for the initiation of DNA synthesis. It is interesting to note that DNA polymerase activity, instead, is not decreased in continuously dividing cells during the G_1 period. A few other findings ought to be mentioned in connection with the G_1 period, namely: (1) Buell and Fahey[8] have shown that in human lymphoid cell lines the synthesis of immunoglobulins begins in late G_1 and continues throughout the S phase up to mitosis; (2) Steward et al.[26] reported that polyribosomes in the cytoplasm are reformed immediately after mitosis using pre-existing mRNA; and (3) in mouse leukemic lymphoblasts Jung and Rothstein[19] showed that at the end of the G_1 period and extending into the very early part of the S phase there is a marked decrease in potassium content of the cell accompanied by an increase in cellular sodium content. These results, although fragmentary, seem to indicate that during the G_1 period there is a series of orderly metabolic events, some of which involve gene expression. There are, in fact, steps that require the synthesis of new proteins and of new RNA molecules.

This series of events, however, is better illustrated in the quiescent cells that can be stimulated to synthesize DNA and divide by an appropriate stimulus. This is because the events are spread over a longer time and can be identified with greater precision. As an illustration of G_0 cells, if one wishes to use this terminology, I would like to take the isoproterenol-stimulated salivary glands in which the acinar cells of the parotid and of the submandibular gland are stimulated to synthesize DNA and then divide by a single administration of isoproterenol, a synthetic catecholamine. The series of metabolic events that occur between the administration of isoproterenol at zero time and the burst of mitoses that occurs 30 hr later has been summarized in a previous paper.[2] There is first an interaction of the hydroxyl groups of the phenyl ring of isoproterenol with a receptor in the salivary gland cell; and after that, a series of metabolic events which include secretion, activation of adenyl cyclase, synthesis of proteins, synthesis of RNA templates, then again a burst of protein synthesis in the free ribosome fraction accompanied by changes in certain enzymes, especially uridylate kinase. Then, accompanied by changes in the concentration of glycogen, there is synthesis of the templates that code for a number of enzymes necessary for the synthesis of DNA. These enzymes appear just before or at the time of the onset of DNA synthesis which, in turn, is accompanied by histone synthesis. Finally, when the genome and the chromosomal proteins have been replicated, the cell is ready for mitosis. It should be stressed that these events have been found to be relevant to the onset of DNA synthesis and mitosis by the appropriate use of inhibitors and by manipulations that clearly showed that the inhibition of these events led to selective inhibition of DNA synthesis and cell division.

A similar sequence of metabolic events has been described in several other models of stimulated DNA synthesis, among which the best known are the regenerating liver after partial hepatectomy and the lymphocyte stimulated by phytohemagglutinin. Notice in the above description the orderly alternation of RNA and protein synthesis like a Ping-Pong mechanism that unlocks the door to the replication of nuclear DNA. Again, in this model as well as in other models of stimulated DNA synthesis, the evidence is substantial that the integrity of the genome is necessary for the triggering of the sequence of metabolic events eventually leading to cell division.

Both the G_1 phase of continuously dividing cells and the extended G_0 phase of quiescent cells stimulated to synthesize DNA and divide are possible target areas for a chemotherapeutic action against tumor growth. At the present moment it goes without saying that we do not have a clue about an effective inhibitor that will not be toxic to normal cells. The remaining part of this discussion will therefore be devoted to an analysis of the regulatory mechanisms of DNA synthesis and cell division in mammalian cells.

A first postulate that is necessary for an intelligent discussion of this problem is, as I have mentioned, based on the considerable amount of evidence that the control of cell division resides in the genetic material in the nucleus. The nucleus receives cytoplasmic signals which determine whether the genes controlling DNA synthesis should be derepressed. This is logical, since cell division obviously must depend on environmental conditions, but it has been made experimentally certain by the work of Henry Harris[17] and co-workers with heterokaryons, and by the work of Graham[15] and Merriam[24] on the activation of brain nuclei inserted into frog eggs. Cytoplasmic signals from the host cell can activate these nuclei and induce in them first RNA synthesis and then DNA synthesis. In addition, Prescott and Goldstein[25] have shown in amoeba that there is a continuous shuttle of proteins between nucleus and cytoplasm and that the cytoplasm of S phase amoeba cells can induce DNA synthesis in transplanted G_2 nuclei. In ordinary circumstances, the nucleus does not receive signals from the cytoplasm calling for DNA synthesis. These signals are proteins which presumably are synthesized de novo in the cytoplasm after stimulation. Acidic nuclear proteins are an excellent candidate for this particular class of proteins that are synthesized de novo in the cytoplasm after stimulation, migrate to the nucleus, and there may derepress that segment of the genome that controls the replication of DNA.[30]

In turn, the translational control of the synthesis of nuclear acidic proteins may be asserted by another class of proteins that are presumably lost from the cytoplasm after a stimulus. That proteins are lost from the cytoplasm in a variety of models of stimulated DNA synthesis is well known. In the regenerating liver after partial hepatectomy there is an increased outpouring of albumin into the circulation.[21] The loss of gamma globulins increases in lymphocytes stimulated with phytohemagglutinin,[11] and in the isoproterenol-stimulated salivary gland the violent secretion produced by the synthetic catecholamine is accompanied by a decided loss of cytoplasmic proteins.[9] In fact, Sudweeks and Hill[27] have been able to induce DNA synthesis in liver cells by plasmaphoresis, that is, by simply removing the plasma proteins from the blood, thus causing an increased secretion of albumin into the blood stream. Loss of cytoplasmic proteins can be controlled in a more subtle way by the permeability of the cell membrane, and a very early loss of intracellular amino acids has been demonstrated by Wiebel and Baserga[29] in stimulated human diploid fibroblasts. The next question is: What changes in the cell cause a loss of cytoplasmic material which, in some cases, can become so imposing as to be revealed by the loss of large macromolecules? Glick and co-workers[14] have shown that removal of sialic acid from the cell surface impedes the secretion of cytoplasmic proteins, and Defendi and Gasic[10] have demonstrated that in transformed cells in culture in which DNA synthesis is stimulated, the amount of sialic acid on the cell surface coat is greatly increased. Several workers have reported an increase in negative charges on the surface of cells stimulated to divide or on the surface of rapidly proliferating cells.[5, 12, 18]

It therefore seems possible to present the following hypothesis on the control of cell division in mammalian cells. While it is a hypothesis, it is also compatible with presently available evidence, and what is not supported by presently available evidence can easily be tested experimentally; therefore it can be quickly either proved or disproved. The hypothesis states that an environmental stimulus causes a change in the cell surface which leads to an increase in the sum of negative charges of the cell surface coat. This is followed by the loss of cytoplasmic material, presumably including some specific repressor materials which inhibit the synthesis of certain acidic proteins. As this repressor material is lost, acidic proteins are synthesized in the cytoplasm (their synthesis being under translational control) and migrate afterwards to the nucleus where they derepress the segment of the genome that controls the initiation of DNA synthesis and therefore of cell division. It seems, therefore, that a profitable area for investigation in the near future will be the identification of the macromolecules that control the expression of the genes that in turn regulate the onset of DNA synthesis and cell division. Since it has been possible to identify and isolate the repressor proteins that control the expression of certain specific genes in bacteria and phage, it is not impossible to hope that a similar achievement in mammalian cells may be possible in the near future. One should not be frightened by the magnitude of the task. The incredible difference in the description of the cell's interphase in textbooks of anatomy or biochemistry of only 10 years ago and what we now know about the cell cycle of cells is indicative of how rapid progress can be.

Acknowledgments

This work was supported by U. S. Public Health Service Research Grants CA-08373 and CA-05222 of the National Cancer Institute, and DE-02678 of the National Institute for Dental Research.

References

1. Baserga, R.: Biochemistry of Cell Division. Charles C Thomas, Springfield, Illinois, 1969.
2. Baserga, R.: Control of DNA Biosynthesis in Mammalian Cells. The Second Annual Biochemistry—PCRI Winter Symposia, Miami, Florida, 1970.
3. Baserga, R., R. D. Estensen, and R. O. Petersen: Proc. Nat. Acad. Sci. USA, 54:1141, 1965.
4. Baserga, R., R. D. Estensen, and R. O. Petersen: J. Cell. Physiol., 68:177, 1966.
5. Ben-Or, S., S. Eisenberg, and F. Doljanski: Nature, 188:1200, 1960.
6. Borun, T. W., M. D. Scharff, and E. Robbins: Proc. Nat. Acad. Sci. USA, 58:1977, 1967.
7. Brent, T. P., J. A. V. Butler, and A. R. Crathorn: Nature, 207:176, 1965.
8. Buell, D. N., and J. L. Fahey: Science, 164: 1524, 1969.
9. Byrt, P.: Nature, 212:1212, 1966.
10. Defendi, V., and G. Gasic: J. Cell. Comp. Physiol., 62:23, 1963.
11. Fisher, D. B., and G. C. Mueller: Proc. Nat. Acad. Sci. USA, 60:1396, 1968.
12. Forrester, J. A., and E. J. Ambrose: Nature, 196:1068, 1962.
13. Gelbard, A. S., J. H. Kim, and A. G. Perez: Biochim. Biophys. Acta, 182:564, 1969.
14. Glick, J. L., A. R. Goldberg, and A. B. Pardee: Cancer Res., 26:1774, 1966.
15. Graham, C. F.: J. Cell Sci., 1:363, 1966.
16. Gurdon, J. B.: Proc. Nat. Acad. Sci. USA, 58:545, 1967.
17. Harris, H.: J. Cell Sci., 2:23, 1967.
18. Heard, D. H., G. F. V. Seaman, and I. Simon-Reuss: Nature, 190:1009, 1961.
19. Jung, C., and A. Rothstein: J. Gen. Physiol., 50:917, 1967.
20. Lark, K. G.: Biochim. Biophys. Acta, 45:121, 1960.
21. Majumdar, C., K. Tsukada, and I. Lieberman: J. Biol. Chem., 242:700, 1967.
22. Martin, D., Jr., G. M. Tomkins, and D. Granner: Proc. Nat. Acad. Sci. USA, 62: 248, 1969.
23. Mendelsohn, N. H., and J. D. Gross: J. Bacteriol., 94:1603, 1967.
24. Merriam, R. W.: J. Cell Sci., 5:333, 1969.
25. Prescott, D. M., and L. Goldstein: Science, 155:469, 1967.
26. Steward, D. L., J. R. Shaeffer, and R. M. Humphrey: Science, 161:791, 1968.
27. Sudweeks, A. D., and R. B. Hill, Jr.: J. Cell Biol., 34:404, 1967.
28. Terasima, T., and M. Yasukawa: Exp. Cell Res., 44:669, 1966.
29. Wiebel, F., and R. Baserga: J. Cell. Physiol., 74:191, 1969.
30. Stein, G., and R. Baserga: Unpublished data.

Gompertz Analysis of Fast- and Slow-Growing Tumor Lines

ANNA KANE LAIRD

Illinois State Psychiatric Institute, Chicago, Illinois, USA

GROWTH OF TUMORS was for many years assumed to be a simple exponential growth process, produced by the free binary fission of the constituent cells. Tumor growth is now known to be considerably retarded in comparison with a simple exponential process; specifically, the retardation of exponential growth is itself an exponential process continuous throughout the growth of the tumor.[2, 3]

Exponential retardation of exponential growth is represented by an equation of the Gompertz type:

$$W(t) = W_o \, e^{\frac{A_o}{\alpha} (1 - e^{-\alpha t})}$$

in which W_0 is the tumor mass or volume at the start of the period of measurement, A_0 is the specific growth rate at the same instant, and α is the rate of exponential decay of A_0.[6]

When the growth rate of a tumor is altered by clinical or experimental manipulation, two theoretically different kinds of change are possible: the time scale of the growth process may have become longer or shorter (the kind of rate change we are familiar with in everyday life), or the degree of retardation of the growth process may have become greater or less, resulting in a change in the steepness of the growth curve so that it resembles exponential growth more or less so than before.

In the present paper, the use of the Gompertz equation for analyzing differences in growth rate observed in a fast- and a slow-growing tumor line is illustrated.

Material and Methods

Data on the growth of individual tumors of their fast and slow tumor lines were kindly furnished by Drs. M. L. Mendelsohn and L. A. Dethlefsen of the University of Pennsylvania.[7] The tumors were isoimplants of C3H mouse mammary tumors selected from spontaneous tumors on the basis of their growth characteristics. The two lines were distinguishable by the second generation, and were maintained for a number of generations.

TABLE 10–4.—GOMPERTZ CONSTANTS OF FAST AND SLOW GROWING TUMORS

ORDINAL NUMBER	FAST a	A_0/a^*	A_N/a^*	SLOW a	$3a$	A_0/a^*	A_N/a^*
1	.011	25.4	22.0	.004	.012	22.0	18.0
2	.012	22.6	17.5	.004	.012	19.0	18.9
3	.016	10.8	4.7	.005	.015	17.5	14.8
4	.018	6.9	5.0	.006	.018	8.0	5.2
5	.023	6.9	3.9	.007	.021	9.4	6.5
6	.028	6.0	3.1	.008	.024	7.0	3.9
7	.029	8.4	4.2	.009	.027	6.4	4.1
8	.031	10.1	5.5	.009	.027	7.5	3.7
9	.037	11.4	7.3	.010	.030	10.4	7.2
10	.039	6.0	3.3	.010	.030	6.5	3.1
11	.040	5.6	.77	.010	.030	8.5	5.1
12	.044	9.3	4.7	.014	.042	5.4	2.6
13	.049	8.9	4.1	.014	.042	7.7	3.9
14	.050	5.7	2.1	.015	.045	5.3	3.4
15	.050	8.8	4.2	.015	.045	6.3	3.7
16	.051	9.2	4.3	.016	.048	8.1	2.8
17	.058	4.5	1.1	.016	.048	7.9	2.4
18	.061	7.6	2.2	.017	.051	5.5	1.8
19	.063	7.4	2.7	.018	.054	6.4	2.0
20	.064	5.1	1.1	.019	.057	5.7	1.4
21	.070	8.2	2.5	.020	.060	4.3	1.2
22	.071	4.4	.39	.021	.063	7.8	2.7
23	.072	8.6	3.1	.024	.072	5.8	.95
24	.075	6.2	2.5	.026	.078	6.2	.99
25	.079	5.9	1.2	.027	.081	6.6	.89
26	.081	6.6	2.0	.031	.093	6.3	.72
27	.096	3.5	.63	.032	.096	5.4	.46
28	.097	7.3	1.7	.036	.108	3.9	.70
29	.101	4.5	.90	.041	.123	5.0	.51
30	.103	5.5	1.3	.041	.123	4.1	.57
31	.110	7.1	1.9	.042	.126	4.1	.46
32	.127	5.0	.85	.048	.144	3.1	.60
33	.128	3.3	.23	.048	.144	2.7	.52
34	.158	4.1	.38	.049	.147	4.3	.30
35	.163	4.7	.78	.068	.204	5.0	.32
36	.195	3.4	.33	.098	.294	3.4	.26

* Values less than 1.0 indicate points lying beyond the inflection point of the growth curve.

Individual tumors were implanted in subcutaneous sites, and were measured at frequent, irregular intervals, never greater than three days. The total number of measurements of each tumor varied from about 10 to more than 30; most tumors were measured 14 or more times. The tumor volume was determined as reported by Dethlefsen, Prewitt and Mendelsohn.[1]

The Gompertz equation was fitted to the set of volume measurements of each tumor; the weighting factor was $1/W^2$, and estimates were obtained of W_0, A_0 and α, with their standard errors. By algebraic manipulation of the growth equation, estimates were also obtained for the value of A_N, the specific growth rate at the time of the last tumor measurement. In all, data on 36 fast and 36 slow tumors were fitted and compared with respect to α, A_0/α, and A_N/α.

Results

The results of fitting the Gompertz equation to these data are shown in Table 10-4. To facilitate the comparison, the tumors of the fast and slow lines were listed in the order of increasing values of α, and then the two lists were matched. The values for α extended over a wide range for both the fast and slow tumors, as can be seen from Table 10-4, but the two lists were very closely matched when the values of α for the slow tumors were multiplied by three. This result indicates that not only were the fast tumors on the average three times faster, but that the two populations consisted of the same representation of variability.

FIG. 10–1.—Gompertz curves fitted to the growth measurements of a fast- and a slow-growing tumor. This is a matched pair of tumors from Table 10-4. The portions of the Gompertz curves shown are corresponding segments of the curves. In this example, the slow-growing tumor was two times as large as the fast tumor when passing through corresponding segments of the curve.

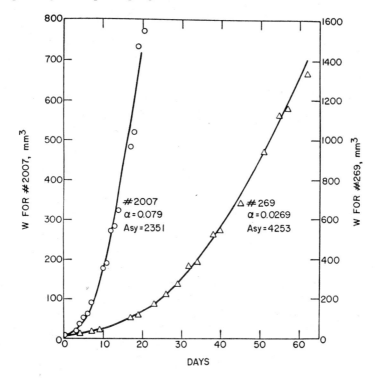

The two tumor lines were then compared with respect to the ratio of A_0/α and A_N/α, also shown in Table 10-4. The much greater scatter of these values is partly an artifact caused by differences in the point on the growth curve at which the first and last tumor measurements fell (since the tumors were measured at intervals of a day or sometimes several days). This scatter is fortunately not so great that it obscures the fact that the two lines are quite similar with respect to the values of A_0/α and A_N/α.

Figure 10-1 shows an example of a matched pair of tumors from the fast and slow tumor lines. The first and last points on the two curves are at very nearly the same position on the curves, and therefore the only difference between the two curves is the time span occupied by the same segment of the growth curve. Incidentally, absolutely the only way any two tumors can be compared is by observing identical segments of the curve; otherwise continuous changes in doubling times, specific growth rates, and absolute growth rates are so rapid that one cannot be sure whether observed differences are real properties of the growth curves, or are simply artifacts attributable to noncorresponding parts of the curve being compared.

Discussion

The present Gompertz analysis of a fast- and a slow-growing tumor line shows that the two lines differ only in the time scale of their growth curves. The degree of retardation, as expressed in the ratio of the retardation to the specific growth rate within the period of measurement, is the same for fast and slow tumors. Hence laboratory selection for fast and slow growth resulted in selection of tumors in terms of the day-to-day time scale of growth, and had no bearing on the exponentiality of the curves.

However, as these experiments show, change in the time scale of growth without change in the degree of deviation from exponential growth requires that the specific growth rate (A_0) and its rate of exponential decay (α) change pari passu, in order for their ratio to remain the same. But in a semilog plot of specific growth rate against time, in which the intercept is A_0, and the slope of the semilog line is α,[5] this coincidence requires that both the intercept and the slope must change in such a way as to keep the numerical ratio between them constant. It is clear that there is no mathematical reason for such a coincidence; it must be biologic. In terms of growth control, these results mean that both cell proliferation and its slowing are somehow bound together in these tumors.

A similar result was found several years ago[4] when data on the fetal growth of a number of birds and mammals were surveyed. In that case also, the time scale differed from species to species, but no significant variation was observed in the degree of departure from exponential

TABLE 10–5.—REGENERATION OF TRICHOGASTER FINS

STUMP % ORIGINAL FIN	W_0	A_0	α	ASYMPTOTE
25%	6.7 mm	.101	.055	42.1 mm
50%	16.8 mm	.046	.051	41.3 mm
75%	26.8 mm	.027	.066	40.2 mm

growth. In contrast, when a variety of tumors of several animal species was studied,[2, 3] tumors of the rat differed consistently from tumors of the mouse with respect to the degree of deviation from exponential growth. Rat tumors came much closer to following exponential growth than did mouse tumors. The species specificity of this effect suggests a genetic control of the relation between specific growth rate and its rate of exponential slowing.

Nevertheless, the constancy of this relation is not universal: simple inspection of the curves comparing regeneration of the fin of the opaline gourami (Trichogaster sp.) from stumps of different relative size[8] shows that in this case the segments of the observed growth curve are quite different. When these data were fitted by the Gompertz equation (unpublished results), the values of α were found to be essentially unchanged, whether the stump represented 25%, 50%, or 75% of the original fin, but the values of A_0, the specific growth rate at the start of regrowth, varied over a wide range, in roughly inverse proportion to the size of the stump (Table 10-5).

Such studies should be extended in the hope that if we understand the biologic nature of the relation between exponential growth and its rate of retardation, we might have a better understanding of growth control mechanisms generally.

References

1. Dethlefsen, L. A., J. M. S. Prewitt, and M. L. Mendelsohn: Analysis of tumor growth curves. J. Nat. Cancer Inst., 40:389-405, 1968.
2. Laird, A. K.: Dynamics of tumor growth. Brit. J. Cancer, 18:490-502, 1964.
3. Laird, A. K.: Dynamics of tumor growth: Comparison of growth rates and extrapolation of growth curves to one cell. Brit. J. Cancer, 19:278-291, 1965.
4. Laird, A. K.: Dynamics of embryonic growth. Growth, 30:263-75, 1966.
5. Laird, A. K.: Dynamics of growth in tumors and in normal organisms. Nat. Cancer Inst. Monogr., 30:15-28, 1969.
6. Laird, A. K., S. A. Tyler, and A. D. Barton: Dynamics of normal growth. Growth, 29:233-248, 1965.
7. Mendelsohn, M. L., and L. A. Dethlefsen: Cell proliferation and volumetric growth of fast line, slow line, and spontaneous C_3H mammary tumors. Proc. Amer. Ass. Cancer Res., 9:47, 1968.
8. Tassava, R. A., and R. J. Goss: Regeneration rate and amputation level in fish fins and lizard tails. Growth, 30:9-21, 1966.

Temporal and Metabolic Aspects of
Tumor Cell Cycles

M. F. RAJEWSKY

*Abteilung Physikalische Biologie, Max-Planck-Institut für
Virusforschung, Tübingen, Germany*

ALTHOUGH MALIGNANT GROWTH may in principle be described as the result of an imbalance between the rates of cell production and cell loss, recent advances in the analysis of the biochemistry of the cell cycle and the kinetics of cell proliferation have provided a basis for more detailed investigation of this complex process. To begin with, it seems necessary to recall that tumors of "clinically" detectable size are the product of multiple selection processes and represent late stages of malignant growth. Clearly, the history of a malignant tumor begins with the initiation and expression of malignant transformation in normal cell systems (if we leave aside the selection for pre-existing malignant cells[41] as a possible cause of cancer), and includes all subsequent stages during which the proliferation of the presumptive tumor cells gradually escapes control by the host. The present report will, therefore, also be concerned with some theoretical and experimental aspects of cell proliferation in relation to carcinogenesis and early malignant growth.

Malignant Tumors

A number of theoretical models have been proposed in order to describe the proliferative behavior of malignant tumors.[36] Basically, the growth rate of a tumor is characterized by the size of its proliferative fraction,[34] by the rate of cell loss from the system,[57] and by the distribution of cell cycle times of the proliferating cells. The growth rate of tumors usually decreases with time in a more or less pronounced manner and, as has been pointed out by Laird[28] and McCredie et al.,[33] can in many cases be approximated by a Gompertzian function.

With the possible exception of leukemic blasts, the mean cell cycle time in primary tumors has been found to be shorter than in the corresponding normal tissues.[5] In general, the proliferative fraction of primary tumors appears to be relatively low.[5] The degree of cell loss (because of cell death, exfoliation, or metastasis) increases with tumor size and is often surprisingly high. In certain tumors, cell loss factors of about 90% have been estimated.[58] Consequently, the observed volume-doubling times of primary tumors usually exceed the potential doubling times calculated on the basis of thymidine labeling or stath-mokinetic data.[58]

Unfortunately, the nonproliferating fraction does not consist only of cells which have irreversibly lost their reproductive capacity. Under certain conditions, nonproliferating cells may apparently re-enter the proliferative compartment.[35] This also implies that so-called "clonogen-ic" tumor cells (malignant stem cells),[6] i.e. cells with a capacity for un-limited multiplication in the host organism, may be present in both the proliferative and nonproliferative fraction of the population. In the latter case, such cells may escape therapeutic treatment when agents are used which are specifically directed against cycling cells or cells in defined stages of the cell cycle.

Although of particular interest, the conditions which enable non-cycling tumor cells to resume proliferation are still largely unknown. Restitution of the nutritional environment to a normal level may be an important factor, and Tannock[63] has found that with increasing dis-tance from a blood vessel, i.e. with decreasing oxygen concentration,[45] the proliferative fraction in a transplantable tumor decreased, where-as the distribution of cell-cycle times remained unchanged. However, other mechanisms, such as the immune response of the host and inter-cellular interactions, may also control the size of the proliferative fraction.

Conversely, there appear to be factors which specifically influence the duration of the different cell-cycle periods. For example, experi-mental data of Bresciani[5] show that high doses of ovarian hormones shorten the mean cell-cycle time in mammary alveolar cells of ovariec-tomized C3H mice by about 75%, while the proliferative fraction of this cell population remains unchanged. Mechanisms of this type may also be operative in cancer cells which have not completely lost their sensitivity to humoral control by the host.

An interesting difference between transplantable tumors grown in solid vs. ascitic form has recently emerged from the studies of several research groups.[17, 29, 63, 64, 68] It was demonstrated that the cell cycle time does not significantly change in the course of solid tumor growth, but increases considerably with age when the tumor is grown in the ascitic form.

The answer to the question of what makes cells leave or re-enter the proliferative compartment of a population ultimately lies in the clarification of the molecular mechanisms involved in the "decision" of a cell to initiate DNA replication and cell division. It is currently believed that this decision marks the "switching on" of a temporal sequence of interrelated gene transcriptions. The order of gene activa-tions in this process is thought to be maintained by the stepwise pro-duction of specific initiator proteins.[37, 42] All that can be said at pres-ent is that cells apparently make the decision to recycle early in the G_1 period, or may even be programmed during the preceding cell cycle.[2, 16, 26, 37] The control of this "decision mechanism" is a function of the genome of the particular cell. Although essential differences between normal and malignant cells may be sought at this level, the respective molecular processes are almost entirely unknown.

Carcinogenesis and Early Malignant Growth

In possible analogy to the differentiation of cells for specialized function,[13, 31, 61, 62, 66] there is evidence (though still indirect and incomplete) suggesting that DNA replication and cell division may play an important role in the process of carcinogenesis. It appears, for example, that under in vivo conditions, malignant growth may not be inducible in cell systems which do not contain proliferating cells or cells that can be triggered back into the cell cycle from a nonproliferative differentiated state. In support of this assumption is the fact that malignant tumors originating from nerve cells or muscle cells of the adult organism are extremely rare or even nonexistent. Conversely, all tissues with a high cancer incidence consist of proliferating cell populations of the steady-state renewing type.[4] Furthermore, the efficiency of many oncogenic agents and viruses seems to be more pronounced in embryonic or neonatal tissues with a high rate of cell proliferation than in the corresponding adult cell systems in steady state.[12, 23, 70]

In general, chemical carcinogens applied in vivo[9, 11, 22, 46, 50] as well as oncogenic viruses applied to cell cultures at high multiplicities[19, 20, 21, 24] seem to share the property of causing an elevated level of DNA synthesis and cell proliferation in the respective target cell populations. One example of this effect is the in vivo response of the parenchymal liver cell population to continuous administration of diethylnitrosamine.[46] The system exhibits the characteristic increase of the fraction of cells synthesizing DNA, following an initial depression. The elevated level, which in this case exceeds the control value by about a factor of three, is maintained until malignant growth becomes apparent in the form of multifocal microcarcinomas. Whether these alterations of proliferative parameters are specific effects of the carcinogenic agents, or rather represent a regenerative response to an increased rate of "toxic" cell inactivation is not clear, although in the case of many chemical carcinogens the latter explanation appears more likely.

Several carcinogenic (or very weakly carcinogenic to noncarcinogenic[67]) agents and viruses have been shown to exhibit a higher tumorigenicity when their application is combined with or followed by an additional stimulation of DNA replication and cell division in the respective target cell populations.[3, 10, 23, 30, 43, 54] Transformation studies in cell cultures using oncogenic viruses, ionizing radiation, or chemical carcinogens suggest that one or more rounds of DNA synthesis and cell division may be required after the initiating treatment before the transformed phenotype is completely established.[1, 8, 20, 52, 65] There is evidence indicating that temporary inhibition of DNA replication and cell division after initiation may result in a reduced transformation frequency.[20] The reduction of the tumorigenic effect of 7,12-dimethyl-benz (a) anthracene by application of actinomycin D shortly before or after treatment with the carcinogen[18] may also be attributable to interference with DNA replication and cell division during and immediately after initiation.

The described observations suggest the following questions: 1. Does the initiation of malignant transformation under in vivo conditions require proliferating cells (and/or "G_0" cells?) , and if so, are specific phases of the cell cycle (DNA replication?) particularly sensitive? 2. Following the initiating event, is a specific proliferative behavior of the target cell population required for the phenotypic expression of malignancy, and for providing the necessary selection pressure in favor of the transformed cells?

In addition to the availability of well-characterized target tissues, an investigation of these problems requires: (1) powerful single-dose "pulse carcinogens" with an in vivo half-life which is short compared with the duration of the cell cycle of the target cells, and (2) the possibility to presynchronize target cell populations in vivo (and to block specific macromolecular syntheses associated with defined cell cycle phases), in order to direct a carcinogen pulse to cells in specific phases of the cell cycle.

There is reason to believe that chemical compounds exist which could qualify as "pulse carcinogens" under in vivo conditions. The characterization of the ultimate reactant metabolites of chemical carcinogens and their kinetics of reaction with cellular targets are of particular importance in this context.

Some of the carcinogenic N-nitroso compounds may not persist in the organism for more than a few hours.[12] An example is the alkylating agent ethylnitrosourea (ENH) which is considered to be a very short-lived compound because of rapid heterolytic decomposition. By absorption measurements at $\lambda = 235$ nm, we have determined the half-life of ENH to be seven to eight min in M/15 phosphate buffer (pH 7.25; 37 C).[49] After administration of a single dose to pregnant rats, ENH has been shown to produce a high yield of malignant tumors in the offspring.[12]

However, the problem of synchronizing cell populations in vivo has not yet been adequately solved. Clearly, this point also has relevance to the analysis of the differential sensitivity of malignant cells during the cell cycle, and to the development of "cell cycle adapted" schemes of tumor therapy. In contrast to the variety of techniques available to produce synchronous or synchronized cell populations in culture,[56] the choice of methods is much more limited in the in vivo situation. On the basis of observations by Newton and Wildy[39] in HeLa cell cultures, the use of temperature changes would appear to be a possibility. This approach has been used by Martin and Schloerb[32] in their interesting study on the induction of mitotic synchrony by intermittent hyperthermia in the Walker 256 rat carcinoma. However, in spite of the encouraging results obtained by these authors, the applicability of temperature shifts for synchronization suffers from the difficulty that the mechanisms underlying the synchronizing effect are insufficiently understood. Conversely, methods based on the selection of a subpopulation of cells in a short fraction of the cell cycle (e.g. mitosis) without interfering with cellular metabolism are difficult to apply in vivo.

We have, therefore, attempted to synchronize proliferating cells for DNA synthesis in several normal tissues and in a transplantable tumor of the rat by temporary specific inhibition of DNA synthesis.[47–49] In the following, some of the results obtained in these experiments will be described.

In Vivo Synchronization of Normal and Malignant Cell Systems by Temporary Inhibition of DNA Synthesis

The procedure used is based on the idea that during the block of DNA synthesis, S cells are prevented from completing DNA synthesis, while cells in G_2, M, and G_1 continue their way through the cell cycle, and accumulate at the G_1-S boundary or in early S. Reversal of the block will then release a partially synchronized population of cells. The degree of synchrony after a single block depends on the duration of the block, on the duration of the S period relative to the cell cycle time, and on the spread of cell cycle times in the population. In addition, the degree of synchrony may be influenced by effects of the inhibitor at the cellular and molecular level; for example, if the inhibitor causes cell inactivation, or changes in the cell cycle parameters of the original asynchronous population.

In the ideal case, both "switching on" and "switching off" of the block should occur as instantaneously as possible. Since the use of hydroxyurea (HU) for specific inhibition of DNA synthesis[48, 69] proved to fulfill these requirements rather well, this agent was exclusively applied in the present studies.

Although the mechanism underlying the inhibitory effect of HU in mammalian cells is still under discussion, there is evidence indicating that the agent may be effective at the level of ribonucleotide reduction.[27] When administered at a dose resulting in a tissue concentration of about 10^{-4} to 10^{-3} moles/10^3 g, HU inhibits DNA synthesis almost completely and instantaneously.[48] The rate of incorporation of ^{3}H-thymidine into different rat tissues during the block was generally between 0.5 and 2.0% of the unblocked control, when measured by liquid scintillation spectrometry after careful elimination of acid-soluble material.[49] As suggested by the short time-constant for the clearance of the agent from the tissues, blocks are reversed almost without delay when the tissue concentration of the inhibitor falls below the critical range.

To analyze the short- and long-term kinetic response to HU blocks of varying duration, a solid transplantable rat mammary tumor (BICR/M1R)[48] was used as a model cell system. This tumor is a subline of the original BICR/M1 tumor,[59] and has been maintained in the author's laboratory since 1965 by transplantation in female isogeneic rats of the Marshall strain. Its cell-cycle parameters were determined by the labeled mitoses method[44] and analyzed with an optimizing computer technique[60] assuming an independent log normal distribution of the phase durations. A recent analysis[60] in the original BICR/M1 line gave almost identical values for the median cell cycle time and for t_{G_2}, but somewhat different values were found for t_S (7.9 ± 2.4 hr) and t_{G_1} (8.3 ± 3.6 hr). The kinetic response of the system following inhibition of DNA synthesis by HU was recorded by measuring the fractions of cells in DNA synthesis and mitosis as a function of time after reversal of the blocks. The data were evaluated by comparison with the kinetics predicted on the basis of the parameters of the asynchronous population.

HU is known to inactivate S cells and cells accumulating at the G_1-S boundary when applied in high concentrations or for extended periods of time.[25, 40, 55] In the latter case, inactivation of cells is likely to be attributable to "unbalanced growth"[14, 51] by excessive dissociation of macromolecular syntheses. The fate of the S and G_1-S subpopulations was therefore followed by prelabeling the cells blocked in S with tritiated thymidine, and recording the passage of labeled and unlabeled cells through their first postblock division.

The short term response of the BICR/M1R system to inhibition of DNA synthesis for five and 10 hr, respectively, was examined. The steep rise in the proportion of cells synthesizing DNA ($n_S^\times/n$) after reversal of a block, and the subsequent wave of mitoses indicated that partial synchronization of the population was achieved. The peak value for $n_S^\times/n$ after a block duration of five hr agreed well with the value expected on the basis of the cell cycle parameters of the asynchronous population. In addition, the cells arrested in S during a five-hr block remained intact, as judged by their capacity to pass through their first postblock mitosis. In contrast to the situation after a block duration of five hr, the peak value obtained for $n_S^\times/n$ after a 10-hr block was clearly too low, indicating that inactivation of a fraction of S and/or G_1-S cells occurred during the block, probably because of the effect of "unbalanced growth." However, in the present case it was also possible that direct toxic effects of HU were involved, since two doses of the inhibitor are necessary to maintain the block for 10 hr.

The data obtained in the BICR/M1R system are consistent with the interpretation that after reversal of a HU block, cells which had been blocked in S complete DNA synthesis faster than under normal conditions. Such an effect would lead to a temporary increase in the rate of cells entering mitosis. It could explain the sharp rise in the curves for n_M/n, as well as the height of the mitotic peaks occurring about seven hr after reversal of the blocks, which considerably exceed the values estimated on the basis of the distributions of cells over the cell cycle expected at this time. The same effect may also be responsible for the separation of two subpopulations of cells (cells arrested in S during the block, and cells accumulating in the G_1-S transition area during the block), as reflected by the two distinct peaks for n_S^x/n observed after the first postblock division. The long term kinetics, as well as the results of similar experiments,[48, 49] indicate that after the first postblock division the cell cycle parameters of the BICR/M1R cells are not significantly different from those of the untreated asynchronous population.

We cannot at present offer an explanation for the assumed acceleration of DNA synthesis. It seems unlikely that the low rate of DNA synthesis maintained during the block, which is probably caused by a small nucleotide pool reserve of the cells, would have this result. However, since HU does not affect the gross syntheses of RNA and protein,[69] it might be argued that the block could lead to an accumulation of "initiator proteins" in the blocked S cells, which after reversal of the block would exert a synchronizing effect on the temporal sequence of replicon initiation in the chromosomes.[42, 48]

Most of the criteria used to specify the degree of synchrony in cell cultures[56] are difficult to apply in the analysis of in vivo experiments. However, since the postblock kinetics of the BICR/M1R system were measured in terms of temporal changes in the proportion of DNA-synthesizing cells, the difference between the peak and the subsequent minimum for n_S^x/n[56] may serve as an "index of synchrony." However, the real degree of synchrony is higher than indicated by this index whenever the fraction of unlabeled cells includes S cells inactivated during the block. Experiments are presently in progress to further improve the degree of synchrony either by precise timing of multiple blocks, or by more complete cell inactivation during the block.

Led by the experience gained with the BICR/M1R system, we have also studied the effect of temporary inhibition of DNA synthesis with HU in a number of normal tissues.[49] It is well known that the parenchymal cell population of adult liver is characterized by extremely low fractions of cells in DNA synthesis and mitosis, and by a very high fraction of apparently noncycling cells which are capable of "re-entering" the cell cycle in the process of liver regeneration.[7] The 30- to 50-fold increase in the proportion of DNA-synthesizing cells following a double block with HU is clearly a "regeneration type" response, i.e. it is essentially caused by triggering nonproliferative cells back into the cell cycle. In analogy to the situation after partial hepatectomy,[7] the fraction of cells in DNA synthesis begins to rise above the control level about 15 hr after the first HU dose. This suggests that already the first dose of HU has exerted a "toxic" effect sufficient to initiate a regenerative response. Interestingly, there was no evidence for cell killing when similar doses of HU were applied to regenerating liver after partial hepatectomy, or to other normally quiescent cell systems stimulated to initiate DNA synthesis, such as folic acid-stimulated kidney or isoproterenol-stimulated salivary gland.[15, 53]

In contrast to the parenchymal cells of the adult liver, the eighteenth day rat embryo may be considered a combination of rapidly proliferating cell systems. Its response to a three-hr transplacental HU block resembles that of the BICR/M1R tumor in that it seems to be of the "kinetic" rather than of the "regenerative" type. The finding that a three-hr block apparently does not affect further development and survival of the embryos[49] argues against any severe toxic cell damage by HU in this system.

Summary and Conclusions

The investigation of the proliferative parameters of malignant tumors is a basic requirement not only for the characterization of malignant growth per se, but also for the development of "cell cycle adapted" schemes of tumor therapy. However, since tumors of clinically detectable size are the products of multiple selection processes, their analysis does not provide information about modifications of cytokinetic parameters associated with early malignant growth and carcinogenesis.

Recent advances in the study of cell population kinetics have led to a more detailed knowledge of the proliferative behavior of malignant tumors. In particular, the significance of parameters such as the proliferative fraction, the distribution of cell cycle times of the proliferating cells, and the degree of cell loss have been recognized. Conversely, there is the enigma of the capacity of a certain proportion of noncycling tumor cells to resume proliferation under conditions which cannot yet be clearly defined.

Various studies have demonstrated the existence of factors affecting proliferative parameters of malignant cell systems, such as the duration of the different phases of the cell cycle, or the size of the proliferative fraction. However, the molecular mechanisms involved in the regulation of the proliferative parameters of cell populations, and particularly in the "decision" of cells to leave or re-enter the cell cycle, are still largely unknown.

Observations in a number of in vivo systems, as well as results of studies performed in cell cultures, suggest that DNA replication and cell division may play an important role in the process of carcinogenesis. It may thus be asked: (1) whether the initiation of malignant transformation requires proliferating cells, and if so, whether specific phases of the cell cycle (DNA replication?) are particularly sensitive, and (2) whether a specific proliferative behavior of the target cell population is needed for the phenotypic expression of malignancy, and for providing the necessary selection pressure in favor of the transformed cells. An investigation of these problems under in vivo conditions requires: (1) well-characterized target tissues, (2) single-dose "pulse carcinogens" whose half-life is short compared with the duration of the cell cycle of the target cells, and (3) the presynchronization of target cell populations in vivo, in order to direct a carcinogen pulse to cells in specific cell cycle phases. Whereas it appears that agents may be available which could qualify as "pulse carcinogens," the problem of synchronizing proliferating cells under in vivo conditions has not been solved.

Results of an experimental study are therefore described which demonstrate that partial synchronization of malignant and normal cell systems in vivo can be achieved by temporary specific inhibition of DNA synthesis with HU. It is hoped that this approach may provide a basis for the investigation of cell cycle-specific events in the process of carcinogenesis, and perhaps be of some interest in the field of tumor therapy.

Acknowledgments

The author is indebted to his colleagues of the European Study Group for Cell Proliferation for many valuable discussions. Special thanks are due to Dr. G. G. Steel, Biophysics Department, Institute of Cancer Research, London, for the computer analysis of the labeled mitoses data, and for encouraging criticism.

Part of the work described in this report was supported by the Deutsche Forschungsgemeinschaft under contract No. Ra 119/3.

References

(References were not submitted; they may be requested directly from the author. Eds.)

Endogenous Growth Regulatory Substances

NANCY L. R. BUCHER

John Collins Warren Laboratories of the Huntington Memorial Hospital of Harvard University at the Massachusetts General Hospital, Boston, Massachusetts, USA

APART FROM THE SECRETIONS of the several endocrine glands, whose growth-promoting effects on specific target organs are well known, definitive information concerning the existence or character of endogenous substances that may regulate growth of the organs and tissues of the body is exceedingly limited. Because of their accessibility and responsiveness to growth stimuli, certain tissues have been extensively studied; mammalian liver, in particular, has served as a model for which endogenous regulatory agents have been intensively sought.

The liver of the adult rat, in which mitosis is a rare event, is endowed with a remarkable latent capacity for growth. A burst of proliferative activity is readily induced by excision of the two main lobes, comprising 68% of the whole organ. The first specific quantifiable index of this growth appears after a 14-hr delay, and consists of an abrupt rise in synthesis of DNA. The rate of DNA synthesis reaches a peak by about 22 hr and then declines; mitosis lags by about six hr, but follows a parallel course, attaining its maximum rate around 28 hr. These events are initially limited to the parenchymal cells, the responses in littoral, ductular and other cells being retarded by about 24 hr. The growth process occurs diffusely throughout the liver remnant and is properly described as a "compensatory hyperplasia," since there is no regrowth of the extirpated lobes. The liver thus affords an attractive system for scrutinizing the transition between latency and active growth, and for searching out the growth-controlling mechanism and its mode of operation.[1-3]

Evidence from several sources[4-8] indicates that control of hepatic regeneration resides outside of the liver and is mediated by a change in composition of the blood. For convenience, we shall refer to this blood-borne regulatory mechanism simply as a "humoral factor," though whether it operates through accrual of a stimulatory agent or dissipation of an inhibitor is not known, nor whether one or several such factors are involved. We have attempted to characterize the factor by establishing cross-circulation of blood between rats, connecting the carotid artery of each partner to the external jugular vein of the other by means of polyethylene cannulas. Under the conditions employed, this procedure permitted a rate of blood exchange between partners of 2 to $2\frac{1}{2}$ ml per min, which was maintained for 19 hr. The partners were then separated, and the rate of DNA synthesis determined at 21 to 22 hr, the time at which it is maximal in livers regenerating normally in control animals. Studies with ^{14}C-thymidine showed that the livers of normal animals were stimulated to synthesize DNA by cross-circulation with partially hepatectomized partners. The response was dose-related in that it was greater in the normal partners of 85% than in those of 68% hepatectomized rats, but it was undetectable in partners of 34% hepatectomized animals. The experimental procedure itself appeared suppressive, since 68% hepatectomized pairs exhibited less than half the activity of 68% hepatectomized single rats. The 68% hepatectomized partners seemed to benefit appreciably from exchange of blood with normal animals.[7]

Although approximately 30% of the blood volumes were exchanged between partners each minute, the humoral agent failed to equilibrate; the activity in the hepatectomized partners was about five-fold greater than in the corresponding normal partners.[7]

When the cross-circulation was discontinued after only 14 or 16 hr instead of 19 hr, the DNA rise expected to occur at 21 hr was still present. If, however, it was discontinued after less than 12 hr, no growth stimulus was demonstrable in the liver of the normal partner. This time requirement seems not merely to reflect the time necessary for a humoral factor in the hepatectomized partner to reach a "critical" concentration, but rather to reflect the need for prolonged exposure to such a factor; normal rats cross-circulated with partners hepatectomized six to seven hr in advance of the start of the exchange still required prolonged exposure before DNA synthesis was initiated. The failure of the humoral factor to equilibrate between partners, coupled with the finding that prolonged exchange is required, suggests that the factor is biologically unstable and rapidly renewed—properties one might reasonably expect in a regulatory agent.[7, 9]

Continuous exchange for at least 14 hr is apparently not required, since a normal partner can respond to cross-circulation with an 85% hepatectomized partner even when the exchange is interrupted for two to four hr during the initial 12- to 14-hr period. These observations suggest that the sequence of events leading to DNA synthesis may progress step-wise, in stages.[9]

Evidence suggests that the very earliest steps in the regenerative process can be initiated nonspecifically, i.e., by means not arising from a liver deficit. During the 14-hr delay which precedes the rise in DNA replication, a number of changes have been observed to occur in the regenerating liver remnant, at least some of which can also be induced by a sham operation. For example, the characteristic increase in rate of synthesis and cellular content of RNA during the first few hours after partial hepatectomy[10, 11] also appears, though to a lesser degree, in livers of sham-hepatectomized control rats. Accompanying the RNA rise is an augmentation in supply of precursor nucleotides, also elicitable to a minor extent by sham operation.[11] Further, it has been shown that laparotomies, or other stressful procedures (such as ip injection of Celite, a mechanical irritant), can cause enhanced synthesis of certain proteins and alterations in adenosine triphosphate metabolism similar to, but of shorter duration than, those induced by partial hepatectomy.[12, 13] Likewise, ip Celite and, to a lesser degree, sham hepatectomy can cause manifold increases in the activity of ornithine decarboxylase, an enzyme that responds in spectacular fashion to the regenerative impetus.[14] It seems that a number of the changes in the liver remnant within the first few hours after partial hepatectomy can

Fig. 10–2.—The effect of surgical or hormonal pretreatment on the response of hepatic DNA synthesis to partial hepatectomy. In control rats, under the experimental conditions employed, the rate of incorporation of ^{14}C-thymidine into DNA in livers regenerating for 14 hr is close to normal. A significant elevation at 14 hr after partial hepatectomy therefore implies that the initial rise, normally seen at 16 to 18 hr, has been accelerated. Values for each type of pretreatment are charted as multiples of the value for "14-hr hepatectomized" controls. The major elevations shown below differ from control values at the 1% significance level.

The number at the top of each bar indicates the number of rats. The times listed at the bottom of the chart for the surgical group represent the interval between the pretreatment indicated and the subsequent partial hepatectomy. In the hormonal group, the adrenal hormones were given four and one-half to eight hr before hepatectomy, growth hormone four and one-half hr before hepatectomy.

Abbreviations: A = "14-hr hepatectomized" controls; B = nonhepatectomized controls; C = nonhepatectomized controls, pretreated with an injection of isotonic saline solution; LAP = laparotomy; ADX = adrenalectomy; SHAM ADX = sham adrenalectomy; CORT = cortisone acetate, 5 mg; HYD = hydrocortisone sodium succinate, 1 to 25 mg; ACTH, 0.75 or 1.50 units.

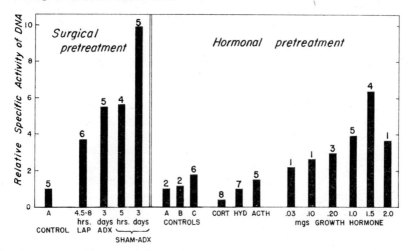

also be brought about by sham operations and certain other procedures which do not involve a liver deficit and do not by themselves cause any rise in DNA synthesis.[14, 15]

In further support of the notion that the initial steps in regeneration may be set in motion by certain forms of duress unrelated to loss of liver substance are the data in Figure 10-2. Figure 10-2 shows that several physical insults, including laparotomy, adrenalectomy, or sham adrenalectomy, applied a few hours or even several days before partial hepatectomy, can significantly shorten the latent period, so that the rise in DNA synthesis occurs two to three hr sooner than in nontraumatized controls.[16] Similar observations have been reported following ip injection of Celite.[17] Conversely, if various insults are applied at the time of partial hepatectomy or during the subsequent course of regeneration, no such acceleration occurs; indeed, a delay is the rule.[9] Although stress may be the common denominator of the various pretreatments tested, the effects are not reproduced by injections of ACTH or adrenal cortical steroids (Figure 10-2). However, bovine growth hormone, injected four or five hr prior to hepatectomy, appeared to shorten the latent period, the effect increasing roughly in proportion to the dose administered (Figure 10-2).[16]

Efforts to evaluate the role of adrenal and pituitary hormones in this acceleration of the DNA response to partial hepatectomy have been seriously hampered by the fact that procedures designed to eliminate the hormones by surgical or pharmacologic means (e.g. by treatment with Metopirone) have in themselves proved stimulatory.[16]

Alternatively, we attempted to probe into the effects of growth hormone on hepatic regeneration by establishing a continuous high endogenous supply through implantation of an active growth hormone-producing strain of rat pituitary tumor cells (GH_3 cells).[18] As shown in Table 10-6 and Figure 10-3, the body growth of animals bearing implants of this tumor far surpassed that of nontumor-bearing controls. Since the rate of incorporation of labeled thymidine into DNA was significantly elevated in the livers of the tumor-bearing rats, (Table 10-6), it was necessary to establish the basal level of activity in each animal. Accordingly, we determined the 1-hr incorporation of ^3H-thy-

TABLE 10–6.—EFFECT OF GROWTH HORMONE-PRODUCING TUMORS ON DNA SYNTHESIS IN REGENERATING RAT LIVER

RATS	BODY WT	^3H DPM PER MG DNA IN A	RATIO × 100 OF DPM PER MG DNA IN B/A AT INTERVALS AFTER HEPATECTOMY						
			8 hr	10 hr	12 hr	13 hr	14 hr	16 hr	18 hr
G.H.T.	320	13,200	3.3 (2.9) *	2.8 (2.5) *		30.0 (20.9) *			
Control	207	6,140		2.5 (2.1) *	3.7 (3.3) *		62.5 (34.9) *	27.1 (18.8) *	142 (107) *

* See Figure 10-3.

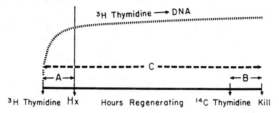

Fig. 10–3.—Experimental design (Table 10-6). ^{3}H-thymidine is injected 1 hr before partial hepatectomy (Hx); the extirpated lobes *(Sample A)* are used to determine the rate of ^{3}H-thymidine incorporation into the intact liver (baseline rate). Rats are killed at intervals after hepatectomy, 1 hr following injection of ^{14}C-thymidine *(liver Sample B)*. The ratio of ^{14}C in the DNA of B to ^{3}H in the DNA of A rises above the normal range (determined to be 2 to 4% in nonhepatectomized control rats) when the rate of DNA synthesis increases in the regenerating liver remnant.

The upper dotted line indicates that approximately 80% of the incorporation of ^{3}H-thymidine occurs during the first hour after injection and therefore the value C (i.e., ^{3}H in the liver at the time of killing) can be substituted for A in situations where no preliminary tissue sample is available. The data in parentheses in Table 10-6 are B/C ratios.

G.H.T. indicates rats bearing the tumor.

midine into DNA in the liver lobes removed at hepatectomy (Sample A in Figure 10-3), and the 1-hr incorporation of ^{14}C-thymidine at intervals during regeneration (Sample B). The ratio of the ^{14}C labeling per mg DNA in the regenerating liver (B) to the ^{3}H labeling per mg DNA in the normal liver (A) fell in the range of about 2 to 4% in livers of nonhepatectomized control animals. This ratio remained unchanged during the first 12 to 13 hr of regeneration in livers of both tumor-bearing and nontumor-bearing rats, after which it rose abruptly in both groups as the regenerative response became manifest.[19] Thus, although the rise in DNA synthesis induced by regeneration is accelerated by several procedures, including single injections of bovine growth hormone, it is relatively unaffected by continuous exposure to elevated levels of the same hormone supplied endogenously. Perhaps prolonged exposure results in metabolic adjustments within the tumor-bearing host that eliminate its effectiveness in the special circumstance of hepatic regeneration, where a sudden change in level may be more important. Although it remains uncertain whether the effects of operation or stress may be mediated through the secretion of growth hormone, a tentative hypothesis is that the several procedures mentioned can in some way stimulate the synthesis of fairly stable molecular species—perhaps enzymes or templates for protein synthesis, or some component of the cell surface—and that liver cells thus "primed" can react faster than normal to the specific stimulus that partial hepatectomy provides.[16]

In a final effort to characterize the humoral agent, we examined its ability to influence the growth rate of a so-called minimal deviation hepatoma, using implants derived from a clonal strain, MH_1C_1, established from the transplantable Morris heptoma, no. 7795.[20] The behavior of these cells in culture has been remarkably stable for many generations; like normal liver cells, they produce albumin in abundance, conjugate steroids with glucuronate or sulfate, bind dyes, and store lipids.[20] We employed a modification of the double-isotope technique used in the preceding experiment (see Figure 10-3). Since under the conditions of these experiments 75% to 80% of the DNA-labeling with ³H-thymidine takes place within the first hour after injection, the ³H in DNA at the time of killing (C) is not grossly different from A, and the ratio of B/C gives data acceptably comparable to B/A; the values in parentheses in Table 10-6 support this contention. The use of B/C was necessitated in the hepatoma experiments by the unavailability of a tumor sample (A) at the time of partial hepatectomy. As before, ³H-thymidine was injected 1 hr before partial hepatectomy, and ¹⁴C-thymidine at intervals thereafter, the rats being killed 1 hr later. Each rat had two subcutaneous hepatoma implants. In Table 10-7, the results expressed as the ratio of ¹⁴C labeling (after hepatectomy) to base line ³H labeling (before hepatectomy) show the complete absence of detectable effect of partial hepatectomy upon the rate of tumor growth; control and tumor values both fall within the range of 1 to 5.5%, in contrast to the very high ratios exhibited by regenerating liver at 22 hr when DNA replication is at its peak. An interesting sidelight is the strikingly close coincidence of values exhibited by the two tumors in each individual rat; this uniformity is all the more remarkable because of the extreme inhomogeneity of the tumors, which contained soft and indurated, hemorrhagic, and necrotic areas in varying proportions.[21] These were pilot experiments, and further studies will be necessary to find whether failure of the hepatoma cells to respond to the regenerative stimulus was actually attributable to their refractoriness to the humoral factor, or whether their growth rate was limited by host-determined factors (such as inadequacy of blood supply), so that no further augmentation was possible. The double-isotope tech-

TABLE 10-7.—EFFECT OF PARTIAL HEPATECTOMY ON DNA SYNTHESIS IN TRANSPLANTED HEPATOMAS

RATIO × 100 OF DPM PER MG DNA IN B/C* AT INTERVALS AFTER HEPATECTOMY

Control Liver	Control Tumors		Hrs after Hepatectomy	Regen. Liver	Tumors after Hepatectomy	
	Left	Right			Left	Right
2.2	1.9	1.2	12.5	3.4	5.1	4.8
2.1	4.5	4.2	22	382.0	2.9	2.9
3.8	5.4		22	304.0	4.8	5.1
			46	65.7	5.4	5.4
mean 2.7	3.4				4.5	

* The experimental design is explained, and the ratio B/C defined in Figure 10-3.

nique selectively measures growth in terms of DNA synthesis in viable cells only; its usefulness in studies of this kind support its broader application to problems relating to carcinogenesis and cancer chemotherapy.

Summary

Regeneration of rat liver serves as a model for investigating mechanisms that regulate organ growth in mammals. The normally quiescent adult liver responds to a surgically induced tissue deficit with a burst of proliferative activity that is shown to depend upon a blood-borne mechanism. This so-called "humoral factor" may be tentatively characterized as follows: it must act over a prolonged period, though exposure may be discontinuous; it is biologically unstable and rapidly renewed; it initiates a stepwise progression of events leading ultimately to DNA synthesis and mitosis. The very earliest steps in the progression (possibly involving RNA and protein synthesis) can be set in motion by a variety of procedures applied several hours, or even several days, in advance of the partial hepatectomy. These pretreatments include surgical manipulations, ip Celite injection, and administrations of bovine growth hormone, but not adrenal cortical hormones. The resulting changes in the liver are presumably reversible and nonspecific, since there is no progression to DNA synthesis without further impetus from the specific humoral factor. The role of growth hormone remains equivocal since growth hormone-secreting tumor implants fail to exert a "priming" effect. Although the humoral factor did not affect growth of minimal deviation hepatoma implants, limitation of response by host factors cannot be ruled out, and further study is required. The first stage of the regeneration process may be a reversible nonspecific tooling-up of biosynthetic machinery that at a later stage is directed specifically and irreversibly to cell reproduction. The implication of these observations is that the very earliest changes in the progression from G_0 or arrested G_1 to S phase do not provide a useful gauge of the blood-borne mechanism, since they are nonspecific and inducible by a variety of means.

Acknowledgments

These studies were performed in association with Drs. Frederick L. Moolten and Theodore R. Schrock and Misses Miriam N. Swaffield and Nancy J. Oakman. In the experiments with growth hormone-producing tumors and hepatomas, we collaborated with Dr. Armen H. Tashjian.

This work was supported by Grant CA 02146 of the National Institutes of Health, U. S. Public Health Service, and Grant P-545 of the American Cancer Society.

This is publication No. 1372 of the Cancer Commission of Harvard University.

References

1. Bucher, N. L. R.: Regeneration of mammalian liver. Int. Rev. Cytol., 15:245-300, 1963.
2. Bucher, N. L. R.: Experimental aspects of hepatic regeneration. New Eng. J. Med., 277:686-696, 738-746, 1967.
3. Bucher, N. L. R., and R. A. Malt: Regeneration of Liver and Kidney. Little, Brown and Co., Boston, Massachusetts. In press.
4. Leong, G. F., J. W. Grisham, B. V. Hole, and M. L. Albright: Effect of partial hepatectomy on DNA synthesis and mitosis in heterotopic partial autografts of rat liver. Cancer Res., 24:1496-1501, 1964.
5. Virolainen, M.: Mitotic response in liver autograft after partial hepatectomy in rat. Exp. Cell Res., 33:588-591, 1964.
6. Sigel, B., F. J. Acevedo, and M. R. Dunn: Effect of partial hepatectomy on auto-transplanted liver tissue. Surg. Gynec. Obst., 117:29-36, 1963.
7. Moolten, F. L., and N. L. R. Bucher: Regeneration of rat liver: Transfer of humoral agent by cross circulation. Science, 158:272-274, 1967.
8. Lieberman, I.: Studies on the control of mammalian deoxyribonucleic acid synthesis. In: *Biochemistry of Cell Division* (R. Baserga, ed.), Charles C Thomas, Springfield, 1969, pp. 119-137.
9. Bucher, N. L. R., T. R. Schrock, and F. L. Moolten: An experimental view of hepatic regeneration. Johns Hopkins Med. J., 125:250-257, 1969.
10. Fujioka, M., M. Koga, and I. Lieberman: Metabolism of ribonucleic acid after partial hepatectomy. J. Biol. Chem., 238:3401-3406, 1963.
11. Bucher, N. L. R., and M. N. Swaffield: Ribonucleic acid synthesis in relation to precursor pools in regenerating rat liver. Biochim. Biophys. Acta, 174:491-502, 1969.
12. Majumdar, C., K. Tsukada, and I. Lieberman: Liver protein synthesis after partial hepatectomy and acute stress. J. Biol. Chem., 242:700-704, 1967.
13. Ove, P., S. Takai, T. Umeda, and I. Lieberman: Adenosine triphosphate in liver after partial hepatectomy and acute stress. J. Biol. Chem., 242:4963-4971, 1967.
14. Schrock, T. R., N. J. Oakman, and N. L. R. Bucher: Ornithine decarboxylase activity in relation to growth of rat liver. Biochim. Biophys. Acta, 204:564-577, 1970.
15. Bucher, N. L. R., and M. N. Swaffield: Unpublished data.
16. Moolten, F. L., N. J. Oakman and N. L. R. Bucher: Accelerated response of hepatic DNA synthesis to partial hepatectomy in rats pretreated with growth hormone or surgical stress. Submitted for publication.
17. Simek, J., Z. Erbenova, F. Deml, and I. Dvorackova: Liver regeneration after partial hepatectomy in rats exposed before the operation to the stress stimulus. Experientia, 24:1166-1167, 1968.
18. Tashjian, A. H., Jr., Y. Yasumura, L. Levine, G. H. Sato, and M. L. Parker: Establishment of clonal strains of rat pituitary tumor cells that secrete growth hormone. Endocrinology, 82:342, 1968.
19. Bucher, N. L. R., M. N. Swaffield, and A. H. Tashjian, Jr.: Unpublished data.
20. Richardson, U. I., A. H. Tashjian, Jr., and L. Levine: Establishment of a clonal strain of hepatoma cells which secrete albumin. J. Cell Biol., 40:236-247, 1969.
21. Bucher, N. L. R., N. J. Oakman, and A. H. Tashjian, Jr.: Unpublished data.

Metastatic Spread of Tumors

B. SYLVÉN

The Cancer Research Division of Radiumhemmet, Karolinska Institute,
Stockholm, Sweden

Introduction

To BRIDGE OVER the gap between my review and the previous topics of this panel could be accomplished by clarifying the significance of invasiveness and metastasis formation. I would like to stress that these two phenomena should be regarded as the best criteria of malignancy. But also, these two phenomena represent quite precise biologic and clinical events, which we might be able to cope with and control long before all primary tumors can be cured, and also before a universal "immunotherapy" of some kind may become a reality and not merely wishfully discussed as a goal. The intriguing problems of invasion and metastasis formation are now partly clarified, as outlined below.

The multiplicity of factors involved in the primary events of metastasis formation appear to present a rather chaotic state of affairs. Several fundamental aspects relating to qualitative and/or quantitative differences between normal and tumor cells have been studied, e.g. membrane structure, mode of adhesion, ameboid movement, contact phenomena, and many other facets extensively reviewed.[1, 2, 19] Some of us may have felt a little uneasy when too far-fetched extrapolations are made from in vitro experiments, since the in vivo conditions sccm more complicated. Certainly a few pathologists still regard our experimental efforts with some doubt, and prefer simple mechanical explanations (internal "growth pressure") as the cause of invasion and destructiveness of tumors directed against surrounding host tissues.

It is, however, gratifying to see that biochemical data on the precise composition and local changes—enzymatic, ionic and others—in the immediate interstitial fluid milieu of solid tumors in vivo are slowly emerging. Such studies may help us to define biochemical features explaining: (1) the detachment of cells, or clusters of cells, from solid tumors, and also (2) the chemical tools responsible for the digestion and removal of ground substances and surrounding fibrous macromolecular proteins of the host. Leaving out all technical details and suggestions as to the local origin of the different components of the interstitial milieu, I will try to present an integrated picture of the most important biochemical factors concerned. Time will permit only a brief account, and, moreover, some factors have previously been discussed,[10-12] including the important role of lactate for the formation of the peripheral edema. It should be stressed further that this presentation refers only to solid (nonleukemic) tumor models devoid of significant homograft reactions; other proteinases possibly derived from leukocytes,[4] and the questionable role of collagenases, hyaluronidases, and other "mucolytic" enzymes are thus omitted.

By direct visual sampling and subsequent analysis of microquantities of cell- and blood-free interstitial fluid (IF) from the peripheral and central parts of solid mouse tumors, a number of biochemical parameters have been ascertained.[13, 16] The factors of possible interest for the detachment of cells are:

1. Lactic acid (lactate): Concentrations ranging from 90 to 160 mg/100 ml with local peak figures up to 320 mg in central tumor IF.

2. Divalent cations: Mainly Ca^{++} and Mg^{++}.

3. -SH groups: Mainly as glutathione (GSH) presenting large and unknown variations in topical concentration.

4. Enzymes: A large host of peptidases, aminopeptidases, and cathepsin B seem of actual interest. In addition, the topical GSH concentration is influenced by the activity level of GSH reductase.[5]

5. Enzyme inhibitors: Trypsin and chymotrypsin inhibitors are most likely present in mammalian IF as well as in the blood. The haptoglobin (Hp) concentration in tumor IF seems generally high enough to prevent all cathepsin B activity at a physiologic pH region.

When the crude tumor IF is assayed for proteinase activity with added cysteine plus EDTA, a peak of activity is generally obtained around pH 4.5 to 5.0. Part of this represents cathepsin B (Figure 10-4). No activity or, in a few cases, a weak activity was occasionally found to extend up to pH 7. Because of its acid range of activity, the role of cathepsin D seems mainly confined to intracellular proteolysis.

Other experiments further suggested that there was a powerful cathepsin B inhibitor in blood and IF. This mystery was solved following the purification and partial characterization of cathepsin B from lysosomal preparations of fresh calf liver by Snellman.[6] This enzyme is both papainlike and trypsinlike; it is activated by thiol groups and slightly inhibited by divalent metal ions like Ca^{++} and Mg^{++} (marked inhibition obtained by Mn^{++} ions). This condition necessitates in vitro assays in the presence of added -SH compounds and simultaneously a chelating agent like EDTA. Suitable substrates were proteins like edestin, serum albumin, and synthetic ones like BANA, BAEE, and LNA.

To identify a cathepsin B inhibitor, all kinds of available serum protein fractions were tested for inhibitory activity on purified cathepsin D and B preparations under carefully standardized conditions.[7] Cohn's fraction IV-b and, still more so, the highly purified Hp fraction

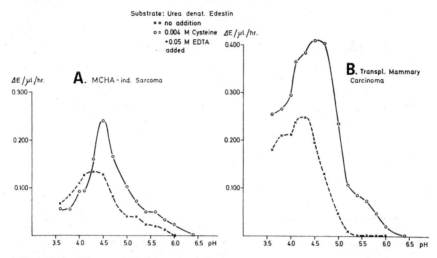

Fɪɢ. 10–4.—The total proteinase activity between pH 3.5 and 7 of interstitial fluid from central and peripheral parts of solid mouse tumors. The dotted curves represent mainly the activity of cathepsin D, while the activity increase, following suitable activation, forms evidence of cathepsin B activity (Hp inhibitor present).

(human source from the KABI Co., Stockholm), mainly Hp Group 2, demonstrated a greatly inhibitory effect against cathepsin B acting on protein substrates. Neither cathepsin D nor trypsin were inhibited by added Hp. The latter was reversibly bound to cathepsin B, but was not hydrolyzed by B as in the case of trypsin.

Further studies on less denatured preparations suggest that the inhibition is brought about by the Hp molecule itself and not by an associated material. Furthermore, the binding site to cathepsin B seemed not the same as in the case of the hemoglobin-Hp linkage.

In rodents, Hp as such (mainly Group 1) is a fairly small molecule of about 70,000 passing through into the extracellular space. In tumor patients and tumor-bearing mice, the serum Hp concentration is generally raised. We have demonstrated the presence of this inhibitor in ascites tumor fluid and IF from solid tumors in mice and rats (Figure 10-5). The Hp inhibitor is thus a reality pertinent to this discussion; it is assumed to protect extracellular proteins as well as other proteins adsorbed to cell surfaces against hydrolysis by active cathepsin B. The Hp 2 still remains to be demonstrated in human tumor IF.

Next, I want to clarify another point of uncertainty, namely whether cathepsin B in an active state is able to disaggregate cells under in vitro conditions. This was shown to be the case; cathepsin B, to some extent activated by added GSH plus lactic acid (about 200 mg/100 ml; see above and reference 15) for chelation of metal ions, rapidly detached C13 hamster fibroblasts (Stoker's line) growing on glass in Ca-

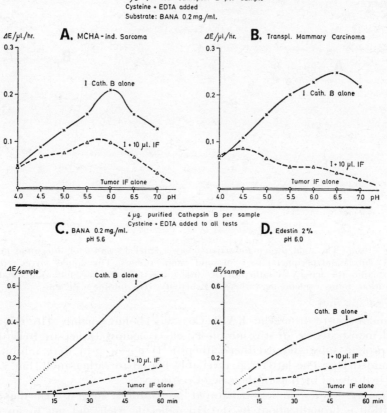

FIG. 10-5.—*A* & *B*. Inhibition of cathepsin B by solid tumor IF. *C* & *D*. Inhibition of cathepsin B by ascites tumor fluid.

and Mg-free Hank's solution. Proper precautions for continuous pH adjustment were taken. The effect was very similar to that of added trypsin, so there is no doubt that this enzyme, once in an active state, will also be able to disaggregate cells in vivo.

Thus, we know the main factors and have also some insight into their biologic interrelationships. I may now try to integrate these factors presenting a coherent approach to the first step of metastasis formation. Starting with cathepsin B in an inactive state entering the interstitial tumor compartment from some cellular source, tumorous or other, the enzyme has to become activated. This may occur first by dissociation of the Hp inhibitor and then activation by GSH plus lactate. The interesting role of lactate as a weak chelating agent cannot be overlooked. We are thus facing a complex series of intermingling reactions where the local pH and microenvironment at cellular or protein surfaces play a role. If some other protein (hemoglobin) would attract the Hp in the IF, then its concentration would decrease. Likewise, the rise in lactate production will locally favor the chelation necessary for enzyme activation and also the chelation of Ca^{++} ions influencing cellular adhesion. The level of GSH reductase is also of significance, as well as all local sources of GSH itself.

From a biologist's point of view, this integration further has one simple point of particularly wide interest, namely that the high rate of glycolysis of tumor cells seems operative also in regard to the mechanisms of invasion, cellular detachment, and metastasis formation. The precise molecular details in the interpretation are, however, not easily approached even by the finest microscale biochemical techniques. Further critical use of histochemical methods would be of value,[14, 18] while macroscale assays on usual homogenates[3] of solid tumors, human or other, can hardly offer useful information.

References

1. Ambrose, E. J., and F. J. C. Roe: The Biology of Cancer. D. van Nostrand Co., Ltd., London, 1966.
2. Curtis, A. S. G.: Cell adhesion: II. The biological evidence. In: The Cell Surface. Academic Press, London, 1967, pp. 125-175.
3. Goldberg, D. M., R. A. McAllister, and A. D. Roy: Proteolytic enzymes in adenocarcinomata of the human colon. Brit. J. Cancer, 23:735-743, 1969.
4. Janoff, A., and J. D. Zeligs: Vascular injury and lysis of basement membrane in vitro by neutral protease of human leukocytes. Science, 161:702-704, 1968.
5. Malmgren, H., and B. Sylvén: The histological distribution of glutathione reductase activity in solid mouse tumor transplants and a comparison with ascites tumors and normal tissues. Cancer Res., 20:204-211, 1960.
6. Snellman, O.: Cathepsin B, the lysosomal Thiol proteinase of calf liver. Biochem. J., 114:673-678, 1969.
7. Snellman, O., and B. Sylvén: Haptoglobin acting as natural inhibitor of cathepsin B activity. Nature, 216:1033, 1967.
8. Sylvén, B.: Some biochemical factors possibly concerned in the destructiveness of malignant growth. In: "Elfde Jaarboek van Kankeronderzoek en Kankerbestrijding in Nederland 1961." J. H. de Bussy, Amsterdam, 1961, pp. 127-133.
9. Sylvén, B.: On the biochemical mechanisms underlying the destructive capacity of malignant cells. Biochem. Biol. Sper. 1:8-20, 1961.
10. Sylvén, B.: The host-tumor interzone and tumor invasion. In: Biological interactions in Normal and Neoplastic Growth, Henry Ford Hospital International Symposium. Little, Brown and Co., Boston, 1962, pp. 635-655.
11. Sylvén, B.: Biochemical factors accompanying growth and invasion. In: Endogenous Factors Influencing Host-Tumor Balance (R. W. Wissler, T. L. Dao, and S. Wood, Jr., eds.) , University of Chicago Press, Chicago, 1967, pp. 267-276.
12. Sylvén, B.: Some factors relating to the invasiveness and destructiveness of solid malignant tumors. In: U.I.C.C. Symposium on the Mechanism of Invasion, Paris, July 1965. Springer-Verlag, 1967, pp. 47-60.
13. Sylvén, B.: Lysosomal enzyme activity in the interstitial fluid of solid mouse tumor transplants. Europ. J. Cancer, 4:463-474, 1968.
14. Sylvén, B.: Studies on the histochemical "leucine aminopeptidase" reaction. VI. The selective demonstration of cathepsin B activity by means of the naphthylamide reaction. Histochemie, 15:150-159, 1968.

15. Sylvén, B.: Cellular detachment by purified lysosomal cathepsin B. Europ. J. Cancer 4:559-562, 1968.
16. Sylvén, B., and I. Bois: Protein content and enzymatic assays of interstitial fluid from some normal tissues and transplanted mouse tumors. Cancer Res. 20:831-836, 1960.
17. Sylvén, B., and H. Malmgren: The histological distribution of proteinase and peptidase activity in solid mouse tumor transplants: A histochemical study on the enzymic characteristics of the different tumor cell types. Acta radiol., Suppl. 154, 1957.
18. Sylvén, B., and O. Snellman: Studies on the histochemical "leucine aminopeptidase" reaction. V. Cathepsin B as a potential effector of LNA hydrolysis. Histochemie, 12:240-243, 1968.
19. Weiss, L.: The Cell Periphery, Metastasis and other Contact Phenomena. North-Holland Publishing Co., Amsterdam, 1967.

11

Interaction of Physical, Chemical, and Viral Agents

The Mediation of X-ray and Chemical Leukemogenesis through Viral Activation

MIRIAM LIEBERMAN

Department of Radiology, Stanford University School of Medicine, Stanford, California, USA

IN THE NEARLY 20 YEARS since their discovery by Gross, the existence of viruses with leukemogenic potential for mice has become a well-documented fact. Leukemogenic viruses have been recovered from a variety of sources: from spontaneous lymphoid tumors of high-leukemia strain mice, from leukemias of various hematologic types induced by physical and chemical carcinogens, and even from several nonleukemic transplantable murine tumors.

In view of the wide distribution of these viruses, one may wonder whether they constitute merely another class of leukemogenic agent to be added to the existing list, or whether they are, in fact, the underlying cause of all of these leukemias. In the latter eventuality, what are the interactions between external carcinogen, virus, and host that bring about leukemia?

A review of radiogenic lymphoma development in mice may serve as a useful model in a discussion of these problems. X-irradiation has the advantage over other carcinogens in that its effect is exerted only during the time of exposure; no residual amounts of carcinogen remain in the animal to introduce an element of uncertainty in the interpretation of results. A further advantage comes from the possibility of limiting radiation exposure to selected parts of the body, which in turn permits investigation of the interaction of various cell types in the neoplastic process.

The experimental animal used in much of this work has been the C57BL mouse. The spontaneous development of leukemia is rare in this strain, and occurs only in quite old animals, yet its frequency rises to nearly 100% within five to six months after x-irradiation under appropriate conditions. Histologically, the neoplasm is a lymphosarcoma, usually of poorly differentiated cell type. It originates in the thymus and its development can be arrested by thymectomy; in such animals, leukemogenesis resumes if they are subsequently given a syngeneic thymus graft.[1] Studies of this phenomenon led to an observation which, together with Gross' finding of a leukemogenic virus in spontaneous lymphomas, suggested the possibility that a virus might be involved in x-ray leukemogenesis as well. It was noted that lymphoid tumors, arising in thymectomized, x-irradiated F_1 hybrid mice bearing a parental strain thymic graft, were frequently of donor genotype.[2] This meant that neoplastic conversion took place in cells which had never been exposed to radiation, hence an indirect induction mechanism must exist, possibly mediated through activation of a latent leukemogenic virus.

A search was instituted for such a virus in radiation-induced lymphomas of C57BL mice, and an active agent was recovered[3] which had the attributes of a virus, subsequently designated the radiation leukemia virus (RadLV). A similar agent was also recovered by Gross from radiation-induced lymphomas of strain C3Hf mice.[4] The activity of RadLV was initially quite low, probably as a result of its low concentration in lymphomatous tissue—where it could not be detected by electron microscopy[5]—and of the insensitivity of the bioassay procedure. Serial passage and direct intrathymic inoculation have augmented the "virulence" of the agent; currently it induces lymphomas with as high a frequency as, and in a shorter time than, x-irradiation.

RadLV has the same morphologic appearance and the same physical and chemical characteristics as other murine leukemia viruses. Antigenically, it is closely related to the Gross virus.[6] However, the Gross virus is essentially nonleukemogenic in C57BL mice; in fact, it renders them resistant to subsequent challenge with RadLV, possibly through an immunologic mechanism.[7]

The isolation of leukemogenic virus from radiogenic lymphoid tumors of C57BL mice was not an isolated occurrence; seven of 10 individual recovery attempts have been successful in our laboratory, and our results have been confirmed elsewhere.[8] It may be inferred from this that RadLV is harbored by all C57BL mice. Moreover, viral particles of characteristic type C morphology have been visualized by electron microscopy in normal C57BL fetal thymus.[9] Similar particles have been described in embryonic tissues of both high-leukemia Ak and low-leukemia C3Hf mice.[10] In addition, leukemogenic activity has been demonstrated in Ak embryos,[11] and susceptibility to leukemia has been maintained in AKR mice derived from the transfer of fertilized AKR ova to low-leukemia C3H females.[12] These findings have contributed to the generally accepted hypothesis that murine leukemia viruses are transmitted from generation to generation through the embryo.

In low-leukemia strains, the infrequency of spontaneous leukemia despite the presence of leukemogenic virus may result from a lack of synchrony between the time when the tissue or blood concentration of virus rises to adequate levels and the time when an abundant population of susceptible cells is present. The target cells for neoplastic transformation, in both x-ray- and virus-induced lymphoma of C57BL mice, are the lymphoid cells of the thymic cortex. Of these, the most exquisitely susceptible cells appear to be the immature lymphoblast-like cells which are normally abundant only during infancy; this may account, in part, for the much higher incidence of lymphomas when leukemogenic viruses are inoculated into mice during the neonatal period, rather than during adult life.[13, 14] At this age, however, the concentration of endogenous virus appears to be very low. It is only in much older mice that attempts to demonstrate the virus by bioassays or immunologic techniques have been successful.[15, 16]

Ionizing radiation upsets the host-virus equilibrium. It produces involution of the thymus, with destruction of most of its lymphoid elements. There follows a period of repair, during which immature, lymphoblast-like cells once again become prevalent.[13] This phase of maturation is fleeting when active bone marrow is preserved by shielding or is injected from syngeneic donors after irradiation. Cytogenetic studies have established that cells from the bone marrow can migrate to the radiation-injured thymus, and contribute to its repopulation and prompt recovery. Following whole-body irradiation, however, a maturation arrest in the immature lymphoblastic stage persists in the thymus for several days. On the basis of this information, Kaplan[17] has postulated that x-irradiation induces lymphomas because: (1) it restores the thymic cortex to the neonatal, virus-susceptible state; (2) it injures the bone marrow, thus preventing the action of a leukemia-inhibiting influence located there; and (3) through an as yet unknown mechanism, it "mobilizes" a latent leukemogenic virus and causes it to reach the susceptible cells in the thymus, probably via the blood stream. Evidence for the latter effect has come from the visualization of viral particles and the appearance of leukemogenic activity in various tissues of mice within a few days after irradiation.[18–20]

It has been postulated[21] that the inhibitory effect of normal marrow may, in part, derive from its capacity to readsorb virus which irradiation has set free in the circulation. Recent evidence from our laboratory[29] supports this hypothesis. Mice were irradiated, either in toto or with thighs shielded, and then given an iv injection of RadLV. Their plasma was tested at intervals for the duration of persistence of leukemogenic activity. In the total-body irradiated groups, activity persisted at a high level for 45 to 60 minutes, whereas in the thigh-shielded groups it was much lower and disappeared rapidly.

By virtue of its destructive effect on the hematopoietic and lymphoid systems, x-irradiation reduces immunologic competence. In the leukemogenic dose range, it has been shown to suppress, temporarily, the homograft reaction in mice.[22] It is conceivable that survival of early neoplastic cells with altered antigenic specificity may be favored by this effect. Reports that either x-irradiation,[23] or the administration of antithymocyte serum,[24] exerts a coleukemogenic effect on viral leukemogenesis provide strong circumstantial evidence that impairment of immunologic responsiveness may contribute to lymphoma development. The role of immunity in radiation-induced leukemia is difficult to evaluate, since the same tissues are involved in both processes.

The hypothesis that RadLV is the causative agent of radiogenic lymphoma, and not merely a passenger virus which proliferates in lymphomatous tissue, has received additional support from recent experiments. A protracted course of interferon injections suppressed virus-induced lymphoma incidence by about 30%. Of greater significance, interferon also inhibited the development of radiation-induced disease by about 60%.[29] The same interferon-sensitive, and therefore presumably viral, mechanism must surely underlie genesis of the disease in both cases. In other experiments, a specific rat anti-RadLV antiserum, which neutralizes the leukemogenic potential of RadLV, has given suggestive evidence of inhibitory activity against the development of radiation-induced C57BL lymphomas.[30]

There is mounting evidence that the series of events which leads to leukemia after exposure to irradiation also takes place when other external leukemogens are used, e.g., the depression of DMBA-induced lymphomas in CFW mice by normal marrow.[25] In C57BL mice, leukemogenic activity has been demonstrated in cell-free extracts prepared from lymphoid tumors induced by several chemical carcinogens,[26-28] and the presence of the group-specific antigen of murine leukemia viruses in chemically induced lymphomas has been reported.[28]

Many questions remain to be answered, but on the basis of the knowledge accumulated so far, a coherent theory of leukemogenesis in mice can be proposed. Latent viruses with neoplastic potential are apparently ubiquitous among mice, and probably among other animals as well. In analogy with the temperate viruses of lysogenic bacteria, they usually remain latent throughout the life of the host, except where some unknown internal event upsets the host-virus equilibrium, as in mice of high-leukemia strains, or where an external physical or chemical stimulus triggers their "activation." When activated and provided with an adequate population of susceptible target cells, these viruses can induce the neoplastic conversion of such cells without the further mediation of external agents, and continue indefinitely to be propagated by, and extractable from, the tumors they induce in the leukemogenically activated state.

References

1. Kaplan, H. S., W. H. Carnes, M. B. Brown, and B. B. Hirsch: Indirect induction of lymphomas in irradiated mice. I. Tumor incidence and morphology in mice bearing non-irradiated thymic grafts. Cancer Res., 16:422-425, 1956.
2. Kaplan, H. S., B. B. Hirsch, and M. B. Brown: Indirect induction of lymphomas in irradiated mice. IV. Genetic evidence of the origin of the tumor cells from the thymic grafts. Cancer Res., 16:434-436, 1956.
3. Lieberman, M., and H. S. Kaplan: Leukemogenic activity of filtrates from radiation-induced lymphoid tumors of mice. Science, 130:387-388, 1959.
4. Gross, L.: Attempt to recover filterable agent from x-ray-induced leukemia. Acta Haematol., 19:353-361, 1958.
5. Dalton, A. J., L. W. Law, J. B. Moloney, and R. A. Manaker: An electron microscopic study of a series of murine lymphoid neoplasms. J. Nat. Cancer Inst., 27: 747-791, 1961.
6. Ferrer, J. F., and H. S. Kaplan: Antigenic characteristics of lymphomas induced by radiation leukemia virus (RadLV) in mice and rats. Cancer Res., 28:2522-2528, 1968.
7. Lieberman, M., and H. S. Kaplan: Interaction between murine leukemia viruses in vivo. Proc. Amer. Ass. Cancer Res., 9:42, 1968.
8. Latarjet, R., and J. F. Duplan: Experiment and discussion on leukemogenesis by cell-free extracts of radiation-induced leukemia in mice. Intern. J. Radiat. Biol., 5:339-344, 1962.
9. Carnes, W. H.: Radiation leukemia virus in embryonic C57BL mouse thymus. Federation Proc., 26:748, 1967.
10. Feldman, D. G., Y. Dreyfuss, and L. Gross: Electron microscopic study of the mouse leukemia virus (Gross) in organs of mouse embryos from virus-injected and normal C3Hf parents. Cancer Res., 27:1792-1804, 1967.
11. Gross, L.: "Spontaneous" leukemia developing in C3H mice following inoculation, in infancy, with Ak leukemic extracts, or Ak embryos. Proc. Soc. Exp. Biol. Med., 76:27-32, 1951.
12. Fekete, E., and H. K. Otis: Observations on leukemia in AKR mice born from transferred ova and nursed by low leukemic mothers. Cancer Res., 14:445-447, 1954.
13. Kaplan, H. S.: The role of cell differentiation as a determinant of susceptibility to virus carcinogenesis. Cancer Res., 21:981-983, 1961.
14. Axelrod, A. A., and H. C. Van der Gaag: Susceptibility to lymphoma induction by Gross passage A virus in C3Hf/Bi mice of different ages: Relation to thymic cell multiplication and differentiation. J. Nat. Cancer Inst., 28:1065-1093, 1962.
15. Rudali, G., and C. Silberman: Apparition de leucémies chez des souris C57BL apres greffe d'organes normaux isologues. Nouvelle Rev. Franc. Hematol., 5:63-68, 1965.
16. Hartley, J. W., W. P. Rowe, W. I. Capps, and R. J. Huebner: Isolation of naturally occurring viruses of the murine leukemia virus group in tissue culture. J. Virol., 3:126-132, 1969.
17. Kaplan, H. S.: The role of radiation in experimental leukemogenesis. Nat. Cancer Inst. Monograph, 14:207-217, 1964.
18. Gross, L., and D. G. Feldman: Electron microscopic studies of radiation-induced leukemia in mice: Virus release following total-body x-ray irradiation. Cancer Res., 28:1677-1685, 1968.
19. Mathe, G., and J. Bernard: Fréquence de leucémies et de tumeurs chez des souris C57BL ayant reçu à la naissance du plasma d'animaux irradiés. Rev. Franc. Etud. Clin. Biol., 3:257-258, 1958.
20. Haran-Ghera, N.: Leukemogenic activity of centrifugates from irradiated mouse thymus and bone marrow. Int. J. Cancer, 1:81-87, 1966.

21. Kaplan, H. S.: On the natural history of the murine leukemias: Presidential address. Cancer Res., 27:1325-1340, 1967.
22. Doell, R. G., C. DeVaux St. Cyr, and P. Grabar: Immune reactivity prior to development of thymic lymphoma in C57BL mice. Int. J. Cancer, 2:103-108, 1967.
23. Haran-Ghera, N.: The mechanism of radiation action in leukaemogenesis: The role of radiation in leukaemia development. Brit. J. Cancer, 21:739-749, 1967.
24. Haran-Ghera, N., and A. Peled: The mechanism of radiation action in leukemogenesis. IV. Immune impairment as a coleukemogenic factor. Israel J. Med. Sci., 4:1181-1187, 1968.
25. Ball, J. K.: Depressive effect of bone marrow on the yield of 7, 12-DMBA induced thymic lymphomas. J. Nat. Cancer Inst., 44:439-445, 1970.
26. Doell, R. G., and W. H. Carnes: Urethan induction of thymic lymphoma in C57BL mice. Nature, 194:588-589, 1962.
27. Haran-Ghera, N.: A leukemogenic filtrable agent from chemically-induced lymphoid leukemia in C57BL mice. Proc. Soc. Exp. Biol. Med., 124:697-699, 1967.
28. Igel, H. J., R. J. Huebner, H. C. Turner, P. Kotin, and H. L. Falk: Mouse leukemia virus activation by chemical carcinogens. Science, 166:1624-1626, 1969.
29. Lieberman, M., and H. S. Kaplan: Unpublished data.
30. Ferrer, J. F., and H. S. Kaplan: Unpublished data.

Interaction of FBJ Osteosarcoma Virus with ^{90}Sr and with ^{90}Sr Osteosarcomas

MIRIAM P. FINKEL, BIRUTE O. BISKIS,
AND CHRISTOPHER A. REILLY, JR.

Argonne National Laboratory, Argonne, Illinois, USA

Introduction

RADIONUCLIDES THAT LOCALIZE in the skeleton produce bone cancer.[1] Because of the potential contamination of man and his environment with radioactive materials, this subject has been intensively studied in atomic energy laboratories throughout the world for many years. Present information is adequate to predict, with some confidence, the consequences of exposure under a variety of conditions, but the basic mechanism of radionuclide oncogenesis remains obscure.

The Experimental Radiation Pathology Group at Argonne National Laboratory has concentrated on the induction of osteosarcomas in mice with ^{90}Sr as a tool for studying radio-oncogenesis.[2] The discovery of a virus (FBJ) that also produces osteosarcomas in mice[3] led to research on the combined action of radiation and virus, which resulted in the hypothesis that radiation induces cancer by inactivating an inhibitor of viral replication.[4] The present experiments were undertaken to provide information on three questions: (1) Can mice be immunized against ^{90}Sr osteosarcomas with FBJ virus? (2) Will irradiating the skeleton increase the susceptibility of adult mice to cancer induction by FBJ virus? (3) Do radiation- and virus-induced bone cancers contain a common viral antigen?

Materials and Methods

Female CF1/Anl (340) mice were used throughout the experiments. Those in the ^{90}Sr-FBJ virus-interaction study, outlined in Table 11-1, were 95-136 days old at the time radiostrontium was injected. They were housed at random in groups of 15 in stainless steel cages a few days before treatment began. The mice were observed daily, and all animals were killed when moribund. Tissues were taken for histopathologic study when necessary for diagnosis.

Roentgenographic examination of the skeleton was begun 28 days after ^{90}Sr treatment, and it was repeated monthly. With this procedure, malignant change could be detected closer to the time when it actually occurred, and bone tumor data were not as seriously influenced by mortality as is the case when tumors are tabulated at death.[5] Also, by watching a lesion develop, it was possible to differentiate between ^{90}Sr-induced and FBJ-induced osteosarcomas with a high degree of accuracy.

[90]Sr was injected intravenously as an equilibrium mixture of [90]Sr-[90]YCl$_2$ in neutral, isotonic solution. [90]Sr has a half-life of 28 years, decaying with a 0.54-Mev beta ray to ^{90}Y, which has a 64-hr half-life and decays with the emission of a 2.27-Mev beta ray to stable zirconium. Deposition within the skeleton occurs very rapidly. Three dosages were used: 1.0, 0.5, and 0.25 μCi/gm body weight. All injections were based on an average weight of 27.5 gm.

FBJ virus was injected ip as a saline extract of FBJ osteosarcomas.[3] The amount of material needed on any one day was pooled from a number of samples in dry ice storage. FBJ virus is a Type C particle, averaging 100 mμ in diameter[6] and belonging to the murine leukemia-sarcoma group of viruses.[7] Originally isolated from a spontaneous osteosarcoma arising in a stock CF1/Anl mouse, the virus is now in its thirty-seventh vertical cell-free passage and continues to produce only parosteal osteosarcomas.

For immunization, 75 mice were initially inoculated with 0.2 ml FBJ-osteosarcoma extract, and 7, 14, and 28 days later they received 0.1 ml extract. Six days after the last injection, 15 of the mice received 1.0 μCi ^{90}Sr/gm, 15 received 0.5 μCi/gm, 15 remained as immunized con-

TABLE 11-1.—EXPERIMENTAL PLAN, SURVIVAL, AND TUMORS OF SOFT TISSUES

| TREATMENT | | | NUMBER OF MICE | Life Expec. (days) | 10% Surv. Time (days) | 0 Surv. Time (days) | TUMORS | | | | |
FBJ Imm.* (ml)	90Sr (µCi/gm)	FBJ† (ml)					Ret. Tis. (%)	Lung (%)	Ovary (%)	Mam. (%)	Other‡ (%)
.5 (4)	0	0	15	483	665	>775	60.0	20.0	0	0	13.3
0	0	.5	15	473	625	665	53.4	13.3	26.6	0	0
0	0	.25	15	443	620	753	40.0	6.7	0	0	0
0	1.0	0	15	192	250	275	26.6	20.0	0	0	0
.5 (4)	1.0	0	15	223	280	315	20.0	13.3	0	0	0
0	1.0	.5	15	202	250	291	26.6	6.7	0	0	0
0	1.0	.25	15	204	235	247	26.6	0	0	6.7	0
0	0.5	0	14	310	385	389	35.6	7.2	0	7.2	0
.5 (4)	0.5	0	15	343	500	728	46.6	13.3	6.7	6.7	0
0	0.5	.5	30	369	480	612	43.3	10.3	0	0	10.0
0	0.5	.25	30	332	470	578	26.7	16.7	6.7	3.3	0
0	0.25	0	30	400	530	602	33.3	10.0	6.7	3.3	3.3
0	0.25	0	30	420	580	658	36.7	33.3	6.7	3.3	0
0	0.25	0	30	437	600	>775	46.6	26.7	3.3	3.3	3.3

* 0.5 ml in 4 fractional doses: 0.2 ml 34 days and 0.1 ml 27 days, 20 days, and 6 days before 90Sr treatment.
† One injection one day after 90Sr.
‡ Hepatomas, hemangiosarcomas, and epidermoid carcinomas.

trols, and 30 were used for serum collection. The pooled serum was tested for antibody by injecting 0.1 ml into neonatal mice $4\frac{1}{2}$ hr before they were inoculated with FBJ-osteosarcoma extract. Another group of neonates were given 0.1 ml serum $4\frac{1}{2}$ hr, 2 days, and 4 days after FBJ extract.

For testing the susceptibility of irradiated mice to FBJ oncogenesis, mice that had received 1.0, 0.5, or 0.25 μCi ^{90}Sr/gm were given 0.5 or 0.25 ml FBJ-osteosarcoma extract one day later. The pooled sample of extract used for these injections was tested for oncogenic potency in 26 neonatal mice; bone cancer had killed three of them by 85 days, and the final incidence was 65%.

Neutralization tests for detecting specific FBJ antibody in ^{90}Sr-induced osteosarcomas are still in progress. They are being conducted by incubating a 1:1 mixture of test plasma and FBJ-osteosarcoma extract for one hour at 37 C before injecting it into neonatal mice. The control test run concurrently consists of incubating a portion of the same extract with saline solution. Plasma rather than serum is used because exsanguination is more successful with heparinized syringes. Recipients of the test samples are examined for bone cancer by palpation twice a week, and all are autopsied when moribund.

Test plasmas were of five general types: (1) from untreated adult CF1/Anl (340) mice, (2) from mice inoculated with FBJ virus at birth and dying with FBJ tumors, (3) from adult mice inoculated with an emulsion of FBJ virus and Freund's incomplete adjuvant four times at four- or five-day intervals and exsanguinated one week after the last injection, (4) from mice bearing transplanted FBJ osteosarcomas, and (5) from mice bearing transplanted ^{90}Sr-induced osteosarcomas.

Four transplant lines have been established from osteosarcomas that appeared in mice treated with 1.0 μCi^{90}Sr/gm alone. (1) Transplant line SF/46 grows successfully in 80% of recipients, but it regresses about 50% of the time. Bony trabeculae appear only occasionally, and the usual appearance of the transplant is that of a fibroblastic osteosarcoma. Test sample SF/46$_1$ was pooled plasma from seven mice that had had first generation transplants that regressed. Pooled plasma from eight mice with fourth generation transplants that had regressed was used as test sample SF/46$_4$. Test sample SF/46$_{16}$ was pooled plasma from mice bearing sixteenth generation transplants. (2) Transplant line SF/48, a well differentiated osteogenic sarcoma, has grown in only 25% of recipients, but it seldom regresses. Plasma was pooled for testing from two mice bearing first generation transplants. (3) Transplant line SF/54, also a well-differentiated osteogenic sarcoma, has grown in 30% of recipients and seldom regresses. Pooled plasma was tested from mice bearing first and third generation transplants. (4) Transplant line CR3/14, another differentiated osteogenic sarcoma, has produced tumors more than 40% of the time, with 50% of the nodules regressing. Test sample CR3/14$_7$ was plasma from one mouse with a seventh generation transplant.

Results

TEST OF IMMUNITY

Pooled serum from the 30 mice inoculated four times in the course of 28 days with FBJ-osteosarcoma extract partially protected neonates against FBJ oncogenesis when it was injected before the virus; 56% (13/23) developed FBJ tumors in contrast to an incidence of 90% (9/10) in the mice not pretreated with serum (Figure 11-1). FBJ-osteosarcoma incidence during the first year after posttreatment with immune serum was similar to the nontreated group, but, when the experiment was terminated at the end of two years, the final incidence was 70% (16/23).

SURVIVAL AND SOFT TISSUE PATHOLOGY

The data on survival and occurrence of soft tissue tumors of the ^{90}Sr-FBJ virus-interaction experiment are summarized in Table 11-1. Life expectancy was associated with ^{90}Sr dosage; the averages were 205 days after the injection of 1.0 μCi/gm, 338 days after 0.5 μCi/gm, and 419 days after 0.25 μCi/gm. With FBJ extract alone, average life expectancy was 466 days. Within each of the ^{90}Sr dosage groups, poorest survival was demonstrated by mice that did not receive FBJ extract, though the difference was marked only with 0.5 μCi/gm, where 10% and 0% survival was reached an average of 100 and 250 days sooner, respectively.

Reticular tissue tumors frequently caused death. They increased with increasing life span (Table 11-1) but otherwise were not influenced

FIG. 11–1.—Cumulative incidence of death with osteosarcoma after neonatal injection of 0.1 ml FBJ-osteosarcoma extract. Pretreatment: 0.1 ml antiserum 4½ hours after FBJ extract. Posttreatment: 0.1 ml antiserum 4½, 53, and 96 hours after FBJ extract.

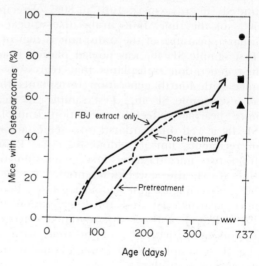

by treatment. Of the mice, 15% had lung tumors, and a few other tumors of soft tissues were observed. There were no serious infectious diseases; 25 cases of dermatitis and seven of abdominal or generalized infection were observed. The major cause of death was osteosarcoma.

MALIGNANT BONE TUMORS

The bone cancer data are summarized in Table 11-2. There were 13 skeletal hemangiosarcomas and five fibrosarcomas of bone. Though these tumors occurred only in irradiated animals, there was no apparent association with dosage of either ^{90}Sr or FBJ virus.

One mouse that had received the immunizing injections of FBJ virus without ^{90}Sr had an osteogenic sarcoma detected roentgenographically as an osteolytic lesion in the proximal metaphysis of the tibia on day 527. Since FBJ osteosarcomas are parosteal, appearing first as periosteal proliferative lesions,[8] this tumor was classified as spontaneous. Histologic examination verified the diagnosis of non-FBJ osteogenic sarcoma.

FBJ OSTEOSARCOMAS.—Immunization with viable FBJ virus (0.5 ml in four fractional injections) induced only one FBJ osteosarcoma in 15 mice. The single injection of 0.5 and 0.25 ml FBJ-osteosarcoma extract induced bone cancer in 6/15 and 2/15 mice, respectively. No FBJ osteosarcomas appeared when 1.0 μCi ^{90}Sr/gm was given, and their number was decreased with both 0.5 and 0.25 μCi/gm.

^{90}SR OSTEOSARCOMAS.—With one exception, the incidence of ^{90}Sr osteosarcomas was associated with the amount of radionuclide given, not with pre- or posttreatment with FBJ virus; 1.0 μCi/gm produced an average of four osteosarcomas per mouse, 0.5 μCi/gm produced 0.92 per mouse, and 0.25 μCi/gm produced 0.48 per mouse. The exception was the group that received 0.5 μCi ^{90}Sr/gm followed by 0.25 ml FBJ-osteosarcoma extract. This group had 1.8 osteosarcomas per mouse, or twice the incidence observed in the other three 0.5 μCi/gm groups.

The ^{90}Sr-osteosarcoma data are plotted in Figure 11-2 as cumulative number of tumors per mouse tallied at the time of roentgenographic diagnosis. The 1.0 μCi/gm groups showed similar tumor incidences until 230 days, when the ^{90}Sr-only group failed to show the same increase. At this dosage level, the immunized mice lived longest and had the most ^{90}Sr bone tumors. A difference appeared among the 0.5 μCi/gm groups at 320 days, when the animals treated with 0.25 ml FBJ extract began to show more osteosarcomas than did the others. No difference occurred among the 0.25 μCi/gm groups.

The anatomic location of the ^{90}Sr osteosarcomas was examined to determine whether it was influenced by treatment. The summary in Table 11-2 shows similarity among groups treated with the same amount of ^{90}Sr but differences between the highest level and the other two. With 1.0 μCi/gm, 48% of the tumors were in long bones and 37% in the

TABLE 11–2—MALIGNANT TUMORS OF BONE

TREATMENT FBJ Imm.* (ml)	TREATMENT ^{90}Sr (µCi/gm)	FBJ† (ml)	OSTEOGENIC SAR. (%)	HEM. SAR. (%)	FIBRO. SAR. (%)	FBJ OSTEO. SAR. (%)	NUMBER PER MOUSE	SR OSTEOSARCOMAS LOCATION (%) Long Bones	Spine	Gird.	Head and Ribs
.5 (4)	0	0	6.7	0	0	6.7	—	—	—	—	—
0	0	.5	0	0	0	40.0	—	—	—	—	—
0	0	.25	0	0	6.7	13.3	—	—	—	—	—
0	1.0	0	0	0	0	—	3.5	52	40	6	2
.5 (4)	1.0	0	0	6.7	0	0	4.4	48.5	32	16.5	3
0	1.0	.5	0	0	6.7	0	3.7	43	41	14	2
0	1.0	.25	0	7.2	0	0	3.9	48	36	14	2
0	0.5	0	0	6.7	0	—	0.93	77	15	8	0
.5 (4)	0.5	0	0	3.3	0	6.7	0.93	79	14	7	0
0	0.5	.5	0	10.0	3.3	6.7	0.90	96	4	0	0
0	0.5	.25	0	10.0	0	3.3	1.8	83	11	6	0
0	0.25	0	0	0	0	—	0.47	86	7	7	0
0	0.25	.5	0	3.3	3.3	10.0	0.57	82.5	6	11.5	0
0	0.25	.25	0	6.7	3.3	3.3	0.40	75	8.3	8.3	8.3

* 0.5 ml in 4 fractional doses: 0.2 ml 34 days and 0.1 ml 27 days, 20 days, and 6 days before ^{90}Sr treatment.

† One injection one day after ^{90}Sr.

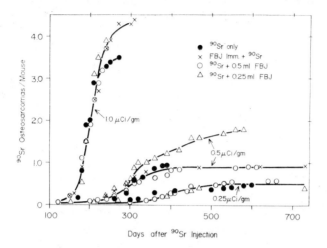

Fig. 11–2.—Cumulative incidence of ^{90}Sr osteosarcomas based on roentgenographic diagnosis as a function of time after injection of 1.0, 0.5, or 0.25 μCi ^{90}Sr/gm. Some groups received ^{90}Sr only, some were immunized with FBJ extract before receiving ^{90}Sr, and some received 0.5 or 0.25 ml FBJ extract one day after receiving ^{90}Sr.

spine; with 0.5 or 0.25 μCi/gm, 83% were in long bones and 9% in the spine.

Data on the length of time between roentgenographic diagnosis of osteosarcoma and death were also examined to determine whether there was an association with treatment. The average time was 19 days in the 1.0 μCi^{90}Sr/gm groups, 41 days in the 0.5 μCi/gm groups, and 57 days in the 0.25 μCi/gm groups. No difference was detected in survival time after diagnosis in the groups treated with FBJ-osteosarcoma extract.

Neutralization Tests

Current results of the tests for the presence of neutralizing antibody to FBJ virus, which are still in progress, are presented in Figure 11-3. The shaded area includes the cumulative mortality from osteosarcoma curves of four separate control tests of FBJ-osteosarcoma extract incubated with saline solution; 50% of the animals inoculated at birth died with bone cancer between 74 and 120 days (an average of 97 days). Plasma from untreated adult CF1/Anl (340) mice gave similar results, 50% incidence being reached at 99 days.

All tests with plasma from animals exposed to FBJ virus were positive (Figure 11-3). Plasma from mice immunized with FBJ virus in Freund's incomplete adjuvant showed high-titered neutralizing antibody, and plasma from mice bearing transplanted FBJ tumors had moderate neutralizing capacity. The most significant protection was

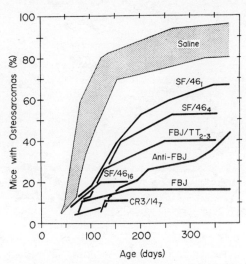

FIG. 11–3.—Cumulative incidence of death with osteosarcoma after neonatal injection of 0.1 ml FBJ-osteosarcoma extract incubated with saline solution or with plasma from mice immunized against FBJ virus (Anti-FBJ), inoculated with FBJ extract at birth and having an osteosarcoma (FBJ), bearing an FBJ-osteosarcoma transplant (FBJ/TT$_{2-3}$), or bearing a ^{90}Sr-osteosarcoma transplant (SF/46$_1$, SF/46$_4$, SF/46$_{16}$, CR3/14$_7$).

obtained with plasma from mice with FBJ tumors induced by the injection of FBJ-osteosarcoma extract at birth.

Plasma from mice carrying four transplant lines of ^{90}Sr osteosarcomas showed varying capacity to neutralize FBJ virus. Test plasmas SF/48 and SF/54 were negative, 50% of the animals inoculated at birth dying with osteosarcoma in 98 and 124 days, respectively. Test plasmas SF/46$_1$ and SF/46$_4$ showed low-titered neutralizing antibody, 50% osteosarcoma-mortality-time being 199 and 250 days, respectively (Figure 11-3). The most recent neutralization test with transplant line SF/46, now in its sixteenth passage, was started 170 days ago, and current results indicate much greater neutralizing capacity than was present in earlier samples. Test plasma CR3/14$_7$, which was also inoculated 170 days ago, appears to contain antibody in very high titer against FBJ virus.

Discussion

The ability of adult CF1/Anl mice to produce antibody against FBJ virus was demonstrated in the passive immunity test, where serum from mice inoculated with FBJ-osteosarcoma extract partially protected newborn mice from FBJ oncogenesis. The beneficial effects of pretreatment were evident immediately, but posttreatment effects did not appear until after one year.

When ^{90}Sr was given, FBJ-immunized mice lived somewhat longer than nonimmunized mice. The reason is not clear since they did not have fewer osteosarcomas or fewer tumors of the reticular tissues. Poorest survival was displayed by mice treated with ^{90}Sr alone. The differences were small in the 1.0 and 0.25 μCi/gm groups, but very striking in the 0.5 μCi/gm group. The reason for this result, also, was not clear since there seemed to be no association within ^{90}Sr groups between life span and osteosarcoma incidence. These results may represent chance variations attributable to small numbers, but the possibility that FBJ virus might have improved the ability of mice to withstand the toxic effects of ^{90}Sr deserves consideration.

The induction of hemangiosarcomas and fibrosarcomas of bone by ^{90}Sr, and the apparent lack of association between their incidence and dose level, have been noted before.[9] FBJ virus seemed to have no relationship to these tumors.

In previous tests, adult mice inoculated with FBJ-osteosarcoma extract had rarely developed bone cancer. Therefore, a low incidence of FBJ tumors was expected in mice treated with virus alone, but it seemed possible that the number might increase when bone was damaged by [90]Sr. Instead, six of 15 adult mice treated with 0.5 ml FBJ extract had FBJ osteosarcomas 128 to 555 days later. Adult mice, therefore, are not resistant to FBJ oncogenesis if the dose is large enough. Radiostrontium decreased, rather than increased, the oncogenic response to FBJ virus. Radiation either damaged the cells that would have responded to viral oncogenesis or damaged the virus. The former explanation is more likely since the amount of radiation from these dosages of ^{90}Sr was significant for cellular damage[10] but insignificant for destruction of virus.

Mice immunized against FBJ virus were not protected against ^{90}Sr oncogenesis. This result suggests that FBJ virus-induced and ^{90}Sr-induced osteosarcomas do not contain a common virus. However, it is possible that similar antigens are involved but that the amount of protective antibody produced was not sufficient to neutralize the antigen resulting from the dosages of ^{90}Sr that were used. Unfortunately, immunized mice were not treated with 0.25 μCi ^{90}Sr/gm.

The group of mice treated with 0.25 ml FBJ-osteosarcoma extract one day after 0.5 μCi[90]Sr/gm had twice as many ^{90}Sr osteosarcomas as the other three 0.5 μCi/gm groups. This kind of result did not occur with other levels of ^{90}Sr, nor when twice as much FBJ extract was given. The animals in this group were the last mice of the 0.5 μCi/gm groups to be treated, and, after eight of the 30 had been done, a different ^{90}Sr solution was used. Therefore, the possibility must be considered that the last 22 mice received more ^{90}Sr than intended. This is unlikely for several reasons, but particularly because the eight mice treated with the original solution had almost as many osteosarcomas as the others: 1.6 per mouse compared to 1.8 per mouse. Nevertheless, this portion of the experiment is to be repeated.

In previous experiments, differences in anatomic location of osteosarcomas depending upon ^{90}Sr dosage had not been noted, probably because diagnosis was not assisted by serial roentgenographic examination.[11] The difference observed in distribution between long bones and spine in this experiment will be helpful in investigations concerned with the amount of absorbed radiation required to produce malignant change in the mouse skeleton.[10]

The demonstration of neutralizing antibody to FBJ virus in the plasma of mice bearing two of the four transplant lines of ^{90}Sr osteosarcomas indicates the presence of FBJ virus, or a very closely related variant, in these tumors. The amount of neutralizing antibody was not associated with histologic type, the fibroblastic osteosarcoma and only one of the three osteoblastic osteosarcomas being positive. However, greater neutralizing capacity was associated with higher incidence of successful growth and with higher incidence of regression. Preliminary electron micrographic examination of the four transplant lines has shown mature Type C particles and buds in both positive transplant lines, SF/46 and CR3/14. The SF/46 tumor also contains Type A cytoplasmic particles, as does SF/54, one of the negative transplant lines. The particles appearing in SF/48, the other negative tumor, have not yet been identified.

The antigen demonstrated in the two ^{90}Sr-osteosarcoma transplant lines does not appear to be a tumor tissue antigen. If it were, the transplant lines with least successful growth would be expected to induce neutralizing antibody in high titer, and this was not the case. If the antigen were a virus, variation in eliciting antibody production could be due to variation in particle maturity, or the virus might be defective, neutralizing antibody being produced in response to a helper virus not necessarily present in all transplant lines. The presence of a defective virus in the ^{90}Sr-induced osteosarcomas would explain why cell-free passage of these tumors has not been successful even though virus particles appear in thin sections.

Neutralization of FBJ osteosarcoma extract with FBJ plasma or with plasma from mice bearing SF/46 and CR3/14 transplant lines only partially protected recipients against FBJ osteosarcomas. Neutralization probably was incomplete, the inoculum containing FBJ virus in low titer. Complete protection should be possible either by increasing the amount of test plasma or by reducing the amount of virus.

Results of the neutralization tests with different samples of transplant line SF/46 suggest that antibody level was higher when the tumor was actively growing than after it had regressed. This result probably is due to greater stimulation of the immune mechanism while antigen is present. Also, neutralizing antibody may play an active role in regression and be left in lower titer after regression. Another possibility is that antigen increased as the tumor was transplanted from generation to generation since the greatest neutralizing capacity was found in the sixteenth transplant generation.

This experiment did not answer many of the questions raised by the first study of the combined action of FBJ virus and ^{90}Sr on the induction of bone cancer in mice.[4] In that study, FBJ virus injected at birth changed the subsequent osteosarcoma response to ^{90}Sr, either shortening the latent period or decreasing the incidence, or both, depending upon the age when ^{90}Sr was injected. In this study, FBJ virus given as fractional immunizing doses to adults during the month preceding ^{90}Sr injection or as a single dose on the day after had very little effect on the induction of ^{90}Sr osteosarcomas. On the contrary, ^{90}Sr prevented the appearance of some FBJ-induced osteosarcomas. The suggestion that immune responses do play a role when FBJ virus and ^{90}Sr are present in the same host is supported, however, by the demonstration of an antigen similar to FBJ virus in some ^{90}Sr-induced osteosarcomas.

Summary

The interaction of FBJ-osteosarcoma virus and ^{90}Sr on the induction of osteosarcomas was studied by immunizing mice against FBJ virus and then treating them with oncogenic amounts of ^{90}Sr and by treating mice with oncogenic amounts of ^{90}Sr and then with FBJ-osteosarcoma virus. Immunization had little effect on the subsequent development of ^{90}Sr osteosarcomas, but treatment with ^{90}Sr before FBJ virus inhibited the development of FBJ osteosarcomas. A beneficial effect of FBJ treatment on ^{90}Sr life-shortening was suggested, and there was an enhancement of the ^{90}Sr-osteosarcoma response when 0.25 ml FBJ extract followed 0.5 μCi ^{90}Sr/gm.

Antigenic relationship between FBJ virus and two ^{90}Sr osteosarcomas was demonstrated by neutralization tests. Both of these tumors, carried as subcutaneous transplants, contained mature and immature Type C particles.

Acknowledgments

This work was supported by the United States Atomic Energy Commission.

We gratefully acknowledge the assistance of our research team: Isabel Greco, Gabriele Rockus, James Knudson, Phylis Dale, Edward Jackson, Leon Stewart, and Mose Burrell.

References

1. Lisco, H., M. P. Finkel, and A. M. Brues: Carcinogenic properties of radioactive fission products and of plutonium. Radiology, 49:361-362, 1947.
2. Finkel, M. P., and B. O. Biskis: Experimental induction of osteosarcomas. Prog. Exper. Tumor Res., 10:72-111, 1968.
3. Finkel, M. P., B. O. Biskis, and P. B. Jinkins: Virus induction of osteosarcomas in mice. Science, 151:698-701, 1966.
4. Finkel, M. P., and B. O. Biskis: Osteosarcomas induced in mice by FBJ virus and ^{90}strontium. In: Delayed Effects of Bone-seeking Radionuclides, Ed. C. W. Mays, et al. Univ. of Utah Press, Salt Lake City, 1969, pp. 417-435.
5. Finkel, M. P., P. J. Bergstrand, and B. O. Biskis: The latent period, incidence, and growth of Sr^{90}-induced osteosarcomas in CF1 and CBA mice. Radiology, 77:269-281, 1961.

6. Biskis, B. O., and M. P. Finkel: Electron microscopy of the FBJ osteosarcoma virus. Proc. Elec. Micr. Soc. Amer., 27th Ann. Meet., 384-385, 1969.
7. Levy, J. A., J. W. Hartley, W. P. Rowe, and R. J. Huebner: Biological characteristics of FBJ osteosarcoma virus. Proc. Amer. Assoc. Cancer Res., 10:50, 1969.
8. Finkel, M. P., P. B. Jinkins, J. Tolle, and B. O. Biskis: Serial radiography of virus-induced osteosarcomas in mice. Radiology 87:333-339, 1966.
9. Finkel, M. P., B. O. Biskis, and G. M. Scribner: The influence of strontium-90 upon life span and neoplasms of mice. In: Progress in Nuclear Energy, Series VI, Vol. 2—Biological Sciences, Pergamon Press, London, 1959, pp. 199-209.
10. Marshall, J. H., and M. P. Finkel: Autoradiographic dosimetry of mouse bones containing Ca^{45}, Sr^{90}, and Ra^{226}. Semiannual Report, Radiological Physics Division, Argonne National Laboratory. ANL-6104:48-65, 1959.
11. Finkel, M. P., and B. O. Biskis: The induction of malignant bone tumors in mice by radioisotopes. Acta Unio internat. contre le cancrum, 15:99-106, 1959.

Interaction of X-ray Treatment, a Chemical Carcinogen, Hormones, and Viruses in Mammary Gland Carcinogenesis

L. M. BOOT, P. BENTVELZEN,
J. CALAFAT, G. RÖPCKE,
AND A. TIMMERMANS

The Netherlands Cancer Institute, Amsterdam, The Netherlands

BESIDES THE WORK on the classic mammary tumor virus (MTV), the hormonal induction of mammary tumors in mice has been one of the main topics of study for a long time in the Biological Department of our institute. On the basis of preliminary experiments by Loeb et al.[1] a technic was developed in which many mammary tumors could be induced by pituitary isografts in otherwise intact female mice of MTV-free strains and hybrids.[2-5] The basic principle involved is relatively simple: an ectopic pituitary, outside the influence of the hypothalamus, produces prolactin continuously, because the hypothalamic neurohumor prolactin inhibiting factor does not reach the general circulation in sufficient quantities to keep the pituitary isograft in check. Con-

TABLE 11–3.—MAMMARY TUMOR INDUCTION IN FEMALE (020 × IF) F_1 MICE
BY ISOGRAFTS OF ONE PITUITARY OF ADULT DONORS
IN SPLEEN OR KIDNEY

| TREATMENT | | | | | WITH TUMOR | | WITHOUT TUMOR |
Site of Implantation	Sex of Donors	No. ANIMALS	No.	%	Av. Age (days)		Av. Age at Death (days)
—	—	41	0	0	—		740
Spleen	♀	52	12	23	697		718
Spleen	♂	50	23	46	580		666
Kidney	♀	51	34	67	561		636
Kidney	♂	51	41	80	507		546

sequently, the mammary gland is exposed to the direct mammo-
trophic action of large amounts of prolactin, in addition to above-
normal quantities of progesterone, through the luteotrophic action of
prolactin on the ovarian corpora lutea. The ultimate results vary, depending on strain of the recipients, site of implantation, and sex and
age of the donors. One example is shown in Table 11-3, in which sex of
the donors and the site of implantation were varied. Male donors generally proved to be more effective than female ones, and the kidney a
better implantation site than the spleen.

At a time it was thought that the pituitary-isografted mice might
serve as a useful model to investigate a possible direct carcinogenic
action of roentgen irradiation or chemical carcinogens on the hormonally stimulated mammary gland. In these and other experiments described below, the routine treatment was to implant one pituitary of
an adult male donor into the left kidney at the age of six to eight
weeks and to apply radiation and/or urethan treatment 14 days later.
No experiment in which local radiation through 1 cm-diameter holes
in a 4 mm-thick lead shield was given to the second left and fourth
right mammary glands resulted in mammary tumor incidences differ-

TABLE 11–4.—MAMMARY TUMOR INDUCTION IN FEMALE (C57BL × C3Hf) F_1
MICE BY X-RAY TREATMENT AND A PITUITARY ISOGRAFT IN THE
KIDNEY, ALONE AND IN COMBINATION

| TREATMENT | | | WITH TUMOR | | WITHOUT TUMOR |
Pit. Isograft in Kidney	Radiation (single dose)	No. ANIMALS	%	Av. Age (days)	Av. Age at Death (days)
—	—	48	0	—	700
—	200 rad. WBR	48	12	520	531
—	400 rad. WBR	43	12	508	518
+	—	98	75	549	613
+	200 rad. WBR	143	85	398	473
+	400 rad. WBR	138	86	387	462
+	200 rad. loc.	92	82	513	563
+	400 rad. loc.	88	78	502	584

TABLE 11–5.—MAMMARY TUMOR INDUCTION IN FEMALE C57BL
MICE BY VARIOUS TREATMENTS

| | TREATMENT | | | WITH TUMOR | | WITHOUT TUMOR |
Pit. Isograft in Kidney	Urethane in Drinking Water	Radiation WBR, 200 rad.	No. ANIMALS	%	Av. Age (days)	Av. Age at Death (days)
—	—	—	193	0	—	621
+	—	—	14	15	570	619
+	—	+	12	41	527	490
+	—	+ (ov. shielded)	11	63	514	503
+	+	—	15	60	369	385
+	+	+	7	43	325	343

ing significantly from those found in the controls. Whole body radiation (WBR, Siemens Isomatix, 250 kv, 8 mA, 1 mm. Cu, FSD 30 cm.; 53,5 rad. min.), however, did have an effect on mammary gland carcinogenesis, as shown in Table 11-4.

Local radiation with 200 or 400 rads hardly increased the mammary tumor incidence or decreased the average tumor age as compared to the controls with pituitary isografts only. Moreover, the tumors were found to be distributed at random, without preference for the irradiated regions. Significant increases in tumor percentages were observed, however, in animals receiving whole body radiation, either with or without pituitary isografts, over those observed in the respective controls. Of interest is the low average tumor age in the irradiated mice with pituitary grafts.

In the following experiments, female MTV- and nodule inducing virus (NIV)-free animals of strains C57BL, 020, and CBA were given pituitary isografts in the kidney and treated with whole body radiation or urethan (0.05% in drinking water), single or in combination (Tables 11-5, 11-6, and 11-7). As was known, pituitary isografts induced but a small number of tumors in the relatively resistant strain C57BL, whereas higher tumor incidence was found in strains 020 and CBA. In all three strains radiation treatment as well as urethan enhanced mammary gland carcinogenesis. Markedly higher tumor incidence was seen

TABLE 11–6.—MAMMARY TUMOR INDUCTION IN FEMALE
020 MICE BY VARIOUS TREATMENTS

| | TREATMENT | | | WITH TUMOR | | WITHOUT TUMOR |
Pit. Isograft in Kidney	Urethane in Drinking Water	Radiation WBR, 200 rad.	No. ANIMALS	%	Av. Age (days)	Av. Age at Death (days)
—	—	—	88	0	—	684
+	—	—	20	60	550	573
+	—	+	15	46	374	402
+	—	+ (ov. shielded)	18	83	347	415
+	+	—	12	66	247	268
+	+	+	15	60	249	273

TABLE 11–7.—MAMMARY TUMOR INDUCTION IN FEMALE CBA
MICE BY VARIOUS TREATMENTS

| | TREATMENT | | | | WITH TUMOR | WITHOUT TUMOR |
Pit. Isograft in Kidney	Urethane in Drinking Water	Radiation WBR, 200 rad.	No. ANIMALS	%	Av. Age (days)	Av. Age at Death (days)
—	—	—	124	2	740	710
+	—	—	14	64	629	684
+	—	+	12	83	402	513
+	—	+ (ov. shielded)	12	91	454	528
+	+	—	15	100	277	263
+	+	+ (ov. shielded)	12	83	319	335

in strains C57BL and CBA, and in all three strains studied the average tumor age was greatly reduced. In the radiation-treated groups, the results were most spectacular when the ovaries were shielded, thus preventing interference with the endocrine mechanism. In the groups treated with urethan, the mammary tumor percentages obtained were depressed by the complication that this drug strongly promoted the occurrence of the type of cancer which each of the strains studied was liable to develop to a certain percentage at a much higher age when not treated with urethan (leukemia in strain C57BL, lung tumors in strain 020, and liver tumors in strain CBA). This is reflected in the relatively low age of the animals which died without mammary tumors in the urethan-treated groups. Naturally many of the animals killed because of a palpable mammary tumor also presented the tumor type characteristic for the particular strain when autopsy was done. In each strain, all animals developing manifest nonmammary gland cancer at an age before the first mammary tumor was found in that particular strain were discarded from the calculations of the mammary tumor incidences.

Routinely a small number of tumors of the various groups were screened by electron microscopy for the presence of B-particles, characteristic for the traditional MTV. Extensive previous investigations of mammary tumors induced by pituitary isografts alone had already shown these particles to be absent from the purely hormonally induced tumors in the three strains studied, whereas they invariably were present when the animals previously had been infected with the MTV from C3H mice. Only in the 020 strain, given the combined treatment of pituitary isografts, irradiation, and urethan, were B-particles found in the tumors. The occurrence of B-particles in mammary tumors of this strain following the combined treatment of whole body radiation, urethan, and subsequent forced breeding has been described previously.[6] The value of the negative results in the other groups is naturally only relative and needs further study.

From the results described above and the literature data, especially those on leukemia induction, it was concluded that it might very well

TABLE 11–8.—MAMMARY TUMOR INDUCTION IN FORCE-BRED MICE BY
IP INJECTION OF WHOLE BLOOD OF IRRADIATED MALE DONORS

RECIPIENT	DONOR	No. ANIMALS	No. ANIMALS WITH TUMOR AT THE AGE OF ONE YEAR
(C57BL × C3Hf) F_1	C57BL	24	3
C3Hf	C3Hf	24	18
(C57BL × C3Hf) F_1	C3Hf	12	2
(C57BL × C3Hf) F_1	(C57BL × C3Hf) F_1	24	3
(020 × DBAf) F_1	C57BL	12	5

NOTE: No mammary tumors were found in untreated force-bred controls before the age of one year.

be that a virus-like agent was involved in the radiation- and/or urethan-induced carcinogenesis in our system. This hypothesis was first tested in the following way: 0.05 ml of whole blood of irradiated male donors (200 rads WBR) was injected ip into six- to eight-week-old female recipients who were later force-bred. The interval between irradiation and collection of blood was 14 days (Table 11-8). The results are indeed highly suggestive for the presence of a viral agent in the blood of irradiated animals, an agent which is not strain-specific.

In the following two experiments, we tried to find more details on the mechanism of action of whole body radiation. Direct irradiation of the exteriorized spleen was as effective in mammary tumor induction in pituitary isograft-bearing animals as whole body radiation with or without shielding of the spleen (Table 11-9). The interval between pituitary isografting and radiation treatment was again 14 days. The spleen thus seems to be one of the organs involved in mammary gland carcinogenesis by whole body radiation, but certainly is not the only organ affected.

When pituitary isograft-bearing animals of strain 020 were injected ip with a suspension of isologous thymus cells (one thymus to 2 ml Tyrode solution, volume injected 0.05 ml), obtained from male animals irradiated (200 rads WBR) 14 days previously, an enhancing action on

TABLE 11–9.—MAMMARY TUMOR INDUCTION IN FEMALE C57BL MICE
BY IRRADIATION OF THE SPLEEN AFTER IMPLANTATION OF A
PITUITARY IN THE KIDNEY

RADIATION TREATMENT	No. ANIMALS	WITH TUMOR %	WITH TUMOR Av. Age (days)	WITHOUT TUMOR Av. Age at Death (days)
—	14	15	570	619
200 rad. WBR	12	41	527	490
200 rad. WBR (spleen shielded)	9	45	500	563
200 rad. to spleen	9	45	540	575
200 rad. to ½ spleen	12	50	540	593

TABLE 11–10.—MAMMARY TUMOR INDUCTION IN FEMALE 020 MICE BY INJECTION OF SUSPENSIONS OF THYMUS CELLS OF IRRADIATED DONORS

Pit. Isograft in Kidney	TREATMENT Thymus Suspension Normal Donor	Irradiated Donor	No. ANIMALS	WITH TUMOR %	Av. Age (days)	WITHOUT TUMOR Av. Age at Death (days)
+	—	—	20	60	550	573
+	—	+	13	90	330	348
+	+	—	15	46	390	395
—	—	+	12	0	—	336
—	+	—	12	0	—	448

mammary tumor formation was again observed (Table 11-10). In animals with no pituitary graft, thymus suspension had no effect on the mammary gland. An as yet unexplained phenomenon is that, at least in strain 020, injection of suspensions of thymus tissue obtained from irradiated as well as normal animals markedly decreased the life span of the treated mice by increasing the occurrence of lung tumors.

Finally it was investigated whether, and if so, in which way, the infective agent induced by irradiation could be transmitted to the offspring. Irradiated female C57BL mice (200 rads, ovaries shielded) were bred to normal C57BL males. In experimental group I, the female offspring of this cross was foster-nursed from birth to the age of three weeks by normal C57BL mothers. In experimental group II, normal newborn C57BL females were foster-nursed by the irradiated mother of the cross mentioned above. In both groups of foster-nursed females, pituitary isografting was performed at the age of eight weeks. Normal females with pituitary isografts served as controls (Table 11-11).

The difference between the experimental groups and the controls is clear. In experimental group II, the radiation-induced infective agent is transmitted with the milk to the foster-nursed offspring. In experimental group I, the offspring of irradiated mothers is already infected at birth, and can not be made agent-free by the foster-nursing technique effective with the classic MTV. In this latter respect, the radia-

TABLE 11–11.—MAMMARY TUMOR INDUCTION IN FEMALE C57BL MICE BY PITUITARY ISOGRAFTS AND AN INFECTIVE AGENT OF IRRADIATED MOTHERS AND FOSTER-MOTHERS

TREATMENT	No. ANIMALS	WITH TUMOR %	Av. Age (days)	WITHOUT TUMOR Av. Age at Death (days)
Controls	14	15	570	619
Exp. group I*	37	48	491	543
Exp. group II*	34	50	510	558

* See text for details.

tion-induced agent resembles the agent found in the GR strain which is also present already in the newborn.[7] Whether the radiation-induced agent can be transmitted by the male as well, as in the GR strain, is under study.

Conclusion

The pituitary isograft-bearing mouse, in which the mammary gland is subjected to excessive hormonal stimulation, appears to be a good model to reveal the presence of a radiation-induced MTV-like agent. In this system, promising results were also obtained after urethan treatment.

References

1. Loeb, L., and M. Moskop Kirtz: Amer. J. Cancer, 36:56-82, 1939.
2. Mühlbock, O., and L. M. Boot: Cancer Res., 19:402-412, 1959.
3. Boot, L. M., O. Mühlbock, G. Röpcke, and W. van Ebbenhorst Tengbergen: Cancer Res., 22:713-727, 1962.
4. Boot, L. M., and G. Röpcke: Cancer Res., 26:1492-1496, 1966.
5. Boot, L. M.: Thesis, Amsterdam, 1969.
   Also published in: Verh. kon. ned. Akad. Wet., afd. Natuurk., tweede reeks, deel LVIII, no. 3. N.V. North-Holland Publishing Company, Amsterdam, 1969.
6. Timmermans, A., P. Bentvelzen, Ph. C. Hageman, and J. Calafat: J. Gen. Virol., 4:619-621, 1969.
7. Bentvelzen, P. A. J.: Thesis, Leiden, 1968.

Effect of Cortisol on HeLa Cell Metabolism and Morphology

N. KELLER, R. E. NORDQUIST,
AND M. J. GRIFFIN

Oklahoma Medical Research Foundation, and Department of Biochemistry, University of Oklahoma School of Medicine, Oklahoma City, Oklahoma, USA

PREVIOUS STUDIES HAVE listed increases in cell water, RNA and protein[1] as well as DNA, RNA, and protein[2] and in sialic acid[3] after short-term cultivation of certain HeLa strains with glucocorticoids such as cortisol. A recent study shows that one HeLa strain, HeLa 71, has an increased G-1 portion of the cell generation cycle, resulting in an increased population doubling time, when grown and subcultured continuously with cortisol (Hcr state).[4] Another strain, HeLa 65, exhibits no long-term growth deterrent with this steroid.[4]

The present study shows that these two HeLa strains have different biochemical, biophysical, and morphologic responses to continuous cultivation with cortisol. Some of the observed biochemical differences may underlie the different growth pattern established in HeLa 71 when cultured with this glucocorticoid. The data compiled to date would appear to indict membranes as one target site of action of hydrocortisone.

Materials and Methods

CELL CULTURE TECHNIQUES

Two HeLa strains were used and are identified by their modal chromosome number.[5] HeLa 65 was originally cloned for suspension culture, and has been adapted for monolayer growth. HeLa 71 is a strain originally cloned for a high level of alkaline phosphatase. Both clones were shown to possess a uniform modal chromosome number over the course of this study, and all biochemical and morphologic results repeatedly investigated were constant over 18 months. Cells were grown in monolayer culture using Eagle's Minimal Essential Medium (MEM) supplemented with 10% Colorado calf serum, 50 units per ml penicillin, and 50 μg/ml each of streptomycin and kanamycin. Cells in the Hcr state received 1.0 μg per ml hydrocortisone (Sigma Chem. Co.) and were grown and subcultured with cortisol for a minimum of three weeks before being studied. Serial subculturing in monolayer was performed by technics previously described.[6] Each experiment utilized replicate Blake cultures including one which was used for counting. Cell counts were routinely obtained on a Coulter Counter (Model B) and were checked with a Brite-Line hemocytometer. All cultures were sacrificed at no more than 70% confluency or less than 50% confluency and represent asynchronous, exponentially growing cell populations. Doubling time determinations utilized T-25 flasks (Falcon) with 4 ml of growth medium.

ASSAYS

Cell volume was measured by the use of a Bauer-Schenck sedimentation tube calibrated in 4 μliter increments. The cells were scraped from the monolayer in medium at room temperature, sedimented in a large tube, resuspended and finally packed in the Bauer-Schenck tube at 1,000 g until the volume was constant (usually 15 min sufficed). The final reading represents the closest packed volume of the cells, since cell deformability excluded essentially all extracellular fluid when packed under these conditions.

For cell water determination, the cells were packed as above, using preweighed conical centrifuge tubes (Ace Glass Co.). The last drop of medium was removed by a fine capillary tube, and the wt thus achieved was taken as the wet wt of the cells. The cells in the tube were vacuum desiccated over P_2O_5 until constant dry wt was obtained.

Ions were determined on cells scraped from the substrate in medium and isolated as described for water determinations. The cell pellet was suspended in a solution 3N in nitric acid and 4N in perchloric acid and hydrolized at 100C for 1 hr. Ca^{2+} and Mg^{2+} were determined by atomic absorption spectroscopy on a Perkin Elmer Model 290B spectrometer, while Na^+ and K^+ were estimated by flame photometry. Zinc was determined on a Perkin Elmer Model 303 Atomic Absorption Spectrophotometer.

Total lipid was determined gravimetrically on cells washed with cold saline buffered with Tris-HCl(5mM), pH 7.4. After extraction of the freshly washed cells with chloroform:methanol (2:1), the organic extractant was evaporated under a stream of nitrogen and the resulting lipid extract desiccated over P_2O_5 to constant wt.

Thin layer chromatography to determine classes of lipids in the two cell strains was performed on glass plates coated with a 250-μ layer of activated silica gel G, and developed in hexane:ether (95:5). Spots were detected by spraying with sulfuric acid and charring. Phospholipid phosphorous was determined by the method of Fiske and Subba-Row.[7]

ATP was determined by the luciferin-luciferase method of Addanki et al.[8] with a Nuclear Chicago Mark I Scintillation Counter. Cells were washed with, and scraped into, cold buffered saline. After centrifugation, 1N perchloric acid was added to the cell pellet at 0C, and insoluble cell material removed by centrifugation. The acid supernatant was exactly neutralized with potassium hydroxide, and the insoluble potassium perchlorate centrifuged and discarded. The supernate was repeatedly frozen and thawed to remove the last traces of perchlorate ions, which inhibit the assay. Filtration of the reconstituted luciferase enzyme preparation (Sigma Chem. Co.) is essential in order to remove interfering fluorescent particulate material before ATP determination.

For glycogen determination, the cell monolayer was washed with buffered saline followed by cell lysis with a small volume of 15% trichloroacetic acid. After sedimentation of insoluble components (used for RNA and DNA analysis), glycogen was precipitated by adjusting the supernate to 80% ethanol and storing a minimum of 15 hr at −20C. The glycogen precipitate was sedimented, hydrolyzed in 1N sulfuric acid for 1 hr at 100C, and glucose determined by the glucose oxidase method.[9, 10]

RNA and DNA estimations were done by hydrolyzing the 15% trichloroacetic acid-insoluble fraction in 1 N perchloric acid at 90C for 30 min. DNA was determined by the diphenylamine method of Burton[11] while RNA was estimated by the orcinol technique.[12] Cell protein was determined by the Lowry method[13] on cells which were washed with saline on the monolayer and lysed in 0.5% sodium deoxycholate.

The half-lysis index was performed using an exponentially growing cell monolayer by counting the number of cells lysed as a function of time. Isotonic saline was used as a medium for the lysing agents, and lysis was defined as penetration of the cell by a 0.05% solution of trypan blue.

All values reported represent an average of at least three experiments with a standard deviation no greater than 8%.

ELECTRON MICROSCOPY

Thin sections were prepared from pelleted cells quickly fixed in 2% glutaraldehyde in 0.1M cacodylate buffer containing 5% sucrose. Some cells were fixed directly on the glass by pouring glutaraldehyde into the tissue culture bottle and incubating at 4C for 2 hr. Following fixation the cells were rinsed in 0.1M cacodylate buffer overnight. The cells were then transferred to 1% osmic acid in 0.1M cacodylate buffer plus 5% sucrose and incubated at 4C for 2 hr. After fixation, cells were dehydrated in graded alcohols, embedded in Cargille's Epoxy Resin (Araldite 6005) or maraglas, and polymerized at 60C for 24 hr. All thin sections were stained with uranyl acetate and lead citrate and photographed at various magnifications on a Hitachi HU-11B. Replicas for electron microscopy were prepared by a special procedure.[14] Whole cells grown on slides were fresh frozen in liquid nitrogen and placed on blocks of dry ice. A large block of brass was then cooled with liquid nitrogen and placed in a Hitachi vacuum evaporator. The slides were transferred to the top of the brass block and the chamber was evacuated to a sufficient vacuum for evaporation. Carbon and palladium were shadowed on the cells from a 45° angle. The replica was removed from the slide by immersion in 10% NaOH at 4C overnight, which also removes most of the organic material. The replica was then rinsed in 3% acetic acid and placed on a copper grid for viewing.

Results

The two cell strains showed marked growth differences in response to cultivation with cortisol. HeLa 65 exhibited no appreciable difference in doubling time (18 hr for both states in this clone) between control cells and those in the Hcr state. When HeLa 71 is cultured with cortisol, its population doubling time is increased 50% (28 hr for Hcr, 18 hr for control).

Cell size is expressed (Table 11-12) in three ways: (a) the average volume measured as described, (b) the average diameter of the living cell as measured from phase-contrast photographs of the monolayers

TABLE 11–12.—CELL SIZE

CELL STRAIN		AVERAGE MEASURED VOLUME $\mu\mu$L/CELL	MONOLAYER AVERAGE DIAMETER μ	AVERAGE DIAMETER CALCULATED FROM AVERAGE VOLUME μ	WATER CONTENT $\mu\mu$G/CELL
HeLa 71	Control	3.7	23.1 ± 1.5	19	3,600
HeLa 71	Hcr	5.9	30.7 ± 1.6	22	5,700
HeLa 65	Control	3.3	22.3 ± 1.8	19	3,200
HeLa 65	Hcr	4.0	23.8 ± 0.2	20	3,700

Cell volume and monolayer diameter measurements were made as described in text. Calculated diameters were computed from the measured average cell volume. Water content was measured as described in text.

using a Unitron 10B inverted microscope, and (c) the average diameter as calculated from the measured volume. It is apparent from these data that the HeLa 71 Hcr cell is much larger than the control cell of the same strain, whereas HeLa 65 showed no significant increase in size when grown in the presence of this steroid. By comparing the calculated diameter with the measured diameter of each of these cells, it can be seen that HeLa 71 Hcr cells grow on the substrate in a more flattened manner compared to the suspended state, than do any of the other three cell types.

The results of measurements of cell water are also recorded in Table 11-12. HeLa 71 Hcr has 50% more water on a per cell basis than its corresponding control cell, in contrast to HeLa 65 which shows only about a 10% increase in the Hcr state. The dry weights are as follows: HeLa 71, 550 $\mu\mu$g/cell; HeLa 71 Hcr, 1000 $\mu\mu$g/cell; HeLa 65, 530 $\mu\mu$g/ cell; HeLa 65 Hcr, 540 $\mu\mu$g/cell. From the above data, we estimated water to represent from 83 to 85% of the measured cell volume for either strain in either state.

An increase in the water content of HeLa 71 Hcr is particularly significant when the cell molar concentration of divalent and monovalent metal ions is examined (Table 11-13). Both strains had increased levels of sodium in the Hcr steady state. Little change was seen in K^+ in

TABLE 11–13.—CELL IONIC CONCENTRATION (mM)

LINES	NA^+	K^+	CA^{2+}	MG^{2+}	ZN^{2+}
HeLa 71	100	38	3.4	7.2	0.21
HeLa 71 Hcr	130	35	4.5	7.6	0.35
HeLa 65	150	54	3.0	6.1	0.22
HeLa 65 Hcr	190	63	2.1	7.5	0.32
MEM	130	6	1.7	0.8	0.01

Intracellular concentrations of ions (mmoles per liter of cell water) for HeLa 71 and HeLa 65 in both control and Hcr states. The bottom line shows the concentration of these ions in complete growth medium. These data are the mean of four determinations and the standard deviation for any value is less than 4%.

TABLE 11–14.—LIPIDS

LINES	TOTAL LIPID $\mu\mu$G/CELL	TOTAL PHOSPHOLIPID PHOSPHOROUS $\mu\mu$MOLES/CELL	PHOSPHOLIPID* $\mu\mu$G/CELL TOTAL LIPID $\mu\mu$G/CELL
HeLa 71	170	0.08	0.34
HeLa 71 Hcr	310	0.13	0.28
HeLa 65	200	0.09	0.28
HeLa 65 Hcr	220	0.12	0.33

* Based on an estimated average molecular weight of 750 for phospholipid.

HeLa 71, while in HeLa 65 a 20% increase was observed in the Hcr state.

Calcium ions increased in HeLa 71 Hcr by 30% whereas they decreased in HeLa 65 Hcr by about 30%. Magnesium ions increased in HeLa 65 Hcr by 23%, but showed no significant change in HeLa 71 from one state to the other. Both strains had about 50% increased levels of Zn^{2+} in asynchronous exponentially growing cell populations in their Hcr states.

Another component of HeLa 71 cells which is increased significantly in the Hcr state is total lipid (Table 11-14). Whereas the cell volume increased only 50% in HeLa 71 Hcr, the lipid increase is 80% (170 $\mu\mu$g/cell versus 310 $\mu\mu$g/cell). Thin layer chromatography of these lipids suggest cholesterol and phospholipid as the major components, with minor amounts of diglycerides and cholesterol esters. An increase in phospholipid phosphorous was observed in the Hcr state of both cell strains; it was more pronounced in HeLa 71 (Table 11-14). Phospholipid to total lipid ratios are not significantly different for either clone in either state.

Results of the DNA assay show no difference for either clone in either state, and were 11 ± 2 $\mu\mu$g/cell. RNA and protein, conversely, show a 30% increase in HeLa 71 Hcr, while HeLa 65 exhibited no significant change in the Hcr state (Table 11-15).

The amount of energy available to an Hcr cell, in the form of ATP, is shown to be more than twice that present in a control cell in both strains (Table 11-15). Though the absolute amounts of ATP differ

TABLE 11–15.—RNA, PROTEIN, ATP AND GLYCOGEN

CELL STRAIN	RNA $\mu\mu$G/CELL	PROTEIN $\mu\mu$G/CELL	ATP $\mu\mu$MOLES/CELL	GLYCOGEN $\mu\mu$G/CELL
HeLa 71 Control	25.2	640	.003	109
HeLa 71 Hcr	33.8	880	.008	210
HeLa 65 Control	25.5	790	.024	157
HeLa 65 Hcr	23.6	730	0.52	320

These values are expressed for exponentially growing asynchronous cells. Based on six determinations these values have a standard deviation no greater than 8%.

TABLE 11–16.—HALF LYSIS INDEX

CONCENTRATION OF LYSING AGENT	HeLa 71 Control	HeLa 71 Hcr	HeLa 65 Control	HeLa 65 Hcr
		Minutes		
0.050% DOC	20	10	10	10
0.040% DOC	20	20	12	40
0.030% DOC	30	30	22	>120
0.020% DOC	>120	>120	>120	>120
0.020% Saponin	3	3	2	3
0.010% Saponin	25	75	36	>120
0.005% Saponin	>120	>120	>120	>120

Results represent the time in minutes required to lyse 50% of the cells, as measured by admittance of trypan blue.

widely between the cell strains, the relative increase from the control to the Hcr state is quite similar, with HeLa 71 showing a proportionally larger increase.

The glycogen assay shows a doubling in this compound in the Hcr state of both strains (Table 11-15).

Table 11-16 shows the results of a study of the effect of lipolytic lysing agents on both strains in both states. HeLa 65 Hcr is more resistant to lysis with both sodium deoxycholate (DOC) and saponin than is the HeLa 65 control. In contrast, little increase in resistance to either agent is evidenced by HeLa 71 Hcr versus its control, though a

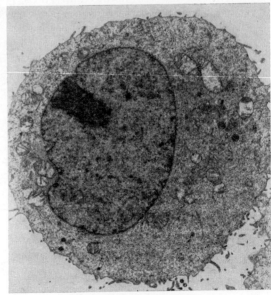

FIG. 11–4.—HeLa 65-Control State. ×6,000.

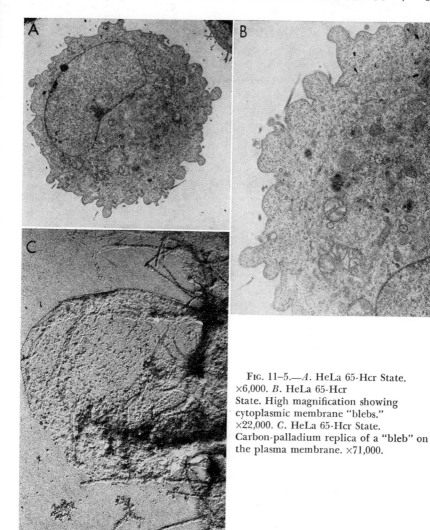

Fig. 11–5.—*A*. HeLa 65-Hcr State.
×6,000. *B*. HeLa 65-Hcr
State. High magnification showing
cytoplasmic membrane "blebs."
×22,000. *C*. HeLa 65-Hcr State.
Carbon-palladium replica of a "bleb" on
the plasma membrane. ×71,000.

slight protection against the uncharged saponin appears to exist for this strain in the Hcr state.

Histochemical results also substantiate biochemical and electron microscopic results. Little difference could be demonstrated between the two states of HeLa 71 and HeLa 65 with regard to DNA, RNA, or protein. But the enhanced glycogen content in the Hcr state of both strains was readily apparent. Two types of glycogen-containing cells in HeLa 71 were demonstrated. In the control culture, there were cells containing some glycogen in large granules and also cells which contained very little glycogen. HeLa 71 Hcr exhibited about 15% of its population as giant cells nearly filled with glycogen. In this culture, there were also large cells which contained fine granules of glycogen and small cells with large granules. These results suggest that glycogen varies qualitatively and quantitatively around the cell cycle.

Histochemically, there were no pools of cholesterol or triglycerides in lipid droplets in the two strains. It is inferred then, that the lipid in the HeLa 65 and HeLa 71 cells is membrane-bound and that the increase in lipid found in HeLa 71 Hcr represents an increase in membrane lipid.

Electron microscopic studies showed the cytoplasm of HeLa 65 contained relatively fewer organelles of all types than that of HeLa 71. For example, mitochondria were fewer in number and lysosomes were relatively smaller and fewer when compared to the other clone (compare Figures 11-4, 11-5A, 11-6, and 11-7A). Golgi zones were adjacent to the nucleus and were small in size. There were short lengths of rough endoplasmic reticulum, but no discernible organization. Smooth endoplasmic reticulum, though sparse, was near the cell's periphery. This clone has a relatively smooth cytoplasmic periphery, in the control state, though occasional cells exhibited "blebs" or evaginations of the plasma membrane, which contained ribosomes or other cytoplasmic organelles. The nuclear membrane of this clone provides a nuclear silhouette that is continuous and smooth, and shows relatively few

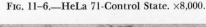

Fig. 11–6.—HeLa 71-Control State. ×8,000.

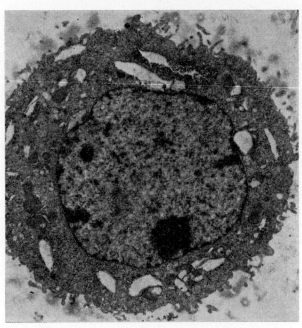

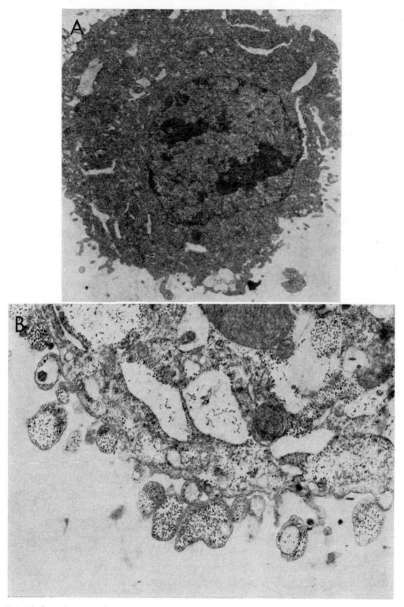

Fig. 11–7.—A. HeLa 71-Hcr State. ×8,000. B. HeLa 71-Hcr State. High magnification showing projections of the plasma membrane which contain glycogen. ×23,000.

microinvaginations as compared to the other clone (Figures 11-4, 11-5A, 11-6, and 11-7A). In the Hcr state, the plasma membrane of HeLa 65 formed large evaginations, some of which contain organelles (Figures 11-5A and B). Figure 11-5C shows a carbon replica of one "bleb."

In the control state, HeLa 71 has a highly crenated outer periphery (Figure 11-6). The cytoplasm contained moderate amounts of glycogen, which were dispersed or found in large vacuoles associated with the rough endoplasmic reticulum. Numerous mitochondria were seen in this strain. Endoplasmic reticulum was abundant but apparently somewhat dilated; in some cells, the lumen was filled with a moderate amount of glycogen (Figure 11-6). In a small number of cells, the plasma membrane had evaginations which contained glycogen.

HeLa 71 had a large increase in glycogen in the Hcr state (Figure 11-7A). The major part of this glycogen was found within large membrane-bound vacuoles some of which were studded with ribosomes. In many fields, topographically separate membrane bound glycogen bodies appeared adjacent to the outer plasma membrane (Figure 11-7B). Similar bodies were seen attached to the plasma membrane.

Discussion

The unbalanced growth of HeLa S_3 cells (herein referred to as HeLa 65) described by Kim et al.[15] is an experimental situation in which synchronized HeLa cells were exposed to DNA inhibitors for varying lengths of time. The resulting loss of cell viability (defined as colony-forming ability) was reversible for up to 16 hr, but prolonged exposure of the cells to these drugs led to their death. Presumably during this initial 16 hr, in which colony-forming ability is recoverable, other physiological alterations are reparable to varying degrees. These alterations still allow cell viability, but recovery processes are uncertain. Lambert et al.[16] describe experiments with HeLa cells treated with excess thymidine. The end result of prolonged treatment with this compound was again cell death. This type of metabolism is also referred to as unbalanced growth. In contrast to inhibitors of cell maturation which are ultimately lethal, the system described in this report affords a continued, though altered, proliferation cycle. Growth of HeLa 71 in the presence of hydrocortisone results in cells capable of continued subculture, but with an increased generation time. This new steady-state growth condition shall be called rebalanced growth (to differentiate between the types of drug-elicited effects on cells). HeLa 65 grown in the presence of hydrocortisone shows only an acute growth response,[4] after which control doubling-time is achieved and retained. Because of the biochemical alterations seen in these cells, this is again rebalanced growth with no alteration in the growth cycle.

The increase in size of the HeLa 71 Hcr cell correlates well with the increases found in cell water in this strain. The predicted cell diameter from measured cell volume is in close agreement with average measured diameter of the living cell. Cell volume increase has also been reported[1, 2] in HeLa S_3 cells treated for 72 hr with hydrocortisone. We studied the acute response of HeLa 65 to growth with hydrocortisone, but this acute response is reversed in the Hcr steady-state condition (after three weeks of growth with hydrocortisone) in this strain. Thus, in HeLa 65, the Hcr cells have a cell volume similar to their corresponding control cells, and also nearly the same water content.

The results of the ion studies become more meaningful when viewed in conjunction with the results of cell water measurements. In both cell strains, intracellular Na^+ concentration is increased when grown in the presence of hydrocortisone, while K^+ concentration is increased only in HeLa 65 Hcr. The increased Na^+ concentration above MEM Na^+ in HeLa 65 cells may represent ions attached at absorptive sites within this cell clone. In HeLa 71 Hcr, the sodium ion content is increased to nearly that of the surrounding medium. No single mechanism of cortisol-mediated inhibition or stimulation of the Na^+, K^+-activated ATPase pump is sufficient to explain all these observations. Increases in Na^+ and K^+ have been reported in rat liver after a two- to four-day treatment in vivo with hydrocortisone.[17]

Of the divalent cations examined, only Zn^{2+} increases significantly in both HeLa 65 and HeLa 71 in the Hcr state. The increase is about 50% for both strains. An increase in Zn^{2+} uptake by both cell strains in the presence of steroid hormones with glucocorticoid activity has been reported[18] in studies done with cells grown in the presence of the steroid for a total of 72 hr. Our steady-state results correlate well with these acute responses. While Mg^{2+} concentration was increased by 23% in HeLa 65 Hcr, there was no significant change in HeLa 71 from one state to the other. In HeLa 65 Hcr, the Ca^{2+} concentration is decreased about 30%, while this ion is increased by 30% in HeLa 71 Hcr. These results for monolayer cultures of HeLa cells contrast with those found by Morrill and Robbins[19] in their studies of HeLa cells in suspension culture. They found a correlation between Ca^{2+} levels and the steady-state level of Na^+ and K^+, but that K^+ levels were higher than Na^+ levels. It is apparent that total amounts of anions must be considered in cation studies since suspension culture medium contains 10 times as much phosphate or bicarbonate ion as the medium used for monolayer culture.

The magnitude of increase in lipid in HeLa 71 Hcr is of interest. Since the surface:volume ratio is a function of the radius squared to the radius cubed, a 50% increase in volume would demand less than 50% total increase in surface membranes of the cytoplasm and the nucleus. The 80% increase seen in lipids in the Hcr state of HeLa 71 cells may indicate that this cell strain responds to hydrocortisone by producing more lipids than would be required just for surface membrane production. The increase in lipid may represent an increase in total membrane production in the Hcr cells, with more membranes per cell. Conversely, it could also represent an increased uptake of lipid in the already existing membrane mosaic. Quantitation of these compounds from membrane fractions will determine which of these alternatives is correct. Rosenberg[20] reported that changes in the gross composition of lipid in membranes may well affect both structure and function of those membranes. The possibility of membrane changes becomes particularly important when it is remembered that Jacob, Brenner, and Cuzin[21] suggested that initiation of DNA replication in bacteria required attachment of the chromosome to the cell membrane, while Comings and Kakefuda[22] suggested that DNA replication in mammalian cells may be initiated at the nuclear membrane. Alteration in the nuclear membrane with altered DNA attachment sites is one possible explanation for the extended generation cycle in HeLa 71 Hcr, since it is believed that the initiation of DNA synthesis is being delayed.

The base line differences in ATP content between the two cell strains may reflect the increase in alkaline pyrophosphatase activity found in HeLa 71,[23] since HeLa 71 possesses high constitutive activity of this enzyme.

A large increase in glycogen was observed in the Hcr cells of both strains. Results also showed more of this material in HeLa 65 than in HeLa 71. This stands in contrast to electron microscopic results of HeLa 65 which showed no particulate glycogen. One possible explanation for the apparent discrepancy between biochemical and electron microscopic results is a difference in glycogen particle size. If the glycogen in the HeLa 65 clones were in the size range of the γ particle (3 $M\mu$) mentioned by Barber et al.,[24] then it would appear ultrastructurally, as diffuse background. By contrast the particles of glycogen in HeLa 71 must be similar to the α particle (200 $M\mu$) these authors have described, and thereby detectable by the electron microscope. Moreover, the biochemical results agree well with reported amounts of glycogen found in liver tissue and muscle.[25, 26]

The increase in glycogen content of these cells in the presence of hydrocortisone suggests a uniform gluconeogenic response much like that exhibited by other organs such as liver, spleen, kidney, etc. In any case, the changes seen in those components involved in energy production for the cell do not seem to be the basis of the growth cycle response of HeLa 71 Hcr, since they are elevated from control levels and do not represent a starvation condition.

Melnykovych[2] and Cox[1] reported increases in RNA and protein in HeLa 65 in the acute state of hydrocortisone treatment. The data presented here for the hydrocortisone regulated state agree well with their observations.

The data with the lysing agents provide further suggestive evidence for different physiological membrane responses of HeLa 71 and HeLa 65 to growth with hydrocortisone. The clone without any growth alterations in the Hcr steady-state, HeLa 65, shows an increased resistance to lipolytic lysing agents. This clone has been shown to gain resistance to deoxycholate lysis by short periods of growth with prednisolone.[27] The cell clone with a permanent growth alteration in the Hcr steady-state, HeLa 71, shows little or no resistance to these lysing agents. The inability to gain resistance when grown with cortisol might result from alterations in membrane lipids to increase the number of lipophilic absorptive sites in HeLa 71 Hcr.

Electron microscopic findings indicate that cellular complexity increases as chromosomal numbers increase. HeLa 65 is a relatively simple cell type which contains few organelles and little if any storage products. HeLa 71 contrasts greatly with HeLa 65 in that the cytoplasm contains many mitochondria, organized golgi zones, extensive lengths of endoplasmic reticulum, and large glycogen particles.

Summary

Two HeLa cell strains, HeLa 65 and HeLa 71, identified by their major modal chromosome numbers, were studied by biochemical and electron microscopic technics in two steady state conditions. Cells cultured continuously with 3×10^{-6} M cortisol were called Hcr (hydrocortisone regulated), while those cultured in medium without added cortisol served as controls. Both strains showed a variety of responses to growth with cortisol. Exponentially growing, asynchronous populations of HeLa 71 show increased amounts of water, lipid, sodium, calcium, zinc, RNA, protein, glycogen, and ATP in the Hcr state. This clone undergoes an increase in doubling time when grown with cortisol. In contrast, HeLa 65, the morphologically more primitive cell by electron microscopy, shows increases in sodium, potassium, zinc, glycogen, and ATP when grown with cortisol. No permanent increase in doubling time is evidenced by this clone in the Hcr state. Ultrastructural studies corroborate some of the biochemical changes elicited in cells grown continuously with cortisol, and suggest alterations in cellular membranes. A study with two lipolytic lysing agents provided further support for this postulation. Physiological differences which may be related to altered growth of HeLa 71 Hcr cells are the increases in water, lipid, protein, RNA and calcium ions, and lack of increase of potassium ions.

Acknowledgments

The authors gratefully acknowledge the aid of Dr. Walter Joel for modifications of the histologic technics and his expert interpretation of these results.

We would like to thank Dr. G. Mark Kollmorgen for helpful discussions, and Mrs. Barbara Warriner and Mrs. Frances Crowell for excellent technical assistance.

This investigation was supported by Public Health Service research grant No. CA-10614 from the National Cancer Institute.

References

1. Cox, R. P., and C. M. MacLeod: Alkaline phosphatase content and the effects of prednisolone on mammalian cells in culture. J. Gen. Phys., 45:439, 1962.
2. Melnykovych, G., and C. F. Bishop: Specificity of prednisolone effect on cell volume, RNA and protein in cell lines with inducible and noninducible alkaline phosphatase. Endocrinology, 81:251, 1967.
3. Carubelli, R., and M. J. Griffin: Sialic acid in HeLa cells: effect of hydrocortisone. Science, 157:693, 1967.
4. Kollmorgen, G. M., and M. J. Griffin: The effects of hydrocortisone on HeLa cell growth. Cell and Tissue Kinetics, 2:111, 1969.
5. Bottomley, R. H., A. L. Trainer, and M. J. Griffin: Enzymatic and chromosomal characterization of HeLa variants. J. Cell Biol., 41:806, 1969.
6. Griffin, M. J., and R. Ber: Cell cycle events in the hydrocortisone regulation of alkaline phosphatase in HeLa S$_3$ cells. J. Cell Biol., 40:297, 1969.
7. Fiske, C. H., and Y. SubbaRow: The colorimetric determination of phosphorus. J. Biol. Chem., 66:375, 1925.
8. Addanki, S., J. F. Sotos, and P. P. Rearick: Rapid determination of picamole quantities of ATP with a liquid scintillation counter. Anal. Biochem., 14:261, 1966.
9. Black, O., and J. H. Anglin: Ultraviolet light alterations of acid maltase activity in epidermis. J. Inves. Derm., 48:252, 1967.
10. Barton, R. R.: A specific method for quantitative determination of glucose. Anal. Biochem., 14:258, 1966.
11. Burton, K.: A study of the conditions and mechanisms of the diphenylamine reaction for the colorimetric estimations of deoxyribonucleic acid. Biochem. J., 62:315, 1956.
12. Ashwell, G.: Colorimetric analysis of sugars. In Methods of Enzymology. S. P. Colowick and N. O. Kaplan, editors. Academic Press, Inc., New York, 3:87, 1957.
13. Lowry, O. H., J. J. Rosebrough, A. L. Farr, and R. J. Randall: Protein measurement with the Folin phenol reagent. J. Biol. Chem., 193:265, 1951.
14. Fisher, H. W., and T. W. Cooper: Electron microscope studies of the microvilli of HeLa cells. J. Cell Biol., 34:569, 1967.
15. Kim, J. H., A. G. Perez, and B. Djordjieric: Studies on unbalanced growth in synchronized HeLa cells. Cancer Res., 28:2443, 1968.
16. Lambert, W. C., and G. P. Studzinski: Recovery from prolonged unbalanced growth induced in HeLa cells by high concentrations of thymidine. Cancer Res., 27:2364, 1967.
17. Ganiev, Kh. G., I. V. Borisendo, L. G. Kaletkina, R. P. Molchagina, V. I. Antonovich, F. S. Ichadzhik, V. I. Rzhevskaya, S. E. Ryndina, G. P. Sokol, and L. V. Shipilova: Effect of steroid hormones on the biochemistry and morphology of intact and carbon tetrachloride-treated rat liver. Aktual. Vop. Patol. Pecheni., 4:179, 1968.
18. Cox, R. P.: Hormonal stimulation of zinc uptake in mammalian cell cultures. Mol. Pharm., 4:510, 1968.
19. Morrill, G. A., and E. Robbins: The role of calcium in the regulation of the steady-state levels of sodium and potassium in the HeLa cell. J. Gen. Phys., 50:781, 1967.
20. Rosenberg, M. D.: Single cell properties—membrane development. In Cell Differentiation. A. V. S. DeReuck and Julie Knight, editors. Little, Brown and Co., Boston, 18, 1967.

21. Jacob, F., S. Brenner, and F. Cuzin: On the regulation of DNA replication in bacteria. Cold Spring Harbor Symposia on Quantitative Biology, 28:329, 1963.
22. Comings, D. E., and T. Kakefuda: Initiation of deoxyribonucleic acid replication at the nuclear membrane in human cells. J. Mol. Biol., 33:225, 1968.
23. Cox, R. P., P. Gilbert, and M. J. Griffin: Alkaline inorganic pyrophosphatase activity of mammalian-cell alkaline phosphatase. Biochem. J., 105:155, 1967.
24. Barber, A. A., W. W. Harris, and U. G. Anderson: Isolation of native glycogen by combined rate-zonal and isopycnic centrifugation. Nat. Cancer Inst. Mono., 21:285, 1966.
25. Bloom, W. L., G. T. Lewis, M. Z. Schumpert, and T.-M. Shen: Glycogen fractions of liver and muscle. J. Biol. Chem., 188:631, 1951.
26. Gaspar, Z. N.: Investigation of the physiologically different glycogen fractions in newborn rabbits. Experientia, 13:113, 1957.
27. Melnykovych, G.: Glucocorticoid-induced resistance to deoxycholate lysis in HeLa cells. Science, 152:1086, 1966.

Resistance to Tumorigenesis Induced by Chemicals and Physical Agents

E. DE MAEYER

Institut du Radium – Biologie, Orsay, France

I SHALL BRIEFLY DISCUSS some attempts using chemical and physical agents to induce resistance to tumorigenesis, and the rationale of this approach. Several examples of virus activation through chemical and physical agents are now available. Most extensively studied has been the activation of the thymic lymphoma virus in C57BL mice through X-irradiation or urethan or a combination of both.[1] X-irradiation and urethan can also activate the mammary tumor virus (MTV)[2] and we had the privilege of hearing more of this provocative work in Dr. Boot's presentation, and the activation of mouse leukemia virus by chemical carcinogens as reviewed by Huebner and Todaro.[3]

The mechanism (s) by which such activation takes place is presently unknown, and it may very well be due to the combined effect of different events. In the case of RLV, it has been proposed that chemical and physical agents influence the number of immature target cells necessary for transformation by the virus.[4] The same agents also sometimes decrease humoral antibodies or cellular immunity[5] and this could favor virus replication as well as acceptance of transformed cells. A more specific mechanism has been proposed by Lwoff 10 years ago, taking as a model his own work on lysogenic induction; ". . . When tumor viruses are involved, and when malignancy is due to the concerted action of a virus and a carcinogen, the role of carcinogens could be the same as when inducers act on lysogenic bacteria: they would upset the balance of the cell virus system by interfering with the synthesis of repressors."[6] Based upon an extensive mendelian analysis of the transmission of MTV in different inbred strains of mice, Bentvelzen recently has interpreted his results as being compatible with the concept of integration of the MTV genome in the cellular genome, with subsequent induction of viral replication by X-rays or chemical carcinogens.[7] Such a model has also been proposed by Huebner and Todaro in the case of mouse leukemia virus.[3] Our own experiments on the effect of chemical carcinogens and UV irradiation on interferon in tissue culture have shown clearly that these agents interfere with the synthesis of interferon, and as a result of this stimulate virus replication.[8] I should like to emphasize that this effect was observed in tissue culture, i.e. in a system where one does not have to invoke decreased antibody formation or cellular immunity in order to explain the stimulation of virus replication. A direct action of the carcinogen on the cell brings the latter in a condition where synthesis of important macromolecules, playing a role in the restriction of virus replication, is inhibited.

The relevance of inhibition of interferon synthesis by chemical and physical carcinogens is twofold. First, it provides a useful model, as well as the first specific example in vertebrate cells, as to how, by interfering with the synthesis of repressor molecules, carcinogens can derange cellular control mechanisms which normally limit expression of genetic material foreign to the cell. Second, it is also possible that inhibition of interferon synthesis does contribute to the stimulation of virus replication by chemical and physical agents in the animal. We have found that X-irradiation and also urethan are very efficient inhibitors of interferon formation in the mouse; the impaired capacity for interferon production can be restored by injecting bone marrow or spleen cells of normal animals.[9, 9a] If stimulation of virus replication plays a role in some forms of chemically and physically induced tumorigenesis, it follows that one should be able to interfere with these forms of carcinogenesis by inhibiting either the replication of this virus or malignant transformation of the cell by the virus. This could theoretically be accomplished through administering preformed interferon before, during, or after exposure to the carcinogen. Such an experiment was carried out by Duplan and Gresser, who kindly allowed me to quote from their unpublished work;[10] C57BL mice, 25 to 30 days old, received ip 40,000 N.I.H. units of mouse interferon daily. Treatment was started 15 days before the first whole body irradiation with 175 R.

The mice were irradiated four times, with a weekly interval between exposures. Interferon treatment continued daily during this period and was extended to 22 days after the last irradiation, accounting for a total of 57 days of interferon treatment with 40,000 N.I.H. units daily. The treatment was not effective in decreasing the incidence of lymphoma in this group as compared to two control groups. A similar experiment was carried out by Jaqueline De Maeyer-Guignard, P. Jullien, and myself. We used mice which were only one week old at the first whole body irradiation of 175 R; interferon was administered three times a week. Again, there was no effect on the incidence of radiation-induced lymphoma. The interpretation of negative results is always delicate, and one can object that maybe not enough interferon was given. Nevertheless, I believe that the results suggest that either RLV is quite insensitive to the antiviral action of interferon, or stimulation of virus replication plays a very limited role in the induction of thymic lymphoma by X-rays.

We know from studies by Gresser et al.,[11] and from our own unpublished work, that the AKR lymphoma virus is quite insensitive to the action of exogenous interferon, since large amounts have to be administered daily in order to obtain some effect; this may explain the negative results obtained in the RLV system. More encouraging results have been obtained by Gelboin and Levy, but in a different system of carcinogenesis. Administration of the synthetic polynucleotide polyriboinosinic-polyribocytidylic acid intraperitoneally into NIH-Swiss mice was capable of significantly inhibiting the formation of skin tumors induced by a single dose of 9,10,dimethylbenzanthracene.[12] Since the known effects of this polynucleotide are enhancement of circulating antibody formation, increase of cellular immunity, and induction of interferon, it is impossible to pinpoint the reason for the protection against the DMBA-induced skin tumor formation, and it is quite possible that the protection was due to a summation of these effects. In conclusion, in spite of the first negative results obtained in the radiation-induced lymphoma system, the attempt of interfering with chemically or physically induced tumorigenesis by administration of antiviral agents, be they interferon or others, merits further attention as a way of elucidating the role of virus stimulation in certain forms of tumorigenesis.

Acknowledgement

The author is indebted to the Ministère des Affaires Etrangeres and the Ligue Nationale Française contre le Cancer for a grant permitting him to attend the Congress.

References

1. Lieberman, M., and H. Kaplan: Science, 130:387-388, 1959.
   Lieberman, M., N. Haran-Ghera, and H. S. Kaplan: Nature, 203:420-422, 1964.

2. Timmermans, A., P. Bentvelzen, Ph. C. Hageman, and J. Calafat: J. Gen. Virol., 4:619-621, 1969.
3. Huebner, R. J., and G. J. Todaro: Proc. Nat. Acad. Sci. USA, 64:1087-1094, 1969.
4. Kaplan, H.: Nat. Cancer Inst. Monogr. No. 4, 141-146, 1960.
   Duplan, J. F., and R. Latarjet: Cancer Res., 26:395-399, 1966.
5. Prehn, R. T.: J. Nat. Cancer Inst., 31:791-805, 1963.
   Malmgren, R. A., B. E. Bennison, and T. W. McKinley: Proc. Soc. Exp. Biol. Med., 79:484-488, 1952.
   Stjernswärd, J.: J. Nat. Cancer Inst., 36:1189-1195, 1966.
   Parmiani, G.: Int. J. Cancer, 5:260-265, 1970.
6. Lwoff, A.: Cancer Res., 20:820-829, 1960.
7. Bentvelzen, P. A.: Thesis, Leiden, 1969.
8. De Maeyer, E., and J. De Maeyer-Guignard: Ciba Foundation Symposium on Interferon, 1967, pp. 218-235.
9. De Maeyer, E., P. Jullien, and J. De Maeyer-Guignard: Int. J. Rad. Biol., 13:417-431, 1967.
9a. De Maeyer-Guignard, J., E. De Maeyer, and P. Jullien: Proc. Nat. Acad. Sci. USA, 63:732-739, 1969.
10. Duplan, J. F., and I. Gresser: Unpublished data.
11. Gresser, I., J. Coppey, and C. Bourali: J. Nat. Cancer Inst., 42:1083-1089, 1969.
12. Gelboin, H. V., and H. B. Levy: Science, 167:205-207, 1970.

12

Myeloma as a Biochemical Model of Cancer: Clinical and Experimental

Experimental Studies

MICHAEL POTTER

*National Cancer Institute, National Institutes of Health,
Bethesda, Maryland, USA*

PLASMA CELL TUMORS are rare forms of neoplasms in both mouse and man. It is, therefore, an extraordinary phenomenon when one can induce plasma cell tumors in high incidence. This can be accomplished in the highly inbred BALB/c strain of mice by injecting ip either various mineral oils or implanting ip plastic discs.[1-3] Plasma cell tumor development in the BALB/c mouse is a complex process that requires several interacting factors. First susceptibility to plasma cell tumor induction appears to be genetically controlled. Initially only in the highly inbred BALB/c strain of mice could these tumors be induced.[1, 3] Very recently Dr. Noel Warner (these proceedings) has been able to induce plasmacytomas in strain NZB mice with mineral oil. Most other strains have been resistant indicating the special sensitivity of the BALB/c. The functions of the genes involved are not known, nor is it known whether these genes are active in the plasma cell itself or whether the genes control components in other cell types that affect plasma cells indirectly.

A second factor in plasma cell tumor development is peritoneal granuloma formation. Peritoneal granulomas that form in the peritoneal connective tissues and on the serosal surfaces have been induced by physically dissimilar agents, e.g. the various light and heavy mineral

459

oils[2, 3] and by plastic discs.[1] Recently, Anderson found a chemically pure substance which is probably present in most light mineral oils called pristane (2,6,10,14-tetramethylpentadecane), which is a highly efficient inducer of plasma cell tumors in BALB/c mice.[4] Three 0.5 ml injections of this oil ip induced plasma cell tumors in 60-70% of mice within 16 months of age, an incidence which is comparable if not somewhat better than mineral oils alone. Pristane is not a specific substance since other pure branched chain hydrocarbons are also effective.[5] The various chemically and physically dissimilar agents share in common the ability to induce the formation of a chronic granulomatous tissue on the peritoneal surfaces. This abnormal tissue environment appears to stimulate plasma cells to develop and grow. Later the plasma cell tumors arise in the peritoneal granuloma. The role of the granuloma is assumed to intensify immune reactions possibly by enhancing the processing and storing of antigens.

A third factor in plasma cell tumor development and the one about which we have recently gained some new information is antigens.[6-16] It has been known for some time that the preponderant heavy chain class expressed in the neoplastic plasma cells of the BALB/c mouse is the IgA class.[1, 17] About 65% of all mouse plasmacytomas that synthesize a complete immunoglobulin (Ig) molecule make an IgA type myeloma protein; in man this figure is roughly 40%. In the mouse as in man and other species, the IgA cells are found in abundance in the lamina propria of the gastrointestinal tract.[18] This fact suggests that antigens of exogenous origin enter the organism via the gastrointestinal tract and stimulate the IgA immune system of cells; or that IgA producing cells are preoccupied with a type of antigen that challenges the organism by entering through the gastrointestinal tract. Evidence that antigens of gastrointestinal origin play an important role in plasma cell tumor development was shown in the experiments of McIntire and Princler[19] who found a greatly reduced incidence of plasma cell tumor development in germ-free BALB/c mice. Germ-free mice lack a gastrointestinal flora and have a poorly developed IgA-producing cell system in their gastrointestinal tissues.[18]

We recently obtained further evidence implicating IgA myeloma proteins with antigens derived from the BALB/c bacterial microflora. Between 5-10% of IgA myeloma proteins were found to precipitate with a specific antigen.[6, 17] These antigens were lipopolysaccharides or teichoic acids from species of bacteria isolated from the BALB/c mouse gut flora. The active IgA myeloma proteins were highly specific and precipitating their respective antigen or agglutinating red blood cells coated with the antigen and in cases where haptens have been identified bound the hapten in equilibrium dialysis.[13, 14]

I would like now to discuss one group of these active myeloma proteins as these exemplify some of the general characteristics of myeloma proteins with antibody-like activity. These are the ones that bind phosphoryl choline-containing antigens. There are now known eight independently induced plasmacytomas that produce an IgA myeloma protein that binds phosphoryl choline-containing antigens. The first protein in this group was described by Dr. Melvin Cohn of the Salk Institute in 1967 and was found to precipitate with the pneumococcus C polysaccharide.[7] Since then, Dr. Cohn has found a second tumor and we have found six tumors in our laboratory that produce IgA myeloma proteins that precipitate with a pneumococcus C polysaccharide.[9-11, 16] It is difficult to say just how many proteins were screened to find these but a reasonable estimate might be between 300-400. Even this frequency is remarkable. The pneumococcus C polysaccharide is not the only antigen that is precipitated by these proteins. We have found, for an example, an antigen produced by a species of *Lactobacillus acidophilus* isolated from the BALB/c gastrointestinal microflora that is also precipitated by these proteins.[10] Leon and Young have shown that precipitation of the pneumococcus C polysaccharide by these myeloma proteins can be inhibited by phosphoryl choline.[9] The precipitation of the *Lactobacillus* antigen by these proteins is also inhibited.

Since the eight myeloma proteins are all of the IgA class and further all of the same genetic origin, that is the inbred BALB/c mouse, it is of interest to ask whether any of these eight proteins structurally resemble each other or whether there are differences. We have examined this problem both antigenically and chemically. In collaboration with Miss Rose Lieberman, National Institute of Allergy and Infectious Diseases, we have prepared individual or M-specific antisera to each of the eight myeloma proteins in this series.[10] It is relatively easy to make a highly specific antiserum to an individual IgA BALB/c myeloma protein by immunization of an appropriate strain of mice. The usual M-specific antiserum prepared in this way identifies a single molecular species of Ig and does not cross-react with any other. We routinely test such antisera with approximately 80 other IgA myeloma proteins and 40 IgG myeloma proteins. The antisera prepared to three of the IgA myeloma proteins that bind phosphoryl choline-containing antigens behaved just this way, that is the antisera were uniquely specific for the immunizing antigen and did not cross-react with other myeloma proteins including myeloma proteins that bind phosphoryl choline-containing antigens. On the basis of antigenic specificities, we identified three different Ig species among the eight.[10] Structural studies of the light polypeptide chains substantiated this finding.[16, 21] One of the molecules was a λ chain, M511, and the two others had unique kappa-chain sequences.[20] When we prepared myeloma specific antisera to any of the other five proteins, we always obtained an antiserum that reacted with all five of the proteins.[10] These antisera nonetheless were highly specific for the group of five IgA phosphoryl choline-binding proteins as they did not precipitate with over 120 other myeloma proteins tested. This was especially remarkable since the myeloma proteins included S63 and S107 from M. Cohn's laboratory as well as three from ours. In collaboration with Dr. Leroy Hood, we have made several structural studies on two of the proteins that share an individual specificity.[21] These are the H8 and T15 proteins. The light chain amino acid sequences from the amino terminus of these two appear to be identical for about 23 residues and, further, the tryptic and thermolysin peptide maps of these light chains appear to be identical.[21] It is possible that as these studies progress, we shall be able to show further identities in these two proteins. Similarities in individual Igs of different cellular origin is evidence in favor of a strict genetic control over antibody specificity.

The finding that myeloma proteins of different structure and of different cellular and host origin identify the same antigen suggests that these antigens must be commonly found in mice and further that the precursors of the neoplastic plasma cells were probably active in making antibody to these antigens. It is of considerable interest that the haptenic group in the case of the phosphoryl choline is a common chemical group in animal lipids, for example the lecithins and sphingomyelins. Normally, however, lecithins and sphingomyelins are not immunogenic in the host and require coupling to a foreign protein to become immunogenic.[22] Such a protein may be derived from a tissue breakdown product and formed in the granuloma itself or the bacterial teichoic acids that contained phosphoryl choline may be complete antigens. It appears that the study of antigens in the myeloma process will yield new information about the development of that process.

Further information on the mechanism of plasma cell tumor formation will require a more extensive understanding of how plasma cell growth is regulated. It is likely that a rather complex mechanism is involved in growth regulation and that in some way all of the influences discussed, genes, antigens, abnormal tissue milieu, act on this pathway. It is possible that the factors regulating intracellular components could be disturbed by "somatic" mutations, or disordered control of the differentiated state, e.g. failure of genes to function properly, and that these events could lead to the increased number of "growth mutants"—we recognize phenotypically as neoplastic cell types.

References

1. Merwin, R. M., and L. W. Redmon: Induction of plasma cell tumors and sarcomas in mice by diffusion chambers placed in the peritoneal cavity. J. Nat. Cancer Inst., 31:997-1017, 1963.
2. Potter, M., and C. R. Boyce: Induction of plasma cell neoplasms in strain BALB/c mice with mineral oil and mineral oil adjuvants. Nature, 193:1086, 1962.
3. Potter, M.: The plasma cell tumors and myeloma proteins of mice. Meth. Cancer Res., 2:105-157, 1967.

4. Anderson, P. N., and M. Potter: Induction of plasma cell tumors in BALB/c mice with 2,6,10,14-tetramethylpentadecane (Pristane). Nature, 222:994-995, 1968.
5. Anderson, P. N.: Plasma cell tumor induction in BALB/c mice. Proc. Amer. Ass. Cancer Res., 11:3, 1970.
6. Potter, M.: Mouse IgA myeloma proteins that bind polysaccharide antigens of enterobacterial origin. Fed. Proc., 29:85-91, 1970.
7. Cohn, M.: Natural history of the myeloma. Cold Spring Harbor Symp. Quant. Biol., 32:211-222, 1967.
8. Cohn, M., G. Notani, and S. A. Rice: Characterization of the antibody to the 6-carbohydrate produced by a transplantable mouse plasmacytoma. Immunochemistry, 6:111-123, 1969.
9. Leon, M. A., and N. M. Young: Six mouse IgA myeloma proteins with phosphoryl choline specificity. Fed. Proc., 29:437, 1970.
10. Potter, M., and R. Lieberman: Common individual specific determinants in five of eight BALB/c IgA myeloma proteins that bind phosphoryl choline. J. Exp. Med. In press.
11. Potter, M., R. Lieberman, L. Hood, and D. J. McKean: Structural and serological studies of six IgA myeloma proteins from BALB/c mice that bind phosphoryl choline. Fed. Proc., 29:437, 1970.
12. Schubert, D., A. Jobe, and M. Cohn: Mouse myelomas producing precipitating antibody to nucleic acid bases and/or nitrophenyl derivatives. Nature, 220:882-885, 1968.
13. Eisen, H. N., E. S. Simms, and M. Potter: Mouse myeloma proteins with anti-hapten antibody activity. The protein produced by plasma cell tumor MOPC 315. Biochemistry, 7:4126-4134, 1968.
14. Eisen, H. N., M. C. Michaelides, B. J. Underdown, E. P. Schulenberg, and E. S. Simms: Myeloma proteins with anti-hapten antibody activity. Fed. Proc., 29:78-84, 1970.
15. Leon, M. A., N. M. Young, and K. R. McIntire: Immunochemical studies of the reaction between a mouse myeloma macroglobulin and dextrans. Biochemistry, 9:1023-1030, 1970.
16. Potter, M., and M. A. Leon: Three IgA myeloma immunoglobulins from the BALB/c mouse: Precipitation and pneumococcal C polysaccharide. Science, 162:369-371, 1968.
17. Potter, M.: Myeloma proteins with antibody-like activity in mice. Proceedings Miami Winter Symposium. In press.
18. Crabbé, P. A., D. R. Nash, H. Bazin, H. Eyssen, and J. F. Heremans: Immuno-histochemical observations on lymphoid tissues from conventional and germ-free mice. Lab. Invest., 22:448-451, 1970.
19. McIntire, K. R., and G. L. Princler: Prolonged adjuvant stimulation in germ-free BALB/c mice development of plasma cell neoplasia. Immunology, 17:481-487, 1969.
20. Hood, L., M. Potter, and D. J. McKean: Submitted for publication.
21. Potter, M., and L. Hood: Unpublished data.
22. Rapport, M. M., and L. Graf: Immunochemical reactions of lipids. Prog. Allergy (Karger, Basel), 13:273-331, 1969.

Structural Studies with Monoclonal Immunoglobulins

N. HILSCHMANN, H. PONSTINGL,

M. HESS, K. BACZKO, D. BRAUN,

S. WATANABE, L. SUTER,

AND H. U. BARNIKOL

Max-Planck-Institut für experimentelle Medizin, Göttingen, Germany

QUITE OFTEN THE STUDY of pathologic conditions is essential in the understanding of normal biochemical processes. This precept has been reconfirmed with paraproteins.

Even the concept of paraproteins has changed in the last five years. Although products of cancer, myelomaglobulins, Waldenström's macroglobulins, and Bence Jones proteins are no longer considered as pathologic or aberrant proteins, but as rather normal constituents of the immunoglobulin spectrum.[1] They are pathologic only in their abnormal increase of production. Furthermore, these proteins are derived from one cell clone and are therefore, contrary to antibody preparations, chemically homogeneous. Today "normal" antibodies are considered as consisting of 10^5 to 10^7 of such monoclonal immunoglobins. These properties made monoclonal proteins an ideal subject for the study of antibody structure.

One of the essential findings resulting from these studies was that the specificity of antibodies is not determined by a different folding of one polypeptide chain, as previously surmised, but by a differing amino acid sequence.

On this basis, the antibody problem, one of the fundamental problems of biology, could be attacked anew. The problem is whether the information for the various antibody specificities is programmed genetically, which means inherited, or whether it has to be acquired during differentiation by a somatic hypermutation process. This question has been raised by several classic hypotheses on the formation of antibodies, but not answered.[2-7] In the last few years, chemical studies on antibody structure have given ample information for discussing this problem in molecular terms.[8-13]

Basic Structure of the Antibody Molecule

According to Fleischman et al.[14] and Edelman,[15] the structure of an IgG (7S) antibody molecule is symmetric and consists of two pairs of subunits, which according to their molecular weights are called light (L) (mol wt 23,000) and heavy (H) (mol wt 50,000) chains. These chains are connected by disulfide bridges and noncovalent bonds. Electromicrographs of Valentine and Greene showed that the molecule is shaped like an Upsilon, whose freely movable arms (the so-called F(ab) fragments) contain the combining sites of the antibody.[16] The Fc fragment has no antigen-binding capacity; it binds complement and is responsible for the skin-sensitizing property of antibodies.

Antibody Heterogeneity

Heterogeneity is one of the predominant features of the immunoglobulins. The exceedingly high number of different specificities indicates the existence of an extremely complex mixture. Since the components of these mixtures are chemically very similar, separation is difficult.

It has been useful to distinguish between three types of heterogeneity: isotypy, allotypy and idiotypy. All of these types of heterogeneity have been characterized serologically.[1]

Isotypy is the class heterogeneity. It is relatively easy to characterize and isolate the different immunoglobulin classes IgG, IgA, IgM, IgE, and IgD by serologic or chemical and physical means.[17]

In these classes, the basic model of the immunoglobulin molecule is modified in several ways. The IgA molecule can occur as monomer and dimer. The IgM molecule is a pentamer and has a molecular weight of 1,000,000. These differences in structure are determined by the H chains. The H chains of the IgG immunoglobulins are of the γ type, those of IgA or IgM molecules of the α or μ type. These chains have a different chemical structure and do not cross-react serologically. In the L chains, two serologically and chemically distinct chain types can be distinguished: η and λ chains. Even if one takes into consideration the various subclasses, like γ_1, γ_2, γ_3 and γ_4, which have been recognized recently, only 20 different variants result from a combination of these H- and L-chain classes and subclasses. This number is much too small to account for antibody specificity. Also, antibodies of the same specificity can be of the IgM and IgG class. This switch in classes is usually observed during the course of immunization. The class heterogeneity is present in every individual.

With allotypy it is quite the opposite. These structural variants, which can be characterized serologically, are inherited markers and of allelic nature. They are, therefore, not present in every individual. In man, we distinguish between the Inv factors which are present on the η

chains, and the Gm system which is distributed on the various sub-classes of the IgG class.[1, 18, 19]

We will characterize these genetic markers in detail in the following section, using the Inv factors as an example. Neither allotypy nor isotypy is sufficient to explain the structural heterogeneity of the antibodies. In man, Inv and Gm factors are not known to have influence on antibody specificity.

It is the idiotypy, the last type of heterogeneity, which is biologically important, because it determines antibody specificity. The characterization of this type of heterogeneity caused the most difficulties because of the chemical similarities of the different chains.

Chemical Characterization of Isotypy and Idiotypy

In order to circumvent the heterogeneity which is observed in every antibody, even when it is prepared most carefully with a homogeneous antigen, monoclonal immunoglobulins were used. These proteins, which are present in patients with multiple myeloma and Waldenström's macroglobulinemia, are homogeneous with respect to all three types of heterogeneity, and are produced in such quantities that they can be isolated in a chemically pure form. By determining the primary structure of two chains which are identical with respect to two types of heterogeneity, the third type can be characterized.

We used for this purpose two L chains of the η type, in order to eliminate structural differences caused by isotypy. These two chains differed so greatly in their amino acid composition that it was to be expected that idiotypic differences should show up very clearly. Ideally, we should have used proteins of the same genetic constitution, which means proteins with the same Inv factor. Although this was not the case, the results of our investigation were clear.

From these comparative sequence studies, it was easy to recognize that the molecule is divided into two parts. Differences in the structure are limited to the N-terminal part of the molecule, which is called variable for that reason. The variability is caused by multiple amino acid exchanges and single deletions of amino acid residues. These exchanges are, however, not so numerous and seldom so radical that the homology (chemical similarity) of this variable part cannot clearly be recognized.[20, 21]

In opposition to it, the amino acid sequence in the C-terminal half of both proteins is identical. It has been called the constant part. A single amino acid replacement in position 191 of the constant part could be recognized as the allotypic variant of the two proteins. Inv a[+] proteins have leucine and Inv b[+] proteins have valine in this position.[20, 22–24]

Therefore, idiotypic variations are identical with the variable parts, which is different in every protein, and which comprised just one half of the molecule in L chains. Allotypic variants cause single amino acid exchanges in the constant part.

This rule is not only valid for η chains, but also for λ chains.[25] Comparative sequence studies with H chains, which are double the length of L chains, revealed also a variable and constant part.[26, 27] The difference is, however, that the constant part is three times as long as in the L chains. The Gm factors are located in this constant part.

Separate Genetic Control of the Variable and Constant Parts

These structural studies have been done with the intention of obtaining insight into the genetic mechanism of antibody formation on a molecular level. As a result of the unique division of the immunoglobulin chains in a variable and a constant part, the genetic control of immunoglobulins is more complicated than with other proteins. This is immediately visualized when one wants to apply the one gene-one protein dogma to this class of proteins.

Assuming there would exist as many complete L-chain genes as variable parts (so far every investigated L chain has a different variable part), the gene responsible for the L chains would look like this: a great number of serially repeated L-chain genes with alternating variable and constant genes. The variable genes then would be modified by evolution; the constant genes, however, must be excluded from an evolutionary change.

This model is, however, completely impossible. A comparison with other animal species, for example with mouse L chains which also have a constant and a variable part,[28] showed that the constant part is not excluded from evolutionary changes, but is almost as variable as the variable part in phylogeny. Furthermore, the genetic markers localized in the constant part (Inv factors) segregate as alleles in a simple mendelian manner.[29, 30] The only possible solution to this is that the constant part is constant because it is present only once in the genome.[31] From these two possibilities an explanation of the variability of the variable part results.

One possibility is that every chain is entirely (variable and constant parts) under the control of one gene for each chain type. A logical consequence of this is that the gene section for the variable part must undergo extensive somatic mutation during differentiation. Several hypotheses for this somatic hypermutation process have been proposed.[32, 33]

Through our investigations these hypotheses have been rendered very unlikely. Instead of this it has to be assumed that the genetic control for the immunoglobulins is separate for the variable and constant parts: one gene for the constant part and many genes for the variable part. These many genes for the variable part are produced during evolution by multiple gene duplications and subsequent muta-

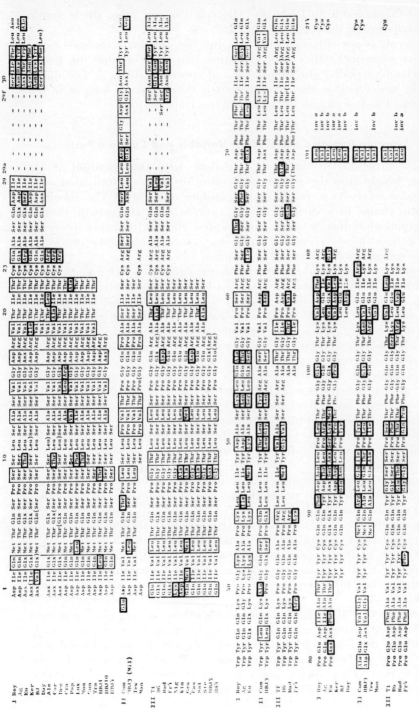

Fig. 12-1.—Comparison of the variable sequences of human η-type L chains of proteins Roy,[12,21] Cum,[12,35] Ti,[36] Ag,[37] Tew,[38] Eu,[39] Ker, BJ, Day, Man,[40] Ale, Car, Dee,[41] B6, Rad, Fr 4,[42] Cra, Pap, Lux, Mon, Tra, Nig, Win, Gra, Cas, Smi,[43] Ste,[44] HBJ 1, HBJ 10, HBJ 4, HBJ 5, HBJ 4,[45] and HBJ 3 (Mil).[46] On the basis of their chemical homology, the proteins are divided in subgroups I to III. Subgroup-specific exchanges are marked by thin, and individual-specific exchanges by thick black boxes, deletions by —. Undetermined sequences are in parentheses.

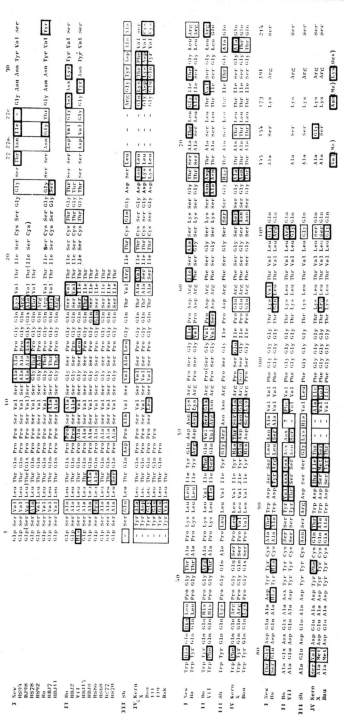

FIG. 12–2.—Comparison of the variable sequences of human λ-type L chains of proteins Kern,[47] New,[48] Vil,[49] Bau,[30,51] 111,[47] 119,[52] Bo, Ha, Sh[55] X,[53] HS 94, 78, 92, 86, 68, 77, 70,[54] BJ 98,[56] HBJ 7, 11, 2, 15, 8,[45] and Rak.[57] On the basis of their chemical homology, the proteins are divided in subgroups I to IV. Signs as in Fig. 12–1.

tions. The variability pattern caused this way is completely different to that which would be the consequence of a somatic hypermutation process. Decisive for this evolutionary model of antibody variability was the finding that the sequences in the variable part can be arrayed in subgroups because of the high regularity with which the amino acid replacements occur.[34]

The Variability Rule (Subgroups)

As already mentioned, there is homology between the variable parts of each chain type. We have investigated the primary sequence of a series of such variable parts of L chains of the η and λ type. In Figures 12-1 and 12-2, the results of these investigations are summarized and compared with the results of other laboratories. The chains are lined up in a way that homologous residues are in identical positions. It can easily be recognized that the variability of these chains is not random, but follows a principle of regularity which finds its expression in subgroups. These subgroups result from the existence of a discriminating gradation in homology between the proteins. The amino acid replacements appear to be much less in proteins within one subgroup (exchange rate up to 25%) than in proteins belonging to different subgroups (exchange rate up to 50%). On the basis of these linked amino acid exchanges, three subgroups could be recognized for the η chains[34, 35, 43] and for the λ chains.[34, 48] Subgroup-specific exchanges are marked by light, individual specific exchanges by dark black boxes in Figures 12-1 and 12-2. Most individual-specific exchanges can be explained by single point mutation.

Since the chains are unequal in length, deletions have to be postulated in different parts of the chains, in order to match homologous positions. Although the number of the deleted amino acid residues varies, it is, however, almost always the same with proteins of one subgroup. Deletions occur in η chains in positions 0 and 29, in λ chains in positions 1, 27, 95/96, and 96. A high degree of variability is observed at the residues C terminal to the cysteines in positions 23 and 88 (87) which are connected by disulfide bonds, and also around position 50. There is evidence that these highly mutable areas participate in the combining site.

Structure and Specificity (Specificity Region)

The forces involved in the formation of the antigen-antibody complex depend upon hydrophobic bonding, hydrogen bridges and, to a lesser extent, electrostatic interaction. Since van der Waal's forces are short-range forces, the combining sites of the antibody have to come into close contact with the surface of the antigen molecule.

The only part of the antibody molecule which can fulfill these requirements is the variable part. This assumption has been confirmed by affinity labeling experiments.[60, 61] According to these experiments, a tyrosine residue in position 86 and a peptide stretching from position 25 to 54 of the variable part of a L chain must participate in or be close to the combining site. These two sites in the chain are close neighbors because of an intrapeptidal SS bridge connecting residues 23 and 88. As will be shown later, these stretches of the variable part show the highest degree of variability.

It is assumed that the variable parts of both the L and the H chains participate in the combining site.

Evolutionary Origin of Antibody Variability

This principle of regularity resulting from a comparison of a greater number of variable parts of η- and λ-type L chains renders a somatic generation of antibody variability highly unlikely. The data, depicted in Figures 12-1 and 12-2, are derived from proteins gained from different individuals. A somatic hypermutation process is supposed to work on a random basis. It cannot lead to an identical pattern of variability in different individuals.

The most likely explanation for this type of antibody variability is that hundreds of millions of years ago, before the vertebrates came into existence, there was only one primordial gene for the variable part. Out of this ancestral gene three or four gene copies have resulted by gene duplication which were then subjected to independent evolution. The results of this process are amino acid replacements at multiple positions and deletions. Each of these copies is serially duplicated, the exchanges and deletions being carried on in evolution. They can be recognized in the form of subgroup-specific sequences which will be superimposed by more recent mutational events. These individual specific exchanges are mostly single-point mutations.

The subgroups can be interpreted as the main branches, the individual proteins as the terminal ramifications of an evolutionary tree.[12, 13]

Variable Parts of H Chains

Similar comparative studies with variable parts of H chains also indicate the existence of subgroups. Data are much more limited than with L chains, but as far as data are available, three subgroup-specific sequences can be recognized.[60, 61]

A most remarkable observation was made when the variable part of a μ chain was compared with that of γ chains. It could clearly be seen that the variable part of this μ chain was more homologous to some of the γ chains than the γ chains themselves.[62] This has given rise to the assumption that all constant parts of the H chains, which means γ, α, and μ chains, have the same set of variable parts.

TABLE 12–1.—N-TERMINAL SEQUENCES OF η-TYPE L-CHAINS OF VARIOUS SPECIES

Human	L	(BJP)	I. Asp Ile Gln Met Thr Gln[34]
			II. Asp Ile Val Met Thr Gln
			III. Glu Ile Val Leu Thr Gln
Mouse	L	(BJP)	Asp Gln Met
			Ile Thr Gln[28, 63]
			PCA Val Leu
Shark	L	(pool)	Asp
			Glu Ile Val Leu Thr[64]
	H,17S	(pool)	Glu Ile Val Leu Thr Gln
	H, 7S	(pool)	Glu Ile Val Leu Thr Gln
Paddlefish	L	(pool)	Asp Ile Val Ile Thr[65]
	H,19S	(pool)	Asp Ile Val Ile Thr

Phylogeny of Antibody Variability

Evolution as the basis of antibody variability makes the points of divergence of the evolutionary tree particularly interesting. Table 12-1 shows a comparison of the N-terminal sequences of L and H chains of man, mouse, shark, and the paddlefish. So far no primitive immunoglobulin has been found without variability. Most likely, such an immunoglobulin would not have the properties of an antibody, since choice between different structures seems to be a necessary requisite of the specific immune response. However, it can be noticed that variability is greatly restricted in the immunoglobulin of the lower vertebrates. This seems to be particularly valid for the immunoglobulins of the paddlefish, where no differences can be seen in the five N-terminal residues of the L and H chains.

The Number of Genes for the Variable Parts

The question arises whether the information for all variable parts of the immunoglobulins is genetically determined. So far there are no two proteins found which had an identical amino acid sequence in their variable parts. It is therefore much too early to make valid calculations on the exact number of genes involved in the genetic control of the variable parts. Linked amino acid replacements within

TABLE 12–2.—NUMBER OF CHEMICALLY DIFFERENT ANTIBODY MOLECULES

DNA content of one haploid human cell[66]	3.25×10^{-12}g
Number of base pairs	3.2×10^9
0.1% thereof	3.2×10^6
Number of variable parts (107 amino acids = 321 base pairs) contained in 0.1%	1×10^4
H-chains (p)	0.5×10^4
L-chains (q)	0.5×10^4
Number of antibody molecules (p × q)	2.5×10^7

subgroup-specific sequences, however, indicate that the number of genes should be very high.

Whether the information for 10^6 different antibodies could be stored in the genome can, however, be calculated. Table 12-2 shows that this could very well be accomplished by even a small percentage of the DNA of a haploid chromosome set. This figure gives the minimal amount of DNA required and has been calculated under the assumption that both the L and the H chains contribute to the combining site. The possible restriction in L- and H-chain combination[67] might decrease the number of variables or increase the number of necessary variable genes.

Serially repeated homologous genes in such a high number seem not to be so unusual. Recent hybridization experiments with mammalian DNA indicate much higher numbers.[68] After all, hemoglobin chains also seem to be controlled by more genes, as had been thought previously.[69, 70]

Somatic Gene Translocation and Fusion Between the Constant and Variable Parts

Since variable and constant parts are expressed in one protein chain, a model consisting of multiple genes for the variable part and one (or a few) genes for the constant part necessarily needs fusion between the constant and one of these variable parts. Fusion on a protein level was excluded by pulse-labeling experiments, which demonstrated that the variable and constant parts are synthesized in one piece proceeding from the N-terminal end.[71] Fusion on the level of the messenger RNA is also very unlikely, since the molecular weight of the messenger and the number of ribosomes attached to it corresponds well with these molecular weights of the L and H chains.[72-75] Therefore, fusion on the DNA level with a proceeding gene translocation has to be assumed.

Gene translocation has also been discussed with reference to the switch of IgM to IgG in the course of immunization. This transition occurs without change in antibody specificity. It is not known, however, whether this so called Nossal switch occurs within one cell.

A Model for Cell Differentiation

The genetic control of antibody synthesis is unique. There is no other class of proteins where one single protein chain is under the genetic control of two separate genes. It might be surmised that this complicated system of information storage might have something to do with the regulation of its expression into protein structure.

One single antibody-forming cell produces antibodies of only one specificity.[76] Further experiments revealed that the immunoglobulins of one cell contain either η- or the λ-type L chains,[77] and that the

γ-type L chains might be either Inv a^+ or b^+ (allelic exclusion).[78] More recently, it was found that the product of a single cell behaves like a monoclonal protein in electrophoreses.[79] Usually these antibodies do not change their specificity or genetic markers. A model with multiple genes for the variable part implies that all the information for every possible antigen is genetically determined. However, in agreement with Burnet's clonal selection hypothesis,[6] only one of these genes per cell should be translated in the sequence of a specific antibody. Therefore, a special control mechanism has to exist, ensuring that only one of the variable genes for every L and H chain becomes functional. One could imagine that this regulation of gene activity might be the task of the gene for the constant part, which is present only once for every chain type. We assume that the fusion of the constant gene with one of the variable genes happens on a random basis before the contact with the antigen. The antigen does not determine or induce the structure of the antibody. It selects, out of several possibilities, one which fits best.

Acknowledgments

Our own work mentioned here was supported in part by the Deutsche Forschungsgemeinschaft. The proteins Roy, Cum, New, and Vil were kindly made available by Dr. Kunkel, New York, the protein Kern by Prof. Bock, Tübingen, the protein Ti by Dr. Naumann, Holzminden, the protein Bau by Dr. Oberdorfer, München, and the proteins 111 and 119 by Dr. van Eijk, Rotterdam. These generous gifts are gratefully acknowledged.

References

1. Kunkel, H. G.: Harvey Lect., 59:219, 1963-1964.
2. Ehrlich, P.: Proc. Roy. Soc. London, Ser. B., 66:424, 1900.
3. Breinl, F., and F. Haurowitz: Hoppe-Seyler's Z. Physiol. Chem., 192:45,1930.
4. Pauling, L.: J. Amer. Chem. Soc., 62:2643, 1940.
5. Jerne, N. K.: Proc. Nat. Acad. Sci. USA, 41:849, 1955.
6. Burnet, F. M.: The Clonal Selection of Aquired Immunity. Vanderbilt University Press, Nashville, 1959.
7. Lederberg, J.: Science, 129:1649, 1959.
8. Killander, J., Ed.: Nobel Symposium III, Gamma Globulins, Structure and Control of Biosynthesis. Almqvist and Wiksell, Stockholm, 1967.
9. Cold Spring Harbor Symp. Quant. Biol., 32, 1967.
10. Cohn, M.: In: Nucleic Acids in Immunology (O. Plescia and W. Braun, eds.), Springer, Berlin, Heidelberg, New York, 1968, p. 671.
11. Edelman, G. M., and W. E. Gall: Ann. Rev. Biochem., 38:415, 1969.
12. Hilschmann, N.: Naturwissenschaften, 56:195, 1969.
13. Hilschmann, N., H. U. Barnikol, M. Hess, B. Langer, H. Ponstingl, M. Steinmetz-Kayne, L. Suter, and S. Watanabe: In: Current Problems in Immunology (Bayer-Symposium I) (O. Westphal, H. E. Bock, and E. Grundmann, eds.), Springer, Berlin, Heidelberg, New York, 1969, p. 69.
14. Fleischman, J. B., R. R. Porter, and E. M. Press: Biochem. J., 88:220, 1963.
15. Edelman, G. M., and J. A. Gally: Proc. Nat. Acad. Sci. USA, 51:846, 1964.
16. Valentine, R. C., and N. M. Greene: J. Mol. Biol., 27:615, 1967.
17. Nomenclature. Bull. World Health Org., 30:447, 1964.
18. Martensson, L., Vox Sang., 11:521, 1966.

19. Steinberg, A. G.: Ann. Rev. Genet., 3:25, 1969.
20. Hilschmann, N., and L. C. Craig: Proc. Nat. Acad. Sci. USA, 53:1403, 1965.
21. Hilschmann, N.: Hoppe-Seyler's Z. Physiol. Chem., 348:1077, 1967.
22. Hilschmann, N.: Proc. 11th Congr. Int. Soc. Blood Transf., Sydney, 1966, Bibl. Haemat., Nr. 29, Part 2, Karger, Basel and New York, 1968, p. 501.
23. Baglioni, C., L. Alescio-Zonta, D. Cioli, and A. Carbonara: Science, 152:1519, 1966.
24. Milstein, C.: Nature, 209:370, 1966.
25. Putnam, F. W., R. Shinoda, K. Titani, and M. Wikler: Science, 157:1050, 1967.
26. Press, E., and N. M. Hogg: Nature, 223:807, 1969.
27. Edelman, G. M., B. A. Cunningham, W. E. Gall, P. D. Gottlieb, U. Rutishauser, and M. J. Waxdal: Proc. Nat. Acad. Sci. USA, 63:78, 1969.
28. Gray, W. R., W. J. Dreyer, and L. Hood: Science, 155:465, 1967.
29. Ropartz, C., J. Lenoir, and L. Rivat: Nature, 189:586, 1961.
30. Steinberg, A. G.: In: Progress in Medical Genetics. Grune and Stratton, New York, London, Vol. 2, 1962, p. 1.
31. Hilschmann, N.: Hoppe-Seyler's Z. Physiol. Chem., 348:1291, 1967.
32. Brenner, S., and C. Milstein: Nature, 211:242, 1966.
33. Smithies, O.: Science, 157:267, 1967.
34. Hilschmann, N., H. U. Barnikol, M. Hess, B. Langer, H. Ponstingl, M. Steinmetz-Kayne, L. Suter and S. Watanabe: Proc. 5th FEBS-Meeting, Prague 1968, FEBS Symposium, Academic Press, Inc., London, Vol. 15, 1969, p. 57.
35. Hilschmann, N.: Hoppe-Seyler's Z. Physiol. Chem., 348:1718, 1967.
36. Suter, L., H. U. Barnikol, S. Watanabe, and N. Hilschmann: Hoppe-Seyler's Z. Physiol. Chem., 350:275, 1969.
37. Titani, K., T. Shinoda, and F. W. Putnam: J. Biol. Chem., 244:3550, 1969.
38. Putnam, F. W.: Science, 163:633, 1969.
39. Cunningham, B. A., P. D. Gottlieb, W. H. Konigsberg, and G. M. Edelman: Biochemistry, 7:1983, 1968.
40. Milstein, C.: Nature, 216:330, 1967.
41. Milstein, C., C. P. Milstein, and A. Feinstein: Nature, 221:151, 1969.
42. Milstein, C.: FEBS-Letters, 2:301, 1969.
43. Niall, H. D., and P. Edman: Nature, 216:262, 1967.
44. Edman, P., and A. G. Cooper: FEBS-Letters, 2:33, 1968.
45. Hood, L., W. R. Gray, B. G. Sanders, and W. J. Dreyer: Cold Spring Harbor Symp. Quant. Biol., 32:133, 1967.
46. Dreyer, W. J., W. R. Gray, and L. Hood: Cold Spring Harbor Symp. Quant. Biol., 32:353, 1967.
47. Ponstingl, H., M. Hess, and N. Hilschmann: Hoppe-Seyler's Z. Physiol. Chem., 349:867, 1968.
48. Langer, B., M. Steinmetz-Kayne, and N. Hilschmann: Hoppe-Seyler's Z. Physiol. Chem., 349:945, 1968.
49. Ponstingl, H., and N. Hilschmann: Hoppe-Seyler's Z. Physiol. Chem., 350:1148,. 1969
50. Baczko, K., D. G. Braun, M. Hess and N. Hilschmann: In preparation.
51. Hilschmann, N., H. Ponstingl, K. Baczko, D. G. Braun, M. Hess, L. Suter, H. U. Barnikol, and S. Watanabe: Proc. 17th Coll. Protides of the Biological fluids. Elsevier, Amsterdam. In press.
52. Hess, M., and N. Hilschmann: Hoppe-Seyler's Z. Physiol. Chem., 351:67, 1970.
53. Milstein, C., J. B. Clegg, and J. M. Jarvis: Biochem. J., 110:631, 1968.
54. Hood, L., and D. Ein: Nature, 220:764, 1968.
55. Wikler, M., K. Titani, T. Shinoda, and F. W. Putnam: J. Biol. Chem., 242:1668, 1967.
56. Baglioni, C.: Biochem. Biophys. Res. Comm., 26:82, 1967.
57. Brackenridge, C. J.: Immunochemistry, 4:227, 1967.
58. Singer, S. J., and N. O. Thorpe: Proc. Nat. Acad. Sci. USA, 60:1371, 1968.
59. Goetzl, E. J., and H. Metzger: Biochemistry, 9:1267, 1970.
60. Cunningham, B. A., M. N. Pflumm, U. Rutishauser, and G. M. Edelman: Proc. Nat. Acad. Sci. USA, 64:997, 1969.

61. Ponstingl, H., and N. Hilschmann: Unpublished data.
62. Wikler, M., H. Köhler, T. Shinoda, and F. W. Putnam: Science, 163:75, 1969.
63. Appella, E., and R. N. Perham: Cold Spring Harbor Symp. Quant. Biol., 32-37, 1967.
64. Suran, A., and B. W. Papermaster: Proc. Nat. Acad. Sci. USA, 58:1619, 1967.
65. Pollara, B., A. Suran, J. Finstad, and R. A. Good: Proc. Nat. Acad. Sci. USA, 59:1307, 1968.
66. Dayhoff, M. O.: Atlas of Protein and Sequence and Structure. National Biomedical Research Foundation, Silver Spring, Vol. 4, 1969, p. 44.
67. Mannik, M.: Biochemistry, 6:134, 1967.
68. Britten, R. J. and D. E. Kohne: Science, 161:529, 1968.
69. Schroeder, W. A., T. H. J. Huisman, J. R. Shelton, J. B. Shelton, E. F. Kleihauer, A. M. Dozy, and B. Robberson: Proc. Nat. Acad. Sci. USA, 60:537, 1968.
70. Hilse, K., and R. A. Popp: Proc. Nat. Acad. Sci. USA, 61:930, 1968.
71. Fleischman, J.: Biochemistry, 6:1311, 1967.
72. Becker, M. J., and A. Rich: Nature, 212:142, 1966.
73. Kuechler, E., and A. Rich: Nature, 222:544, 1969.
74. Williamson, A. R., and B. A. Askonas: J. Mol. Biol., 23:201, 1967.
75. Shapiro, A. L., M. D. Scharff, J. V. Maizel, and J. V. Uhr: Proc. Nat. Acad. Sci. USA, 56:216, 1966.
76. Nossal, G. J. V., and O. Mäkelä: Ann. Rev. Microbiol., 16:53, 1962.
77. Cebra, J. J., J. E. Colberg, and S. Dray: J. Exp. Med., 123:547, 1966.
78. Pernis, B. G., G. Chiappino, A. S. Kelus, and B. G. H. Gell: J. Exp. Med., 122:853, 1965.
79. Marchalonis, J. J., and G. J. V. Nossal: Proc. Nat. Acad. Sci. USA, 61:860, 1968.

Molecular Biology of Myeloma

BERNARD MACH

Institute of Molecular Biology, University of Geneva,
Geneva, Switzerland

Introduction

MOLECULAR BIOLOGY IS, generally speaking, a biochemical approach to biology. The term is, in fact, frequently used in a more restricted sense and concerns the study of the transfer of genetic information responsible for the orderly synthesis of biologic material and for cell growth. A discussion on molecular biology of myeloma must consider at the same time the contribution of molecular biology to our understanding of myeloma and the contribution of myeloma, as a biologic tool, to molecular biology. The importance of this second aspect is illustrated by the fact that myeloma tissue has been used in the study of several problems of molecular biology. One of the reasons for this interest is that this tissue consists of a highly homogeneous cell population, which synthesizes in large amount a unique protein product—the specific γ-globulin of each myeloma.

| Replication | Transcription | Translation | Secretion |

$$\boxed{} \longrightarrow DNA \longrightarrow RNA \longrightarrow PROTEIN \longrightarrow$$

The first steps in this transfer of genetic information (replication and transcription) have not yet been studied extensively in the case of myeloma. The viruslike particles observed in myeloma cells are studied by several groups, but there is not evidence of any relationship between those particles and either the abnormal growth pattern or the production of γ-globulins.[1] Protein synthesis, however, and in particular the synthesis of specific γ-globulin molecules, has been studied in detail in myeloma. The process of storage and secretion of the γ-globulins produced has also been thoroughly investigated.

Studies of Protein Synthesis and Secretion in Myeloma

Various aspects of the general problem of protein synthesis and secretion in myeloma have been studied in detail. These studies were made possible by the use of transplantable myeloma tumors of the mouse, an experimental tool developed mainly by the pioneer work of Dr. M. Potter at the National Institutes of Health.[2]

THE CELL-FREE SYNTHESIS OF SPECIFIC GLOBULIN[3, 4]

Subcellular fractions were prepared from mouse plasmocytoma tumors (microsomes, "pH 5" or crude activating enzymes, tRNA), and a cell-free system highly active in protein synthesis was developed. It could then be shown that the protein product of this microsomal system was a polypeptide chain showing the same chemical specificity (at the level of tryptic peptide analysis) as the γ-globulin L chain produced by the particular myeloma used in the study.

DIRECT TEST OF THE "TRANSLATIONAL CONTROL THEORY"

It had been suggested[3, 5, 6] that the specific amino acid substitutions responsible for the structural and biologic specificity of antibody molecules could be introduced, during the process of translation, by specific tRNA or activating enzymes, modified as the result of mutations. Such a theory could account for some of the features of the amino acid sequence variability observed among different immunoglobulins. It has also the merit of being a theory which can be tested experimentally, a property not shared by most of the proposals concerning the generation of antibody diversity. The cell-free system described above has been used to investigate the translation of mRNA from a given myeloma tumor in the presence of tRNA prepared from another myeloma. In the case of three different myelomas, it could be shown that none of the amino acid substitutions detectable by the tryptic peptide analysis was determined or influenced by the translation machinery of another myeloma.[7]

SYNTHESIS OF γ-GLOBULIN BY FREE RIBOSOMES

It has been postulated that proteins which are secreted out of a cell are synthesized exclusively on polysomes bound to the endoplasmic reticulum, whereas proteins which are used inside the cell are made on membrane-free ribosomes.[8] In the case of myeloma tumors, however, it was found that free ribosomes were capable of synthesizing the same immunoglobulin chains that the microsomal cell-free system just described produced.[9, 10] Several important questions are raised by this finding. Although under normal conditions γ-globulins are thought to be secreted out of the cell in which they have been synthesized, it is not known whether those γ-globulins which are made on membrane-free ribosomes ever leave the cell. We think that it is important to consider that a cell which might not have an endoplasmic reticulum and the possibility to secrete γ-globulin, might nevertheless be considered as a γ-globulin-producing cell. The product, in that case, presumably would never leave the cell or its surface.

DIFFERENCE IN ISOACCEPTING tRNA AMONG DIFFERENT MYELOMAS IN THE CASE OF SEVERAL AMINO ACIDS

Although the γ-globulin mRNA from a given myeloma can be faithfully translated by tRNAs from other myelomas, the tRNAs from different myelomas are strikingly different. These differences were first demonstrated (in the case of threonine and leucine) when the various isoaccepting tRNA species, specific for a given amino acid, were analyzed by chromatography on methylated albumin kieselguhr.[3] This analysis can be performed with a better resolution by reverse-phase chromatography, and with this method tRNA differences have been shown in the case of serine,[11] leucine,[12] and of five amino acids compared on four different myelomas as well as between myeloma and normal tissue.[10, 13] It is important to consider these differences in specific tRNA species in the light of the observed modification induced in certain tRNAs of host cells by either bacteriophage or animal viruses.[14, 15, 16, 17]

DETAILED STUDY OF THE RIBOSOMAL SUBUNITS OF MYELOMA

A systematic study of ribosomes and ribosomal subunits, from the structural and functional point of view, has been undertaken with mouse myeloma ribosomes. The availability of a homogeneous tissue was important for this study, which has resulted in the description of a preparation of subunits showing a more active response to added template RNA than those previously described.[18]

STUDY OF THE TRANSPORT AND SECRETION OF γ-GLOBULIN MADE IN MYELOMA CELLS

Largely through the work of Knopf and Melchers,[19, 20, 21] great progress has been made in understanding the transport and secretion of γ-globulin made in myeloma cells. Kinetic studies[20] have established that γ-globulin, after a short stay in the "rough endoplasmic reticulum," are transported to the "smooth endoplasmic reticulum" fraction of the plasmocyte, and then, in another step, are excreted out of the cell. The relationship between the attachment of the carbohydrate residues and this transport and secretion process has been investigated by Melchers.[21] In the case of a light chain-producing myeloma, it was found that the γ-globulin chain "acquired its carbohydrate group step by step at different subcellular sites within the plasma cell."[21] There is, however, no proof that this attachment is a prerequisite for transport and secretion.

Synthesis and Secretion of γ-Globulin and Different Types of Myelomas

A number of induced and transplantable mouse myeloma tumors do not secrete any γ-globulins. Furthermore, in the life history of certain "secreting" mouse myelomas, one can observe (usually after a number of generations) the cessation of the production of γ-globulin while the tumor continues to grow, apparently unaffected. Whatever the level of the block responsible for the absence of γ-globulin secretion, it seems from these two examples that the secretory activity of the myeloma cell is not directly related to the uncontrolled growth of the tissue.

It is evident, from our knowledge of the mechanism of protein synthesis, and of the process of transport and secretion of γ-globulins, that the absence of extracellular γ-globulin could result from blocks at a variety of levels. It is thus theoretically conceivable that different kinds of myelomas might exist, depending on whether they secrete intracellular γ-globulin (or either light or heavy chains alone) and whether they synthesize γ-globulin (or either chain alone). A group of mouse myeloma variants with secretion of L chains only, and with intracellular synthesis of H chains has been described.[22] A class of myeloma with intracellular synthesis of γ-globulin but with no secretion ("pseudo nonproducers") could result from a variety of possible blocks in the complicated secretion process, or possibly from the inactivation or even the absence of endoplasmic reticulum. "True nonproducers," on the other hand, would be myelomas without synthesis and obviously without secretion. Again, many different possibilities can be envisaged which would result in the absence of γ-globulin synthesis.

On the basis of this distinction between block in synthesis and block in secretion, and of existing information concerning myelomas producing either L chain alone[1] or incomplete heavy chains,[23, 24] one can group myelomas as follows:

1. Producers: Myeloma with synthesis and secretion of γ-globulin.

2. Partial producers: Myeloma with synthesis and secretion of only a portion of γ-globulin molecule: (a) only one of the two chains;[22] (b) only a portion of a chain (incomplete chain and absence of the other chain?).

3. Pseudo nonproducers: Myeloma with synthesis of γ-globulin but without secretion (block in secretion).

4. True nonproducers: Myeloma without synthesis.

References

1. Cohn, M.: Cold Spring Harbor Symp. Quant. Biol., 31:211, 1967.
2. Potter, M.: Meth. Cancer Res., 2:106, 1966.
3. Mach, B., H. Koblet, and D. Gros: Cold Spring Harbor Symp. Quant. Biol., 31:269, 1967.
4. Mach, B., H. Koblet, and D. Gros: Proc. Nat. Acad. Sci. USA, 59:445, 1968.
5. Potter, M., E. Appella, and S. Geisser: J. Mol. Biol., 14:361, 1965.
6. Campbell, J.: J. Theoret. Biol., 16:321, 1967.
7. Mach, B.: In preparation.
8. Siekevitz, P., and G. E. Palade: J. Biophys. Biochem. Cytol., 7:619, 1960.
9. Lisowska-Bernstein, B., M. E. Lam, and P. Vassalli: Proc. Nat. Acad. Sci. USA. In press.
10. Mach, B.: In preparation.
11. Yang, W.-K., and G. D. Novelli: Proc. Nat. Acad. Sci. USA, 59:208, 1968.
12. Mushinski, J. F., and M. Potter: Biochemistry, 8:1684, 1969.
13. Mach, B.: Behringwerk-Mitteil., 49:144, 1969.
14. Kano-Sueoka, T., and N. Sueoka: J. Mol. Biol., 20:183, 1966.
15. Waters, L. C., and G. D. Novelli: Proc. Nat. Acad. Sci. USA, 57:979, 1967.
16. Hung, P. P., and L. R. Overby: J. Biol. Chem., 243:5525, 1968.
17. Subak-Sharpe, et al.: Cold Spring Harbor Symp. Quant. Biol., 31:583, 1966.
18. Mechler, B., and B. Mach: In preparation.
19. Melchers, F., and P. M. Knopf: Cold Spring Harbor Symp. Quant. Biol., 32:255, 1967.
20. Knopf, P. M., Y. S. Choi, and E. S. Lennox: Behringwerk-Mitteil., 49:155, 1969.
21. Melchers, F.: Behringwerk-Mitteil., 49:169, 1969.
22. Schubert, D., and M. Cohn: J. Mol. Biol., 38:273, 1968.
23. Franklin, E. C.: J. Exp. Med., 120:691, 1964.
24. Seligmann, M., et al.: Science, 162:1396, 1968.

Clinical and Biochemical Studies Associated with Immunoglobulin Abnormalities

M. SELIGMANN

Laboratory of Immunochemistry, Research Institute on Blood Diseases, Hôpital Saint-Louis, Paris, France

MANY AUTHORS HAVE CONSIDERED that human monoclonal immunoglobulins (MIg) were truly abnormal globulins synthesized by malignant plasmocytes or lymphoid cells. Current evidence strongly suggests that MIg represent a selected population of normal immunoglobulin molecules. For instance, experiments with antisera to individual MIg have shown that these proteins contain antigenic determinants which appear to be characteristic of each MIg. This finding has been interpreted as evidence in favor of their "abnormal" nature. More recent studies on this individual antigenic specificity of myeloma globulins[1-3] have shown that antigenic determinants similar to most individual specific antigens of myeloma proteins are present in minor populations of normal immunoglobulin molecules.

MIg may be defined as abnormally homogeneous populations of immunoglobulin molecules. This homogeneity is in contrast with the extreme heterogeneity of the normal immunoglobulin molecules. The structural homogeneity of MIg is reflected in the characteristic electrophoretic spike and in the presence of a single type of light and/or heavy polypeptide chains in all the molecules. This homogeneous character presumably reflects their synthesis by a single clone of immunoglobulin-producing cells.

In this context, one must emphasize the close analogies between MIg and purified antibodies of restricted specificity[4] which are characterized by limited electrophoretic heterogeneity, selective occurrence of one type or subclass of polypeptide chains, and individual antigenic specificity. Moreover, immunization of some animals by bacterial carbohydrate antigens leads to the production of antibodies with MIg characteristics.[5]

Several antibody activities (such as antierythrocytic antigen I, antistreptolysin, anti-IgG, antinitrophenyl) have now been recognized in a number of human MIg (reviewed in Reference 6). Actually, all MIg may well be individual antibodies.

Homogeneous MIg have been demonstrated in a large number of

patients with diseases other than myeloma and in apparently healthy persons.[7-11] In a few well-documented cases, the MIg have been shown to be transient,[10] and this spontaneous disappearance is hardly compatible with the hypothesis of a malignant proliferation. A great diversity of clinical patterns associated with MIg in the absence of overt myeloma has been documented. Some very uncommon diseases, such as Gaucher's disease and lichen myxoedematosus, are frequently associated with MIg, and the relationship remains obscure. One may also emphasize that homogeneous MIg may be found in the serum of infants with primary immunologic deficiencies[10] and also in such infants after therapeutic graft of lymphoid cells.[12]

These considerations imply that MIg should be considered as structurally and functionally normal immunoglobulin molecules and that the finding of such homogeneous immunoglobulins does not necessarily imply that a malignant proliferation has taken place. However, the presence of an appreciable amount of Bence Jones protein is very seldom encountered in nonmalignant cases, and the unbalanced synthesis with a great excess of light chains might be a characteristic feature of the malignant plasma cell. Another group of diseases characterized by a profound abnormality in the synthesis of monoclonal immunoglobulins, namely heavy-chain diseases, seems to be always associated with a malignant proliferation and deserves further consideration.

Heavy-chain diseases are characterized by the presence in serum of an "abnormal" immunoglobulin (which seems to have no counterpart in normal serum) devoid of light chains, related to only one subclass of heavy chains and representing only a portion of the heavy chain including the Fc fragment. Heavy-chain diseases have now been found for each of the three major classes of immunoglobulins: γ-chain disease,[13, 14] α-chain disease,[15, 16] and μ-chain disease.[17]

Alpha-chain disease is probably not an uncommon condition, since in the past two years five cases have been detected in Paris and, in addition, 12 foreign cases have been authenticated in our laboratory. The immunoglobulin abnormality can escape routine protein studies because (1) the abnormal electrophoretic band, when present, is very broad and there is no spike; (2) in half of the cases, no abnormal band is detectable in the serum electrophoretic pattern; (3) moreover, the abnormal γA precipitin line is sometimes barely visible at immunoelectrophoretic analysis when using polyvalent antisera and is detected only when using monospecific antisera to γA. The absence of precipitation of the abnormal γA protein with antisera to light chains is not a sufficient criterion for diagnosis, since such a failure to precipitate has been encountered with several γA myeloma proteins. The lack of light chains has to be demonstrated by chemical methods or by special immunologic studies using antisera containing antibodies which give precipitin reactions only when light and α heavy chains are combined. In view of their considerable electrophoretic heterogeneity, the "mono-clonal" character of the α-chain disease proteins had to be proved by their structural and antigenic homogeneity. All studied proteins belonged exclusively to the α_1 subclass, which constitutes about 85% of the normal γA molecules. These proteins have a very high tendency to polymerize. The polymers, held together by noncovalent forces in addition to disulfide bonds, were shown to occur in vivo, and this may explain the low output of the anomalous protein in urine. Molecular weight determinations have been performed for three purified proteins. The molecular weights of the monomer were 34,500, 36,900, and 38,600 as compared with 56,600 for a myeloma α_1 chain.[18] Two of these proteins have a very high carbohydrate content, especially for sialic acid and galactosamine. If allowance is made for carbohydrates, the molecular weight of the polypeptide portion of the proteins is identical for two of them (29,300 and 29,500), but larger for the third protein (34,200). Chemical and immunologic studies have shown that, as in γ-heavy chain disease,[19] these α-chain disease proteins include the Fc fragment. Therefore, more than half of the Fd piece is lacking. Structural studies are in progress in order to determine precisely the length and location of the segment of Fd piece which is missing in these proteins. The study of the NH2-terminal region of γ-heavy chain disease proteins has led to diverging data. In one of these proteins the N terminus is identical to that of complete γ chains,[20] and sequence data clearly indicate a deletion;[21] whereas in two other γ-chain disease proteins, the N-terminal portion of the variable part of the normal γ-chain is missing.[22] Sequence studies of the NH2-terminal region of all heavy-chain disease proteins are clearly of the utmost importance in order to determine if a deletion at the level of the genes coding for heavy chain is a constant feature. Furthermore, since, to date, no light-chain synthesis has been detected at the intracellular level,[15, 22] the findings suggest that, in addition to the heavy-chain gene abnormality, the genes coding for light chains are not expressed in these tumor cells. If these data are confirmed by more sophisticated biosynthetic studies, we are faced with a puzzling problem of molecular biology.

The clinicopathologic features were remarkably similar in patients with α-chain disease. All but one were affected with a neoplastic and mostly plasmacytic proliferation involving primarily the whole length of the small intestine and the mesenteric nodes, and all of these patients exhibited a severe malabsorption syndrome. That α-chain disease primarily involves the intestinal tract is not an unexpected finding, in view of the importance of the digestive lymphoid tissue in the γA synthesis.[23] However, it is in contrast to the rarity of intestinal involvement in γA myeloma. These patients also differ from myeloma patients by their young age (12 to 30 years old). Even if we assume that an enteral antigenic stimulus is a triggering factor in the production of the malignant proliferation, the reason why it leads to α-chain disease occurring early in life and not to myeloma remains obscure. In addition, α-chain disease shows a striking predilection for some populations. Two of the five patients detected in Paris were Arabs, two others were Kabyls from Algeria, and the fifth was a Eurasian. Among the 12 other cases authenticated in our laboratory, three were Arabs, three Sephardim Jews, two Kabyls, two South Italians, and one from south of Spain. This may be a result of the action of environmental factors such as intestinal microorganisms, or of a genetic predisposition similar to that found in Waldenström macroglobulinemia,[24] or of both. These findings do, of course, remind one of the mouse situation for induced myelomas and the genetic factors possibly involved in the production of monoclonal antibodies to streptococcal carbohydrates in rabbits.[5]

Another topic pertinent to this symposium should be briefly approached, namely nonsecretory human myeloma. A few well-documented cases of multiple myeloma without any monoclonal immunglobulin in either serum or urine have been reported. The incidence of such cases is about 1% of myeloma patients.[25] Whether in such instances the neoplastic plasma cells do not synthesize or do not secrete immunoglobulin had not yet been established with convincing evidence. In five such consecutive cases of nonsecretory human myeloma, we have been able to demonstrate by immunofluorescence the presence within the plasma cells of nonsecreted monoclonal immunoglobulin chains.[26] In two of these patients, the plasma cells showed numerous brightly fluorescent nuclear inclusions. Furthermore, similar findings have been demonstrated in our laboratory for two patients with "nonsecretory macroglobulinemia." The first patient had numerous small cytoplasmic inclusions in some lymphocytes and Russell body-type inclusions in plasma cells. All of these inclusions stained brilliantly with fluorescent antisera specific for μ and η chains.[27] The other patient had a chronic lymphocytic leukemia with crystalline inclusions in many lymphocytes; these crystals were positive for μ and λ chains with labeled antisera.[28] The mechanism of the nonsecretion phenomenon in such cases remains unknown and may not be univocal. The hypothesis of a block in the secretion process is, however, suggested by the cytologic features.

References

1. Seligmann, M., G. Meshaka, D. Hurez, and C. Mihaesco: Studies on the reaction of individual antigenic specificity of γG type myeloma globulins. In: Immunopathology, IVth International Symposium, Monaco, 1965 (B. Schwabe, ed.), Vol. 1, 1965, 229 pp.
2. Grey, H. M., M. Mannik, and H. G. Kunkel: Individual antigenic specificity of myeloma proteins. Characteristics and localization to subunits. J. Exp. Med., 121: 561, 1965.
3. Hurez, D., G. Meshaka, C. Mihaesco, and M. Seligmann: The inhibition by normal IgG globulins of individual specific antibodies to IgG myeloma globulins. J. Immunol., 100:69, 1968.

4. Kunkel, H. G.: Myeloma proteins and antibodies. Harvey Lect., S. 59:219, 1964.
5. Braun, D. G., K. Eichmann, and R. M. Krause: Rabbit antibodies to streptococcal carbohydrates. Influence of primary and secondary immunization and of possible genetic factors on the antibody response. J. Exp. Med., 129:809, 1969.
6. Metzger, H.: Myeloma proteins and antibodies. Amer. J. Med., 47:837, 1969.
7. Waldenström, J., S. Winblad, J. Hallen, and S. Liungman: The occurrence of benign, essential monoclonal (M type), nonmacromolecular hyperglobulinemia and its differential diagnosis. IV. Studies in the gammapathies. Acta Med. Scand., 176:345, 1964.
8. Osserman, E. F., and K. Takatsuki: Considerations regarding the pathogenesis of the plasmacytic dyscrasias. Series Haemat., 4:28, 1965.
9. Hallen, J.: Discrete gammaglobulin (M-components) in serum. Clinical study of 150 subjects without myelomatosis. Acta Med. Scand., Suppl. 462, 1966.
10. Danon, F., J. P. Clauvel, and M. Seligmann: Les "paraprotéines" de type IgG et IgA en dehors de la maladie de Kahler. Rev. Franc. Etud. Clin. Biol., 12:681, 1967.
11. Hobbs, J. R.: Paraproteins, benign or malignant? Brit. Med. J., 3:699, 1967.
12. De Koning, J., L. J. Dooren, D. W. Van Bekkum, J. J. Van Rood, K. A. Dicke, and J. Radl: Transplantation of bone marrow cells and fetal thymus in an infant with lymphopenic immunological deficiency. Lancet, 1:1223, 1969.
13. Franklin, E. C., J. Lowenstein, B. Bigelow, and M. Metzger: Heavy chain disease: A new disorder of serum γ-globulins. Report of the first case. Amer. J. Med., 37:332, 1964.
14. Osserman, E. F., and K. Takatsuki: Clinical and immunochemical studies of four cases of heavy ($H\gamma^2$) chain disease. Amer. J. Med., 37:351, 1964.
15. Seligmann, M., F. Danon, D. Hurez, E. Mihaesco, and J. L. Preud'homme: Alpha-chain disease: A new immunoglobulin abnormality. Science, 162:1396, 1968.
16. Seligmann, M., E. Mihaesco, D. Hurez, C. Mihaesco, J. L. Preud'homme, and J. C. Rambaud: Immunochemical studies in four cases of alpha chain disease. J. Clin. Invest., 48:2374, 1969.
17. Forte, F. A., F. Prelli, W. Yount, S. Kochwa, E. C. Franklin, and H. Kunkel: Heavy chain disease of the mu type; report of the first case. Blood, 34:abstr. 19, 1969.
18. Dorrington, K. J., E. Mihaesco, and M. Seligmann: The molecular size of three α-chain disease proteins. Biochim. Biophys. Acta. In press.
19. Franklin, E. C.: Structural studies of human 7S γ-globulin (G-immunoglobulin). Further observations of a naturally occurring protein related to the crystallisable (fast) fragment. J. Exp. Med., 120:691, 1964.
20. Prahl, J. W.: N- and C-terminal sequences of a heavy chain disease protein and its genetic implications. Nature, 215:1386, 1967.
21. Frangione, B., and C. Milstein: Partial deletion in the heavy chain disease protein ZUC. Nature, 224:597, 1969.
22. Ein, D., D. N. Buell, and J. L. Fahey: Biosynthetic and structural studies of a heavy chain disease protein. J. Clin. Invest., 48:785, 1969.
23. Crabbe, P. A., and J. F. Heremans: Étude immunohistochimique des plasmocytes de la muqueuse intestinale humaine normale. Rev. Franc. Etud. Clin. Biol., 11: 484, 1966.
24. Seligmann, M.: A genetic predisposition to Waldenström's macroglobulinaemia. Acta Med. Scand., 179 (Suppl. 445) :140, 1966.
25. Osserman, E. F., and K. Takatsuki: Plasma cell myeloma: Gamma globulin synthesis and structure. A review of biochemical and clinical data, with the description of a newly-recognized and related syndrome, "H γ2-chain (Franklin's) disease." Medicine, 42:357, 1963.
26. Hurez, D., J. L. Preud'homme, and M. Seligmann: Intracellular "monoclonal" immunoglobulin in non secretory human myeloma. J. Immunol., 104:263, 1970.
27. Seligmann, M., D. Hurez, et al.: In preparation.
28. Hurez, D., and G. Flandrin: In preparation.

Myeloma as the Biochemical Model of Cancer: Clinical Studies

DANIEL E. BERGSAGEL

University of Toronto, and Princess Margaret Hospital, Toronto, Ontario, Canada

ANTIBODY-PRODUCING CELLS are derived from a cell renewal series which includes undifferentiated stem cells and differentiated antigen-sensitive cells. Antigen-sensitive cells are stimulated to proliferate by contact with an antigen, and each cell is restricted in the number of antigens to which it can respond.[1] Thus, antigen-sensitive cells have differentiated to the stage that they are committed to produce a specific type of immunoglobulin which has antibody activity for a specific antigen. I have always been attracted by the hypothesis that a malignant transformation may affect the cells of this series, which are capable of proliferating at any stage of differentiation, and that the plasma cell neoplasm which results would be characterized by a distinctive pattern of protein synthesis. The cells at each stage of differentiation probably have distinctive properties, and for this reason a classification of plasma cell neoplasms based on the pattern of protein synthesis should be useful for grouping tumors with similar growth rates, similar clinical manifestations and similar clinical courses.

In this paper, I will present some clinical evidence which supports this hypothesis. I will also consider studies of the synthesis of myeloma proteins which have been used to estimate tumor size, growth rate, and the effects of treatment on the neoplasm.

Plasma Cell Differentiation and the Frequency of Neoplasia

A concept of the stages in plasma cell differentiation is illustrated in Figure 12-3. It seems likely that there are uncommitted, undifferentiated stem cells which proliferate so as to maintain the size of the stem cell pool constant; one would not expect this primitive cell to synthesize either light or heavy polypeptide chains. Since all immunoglobulins contain light chains, it seems likely that one of the initial stages in differentiation requires a decision as to whether the cell will produce type K or type L light chains. The next stage involves the selection of the type of heavy chain to be produced, of which the five antigenic types listed on the right have been recognized. These committed cells will produce both light and heavy chains.

Differentiation in a cell series is usually associated with extensive proliferation, so that increasing numbers of cells are present at each successive stage. One would expect that the majority of plasma cells would be differentiated cells that have been programmed to produce both light and heavy chains.

Malignant transformations probably occur only in cells that are capable of proliferation. It seems likely that the cells at each stage of differentiation represented in this diagram are capable of proliferation.

If the hypothesis which I stated earlier is correct, and the cells at each stage of differentiation are equally susceptible to a malignant transformation, one would expect to find that most plasma-cell neoplasms produce both light and heavy chains, and that tumors producing only light chains would occur more frequently than tumors which produce no protein. This, in fact, is what has been observed. The figures shown in Figure 12-3 represent the protein synthesis patterns of 985 patients with plasma-cell neoplasms studied by three groups of investigators.[2-5] These observations are compatible with the hypothesis that malignant transformations may affect plasma cells at different stages of differentiation, but it must be recognized that mutations could also explain the occurrence of tumors which produce only light chains or no protein. Studies of mutant mouse myelomas which have lost the ability to secrete complete immunoglobulins have revealed that some of these tumors continue to synthesize both light and heavy chains, but only the light chains are secreted.[6] It is postulated that these tumors have lost one, or more, of the enzymes required for assembling light and heavy chains, and that linkage of the heavy to the light chain is essential for the secretion of the heavy chain. It is possible that some human plasma cell tumors which secrete only light chains may have similar defects, and more detailed studies are required to determine whether these tumors produce heavy chains that are not secreted.

Mannik and Kunkel[7] noted that the 60:30 ratio of kappa to lambda

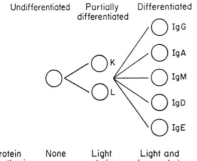

FIG. 12-3.—Scheme relating hypothetical stages in plasma cell differentiation, the protein synthesis pattern at each stage, and the frequency of neoplasms secreting no protein, light chains only, and complete immunoglobulins in 985 patients with plasma cell neoplasms.[2-5]

330/70

TABLE 12–3.—PROTEIN SYNTHESIS BY PLASMA CELL NEOPLASMS

M-PROTEIN CLASS	OSSERMAN & TAKATSUKI[2]	HOBBS[3, 4]	PRUZANSKI[5]	TOTAL	%
IgG	142	238	133	513	52.1
IgA	58	94	31	183	18.6
IgM	41	42	24	107	10.9
IgD	—	4	5	9	0.9
IgE	—	—	—	—	<0.01
Light chains (K or L only)	59	52	37	148	15.0
2 or more M-Proteins	—	8	5	13	1.3
No M-Protein	3	6	3	12	1.2
Totals	303	444	238	985	100.0

light chains in normal serum immunoglobulin was almost identical to the ratio of kappa to lambda light chains in myeloma proteins. If one assumes that the serum levels reflect the number of plasma cells producing these two types of light chains, this observation would suggest that the cells producing kappa and lambda light chains are equally susceptible to malignant transformations. Hobbs[3] has extended these observations with an analysis of the frequency of the heavy-chain classes in myeloma proteins. In this analysis, he postulated that the proportion of normal immunoglobulin produced per day reflects the numbers of plasma cells producing each class of immunoglobulin. He found a surprisingly good correlation between the frequency of neoplasms producing each class of immunoglobulin and the normal production rate for that immunoglobulin. These observations support the view that the classes of plasma cells which produce the various types of immunoglobulins are equally susceptible to malignant transformations. The proteins produced by 985 patients with plasma cell neoplasms[2–5] are shown in Table 12-3.

M-Protein Studies to Estimate Tumor Size, Growth Rate and the Response to Therapy

TUMOR SIZE

Studies of mouse plasma cell tumors suggest that all of the tumor cells synthesize the myeloma protein.[6] The development of methods for estimating the M-protein synthesis rate in vivo and in vitro has permitted estimates to be made of the total plasma cell tumor mass in four patients with IgG myeloma.[8] The principle of this method is shown in Table 12-4. The calculated total tumor cell mass in the four patients studied ranged from 6×10^{11} to 8×10^{12}. Studies of a mouse plasma cell tumor[9] have shown that 4.4% of the tumor cells have the proliferative capacity to form tumor colonies and perpetuate the tumor; the remaining cells appear to be end-stage cells. The tumor stem cell fraction has not been estimated in patients, but it seems

TABLE 12–4.—PLASMA CELL NEOPLASMS

ESTIMATION OF TOTAL BODY TUMOR CELL MASS

Measure M-Protein synthesis rates:

$$\frac{\text{Total} \quad \text{(in vivo)}}{\text{per cell (in vitro)}} = \text{Total M-protein producing cells}$$

Salmon & Smith, Clin. Res. 17:407, 1969

IgG myeloma $6 \times 10^{11} - 8 \times 10^{12}$ cells

likely that this fraction is at least one to two orders of magnitude smaller than the total tumor cell mass.

GROWTH RATE

Early studies relating the increase in the weight of mouse plasma cell tumors to the serum M-protein concentration revealed that the rate of increase in the M-protein parallels the rate of increase in tumor mass.[10, 11] Several investigators have followed M-protein changes in patients with plasma cell neoplasms, and shown that the rate of increase is exponential.[12–15] In Figure 12-4, I have plotted the serum con-

FIG. 12–4.—Estimation of the tumor cell kill resulting from 14 courses of melphalan therapy from the time required for the tumor to regrow to its original size (i.e., produce the original M-protein serum concentration) and the tumor-doubling time, estimated from the time required for the serum M-protein concentration to double.

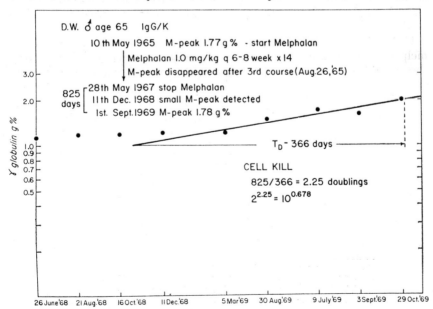

centration of an IgG/K M-protein in a patient who had discontinued melphalan after achieving a good remission. This protein increased exponentially with a doubling time of 366 days. It will be noted that this patient responded very well to melphalan therapy, in that the M-protein disappeared completely from the serum electrophoresis pattern, and could not be detected by immunoelectrophoresis. For this reason, melphalan therapy was stopped after 14 courses had been given, and it took 825 days for the M-protein to return to the pretreatment concentration. If one assumes that the tumor growth rate was constant after melphalan therapy was discontinued, it is possible to estimate the tumor cell kill from the interval required for the tumor to regenerate to its original size divided by the estimated tumor doubling time. This calculation indicates that 14 courses of melphalan therapy reduced the tumor by the equivalent of 2.25 doublings, or 68%. Thus, although melphalan therapy caused the M-protein to disappear completely from the serum of this patient, the cell kill estimates would suggest that there were more than 10^{11} tumor cells remaining when therapy was discontinued, if the original tumor cell mass is assumed to be 10^{12} as suggested by the experiments mentioned above.

Hobbs[15] has measured the M-protein doubling time in patients producing different classes of myeloma protein (Table 12-5). The patients in this study were not responding to therapy with melphalan or cyclophosphamide. In addition, Hobbs[16] has reported the doubling time of a patient with IgM/K macroglobulinemia who was followed for 12 years without any therapy. The doubling time varied for each group of patients, being shortest with tumors producing only light-chain proteins and longest for the patient producing the macroglobulin (Table 12-5).

If the classification of plasma cell tumors on the basis of the class of M-protein does group tumors with significantly different growth rates, one would expect that the tumors with the shortest growth rate would be more aggressive, occur in a younger age group, and have a shorter survival. Hobbs[4] has shown that the age at diagnosis for patients with tumors producing only light chains is significantly younger

TABLE 12–5.—AGE AND MEAN M-PROTEIN DOUBLING TIMES*

M-PROTEIN	NUMBER	MEAN AGE (YRS.)	M-PROTEIN DOUBLING TIME (MONTHS)	
			Mean	Range
Light chains only	11	55.5	3.4	1-7
IgA	17	63.1	6.3	2-14
IgG	24	62.1	10.1	3-24
IgM	51	62.9†	72‡	72‡

* From data reported by Hobbs.[15]
† Mean age calculated for 51 patients reported in references 17-21.
‡ M-protein doubling time for one untreated patient with IgM/K.[16]

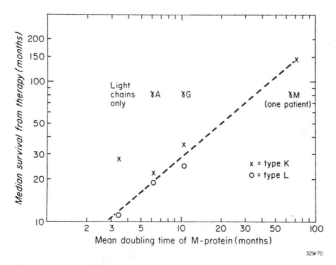

329/70

Fig. 12–5.—Mean M-protein doubling times (see Table 12-5) and the median survival of patients with plasma cell tumors producing different classes of immunoglobulins.[22]

than for those with tumors producing IgG and IgA, and that skeletal lesions and hypercalcemia occur significantly more frequently in patients producing only light-chain proteins. The age at diagnosis for IgM shown in Table 12-5 is for a series of 51 patients with macroglobulinemia reported in the literature,[17–21] and does not differ from the mean age of patients with IgA or IgG myeloma.

The M-protein doubling times shown in Table 12-5 and the median survival from the start of melphalan therapy reported by the Southwest Cancer Chemotherapy Study Group[22] have been plotted on double logarithmic paper in Figure 12-5. It will be noted that there does appear to be a correlation between the mean M-protein doubling time and survival for these groups of patients. The survival of patients producing only kappa light-chain proteins, however, is significantly better than one would expect if the tumor doubling time is only 3.4 months. It will be recalled that Hobbs[15] measured the M-protein doubling time on patients who failed to respond, or were relapsing, while on treatment with melphalan or cyclophosphamide, and it is possible that this group contained mainly patients producing type L light-chain proteins, since it has been reported[22, 23] that patients producing only type K light-chain proteins respond more frequently to therapy and survive longer than those producing only type L light-chain proteins. It would be of considerable interest to determine the doubling time of patients producing only type K or type L light chains prior to the onset of therapy to determine whether the growth rate is slower for type K than for type L.

Summary

Clinical observations are presented which support the hypothesis that malignant transformations may affect precursors of antibody-producing cells at different stages of differentiation. The antigen-sensitive cells which are committed to produce each class of immunoglobulin appear to be equally susceptible to malignant transformation. A classification of plasma cell neoplasms on the basis of the immunoglobulin produced by the tumor appears to group patients with similar growth rates, clinical manifestations, and prognoses. Because of the slow growth rate of some of these tumors, it is possible to achieve good clinical remissions with treatments that reduce the tumor cell mass by less than 1 log.

References

1. Osoba, D.: Restriction of the capacity to respond to two antigens by single precursors of antibody-producing cells in culture. J. Exp. Med., 129:141-152, 1969.
2. Osserman, E. F., and K. Takatsuki: Plasma cell myeloma; γ-globulin synthesis and structure. A review of biochemical and clinical data with the description of a newly-recognized and related syndrome "H-γ²-chain (Franklin's) disease." Medicine, 42:357-384, 1963.
3. Hobbs, J. R.: Monoclonal immunoglobulins from random mutations. Brit. J. Cancer, 22:717-719, 1968.
4. Hobbs, J. R.: Immunochemical classes of myelomatosis. Brit. J. Haemat., 16:599-606, 1969.
5. Pruzanski, W., and M. A. Ogryzlo: Abnormal urinary proteins in malignant diseases. In: Advances in Clinical Chemistry, Academic Press, New York and London, Vol. 15. In press.
6. Cohn, M.: Natural history of myeloma. Cold Spring Harbor Symp. Quant. Biol., 32:211-221, 1967.
7. Mannik, M., and H. G. Kunkel: Two major types of normal 7S γ-globulin. J. Exp. Med., 117:213-230, 1963.
8. Salmon, S. E., and B. A. Smith: Multiple Myeloma: Plasma cell gammaglobulin synthesis and total body tumor cell mass. Clin. Res., 17:407, 1969.
9. Bergsagel, D. E., and F. A. Valeriote: Growth characteristics of a mouse plasma cell tumor. Cancer Res., 28:2187-2196, 1968.
10. Nathans, D., J. L. Fahey, and M. Potter: The formation of myeloma protein by a mouse plasma cell tumor. J. Exp. Med., 108:121-130, 1958.
11. Osserman, E. F., R. A. Rifkind, K. Takatsuki, and D. P. Lawlor: Studies of morphogenesis and protein synthesis in three mouse plasma cell tumors. Ann. N. Y. Acad. Sci., 113:627-641, 1964.
12. Waldenström, J.: The occurrence of benign essential monoclonal (M-type) non-macromolecular hyperglobulinemia and its differential diagnosis. IV. Studies in the gammapathies. Acta Med. Scand., 176:345-365, 1964.
13. Hällén, J.: Discrete gammaglobulin (M-) components in serum. Clinical study of 150 subjects without myelomatosis. Acta Med. Scand., Suppl. 462, 1966.
14. Hobbs, J. R.: Paraproteins, benign or malignant? Brit. Med. J., 3:699-704, 1967.
15. Hobbs, J. R.: Growth rates and responses to treatment in human myelomatosis. Brit. J. Haemat., 16:607-617, 1969.
16. Clinicopathological Conference: A case of Waldenström's macroglobulinemia with slow progression. Brit. Med. J., 2:237-242, 1968.
17. Kappeler, V. R., A. Krebs, and G. Riva: Klinik der Makroglobulinämie Walden-

ström: Beschreibung von 21 Fällen und Übersicht der Literatur. Helvetica Med. Acta, 25:55-152, 1958.

18. Klemm, D., H. Schubothe, P. Obrecht, and H. Langendorff: Über der therapeutische Beeinflussung makroglobulinämischer Krankheitsbilder. Klin. Wochenschr., 41:805-809, 1963.

19. Fahey, J. L., R. Scoggins, J. P. Utz, and C. F. Szwed: Infection, antibody response and gammaglobulin components in multiple myeloma and macroglobulinemia. Amer. J. Med., 35:698-707, 1963.

20. Waldenström, J.: Macroglobulinemia. Adv. Metabol. Disorders, 2:115-185, 1965.

21. Houston, E. W., S. E. Ritzmann, and W. C. Levin: Chromosomal aberrations common to three types of monoclonal gammapathies. Blood, 29:214-232, 1967.

22. Alexanian, R., A. Haut, A. U. Khan, M. Lane, E. M. McKelvey, P. J. Migliore, W. J. Stuckey, Jr., and H. E. Wilson: Treatment for Multiple Myeloma. J. Amer. Med. Ass., 208:1680-1685, 1969.

23. Bergsagel, D. E., P. J. Migliore, and K. M. Griffith: Myeloma proteins and the clinical response to Melphalan therapy. Science, 148:376-377, 1965.

13

Modern Interpretations of Biochemical Theories of Cancer

Temporal Studies of the Biosynthesis of Chromatin in Synchronized Mammalian Cell Cultures

MICHAEL E. McCLURE AND

LUBOMIR S. HNILICA

Department of Biochemistry, The University of Texas M. D. Anderson Hospital and Tumor Institute at Houston, Houston, Texas, USA

Introduction

THE MECHANISM OF GENE regulation in eukaryotic cells is unknown. Certain chromosomal proteins have, however, been suggested to serve a role in regulating genetic activity.[1, 2] The acid-soluble chromosomal proteins (histones) have commanded much attention in this respect. The syntheses of histones and DNA are closely coupled events in eukaryotic cells.[3] It remains controversial, however, as to whether histone synthesis is strictly confined to the cell cycle period characterized by active DNA synthesis (S period). In particular, evidence exists suggesting the synthesis of histone during the G_1 period of the cell cycle.[4, 5] Such evidence could indicate a turnover of histones associated with genetic activity. Even if histone synthesis occurs exclusively during the S period, histones may still play a role in gene regulation by maintaining developmentally dictated genetic inactivation in certain

494

genomic regions of differentiated tissues. An example of this latter possibility might be found in the euchromatin-heterochromatin concept. These two forms of chromatin synthesize their DNA content during temporally segregated portions of the cell cycle,[6] and are known to represent active and inactivated chromatin, respectively.[7] Since the synthesis of a new genome during the S period entails the association of newly synthesized histone and DNA, a major difference in histone content of early S (euchromatin) and late S (heterochromatin) chromatin should be demonstrated by the accumulation kinetics for the various histone fractions. This approach is equally valid for studies of nonhistone chromosomal protein accumulation into chromatin during the cell cycle. In the present study, the temporal relationship of the synthesis of DNA, histones, and nonhistone chromosomal proteins during the mammalian cell cycle is described.

Materials and Methods

CELL CULTURE

Cultures of a cloned cell strain (Don-C) of an established male Chinese hamster *(Cricetulus griseus)* fibroblast cell line were grown under 10% CO_2 in McCoy's 5 A medium supplemented with 0.08 gm/liter of lactalbumin hydrolysate and 10% fetal calf serum. For experimental purposes, Don-C cultures were grown as monolayers in rotary cultures using 1700 cm^2 Bellco Cell Production Vessels (CPVs) and a specially constructed culture mill. Each culture was seeded with about 100×10^6 cells in 250 cc of growth medium, rotated at 0.063 rpm for one to two hours, and rotated at 0.240 rpm thereafter. Under these conditions, the cultures increased numerically at a rate similar to that observed for stationary cultures.

CELL SYNCHRONIZATION

The Colcemid (CIBA Pharmaceuticals) blockage of cell division (0.06 $\mu g/ml$, three hours) and harvest of metaphase cells by selective dislodgement followed (essentially) the procedure described by Stubblefield and Klevecz.[8] The 12 CPVs provided 14 square feet of growing surface with yields of 0.8 to 1.1 cc of pelleted metaphase cells (240-330 $\times 10^6$ cells) and synchrony levels of 96% or better. Such cells were "reversed" from blockage by dispersal into 37C growth medium, and were cultured in Roux flasks (about 1.5×10^6 cells per ml of medium).

ADMINISTRATION OF ISOTOPIC PRECURSORS

The kinetics of DNA synthesis were studied by pulse labeling (15-min labeling interval) and continuous labeling (cumulative) experiments using ³H-[methyl]-thymidine (Schwartz BioResearch, S.A. 11 c/mm) at 1 μc/ml final concentration. In both cases, termination of the ³H-thymidine (³H-TdR) experiments followed the procedure described by Stubblefield et al.[9] for scintillation analysis. Aliquots of the 0.1 N NaOH hydrolysate of the monolayer were counted in a modified Bray's solution, consisting of 1,4-dioxane (500 ml), toluene (500 ml), methanol (300 ml), napthalene (100 gm), PPO (5 gm), and POPOP (0.1 gm) by a Packard Liquid Scintillation Spectrometer (Model 3003). The counting system required 10 hours of dark adaptation because of chemiluminescence and, thereafter, counted ¹⁴C at 85% efficiency with minimal quenching.

RNA synthesis was studied by continuous labeling experiments using 5 μg/ml of ³H-uridine (Nuclear Chicago, S.A. 17.3 c/mm). The cultures were harvested and prepared for radioautographic analysis according to methods described by Schmid.[10]

Protein synthesis was studied by pulse labeling cultures (one-hr labeling period) with a ¹⁴C-amino acid mixture (Schwartz BioResearch, lot no. 6703 and 6802) contained in 37C Hank's balanced salt solution at a final concentration of 1 μc/ml. Control experiments showed that this procedure did not affect the rate of DNA synthesis or the proportional distribution of label into five different protein fractions. The labeling period was terminated by rinsing the cultures one time with a 4C solution of 0.075 M NaCl + 0.024 M Na-EDTA (saline-EDTA), removing the cells from the glass surface by a four- to six-minute treatment with the cold saline-EDTA solution, suspending the collected pellet in two to three volumes of 4C McCoy's 5a + 5% glycerol, and freezing the cells (–100C) until used for analysis.

ISOLATION OF CHROMATIN

Chromatin isolation initially followed the method reported by Marushige and Bonner.[11] All isolation steps occurred at 0 to 4C. The method was adjusted to the small sample volumes available by the reduction of the solution volumes employed. In general, cells suspended in 35 cc of cold saline-EDTA + 0.1 cc of octanol were blended and stirred, as described by the above authors, in an ice-bath cooled 250 cc stainless-steel miniblender (Eberbach Corp.) using a Waring blender motor unit and a Variac voltage controller. The crude chromatin pellet obtained was hand-homogenized and centrifugally "washed" (successively) in saline-EDTA, Tris buffer, and 1.7 M sucrose according to the original method. The resultant chromatin pellet was not resheared for solubilization, but was, instead, hand-homogenized and centrifugally "washed" (successively) twice in 2 cc volumes of 0.14 M NaCl + 0.01 M Na-citrate (pH 7.6) and twice in 2 cc volumes of 0.1 M Tris-HCl buffer (pH 7.6) as described previously for nuclei.[12] The final pellet was designated as stage three chromatin.

Compositional analysis for DNA[13] and protein[14] demonstrated acid-soluble protein to DNA ratios of about 1.20.

FRACTIONATION OF CHROMATIN

Acid-soluble proteins were extracted from stage three chromatin by hand-homogenization in 1 cc volumes of 0.4 N H_2SO_4 (0-4C) and centrifugally clarified (10,000 × g, 15 min). The thrice extracted residue was saved and the three supernates were pooled, dialyzed against 4C deionized water, shell frozen, and lyophilized. The lyophylate was termed crude whole histone.

Dehistoned chromatin was extracted three times in 0.1 N NaOH (4C) by methodology similar to the acid extraction procedure. The lyophylate contained 97% of the total chromatin DNA, 86% of the RNA (determined by the orcinol method[15]) and about 45% of the acid-insoluble protein. The nucleic acids were removed by a conventional perchloric acid (PCA) hydrolysis procedure (100C, 15 min) before further analysis. The protein pellet obtained was designated as the cold 0.1 N NaOH soluble (CNS) fraction.

The residue remaining after cold acid and cold base extraction was subjected to PCA hydrolysis to remove nucleic acids. The protein product was solubilized in 1 N NaOH (100C, 15 min) and centrifugally clarified. The final hydrolysate was termed the hot 1 N NaOH soluble (HNS) fraction and contained about 50% of the acid-insoluble protein in dehistoned chromatin. The totally insoluble residue (TIR) fraction remaining after all of the above steps contained radioactivity and protein, and represented 5 to 6% of the total chromatin mass.

FRACTIONATION OF THE HISTONES

Crude whole histone was electrophoretically fractionated in 15% polyacrylamide gels according to the methodology described recently by Bonner and co-workers.[16] In the present study, the 15% urea-gel solution was loaded into 0.6 × 8 cm glass columns (chromic acid cleaned) to a height of 6.0 cm. Whole histone lyophylates were dissolved in 10 M urea (60 min) and applied (25 or 50 μliter volume) to the polymerized gel columns. The load concentration did not exceed 80 μg per column. The samples were electrophoresed for three hr at 5 ma per column constant current (Spinco Duostat) in a home-made apparatus. The gels were reamed free, stained in 1% Naphthol Blue Black (Allied Chemical Co.) in 40% ethanol-7% aqueous acetic acid for at least eight hr, and destained electrophoretically (ca. two hours) using a 24-v (10 amp) Allstate battery charger.

The banding patterns of whole histone preparations from rat liver, rat ascites cells, Chinese hamster cells, and calf thymus cells were remarkably similar. The various fractions were identified by comparison with the individual protein band positions attained by isolated calf thymus histone fractions (prepared as described previously[17]) .

QUANTITATIVE ANALYSIS OF THE AMOUNT AND RADIOACTIVE CONTENT OF CHROMOSOMAL PROTEINS

The amount of protein contained in both the CNS and HNS chromosomal protein fractions was determined by Lowry analysis,[14] using a bovine serum albumin standard and appropriate solvents. The radioactivity content in such proteins was determined by scintillation analysis of sample aliquots in the Bray's counting solution. The radioactivity measurement was corrected for background counts, efficiency, and quenching to disintegrations per minute (dpm). The over-all results were expressed as a specific activity (dpm per unit weight of protein) for each fraction.

The gel-fractionated histone fractions were quantitated densitometrically using a modified Photovolt Model 530 densitometer (0.1 × 3 mm slits) equipped with a Photovolt Model 42B variable-response recorder (1:4 expansion) and a Photovolt Model 49A electronic integrator. The recorder was operated at a response setting of five. The scanning wave-length (610 mμ) was controlled by an interference filter (half-width 10 mμ). The relative amount of protein in each histone fraction was expressed as a fractional proportion of the whole histone weight.

The radioactivity content of each histone fraction was determined by mechanically slicing the entire gel column (sequentially) into 1-mm discs. The discs were depolymerized by a method similar to that reported by Tishler and Epstein[18] and counted in the Bray's solution described earlier. The radioactivity content and the relative weight value obtained for each histone were expressed as a specific activity value (dpm per unit weight of protein).

Results

CHARACTERIZATION OF THE SYNCHRONIZED CELL CYCLE

The initial point (zero hr time point) in the studies to be reported was the moment of dispersal of the synchronized metaphase cell population into 37C medium. This was designated as the "reversal" point, and all subsequent time points were denoted as the "hour after reversal."

The reinitiation of cell division was studied cytologically in slides prepared from samples collected successively later than the initial reversal point. The results (Figure 13-1) showed anticipated patterns of cell division. Following an initial period of time (about 15 min) required to reverse the Colcemid effect, the synchronized population demonstrated an orderly progression through the remaining phases of mitosis. It was noted that some metaphase cells reinitiated division

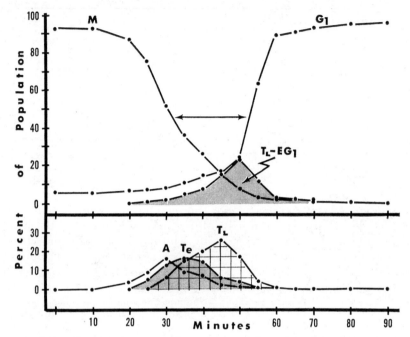

FIG. 13–1.—The duration of cytologic stages during reinitiated cell division. Synchronized cell cultures were harvested, fixed in 50% aqueous acetic acid (without prior hypotonic treatment), stained in 1% aceto-orcein, and prepared for study by the conventional squash procedure. The cytologic stages scored were metaphase (M), anaphase (A), early telophase (T_e), late telophase (T_L), late telophase-early G_1 (T_L-EG_1), and G_1. Double-headed arrows mark the interval used to estimate the average duration of division. Cell counts of at least 500 cells were made for each time point sampled.

earlier than others, and hence the division categories scored appeared as a distribution about an average value instead of a sharp "step" event. This variation apparently persisted throughout the synchronized cell cycle, since other workers reported a nonstep entrance into the subsequent mitotic period.[9]

The average duration of the reinitiated division process (20 min) was estimated by measuring the interval between the metaphase depletion curve and the nucleated G_1 cell appearance curve at the midway point (in this case, 46%). This value summed with the known duration of prophase (6.5 to 7.7 min) suggested a mitotic interval of 27 to 28 min, which closely agreed with the 26- to 28-min interval normally attributed to Don-C cell cultures, and indicated that reinitiated division proceeded at a nearly normal rate.

In cultures reversed into 5 μc/ml of ³H-UR, chromosomal sites of RNA synthesis (grain foci) were first detected by radioautography in late telophase cells. That RNA synthesis resumed in late telophase

TABLE 13-1.—INCORPORATION OF H³-UR INTO DIVIDING DON-C CELLS

CELL STAGE	ANAPHASE	EARLY TELOPHASE	LATE TELOPHASE	LATE TELOPHASE TO EARLY G₁
Ratio*	4.8 ± 0.5	4.6 ± 0.7	8.5 ± 0.5	10.6 ± 1.2
Normalized to Anaphase	1.0	1.0	1.8	2.2

* The ratio of grains counted over the cells to the background count was determined from the results of three separate counting periods for each category (75 cells total). The 95% confidence interval was determined from the results.

cells was also shown by the results of grain count analysis (Table 13-1). Such data were consistent with the report that RNA synthesis began one hour after reversal in this system.[9]

Cumulative DNA synthesis and concomitant net protein synthesis were monitored in synchronized cultures reversed into growth medium containing 1 μc/ml of ³H-TdR by scintillation analysis and chemical analysis, respectively. The rate of DNA synthesis and concomitant

FIG. 13-2.—Kinetic analysis of DNA and protein synthesis during the cell cycle. Each point plotted is the average value of duplicate determinations from a sample hydrolysate. Lowry-analyzed protein (solid triangles, open circles), cumulative DNA synthesis (solid circles), and the DNA synthetic rate estimates (open squares) are represented. The methodology employed is described in the text. The assigned cell cycle intervals appear in the central portion of the figure.

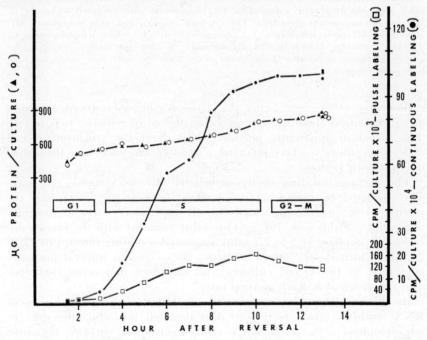

net protein synthesis were simultaneously monitored in a concurrent replicate culture series pulse labeled with ^{3}H-TdR (1 μc/ml). The results (Figure 13-2) showed that the net protein content per culture approximately doubled during the cell cycle, in agreement with earlier reports.[9, 19] The temporal pattern of net protein accumulation was similar to that reported by Stubblefield et al.[9] Although a minor accumulation of ^{3}H-TdR into DNA was observed to begin at two hr after reversal, major incorporation of ^{3}H-TdR was not observed until three hr after reversal. A pause in the accumulation of ^{3}H-TdR occurred between six and seven hr after reversal. A similar pause has been noted previously.[9, 20] This pause was also noted in the DNA rate-curve of Figure 13-2. Although the rate-curve pause was minimally shown in Figure 13-2, a recent report demonstrated a marked depression at this point in a similar curve.[21]

The kinetic events described above permitted a temporal definition of the various cell cycle periods in this synchrony system. In Figure 13-2 and all subsequent temporal figures, we considered zero to one hr after reversal as reinitiated mitosis, one hr to two and one-half hr as G_1, two and one-half to 10 hr as S, and 10 to 12 hr as G_2-mitosis. It was apparent that the cell cycle of bulk-produced, synchronized cultures evidenced growth characteristics remarkably similar to those reported previously for small-scale systems. In agreement with earlier workers using the small-scale systems, we considered it unlikely that serious biochemical imbalances occurred in the synchronized cell population. Indeed, synchronized cultures proved viable under routine culture conditions for periods of time similar to standard random cultures.

CHROMOSOMAL PROTEIN (HISTONE) ACCUMULATION DURING CHROMATIN BIOSYNTHESIS

The synchronization procedure described permitted studies on the rate of accumulation of histones into chromatin during defined intervals of the cell cycle of Don-C cells. Each time point analyzed represented a pooled sample of at least two independent synchrony preparations. The degree of progress into the cell cycle was monitored by the determination of the rate of DNA synthesis and net protein increase in an aliquot culture established from the synchrony preparation. The ratio of the level of DNA labeling to the net protein content for each experimental point was compared to a standard curve compiled from a continuous synchrony assay (Figure 13-3).

The temporal pattern of whole histone accumulation into chromatin was determined from the specific radioactivity of the various gel-separated histone fractions (Figure 13-4). An isolated metaphase cell population (95% final synchrony) was labeled in the presence of Colcemid and was found to demonstrate low levels of radioactive histone accumulation into chromatin. Despite the low level of radioactivity in this temporal sample, it was possible to analyze the distribution of radioactivity among the histone fractions. Since radioautography previously has shown that a 95% metaphase population had no more than 5% of the total cell population engaged in DNA synthesis, it was expected that this metaphase sample would demonstrate a level of histone accumulation no greater than 5% of the average S period level. The level observed (about 2% of the S period rate) was considered, therefore, to be attributable to the interphase cells contaminating the metaphase population. The metaphase sample thus served to indicate a minimal "background" level of histone accumulation caused by asynchronous elements in the synchronous population. Indeed, the small increase in the rate of accumulation in the G_1 sample (one and one-half hr) appeared to be adequately explained by the contributions made by asynchronous interphase cells and a small number of cells in the synchronous population which began DNA synthesis earlier than the rest of the synchronized cell population. It was clear that no major accumulation of histone into chromatin occurred during G_1.

FIG. 13–3.—The rate of DNA synthesis relative to the net protein content in synchronized cell cultures. The ratio of ³H-TdR incorporated during a 15-min pulse interval to the net protein content in the cultures was compiled from the data in Figure 13-2. The standard curve obtained (solid circles) was consistent with earlier results on the timing of cell cycle intervals and served as a convenient means of monitoring cell cycle progress. The experimental points (triangles) compared to the standard curve represented the G_1 (one to two hr), G_1-S_e (two to three hr), S_e (five to six hr), S_1 (eight and one-half to nine and one-half hr) and the G_2-M (11 to 12 hr) cultures reported in subsequent portions of this paper.

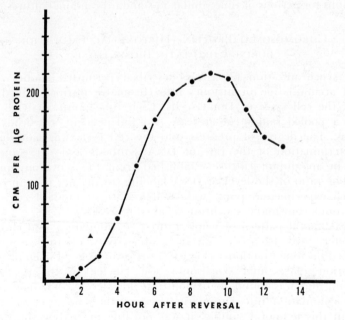

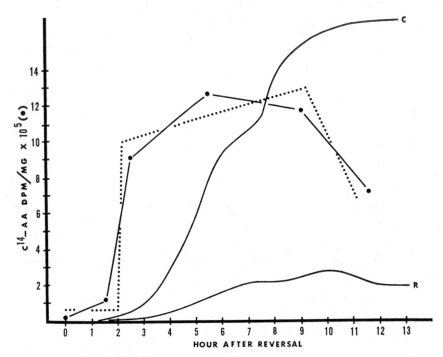

FIG. 13–4.—The accumulation of newly synthesized histone into chromatin during synchronous culture growth. The calculated rates of whole histone accumulation were plotted relative to the degree of progress through the cell cycle. The temporal pattern of histone accumulation (solid circles) was compared to the rate of DNA synthesis (R curve) and the relative net accumulation of DNA (C curve) from Figure 13-2. The dotted profile curve represents the expected accumulation profile for histone assuming: (1) no histone accumulation during G_1, (2) an increase in histone accumulation corresponding to the observed increase in the rate of DNA synthesis during the cell cycle, and (3) the cessation of histone accumulation with the completion of DNA synthesis (blurred by synchrony decay).

The major period of the accumulation of newly synthesized histone into chromatin decidedly occurred during the S period and declined with the cessation of DNA synthesis at the end of the S period (Figure 13-4). The accumulation curve for histone, in fact, resembled the curve reported by Klevecz and Stubblefield[20] for the temporal pattern of increase and decrease in the number of cell nuclei engaged in DNA synthesis. Moreover, if a correction was applied for the faster rate of late S (heterochromatin) DNA synthesis,[22, 23] a "step" type curve could be constructed in agreement with the plotted data.

To compare the temporal patterns of accumulation of the various histone fractions, the specific activity value for each fraction was compared to the average whole-histone specific activity as a ratio to demonstrate the variation from the over-all average value for each fraction

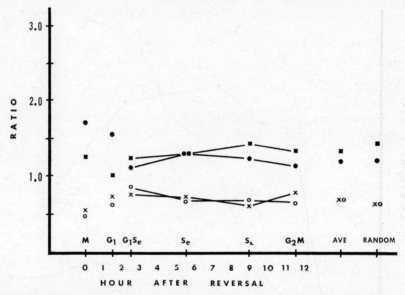

Fig. 13–5.—Proportional relationships for the accumulation of the various histone fractions into chromatin during synchronous culture growth. Conditions are as described in the text. The fractions that appear in the figure are the f1 (solid square), f3 (solid circle), f2b-f2a2 (open circle) and f2a1 (X). The ordinate value represents the ratio of each fraction to the average whole-histone value.

(Figure 13-5). It was immediately obvious that the histone fraction specific activities could be classified into two groupings. The first group (f1 and f3) consistently demonstrated specific activities about twofold higher than the second grouping (f23-f2b and f2a1). This relationship was observed in cell samples from particular periods of the cell cycle as well as in random cell samples. Indeed, the summation of the individual cell cycle period patterns strongly resembled, as it should have, the random cell pattern. It is also obvious from these data that no histone fraction was selectively accumulated (or not accumulated) at any particular time during chromatin biosynthesis (the S period). Moreover, no major increase or decrease in the accumulation of one or more histones occurred during the S period. The expected specific activity for each histone was calculated assuming maximal labeling of the histone molecules by the ^{14}C amino acid mixture employed. With the exception of the f1 histone, all of the fractions demonstrated similar specific activities (2.1×10^4 dpm/mg amino acids). The f1 histone showed a calculated specific activity (2.3×10^4 dpm/mg amino acids) higher than the other fractions by about 9%. This value agreed reasonably well with the 11% (average) difference in specific activity observed between the f1 and f3 histones of the synchronous population. This line of reasoning showed that the labeling mixture used would explain the differences between f1 and f3 in the group-one specific activities, but failed to explain the twofold difference between the group-one (f1 + f3) and group-two (f2b-f2a3 and f2a1) specific activities.

Since the specific activities of the metaphase histone reflected the values for the asynchronous contaminating interphase cells, the unusual relationship of the metaphase and G_1 histone fractions might represent the kinetics of histone accumulation corresponding to the recovery from Colcemid toxicity in these cells, the recovery from "lag" growth, or both. Under these assumptions, it was expected that the G_1 pattern should show a tendency to approach the expected relationships. Such an effect was noted (Figure 13-5). It must be stressed that the period from G_1-S_e (two to three hr) to G_2-M (11 to 12 hr) represented the temporal pattern of the synchronous culture, and that the 3% contribution by asynchronous or "lag" affected population elements to the accumulation kinetics would be overwhelmed by the histone accumulation by 97% of the population during this interval.

FIG. 13–6.—The accumulation of newly synthesized nonhistone proteins into chromatin during synchronous culture growth. The 0.1 N NaOH soluble (CNS) and 1.0 N NaOH soluble (HNS) protein fractions appear in the figure. The CNS nonhistone protein (solid circles) and the HNS nonhistone protein (solid squares) are compared to the relative net DNA accumulation curve (C curve) and the DNA rate curve (R curve), as described in Figure 13-4.

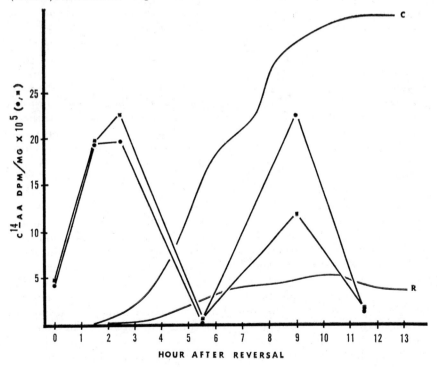

CHROMOSOMAL PROTEIN (NONHISTONE) ACCUMULATION DURING CHROMATIN BIOSYNTHESIS

Unlike histones, both the 0.1 N NaOH (cold) soluble (CNS) protein fraction associated with DNA and the 1 N (hot) soluble (HNS) protein fraction evidenced high rates of accumulation into chromatin during the G_1 and G_1-S_e periods of the cell cycle (Figure 13-6). The rate declined dramatically after the initiation of DNA synthesis in the synchronous population. Nonhistone protein accumulation achieved significant levels again during late S. Both fractions declined during the G_2-M period, as predicted by the initial metaphase sample (M) data. Since the two fractions demonstrated similar levels of accumulation during G_1, the departure from similarity noted during late S might reflect either a twofold increase in the CNS fraction kinetics (relative to HNS protein) or a twofold decrease in HNS kinetics (relative to CNS proteins). In general, the temporal patterns of accumulation into chromatin of histone and nonhistone proteins were observed to be inversely correlated, i.e., periods of active histone accumulation were characterized by low rates of nonhistone protein accumulation and vice versa.

Discussion

The temporal assignment of the term G_1 or G_2 to synchronous cell cycle intervals by an investigator in no way forces asynchronous cells synthesizing DNA and histones during these intervals to cease these activities. Since the analytic procedures employed by current workers are of sufficient resolution to detect the biosynthetic activities of such "contaminating" cells, they must be given adequate consideration in the interpretation of the data obtained. In the present study, the synchronized (95%) metaphase population clearly showed net histone synthesis and accumulation into chromatin. Although histone synthesis in metaphase cells cannot presently be excluded, it is, indeed, highly unlikely that newly synthesized histones accumulate in metaphase chromatin. The accumulation into chromatin in the "metaphase" sample was most certainly attributable to the asynchronous interphase cells (5%) contained in the sample. A similar qualification must necessarily be applied to the results obtained in our studies of the G_1 interval in the mammalian cell cycle. In view of the low level of histone accumulation observed, the known content of asynchronous population elements, and the early entrance of a small proportion of the asynchronous population into the S period, we concluded from our data (Figure 13-4) that there was no appreciable accumulation of histone into G_1 chromatin in our system. This conclusion contrasted with a recent report of G_1 histone accumulation into chromatin,[5] but was supported by an early study by Robbins and Borun,[24] by recent studies on the nature of the "coupling" of DNA and histone synthesis[25] and, in particular, by the "turnover" studies of Byvoet[26] and Hancock.[27]

Our studies on the accumulation of newly synthesized histone fractions into chromatin showed several interesting relationships (Figure 13-5). It was noted that there was little variation in the proportions of the histone fractions accumulated during the S period. These results failed, therefore, to demonstrate major variations in histone content correlated with either the biosynthesis of genetically active euchromatin during early S or the biosynthesis of genetically inactive heterochromatin during late S. Such evidence supports the suggestion that the histone contents of the two chromatin states are (at the least) quite similar. It also was observed that the f1 and f3 fractions showed specific activities about two times higher than the f2b-f2a2 and f2a1 histone fractions. The nearly constant twofold difference noted presumably reflected either different synthesis rates, different synthesis mechanisms, or synthesis from different intracellular amino acid pools. Such differences (two- to threefold) have also been reported in other systems,[28] although another study was not in agreement.[4]

The high rate of nonhistone protein accumulation into chromatin during G_1 and late S proved of great interest. It was possible that such activity might reflect periods of intense genetic activity, since excessive nonhistone accumulation into chromatin has been correlated with sites of active RNA synthesis.[29-31] The second accumulation peak is of particular interest since it occurred during the interval of heterochromatin biosynthesis. Leveson and Peacocke[32] have demonstrated a number of acidic protein-DNA complexes which appear to be unique to heterochromatin. Moreover, the second peak of nonhistone accumulation occurred during a temporal interval which coincided with the second peak in the DNA synthesis rate curve. It was during this interval that heterochromatin was synthesized at an accelerated rate.[22, 23] Although a clear interpretation of the accumulation kinetics for nonhistone proteins awaited further resolution, it was clear that these proteins were actively accumulated during relatively "slack" periods of histone accumulation and were, in some way, integrally concerned with functional chromatin activity.

Summary

Synchronous cultures of Chinese hamster cells (Don-C) were established from a selectively dislodged metaphase cell population. Such cultures demonstrated temporal patterns of DNA, RNA, and net protein synthesis not unlike those predicted from untreated cells. Studies conducted to determine the temporal patterns of accumulation of newly synthesized chromosomal proteins into chromatin during synchronous culture growth demonstrated: (1) the absence of appreciable histone accumulation into mitotic and G_1 chromatin, (2) a major period of histone accumulation into chromatin during the S period, (3) similar proportions of accumulation of histone fractions into chromatin in both synchronized and random cell samples, (4) a twofold difference in the specific activities of f1 and f3 relative to f2b-f2a2 and f2a1 histones, (5) two major periods of accumulation of nonhistone proteins into chromatin, (6) a twofold difference in the specific activities of two different nonhistone protein fractions during late S of the cell cycle, and (7) an inverse relationship between the temporal accumulation patterns of histones and nonhistone chromosomal proteins.

Acknowledgments

This investigation was supported by grants from the American Cancer Society (E-388), the U. S. Public Health Service (CA-07746), The Robert A. Welch Foundation (G-138), and an Institutional Grant (FR 05511-07-IN-88).

References

1. Huang, R., and J. Bonner: Histone, a suppressor of chromosomal RNA synthesis. Proc. Nat. Acad. Sci. USA, 48:1216, 1967.
2. Paul, J., and R. S. Gilmour: Organ-specific restriction of transcription in mammalian chromatin. J. Mol. Biol., 34:305, 1968.
3. Hardin, J., G. Enim, and D. Lindsay: Simultaneous synthesis of histone and DNA in synchronously dividing Tetrahymena pyriformis. J. Cell. Biol., 32:709, 1967.
4. Gurley, L., and J. Hardin: The metabolism of histone fractions. I. Synthesis of histone fractions during the life cycle of mammalian cells. Arch. Biochem. Biophys., 128:285, 1968.
5. Sadgopal, A., and J. Bonner: The relationship between histone and DNA synthesis in Hela cells. Biochim. Biophys. Acta, 186:349, 1969.
6. Pera, F.: Dauer der DNS-Replikation von eu- und hetero-chromatin bei Microtus agrestis. Chromosoma, 25:21, 1968.
7. Brown, S.: Heterochromatin. Science, 151:417, 1966.
8. Stubblefield, E., and R. Klevecz: Synchronization of Chinese hamster cells by reversal of colcemid inhibition. Exp. Cell Res., 40:660, 1969.
9. Stubblefield, E., R. Klevecz, and L. Deaven: Synchronized mammalian cell cultures. I. Cell replication cycle and macromolecular synthesis following brief Colcemid arrest of mitosis. J. Cell Physiol., 69:345, 1967.
10. Schmid, W.: In: Human Chromosome Methodology (J. Junis, ed.), Academic Press, New York, 1965, p. 91.
11. Marushige, K., and J. Bonner: Template properties of liver chromatin. J. Mol. Biol., 15:160, 1966.
12. Hnilica, L. S.: Proteins of the cell nucleus. Prog. Nucl. Acid Res. Mol. Biol., 7:28, 1967.
13. Burton, K.: A study of the conditions and mechanism of the diphenylamine reaction for the colorimetric estimation of deoxyribonucleic acid. Biochem. J., 62:315, 1956.
14. Lowry, O., N. Rosebrough, A. Farr, and R. Randall: Protein measurement with the folin phenol reagent. J. Biol. Chem., 193:265, 1951.
15. Hurlbert, R. B., H. Schmitz, A. Brumm, and V. Potter: Nucleotide metabolism II. Chromatographic separation of acid-soluble nucleotides. J. Biol. Chem., 209:23, 1954.
16. Bonner, J., G. Chalkley, M. Dahmus, D. Fambrough, F. Fujimura, R. Huang, J. Huberman, R. Jensen, K. Marushige, H. Ohlenbusch, B. Olivera, and J. Widholm: In: Methods in Enzymology (L. Grossman and K. Moldave, eds.), Academic Press, New York, 1968, p. 82.
17. Hnilica, L. S.: Studies on nuclear protein I. Observations on the tissue and species

specificity of the moderately lysine rich-histone fraction 2b. Biochim. Biophys. Acta, 117:163, 1966.

18. Tishler, P. V., and C. J. Epstein: A convenient method of preparing polyacrylamide gels for liquid scintillation spectrometry. Anal. Biochem., 22:89, 1968.

19. Killander, D., and A. Zetterberg: Quantitative cytochemical studies on interphase growth. I. Determination of DNA, RNA, and mass of age determined fibroblast *in vitro* and of intercellular variation in generation time. Exp. Cell Res., 38:272, 1965.

20. Klevecz, R., and E. Stubblefield: RNA synthesis in relation to DNA replication in synchronized Chinese hamster cell cultures. J. Exp. Zool., 165:259, 1967.

21. Klevecz, R.: Temporal coordination of DNA replication with enzyme synthesis in diploid and heteroploid cells. Science, 166:1536, 1969.

22. Ockey, C.: In: Chromosomes Today (C. Darlington and K. Lewis, eds.), Oliver and Boyd Ltd., London, England, 1966, p. 226.

23. McClure, M.: M. S. Thesis, The University of Texas at Houston, Houston, Texas, 1966.

24. Robbins, E., and T. Borun: The cytoplasmic synthesis of histones in hela cells and its temporal relationship to DNA replication. Proc. Nat. Acad. Sci. USA, 57:409, 1967.

25. Mueller, G.: Biochemical events in the animal cell cycle. Fed. Proc., 28:1780, 1969.

26. Byvoet, P.: Metabolic integrity of deoxyribonucleohistones. J. Mol. Biol., 17:311, 1966.

27. Hancock, R.: Conservation of histones in chromatin during growth and mitosis *in vitro*. J. Mol. Biol., 40:457, 1969.

28. Stellwagen, R., and R. Cole: Chromosomal proteins. Ann. Rev. Biochem., 38:968, 1969.

29. Beerman, W.: Cytological aspects of information transfer in cellular differentiation. Amer. Zool., 3:23, 1963.

30. Swift, H.: In: The Molecular Control of Cellular Activity (J. M. Allen, ed.), McGraw-Hill Book Co., New York, 1962, p. 73.

31. Frenster, J.: Nuclear polyanions as de-repressors of synthesis of ribonucleic acid. Nature, 206:680, 1965.

32. Leveson, J. E., and A. R. Peacocke: Complexes of non-histone protein in calf thymus chromatin. Biochim. Biophys. Acta, 117:163, 1967.

Role of Metabolic Imbalance in Neoplasia

GEORGE WEBER, JOHN A.
FERDINANDUS, AND SHERRY
I. F. QUEENER

Department of Pharmacology, Indiana University School of Medicine,
Indianapolis, Indiana, USA

Introduction and Conceptual Background

CANCER FORMATION RESULTS in heritable changes in the control of cellular multiplication. When liver cancer cells were examined for the activity and behavior of various key enzymes and opposing metabolic pathways of synthesis and degradation, a marked alteration in the balance of opposing enzymes and metabolic pathways was recognized.[1-3] When in a spectrum of hepatomas the rate of proliferation of the different lines and the biochemical properties were compared, it was discovered that the pattern of metabolic alterations exhibited a close relation to cell proliferation rate.[4-6] The linking of cell proliferation rate and metabolic imbalance suggests that the genetic alterations underlying the progressive expression of the increased growth rate and the extent of metabolic imbalance are at the core of the neoplastic transformation. These genetic changes are expressed in a network of interrelated, gradual alterations in key enzyme activities, isozyme pattern, metabolic imbalance, and growth rate of the different lines of tumors in the hepatoma spectrum.

The purpose of this paper is to provide a brief documentation of the use of the molecular correlation concept and the hepatoma spectrum for probing gene expression in terms of cell replication rate and enzymatic and metabolic imbalance.

THE MOLECULAR CORRELATION CONCEPT AS A CONCEPTUAL AND EXPERIMENTAL METHOD FOR IDENTIFICATION OF THE PATTERN OF GENE EXPRESSION IN CANCER CELLS

The molecular correlation concept postulated that there is a pattern of metabolic alterations in tumors that may be identifiable, provided that a number of preconditions are met which allow detection of the

TABLE 13–2.—Prerequisites for Understanding the Molecular
Pattern of Cancer Cells

1. *A suitable tumor system which should have the following properties:*
   (a) Should provide a spectrum of the same cell type where the molecular signs of cancer can be studied in a graded, quantitative manner.
   (b) Should allow repeatability at will in any laboratory.
   (c) Should have homologous normal resting and rapidly proliferating normal tissues for control studies.
2. *Identification of key enzymes in the synthetic and catabolic pathways for each metabolic pathway.*
3. *An understanding of the control of metabolic homeostasis through gaining an insight into enzyme regulation:*
   (a) Elucidation of factors that regulate the activity of the enzymes.
   (b) Elucidation of factors that regulate the synthesis and degradation of enzymes.
4. *Establishment of the relevance of the metabolic pattern observed in cancer cells to the core of the neoplastic process:*
   (a) Determine which alterations are essential to neoplasia.
   (b) Determine which alterations are coincidental to neoplasia.

pattern amid an apparent diversity of biochemical changes.[4–6] Table 13-2 shows the main prerequisites for an understanding of the molecular pattern of cancer cells.[6]

The availability of a number of lines of hepatomas that exhibited different growth rates[7] met the prerequisites for a model system. With the identification of key enzymes, their role in the pathways, and some of their regulatory properties, it has become possible to recognize the alterations in gene expression manifested in alteration of the amount of gene products or enzymes and their relationship with tumor proliferation rate.

The molecular correlation concept, based on work in our laboratories and on published data from other centers, suggested that metabolic alterations can be classified into three groups according to their relation to hepatoma growth rates.[4–6] Table 13-3 shows the classification recommended for identifying the linkage of the extent of enzymatic and metabolic alterations with growth rate.

In Class 1 belong biochemical parameters that correlate positively

TABLE 13–3.—The Molecular Correlation Concept

(A Conceptual and Experimental Approach: To Elucidate and Interpret the Molecular Basis of Altered Gene Expression and Metabolic Pattern in Cancer Cells)

Relation of Metabolic Parameter with Growth Rate	Significance of Change
Class 1. Correlates with growth rate	Essential
Class 2. Altered in same direction in all tumors	Ubiquitous
Class 3. No relationship	Irrelevant, coincidental

The biochemical parameters are grouped into 3 classes according to their correlation with the biological behavior and growth rate of neoplasms.

or negatively with tumor growth rate; in Class 2, those that are increased or decreased in all hepatomas; in Class 3, those that show no relation to growth rate.[4-6]

GROWTH RATE AS ALTERATION OF GENE EXPRESSION AND AS AN EXPERIMENTAL TOOL

The biologic behavior of the cancer cell involves alterations in the information coded in DNA which is expressed phenotypically by a loss of control of cell multiplication. This is expressed to different degrees, resulting in different rates of cell proliferation. Thus, growth rate may directly reflect the extent of genomic alterations in a cell line. Growth rate is also useful to the investigator as a parameter characterizing malignancy because it can be quantitated with a good degree of accuracy (Table 13-4).

The use of growth rate as a quantifiable parameter of the biologic behavior of tumors does not mean that one loses sight of the clinical importance of other characteristics of neoplastic cells such as invasiveness or ability to disseminate. However, these latter properties are difficult to measure with precision.

Moreover, growth rate is also relevant because it enters in the diagnosis and the prognosis of all cancer cases, and it plays a role in the design and the evaluation of the effectiveness of radiation and chemotherapy. The investigations carried out with the aid of the molecular correlation concept are designed to identify the correlation of gene expression, in terms of metabolic behavior, with the altered expression of the genome as manifested in different growth rates in the different lines of the hepatoma spectrum.

TABLE 13-4.—MEASURING METHODS FOR RANKING TUMORS OF THE HEPATOMA SPECTRUM BY GROWTH RATE

GROWTH RATE: MEASURABLE WITH PRECISION WITH ONE OR SEVERAL OF THE FOLLOWING METHODS WHICH ALL GIVE SIMILAR RANKING:

1. *Biological* — (a) Tumor size and volume
   (b) Tumor weight
   (c) Average time between transplantations
   (d) Time required to kill host
2. *Cytological* — Mitotic counts
3. *Biochemical*— Incorporation of Thymidine (Tdr) into DNA
   In Vivo (a) Injection of Tdr; extraction and counting of DNA
   In Vitro (b) Using Tdr in autoradiography
   (c) Incubation of tissue slices with Tdr; counting incorporation into DNA
   (d) Incubation of slices with Tdr; studying ratios of Tdr to DNA/ Tdr to CO_2

TABLE 13–5.—SIGNIFICANT PROPERTIES OF MORRIS HEPATOMA SPECTRUM

PROPERTIES	PARAMETERS	EXTENT OF CHANGE FROM NORMAL		
		Slight	Intermediate	Normal
Biological behavior	Growth rate	Low	Medium	Rapid
Morphology	Differentiation	Near normal	Medium	Poor
Genetic apparatus	Chromosome number	Normal	Increased	High
	Chromosome karyotype	Normal	Nearly normal	Abnormal
Energy generation	Respiration	Normal	Moderate	Moderately low
	Glycolysis	Low	Normal or increased	High
Replication and functions	Imbalance of opposing pathways of synthesis and degradation	Moderate	Pronounced	Extensive

SIGNIFICANT PROPERTIES OF THE HEPATOMA SPECTRUM

There are now about 40 different lines of transplantable hepatomas that were induced originally by the feeding of various carcinogens, and the biologic properties of these tumors have been described.[7] To provide an assessment of the current situation, we have summarized some of the significant properties of the hepatoma spectrum from the point of view of the molecular correlation concept (Table 13-5).

For the various properties listed, the extent of changes from normal is slight or moderate in the slowly growing hepatomas, more pronounced in those with intermediate growth rate, and extensive in the rapidly growing tumors. In the following parts of the presentation, we will discuss alterations in gene expression in the various metabolic pathways in the hepatoma spectrum. To place these changes in proper perspective, alterations in differentiation and regeneration will also be brought into the frame of reference.

Materials and Methods

The animals were kept in separate cages and illuminated daily from 6 AM to 7 PM. Purina laboratory chow and water were available ad libitum.

STUDIES ON REGENERATING LIVER

For studies on regenerating liver, male Wistar albino rats weighing 180 to 200 gm were obtained from Harlan Industries, Inc., Cumberland, Indiana. The rats were partially hepatectomized under light ether anesthesia by removal of 66% of the liver.[8] Sham-operated animals were used as controls.

STUDIES ON DIFFERENTIATING LIVER

Pregnant rats were also purchased from Harlan Industries. The litters were allowed to stay in the same cage with the mother for 18 days after birth; then they were placed in individual cages with Purina chow and water available ad libitum.

TUMOR-BEARING AND CONTROL ANIMALS

Male Buffalo strain and ACI/N rats were used in these experiments. Normal rats of the same strain, sex, age, and weight were used for controls and were sacrificed along with the tumor-bearing rats under the same conditions. The tumor-bearing and control rats were shipped by air express from Dr. H. P. Morris, Department of Biochemistry, Howard University College of Medicine, Washington, D. C., to Indiana University School of Medicine, Indianapolis, Indiana. The collaboration of Dr. Morris in the tumor experiments in gratefully acknowledged, and the details of these experiments will be reported in full elsewhere. We used a number of tumor lines, but concentrated on hepatomas which included the slow-growing 9618-A and 9618-B, hepatomas which now are considered of intermediate growth rate such as 7800 and 5123-D, and rapidly growing hepatomas 3924-A, 7777, and 3683. The tumors were transplanted bilaterally in a subcutaneous position, and they were allowed to grow to a diameter of about one inch, at which time they were harvested. The biologic and growth properties of the hepatoma spectrum were previously described.[7]

EXPERIMENTAL PROCEDURES

The rats were stunned, decapitated, and exsanguinated. Livers and tumors were rapidly removed and placed in beakers which stood on crushed ice. Tissues were carefully dissected free of necrotic, hemorrhagic, and nontumorous material.

For studies on thymidine utilization, the tissues were sectioned into 1- to 2-cm cubes, and slices were cut to uniform thickness of about 1 to 2 mm by a Stadie-Riggs slicer. Fifty mg of tissue slices were placed in separate 25-ml Erlenmeyer flasks containing 5 ml of Krebs-Ringer phosphate buffer (pH 7.4), 12.5 mM glucose, 20 mM glycylglycine, and 0.5 μCi of 2-^{14}C-thymidine (specific activity 43.7 mc/mM, New England Nuclear). Each flask was capped with a rubber stopper (No. 8826 Rubber Stoppers, 13 mm, Arthur H. Thomas Co.), from which was suspended, by a straight pin, a glass fiber filter strip (934AH glass fiber filter, 2.4 cm, Reeve Angel) cut to the dimensions of 1 × 2.4 cm.

Flasks were incubated at 37C and shaken at 72 rpm in a Dubnoff metabolic shaker. The reaction was terminated after incubation times of 0, 45, and 90 min by first injecting 50 ml of hyamine hydroxide through the rubber stopper (Hydroxide of Hyamine 10-X, Packard Co.) onto the glass fiber filter strip, then injecting 1 ml of 50% trichloroacetic acid (TCA) into the bottom of the flask. The flasks were shaken an additional 30 min at 37C, after which the rubber stoppers were removed and the filter strips placed in scintillation vials. Ten ml of scintillator fluid (0.03% POPOP and 0.5% PPO in toluene from New England Nuclear) were added to each vial. The vials were counted for radioactive CO_2 on a Packard Tri Carb liquid scintillation spectrometer (model 314 EX).

For determining thymidine incorporation into DNA, the remaining contents of the flasks were homogenized and transferred to 10-ml volumetrics and brought to volume with distilled water. The volumetrics were shaken vigorously for 30 sec, and aliquots of 0.3 and 0.6 ml were pipetted into separate Millipore filter apparatus which contained glass fiber filter discs (934AH glass fiber filter, 2.4 cm, Reeve Angel) and 5 ml of 10% ice-cold TCA. Suction was applied and the filter discs washed successively with cold 10-ml portions of 10% TCA, alcoholether (1:1), and ether. The filters were air dried for one min by suction, then placed in scintillation vials to which were added 10 ml of scintillator fluid.

EXPRESSION AND EVALUATION OF RESULTS

The incorporation of thymidine into DNA and degradation of thymidine to CO_2 were expressed as dpm/gm of tissue/hr. The counts obtained for incorporation of thymidine into DNA were corrected for self-adsorption by extrapolating cpm/gm of tissue to infinite dilution.[9]

The results were subjected to statistical evaluation by means of the t test for small samples. Differences between means giving a probability of less than 5% were considered to be significant.

ASSAY METHOD FOR DIHYDROURACIL DEHYDROGENASE (E.C. 1.3.1.2)

For this enzyme assay, 20 or 30% homogenates were prepared from livers or hepatomas. The homogenizing medium contained 0.25 M sucrose and 1 mM cysteine, and the solution was adjusted to pH 7.4. The cysteine was freshly prepared and added to the homogenizing medium before it was used. The homogenate was centrifuged at 0C at 100,000 $\times$ g for 30 min in a Model L Spinco ultracentrifuge. The resulting supernatant fluid was used as obtained or, in certain cases, it was subjected to further purification steps. In most cases, for routine comparison, the 100,000 $\times$ g supernatant was used for the enzyme determinations.

The assay system followed the uracil-dependent NADPH oxidation at 37C in the following reaction mixture: potassium phosphate buffer, pH 7.4, 100 μmoles; NADPH, 0.70 μmoles; uracil, 0.01 μmoles; enzyme,

0.05 to 0.30 ml of a 20% supernatant fluid; distilled water to complete to a final volume of 3.0 ml. The reaction was initiated with the substrate, uracil, and the rate was recorded at 340 mμ in a Gilford Model 2000 recording spectrophotometer. A blank consisting of an identical reaction mixture without uracil was recorded simultaneously. The difference between the rate of the blank and of the full reaction mixture was taken as the activity of the dihydrouracil dehydrogenase.

Careful kinetic studies were carried out to establish optimum conditions for the system where only the amount of enzyme protein was rate-limiting. As a result of such studies, which will be published in detail elsewhere,[17] it became possible to perform the enzyme reaction at optimum uracil and NADPH concentrations. Under these conditions, the enzyme activity was proportionate with enzyme amount added and reaction time for a period of at least five min. The enzyme activity was expressed in μmoles of substrate metabolized/hr per g tissue wet weight or per mg protein of the extract or per average cell.

Results and Discussion

GENE EXPRESSION AND ITS REGULATION IN CARBOHYDRATE METABOLISM

An outstanding characteristic of hepatic carbohydrate metabolism is that the biosynthetic pathway of glucose formation from lactate, gluconeogenesis, is opposed by the catabolic pathway of glucose, glycolysis.

FIG. 13–7.—Repression and derepression of anabolic and catabolic enzymes in differentiation, diabetes, and insulin treatment.

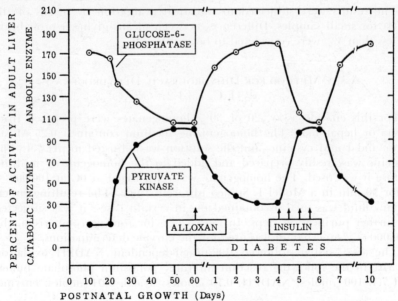

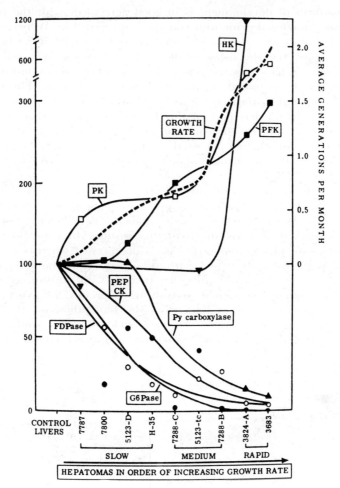

FIG. 13–8.—Correlation of the activities of key glycolytic and key gluconeogenic enzymes with hepatoma growth rate. Percentages based on normal control livers.

The regulation of the balance of the opposing pathways of gluconeogenesis and glycolysis is exerted chiefly through control of the activities and biosynthesis of a quartet of key gluconeogenic enzymes that are opposed by a triad of key glycolytic enzymes.

The developmental pattern of the key glycolytic enzymes (glucokinase, phosphofructokinase, pyruvate kinase) follows an upswinging line from low values after birth to high activities in the adult rat liver. In contrast, the hepatic key gluconeogenic enzymes (glucose-6-phosphatase, fructose 1,6-diphosphatase, phosphoenolpyruvate carboxykinase and pyruvate carboxylase) exhibit a rapid rise to high values after delivery and a decrease to somewhat lower values in the adult rat. That the key gluconeogenic and the key glycolytic enzymes follow specific patterns of development is in good agreement with the predictions of the functional genic unit concept as proposed by Weber et al.[10] Figure 13-7 illustrates results obtained in our laboratories, where in order to characterize the behavior of the key gluconeogenic and glycolytic enzymes we have selected one from each group for examining developmental and hormonal regulation of gene expression. The opposing developmental pattern of glucose-6-phosphatase and pyruvate kinase is shown in the left part of this Figure. It appears that gene expression involves the partial repression of the expression of the glucose 6-phosphatase synthesizing potential of the genome and the gradual derepression of the pyruvate kinase synthesizing capacity of the genome.

We have shown previously that insulin functions as an inducer of hepatic pyruvate kinase[11] and as a suppressor of glucose 6-phosphatase biosynthesis.[12] When rats are made diabetic by alloxan injection, there is a marked decrease in circulating insulin. In consequence, in the diabetic rats, glucose 6-phosphatase is derepressed whereas pyruvate kinase biosynthesis is decreased with the decrease in the level of its inducer. In turn, when the rats are treated with insulin, gene expression is returned to normal as insulin suppresses the synthesis of the gluconeogenic enzyme and increases the biosynthesis of the glycolytic one. This may be considered as a model system for studying the sequential development of gene expression in differentiation and hormonal regulation.

Fig. 13–9.—Correlation of ratios of key glycolytic/gluconeogenic enzymes with hepatoma growth rate.

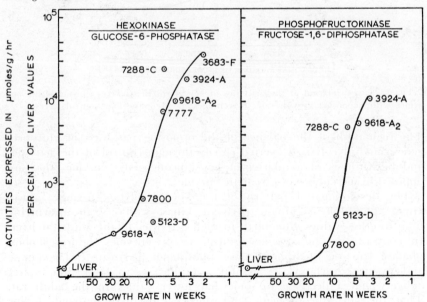

The opposite behavior of the key gluconeogenic and key glycolytic enzymes observed in differentiation and in diabetes is also reflected in the behavior of these enzymes in the hepatoma spectrum. Figure 13-8 shows that parallel with the increasing growth rate, the key gluconeogenic enzymes decrease and the key glycolytic ones increase. It appears that the glycolytic enzymes become derepressed, whereas the gluconeogenic ones are gradually repressed. The ratio of the glycolytic/gluconeogenic enzymes correlates closely with the proliferation rate of the different cell lines (Figure 13-9). Taking the ratio of these enzymes in the normal liver as 100, there is a nearly 1,000-fold increase in the rapidly growing tumors. The alterations in the ratios of the opposing enzymes of the antagonistic pathways that parallel the hepatoma growth rate reflect the gradually emerging metabolic imbalance that is linked with the proliferation rate of the different hepatoma lines. Thus, the neoplastic transformation that is expressed in the replicative cycle as an increased rate of growth is expressed concurrently in the extent of progressive imbalance in the ratios of the opposing key enzymes of glycolysis and gluconeogenesis. Consequently, as first shown in this laboratory,[13] there is a gradual increase in aerobic glycolysis that correlates with the growth rate of the hepatomas.

Gene Expression and Its Regulation in Nucleic Acid Metabolism

In order to detect the control points and key enzymes in pyrimidine and nucleic acid metabolism we have attempted to identify the opposing metabolic pathways and key enzymes that may play a strategic role in neoplasia.

Opposing Pathways of Synthesis and Breakdown in Pyrimidine Metabolism: Relation to Hepatoma Growth Rate.—Consideration of the biosynthetic pathway leading to UMP and the catabolic pathway from UMP to its breakdown products reveals that in the adult liver the biosynthetic pathway has low activity whereas the catabolic one is highly active and should be predominant. Investigations of Sweeney et al.[14] showed that the activities of the initial enzymes of UMP biosynthesis, aspartate transcarbamylase and dihydroorotase, were progressively elevated with the increase in growth rate in the hepatoma spectrum. This suggested that the increased rate of UMP formation is related in part to a rise in biosynthetic enzymes. In analyzing data in the literature, we noted that there was a decrease in the catabolism of the metabolites of UMP, since a decrease in the degradation of uracil to CO_2 in the hepatomas was reported.[15, 16] It seemed to us that the decrease was parallel with the increase in hepatoma growth rate.

Since dihydrouracil dehydrogenase appears to be the rate-limiting enzyme and is the starting step in uracil degradation,[23] studies were performed in our laboratories to ascertain whether this enzyme decreased in hepatomas and whether its decrease was linked with the in-

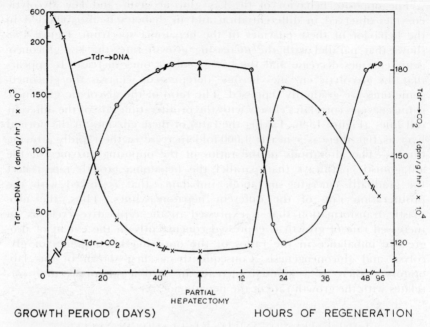

GROWTH PERIOD (DAYS)   HOURS OF REGENERATION

FIG. 13–10.—Repression and derepression of synthetic and degradative pathways of thymidine in liver in differentiation and in induced proliferation.

creased proliferation rate in the tumors. The kinetic parameters of dihydrouracil dehydrogenase were worked out, and the conditions for the assay were applied to rat liver and hepatoma systems.[17] The results showed that this enzyme activity decreased roughly parallel with the increase in hepatoma growth rate, and that there was very low activity of this enzyme in the very rapidly growing hepatoma.

The sum of results suggests that with the increasing growth rate of the hepatomas as the biosynthetic pathway of UMP increases, the catabolic one decreases. The activities of the two biosynthetic enzymes and the one catabolic enzyme examined provide an explanation, at least in part, for this phenomenon. Whether only the activities of the key enzymes will be altered in a reciprocal fashion or whether other enzymes in these pathways will also change in this way is under investigation.

OPPOSING PATHWAYS OF SYNTHETIC AND CATABOLIC UTILIZATION OF THYMIDINE: BEHAVIOR IN DIFFERENTIATION.—To examine the pathways responsible for the channeling of thymidine into DNA (biosynthetic utilization) and the channeling of thymidine into CO_2 (the degradative pathway), an in vitro technique was worked out that allows the simultaneous assay of the incorporation of thymidine to DNA and its degradation to CO_2 in an in vitro tissue slice system. The details are given in the Materials and Methods section.

Utilizing this technique, the behavior of the synthetic and the degradative pathways was followed in rats of different age groups from the early postnatal time to adulthood. These studies then deal with the behavior of the opposing pathways of hepatic thymidine utilization during differentiation. The results shown in Figure 13-10 indicate that the incorporation of thymidine into DNA is high in liver of very young rats, whereas the opposing pathway, the degradation of thymidine to CO_2, is low. During subsequent development, the thymidine biosynthetic pathway decreases, reaching very low levels in the liver of adult rats, while the catabolic pathway increases to high levels. These results can be interpreted as the sequential derepression of the genes governing the degradative pathway and the gradual repression of those for the biosynthetic pathway of thymidine during differentiation and development in rat liver. In the adult rat, the hepatic ratio of the biosynthetic/catabolic pathway is very low; this favors the catabolic utilization of thymidine. The steady state of the opposing enzymes is reflected in the resting state of DNA metabolism and replication in adult rat liver.

EFFECT OF ACTINOMYCIN D ON THE BEHAVIOR OF THE CATABOLIC PATHWAY IN DEVELOPING RAT LIVER.—The progressive derepression of the degradative pathway of thymidine can be inhibited by administration of actinomycin D. As shown in Table 13-6 degradation of thymidine into CO_2 rises during the postnatal period in the rat liver. Actinomycin D administration is capable of preventing or interrupting this rise. These results are in line with the suggestion that the increase of the catabolic pathway during development entails an increase in the biosynthesis of some of the key enzymes involved, and that this process requires the production of new RNA.

OPPOSING PATHWAYS OF SYNTHETIC AND CATABOLIC UTILIZATION OF THYMIDINE: BEHAVIOR IN REGENERATING LIVER.—The potential for altered gene expression remains present in normal liver, and can be un-

TABLE 13–6.—EFFECT OF ACTINOMYCIN D ON THYMIDINE DEGRADATION TO CO_2 IN DEVELOPING RAT LIVER*

RATS	POST-NATAL AGE OF RATS IN DAYS		
	1	3	5
Controls	824 ± 65	1,211 ± 74	1,389 ± 43
	(100)	(147) [†]	(169) [†]
Actinomycin treated	—	600 ± 92	870 ± 113
		(73) [‡]	(105) [‡]

* The mean values and standard errors represent four or more animals in each group. Activities are expressed as $dpm/g/hr \times 10^{-3}$. Actinomycin D was injected intraperitoneally twice daily (8 a.m. and 8 p.m.) at a dose of 50 $\mu g/kg$; controls were injected with distilled water. Percentages of 1-day control values are given in parentheses.

† Statistically significant difference as compared with values of 1-day-old rats ($p = < 0.05$).

‡ Statistically significant difference as compared with values of untreated rats of the same age groups ($p = < 0.05$).

leashed by suitable physiologic signal systems. This can be accomplished by performing partial hepatectomy on the rats, which leads to waves of mitosis and a rise in cell replicative function, causing an increase in the number of cells and liver weight until the previous liver/body weight ratio, liver weight, and total liver cellularity are re-established.[8] Examination of the behavior of opposing pathways of thymidine utilization and breakdown revealed that partial hepatectomy resulted in a decrease in CO_2 production from thymidine and an increase in the incorporation of thymidine into DNA, reaching a maximum imbalance at about 24 hr after operation. Thus, the ratio of thymidine into DNA/thymidine into CO_2 reaches a peak at 24 hr. The activities of the pathways of opposing utilization of thymidine return to normal range, reaching the previous adult levels at about 96 hr.

Thus, differentiation entails a sequential repression and derepression of genes controlling opposing pathways of thymidine utilization. By partial hepatectomy it is possible to unleash the genomic potential in the adult rat, resulting in a repression of the derepressed pathway of thymidine catabolism and a derepression of the repressed pathway of utilization of thymidine for biosynthesis. The forces that operate in a reciprocal fashion in controlling the opposing pathways of thymidine utilization restore the balance after the wave of regeneration reaches completion.

BEHAVIOR OF THE OPPOSING METABOLIC PATHWAYS AND SOME OF THE ENZYMES OF THE SYNTHETIC AND CATABOLIC UTILIZATION OF THYMIDINE IN DIFFERENTIATION.—To gain further insight into the sequence of gene expression during differentiation, the behavior of the opposing metabolic pathways controlling thymidine metabolism in rat liver during differentiation (Table 13-7) was compared with that of some of the enzymes involved in the channeling of thymidine into the biosynthetic

TABLE 13–7.—THYMIDINE METABOLISM IN RAT LIVER DURING DIFFERENTIATION*

AGE (DAYS)	THYMIDINE INTO DNA DPM/G/HR $\times 10^3$	THYMIDINE TO CO_2 DPM/G/HR $\times 10^3$	THYMIDINE INTO DNA THYMIDINE TO $CO_2 \times 10^{-3}$
1†	598 ± 50 (3,000)	844 ± 66 (45)	670 ± 80 (7,300)
2	384 ± 24 (2,260)	1,123 ± 58 (60)	350 ± 10 (3,800)
3	306 ± 19 (1,800)	1,128 ± 63 (60)	260 ± 20 (2,800)
4	273 ± 19 (1,600)	1,185 ± 131 (64)	230 ± 30 (2,500)
6	708 ± 19 (1,200)	1,273 ± 73 (69)	160 ± 10 (1,750)
18	84 ± 3 (500)	1,573 ± 72 (85)	54 ± 5 (590)
22	70 ± 15 (410)	1,647 ± 134 (89)	42 ± 8 (450)
24	51 ± 6 (300)	1,655 ± 49 (89)	34 ± 4 (370)
25	45 ± 2 (260)	1,680 ± 50 (90)	27 ± 1 (290)
30	39 ± 4 (230)	1,690 ± 184 (91)	24 ± 3 (260)
Adult	17 ± 1 (100)	1,859 ± 27 (100)	9 ± 4 (100)

* Means and standard errors are given with the percentages of adult values in brackets.
† Three or more rats were used for each age group.

TABLE 13–8.—DNA BIOSYNTHETIC PATHWAY AND ENZYMES IN DIFFERENTIATION*

	AGE (DAYS)	THYMIDINE INTO DNA	DNA POLYMERASE[†]	THYMIDINE[‡] KINASE
Fetus	15		6,171	
	17			15,289
	18		1,271	
	19			9,122
	20		1,143	
	21			2,844
Newborn	1	3,000	1,457	
	2	2,260	1,157	2,544
	3	1,800		
	4	1,600		
	6	1,200	900	
	7			1,522
	12		557	
	14			600
	18	500		
	22	410		
	24	300	314	
	25	260		
	30	230		
	35			200
Adult	180	100	100	100

* Data are expressed as percentages of adult rat liver values.
† Ove et al., Cancer Res. 30:535, 1969.
‡ Klemperer and Haynes, Biochem. J. 108:541, 1968.

and catabolic pathways. Table 13-7 shows the results of studies on incorporation of thymidine into DNA, of degradation of thymidine to CO_2, and the ratios of the two pathways during differentiation. The incorporation of thymidine into DNA is 30 times higher in the one-day-old rat than in the adult. The degradation of thymidine to CO_2 is 45% of the adult value. The ratio of synthetic/catabolic utilization of thymidine in the newborn rat liver is 73 times that observed at the end of the differentiation of the adult rat liver.

Table 13-8 shows that in the liver of very young rats, concurrently with the high values of incorporation of thymidine to DNA, the DNA polymerase[18] and thymidine kinase[19] (key enzymes of DNA biosynthesis) also exhibit high activities. The polymerase is 61 times, and the thymidine kinase 152 times, greater than the activities observed in adult rat liver.

Along with the increase in the degradation of thymidine to CO_2 pathway, there is also a rise in the activities of enzymes involved in the degradative pathway, such as thymidine phosphorylase and uridine phosphorylase,[20] and in dihydrouracil dehydrogenase (Table 13-9).

Thus the data tabulated in Tables 13-8 and 13-9 indicate that certain enzymes involved in the behavior of the opposing pathways of thy-

TABLE 13–9.—BEHAVIOR OF DNA CATABOLIC PATHWAY AND ENZYMES
IN DIFFERENTIATION*

	AGE (DAYS)	THYMIDINE TO CO_2	THYMIDINE PHOSPHORYLASE[†]	URIDINE PHOSPHORYLASE[†]	DIHYDROURACIL DEHYDROGENASE
Fetus	19-20			20	
Newborn	1	45	25	9	
	2	60			
	3	60	50	30	28
	4	64			50
	6	69			
	7		65		
	14		91		
	18	85			
	22	89			
	24	89			40
	25	90			
	30	91			
Adult	180	100	100	100	82
	>180				100

* Data are expressed as percentages of the adult rat liver values.
† Stevens and Stocken, Biochem. J., 87:12, 1963.

midine utilization and breakdown closely relate to the behavior of the over-all metabolic pathways. These results suggest that the genic expression for these enzymes in opposing pathways of synthesis and breakdown is under reciprocal control mechanisms.

BEHAVIOR OF ENZYMES IN REGENERATING LIVER.—According to recent studies of Labow et al.[21] the key enzymes of DNA biosynthesis increase in the regenerating liver, reaching a peak 24 to 48 hr after operation. We calculated from their data that the activities of DNA polymerase, dTMP synthetase, dTMP kinase, TdR kinase, and dCMP deaminase reach a level in activity at 48 hr after operation, which is roughly 10, 12, 16, 8, and 7 times greater, respectively, than the activity found in normal resting liver. The rise in these activities is in line with the elevation in the incorporation of thymidine into DNA and apparently it is linked with the increase in gene expression that is manifested in the rise of cell replication in the regenerating liver.

The behavior of thymidine metabolism in regenerating rat liver is shown in Table 13-10. The peak in the rise of the biosynthetic utilization of thymidine is reached at 24 hr after operation when there is a ninefold rise in the incorporation of thymidine into DNA. Concurrently, there is a decrease of only 36% in the degradative pathway. These reciprocal alterations show up in the ratios of the synthetic/catabolic pathways in a 14-fold rise at 24 hr after partial hepatectomy. It is important that, in the regenerating liver, the high replicative activity is achieved chiefly with a derepression of the synthetic enzymes and the over-all metabolic pathway of DNA synthesis. At the same time, there

TABLE 13–10.—Thymidine Metabolism in Regenerating Rat Liver

Hours After Partial Hepx.	Thymidine into DNA dpm/g/hr $\times 10^3$		Thymidine to CO_2 dpm/g/hr $\times 10^3$		Thymidine to DNA Thymidine to $CO_2 \times 10^{-3}$	
Control 0	17 ± 1	(100)	1,859 ± 27	(100)	9.2 ± 0.4	(100)
15	19 ± 2	(112)	1,798 ± 96	(97)	9.8 ± 0.8	(107)
18	84 ± 5	(500)	1,526 ± 107	(82)	56.0 ± 7.0	(610)
21	128 ± 6	(750)	1,278 ± 74	(69)	106.0 ± 5.0	(1,060)
24	155 ± 12	(912)	1,197 ± 49	(64)	133.0 ± 10.0	(1,450)
36	132 ± 4	(780)	1,346 ± 112	(72)	99.0 ± 7.0	(1,070)
48	76 ± 3	(450)	1,809 ± 77	(97)	44.0 ± 2.0	(480)
96	50 ± 3	(290)	1,843 ± 54	(99)	28.0 ± 2.0	(300)

Means and standard errors are given with the percentages of control values in parentheses. Three or more rats were used for each time period.

is a relatively small decrease in the degradative path, and in the activity of dihydrouracil dehydrogenase.

OPPOSING PATHWAYS OF SYNTHETIC AND CATABOLIC UTILIZATION OF THYMIDINE: RELATION TO HEPATOMA GROWTH RATE.—In Table 13-11, the hepatomas are listed in order of increasing growth rate, and the synthetic and catabolic utilization of thymidine and the ratio of the opposing pathways are tabulated. Even in the slowest growing tumor in this spectrum, the incorporation of thymidine into DNA increased nearly threefold, and the degradation of thymidine into CO_2 decreased to 49%; the ratio increased sixfold over the value found in the liver of control rats. The opposing behavior of these antagonistic pathways is gradually emphasized with the increase in growth rate. In the most rapidly growing tumor in this series, the 9618-A$_2$, the incorporation of thymidine into DNA increased 31-fold, whereas the degradation de-

TABLE 13–11.—Correlation of Synthetic and Degradative Pathways of Thymidine with Hepatoma Growth Rate*

	Thymidine to DNA	Thymidine to CO_2	Thymidine to DNA Thymidine to CO_2
Liver†	100	100	100
Hepatomas			
9618-A	280	49	615
9618-B	292	36	810
7800	370	6.9	5,750
5123-D	706	6.5	13,500
3924-A	1,890	0.094	2,210,000
7288-C	2,360	0.050	5,620,000
7777	4,520	0.064	8,700,000
3683-F	3,900	0.045	11,500,000
9618-A$_2$	3,180	0.041	13,900,000

* Data are expressed as percentages of normal liver values.†
† Normal liver values: Tdr to DNA = 11,330 ± 250; Tdr to CO_2 = 1,065,000 ± 17,000 in dpm/gm/hr.

creased to 0.041% of the values of normal control rat liver. The ratio in this rapidly growing tumor increased nearly 14-million fold. The widening gap between the synthetic and catabolic utilization of thymidine, the resultant preponderance of the synthetic above the catabolic pathway, and the relationship of the tumor growth rate are shown in Figures 13-11 and 13-12. It is important to note that the gradual imbalance which is linked to the increase in proliferation rate in the hepatomas is much more marked than that in the regenerating

FIG. 13–11.—Correlation of opposing pathways of synthetic and degradative utilization of thymidine with hepatoma growth rate.

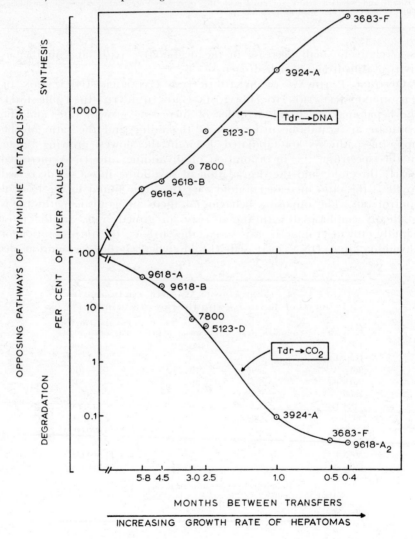

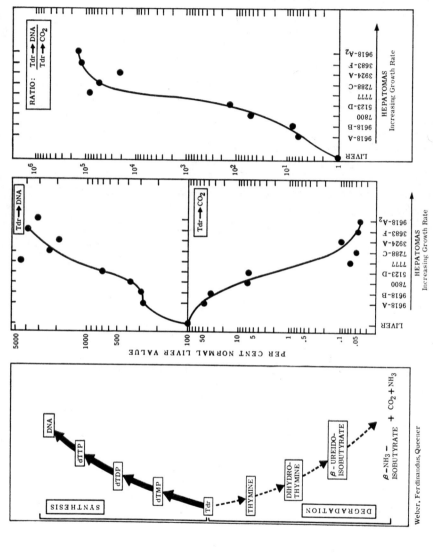

Fig. 13–12.—Behavior of synthetic and degradative utilization of thymidine and the ratios of the two pathways in hepatomas of different growth rates.

liver. The hepatomas are characterized by a sharp decrease in the catabolic pathway, resulting in an enormous increase in the ratios; in contrast, the alterations are much smaller in the regenerating liver where the degradative pathway decreased only to a minor extent.

BEHAVIOR OF KEY ENZYMES IN THE SYNTHETIC AND DEGRADATIVE PATHWAYS OF NUCLEIC ACID METABOLISM IN HEPATOMAS OF DIFFERENT GROWTH RATES

In Figure 13-13 we assembled the evidence demonstrating the correlation of DNA metabolic pathways and key enzyme activities with the increase in hepatoma growth rate. In the upper left panel is shown the increase in growth rate in the hepatomas, as determined by Dr. Morris according to the average months between tumor transfers. The ratios of incorporation of thymidine into DNA/degradation of thy-

FIG. 13–13.—Correlation of DNA metabolic pathways and enzyme activities with hepatoma growth rate.

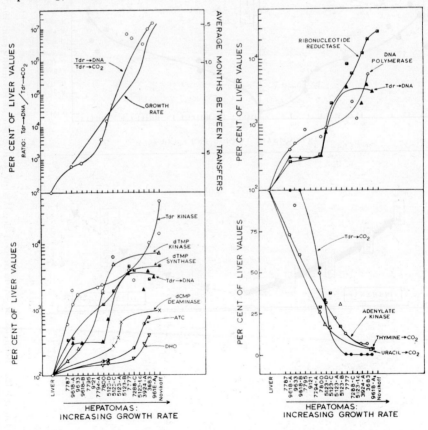

midine to CO^2 are given as determined in our laboratories. Close agreement between the biologic and chemical assay of growth rate is observed, and attention is drawn to the fact that the ratio correlates with cell replication rate over a million-fold range. This then is the most sensitive measure for detecting neoplastic alterations in the tumors.

In the right upper panel are shown the results of Elford et al. who discovered the correlation of ribonucleotide reductase activity with hepatoma growth rate,[22] and those of Laszlo and his group who recognized the correlation of DNA polymerase activity with hepatoma growth rate.[18] For comparison, the incorporation of thymidine into DNA, as reported from our laboratories, is also shown in that panel.

In the left lower panel are the results of Sweeney et al.[14] who reported the correlation of aspartate transcarbamylase and dihydro-orotase with hepatoma growth rate, and in this panel we have reorganized and plotted in the order of hepatoma growth rate the results published by Sneider et al.[16] These data indicate to us that the activities of Tdr kinase, dTMP kinase, dTMP synthetase, and dCMP deaminase correlate positively with hepatoma growth rate. It seems that there is a rough correlation between the extent of the rise that occurs in the enzyme activities and the activity level of the enzyme observed in the resting liver. For instance, in normal liver, the very lowest activities are observed for ribonucleotide reductase, DNA polymerase, dTMP synthetase, and dTMP kinase. These are the enzymes with the greatest extent of rise in the hepatomas and also in regenerating liver. The enzyme dCMP deaminase which exhibits the highest activity in normal liver is among those showing the smallest rise in the regenerating and neoplastic liver.

The lower right panel shows the progressive decline in the degradation of thymine, thymidine and uracil into CO_2, and the decrease in adenylate kinase activity, along with the increase in hepatoma growth rate. The decrease in the degradative pathway reflects an approximate mirror picture of the progressive increase in the biosynthetic pathway.

AN INTEGRATED PICTURE OF THE METABOLIC IMBALANCE AND THE RELATION TO HEPATOMA GROWTH RATE.—We have recognized the antagonistic behavior of opposing pathways of synthesis and catabolism and some of their key enzymes in hepatic differentiation and in regeneration. Figure 13-14 shows the imbalance of synthesis and catabolism in pyrimidine and nucleic acid metabolism in the hepatoma spectrum. With the increase in tumor growth rate, there is a progressive increase in the imbalance of the opposing pathways of synthesis to degradation in pyrimidine metabolism and in the synthetic and catabolic utilization of thymidine. There is a progressive increase in the activities of key enzymes leading to DNA biosynthesis, paralleled by a concurrent decrease in the enzymes and pathways of pyrimidine and nucleic acid degradation.

These events indicate a close linkage in the expression of the repli-

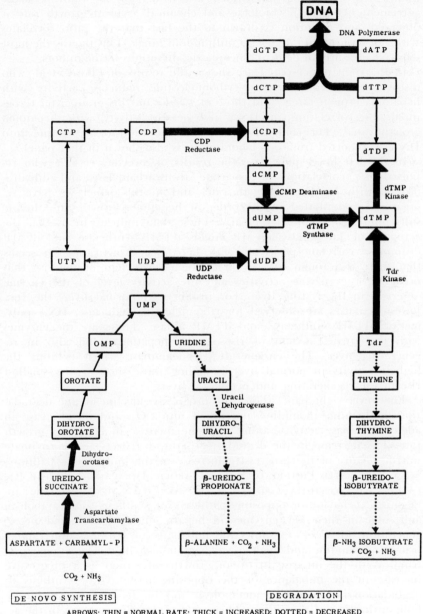

ARROWS: THIN = NORMAL RATE; THICK = INCREASED; DOTTED = DECREASED

Weber and Queener

FIG. 13–14.—Imbalance of synthetic and catabolic pathways of pyrimidine and DNA metabolism in hepatomas.

cative potential of the genome with the extent of the progressive imbalance in DNA metabolism and, as described earlier, in carbohydrate metabolism. The results underline the importance of ratios as indicators of the link between replicative and translative and transcriptive expression of the altered genome in neoplasia. As has been previously pointed out,[4-6] no similar imbalance has been observed in the regenerating liver; thus, the alterations observed in the metabolic imbalance in hepatomas are specific and characteristic of neoplasia.

Summary

The role of metabolic imbalance in neoplasia was discussed in a spectrum of hepatomas of different growth rates. The neoplastic transformation involves an alteration in gene expression as manifested through progressive alterations in the balance of opposing metabolic pathways. The gradual shift in the balance of these opposing pathways is associated with progressive alterations in the growth rate of the different hepatoma lines. The close linking of cell proliferation rate and biochemical changes reveals quantitative and qualitative lesions that are specific to neoplasia.

The alterations in gene expression were evaluated in the light of the behavior of the opposing pathways of metabolism in differentiating and in regenerating liver.

The close linking of biochemical imbalance to growth rate now permits the integration of the biochemical changes in a meaningful pattern in cancer cells.

Acknowledgments

Supported by grants from the United States Public Health Service (National Cancer Institute Grant No. CA-05034), American Cancer Society, and Damon Runyon Memorial Fund, Inc.

References

1. Weber, G., and A. Cantero: Cancer Res., 15:679, 1955.
2. Weber, G., and A. Cantero: Cancer Res., 19:763, 1959.
3. Weber, G.: Advances Cancer Res., 6:403, 1961.
4. Weber, G.: Gann Monograph, 1:151, 1966.
5. Weber, G., and M. A. Lea: Methods Cancer Res., 2:523, 1967.
6. Weber, G.: Naturwissenschaften, 55:418, 1968.
7. Morris, H. P.: Advances Cancer Res., 9:227, 1965.
8. Higgins, G. M., and R. M. Anderson: Arch. Pathol., 12:186, 1931.
9. Perg, C. T.: Advances Tracer Methods, 3:81, 1966.
10. Weber, G., R. L. Singhal, N. B. Stamm, and S. K. Srivastava: Fed. Proc., 24:745, 1965.
11. Weber, G., N. B. Stamm, and E. A. Fisher: Science, 149:65, 1965.
12. Weber, G., R. L. Singhal, and S. K. Srivastava: Proc. Nat. Acad. Sci. USA, 53:96, 1965.
13. Sweeney, M. J., J. Ashmore, H. P. Morris, and G. Weber: Cancer Res., 23:995, 1963.

14. Sweeney, M. J., D. H. Hoffman, and G. A. Poore: Proc. Amer. Ass. Cancer Res., 8:66, 1967.
15. Ono, T., and V. R. Potter: Cancer Res., 23:240, 1963.
16. Sneider, T. W., V. R. Potter, and H. P. Morris: Cancer Res., 29:40, 1969.
17. Queener, S. I., and G. Weber: To be published.
18. Ove, P., M. D. Jenkins, and J. Laszlo: Cancer Res., 30:535, 1970.
19. Klemperer, H. G., and G. R. Haynes: Biochem. J., 108:541, 1968.
20. Stevens, L., and L. A. Stocken: Biochem. J., 87:12, 1963.
21. Labow, R., G. F. Maley, and F. Maley: Cancer Res., 29:366, 1969.
22. Elford, H. L.: Fed. Proc., 27:300, 1968.
23. Fritzson, P., and U. Spaeren: J. Biol. Chem., 235:719, 1960.

A Geneticist Looks at Cancer

ANDRÉ LWOFF

Institut de Recherches Scientifiques sur le Cancer, Villejuif, France

NEVER DID I THINK of myself as a geneticist. But, as a director of a cancer institute, I am on duty. So I have accepted most humbly the title of the paper and the label "geneticist" which has been pinned on me by the congress pentagone. For I am, like every Frenchman, highly disciplined. The real title should be "A director of a cancer institute discovers cancer." There are many ways of looking at cancer and the one selected is necessarily arbitrary.

Throughout the living world, the organization and functioning of the cellular machine is remarkable by its unity. The structure of genetic material, the transfer RNA and ribosomes, the mechanics of replication, transcription, and transduction, the control of expression, the biosynthesis of essential metabolites, and the movements of energy are all essentially the same. However, protists or microbes, or multicellular organisms, if united by physiology, are separated by pathology and especially by cancer. The unicellular protists are independent organisms. Their growth and division are controlled by food. The metazoan cells are interdependent parts of an organism. Their growth and division are controlled by the organism as a whole. The general cellular balance results from an interplay of inhibitions and stimulations. When a cell loses its sensitivity to the factors of coordination, it becomes malignant, and cancer develops.

A malignant cell is, by definition, a cell able to cause cancer, and it is a truism that there is no cancer without a malignant cell. Everyone knows that chemical carcinogens and oncogenic viruses are capable of converting in vitro a normal cell into an abnormal, transformed one, and of causing cancer in animals. So, transformation is often equated with cancer. This viewpoint will be discussed. In doing so, I will not forget my assignment, and will try to understand how genetics comes into the picture. Maybe I should add that the obligation to write this paper has been the source of a lot of worries, until I succeeded in convincing myself that I was not expected to solve the cancer problem.

A geneticist considering leukemia in mice is struck by the existence of two types of strains: low incidence and high incidence strains. It seems as though leukemia may be controlled by the genetic make-up of the host. This is exciting.

Seventeen years ago, in 1953, as a by-product of the study of lysogeny and of the discovery of induction, two hypotheses were proposed: (1) the potentiality of a cell to become malignant is perpetuated in the form of viral genetic material, and (2) carcinogenic agents act by inducing the expression of a repressed virus. Robert Huebner and his group seem to be convinced that this is reality. In fact, all strains of mice harbor a leukemogenic virus which is transmitted vertically and is responsible for the malignant transformation of blood cells. It is fortunate for the geneticist that these viruses, just as others, undergo mutations: some viral strains are of low leukemogenic activity, whereas others induce leukemia rapidly in a large fraction of the infected animals. So the geneticist is faced with a genetically fascinating situation where genetically different viruses interact with genetically different mice, the outcome of this genetic web being either health or disease.

Virus is present in a low-incidence strain, but cancer develops only in a small fraction of the population. The incidence of the disease is precipitated by x rays which, as revealed by electron microscopy and immunofluorescence, induce viral development. The virus here seems to be the determining factor. From a low-virulent strain of leukemogenic virus, mutants can be selected by rapid repeated transfers in animals. These viruses, injected into mice of low-incidence strain, induce the rapid development of leukemia in a large fraction of the animals.

The virulence of a leukemogenic virus, its ability to elicit cancer in an animal, is obviously related to its rate of multiplication which determines the rate of transformation and the number of transformed cells present in the animal. Viral virulence can only be determined by the genetic constitution of the virus. How does the genetic constitution of the host come into the picture? It is known[9] that the immune status of the host is a major determinant in the development of tumors. It is known also that it is cell-mediated. In fact, the growth of many tumors is retarded or even suppressed by the injection of sensitized lymphocytes.

The defense mechanisms of an animal are operative throughout life, but the importance of the immune response, at least in mice, decreases greatly with age. And with age, the incidence of leukemia increases greatly.

Virus-induced malignant cells exhibit virus-specific antigens able to evoke immune responses in the host. These responses, which determine the fate of the animal, are not mediated by antibodies but by cells. Antilymphocytic serum (ALS) greatly increases the oncogenic potentiality of viruses. Polyoma virus and SV-40 produce tumors only if injected into newborn mice. But if these viruses are injected into three-week-old animals treated with ALS, tumors develop. The oncogenicity of adenovirus 12 is increased by treatment with ALS. ALS also increases the oncogenic activity of murine sarcoma virus.[2, 7] Treatment of mice with ALS alone induces the appearance of various types of tumors for which the spontaneous infection by polyoma virus was found to be responsible. ALS shortens the latent period in mice injected with Moloney virus.[9] Finally, the effects of ALS on the development of murine leukemia is suppressed by the injection of sensitized lymphocytes.[9]

BCG enhances the immune response and resistance to various infections. In mice, it inhibits the growth of various tumors, whether spontaneous or induced by carcinogens.[6]

The induction of leukemia in mice by x rays is sometimes attributed to the induction of viral development. However, like many carcinogens, x rays have an immune suppressive activity. It seems probable that both viral induction and depression of the immune response are operative in the x-ray induction of leukemia. This dual effect probably accounts for their high carcinogenic activity.

In a given species, the importance of the immune response varies greatly with individuals. As shown by Benacerraf, certain strains are even unable to perform given specific immune responses which are controlled by specific autosomal dominant genes.

The question is naturally posed as to whether the low or high incidence of leukemia could not depend on the intensity of the immune response. Whatever the case may be, cell-mediated immunity undoubtedly is an essential defense mechanism against virus-induced tumors. Moreover, in some cases, the cell transformed by chemical carcinogens is malignant. Yet the ultimate genetic and molecular mechanism by which a chemical carcinogen acts is not known. In a virus-transformed malignant cell, the metabolism and the behavior are altered, but the basic mechanism of viral carcinogenesis is also unknown. However, a large number of hypotheses are available.

All the data duly considered, it seems as though the development of tumors involves two essential though different steps: the transformation of the cell, which is of course a prerequisite for cancer, and the multiplication of the malignant cell in the host.

Maybe one should recall that an oncogenic virus can transform cells in vitro with a probability close to one. This is also sometimes the case for some chemical carcinogens. Transformation should not be equated with cancer. Transformation is a feature of the cell and cancer is a disease of the organism. The fate of an animal depends on the outcome of the fight against foreign entities, whether microbes or transformed cells. Immunity against tumor cells is generally low, so that injected transformed cells are destroyed only when they are few and multiply if the implant is heavy. Things happen as if the development of leukemia would depend on the relative number of malignant cells and the relative intensity of the immune response. The number of malignant cells is controlled by the genetic constitution of the virus. The level of the immune response depends on the quality and amount of the viral transplantation antigen, but is under the command of the genetic constitution of the host. The genetic constitution of the virus and of the host interacts in the most conspicuous way. In addition, any factor able to influence the multiplication of the malignant cell can shift the balance in one direction or in another. This is the case for interferon which, as shown by Ion Gresser, depresses and even prevents the development of leukemic cells in mice.

The immune response is controlled by the host genotype, but its expression may be depressed or enhanced by extrinsic factors. Here, like anywhere else, the phenotype is the result of the interplay of heredity and environment. This can only please the geneticist who concludes that genes are important in virus-induced cancers as everywhere else, and even more so.

On the whole, it is remarkable how much we know and how little we understand. If I have accepted to give this paper, it is because I felt unable to refuse the challenge. Yet, as foreseen, nothing new emerges from all this except the conclusion which was reinforced while I attended these congress sessions: cancer, in addition to being a disease, is also a problem.

References

1. Alexander, P.: Immunotherapy of cancer: Experiments with primary tumours and syngeneic tumour grafts. Prog. Exp. Tumor Res., 10:23-71, 1970.
2. Allison, A. C.: Effects of antilymphocytic serum on bacterial and viral infections and virus oncogenesis. Fed. Proc., 29:167-168, 1970.
3. Allison, A. C.: Immune responses to virus-induced tumours. Proc. Roy. Soc. Med., 62 (9) :956-958, 1969.
4. Allison, A. C., L. D. Berman, and R. H. Levey: Increased tumour induction by adenovirus type 12 in thymectomized mice and mice treated with anti-lymphocyte serum. Nature, 215:185-187, 1967.
5. Allison, A. C., and L. W. Law: Effects of antilymphocyte serum on virus oncogenesis (32657) . Proc. Soc. Exp. Biol. Med., 127:207-212, 1968.
6. Benacerraf, B.: The effect of enhancement of natural resistance upon tumor rejection. Acta Unio Int. Contra Cancrum, 19:73-76, 1963.

7. Hirsch, M. S.: Effects of antilymphocytic serum on host responses to infectious agents. Fed. Proc., 29:169-170, 1970.
8. Hugh, O., M. Devitt, and B. Benacerraf: Genetic control of specific immune responses. Adv. Immunol., 11:31-74, 1969.
9. Law, L. W.: Effects of antilymphocyte serum on the induction of neoplasms of lymphoreticular tissues. Fed. Proc., 29:171-176, 1970.

Differentiation and Cancer

G. BARRY PIERCE AND
CAROL WALLACE

*Department of Pathology, University of Colorado School of Medicine,
Denver, Colorado, USA*

THE IDEA THAT many of the cells in a cancer are benign has not been widely appreciated, although great heterogeneity of cellular structure of cancers has long been recognized light microscopically. Some parts of a tumor may closely resemble normal tissues, while others vary remarkably from the normal appearance. For example, skin cancers may have "pearls" of well-differentiated squamous cells, surrounded by large masses of undifferentiated cancer cells. Osteosarcomas or chondrosarcomas may have foci of recognizable bone or cartilage, respectively, embedded in masses of highly malignant cells. Two theories have been proposed to explain this heterogeneity of structure. The older, and now less favored, is based on the assumption that fully differentiated normal cells are the target in carcinogenesis, which, as a result of mutation are incorporation of viral DNA into the genome or some other mechanism, dedifferentiate and lose overt manifestations of the particular differentiation. If dedifferentiation were extreme, marked departure from normal structure and function would develop[8, 12]—with the evolution of a highly malignant tumor; and if it were minimal, a more normal appearance would be preserved and a less malignant tumor would be the result. Various degrees of dedifferentiation in a single tumor would account for the heterogeneity described here.

Although the idea of dedifferentiation has never been disproved, there are many theoretical faults with the concept, and oncologists have recently turned to the notion that tumors retain capacity for differentiation of the parent tissue. This concept could account for the heterogeneity found in tumors, but unequivocal documentation of the process of differentiation in cancers has been unobtainable until recently.[1, 4, 7, 13–17, 21]

Evidence from four tumors which we have studied bears upon these ideas. The first was teratocarcinoma of the testis of strain 129 mice which was first isolated by Stevens and Little,[23] and later shown by Stevens to originate from primordial germ cells early in fetal development.[24] These are bizarre tumors[13, 15] which contain a heterogeneous mixture of at least 12 somatic tissues, including muscle, glands, brain, bone, and cartilage, chaotically arranged and intermixed with highly malignant cancer cells. These cancerous areas resemble embryonic epithelium and have been named embryonal carcinoma.

Teratocarcinomas were ideally suited for studies to determine whether cancer cells could differentiate, because if embryonal carcinoma differentiated into cartilage, for example, the transition ought to be easily recognized. A means of isolating embryonal carcinoma was developed, and the carcinoma cells were dissociated enzymatically and cloned in vivo. Of 372 single cells, each transferred to the intraperitoneum of a strain of 129 mouse, 11% gave rise to teratocarcinomas.[7] These tumors varied remarkably in their growth rates, ability to produce embryoid bodies, and their ability to produce differentiated tissues in kind and amount. Nevertheless, they were teratocarcinomas, and the data indicated that single embryonal carcinoma cells had the capacity to differentiate into the somatic tissues of this tumor.

Although the somatic tissues that differentiated from embryonal carcinoma appeared benign, many pathologists considered them to be malignant, although not as malignant as embryonal carcinoma. Thus it was necessary to establish whether they were benign or malignant. Since malignancy is a clinical concept, the somatic tissues were isolated and their effect upon an animal host was determined. Transplants free of embryonal carcinoma developed into small cystic structures at the site of transplantation.[16] On serial section, these cysts proved to be the equivalent of benign dermoid cysts of the ovary and contained a multiplicity of well-differentiated tissues. Animals bearing these transplants were set aside to observe the effect on the host, and in a period of six months, neither progressive growth of the transplants nor death of the animals occurred. Since six months is a long interval of time in the life span of a mouse, it was concluded that the tissues derived from embryonal carcinoma were biologically benign.[16]

This was the most convincing demonstration of the capacity for differentiation of malignant stem cells of mammals and supports the observation of Braun,[1] who, by selective transplantation and culture of shoots from teratomas of plants, obtained normal plants capable of bearing fertile seed. We have been unable to develop fertile mice in our transplants, although replicas of 7- to 8-day-old mouse embryos have been obtained.[15, 16] Then organization apparently breaks down.

In a further test of the concept that stem cells have the ability to differentiate, we have studied a transplantable squamous cell carcinoma of Irish rats. The tumor, obtained from Dr. Katherine Snell,[5] was slowly growing and required a large inoculum to ensure 100% transplantability. The grafts grew to a diameter of 2 to 3 cm in about three months, and were composed of numerous squamous pearls separated from each other by masses of undifferentiated cancer cells. The tumor did not metastasize, but destroyed its host by cachexia and infection.

Animals bearing transplants of this tumor were injected with tritium-labeled thymidine, and the cells capable of synthesizing DNA were determined by radioautography with the light microscope.[14, 17] At two hr, labeled cells were found in the undifferentiated portions of the tumor, whereas at 50 and 96 hr after the injection of a pulse-dose of tritium-labeled thymidine, many labeled cells were found in the pearls.[17] The data are summarized in Table 13-12. When 5,410 consecutive labeled undifferentiated cells were counted, 779 pearls were encountered. These contained only five labeled nuclei. At 96 hours, in a survey of 733 pearls, 219 labeled nuclei were counted. It was concluded from this study, in accord with the deductions of Frankfurt,[2] that the growth of the tumor was dependent upon proliferation of undifferentiated cells. It was tempting to postulate that the growth of the pearls was dependent upon incorporation and differentiation of undifferentiated cells, but since malignant cells can invade, it was necessary to demonstrate that the labeled cells in the pearls had differentiated into squamous cells. The experiments were repeated using the resolution of radioautography with the electron microscope to determine the degree of differentiation of the labeled cells.

Cells labeled at two hr lacked desmosomes with little or no interdigitation of plasma membranes between adjacent cells.[14, 17] Ribosomes, both free and in polysomal configuration, were the dominant organelle of the cytoplasm, although a few profiles of attenuated rough endoplasmic reticulum were present. Microtubules and filaments were rare. Osmophilic inclusions and single Golgi complexes were occa-

TABLE 13–12.—INCORPORATION OF ³H-THYMIDINE BY SQUAMOUS CELL CARCINOMA

TIME	NO. LABELED UNDIFFERENTIATED CELLS	NO. PEARLS	NO. LABELED CELLS IN PEARLS	LABELED CELLS/PEARL
2	5410	779	5	0.005
14	7813	1025	18	0.018
50	3358	535	56	0.11
96	2867	733	219	0.29

TABLE 13–13.—TUMOR FORMING ABILITY OF UNDIFFERENTIATED
SQUAMOUS CELL CARCINOMA AND PEARLS

No. Transplants	Type of Tissue	No. Tumors
84	Undifferentiated	27
78	Pearls	0

sionally visualized, but the over-all impression gained was that this was an undifferentiated cytoplasm characteristic of rapidly proliferating stem cells.[25]

In contrast, at 96 hr, the labeled cells in the pearls were extremely well differentiated.[14, 17] Those at the outermost margin of the pearl resembled basal cells, and there were all degrees of differentiation to mature squamous cells. The latter had numerous desmosomes with many tonofibrils. In addition, the rough endoplasmic reticulum was well developed and there were many membrane lining granules, and large keratohyaline granules, especially in cells near the center of the pearl. Consequently, it could be assumed that labeled cells in the pearls had differentiated. As further evidence of their differentiated state and benign nature, pearls composed mainly of these morphologically well-differentiated cells and minimal keratin were dissected from the tumors and selectively transplanted subcutaneously in the appropriate strain of rats.[14, 17] The differentiated cells were incapable of forming a tumor (Table 13-13). Thus it would appear that the stem cell of this nongerminal tumor, like its germinal counterpart,[7] had a capacity for differentiation which could lead to the evolution of well-differentiated postmitotic and apparently benign cells.[17]

Experiments now in progress indicate that the mature-appearing areas of chondrosarcoma and osteosarcoma also arise by differentiation of malignant stem cells.

Since many pathologists would have anticipated these results on the basis of light microscopic examination of these tumors, we studied monocellular and extremely malignant cancers with the electron microscope to determine whether ultrastructural evidence of differentiation was present.[13] This proved to be the case, and in ultrastructural studies of a wide variety of tumors reported by others, superb caricatures of differentiation of the normal have been found.[3, 8, 11, 19] Some authors attributed their observations to dedifferentiation;[8] others, to differentiation.[3, 11]

The data on differentiation of cancer cells are particularly important to the understanding of the cellular kinetics of tumors. Mendelsohn,[9] for example, has produced convincing evidence that as many as 45% of the cells of undifferentiated mammary carcinomas are not synthesizing DNA and are "senile." One could logically ask, are these cells senescent because of limitations imposed upon them by their environment, or have they in fact differentiated to postmitotic benign forms? The data from our studies support the idea that postmitotic cells in tumors are the result of differentiation of some of the progeny of the stem cells, and as such should be benign.

Rabinowitz and Sachs[18] have cloned polyoma-induced fibroblastic cells, and have isolated variants from these clones that display contact inhibition, epithelioid morphology, decreased tumorigenicity, and loss of polyoma viral transplantation antigen. These cells still contain polyoma viral genome. It would be interesting to know if the abortive processes of differentiation which we have demonstrated in cancer cells might be able to "control" the polyoma genome, allowing for evolution of benign cells.

Behind all of these studies in differentiation and cancer is the hope that it will be possible to direct the differentiation of malignant to benign cells as a means of clinical therapy.[14, 15] Recently, Silagi and Bruce[22] observed that BUdR in low concentration had little effect on growth rate of melanoma cells in vitro, but the cells were contact inhibited and lost tumorigenicity. In a similar vein, Saffiotti et al.[20] have shown that vitamin A, which is known to convert squamous to glandular epithelium in vitro, greatly reduces the incidence of squamous cell carcinoma of the bronchus in animals given carcinogen via the trachea.

The mode and pattern of development of benign tissues from the malignant stem cells of these tumors is reminiscent of normal differentiation and supports the concept that cancer is an aberration of tissue renewal.[14] Tissues are normally renewed by proliferation of stem cells with differentiation of the progeny. These activities are controlled and coordinated to meet the needs of the host. Aberration of the controls could lead to the expression of the malignant phenotype as postulated by others.[6]

The idea that many of the cells of a cancer are postmitotic and apparently well-differentiated and benign imposes problems for the molecular biologists who are attempting to understand the process of carcinogenesis. To date, most of their effort has been directed at the biochemical examination of cancers, which may contain few malignant cells. Since carcinogenesis is a process, it is unlikely that study of the end product will lead to many insights into the process. A fruitful area for studying the process of carcinogenesis would be the in vitro systems in which apparently normal cells are transformed by virus in a few hours. Sequential studies during the period of conversion should elicit important information on the aberrations of control mechanisms which allow for the expressions of the malignant phenotype.

Acknowledgments

The authors wish to acknowledge with thanks the technical assistance of Mr. Alan Jones and Mrs. Elizabeth Saunders.

These studies were supported by Grants E105L from the American Cancer Society and AM 13112 from the U. S. Public Health Service.

References

1. Braun, A. C.: The plant tumor cell as an experimental tool for studies on the nature of autonomous growth. Canad. Cancer Conf., 4:89-98, 1961.
2. Frankfurt, O. S.: Mitotic cycle and cell differentiation in squamous cell carcinomas. Int. J. Cancer, 2:304-310, 1967.
3. Friedmann, I., and E. S. Berg: Electron microscopic investigation of experimental rhabdomyosarcoma. J. Path., 97:375-382, 1969.
4. Goldstein, M. N., J. A. Burdman, and L. J. Journey: Long term tissue culture of neuroblastomas. II. Morphologic evidence for differentiation and maturation. J. Nat. Cancer Inst., 32:165-200, 1964.
5. How, S.-W., and K. C. Snell: Skin tumors induced in rats by the dietary administration of N,N'-2,7-fluorenylenebisacetamide. J. Nat. Cancer Inst., 38:407-434, 1967.
6. Jacob, F., and J. Monod: Genetic repression, allosteric inhibition, and cellular differentiation. In: Cytodifferentiation and Macromolecular Synthesis (M. Locke, ed.) , Academic Press, Inc., New York, 1963, p. 30.
7. Kleinsmith, L. J., and G. B. Pierce: Multipotentiality of single embryonal carcinoma cells. Cancer Res., 24:1544-1551, 1964.
8. Lin, H.-S., C.-S. Lin, S. Yeh, and S.-M. Tu: Fine structure of nasopharyngeal carcinoma with special reference to the anaplastic type. Cancer, 23:390-405, 1969.
9. Mendelsohn, M. L.: Autoradiographic analysis of cell proliferation in spontaneous breast cancer of C3H mouse. III. The growth fraction. J. Nat. Cancer Inst., 28:1015-1028, 1962.
10. Nameroff, M. A., M. Reznik, P. Anderson, and J. L. Hansen: Differentiation and control of mitosis in a skeletal muscle tumor. Cancer Res., 30:596-600, 1970.
11. Nameroff, M. A., M. Reznik, P. Anderson, and J. L. Hansen: Ultrastructure of a transplantable murine rhabdomyosarcoma. Cancer Res., 30:601-610, 1970.
12. Oberling, C., and W. Bernhard: The morphology of the cancer cells. In: The Cell (J. Brachet and A. E. Mirsky, eds.) , Academic Press, Inc., New York, 1961, p. 405.
13. Pierce, G. B.: Ultrastructure of human testicular tumors. Cancer, 19:1963-1983, 1966.
14. Pierce, G. B.: Differentiation of normal and malignant cells. Fed. Proc., 29:1248-1254, 1970.
15. Pierce, G, B., and F. J. Dixon: The demonstration of teratogenesis by metamorphosis of multipotential cells. Cancer, 12:573-583, 1959.
16. Pierce, G. B., F. J. Dixon, and E. L. Verney: Teratocarcinogenic and tissue forming potentials of the cell types comprising neoplastic embryoid bodies. Lab. Invest., 9:583-602, 1960.
17. Pierce, G. B., and C. Wallace: In preparation.
18. Rabinowitz, Z., and L. Sachs: Control of reversion of properties in transformed cells. Nature, 225:136-139, 1970.
19. Rosai, J., K. Khodadoust, and I. Silver: Spermatocytic seminoma. II. Ultrastructural study. Cancer, 24:103-116, 1969.
20. Saffiotti, J., R. Montesano, A. R. Sellakumar, and S. A. Borg: Experimental cancer of the lung, inhibition by vitamin A of the induction of tracheobronchial squamous metaplasia and squamous cell tumors. Cancer, 20:857-864, 1967.
21. Seilern-Aspang, F., and K. Kratochwill: Induction and differentiation of an epithelial tumor in the newt (Triturus cristatus) . J. Embryol. Exp. Morphol., 10:337-356, 1962.
22. Silagi, S., and S. A. Bruce: Suppression of malignancy and differentiation in melanotic melanoma cells. Proc. Nat. Acad. Sci. USA, 66:72-78, 1970.

23. Stevens, L. C., and C. C. Little: Spontaneous testicular tumors in an inbred strain of mice. Proc. Nat. Acad. Sci. USA, 40:1080-1087, 1954.
24. Stevens, L. C.: Origin of testicular teratomas from primordial germ cells in mice. J. Nat. Cancer Inst., 39:549-552, 1967.
25. Waddington, G. H.: Ultrastructure aspects of cellular differentiation. Symp. Soc. Exp. Biol., XVII, Cell Differentiation, pp. 85-97, 1963.

Cell Surface and Cancer

GEORGE KLEIN

Department of Tumor Biology, Karolinska Institute,
Medical Faculty, Stockholm, Sweden

THE SIGNIFICANCE OF cell surface changes for neoplastic growth first became apparent when the behavior of normal and neoplastic cells was compared in tissue culture. Changes in contact inhibition[1] and electronegative surface charge[2] were speculatively related to the invasive behavior of cancer cells in vivo. The exact relationship between the changed in vitro behavior, particularly the relative resistance of transformed cells to contact inhibition of division, and tumorigenic behavior in vivo is still not known; in fact, the picture seems to become more complicated with time. Recently, Rabinowitz and Sachs[3] have isolated a number of "revertants" from polyoma-transformed cell lines that showed a contact-inhibited behavior in monolayer cultures. Although this behavior resembled the original, nontransformed line and differed sharply from the relatively uninhibited transformants, the revertants nevertheless continued to show highly tumorigenic behavior in vivo. When a number of other changed properties, characteristic of the transformed line, were compared in the revertants, it was found, moreover, that the various properties could all undergo "reversion," but independently of each other and of tumorigenicity in vivo. It is well known that the latter can undergo reversion on its own, in that highly tumorigenic lines may become low-tumorigenic on continuous culture.

The independent change of different measurable parameters of cell behavior in vitro is strongly reminiscent of the "independent progression of unit characteristics" used to describe the natural history of tumor development in vivo. As Foulds formulated it clearly a number of years ago,[4] a number of more or less well defined in vivo characteristics, such as hormone dependence, invasiveness, ability to metastasize, growth rate, and various morphologic properties, change independently of each other in the course of tumor progression.

It is conceivable that while the same chemical and viral agents can "transform" monolayer-grown cells into less contact-inhibited cells and normal cells in vivo into malignant variants, different cellular changes are responsible. Resistance to contact inhibition is probably the most important mechanism in monolayer cultures where contact inhibition is the main growth-limiting factor, whereas quite different properties will be decisive in vivo if homeostasis functions through other mechanisms. Sometimes, both properties would be acquired at the same time, but this would not be necessary. The segregation of the relevant characteristics and their determination mechanisms might be studied in somatic cell hybrids (vide infra).

Cell Surface Changes Associated with Malignant Transformation

One type of cell surface change, consistently associated with transformed behavior in vitro, is expressed by the agglutinability with certain plant agglutinins, such as wheat germ lipase or concavalin A.[5-7] This is probably attributable to a change in the arrangement or the availability of certain carbohydrate groups of the outer cell surface. As a rule, nontransformed, i.e. contact-inhibited, cells do not agglutinate, whereas transformed cells agglutinate, irrespectively of the mode of transformation; this includes oncogenic RNA and DNA viruses, chemical carcinogens and x irradiation. It is also important that nontransformed cells become agglutinable after gentle trypsinization. This is probably caused by the unmasking of the relevant carbohydrate receptors after the removal of some proteolysis-sensitive outer surface components. This has led to the concept of unmasking of normal membrane constituents in the course of transformation, i.e. a kind of loss mechanism at the cell surface level.

The biochemical study of cell membranes in relation to transformation is in its earliest stage of development. Interesting changes have been reported recently in the ganglioside composition of transformed cells by Hakomori et al.[8] In a different system, Mora et al.[9] found a considerable decrease of certain high-molecular gangliosides (although not the same compounds as in Hakomori's experiments) in SV40- and polyoma-transformed mouse fibroblasts, but not in a spontaneously transformed line.

Expression of the Malignant Trait in Cell Hybrids

The loss of trypsin-sensitive "masking substances," covering the phytoagglutinin receptors and the possible loss of certain gangliosides from transformed cells, is reminiscent of earlier deletion theories of carcinogenesis, although with less emphasis on the cell interior and more on the cell surface. On a deletion basis, nontransformed or non-tumorigenic behavior should dominate over transformed or tumori-genic behavior, respectively, in somatic cell hybrids. Previously, the opposite appeared to be true.[10-12] Recently, Henry Harris and our group performed some collaborative experiments, leading to a differ-ent conclusion, however. In the first series,[13] a low-tumorigenic, 8-azaguanine resistant L-cell subline (A9) was hybridized with three different highly malignant ascites tumors, the long-transplanted Ehr-lich carcinoma, the polyoma-induced SEWA sarcoma, and the methyl-cholanthrene-induced MSWBS sarcoma. All three hybrids were low-tumorigenic, even after inoculation into newborn, x-irradiated (400 r) recipients. In the case of the A9-Ehrlich combination, all five inde-pendently fused hybrid clones showed a low-tumorigenic behavior. Highly malignant "segregants" grew out in a minority of the inocu-lated animals. These could be maintained subsequently by serial transplantation in vivo and gave a high incidence of takes. In com-parison with the low-tumorigenic hybrid line maintained in vitro, all such "high-malignant segregants" were characterized by considerable chromosome losses.

Since A9 is deficient with regard to inosinic acid pyrophosphorylase (IMP[14]), an IMP-positive "revertant" line (A9-RI) and another, thy-midine kinase-deficient, IMP-positive L-cell subline (B82) were also tested. Both lines suppressed the high tumorigenicity of their Ehrlich partner.[15] It was therefore concluded that the IMP deficiency as such could not be responsible for the suppression of high-malignant be-havior by the L-cell sublines. High-tumorigenic segregants were iso-lated after in vivo inoculation of the A9 RI-Ehrlich and the B82 Ehrlich hybrids in the same way as from A9-Ehrlich, and were also charac-terized by extensive chromosome losses.

Still another high-malignant cell was tested after fusion with the A9 cell; the Moloney ascites lymphoma YAC and its YAC-IR subline. Both the YAC-A9 and the YACIR-A9 hybrid were practically devoid of tumorigenic ability.

The question may be raised whether the low tumorigenicity of these hybrids was attributable to a relative histoincompatibility rather than to any intrinsic inability to grow as malignant tumors. The L-cell line was derived from the C3H mouse strain several decades ago, and al-though it still carries the C3H-derived H-2^k isoantigen complex,[13] ap-parently with an unchanged composition,[16] it obviously cannot be fully compatible with any C3H strain presently maintained. Since such in-compatibility would be restricted to the relatively weak non-H-2 anti-gens, and in view of the fact that the hybrids failed to grow in more than a minority of newborn, irradiated C3H mice, the immunologic explanation did not appear likely. This was further emphasized by the finding[13, 17] that the Ehrlich cell suppressed the antigenic expression of its partners. This suppression affected both the genetically determined H-2^k isoantigen complex and the surface antigen determined by the L-cell virion, a C-type virus carried by the various L-cell sublines.[18] In some of the high-malignant A9-Ehrlich segregants, antigen suppression was again replaced by full expression, after substantial chromosome losses, whereas others maintained a low membrane antigen level. The point is, however, that the "full" A9-Ehrlich hybrid had the lowest expression of both genetically and virally determined membrane antigens. This further reduces the probability that its low tumorigenic behavior was caused by histoincompatibility.

The L-cell and its different variants are highly aneuploid, and this may be relevant for its suppression of tumorigenic behavior. This was tested by fusing diploid fibroblasts from primary explants, derived from our own inbred lines, with high-malignant partners and testing the hybrid cells for malignant growth in newborn, irradiated recipients of the most closely compatible genotype. In the first series, three hybrid cell populations were tested, derived from independent fusion events between normal diploid CBA/T6T6 fibroblasts and Ehrlich ascites tumor cells. In addition, 10 different clones were isolated from one of the three mass cultures. Although there were minor differences between the different clones with regard to their latency period after inoculation and the minimum cell dose required for a take, by and large, all three mass cultures and all derived clones were highly tumorigenic in newborn, 400 r x-irradiated CBA recipients, i.e. a genotype compatible with the CBA/T6T6, but not with the Ehrlich parental cell.[19] Chromosomal examination showed, however, that all hybrid lines and clones have suffered extensive chromosome losses prior to inoculation. This may be related to the fact that neither parental cell was preadopted to tissue culture.

In the next step, a series of hybrids were produced by fusing the polyoma-induced mouse ascites tumor SEWA (of ASW origin) with primary CBA/T6T6 fibroblasts. This time, a strictly histocompatible host was available (ASW × CBA F$_1$ hybrid). Of 15 clones, 13 were highly tumorigenic, and grew in nearly 100%, whereas two clones gave only 40 to 50% tumors even with high cell doses. Chromosomal examination showed[20] that the two low-tumorigenic clones, and one additional high-tumorigenic clone, had the highest chromosome number in the whole series and came closest to a complete hybrid. Whenever tumors arose from these three clones, they showed a drastic reduction of their chromosome number. The other high-tumorigenic clones already had strongly reduced chromosome numbers in vitro, prior to inoculation.

Presently, still another hybrid, of a similar kind, is being tested. The ascites line of a TA3, a mammary adenocarcinoma of strain A origin, was fused with normal diploid fibroblasts derived from the ACA strain. The hybrid was relatively low-tumorigenic; approximately 40% progressively growing tumors were obtained in genetically compatible newborn, irradiated A × ACA F_1 hybrids. Interestingly, high tumorigenic variants that arose after in vivo passage, in this case as well, on further testing, grew more frequently in the parental A strain (i.e. the strain of the highly malignant TA3 parent cell) than in the opposite, ACA strain. Since A and ACA are congenic resistant strains that differ at the H-2 locus only,[21] this suggests preferential elimination of the ACA-derived (i.e. normal) genome from the high-tumorigenic variant subline.

These findings thus showed that even normal diploid cells can suppress the tumorigenic capacity of highly malignant fusion partners. Subsequently, the suppressor can be lost, in parallel with extensive chromosome losses from the hybrid. This either means that it is directly specified as the DNA level or, if controlled, a more peripheral, episomal level, that this level is under indirect chromosomal control.

Previous reports[10–12, 22] have suggested that hybridization of low- and high-tumorigenic lines regularly leads to the dominance of the high-tumorigenic partner. In several such studies, the chromosomal constitution of the hybrid cells and the resulting tumors was not critically compared, however, and it cannot be decided on the basis of available data whether chromosomal reduction in vitro, prior to inoculation, or in the resulting in vivo tumors may have accompanied progressive growth in vivo, as we have seen it frequently in our material. There are other differences between the cell lines hybridized and tested in different laboratories. In the experiments of Barski, for instance, high- and low-tumorigenic lines of the same cell type have been hybridized with each other.

Conceivably, whatever change is responsible for the behavior of the high-tumorigenic line and at whatever level (e.g. viral or cellular nucleic acid) it is specified, this could be readily imposed on another cell of the same differentiation history, whereas a low-tumorigenic cell of a different history may impose its own, more restrictive behavior. It is interesting to note, in this connection, that sensitivity to contact inhibition was dominant over resistance in two different fusion series.[23, 24]

One further point, concerning our series, is of interest in the present context. When we fused the polyoma tumor SEWA with A9 or with primary, diploid fibroblasts, several of the resulting hybrids were low-tumorigenic, as already mentioned. Such hybrids maintained the polyoma-induced transplantation antigen and were still fully capable of immunizing allogeneic or syngeneic mice against established polyoma tumor isografts.[25] It may be assumed that the constitution of the partner cell rendered the hybrid insusceptible to the oncogenic action of the virus. It also follows that the presence of the virally determined transplantation antigen is not sufficient for neoplastic behavior, and the membrane change (s) it expresses, although perhaps necessary, are not by themselves sufficient for progressive growth. The full neoplastic potentialities are only realized after some suppressor, contributed by the partner, has been lost by chromosomal segregation.

Tumor-Associated Changes in Surface Antigens

Perhaps the most consistent change associated with tumor development in vivo and neoplastic transformation in vitro is the appearance of new surface antigens. Although the strength of antigenicity and the cross-reactivity patterns vary widely from system to system, it can be stated that the curiously oscillating history of tumor immunology has presently been reduced to the acceptance of at least a relatively weak, tumor-associated, potentially rejection-inducing immunogenicity in most experimental tumors adequately studied.[26-29] The antigens are often referred to as TSTA (tumor specific transplantation antigens). At least in oncogenic virus systems, the distribution of these antigens is not restricted to the tumor cells, however. "Tumor associated transplantation antigen" or TATA would be, therefore, a more adequate designation.

It is frequently assumed that all transplantation-type antigens, i.e. antigens capable of inducing rejection reactions in autochthonous, syngeneic, or allogeneic hosts, must be localized on the outer cell surface. This is a reasonable generalization, since it is hard to see how a living target cell could be attacked, either by humoral antibody or by cell-mediated host reactions, unless the responsible antigenic receptor site (s) are exposed on the outer cell membrane. For many systems, there is experimental evidence to confirm this, by demonstrating the presence of tumor associated transplantation-type antigens on the outer cell membrane. The reactions include membrane fluorescence,[30-34] immediate[35-37] or delayed cytotoxicity, the latter measured by colony inhibition,[38-40] immune adherence,[41-43] and mixed hemadsorption,[44-46] performed with living target cells. Furthermore, the absorbing capacity of whole, intact, viable ascites tumor cells was of the same order as of cell homogenates, whenever a critical comparison has been made.[47, 48, 76]

Whereas transplantation antigens are thus obviously membrane-expressed, it does not follow that all membrane-expressed antigens are necessarily immunogenic in autochthonous or syngeneic hosts. Obviously, genetically determined isoantigens are not, since they are present on all tissues and appear early during embryonic life. Other membrane antigens are specified by cell differentiation. This category includes the antigens characteristic for various types of lymphoid cells, such as TL,[49] theta,[50] LY,[51] etc. Antigens of this category can be detected by allogeneic sera, since they exist in different allotypic forms. Other antigens can be detected by heteroimmunization, like the

MSLA system associated with certain types of mouse lymphoid cells[52] or the IgM-kappa type molecules built into the membrane of certain human lymphoma cells.[53] The various differentiation-related antigens do not act as autoantigens; they are obviously regarded as "self" by the immune system. In order to act as an autoantigen, a tissue constituent must obviously meet some special conditions, such as compartmentalization or binding to appropriate carriers.[108]

The two major categories of membrane-localized, transplantation-type antigens that can act as autoantigens in autochthonous and syngeneic hosts are the virally determined, tumor-associated antigens, and the tumor-associated antigens present on chemically induced or spontaneous tumors.

One of the most important questions that can be considered in relation to these antigens is the role they may play in expressing a membrane change that could be related to the resistance of the tumor cell to growth regulation, i.e. its neoplastic behavior. The surface antigens determined by small oncogenic DNA viruses, such as polyoma or SV40, are particularly interesting in this respect. Since these viruses carry very little genetic information, any cellular change that is consistently and regularly associated with the transformation induced by them is likely to play an essential part in the transformation process. The polyoma-induced transplantation antigen is not part of the virion.[54] Inactive virus can induce antiviral antibodies, but no transplantation resistance, whereas allogeneic, nonvirus-producing tumor cells induce specific transplantation resistance against polyoma tumor isografts, but no antiviral antibodies. The cell-associated polyoma-induced transplantation antigen is solidly maintained during serial passage in vivo, even if it is provided with a negative selective value, by forcing the tumor through specifically preimmunized hosts.[55]

One important question is whether the polyoma-induced or the relatively similar (although not cross-reactive) SV40-induced transplantation antigen is under the direct control of the viral genome, known to be integrated with the cell genome[56] and at least partially transcribed in transformed cells,[57, 58] or represents some more indirect consequence of the neoplastic transformation, perhaps similar to the unmasking of normal cell membrane constituents, in analogy with the phytoagglutinin receptors discussed earlier. Another model would be the reappearance of embryonic antigens in relation to tumorigenesis, like the fetal alpha-globulin in hepatomas[59] or the carcinoembryonic antigen (CEA) present in colonic and other gastrointestinal tumors.[60]

No decisive evidence is available about this problem, but a virally coded antigen seems a more attractive possibility, for the following reasons: (1) All in vivo and in vitro transformants induced by the same virus, share the same antigenic specificity, even if they are of quite different histologic types, whereas tumors induced by different viruses do not cross-react, even if they are of similar histologic types.

This is quite different from the changes in agglutinability or in cellular gangliosides, where the same type of membrane alteration is shared among tumor cells induced by different viruses; (2) if the antigens would be present on normal cells in a masked form that could be unmasked, e.g. by proteolytic enzymes, it is hard to see how such an unmasking could be avoided in the normal organism. If antigen would be released regularly, it would either have to induce tolerance—and this would not be compatible with the immunogenicity of the transformants—or sensitization, which is not the case either; (3) the embryonic antigens so far discovered in tumors are strictly tissue-specific, whereas the virus-induced transplantation antigens are not tissue, but virus-specific, as already mentioned; and (4) the virally induced transplantation antigens cross-react between the cells of different species, transformed by the same virus. This has been shown e.g. for polyoma transformed mouse and hamster cells,[61] and for SV40-transformed cells of different species.[62] A virus-specific unmasking of the same cellular constituent in different species and in different tissues is more difficult to imagine than the appearance of virally coded (and, therefore, virus-specific) materials.

An interesting distinction between a "derepressed" embryonic antigen and a rejection-inducing, transplantation antigen is provided by the study of Baldwin[34] on rat hepatomas. Although an intracellular fetal globulin is present in many azo-dye-induced hepatomas, giving completely cross-reactive immunodiffusion patterns, their tumor-associated rejection-inducing antigens are individually distinct, like in other chemically-induced tumors.

Whether the virally induced transplantation antigen is coded by the viral or the virally altered cellular genome, the question whether it plays an essential or a purely trivial role in relation to the neoplastic change remains the same. Its maintenance in spite of adverse selection speaks in favor of some important function in relation to neoplastic behavior. Tumor cell populations are very plastic, and chromosomal and other variants arise all the time, providing a broad background for selection. Isoantigenic variants can be readily selected when tumors are grown in the presence of long-maintained immunologic pressures against antigens that can be lost without serious harm to continued cell life and proliferation.[63, 64]

Occasionally, it has been claimed that the polyoma-induced transplantation antigen can be lost from polyoma tumors, but, as a rule, these claims have been restricted to the hamster system and no distinction was made between a loss of immunogenicity and the development of immunoresistance. The latter, i.e. the ability to evade the rejection reaction, frequently evolves without a corresponding loss of the antigen, as judged by the persistence of immunogenicity in the rejection test or the ability to elicit the formation of specific antibody.[65] In view of this, it is important to document alleged losses, even in terms of immunogenicity, before drawing the conclusion that they reflect a disappearance of the antigenic site.

The opposite phenomenon, preservation of the virally determined surface antigen in the course of "reversion" from the transformed to nontransformed state, has been demonstrated, as already mentioned.[3, 66, 67] The maintenance of the polyoma-specific transplantation antigen in the low-tumorigenic hybrids produced by the fusion of a polyoma-induced tumor (SEWA) with the A9 cell line and with normal diploid (CBA6T6) fibroblasts, also discussed above, is another case in point.

The appearance of new, transplantation-type antigens in connection with viral oncogenesis is not restricted to DNA-virus-induced tumors. RNA-virus systems, including nonpermissive transformants, show a fully analogous phenomenon: new transplantation antigens appear, characteristic for the group of tumors induced by the same virus, and not dependent on the release of infectious virus. Previously, this has been demonstrated for mouse tumors induced by the Rous sarcoma virus.[68] More recently, similar findings have been reported by Ting and Law, for a nonvirus releasing, murine sarcoma virus (MSV)-induced tumor.[69]

The contention, implicit in much of the reasoning above, that the appearance of the surface change expressed by the virus-induced transplantation antigen is not sufficient to make a cell neoplastic by itself, is affirmed by the finding of Bauer et al.[70] that avian myeloblastosis virus (AMV), although nononcogenic in mice, can nevertheless immunize them against RSV-sarcoma isografts. In other words, the induction of an antigen identical or cross-reactive with the antigen characteristic for mammalian RSV sarcomas is not sufficient to allow neoplastic growth in the AMV-inoculated animals. This does not exclude, however, that the antigen could be essential for the RSV-transformed tumor cells. Conceivably, the virus may produce a surface change that makes certain cells disobedient to their growth control. Depending on whether the viral genome is maintained in the cell lineage, either by some form of integration with the cell genome or by its reproduction at a speed compatible with cell division, the change will be transmitted to the progeny; otherwise it will be aborted. In line with this picture, temporary appearance and subsequent disappearance of the polyoma-induced surface antigen has been demonstrated during abortive polyoma-induced transformation.[71, 72] It is also highly likely that certain types of surface change, expressed as new surface antigens, may render cells with a certain kind of differentiation disobedient to their superimposed growth regulation, whereas in other cells, subject to other kinds of growth control, the same change may be quite innocuous. Mouse leukemia viruses (MLV) may be mentioned as an example: they induce the same or closely cross-reactive antigens on fibroblasts and on the leukemia cells, but the fibroblasts do not turn neoplastic unless a sarcomagenic viral genome (MSV) is added to the system. Whether the MSV genome specifies any additional surface antigen, not already specified by MLV, that functions in a "helper capacity" is not known; existing evidence points to very strong cross-reactivity, if not identity.[73] The target cell specificity of other oncogenic viruses is well known, and there are many other cases of antigenic conversion of the "wrong," i.e. non-transformant, cell type.

The permissive, virus-releasing, oncogenic RNA virus systems are also of considerable interest for the present discussion. Their distinctive transplantation and surface antigens were among the first to be studied.[35, 74, 75] Frequently, the virus-associated antigens present on the surfaces of murine leukemia cells, for example, were merely believed to reflect the budding of infectious virus from the cell membrane. In our view, this was unlikely,[76] because virus release and surface antigen concentration, measured by a number of tests, did not correlate in a series of Moloney virus-induced lymphomas. The formal proof that the virally determined surface antigen is distinct from budding virus, both with regard to localization and specificity, was recently provided by the elegant ferritin-labeling studies of Aoki et al.[77]

All this leads to a remarkably unified picture; without exception, all known oncogenic viruses change the cell membrane in a specific way (common for different tumors induced by the same virus, different for tumors induced by different viruses), no matter whether the virus buds from the cell membrane or not. It is most remarkable that such a generalization can be made at all, and one may, in fact, ask whether a virus that would not change the cell surface could play an oncogenic role at all.

Visualizing the cell membrane as the main target of viral oncogenic action is rather attractive for other reasons as well. It is quite true that many viruses influence the macromolecular syntheses of their host cell quite drastically. In fact, these effects are so drastic, as a rule, that they are often not detected until and unless the cell undergoes a lytic, cytocidal, i.e. by definition nononcogenic, interaction with the virus. The concept that the virus interferes with regulation processes in the transformed cell in a more subtle way, at some more peripheral level, such as by disturbing the function of membrane localized growth regulation receptors, for example, is simpler and can be more easily conceived as compatible with continued cell life and proliferation.

The new transplantation antigens associated with chemically induced tumors are also of great interest, but in somewhat different ways. The large number of individually distinct specificities, different for different tumors induced by the same agent, including multiple tumors arising in the same individual host,[78] is very puzzling. No claims of cross-reactions have stood the test of time, and a critical study by one of the pioneers of this field adds recent confirmation to this.[79] The largest number of cross-tested tumors of one kind is probably represented by the study of Baldwin[34] on a series of azo dye-induced hepatomas; it has led to the same conclusion of individually distinct specificities. To me, the assumption that chemical carcinogenesis involves the activation of latent oncogenic viruses and the additional postulate that these could be different in the different tumors and sufficiently numerous to account for the individually distinct antigenic specificities, appears rather unreasonable, and, if extended to include different primary tumors in the same animal, most unlikely.

Although tumors induced by known viruses carry cross-reacting, group-specific transplantation antigens, the recent work of Morton[80] and Vaage[81] indicates that, at least in the MTV-associated mouse mammary carcinoma system, weak and individually distinct antigenic specificities are superimposed on the common group-specific antigen. In the ordinary cross-immunization test, they are masked by the common antigen, but can be revealed if tolerance is induced against the latter. It is possible that the group-specific common antigen covers a similar individual variability in other virus-induced tumor systems, where the tolerance method has not been applied to study the question.

Does the individual specificity of chemically induced tumors reflect a preexisting clonal variation, as recently postulated,[82] or is it related to the interaction of the chemical carcinogen with the cell genome? Tumors induced by the implantation of cell-impermeable films are only very weakly antigenic,[83, 84] in sharp contrast to histologically similar tumors induced by chemical carcinogens. Since they appear after very long latency periods, this was previously attributed to immunoselection by the surveillance mechanism. Very recently, it has been shown, however, that such tumors are very weakly antigenic, even if they are allowed to develop within a diffusion chamber, i.e. sheltered from the host response.[85] In view of this, it is more likely that the relatively strong antigenicity of the chemically induced tumors is attributable to the interaction of the chemical carcinogen with the cell genome. This is also supported by the fact that the "strength" of antigenicity is different in tumors induced by different chemical agents.[84, 86]

It is even more difficult to speculate about the relative importance of membrane antigenicity for malignant misbehavior in the chemically induced tumors than in the viral systems. The individuality of the antigens does not exclude that they may play an important role. They may reflect slightly different changes of the same basic membrane structure, similar in one respect (nonfunctionality in relation to growth regulation), but different in fine detail. It is also possible, however, that they reflect characteristics secondary to the neoplastic change. The relative stability of antigens in chemically induced tumors is not well known. Occasionally it has been reported that antigenicity decreased or disappeared during serial passage. There was no attempt to distinguish between changes in immunogenicity and the development of immunoresistance, however. Because of the individually distinct antigenicity of the different tumors, such experiments must be performed with the help of a frozen tumor bank. In an unpublished experiment, we have compared a late and an early generation of the same methylcholanthrene-induced sarcoma for immunogenicity and immunosensitivity in cross-immunization-rejection type experiments. An apparent decrease in antigenicity during serial passage was, in this case, entirely caused by the development of immunoresistance and not by a decline in immunogenicity, since the heavily irradiated cells of the late tumor immunized equally well against challenge with graded doses of viable cells from the early tumor as the early tumor itself, whereas the late tumor was not rejected equally well, no matter whether immunization was performed with the early or the late tumor. Since serial passage in immunologically competent animals tends to favor immunoresistant cells and since immunoresistance can develop without antigenic loss,[65, 87] this is not surprising. The persistence of the immunogenic antigen would be compatible with its postulated importance for the neoplastic cell.

Some Perspectives

For further meaningful development of this field, and particularly for a better understanding of the meaning of the membrane changes expressed through the immunologic language of new antigens and their possible relevance for potentially or fully neoplastic behavior, two approaches seem to be very important. One is the isolation and chemical characterization of the membrane structures involved (and the earliest beginnings of this can be visualized in references 8, 9, and 88), and the other is the establishment of links between membrane antigen changes and cellular behavior. A start in the latter direction has been made by Borek and Sachs,[89] but the methodologic difficulties are still very great. It can also be noted that in a system with no known oncogenic component, herpes simplex virus (HSV) infection of monolayer cultures, Roizman[90] found that different viral envelope mutants induce different membrane changes. This can, in turn, be related to changes in the pattern of "social behavior" of the infected cells, characteristic for each mutant.[90] Since some herpes-type viruses are oncogenic in animals[91–93] and others are suspected for possible oncogenic or cocarcinogenic effects in man,[94–98] Roizman's observation may have considerable relevance. In two pertinent systems, Marek's disease in chickens and EBV infection of human lymphoblastoid cell lines, virus-induced membrane antigens could be demonstrated in carrier cultures,[99, 100] and as far as Burkitt's lymphoma is concerned, in biopsies as well.[101]

Finally, a word may be said about new membrane antigens in human tumors. These are in a very preliminary state of exploration, but interesting results are emerging. They may give etiologic clues and also contribute new information to the understanding of neoplastic cell behavior. There are, of course, many immunotherapeutic and preventive aspects as well, but these are much too complex to be dealt with in the present context.

In the human tumors so far studied, certain membrane alterations have been found by immunologic methods that may reflect a viral association, in view of the cross-reactivity patterns obtained. This category includes Burkitt's lymphoma and nasopharyngeal carcinoma, in their relation to EBV-determined antigens, as already mentioned.[94-97] Cross-reactive antigens have also been found in human osteosarcoma,[102] neuroblastoma,[103] and cancer of the colon and of the breast.[104, 105] Noncrossreactive antigens, found in melanoma, however, argue against a viral association.[106, 107] These developments are encouraging, but their interpretation is still very difficult and beset with potential pitfalls. Obviously, indirect evidence of many different types will have to be gathered before firm etiologic conclusions can be drawn.

References

1. Abercrombie, M., and E. J. Ambrose: Cancer Res., 22:525, 1962.
2. Ambrose, E. J.: J. Microsc. Soc., 80:47, 1961.
3. Rabinowitz, Z., and L. Sachs: Virology, 40:193, 1970.
4. Foulds, L.: J. Chron. Dis., 8:2, 1958.
5. Aub, J. C., C. Tieslau, and A. Lankester: Proc. Nat. Acad. Sci. USA, 50:613, 1963.
6. Burger, M. M.: Proc. Nat. Acad. Sci. USA, 62:994, 1969.
7. Inbar, M., and L. Sachs: Nature, 223:710, 1969.
8. Hakomori, S., and W. T. Murakami: Proc. Nat. Acad. Sci. USA, 59:254, 1968.
9. Mora, P. T., R. O. Brady, R. M. Bradley, and V. W. McFarland: Proc. Nat. Acad. Sci. USA, 63:1290, 1969.
10. Scaletta, L. J., and B. Ephrussi: Nature, 205:1169, 1965.
11. Barski, G., and F. Cornefert: J. Nat. Cancer Inst., 28:801, 1962.
12. Marin, G., and J. W. Littlefield: J. Virology, 2:69, 1968.
13. Harris, H., O. J. Miller, G. Klein, P. Worst, and T. Tachibana: Nature, 223:363, 1969.
14. Littlefield, J. W.: Science, 145:709, 1964.
15. Harris, H., and G. Klein: Nature, 224:1314, 1969.
16. Klein, D., D. J. Merchand, J. Klein, and D. C. Shreffler: J. Nat. Cancer Inst., 44:1149, 1970.
17. Klein, G., U. Gars, and H. Harris: Exp. Cell Res. In press.
18. Leclerc, J. C., J. P. Levy, B. Varet, and S. Oppenheim: Seanc. Acad. Sci., 266:2206, 1968.
19. Bregula, U., G. Klein, and H. Harris: In preparation.
20. Wiener, F., G. Klein, and H. Harris: In preparation.
21. Snell, G. D.: Meth. Med. Res., 10:8, 1964.
22. Defendi, V., B. Ephrussi, H. Koprowski, and M. C. Yoshida: Proc. Nat. Acad. Sci. USA, 57:299, 1967.
23. Weiss, M. C., G. J. Todaro, and H. Green: J. Cell Physiol., 71:105, 1968.
24. Weiss, M. C.: Proc. Nat. Acad. Sci. USA, 66:79, 1970.
25. Klein, G.: Unpublished data.
26. Klein, G.: Fed. Proc., 28:1739, 1969.
27. Old, L. J., and E. A. Boyse: Ann. Rev. Med., 15:167, 1964.

28. Sjögren, H. O.: Prog. Exp. Tumor Res., 6:289, 1965.
29. Klein, G.: Ann. Rev. Microbiol., 20:223, 1966.
30. Möller, G.: J. Exp. Med., 114:415, 1961.
31. Klein, E., and G. Klein: J. Nat. Cancer Inst., 32:547, 1964.
32. Tevethia, S. S., A. L. Couvillion, and F. Rapp: J. Immunol., 100:358, 1968.
33. Irlin, I. S.: Virology, 32:725, 1967.
34. Baldwin, R. W., and M. Moore: Int. J. Cancer, 4:753, 1969.
35. Slettenmark, B., and E. Klein: Cancer Res., 22:947, 1962.
36. Old, L. J., E. A. Boyse, and E. Stockert: Nature, 201:777, 1964.
37. Old, L. J., E. A. Boyse, D. A. Clarke, and E. A. Carswell: Ann. N.Y. Acad. Sci., 101:80, 1962.
38. Hellström, K. E., and I. Hellström: Adv. Cancer Res., 12:167, 1969.
39. Hellström, I., K. E. Hellström, and G. E. Pierce: Int. J. Cancer, 3:467, 1968.
40. Hellström, I., and K. E. Hellström: Int. J. Cancer, 4:587, 1969.
41. Nishioka, K., R. F. Irie, T. Kawana, and S. Takeuchi: Int. J. Cancer, 4:139, 1969.
42. Nordenskjöld, B., E. Klein, T. Tachibana, and E. M. Fenyö: J. Nat. Cancer Inst., 44:403, 1970.
43. Tachibana, T., and E. Klein: Immunology. In press.
44. Barth, R. F., Å. J. Espmark, and A. Fagraeus: J. Immunol., 98:888, 1967.
45. Metzgar, R. S., and S. R. Oleinick: Cancer Res., 28:1366, 1968.
46. Tachibana, T., P. Worst, and E. Klein: Immunology. In press.
47. Haughton, G.: Transplantation, 4:238, 1966.
48. McKhann, C. H. F.: Wistar Inst. Symp. Monogr. No. 3, Isoantigens and Cell Interactions, The Wistar Institute Press, 1965, p. 34.
49. Boyse, E. A., E. Stockert, and L. J. Old: J. Exp. Med., 128:85, 1968.
50. Reif, A. E., and J. M. V. Allen: Nature, 203:886, 1964.
51. Boyse, E. A., and L. J. Old: Ann. Rev. Genet., 3:269, 1969.
52. Shigeno, N., C. Arpels, U. Hämmerling, E. A. Boyse, and L. J. Old: Lancet, p. 320, 1968.
53. Klein, E., G. Klein, J. Nadkarni, J. Nadkarni, H. Wigzell, and P. Clifford: Cancer Res., 28:1300, 1968.
54. Sjögren, H. O.: J. Nat. Cancer Inst., 32:645, 1964.
55. Sjögren, H. O.: J. Nat. Cancer Inst., 32:661, 1964.
56. Westphal, H., and R. Dulbecco: Proc. Nat. Acad. Sci. USA, 59:1158, 1968.
57. Benjamin, T. L.: J. Mol. Biol., 16:359, 1966.
58. Aloni, Y., E. Winocour, and L. Sachs: J. Mol. Biol., 31:415, 1968.
59. Abelev, G. I.: Cancer Res., 28:1344, 1968.
60. Gold, P., and S. O. Freedman: J. Exp. Med., 122:467, 1965.
61. Hellström, I., and H. O. Sjögren: Int. J. Cancer, 1:481, 1966.
62. Girardi, A. J., and R. A. Roosa: J. Immunol., 99:1217, 1967.
63. Klein, E., G. Klein, and K. E. Hellström: J. Nat. Cancer Inst., 25:271, 1960.
64. Bjaring, B., and G. Klein: J. Nat. Cancer Inst., 41:1411, 1968.
65. Fenyö, E. M., E. Klein, G. Klein, and K. Swiech: J. Nat. Cancer Inst., 40:69, 1968.
66. Macpherson, I.: Adv. Cancer Res., 13. In press.
67. Pollack, R. E., H. Green, and G. J. Todaro: Proc. Nat. Acad. Sci. USA, 60:126, 1968.
68. Jonsson, N., and H. O. Sjögren: J. Exp. Med., 123:487, 1966.
69. Law, L. W., and R. C. Ting: Proc. Soc. Exp. Biol. Med., 131:960, 1969.
70. Bauer, H., J. Bubenik, T. Graf, and C. Allgaier: Virology, 39:482, 1969.
71. Stoker, M.: Nature, 218:234, 1968.
72. Meyer, G., F. Birg, and H. Bonneau: Compt. Rend. Acad. Sci., 268:2848, 1969.
73. Chuat, J. C., L. Berman, P. Gunvén, and E. Klein: Int. J. Cancer, 4:416, 1969.
74. Klein, G., H. O. Sjögren, and E. Klein: Cancer Res., 22:955, 1962.
75. Old, L. J., E. A. Boyse, and F. Lilly: Cancer Res., 23:1063, 1963.
76. Klein, G., E. Klein, and G. Haughton: J. Nat. Cancer Inst., 36:607, 1966.
77. Aoki, T., E. A. Boyse, L. J. Old, E. de Harven, U. Hammerling, and H. A. Wood: Proc. Nat. Acad. Sci. USA, 65:569, 1970.

78. Globerson, A., and M. Feldman: J. Nat. Cancer Inst., 32:1229, 1964.
79. Basombrio, M. A., and R. T. Prehn: Proc. Amer. Ass. Cancer Res., 11:6, 1970.
80. Morton, D. L., G. F. Miller, and D. A. Wood: J. Nat. Cancer Inst., 42:289, 1969.
81. Vaage, J.: Cancer Res., 28:2477, 1968.
82. Burnet, F. M.: Nature, 226:123, 1970.
83. Klein, G., H. O. Sjögren, and E. Klein: Cancer Res., 23:84, 1963.
84. Prehn, R. T.: M. D. Anderson Hosp. Symp. Fund. Cancer Res., 16:475, 1962.
85. Bartlett, G. L.: Proc. Amer. Ass. Cancer Res., 11:5, 1970.
86. Prehn, R. T.: Ann. N.Y. Acad. Sci., 164:449, 1969.
87. Klein, E., and E. Möller: J. Nat. Cancer Inst., 31:347, 1963.
88. Smith, R. W., J. Morganroth, and P. T. Mora: Nature, 227:141, 1970.
89. Borek, C., and L. Sachs: Proc. Nat. Acad. Sci. USA, 56:1705, 1966.
90. Roizman, B., and S. B. Spring: In: Proceedings of the Conference on Cross Reacting Antigens and Neoantigens. (J. J. Trenting, ed.), Williams and Wilkins Co., Baltimore, 1967, p. 85.
91. Churchill, A. E., and P. M. Biggs: J. Nat. Cancer Inst., 41:951, 1968.
92. Mizell, M., I. Toplin, and J. J. Isaacs: Science, 165:1134, 1969.
93. Meléndez, I. V., M. D. Daniel, R. D. Hunt, C. E. O. Fraser, F. G. Carcia, N. W. King, and M. E. Williamson: J. Nat. Cancer Inst., 44:1175, 1970.
94. Klein, G., G. Pearson, G. Henle, W. Henle, G. Goldstein, and P. Clifford: J. Exp. Med., 129:697, 1969.
95. Klein, G., P. Clifford, G. Henle, W. Henle, G. Geering, and L. J. Old: Int. J. Cancer, 4:416, 1969.
96. Schryver, A. de, S. Friberg, Jr., G. Klein, W. Henle, G. Henle, G. de Thé, P. Clifford, and H. C. Ho: Clin. Exp. Immunol., 5:443, 1969.
97. Henle, G., W. Henle, P. Clifford, V. Diehl, G. W. Kafuko, B. G. Kirya, G. Klein, R. H. Morrow, G. M. R. Munube, P. Pike, P. M. Tukei, and J. L. Ziegler: J. Nat. Cancer Inst., 43:1147, 1969.
98. Naib, Z. M., A. J. Nahmias, W. E. Josey, and J. H. Kramer: Cancer, 23:940, 1969.
99. Chen, J. H., and H. G. Purchase: Virology, 40:410, 1970.
100. Klein, G., G. Pearson, J. S. Nadkarni, J. J. Nadkarni, E. Klein, G. Henle, W. Henle, P. Clifford: J. Exp. Med., 128:1011, 1968.
101. Klein, G., P. Clifford, E. Klein, and J. Stjernswärd: Proc. Nat. Acad. Sci. USA, 55:1628, 1966.
102. Morton, D. L., and R. A. Malmgren: Science, 162:1279, 1968.
103. Hellström, I. E., K. E. Hellström, G. E. Pierce, and A. H. Bill: Proc. Nat. Acad. Sci. USA, 60:1231, 1968.
104. Hellström, I., K. E. Hellström, G. E. Pierce, and J. P. S. Yang: Nature, 220:1352, 1968.
105. Hellström, I., K. E. Hellström, C. A. Evans, G. H. Heppner, G. E. Pierce, and J. P. S. Yang: Proc. Nat. Acad. Sci. USA, 62. In press.
106. Morton, D. L., R. A. Malmgren, C. Holmes, and A. S. Ketcham: Surgery, 64:233, 1968.
107. Lewis, M. G., R. L. Ikonopisov, R. C. Nairn, T. M. Phillips, G. Hamilton-Fairley, D. C. Bodenham, and P. Alexander: Brit. Med. J., 3:547, 1969.
108. Iverson, G. M., and D. W. Dresser: Nature, 227:274, 1970.

Comparative Studies of the Surface of Cells in Tissue Culture Before and After Transformation with Oncogenic Viruses

C. A. BUCK, M. C. GLICK,

J. F. HARTMANN, AND L. WARREN

Department of Therapeutic Research, School of Medicine, University of Pennsylvania, Philadelphia, Pennsylvania, USA

THERE IS A RAPIDLY growing interest in the role of the cell surface and the surface membrane in cell behavior. Logic dictates that such processes as intercellular adhesiveness and "contact inhibition" of motion[1] and metabolism[14] must involve the cell surface. The threat of the malignant cell lies in its loss of control. Since it is quite possible that an important component of control may reside in the cell surface, this structure may be examined in the normal and malignant cell with some hope that significant differences will be found.

Coman[6] showed several years ago that there was a decreased adhesiveness between neoplastic, squamous cells (V2 carcinoma) as compared to their normal counterpart, and De Long et al.[10] provided evidence that cancer cells were unable to bind calcium ions as well as normal cells. Later Coman[7] was able to show that while malignant cells showed less mutual adhesiveness toward each other than normal, they displayed an increased stickiness to foreign objects. These striking observations, whatever the underlying mechanisms, can best be explained by a change in the surface structure of the malignant cell. This change could be, in part, the basis for the formation of metastases.

There is further evidence of differences in the surfaces of normal and malignant cells. It has been shown that virus-transformed tissue culture cells display sites on their surface which combine with a wheat germ agglutinin[5] or with another plant agglutinin, concanavalin A.[12] These sites are also present on cells before they are transformed, but they are covered with a material that can be removed by trypsin, i.e. normal cells are reactive only after treatment with trypsin. Changes in glycolipids have also been observed in virus-transformed cells by Hakomori et al.[11] and Mora et al.[16]

This brief selection of information from the literature would suggest that it would be profitable to look further for differences between the normal and the malignant cell surface. Our approach is biochemical, and the glycoproteins are our focus of interest.

Two lines of work in progress in our laboratory will be described: (1) the carbohydrate content of tissue culture cells before and after transformation by RNA and DNA oncogenic viruses, and (2) comparison of glycoproteins from the cell surface of tissue culture cells before and after viral transformation.

The Carbohydrate Content of Tissue Culture Cells Before and After Viral Transformation

Analyses of the sugars found in glycoproteins and glycolipids of whole animal cells have been done preliminary to an investigation of the sugar content of the surface membranes. However, it is likely that changes in the sugar content of whole cells reflect changes in the cell surface, since a major portion of most sugars resides in the cell surface[22] (Table 13-14).

L-Fucose, D-galactose, D-mannose, N-acetylglucosamine and N-acetylgalactosamine were measured by gas liquid chromatography by the method of Lehnhardt and Winzler.[13] In some instances, the hexosamines were measured by the method of Boas,[3] while sialic acid was measured by the thiobarbituric acid assay[19] after passing the hydrolysate through a small column of Dowex-1-acetate.[18]

It has been shown by Wu et al.[21] that the carbohydrate content of various membrane systems of the mouse fibroblast, 3T3, transformed by polyoma virus is lower than in nontransformed 3T3. Our measurements on normal and DNA virus-transformed cells are in agreement with the findings of Wu et al.[21] In Table 13-15A are seen the results of an experiment in which L-fucose, D-mannose, and D-galactose were measured in a cell line derived from a Chinese hamster, and cells from this line transformed by either polyoma or SV40 viruses. (Work with Chinese hamster cells was done in collaboration with Dr. V. Defendi, Wistar Institute, Philadelphia.) It can be seen that the

TABLE 13–14.—THE CARBOHYDRATE CONTENT OF SURFACE MEMBRANES AND WHOLE L CELLS*

	WHOLE CELL μMOLE $\times 10^{-10}$	SURFACE MEMBRANE μMOLE $\times 10^{-10}$	PERCENT OF TOTAL IN SURFACE MEMBRANE
L-Fucose	6.3 ± 3.8	2.3 ± 2.2	36
D-Mannose	52.8 ± 12.0	8.5 ± 2.5	16
D-Galactose	32.8 ± 4.6	21.6 ± 2.9	66
D-Hexosamine	58.3 ± 17.3	25.9 ± 5.5	44
Sialic acid	8.9 ± 1.7	6.5 ± 1.4	73

* Values represent means ± standard deviation. Whole cells, N = 12. Membranes isolated by zinc ion method; N = 7.

TABLE 13–15.—CONTENT OF SUGARS IN NORMAL CHINESE HAMSTER
AND SV40 OR POLYOMA TRANSFORMED CELLS

	CONTROL μmole/mg Protein $\times 10^{-4}$	SV40 TRANSFORMED μmole/mg Protein $\times 10^{-4}$	% Change	POLYOMA TRANSFORMED μmole/mg Protein $\times 10^{-4}$	% Change
A. Cells					
L-Fucose	23 ± 3	12 ± 3	−58	8 ± 2	−65
D-Mannose	165 ± 21	101 ± 18	−39	115 ± 28	−30
D-Galactose	149 ± 13	88 ± 17	−41	90 ± 16	−30
B. Cells + Wash					
L-Fucose	24 ± 9	15 ± 9	−38	10 ± 2	−58
D-Mannose	196 ± 13	165 ± 28	−16	184 ± 29	−6
D-Galactose	221 ± 32	217 ± 3	−2	198 ± 63	−10

Mean ± standard deviation of 3 experiments, each done with 3 separate cell cultures, in duplicate.

transformed cells contain less of the three sugars (μmole sugar per mg protein) than does the normal control. These three sugars are found in the glycoproteins and glycolipids of the cell and are, on the whole, bound to membrane.

In Table 13-16, the carbohydrates of cells in tissue culture derived from baby hamster kidney (BHK21/C_{13}) are compared to BHK21/C_{13} cells transformed by either the Bryan strain or Schmidt-Ruppin strain of Rous sarcoma virus. (Cell lines of early passage were kindly supplied by Dr. I. A. Macpherson, Imperial Cancer Research Fund, London.) Here a different picture is seen; the fucose concentration is lower in the transformants. The other carbohydrates show no change or are elevated. In Table 13-17, it can be seen that upon transformation of another cell type, chick embryo fibroblasts with Rous virus, the fucose concentration decreases while other carbohydrates generally show little change or are elevated.

As data on the carbohydrate levels of the three systems described accumulate, certain general patterns emerge, and some tentative conclusions can be suggested.

TABLE 13–16.—CONTENT OF SUGARS IN BHK21/C_{13}, C_{13}/B_4
AND C_{13}/SR_7 CELLS

	BHK21/C_{13} μmole/mg Protein $\times 10^{-4}$	C_{13}/B_4 (BRYAN STRAIN) μmole/mg Protein $\times 10^{-4}$	% Change	C_{13}/SR_7 (SCHMIDT-RUPPIN STRAINS) μmole/ mg Protein $\times 10^{-4}$	% Change
L-Fucose	26	15	−42	16	−38
D-Mannose	114	126	+11	148	+30
D-Galactose	82	77	−6	81	−1
N-acetyl-D-glucosamine	121	181	+50	191	+58
N-acetyl-D-galactosamine	20	68	+240	59	+195
Sialic acid	67	68	+1	69	+3

One of two experiments which show essentially the same results.

TABLE 13–17.—CONTENT OF SUGARS IN NORMAL AND
RSV-TRANSFORMED CHICK EMBRYO FIBROBLASTS

	CHICK EMBRYO FIBROBLASTS μMOLE/MG PROTEIN $\times 10^{-4}$	TRANSFORMED μMOLE/MG PROTEIN $\times 10^{-4}$	% CHANGE
L-Fucose	45	26	−42
D-Mannose	213	224	+ 5
D-Galactose	158	232	+47
N-acetyl-D-glucosamine	327	358	+ 9
N-acetyl-D-galactosamine	83	72	−13
Sialic acid	244	326	+34

Schmidt-Ruppin strain of RSV used. One of 5 experiments each of which shows that the concentration of L-fucose is lower in the transformed cell (mean reduction 44%).

1. It would seem from Table 13-15A that cells transformed by DNA viruses (polyoma, SV40) have consistently lower concentrations of sugars than do cells transformed by RNA viruses. However, the cells have been washed during their preparation, and the material removed from the cells during washing must be taken into account. Operationally, the cells are grown on glass and upon harvesting, the medium is poured off and the cells are gently washed with salt solution to remove the medium. The cells are then scraped off, saline solution is added, and the cells are poured into a tube. After centrifugation, a pellet and clear supernatant solution (wash) are obtained. The data in Table 13-15A were obtained using the pellet from the washed cells. Examination of the supernatant after dialysis reveals it to be very rich in bound carbohydrate. When the over-all carbohydrate concentration of the entire system (cells plus wash) is calculated, it is found that the transformed cells contain as much or even more carbohydrate-containing macromolecules than the parent cell, except for L-fucose which still tends to remain low (Table 13-15B). It would seem that transformed cells shed glycoproteins upon agitation more readily than do the nontransformed.

RSV transformed cells in comparison to normal cells have similar or elevated levels of carbohydrates. These cells do not seem to lose large amounts of carbohydrate-rich materials upon washing. Therefore, when the carbohydrate values for cells and washes are combined, there is relatively little change.

2. The most consistent finding we have is that upon transformation with either RNA or DNA viruses the levels of L-fucose are greatly decreased. Whether L-fucose on glycoproteins and glycolipids within the cell or on the surface plays a special role in malignancy or in cell growth is an intriguing problem. It has been shown by Cox and Gesner[8, 9] that L-fucose (and D-mannose in some systems) added to the medium of certain cells in tissue culture alters their morphology

and growth pattern. Other sugars at the same concentrations had no effect. In contrast to L-fucose, the pattern of change of sialic acid, which, like L-fucose, is found terminally in glycoproteins, can be lowered, the same (Table 13-16), or elevated (Table 13-17) in transformed cells.

3. There is considerable variation in the levels of carbohydrates in cells in tissue culture. The levels vary with rate of division of the cell or whether the cell is in log or plateau phase of growth. The levels also change in a regular pattern during the division cycle, as studied in synchronized cultures of KB cells.[22] Work in this laboratory has also shown that the carbohydrate levels are decreased when cells are grown in tissue culture in the absence of protein in the medium.

Although the changes described above may very well reflect changes in the surface of the cell, this is certainly not proved, and it will now be necessary to isolate the surface structure of these cells, and analyze and compare them. We hope that correlations can be made between changes in the levels of sugars in the cell and changes in their metabolic and social behavior. Most of the sugars of the cell are found in glycoproteins. The studies described above are essentially surveys preliminary to an examination of larger components of the cell, the glycoproteins. It is in these macromolecules (as well as in glycolipids) that groups of sugars are held, in a specific manner to exert, perhaps, specific and important effects. A study of the glycoproteins of the surface of cells will now be described.

Comparison of Glycoproteins of the Surface of Cells in Tissue Culture Before and After Virus Transformation

The surface structures of morphologically normal BHK21/C_{13} cells were compared with BHK21/C_{13} cells after they had been transformed with the Bryan strain (C_{13}/B_4) or the Schmidt-Ruppin strain ($C_{13}SR_7$) of Rous sarcoma virus, and with the oncogenic polyoma virus. Thus, in this study the effects of RSV transformation have been studied and some data have also been obtained using these same cells transformed by polyoma virus.

In these studies, the double-label method was used. Control cells were labeled with either ^{14}C amino acids, L-fucose, or D-glucosamine, while transformed cells were labeled with the ^3H precursor. In all experiments, the labeling was also reversed. Isotopic precursor was added to the medium of rapidly dividing cells over a 72-hour period. The medium was then poured off, the cells were gently washed, and the cells, on glass, were exposed to trypsin for 15 min at 37°. Soybean trypsin inhibitor was added, and the cells, now free, were centrifuged. The supernatant solution containing the material removed from the surface of the cells by trypsin will be referred to as "trypsinate." Surface membranes were obtained from the cells by the zinc ion method.[20]

Trypsinization removed approximately 15 to 25% of the total isotope (fucose or glucosamine) and 18 to 24% of the total sialic acid from the cells, as measured by the thiobarbituric acid assay.[19] When fucose was used as a radioactive precursor and was incorporated into cells, virtually all of the radioactivity could be recovered as fucose. No other radioactive materials were found. The specific activities of the fucose in the various types of cells were approximately the same.

In the double-labeling method, a ^{14}C-labeled trypsinate from one kind of cell was mixed with a ^{3}H-labeled trypsinate from another kind of cell, both isotopes being derived from the same precursor, e.g. [14]C and ^{3}H-fucose. The trypsinate mixture was applied to a column of Sephadex G-200, and the column was developed with buffer. Each fraction from the column was counted for both ^{3}H and ^{14}C in a liquid scintillation spectrometer. In other experiments, the mixed trypsinate or mixed membranes were treated with pronase for five days according to the method of Spiro,[17] and fractionated on columns of Sephadex G-50.

In these experiments, the results obtained with ^{14}C and ^{3}H fucose showed clear-cut differences between normal and transformed cells. In an experiment where normal cells were labeled with ^{14}C-fucose and C_{13}/B_4 (transformed) cells were labeled with ^{3}H-fucose, chromatography of the membranes on Sephadex G-200 showed that both peaks from the C_{13}/B_4 cells moved ahead of the corresponding peaks of that of the $BHK21/C_{13}$ cells. A comparison of the fucose-labeled trypsinates fractionated on columns of Sephadex G-200 revealed again a marked difference between material from $BHK21/C_{13}$ and C_{13}/B_4 cells, with a proportionately larger amount of radioactivity derived from C_{13}/B_4 in the higher molecular weight region.

Surface membranes of $BHK21/C_{13}$ and C_{13}/B_4 were digested with pronase and chromatographed on columns of Sephadex G-50. A fucose-containing material of higher molecular weight was found in the surface membrane of the transformed cell. However, the membrane of the normal cell also appeared to have a small amount of this material, as evidenced by a slight shoulder in this region.

When trypsinates of normal and transformed cells labeled with fucose were treated with pronase and chromatographed on columns of Sephadex G-50, a distinct peak of fucose-containing material was seen in the elution pattern of C_{13}/B_4 and C_{13}/SR_7 cells, while only a trace of a peak was seen in the same region in the elution pattern of normal cells. When the isotopic labels were reversed, similar patterns and differences were found. When a trypsinate from C_{13}/B_4 cells labeled with ^{14}C-fucose was co-chromatographed on Sephadex G-50 with a trypsinate from C_{13}/SR_7 labeled with ^{3}H-fucose, the fucose-containing peaks of the two transformed cells eluted in precisely the same area. In many experiments, this peak has always been observed, but it has been noted that there is some variation in its shape. Undoubtedly its composition is rather complex.

Digestion of trypsinates and membranes by pronase removes the vast bulk of protein, leaving polysaccharides and oligosaccharides attached to short polypeptide chains. To show that the patterns described above were not the result of incomplete or differential digestion by pronase, cells were labeled with ^{14}C- or ^{3}H-labeled phenylalanine, leucine, and valine; the trypsinates of these cells were digested with pronase and then chromatographed on Sephadex G-50. No radioactivity remained in the area where differences were seen in fucose-containing peaks. Similar results have been obtained using amino acid-labeled membranes.

The experiments in which fucose was employed have shown a clear difference between the surface structures of dividing cells before and after transformation with two strains of Rous virus. As stated before, essentially all of the radioactive fucose was recovered as such. Further, fucose has a limited discrete distribution. These two factors probably aided in the detection of the distinct and reproducible changes described.

Experiments similar to those detailed above have been done using ^{14}C- and ^{3}H-glucosamine, and here the results are not as clear. Glucosamine can be converted to galactosamine and sialic acids, and some might be deaminated. The hexosamines have a widespread distribution in glycoproteins and in mucopolysaccharides. Labeling with this isotope may, therefore, result in a complex elution pattern.

Comparisons of surface membranes from trypsinized cells labeled with ^{14}C- and ^{3}H-glucosamine and dissolved in SDS and chromatographed on Sephadex G-200 show that the material from C_{13}/B_4 is of larger size and comes off the column earlier than that from BHK21/C_{13}. Cochromatography of the trypsinates on columns of Sephadex G-200 shows a peak of the material completely excluded from the column. This peak consists largely of mucopolysaccharide, because treatment with hyaluronidase reduces it by half. A second peak follows in which the material from C_{13}/B_4 tends to migrate ahead of the corresponding material derived from BHK21/C_{13}. This shift was not clearly seen when material from C_{13}/SR_7 cells was compared with that from BHK-21/C_{13} cells. In other experiments, the trypsinates of BHK21/C_{13} cells grown with ^{14}C-glucosamine and of virus-transformed cells grown in the presence of ^{3}H-glucosamine were digested with pronase and cochromatographed on columns of Sephadex G-50. An initial hyaluronidase-sensitive material was completely excluded by the column migrating with blue dextran. In a second region, the material derived from C_{13}/B_4 migrated ahead of that from BHK21/C_{13}. The material in this region cochromatographed with the high molecular weight, fucose-containing peak present in growing virus-transformed cells. A third region consisted of small material migrating just ahead of the phenol red marker.

There was some variability in the elution pattern when various preparations of glucosamine-labeled material were used. However, the more rapid migration of the material from C_{13}/B_4 was always seen in the middle region of the runs. When one preparation was cochromatographed on several occasions, it always gave the same pattern. Elution patterns of pronase digests of glucosamine-labeled membranes were very complex, making it difficult to resolve any major differences.

Experiments have been done in which normal and virus-transformed cells were labeled with phenylalanine, leucine, and valine (^{14}C and ^{3}H), and their trypsinates and membranes compared by cochromatography on columns of Sephadex G-200. The elution patterns of the normal and transformed cells were very similar, and no real differences were found. It cannot be concluded from these results that the protein populations are identical. This problem will have to be resolved using more sensitive methods of protein fractionation than size-distribution on Sephadex columns.

In these studies, peaks of materials eluting with the phenol red marker at the end of the column run were always seen, regardless of the isotopic precursor used. This low molecular weight was variable in quantity. Neither the size, pattern, nor position of this material could be correlated with viral transformation.

To see whether the changes observed in cells transformed by Rous virus (C_{13}/B_4) were peculiar to this system or were of a more general nature, dividing C_{13}/B_4 cells and C_{13}/PyY cells (kindly supplied by Dr. R. A. Roosa, Wistar Institute, Philadelphia) (transformed by polyoma virus) were labeled with ^{14}C- and ^{3}H-fucose, respectively, and trypsinized. The trypsinates were mixed and digested with pronase and cochromatographed on columns of Sephadex G-50. A radioactive peak was seen in the elution pattern of material derived from C_{13}/PyY cells that was in the same location as that of the early-eluting peak from C_{13}/B_4 cells. Experiments have been done with the mouse cell line, Balb/3T3,[2] and with its counterpart RSV-3T3, transformed by Rous sarcoma virus (cell lines kindly supplied by Dr. G. J. Todaro, National Institutes of Health, Bethesda). Here a fucose-containing peak appears in the transformed cells which is not detected in the normal counterpart.

We can therefore conclude that upon transformation of baby hamster kidney cells (BHK21/C_{13}) with two strains of Rous virus (RNA virus), or with polyoma virus (DNA virus), or upon transforming a mouse cell with RSV (RNA virus), one or more macromolecules containing fucose localized on the cell surface and in the surface membrane appear in relatively large quantity. The evidence suggests that there is some heterogeneity in the "fucose peak" that appears. There is also evidence that there are similar fucose-containing materials present in cells before viral transformation but in small and variable quantities. This is indicated by the presence of a shoulder in the elution pattern of material of normal cells in the same region in which appears the distinct fucose-containing peak of transformed cells.

In the experiments described, cells were labeled only when they were actively dividing. To see whether the same elution patterns would be obtained with materials from cells when not dividing, experiments have been done in which cells were labeled with ^{14}C- and ^{3}H-fucose only after they had reached confluency and were in a plateau phase of growth. The pronase digests of either trypsinates or membranes, in various combinations, were cochromatographed on columns of Sephadex G-50. The results show that trypsinates and membranes from C_{13}/B_4 cells in plateau phase contain much less of the large, fucose-containing material than is present in the same cells when actively dividing. The peak is undetectable in the membrane, although it is still detectable in the trypsinate. Little or none of this material is seen in nondividing, normal cells (BHK21/C_{13}). However, even in actively dividing normal cells, there is only a small amount present. From the data, it would seem that the quantity of the fucose-containing material in the surface of transformed cells is growth-dependent. It is clearly present in actively dividing, transformed cells, and, to some extent, in actively dividing normal cells. When the cell stops dividing, it decreases sharply in amount. At the present time, the significance of these findings is unknown.

It is not possible to say at this time how this material arises. The peak itself could consist of one or more materials, most probably glycoprotein, containing L-fucose, and probably D-glucosamine and its derivatives, D-galactosamine and sialic acids. It might simply be synthesized in greater amounts in the transformed cell and incorporated to a greater extent into the surface membrane. It might also be degraded at a slower rate in transformed cells. Finally, it is possible that the protein is always there, but upon transformation (or during mitosis), new sugars such as L-fucose are added to pre-existing structures. The new additions of sugars might occur because new specific glycosyl transferases are formed or are activated. If this is so, the material in the "fucose peak" area could provide specific acceptor substrate for the transferase (s). It has been shown by Bosmann et al.[4] that upon transformation of 3T3 by polyoma virus, the activity of several glycosyl transferases increases. At the present time, efforts are being made to purify and analyze the material(s) in the "fucose peak" area.

Acknowledgments

This work was supported by U. S. Public Health Service Grant 5P01 AI07005-05, and American Cancer Society Grants PRP-28, E-539, and PRA-68.

References

1. Abercrombie, M., and J. E. M. Heaysman: Expl. Cell Res., 6:293, 1954.
2. Aaronson, S. A., and G. J. Todaro: J. Cell Physiol., 72:141, 1968.
3. Boas, N. F.: J. Biol. Chem., 204:353, 1953.
4. Bosmann, H. B., A. Hagopian, and E. H. Eylar: J. Cell Physiol., 72:81, 1968.

5. Burger, M. M.: Nature, 219:499, 1968.
6. Coman, D. R.: Cancer Res., 4:625, 1944.
7. Coman, D. R.: Cancer Res., 21:1436, 1961.
8. Cox, R. P., and B. M. Gesner: Proc. Nat. Acad. Sci. USA, 54:1571, 1965.
9. Cox, R. P., and B. M. Gesner: Cancer Res., 28:1162, 1968.
10. DeLong, R. P., D. R. Coman, and F. Zeidman: Cancer, 3:718, 1950.
11. Hakomori, S. I., C. Teather, and H. Andres: Biochem. Biophys. Res. Com., 33:563, 1968.
12. Inbar, M., and L. Sachs: Nature, 223:710, 1969.
13. Lenhardt, W. F., and R. J. Winzler: J. Chromotog., 34:471, 1968.
14. Levine, M., Y. Becker, C. W. Boone, and H. Eagle: Proc. Nat. Acad. Sci. USA, 53:350, 1965.
15. Meezan, E., H. C. Wu, P. M. Black, and P. W. Robbins: Biochemistry, 8:2518, 1969.
16. Mora, P. T., R. O. Brady, R. M. Bradley, and V. W. McFarland: Proc. Nat. Acad. Sci. USA, 63:1290.
17. Spiro, R. G.: J. Biol. Chem., 240:1603, 1965.
18. Svennerholm, L.: Acta Chem. Scand., 12:547, 1958.
19. Warren, L.: J. Biol. Chem., 234:1971, 1959.
20. Warren, L., and M. C. Glick: In: Fundamental Techniques in Virology (K. Habel and N. P. Salzman, eds.) , Academic Press, New York, 1969, p. 66.
21. Wu, H. C., L. Meezan, P. H. Black, and P. W. Robbins: Biochemistry, 8:2509, 1969.
22. Glick, M. C., et al.: In preparation.

14

Cellular and Molecular Mechanisms of Carcinogenesis: A Rapporteur Report

Carcinogenesis — Cellular and Molecular Mechanisms

R. J. C. HARRIS

Department of Environmental Carcinogenesis,
Imperial Cancer Research Fund, London, England

Reactive Forms of Chemical Carcinogens and Their Interactions with Tissue Components

IT IS EXACTLY 40 years, said Elizabeth Miller in her introductory paper, since Kennaway and Hieger announced the carcinogenicity of 1:2:5:6-dibenzanthracene (the first synthetic polycyclic hydrocarbon) for mouse skin, and only now were we approaching a unified view of chemical carcinogenesis—the idea that most, if not all, the ultimate reactive forms are strong electrophiles and attack the nucleophilic sites in the cell such as are found in nucleic acids and proteins.

Figure 14-1 (which I have adapted from a diagram from the article on Ribosomes by M. Nomura in Scientific American, October, 1969) shows the categories of DNA, RNA, and protein. The DNA genetic code is transcribed as messenger (m) RNA and this is translated into protein by the ribosome-tRNA synthesizing system.

The first target for agents which produce heritable changes in cells is obviously DNA. Philip Lawley presented the evidence for himself and his colleagues that alkylating agents can react, for example, at guanine-N-7, or O-6 or C-8. The alteration in purine and pyrimidine bases can result in depurination of the DNA, in mispairing during replication, and in changes in conformation of the DNA molecule. Reactive forms of the carcinogenic hydrocarbons, aminoazo dyes, and aromatic amines and amides all react with DNA, but the exact sites of reaction and the relationship between them remain to be determined, and so does the extent to which repair processes can excise the damaged bases and reconstitute the molecule. I. Bernard Weinstein found no direct evidence for a somatic mutation theory of carcinogenesis presumed by proponents of heritable changes. Carcinogens may change the cytoplasmic environment, for example, by modification of RNA, and interrupt the "genetic message" in this way. N-Acetoxyacetylaminofluorene, for example, may select guanosine residues in single-strand loops of tRNA and thus change the conformation of the molecule, the nature of this change being influenced by the base sequences adjacent to guanosine. Such disturbances in RNA translation could have secondary consequences with respect to cell differentiation, regulation, and autonomy.

Carcinogen-protein interactions have been studied since the first report of James and Elizabeth Miller in 1947. Hiroshi Terayama has isolated a series of polar dyes from the livers of rats treated either acutely or continuously with azo dye. The polar dyes are compounds of dye metabolite and an amino acid, and are extractable with butanol from pronase digests of total liver proteins. Cysteine, tyrosine, and methionine derivatives have been characterized. Liver arginase was first postulated as the dye-binding protein. However, the most efficient receptor is a nonbasic cell-sap protein which is deleted from the liver during the early period of dye feeding. Later, though, another dye-binding protein appears.

Tumor cells do not spring unheralded from normal cells, at least not in vivo, and so the consequences of carcinogen interaction with cell macromolecules should be apparent in the initiation of the carcinogenic process. Emmanuel Farber and his colleagues have studied the hyperplastic liver nodules which first arise when acetylaminofluorene (or aflatoxin or ethionine) are fed to rats. These cells are the precursors of the tumors, and the population may be distinguished both structurally and biochemically from surrounding normal liver. There is an aberrant glycogen in these cells (possibly with bound carcinogen) and an "altered" DNA. The nodules may be cultivated in vitro (unlike normal rat-liver) and will there differentiate into ducts.

Not only do we now see common pathways in the enzymic conversion of carcinogens to active forms, but we have an explanation for such refractory species of animals as guinea pigs and, possibly, for more resistant individuals. It is conceivable that the heavy cigarette smokers who do not contract lung cancer are protected by cellular enzyme systems which, on balance, convert the carcinogens to inactive metabolites rather than to active forms.

Chemical Carcinogenesis In Vitro

Leo Sachs described the characteristics of hamster embryo cells transformed in vitro by carcinogens. The new clones, whether produced by chemical, physical, or viral carcinogens, had a similar phenotype, including continuous growth in vitro (normal cells grow for only limited periods) and the production of tumors in vivo. The transformed cells also showed characteristic changes in cell surface membranes: the exposure of agglutinable sites and the induction of specific neoantigens.

Katherine Sanford believes that almost all cell lines (embryonic, neonatal, or adult from rats, mice, or hamsters) will, in time, transform spontaneously without deliberate addition of a known carcinogen. C3H mouse embryo cells, grown by Evans and Andersen in a chemically-defined medium with either gelding horse or fetal calf serum, transformed within 90 to 180 days in the horse-serum medium but required several years in the fetal calf. Three spontaneously transformed lines studied were cross-reactive antigenically and were found to contain "C type" particles.

Charles Heidelberger, Sukdeb Mondal, and their colleagues have differed from other groups who have used embryo cells in deriving a quantitative system for transforming a permanent line of C3H adult mouse prostate cells with polycyclic hydrocarbon carcinogens. They found first that the dose-response curves for toxicity and transformation were quite different and second, that it was possible to transform single cells with methylcholanthrene with 100% efficiency. This appears to answer two of the three possible questions related to cellular mechanisms of carcinogenesis in vitro: first, whether transformation is direct, and second, whether (pre)transformed cells are selected from a mixed population by differential toxicity. The third possibility, activation of a latent virus, still remains open, although antigens associated with the murine sarcoma-leukemia group were not found. The transformed cell clones grew like tumors in C3H mice and, moreover, although 14 of 17 clones were immunogenic in seven pairs studied, the immunity was not cross-reactive.

Japanese investigators of carcinogenesis in vitro have preferred to use 4-nitroquinoline-N-oxide (4NQO). Toshio Kuroki defined "transformation" of his hamster cells as the continuous proliferation of cells in vitro forming piled-up, dense layers. In the presence of even very low concentrations of 4NQO, or its metabolites, transformation in this sense took only 20 to 40 days. Progression to malignancy required several further passages of the cells, which then produced fibrosarcomas in hamsters. Two of 12 control cell lines transformed after 260 days in vitro.

Hajim Katsuta used a line of liver parenchymal cells, derived from two- to three-week-old rats, and the age was critical. They were transformed by 4NQO within 25 days, and after four months in culture gave tumors on transplantation into rats. Control lines also became malignant, but only after 17 months.

There was much discussion of the question of phenotype reversion. Sachs found that chemically-transformed hamster cells could lose all their "markers" and revert to normal (virally transformed cells retained their capacity for continuous cultivation in vitro)—but then are cells in vitro normal, or half-transformed? Most will transform spontaneously if given enough time (and loving care). Revertants, in Sachs' system, first gained extra chromosomes, and then lost some of these selectively. Whether such processes can be found to occur in tumors in vivo remains to be discovered.

Charles Heidelberger recorded one other fascinating observation. When the prostate cell number is increased from one to 1,000, the efficiency of transformation is reduced from 100% to 10%. Do transformed cells inhibit each other? Is this why tumors arising from carcinogens in vivo appear to originate from very few cells?—a query raised by Donald Metcalf.

These must be regarded as model systems, but as such, may enable chemical carcinogenesis to catch up with viral carcinogenesis since, despite their lead, says Heidelberger, virologists still do not fully understand the mechanisms of viral oncogenesis.

Biologic Aspects of Cell-Virus Interaction

Just how much understanding of viral oncogenesis the virologists have, we discovered in the next two sessions.

Hilary Koprowski is investigating vertical transmission of viruses (so important a concept in murine and avian leukemia) by infecting mouse eggs and sperm. In the course of this, not only has he shown that the spermatozoa could "integrate" SV40 DNA but also that, in SV40 virus-transformed mouse cells, an "embryonic" species-specific antigen appeared, probably as a result of derepression.

In the near future, he believes, there should be an investigation of the part played by pseudovirions (which encapsidate normal DNA) in transduction. Moreover, we had all been thinking in terms of one cell-one virus, and we should have to turn our attention to interactions between viruses (some of them latent) in the same cell.

There were, said Michael Stoker, three essential criteria for viral transformation by polyoma and SV40 viruses. First, continued cell survival and multiplication; second, expression of the transforming genes; and third, stable perpetuation of the viral genome. These he illustrated by reference to his own polyoma: BHK21 cell system. The first requirement (cell survival) implied that cytocidal ("late") genes of the virus must not be expressed—so that no virus is produced by the transformed cells. It is possible that permissive cells (e.g. mouse, for polyoma virus) are transformed by mutant viruses—defective for "late" gene functions. Only 2 to 4% of BHK21 cells undergo stable transformation by polyoma. The remainder (at very high multiplicities) possibly undergo an abortive transformation. These cells grow to clones of about 32 cells (with the characteristics of stable transformation) but then revert to normal. It appears, therefore, that the second criterion (expression of the transforming genes) is inadequate by itself unless it is followed by the third (stable perpetuation). An important feature of viral transformation may be that the transformants require less of a serum factor to initiate the cell cycle and thus have a survival advantage in conditions of high density (or in suspension). Revertants also occurred in this system, but these could be differentiated from abortants.

The oncogenic DNA viruses can apparently contribute more than viral genes, since Sachs has found that lethally-irradiated cells could be "restored" by infection with oncogenic DNA viruses. Is this perhaps where the transducing pseudovirions play a role?

The failure of "late" genes to be expressed in transformation may be a result of inhibition by specific cellular factors. Roland Cassingena has identified a "repressor" in extracts of SV40-transformed hamster, mouse, or cat cells. It inhibits plaque formation by SV40 in infected monkey cells, at suitable dilution and in the presence of basic proteins such as poly-L-lysine or poly-L-ornithine, which stimulate pinocytosis. "Repressor" is not found in cells transformed by adenovirus 12, polyoma, or methylcholanthrene, and it does not inhibit VS, polio I, vaccinia, or herpesvirus in the monkey cells. Small quantities of "repressor," which has the properties of a protein, are found in cells productively infected by SV40, and uninfected permissive cells contain a substance which neutralizes its activity.

Molecular Aspects of Cell-Virus Interaction

The transcription of SV40 genome, i.e. from DNA to mRNA (Figure 14-1), was discussed by Gerhard Sauer. In productively-infected cells, it occurs sequentially. By six hours after infection, "early mRNAs" are being synthesized and by seventeen hours, "late mRNA" transcription begins. SV40 virus-transformed 3T3 mouse cells contain mRNA with 40% homology with mRNA from productively infected cells, and most of this was with "early-mRNA." All of the viral genes necessary for transformation and virus replication are present in SV40-3T3 cells, since fusion with permissive cells leads to production of fully infectious SV40 virus. The degree of function of the viral genome in the transformed cells may thus be important, and this may be controlled by cellular factors—for example, by something like Cassingena's "repressor" molecules.

Other cellular factors (SV40 essential replicative factor—acronym,

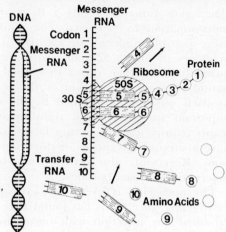

FIG. 14–1.—DNA, RNA, and protein categories. (Adapted from M. Nomura, Scientific American, October, 1969).

SERF) were described by Saul Kit in SV40-permissive cell lines, in rabbit kidney cell lines, and in some primary hamster and human cells. When SV40 is "rescued" from transformed mouse or hamster cells by fusion with susceptible monkey kidney cells, virus appears first in the nucleus of the transformed cell and then infects the susceptible cell, which provides SERF. The decisive step is the release of the SV40 DNA from integration (excision) and, in some transformed hamster cell lines, this may be achieved directly, e.g. with mitomycin C. One may speculate as to how far this process of excision is the opposite of integration, and to what extent abortive transformation (a far more common event than true transformation, as Stoker has shown) is regulated by similar factors. The possibility that SERF inactivates repressor was suggested by Fred Rapp, who could not detect repressor in a variety of SV40-transformed cells.

An important question for the small oncogenic DNA viruses is how much of the virus genome is occupied in coding for the manufacture of virus itself, for this may determine (in the simplest manner) how much is "left over" for transformation. William Murakami presented some elegant analyses of viral polypeptides for polyoma, SV40, and an adenovirus. Fortunately, oncogenic viruses can, even if present in only a single copy, provide at least one "gene" for transformation as well as providing for their own synthesis.

The RNA of the avian tumor viruses is more complex. Some low molecular weight (4S) RNA is associated, in the virus, with 70S. This 4S RNA has been shown to act as tRNA for at least 15 amino acids. Some of the coat molecules of the avian tumor viruses act as type-specific antigens mediating host-cell range and interference between subgroups. An internal component contributes a group-specific antigen

(Cofal). William Robinson could distinguish six proteins for RSV (O) $_\beta$. In comparison with RAV1, two of these were different and four indistinguishable. A group-specific antigen had also been found in leukosis-free chick embryo cells, confirming an earlier report by Dougherty and DiStefano.

Let me summarize these two sessions very briefly in terms of the, as yet, unanswered questions: Are the oncogenic DNA viruses which transform cells actually defective for "late" functions, or are these excluded or inhibited in some way? What determines whether the DNA is integrated? What determines the induction of new antigens which may, or may not, be demonstrable? What determines the "excision" of the DNA—apparently the prerequisite for viral synthesis in heterokaryons? As Charles Heidelberger says, the virologists have indeed a long way still to go.

Tumor-Specific Antigens

So that we may all agree on our terminology, Figure 14-2 is a summary of the relationship between a transforming (DNA) virus and the tumor-specific antigens. For most oncogenic DNA viruses, no virus synthesis occurs, and viral antigens (as distinct from virus-specified antigens) are not found. This simple picture may not be true for all DNA viruses and is inaccurate for oncogenic RNA viruses, also, since direct integration of RNA into the cell's genome is impossible and, where the malignant cells synthesize virus, viral antigens will appear in membranes and intracellular fluids.

Werner Henle outlined the properties of the herpeslike (EB) virus first discovered by Epstein and Barr in cultures of Burkitt lymphoma cells. EB virus has apparently a world-wide distribution, and it was a great step forward when Werner and Gertrude Henle showed that it was a cause of infectious mononucleosis in young Caucasian adults. Three methods of investigation of sera and cells from patients and controls each utilize virus-specified antigens. The first, devised by the Henles, visualizes viral capsid antigens; the second, on cell cultures in-

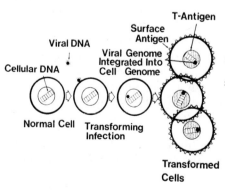

FIG. 14–2.—Summary of the relationship between a transforming (DNA) virus and the tumor-specific antigens.

fected with virus, early induced antigens; and the third (from the Klein's Laboratory), cell membrane antigens specified by the virus. The sera from Burkitt lymphoma patients score in all three tests. Recently, similar antibodies to a similar virus and its specified antigens have been found in patients with carcinoma of the postnasal space. Despite the widespread occurrence of the virus, Burkitt lymphoma patients have a much higher antibody titer to capsid and membrane antigens than do normal controls. Some patients with chronic lymphatic leukemia or Hodgkin's disease also have high titers. Significantly, the long-term survival of the lymphoma patients correlated well with their antibody titers to the early antigens.

Similar herpeslike viruses have been found in association with lymphoid cell lines from apparently normal individuals, as well as those with leukemia. A herpeslike virus is the cause of Marek's disease of chickens (a malignant lymphoproliferative disease), and of kidney tumors in leopard frogs.

An unrelated herpesvirus (2) has recently been found in association with cervical carcinoma, especially in promiscuous women, but its etiologic significance also remains to be determined.

EB virus has not produced tumors in experimental animals, but transformation of lymphoid cells in vitro has been observed by Paul Gerber, by the Henles, and by John Pope.

In the light of spontaneous transformation of mouse cells in vitro, of the possibilities of virus interaction, and of the recently propounded theory of oncogenes and type-C particles (Huebner and Todaro), what Janet Hartley had to say about the detection of murine leukemia virus-induced antigens was most timely. The viruses (Type C particles) all form members of one large group. Most of them are produced in, and bud from, external or internal membranes of infected cells, so there are virus-specified cell membrane antigens and also viral membrane antigens (where virus develops). Soluble envelope protein antigens are found in plasma and tissue extracts which, like the surface antigens, are virus type-specific. A soluble group-specific antigen may be detected by immunodiffusion, complement fixation, or immune fluorescence. This is always associated with the appearance of infectious virus. All naturally occurring strains of mouse leukemia virus are found in one subgroup, and all are neutralized by rat antiserum to Gross passage A virus, but not normally by antiserum to the second subgroup FMR (Friend, Moloney, Rauscher). Graffi's virus appears to be distinct from these, and may represent a third subgroup.

The problem of cross-reactivity in immunogenic methylcholanthrene-induced mouse sarcomas was raised again by Charles McKhann. Fifteen tumors gave no cross-reaction by transplantation tests, but two of five showed similarities in an anti-mouse globulin test, and 20 to 30% in more extensive tests by the colony-inhibition technique of Hellström and Sjögren. The amounts of seven normal H-2 antigens were found to vary (but not as between them) in five tumors examined, and the lower the amount of the normal antigens, the higher the amount of tumor-specific antigens. Moreover, and this was quite unexpected, the tendency of the tumor to metastasize paralleled the H-2 antigens and not the others. The author speculated on the distribution of the tumor-specific antigens in the light of the recent results from Aoki, Boyse, Old, and their colleagues on the distribution of H-2 antigens in clusters on the cell surface.

The final paper, by Paul Black, also showed quite clearly that the cell membranes are not only (now that the molecular biology of DNA-RNA-protein transcription and translation have been analyzed) the next cell organelles for investigation but, more important, the methods for doing this are now being developed.

New surface antigens on, or in, cancer cells can arise not only by derepression—the carcinoembryonic antigens of colon carcinoma (Gold) and the α-fetoproteins of hepatoma are examples of this—but also by failure of synthesis. Thus the colon adenocarcinoma which failed to show blood group A substance could not synthesize A from H (O) by addition of terminal sugars. In an analogous way, Forssman antigens appear in polyoma-transformed hamster cells because the synthesis of A substance fails. Similarly, cytolipin replaces hematoside. There is biochemical evidence that the necessary sugars are not transferred to the membrane because of a deficiency in the transferase enzymes responsible.

In his opening address to this session, Richmond Prehn warned against an easy optimism. "Tumor antigens," he said, "are, this time, here to stay," but "enthusiasm for the immunologic approach to cancer prevention, diagnosis and therapy may eventually, again, be somewhat dampened. It is safer to assume," he went on, "that most 'spontaneous' and some experimentally-induced tumors have little or no measurable immunogenicity."

The induction of tumors in immunologically deprived animals is still not clear experimentally. In discussion, some examples were given. Trainin found more spontaneous lung adenomas in mice treated with antilymphocyte serum (ALS). However, another discussant had found no difference in spontaneous tumor incidence in a large group of mice treated with ALS. Thymectomized mice were more susceptible to adenovirus 12 (Yohn) and to polyoma (Defendi). Immunologically incompetent individuals usually seem (in half the cases) to get leukemia or lymphomas—and one might wonder which came first?

The most clinically promising approach, said Prehn, is the nonspecific stimulation of host response, but there is a danger that overconcentration on immunity may reduce the attention given to other homeostatic mechanisms which may be far more important for the control of early tumors.

Chemical carcinogenesis appears at last to be approaching uniformity in terms of the nature of the reactive intermediates. The types of interaction of chemical carcinogens with DNA, RNA, and protein targets can now be envisaged and, as homeostatic mechanisms in mammalian cells are increasingly understood in molecular terms, we can anticipate understanding both chemical and viral carcinogenesis at the molecular level. The in vitro systems that will make this possible now exist for both chemicals and viruses. At the same time, increasing knowledge of the structure of cell membranes and of pathways of membrane biosynthesis will enable us to analyze the molecular changes which occur in tumor cell membranes, changes which at present we can only recognize immunologically.

This has been a conference in which everyone will have learned something, and I should like to pay tribute to James Miller, the Chairman, for his meticulous handling of it.

Acknowledgments

I gratefully acknowledge the help of Mr. D. Auger, F.R.P.S., who prepared the figures (and slides therefrom).

Part B

REGULATION OF GENE EXPRESSION

15

Molecular Biology of the Gene

Historical Perspectives

WENDELL M. STANLEY

Departments of Biochemistry and Molecular Biology and the Virus Laboratory, University of California, Berkeley, California, USA

A NEW SCIENCE within biology began to emerge about 30 years ago involving interactions between the chemical, physical, immunologic, and genetic aspects of biology. Although this new area of science was recognized and selected by Warren Weaver for special and continuing support by the Rockefeller Foundation in 1933, and a section entitled "Molecular Biology" appeared in a Foundation report in 1938, the expression "Experimental Biology" continued to be used to describe this activity in Foundation reports. In a 1951 report it was stated that experimental biology had become molecular biology, and in 1957 the term "molecular biology" was used in the Foundation Annual Report to describe this activity. By this time molecular biology was in full flower, with important discoveries being made with increasing frequency and with departments or institutes of molecular biology being organized within universities. The concept of molecular biology had arrived, and its usefulness as a special approach to many important problems was widely recognized. Studies on the molecular biology of the gene have probably yielded more important advances and useful knowledge than in any other area. This information, as well as special concepts that have been developed from this information, are now beginning to be applied to the cancer problem. I shall review some of these advances involving the molecular biology of the gene, and then discuss the applications, currently being made to the tumor viruses, which seem to me to be especially promising in connection with an understanding of the problem of cancer in man.

Perhaps the first time gene action was thought of in terms of a biochemical action was in the description by the English physician, Sir

Archibald Garrod, in 1909, of the disease alkaptonuria. He considered that a change in a gene resulted in the failure to produce an enzyme, and this caused the disease. Unfortunately, his idea failed to attract attention and was overlooked until the work of Beadle and Tatum in 1941 on neurospora which firmly established the one-gene, one-enzyme concept. About this time Delbrück, Hershey, and Luria took up the study of bacterial viruses and started what came to be known as the "phage group." This group and the adherents it attracted over the years made brilliant discoveries having to do with the manner of growth, mechanism of replication of DNA, mechanics of mutation and of genetic recombination, temperature-sensitive mutants, and genetic fine structure within the bacterial viruses. This work did much to bring enthusiasm and to secure support for molecular biology.

A few years earlier, I had isolated tobacco mosaic virus in the form of a crystallizable material which was soon shown to be a nucleoprotein. Although there was a considerable amount of reluctance on the part of many scientists, especially those medically trained, to accept the fact that virus activity could reside in a crystallizable nucleoprotein, the tobacco mosaic work did start a stream of molecular biologic research that has continued to grow. It was realized that viruses were literally bits of genetic material encased in a protective coat made up largely of protein that displayed their biologic activity only within certain susceptible cells, and in so doing altered the metabolism of such cells.

In 1944, Avery, MacLeod, and McCarty reported their isolation of the transforming principle of pneumococci in the form of DNA, thus establishing for the first time the most significant and very important fact that DNA could possess and transmit genetic information. Unfortunately, because many scientists considered proteins to be important in genetic transmission and because of the general acceptance of the tetranucleotide theory for the structure of DNA, the scientific climate was such that the significance of this great discovery remained virtually unrecognized, and it was some years before it affected the trend of science. Two events of 1951 that were to have an effect on subsequent developments were the discovery of transduction by Lederberg and Zinder and the description by Pauling of the α helix for the structure of peptides and proteins. It was not until 1952, when Hershey and Chase published their famous experiments showing that the genetic information of bacterial viruses was carried in their DNA, that there started a gradual acceptance of DNA as the carrier and transmitter of genetic information. Also in 1952, Schachman, Pardee, and Stanier reported on the isolation of ribosomes and the fact that they contained RNA and not DNA. In 1956, Fraenkel-Conrat and Gierer and Schramm made the important discovery that virus activity of tobacco mosaic virus nucleoprotein was carried solely by the RNA of the virus, thus proving for the first time that RNA could also carry and transmit genetic information. Earlier Markham had, on the basis of work with turnip yellow mosaic virus, expressed the view "that the nucleic acid is in fact the substance directly controlling virus multiplication," but the evidence was not as convincing as that which came later.

Watson and Crick revolutionized scientific thought by their presentation, in 1953, of the double helix for the structure of DNA and the implications for the mechanism of replication which were obvious from that structure. Conceptually, this represented a great forward step that brought forth an avalanche of new and exciting discoveries related to the replication and functioning of both types of nucleic acids, the storage and transfer of genetic information, and cellular control mechanisms. DNA and RNA were synthesized in vitro, messenger RNA was discovered, the genetic code was broken, and a gene and gene repressor were isolated. The genetics and control mechanisms, at least within the bacterial cell *Escherichia coli,* were pretty well worked out and understood, and openings were made for similar studies on the more important and much more complex mammalian cells.

Molecular biology had made monumental advances and was now ready to move on to the remaining important problems such as differentiation, control mechanisms within mammalian cells, including inborn errors of metabolism and cancer, and to problems involving the nervous system and the mind. Of these, I now propose to concentrate on a special approach to the cancer problem which is provided by the viruses.

Just before the turn of the century, and about the time of the discovery of viruses, Sanarelli found that a tumor of rabbits called myxoma was caused by an agent which Moses proved in 1911 to be a virus. Then, in 1908, Ellermann and Bang reported that a virus was responsible for fowl leukemia. Rous discovered, in 1911, the virus of chickens which came to be known as the Rous sarcoma virus. A year earlier Fujinami and Inamoto described a myxosarcoma of chickens which, in 1914, they proved to be caused by a virus. A controversy developed as to whether such growths were true cancers. It was thought by many that if the sarcoma was a real cancer it could not possibly be caused by a virus. As a result, the real significance of these discoveries was not recognized until many years later. Even when Shope, in 1932, described two new rabbit viruses, one causing papillomas and the other fibromas, when Lucke, also in 1932, found than an adenocarcinoma of the kidney of the leopard frog was caused by a virus, and Bittner reported on his mouse mammary cancer agent in 1936, the time was still not ripe for general acceptance of the significance of this work.

Extensive documentation of work on viral cancers and a thorough exposition of the real and potential significance of this work was published by Rous in 1936, but this splendid presentation fell on deaf ears. For a period of over 15 years only a few investigators worked on virus-cancer relationships. The field attracted attention in 1951 when

Gross obtained a viral preparation which caused leukemia when injected into newborn mice. He noted, in 1953, that his viral preparations would also cause growth in the salivary glands and concluded, from heat inactivation and differential filtration experiments, that these were caused by a virus different from the leukemia virus. About this time I became interested in the relationships between viruses and cancer, and in a general sessions address before the Second National Cancer Conference in 1952 I stated the following: "Twenty years ago the relationship between viruses and cancer was scarcely mentioned and when it was, one had to speak softly. Today large and well-attended conferences are held on this same subject and virus-induced tumors in animals and plants are accepted generally. It is timely, therefore, to focus our attention on viruses and the cancer problem despite great gaps in our information. . . . I shall concentrate on those properties of viruses which I believe to be most pertinent to the cancer problem. I refer to mutation, to the latency phenomenon of viruses in their hosts, to the incubation period of viruses in their vectors, to the masking of viruses in their hosts, to the phenomenon of interference, to the problem of the origin of viruses including particularly the question as to whether they can arise from normal constituents of cells, to the lysogenic bacteria story and to the role which the concept of cells literally growing away from a virus, may play." I ended the address with the following: "Because viruses are marked by a special activity, which in some cases results in tumors, and in other cases in the regression of tumors, because some, at least, are stable and crystallizable nucleoproteins, because they can enter into and direct the metabolic chain of events within cells and because they can mutate with marked changes in properties, they afford a most attractive experimental approach to the cancer problem. The viruses provide a major and several minor keys to the hearts of cells, and the innermost secrets of cells, including the cancer problem, are ours if we but ask the correct questions."

In 1957, Stewart and Eddy grew the salivary gland virus of Gross to high titers in tissue culture and, because it caused a variety of tumors in mice, they called it polyoma virus. Huebner and associates found that polyoma was essentially a natural infection of mice, generally causing few symptoms in nature, but the virus could cause cancer in rats and hamsters. An early significant finding was that the virus seemed to disappear from the transformed hamster cells. In 1962, Enders found that a virus isolated from monkey kidney cells by Hillemann, and called SV40, would grow in, and cause transformation of, human cells, and Trentin found that some human adenoviruses would grow in hamsters and cause cancer. A variety of mouse and avian tumor or leukemia viruses were isolated and subjected to investigation by dozens of investigators. Thus, within a 10-year period, numerous investigators had been attracted to the virus-cancer field. But at the Third National Cancer Conference in 1956 I noted that ". . . I must say that I continue to be amazed at the willingness of so many investigators to accept viruses as etiologic agents for animal cancers and their unwillingness to consider them of etiologic importance in cancers of man. Cancer is a biologic and not a theologic problem. The fact that only two little studied and benign virus-induced tumors of man are known and that viruses have not yet been seriously implicated in human cancer does not mean that they are not there and that they are not of etiologic importance. It could mean only that, with the exceptions noted, the very few really serious attempts to prove the presence of a virus were unsuccessful for one reason or another. Basic biologic phenomena generally do not differ strikingly as one goes from one species to another, and I regard the fact, now proved beyond contention, that viruses can cause cancer in animals to be directly pertinent to the human cancer problem. I believe that recent advances in the cultivation of human cells in vitro and especially the newer knowledge of certain properties of viruses warrant today a marked change in our thinking on the problem of human cancer. I believe the time has come when we should assume that viruses are responsible for most, if not all, kinds of cancer, including cancer in man, and design and execute our experiments accordingly. Cancer is basically a problem in growth, and there is no reason to believe that the growth of most human cells is different basically from the growth of most animal cells. Acceptance of the viral etiology of human cancer as a working hypothesis will involve a marked change in attitude on the part of many investigators, but this is necessary if the right approach and the right design of experimentation are to result. What we do depends in large measure upon what we think."

In 1963, the Hanafusas and Rubin made a discovery which was to have a very profound effect on the direction of research on virus-cancer relationships. The high-titer Bryan strain of Rous sarcoma virus commonly used was found to consist of a mixture of a high concentration of a leukemia virus, which would multiply in, but not cause transformation of, chick embryo cells, and a low concentration of a sarcoma virus that would cause transformation, but did not appear to yield infectious virus, unless subsequently the leukemia virus was added as a helper virus to the transformed cells. Although there are strains of avian sarcoma virus that can grow in chicken cells without helper virus, this strain of Rous sarcoma virus was thought to be defective by lacking the full information for making a complete protein coat, information which was provided by the helper leukemia virus. Extensive additional work by several investigators has provided evidence that the phenomenon, while basically true, is caused by complex virus-host relationships. Differences in the surface determinants of the virus and in genetically determined receptors of the cell result in differing susceptibilities of different host cells. Thus, some Rous sarcoma virus-transformed avian cells which appeared to be producing no infectious virus were actually producing viral particles, but these possessed a different host range. They would not infect most chick embryo cells, but were found infectious for Japanese quail embryo cells. By contrast, Rous sarcoma virus-transformed mammalian cells generally fail to produce infectious particles. This situation is similar to transformation caused by DNA tumor viruses, where transformation and virus production appear to be mutually exclusive.

The work on interactions between two different viruses stimulated exploration with other combinations, and significant information continues to be forthcoming. Huebner, Rowe, Melnick, Rapp, and associates made a variety of hybrids from different adenoviruses and SV40 which appeared to consist of a "defective" SV40 genome linked to adenovirus DNA enclosed in an adenovirus capsid provided by a helper adenovirus that could cause transformation of hamster cells with production of T antigens specific to both viruses but with no infectious adenovirus or SV40 virus. The ramifications of these investigations are large indeed. Just recently, Fischinger and O'Connor extended their observation that infection with an aggregate produced by centrifugation of "defective" mouse sarcoma virus and mouse leukemia virus produced a competent mouse sarcoma virus, to include a virus from another species. They centrifuged cat leukemia virus with the "defective" mouse sarcoma virus and obtained a focus-forming virus capable of indefinite propagation in cat cells but not in mouse cells. They also found that this virus, even after several passages in cat cells, could be caused to regain the ability to grow in mouse cells merely by centrifuging it with mouse leukemia virus. Huebner and associates extended this work by the trans-species rescue of defective mouse sarcoma virus with leukemia virus derived from cats. Hamster tumor cells, produced by the defective mouse sarcoma virus, were grown with cat embryo cells in the presence of cat leukemia virus. Later, suggestive evidence for the presence in hamsters of an indigenous C-type virus was obtained. The potential for investigating the interactions between different viral genomes and different viral capsids is great indeed, and many investigators are presently busily engaged in this work. The application to putative human cancer viruses is obvious, and this area is, of course, not being overlooked.

The actual state of the viral nucleic acid in transformed cells has intrigued scientists ever since the early observation by Shope that papillomas in wild rabbits yielded much infectious virus, whereas papillomas in domestic rabbits yielded little or no infectious virus. Later Ito found that virus activity was actually present in the papillomas of domestic rabbits, but in the form of nucleic acid with little or no protein coat since the production of the viral capsid was inefficient in this host.

The state of virus nucleic acid in hamster and mouse cells transformed by polyoma and SV40 viruses has been studied by several investigators. These viruses have ring-shaped DNA of a molecular weight of three million, equal to about six to 10 genes, of which at least one third are needed for the protein components. Dulbecco has evidence that in the 3T3 line of mouse cells transformed by polyoma or SV40 viruses there are about five and 20 viral DNA molecular equivalents, respectively, per cell and that this viral DNA is integrated in the cellular DNA. Evidence has also been obtained that detachment of integrated viral DNA can be accomplished by fusion with permissive cells in the case of SV40 virus, but as yet not in the case of polyoma. Studies on the transcription of the viral DNA indicate that no more than one third is necessary for transformation, hence no more than two or three genes may be involved. It is obvious that an understanding of the mechanism involved in one type of transformation is close at hand. Perhaps via the use of temperature-sensitive viral mutants the door will soon be opened.

How soon will it be possible to apply information gained from these model studies to human cancer? Since 1957, when Dmochowski reported the presence of unusual particles in sections from human lymphoma, particles resembling those which Bernhard and Guérin first clearly described and called C-type particles in 1958, increasing attention has been given to human cancer. DNA herpes-type virus has been isolated and grown in tissue culture from hundreds of patients with leukemia and lymphoma. These viral isolations are presently under intensive study. A virus responsible for malignant lymphomas in African and other children seems to be the causative agent for mononucleosis, and this relationship is under intensive study. When cultured human cells from patients with nonmalignant diseases such as Fanconi's anemia or Down's syndrome, which nevertheless increase the risk to cancer, are infected with SV40 or adenovirus 12, the probability of malignant transformation is much greater than with normal cells. RNA C-type viral particles are being found repeatedly in human leukemias and in some carcinomas. Although repeated attempts were made to grow such particles in cell culture, none was successful until recently when C-type virus from a human liposarcoma was grown by Morton, Hall and Malmgren. Antibodies in the serum of the patient from whom the culture was obtained reacted specifically with cytoplasmic antigens in the original liposarcoma and in the cultured cells.

Recently Huebner, Todaro, and co-workers have suggested that the cells of most or all vertebrate species, including man, have C-type RNA tumor virus genomes that are most commonly vertically transmitted from parent to offspring in a covert form. Depending upon host genotype and various modifying environmental factors, either virus production or tumor formation or both may develop in the host. They believe that carcinogens, irradiation, and the normal aging process all favor the partial or complete activation of these genes. They believe that the ultimate control of cancer may depend on the delineation of factors responsible for derepression of virus expression and of the nature of repressors involved. Certainly great progress is already being made, not only with model systems but also with potential tumor viruses isolated from man in animal test systems and in hybridization and serologic studies. Excellent leadership is being provided by the National Cancer Institute, mainly through its special virus-cancer program, and the bountiful harvest of knowledge from molecular biology is now starting to be applied to the human cancer problem. Much remains to be done, but potentially productive approaches are clear and the future is indeed rich with promise.

Biosynthesis of DNA

ROBERT L. SINSHEIMER

Division of Biology, California Institute of Technology,
Pasadena, California, USA

THE FAMOUS COMPLEMENTARY double helical structure for DNA of Watson and Crick immediately suggested a scheme for DNA replication[1] often referred to as the "Y" or fork model. The classical experiment of Meselson and Stahl,[2] since confirmed in a variety of organisms, established the validity of a fundamental element of this scheme—the separation of the two parental strands in a semiconservative process, one going to each daughter DNA molecule. The semiconservative nature of DNA replication has since been found to be correct even for single-strand DNA synthesis.

The validity of the base pairing concept has been repeatedly established in in vivo and in vitro[3] experiments. Enzymatic research has demonstrated that the nucleotide precursors of the DNA strands are the 5′-deoxyribonucleoside triphosphates, and synthetases have been extensively purified which are able to extend polynucleotide chains by addition of nucleotides to a 3′ end in accordance with the base sequence of another DNA strand as complementary template.[4] The most dramatic illustration of this biochemical competence and our understanding of these processes has been the in vitro replication of a single-stranded viral DNA to yield infective copies—a tribute to the fidelity of the replication.[5]

However, it has not thus far been possible to obtain any sustained replication of double-stranded DNA in in vitro systems, and it is becoming increasingly clear that this most fundamental process is considerably more intricate than was originally envisioned. It most likely involves a complex of enzymes and factors usually clustered, perhaps in an ordered array, on a membrane surface, and these factors very likely perform a variety of functions in addition to simple chain elongation. These may include the introduction of specific chain nicks, the facilitation of chain separation, the ligation of cut chains, the introduction of methyl groups, the initiation of de novo chains, etc. Unfortunately our knowledge of these presumed factors and their integrated action is as yet scant.

A most basic question concerns the direction of chain synthesis. The two strands of the Watson-Crick helix are opposite in polarity. As a consequence, the synthesis of the two new strands in a fork model requires that, over-all, one be extended in a 5′ to 3′ direction and the other in a 3′ to 5′ direction. All of the polymerases thus far identified extend chains only in the 5′ to 3′ direction. Extensive and ingenious searches for enzymes that might extend chains in the 3′ to 5′ direction or that might use deoxyribonucleoside 3′-triphosphates rather than 5′-triphosphates have so far been fruitless.

In consequence, various ingenious mechanisms have been proposed that, by postulating appropriate enzymatic machinery at the replication site, accomplish the net synthesis of two strands of opposite polarity, while actually making use only of synthesis in the 5′ to 3′ direction.

Some of these proposals[6] require repeated de novo initiation of the chain to be extended in the 3′ to 5′ direction; the chain is thereby made in short segments which are subsequently joined. Another proposal[7] avoids the problem of de novo initiation but introduces a requirement for a specific endonuclease at the fork.

Both proposals account for the observations of Okazaki[8] that the label incorporated into DNA during brief pulses is found, after denaturation, in short segments, 1,000 to 2,000 nucleotides in length. Both require that there be periodic signals along the DNA for chain initiation and termination or for chain cutting. Such signals might be related to those presumably employed during transcription for cistron initiation or termination. The ubiquitous presence of methylated bases[9, 10] (5-methylcytosine or 6-methylaminopurine) in generally minute proportions in DNA has led to suggestions that they may play a role in such punctuation. It is relevant that if DNA methylation is prevented, DNA synthesis stops after completion of one full round—i.e. as soon as a DNA lacking methylated bases on both strands would be formed at a fork.[10, 11]

Okazaki[6] and others[12] have also shown that upon extraction a significant portion of the freshly nascent DNA is found in a single-stranded state. However it is not yet clear to what extent this observation reflects the in vivo condition, and to what extent it is a consequence of the effect of the extraction conditions upon the necessarily complex structure that must exist at the replication fork.

Proposals which involve scission, even if transient, of the parental strands resolve conceptually another long-standing difficulty of the fork model—that the two parental strands must be unwound at a rate of one turn per 10 nucleotide pairs replicated. In *Escherichia coli,* this rate would correspond to several thousand revolutions per minute. It has been difficult to envision the entire DNA chain rotating at this rate back to a postulated swivel point at the origin of replication.[13] The introduction of transient scissions, of course, introduces local swivel points.

It is well known that the thermal melting points for DNA—the in vitro temperatures for denaturation and chain separations—are often 30 to 50° higher than in vivo temperatures, under ionic conditions comparable to those found in cells. While the energy for denaturation and chain unwinding can readily be derived from the energy released upon hydrolysis of the triphosphate groups, some means to catalyze the chain separation has seemed likely. Bruce Alberts[14] has recently discovered a protein, the gene 32 product of bacteriophage T4, that may play exactly this role. This protein, 35,000 mol wt, binds specifically and in a highly cooperative manner to single-stranded DNA. In its presence, the thermal melting point for double-stranded DNA is reduced nearly 30°. In infections with mutants lacking this protein, both DNA synthesis and genetic recombination are blocked.

The models I have discussed have implicitly assumed that both parental strands provide information of the daughter strands, i.e. that each serves as a template for one daughter strand. Models have been proposed[15] which introduce the concept of a master strand—a chosen member of the parental pair which serves as the sole source of transferred information. In such models, this strand serves as template for its complement, which in turn serves as template for the complement of the other parental strand.

The evidence for such models is indirect and in my view not compelling; but, conversely, such models cannot be rigorously excluded in our crude state of knowledge.

I would like to illustrate some of these concepts and questions by a brief description of our current knowledge of the manner of replication of the single-stranded DNA of the bacteriophage ΦX 174.

The DNA of this virus is a single-stranded ring of 1.7 million mol wt. In normal infection, as soon as this DNA is introduced into the bacterial cell it is converted to a double-stranded DNA ring in which the parental strand remains integral.[16] This process, which manifestly requires a de novo initiation of the complementary strand, is performed by pre-existent host enzymes. We do not know the nature of these enzymes, but it is noteworthy that when host mutants of the Bon-hoeffer type[17]—defective in DNA synthesis at elevated temperatures—are infected at such temperatures, conversion of the ΦX DNA to the double-stranded form is blocked. Unfortunately, the defect in these host mutants is not known, although it does not seem to concern the supply of deoxyribonucleoside triphosphates.

After formation of the double-stranded or replicative form (RF), this becomes associated with a pre-existent site on the bacterial membrane, at which it is first transcribed and subsequently replicated to make daughter double-stranded DNA rings. This replication, which requires the participation of both virus-specified and host-specified factors, is semiconservative in such a manner that of the two daughter double-stranded rings, the one with the original parental viral DNA strand remains at the membrane site while the other progeny ring is released into the cytoplasm.[18]

To reproduce a double-stranded DNA ring semiconservatively, one strand at least must be opened. If we isolate the ΦX RF from the membrane site, we find that the parental viral DNA ring remains closed while the complementary strand of the ring is nicked.

The RF DNA which remains at the membrane site continues to replicate, while the progeny released into the cytoplasm at this stage simply accumulate. Replication of the RF is relatively leisurely; the net rate is one doubling every 40 sec although the actual time for ring synthesis is very brief, certainly less than 10 sec. We have no knowledge of the means of control of initiation of the DNA replication nor of the means by which transcription and replication are somehow interleaved so as not to interfere.

We have been able to isolate RF DNAs in the process of replication and study their structure.[19] In the electron microscope, we see Cairns-type structures and branch structures. More detailed analysis indicates that the replicating structure involves an extension and elongation of the 3′ end of the complementary strand with displacement of the 5′ end of the same strand, while at the same time a new viral strand is laid down along the displaced strand. Almost any of the previously described schemes can be adapted to explain the events at the fork, if appropriate nucleases, ligases, polymerases, and other factors are postulated.

Evidently a rather intricate series of events must also be postulated at the conclusion of a round of replication when the nascent ring must be closed and separated.

At about 12 min after infection when some 10 to 15 progeny double-strand rings have accumulated within the cell, there is an abrupt transition to a new pattern of DNA synthesis. Host DNA synthesis which had continued unperturbed is now turned off by unknown means. Replication of the RF at the membrane site is similarly almost completely turned off. The double-stranded DNA rings which had accumulated as completely closed rings in the cytoplasm are now used as templates for the formation of the single-stranded DNAs of the progeny particles.

This process involves a curious and illuminating revision of the previous mode of RF replication. The progeny RF are first nicked at a specific site in the viral strand. In the process, the phosphate ligand at the nick is removed. The viral strand is then elongated, using the closed complementary strand as template and displacing its own 5′ end. This end presumably does not dangle freely, but must be held near the origin so that when the synthesis has proceeded around, a join can be made to close a single-stranded viral DNA.[20] A possible mode of making such a join involves a self-pairing nucleotide sequence.

This synthesis of the viral single-stranded DNA involves again the participation of both virus-specified and host-specified factors. We have recently isolated a viral mutant that appears to be defective in the later stage either of cutting off the nascent single strand or of making the ring join. Another viral cistron is known which appears to direct the synthesis of a protein which may play a role analogous to that of Alberts' in denaturation.

In addition, it is known that the process of single-strand synthesis is a carefully integrated act. The presence of several components of the ΦX viral coat is required for single-strand synthesis. The single strand appears to be wrapped up as it is made; free single strands are never found in the cell. And if it cannot be encapsulated, it is simply not made. The mechanism of this integration is as yet obscure.

While there is distinct progress, it is clear that we do not as yet understand the details of double-strand DNA replication. Nor do we comprehend the controls which evidently exist upon its initiation and termination. The viral systems which have well-defined DNA substrates and which afford numerous opportunities for experimental manipulation seem to offer the best approach toward early resolution of these questions. The relevance of these issues to the understanding of cancer and uncontrolled cell growth is self-evident.

References

1. Watson, J. D., and F. H. C. Crick: Nature, 171:964, 1953.
2. Meselson, M., and F. W. Stahl: Proc. Nat. Acad. Sci. USA, 44:671, 1958.
3. Lehman, I. R., S. B. Zimmerman, J. Adler, M. J. Bessman, E. S. Simms, and A. Kornberg: Proc. Nat. Acad. Sci. USA, 44:1191, 1958.
4. Englund, P. T., M. P. Deutscher, T. M. Jovin, R. B. Kelly, N. R. Cozzonelli, and A. Kornberg: Cold Spring Harbor Symp. Quant. Biol., 33:1, 1968.
5. Goulian, M., A. Kornberg, and R. L. Sinsheimer: Proc. Nat. Acad. Sci. USA, 58: 2321, 1967.
6. Okazaki, R., T. Okazaki, K. Sakabe, K. Sugimoto, R. Kainuma, A. Sugino, and N. Iwatsuki: Cold Spring Harbor Symp. Quant. Biol., 33:129, 1968.
7. Kornberg, A.: Science, 163:1410, 1969.
8. Okazaki, R., T. Okajobi, K. Sakabe, K. Sugimoto, and A. Sugino: Proc. Nat. Acad. Sci. USA, 59:598, 1968.

9. Doskocil, J., and Z. Sormova: Biochim. Biophys. Acta, 95:513, 1965.
10. Bellen, D.: J. Mol. Biol., 31:477, 1968.
11. Lark, C.: J. Mol. Biol., 31:401, 1968.
12. Oishi, M.: Proc. Nat. Acad. Sci. USA, 60:329, 1968.
13. Cairns, J.: J. Mol. Biol., 6:208, 1963.
14. Alberts, B. M.: Fed. Proc. In press.
15. Kubitschek, H. E., and T. R. Henderson: Proc. Nat. Acad. Sci. USA, 55:512, 1966.
16. Sinsheimer, R.: Prog. Nucl. Acid Res. Mol. Biol., 8:115, 1968.
17. Bonhoeffer, F.: Z. Vererbungsl., 98:141, 1966.
18. Knippers, R., and R. L. Sinsheimer: J. Mol. Biol., 34:17, 1968.
19. Knippers, R., J. M. Whalley, and R. L. Sinsheimer: Proc. Nat. Acad. Sci. USA, 64:275, 1969.
20. Knippers, R., A. Razin, R. Davis, and R. L. Sinsheimer: J. Mol. Biol., 45:237, 1969.

Human Spleen tRNA in Normal Subjects and Malignant Lymphoma Patients: Major and Minor Nucleoside Contrast

ARNOLD MITTELMAN, GIRISH B. CHHEDA, AND JOHN M. LUCH

General Clinical Research Center, Roswell Park Memorial Institute, Buffalo, New York, USA

Introduction

THE DEVELOPMENT OF the nucleic acid-protein theory has demonstrated the important relationship of transfer-RNA (tRNA) to the general physiologic state of the tissue. The profiles of the specific amino acid-accepting ability of tRNAs of both neoplastic and normal tissues have therefore been studied and compared. Taylor et al.[17] examined differences of specific tRNAs from tumor tissue and nonneoplastic tissue from mouse. Goldman et al.[9] discovered differences in phenylalanine tRNA from tissue of rat liver and ascites tumor cells. Holland et al.[13] found a new species of tyrosyl tRNA in simian virus 40 (SV40) tumors.

A possible explanation of this difference of amino acid-accepting abilities of neoplastic and nonneoplastic tRNA is an alteration in recognition sites of the RNA. It has been speculated that methylation of bases may provide for a recognition mechanism.[8] Mittelman et al.[16] found that extracts of SV40 are capable of hypermethylating homologous tRNA extracted from normal liver, whereas extracts of normal tissue cannot. Berquist and Matthews[2] found a higher content of methylated guanines and methylated adenines in a CH3 mouse spontaneous mammary adenocarcinoma and in an S 180 ascites tumor as compared with mouse liver and spleen. Other recent reports of high RNA methylation in tumors have appeared.[14, 18]

The extraction of tRNA from human spleen tissue and the isolation and analysis of the constituent nucleosides of the tRNA are described in this report. The major and minor nucleoside content of tRNAs of both neoplastic and nonneoplastic tissues was determined and compared. Any alteration in the nucleoside content with neoplasm could therefore be examined.

Materials and Methods

MATERIALS

All chemicals used were reagent grade. Crude venom phosphodiesterase of *Crotalus adamenteus* was purchased from Ross Allen Reptile Farm. The enzyme was purified in our laboratory by acetone fractionation[19] and treatment with an ion exchange resin.[15] Purified bacterial alkaline phosphatase was purchased from Worthington Company. Chelex-100 resin, 200-400 mesh, was purchased from Bio-Rad and converted to a copper form by the method of Goldstein.[10] Standard markers of the minor (modified) nucleosides were obtained from the laboratory of Dr. Ross Hall, Roswell Park Memorial Institute.

The human spleen was the source of the tRNA analyzed in this work. Four spleens from patients with nonneoplastic diseases were used, along with two spleens from patients with Hodgkin's disease and two spleens which were infiltrated with a chronic lymphatic leukemia. The spleens varied in weight from 225 g to 1,500 g.

ISOLATION OF tRNA

The tRNA extraction was a modification of the procedure of Brunngraber.[4] The procedure was started approximately 20 min after blood was clamped off from the spleen during operation. All work was done at 4 C unless otherwise specified.

Two hundred grams of tissue were homogenized in a Waring blender with 300 ml of water-saturated phenol and 300 ml of 1.0 M NaCl, .005 M EDTA in .1 M tris-HCl, pH 7.5. Homogenization was continued approximately two min until a thick, dark brown homogenate was obtained. The homogenate was centrifuged at 10,000 rpm for 10 min, and the aqueous layer was carefully decanted off. Two and one-half volumes of cold 95% ethanol were added, and the DNA which immediately precipitated was wound out of the solution with a stirring rod and lyophilized. The solution was kept at 4 C for 16 hr until RNA precipitation was complete.

PURIFICATION OF tRNA

The tRNA precipitate was pelleted by centrifugation at 10,000 rpm for 10 min. Removal of residual DNA and purification of tRNA was done according to the procedure of Zubay.[21] The tRNA was dissolved in .3 M sodium acetate (pH 7.0). Isopropanol was added (.54 vol) with stirring, and the temperature was adjusted to 25 C. The suspension was centrifuged at 8,000 rpm for five min at room temperature. The supernatant was saved, while the precipitate was dissolved in .3 M sodium acetate buffer and again treated with .54 vol isopropanol. This suspension was centrifuged at 8,000 rpm for five min at room temperature, and the supernatant saved. The combined supernatants were treated with additional .54 vol isopropanol. The temperature of the suspension was adjusted to 40 C and centrifuged at 40 C for 10 min at 10,000 rpm. The tRNA precipitate pellet was dissolved in distilled water, and the solution was dialyzed against distilled water overnight. The yield of tRNA was approximately 150 mg/kg of spleen tissue.

ENZYMIC HYDROLYSIS OF tRNA

The tRNA was hydrolyzed to its constituent nucleosides by the method of Hall.[11] One hundred milligrams of tRNA were dissolved in 10 ml of .001 M $MgSO_4$. Two units of purified snake venom phosphodiesterase, 2 units of bacterial alkaline phosphatase, and 3 drops of toluene were added. The mixture was incubated at 37 C for approximately seven hr or until hydrolysis was complete. The pH of the mixture was adjusted to 9.2 at the beginning and periodically throughout the incubation period. The solution was then neutralized and lyophilized.

LIGAND EXCHANGE CHROMATOGRAPHY

Ligand exchange chromatography was used for the gross separation of the major nucleosides. A 65 cm $\times$ 1 cm column of Chelex-100 copper resin was packed and washed with water. Then 75 mg of tRNA were dissolved in 2 ml of water, and the sample was applied to the column. The first eluting agent used was water, which eluted the nucleotides and pyrimidine nucleosides. These elutions were complete with 475 ml of water. Then 500 ml of 1N NH_4OH was passed through the column to elute the majority of the purine nucleosides. Total O.D. recovery from the column was 92%.

PAPER CHROMATOGRAPHY

Each of the major peaks from the column were lyophilized, and the nucleosides were further resolved by paper chromatography. Descending solvent chromatography was employed with Whatman 3 MM chromatography paper for isolation of nucleosides and Whatman 1 MM paper for comparative identification. Standard markers were used to identify nucleosides.

SOLVENTS USED

The solvents used were: (A) ethyl acetate-isopropanol-water, 4-1-2; (B) isopropanol-water-concentrated ammonium hydroxide, 7-2-1; (C) ethyl acetate-2 ethoxyethanol-16% formic acid, 4-1-2 (upper phase); (D) normal butanol-water-concentrated ammonium hydroxide, 86-14-5; (E) .05 M. glycine, pH 9.2; and (F) .05 M. glycine-.05 glycine-.05 M. borate, pH 9.2.

FURTHER ANALYSIS

The 2′0 methylated nucleosides were also subjected to high-voltage electrophoresis for identification purpose (solvent E and solvent F, 20v/ cm, two hr). The UV absorption spectrum of each nucleoside isolated was compared with standard spectra.

The mole per cent of each nucleoside was calculated. A comparison of mole per cent of nucleosides of RNA from both neoplastic and non-neoplastic tissues was then made.

Results

The isolation and purification of tRNA by the Brunngraber method specifies a purification of the RNA by use of a DEAE cellulose column.

FIG. 15–1.—Sucrose gradient analysis of the final tRNA product. Gradient consisted of 30 ml of a 5% to 20% sucrose in .05M NaCl, .001M $MgCl_2$, .01M CH_3COONa, pH 5.1. One milligram tRNA was analyzed. Tube collections of .75 ml were made.

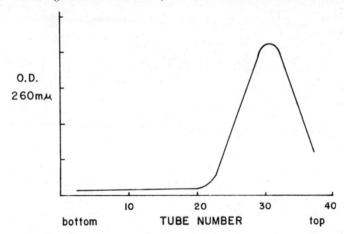

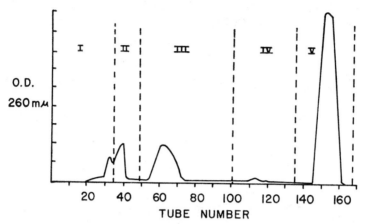

Fig. 15–2.—Fractionation of hydrolyzed tRNA on Chelex-100, copper form resin column. Tube collections of 5.0 ml were made.

This separates the tRNA from the large amount of glycogen found in liver tissue. This purification step was unnecessary in working with spleen tissue, since it has a minimal glycogen content. The DNA content of the spleen was very large (5 g/kg spleen tissue). Therefore the RNA purification of Zubay was used to eliminate all DNA. Sucrose gradient of the final tRNA product revealed a pure 4-S peak, as shown in Figure 15-1. Treating the tRNA with diphenylamine reagent[5] revealed no deoxy-sugar moieties.

TABLE 15 1.—ISOLATION OF NUCLEOSIDES BY PAPER CHROMATOGRAPHY

MAJOR FRACTION FROM COLUMN	SOLVENT SYSTEM	TIME (HOURS)	COMPOUNDS ISOLATED
I	B,C	16,8	oligonuclcotides
			nucleotides (uridine and cytidine phosphate)
II	A,B	60,16	uridine
			pseudouridine
			2′0 Methyluridine
			other uridine derivatives
III	B,C	16,8	cytidine
			2′0 Methylcytidine
			PCTR
			other cytidine derivatives
IV	B	16	phosphodiesterase contaminant
V	B,C	16,8	adenosine
			guanosine
			2′0 Methyladenosine
			2′0 Methylguanosine
			6-methylaminopurineriboside
			7-methylguanosine
			other adenosine derivatives
			other guanosine derivatives

TABLE 15–2.—Rf Values of Nucleosides in Paper Chromatography

Compound	Solvent System			
	A	B	C	D
adenosine	.37	.54	.61	.26
guanosine	.14	.25	.29	.05
uridine	.29	.25	.42	.09
cytidine	.09	.10	.32	.16
pseudouridine	.10	.29	.15	.04
6-MAPR		.69	.54	.37
2′0 Me Cytidine	.19	.20	.35	.32
2′0 Me Guanosine	.30	.14	.34	.20
2′0 Me Adenosine	.55	.70	.65	.48
2′0 Me Uridine	.55	.58	.46	.30
7-Me Guanosine		.35		.04
PCTR	.01	.23	.24	

The tRNA digest was first separated into major fractions, as shown in Figure 15-2. Fraction I was composed of partially hydrolyzed oligo-nucleotides and nucleotides. Fraction IV was composed of impurities of the snake venom phosphodiesterase preparation. The other three fractions represented the major nucleosides along with their modified minor derivatives. These minor nucleosides were isolated well by paper chromatography, as shown in Table 15-1. The Rf values of nucleosides isolated by paper chromatography, shown in Table 15-2, compared well with those of the nucleosides of tRNA described by Hall.[12] The 2′0

TABLE 15–3.—Mole Percent Values of Nucleosides of Human Spleen tRNA

Compound	tRNA Extractions*						
	Chesbro 1	Snyder 2	Boghell 3	4	5	6	7
uridine	15.6	14.6	15.9	13.1	15.7	16.7	14.1
2′0 Me Uridine		.68		2.5	.89	1.9	1.1
pseudouridine	1.5	.7	1.9	5.0	3.0	5.6	6.7
other uridine derivatives	1.0	.7	3.2	1.3	3.0		
cytidine	33.5	26.9	33.2	31.8	14.3	20.4	22.2
2′0 Me cytidine	1.0	.53			.3		1.2
other cytidine derivatives		.1	1.3	1.3	1.3	1.9	2.2
guanosine	23.5	26.5	22.4	27.5	22.5	25.9	25.9
2′0 Me guanosine		2.0					
7-Me guanosine					1.4		
other guanosine derivatives	3.6	2.7	1.9		4.7	1.9	2.3
adenosine	15.4	23.3	18.6	18.8	21.6	24.1	25.6
2′0 Me adenosine		.5					.3
6-MAPR	.51	.56	.64	1.1	.89	1.9	.5
PCTR		0.1					
other adenosine derivatives		.33			1.0		.84

* Extraction 1, 2, 3: normal. Extraction 5, 6: Hodgkin's disease. Extraction 7, 8: lymphatic leukemia.

ribose methylated compounds subjected to electrophoresis did not show any change in mobility with the addition of borate to the buffer, whereas the mobility of other nucleosides did change. This observation was described by Hall.[11] Ultraviolet spectra of the isolated derivatives compared well with those of spectra from standard marker nucleosides.

The four major nucleosides along with their minor modified derivatives were purified sufficiently to calculate their mole per cent of the total RNA molecule, as shown in Table 15-3. It is seen from Table 15-1 that cytidine and uridine nucleotides appeared at breakthrough volume from the Chelex-100 column. These phosphates were believed to be caused by an incomplete hydrolysis of the tRNA. Therefore, the phosphate mole per cent values were added to the mole per cent of their respective major nucleosides.

Discussion

Human tRNA resembles well the tRNA of lower organisms, as seen in Table 15-4. The spleen RNA has a high $\frac{GG}{AU}$ ratio, and the ratio $\frac{A + U + \text{pseudouridine}}{G + C}$ falls within the range of .6 to .7. These characteristics are common of tRNAs isolated from a wide variety of sources from a broad range of the phylogenetic spectrum, as reported by Brown.[3]

Brown also states that another common characteristic of a wide variety of tRNAs is an $\frac{A}{U}$ and $\frac{G}{C}$ ratio close to unity. In human spleen tRNA, however, the nonneoplastic and neoplastic $\frac{A}{U}$ ratios were .78 and .64, respectively, and the $\frac{G}{C}$ ratios were .72 and 1.13 respectively. These ratios could suggest a unique feature of the RNA isolated, but more data from different human tissues and from different experimental procedures would have to be examined before a general statement of $\frac{G}{C}$ and $\frac{A}{U}$ ratios of human tRNA could be formulated.

It was of interest to calculate the mole per cent of the total minor

TABLE 15–4.—MOLE PERCENT COMPARISONS OF
NUCLEOSIDES OF DIFFERENT RNA TYPES

| | MOLE PERCENT | | |
COMPOUND	Human Nonneoplastic	Human Neoplastic	Yeast
adenosine	18	22	17
uridine	14	14	17
guanosine	23	27	26
cytidine	32	24	29
pseudouridine	2.0	5.5	3.0
6-MAPR	.6	1.6	
2′0 Me uridine	.8	1.6	
2′0 Me cytidine	.7	.7	

nucleosides in the tRNA. There is good evidence of an increase in degree of methylation of bases as we advance in the phylogenetic scheme. Zachau[20] describes this "refining of modification in evolution" by stating that animal tRNA has more minor nucleosides than yeast tRNA, while yeast tRNA is more highly modified than bacterial RNA. Bell[1] reports a modified nucleoside level of 4 mole % from yeast tRNA, while Cantoni[6] reports that modified nucleosides make up 10 mole % of rat liver tRNA.

Human spleen tRNA analyzed in this work supports this contention of increased modification in evolution. Minor modified nucleosides made up 13% of the total nucleoside level of the tRNA. Although this increase in methylation in evolution has been well documented, no conclusive statements have yet been made as to the function of the modified bases from a phylogenetic standpoint.

Due to the amount of tRNA analyzed, and the small mole per cent of each minor nucleoside in the tRNA, many minor nucleosides could not be isolated and purified sufficiently to give an accurate indication of their mole per cent value in the tRNA. Pseudouridine and 6-methylaminopurine riboside were isolated easily by the procedures used, and a direct comparison of these two nucleosides was done. Each showed a higher mole per cent value in neoplastic tRNA compared with nonneoplastic tRNA. 2-0-Methyluridine was also slightly higher. Mole per cents of the 2-0-methylcytidines were approximately equal in the neoplastic and nonneoplastic tRNA. Since these were the only minor nucleosides compared, it would be interesting to speculate on a general phenomenon of increases in other modified nucleosides in tRNA of neoplastic tissue.

The absence of N-(purin-6-ylcarbamoyl)threonine riboside in neoplastic tRNA is an interesting observation. This, however, may be artifactual. This modified nucleoside was recently discovered by Chheda,[7] and appears next to the anticodon of the tRNA molecule. This nucleoside also appears to have cytokinine activity. The importance of this nucleoside in the physiologic control of the cell by tRNA is being studied.

Acknowledgment

This study was supported by Research Grant 1 MO1 FR00262-05 from the Institute of General Medicinal Sciences, U. S. Public Health Service.

References

1. Bell, D. B., R. V. Tomlinson, and G. M. Tener: Biochemistry, 3:317, 1964.
2. Berquist, and Matthews: Biochem. J., 85:305, 1962.
3. Brown, G. L.: Progr. Nucl. Acid Res., 2:259, 1963.
4. Brunngraber, E. F.: Biochem. Biophys. Res. Comm., 8:1, 1962.
5. Burton, K.: Biochem. J., 62:315, 1956.
6. Cantoni, G. L., H. H. Richards, M. F. Singer, and H. V. Gelboin: Biochim. Biophys. Acta, 61:354, 1962.

7. Chheda, G. B.: Life Sci., 8 (Part II) :979, 1969.
8. Gold, M., R. Hausmann, U. Maitra, and J. Hurwitz: Proc. Nat. Acad. Sci. USA, 52:292, 1964.
9. Goldman, M., W. M. Johnston, and C. A. Griffin: Cancer Res., 29:1051, 1969.
10. Goldstein, G.: Analyt. Biochem., 20:477, 1967.
11. Hall, R. H.: Biochim. Biophys. Acta, 68:278,1963.
12. Hall, R. H.: Biochemistry, 4:661, 1965.
13. Holland, J. J., M. W. Taylor, and C. A. Buck: Proc. Nat. Acad. Sci. USA, 58:2437, 1967.
14. Karge, A. M., B. Fredlender, and R. Saloman: Israel J. Chem., 3:78, 1966.
15. Keller, E. B.: Biochem. Biophys. Res. Comm., 17:412, 1964.
16. Mittelman, A., R. H. Hall, D. S. Yohn, and J. J. Grace, Jr.: Cancer Res., 27:1409, 1967.
17. Taylor, N. W., G. A. Granger, C. A. Buck, and J. J. Holland: Proc. Nat. Acad. Sci. USA, 57:1712, 1967.
18. Tsutsui, E., P. R. Srinivasan, and E. Borek: Proc. Nat. Acad. Sci. USA, 56:1003, 1966.
19. Williams, E. J., S. C. Sung, and M. Laskowski, Sr.: J. Biol. Chem., 236:1130, 1961.
20. Zachau, H. G.: Angew. Chem., 81:645, 1969.
21. Zubay: J. Mol. Biol., 4:347, 1962.

16

Regulatory Behavior of Organelles in Normal and Cancer Cells: Cell Function and Multiplication

The Interphase Nucleus: Problems of Structure and Function in 1970

W. BERNHARD

Institut de Recherches sur le Cancer, Villejuif, France

LIFE SEEMS TO HAVE existed for about three billion years, but only at the beginning of the last third of this time did cells appear with nuclei.[63] The transition from prokaryotes to eukaryotes was soon followed by the evolution from unicellular organisms to metazoa and, afterward, by the rapid ramification of many species with explosive growth (Figure 16-1). The phylogenetic importance of the acquisition of a nucleus, together with chloroplasts and mitochondria, can hardly be overestimated. One may wonder why it was advantageous to locate the carriers of genetic information within a specialized compartment, the nucleus. In the bacterial cell, there exists no nuclear membrane and no nucleolus. Transcription is rapidly followed by translation. In eukaryotes, on the contrary, there is a complex system of processing of the transcribed rRNA and probably also of mRNA which delays the end result, namely protein synthesis. In addition, the pores of the nuclear membrane which are used as passage for nuclear RNP into the cytoplasm are likely to be capable of regulating the flow of material in both ways. Means of accelerating, delaying, or stopping this trans-

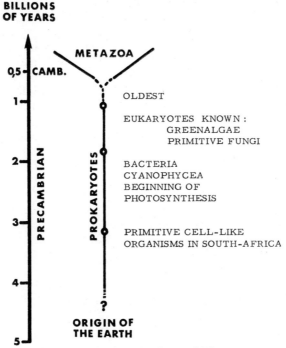

BILLIONS OF YEARS

METAZOA

0,5 — CAMB.

1 —   OLDEST

EUKARYOTES KNOWN :
GREENALGAE
PRIMITIVE FUNGI

2 —   BACTERIA
CYANOPHYCEA
BEGINNING OF
PHOTOSYNTHESIS

3 —   PRIMITIVE CELL-LIKE
ORGANISMS IN SOUTH-AFRICA

4 —

?

ORIGIN OF
THE EARTH

5 —

PRECAMBRIAN

PROKARYOTES

Fig. 16–1.—Early history of life.

port probably represent additional controls. Further epigenetic controls are assumed to exist in the cytoplasm. The complexity of these mechanisms of processing the genetic copies can easily explain the much greater flexibility and diversity in the reaction of the eukaryote cell toward environmental factors. The maintenance of the chromatin in a separate compartment is also likely to guarantee a better homeostasis for gene activation and function. Finally, there may be more than a mere quantitative difference between storing the 2,000 to 4,000 genes of the bacterial cell, and the five to 10,000,000 of the cell of higher organisms; the bacterial DNA has no histones and no residual proteins linked with the genophor as in the case of the eukaryote.[49]

The nucleus, therefore not only appears as the supreme legislator of the cell with an exceptionally long and conservative memory, but it also has a certain degree of executive power in the way it processes, accelerates, or delays the information eventually shifted to the cytoplasm. However, the switch on of nuclear function appears to be regulated by cytoplasmic signals.[31, 33]

The Chromatin

Chromatin is most easily visualized in electron micrographs of interphase nuclei as condensed chromatin (heterochromatin). About 80 to

90% of the total nucleohistone content of the nucleus is, indeed, densely packed and considered as nonfunctional.[25, 49] It is mainly found along the nuclear membrane, sometimes in lamellar orientation[20] and associated with the nucleolus. The unraveled chromatin (euchromatin) is more difficult to reveal, as its uncoiled fibrils may be easily confused with the transcribed RNA which has the same contrast if the classic staining methods of electron microscopy are applied. However, a new staining procedure, recently described, bleaches all DNP, by means of EDTA, but does not alter the contrast of RNP[7] (Figure 16-2). Although this method is not really specific, it allows the distinction of

FIG. 16-2.—Liver cell nucleus, stained with the preferential RNP staining. All the chromatin appears bleached, which allows better visualization of nuclear ribonucleoproteins. ×25,000. (Courtesy of Dr. P. Petrov.)

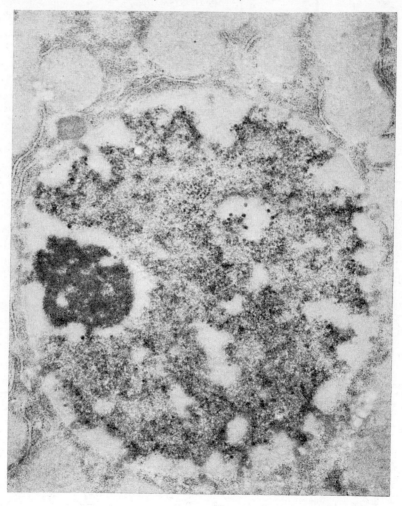

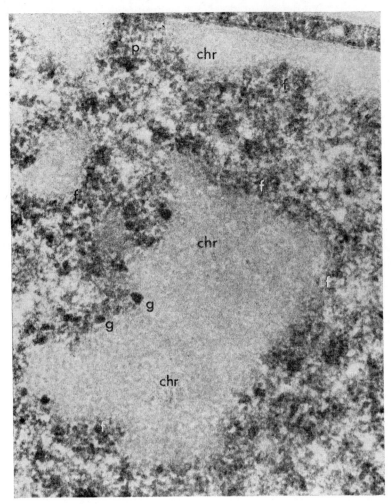

Fig. 16-3.—Higher magnification of a liver cell nucleus, treated with the preferential RNP stain. Bleached chromatin (chr), perichromatin fibrils (f), perichromatin granules (g), nuclear pore (p). ×60,000.

both types of nucleoproteins. The unraveled, functional chromatin is most frequently found at the surface of the condensed areas, or in between them (interchromatin space) (Figure 16-3).

According to Ris,[49] the native structure of chromatin fibers, as revealed in the hydrated nucleus by freeze-etching, measures 250 A in diameter. The basic unit, however, visualized after complexing the bivalent metal ions, seems to be a nucleohistone fiber of 100 A in diameter. Still smaller units, about 40 A thick, have also been shown, which may represent a single double-stranded DNA helix linked with histones.[34, 50] The length of the DNA molecules depends very much on the isolation method, but molecular weights up to 500 million have been measured. There is good evidence that these molecules are linear;[49] the only known exception is the extrachromosomal nucleolar DNA in amphibian oocytes, which is circular.[40]

Britten and Kohne[13] recently have shown that, depending on the species, a variable amount of chromatin (up to 60% at least) contains repetitious DNA. This means that the same nucleotide sequences are scattered throughout the genome in many hundreds or thousands, perhaps millions of copies, most of which are probably never transcribed. It is assumed that the accumulated inert DNA plays an important phylogenetic role in the appearance and diversification of new families, but the exact mechanism of this phenomenon is not yet understood. In the case of the nucleolar organizer chromosome, there also exists a high redundancy or amplification[14] of the same clustered DNA cistrons, e.g. in *Xenopus* there are more than 1,000 identical copies.[12] These identical nucleotide sequences (rDNA) are preparing the ribosomal precursor RNA (45S rRNA) [19, 46, 54] and still heavier forms.[56] Normally, all of the copies are capable of functioning, which obviously allows a very rapid ribosome synthesis when this is a top requirement of the cell.

Chromatin Activation and Transcription

Ringertz[48] has proposed the term "chromatin activation reaction," which he believes to be a multistep phenomenon leading to specific gene derepression. The earliest changes are physicochemical alterations of the chromatin, probably to the metal ions (Ca, Mg), inducing unmasking of phosphate groups and being accompanied by increased binding of acridine orange or actinomycin D. The second step is characterized by enzymatic modification of chromatin which leads to acetylation of histones.[3] Methylation, thiolation, or phosphorylation may also occur. This change is immediately followed by early RNA synthesis outside the nucleolus. However, this RNA does not migrate into the cytoplasm, but is metabolized in situ. Meanwhile, the size of the nucleus is considerably increased because of migration of proteins from the cytoplasm into the nucleoplasm. DNA synthesis, as well as nucleolar RNA synthesis, is now switched on. Increased nucleolar activity is followed by the appearance of new ribosomes in the cytoplasm, and finally, the synthesis of specific proteins. One can conclude that gene expression is initiated and controlled at many different levels, most of which do not act directly on transcription as in bacterial systems.[28, 55, 60]

Visualization of the Transcription Sites

The most important transcription site, already visible in the light microscope, is, of course, the nucleolus, which can be considered as a permanent gene product, containing ribosomal RNA in the heavy precursor form (45S), as well as 28S and 18S, with cleavage intermediates. All forms are linked with proteins.[19, 47, 54] The different ribosomal RNAs, as well as mRNA, have been visualized in purified fractions and their length has been measured directly with the electron microscope by Granboulan and Scherrer.[30] The problems of the nucleolus have been reviewed elsewhere,[10] and will be treated separately by Dr. Muramatsu in this Congress. Therefore, we shall not mention them here.

The EDTA-staining method has enabled us to demonstrate hitherto unknown RNP components of the nucleoplasm which are found in close contact with certain chromatin areas. We called them "perichromatin fibrils."[43] These are densely stained fibrillar elements, from 30 A to 200 A thick, irregularly coiled; they are sparse in some areas but accumulate into dense aggregates in other regions. It can be shown that incorporation of RNA precursors takes place precisely at these sites, as revealed by high resolution radioautography.[21] This newly synthesized RNA is nonrandomly distributed throughout the nucleoplasm, and is thought to translate the degree of localized gene activity. Digestion experiments with proteases indicate that these fibrils are rapidly complexed with proteins.

Perichromatin Granules

First described in the early 1960s by Swift[64] and by Watson,[66] these components seem to be universally present in all cells. They are located in the peripheral portions of the condensed chromatin, and clearly have a structural relationship with perichromatin fibrils from which they probably arise. They are, indeed, composed of similar closely packed fibrils of about 30 to 50 A in thickness and of a voluminous protein matrix of low contrast. Their number varies considerably, according to the functional state of the cell. They may be found close to the nuclear pores, or even within them, where they undergo a configurational change. Indeed, they have never been found to cross the pores as such, but they are dissolved into their fibrillar components. These granules seem to have a carrier function, and it was suggested that they might represent the morphologic substrate of some type of messenger RNA.[43] This assumption is based on the fact that their cytochemical behavior is very similar to that of Balbiani granules in giant Dipteran chromosomes, components which are likely to carry messenger RNA.[5] We have only proposed this hypothesis, it has yet to be proved. The messenger function of perichromatin granules can only be demonstrated after they have been purified and analyzed biochemically.

Interchromatin Granules and Unidentified RNA Species

Interchromatin granules of an average diameter of 200 to 250 A are present in all cells in the interchromatin areas,[9] where they are always interconnected by tiny fibrils to form chains which, in turn, are grouped in loose clusters. They probably form a contiguous network throughout the nucleoplasm.[57] They certainly contain RNA and protein, but there always remains a residue after combined protease and RNase digestion. They may correspond to the 30S or 40S RNP granules isolated in a special nuclear fraction known to contain a large amount of proteins and a short-chain RNA.[42, 53] It is significant that these particles called "nuclear ribosomes" by some authors,[2, 52] have not revealed ultrastructural features comparable to those of cytoplasmic ribosomes. Their function remains totally unknown. They are slowly labeled, relatively stable structures, and certainly do not migrate into the cytoplasm. They are frequently more prominent after virus infection and in cells treated with a variety of antimetabolites and other drugs. It is unlikely that they are carriers of the rapidly labeled, still mysterious heterogeneous (Hn)[44] or messenger-like nuclear RNA, most of which does not leave the nucleoplasm but is metabolized in situ.[19, 55, 59]

It is not as yet understood why the nucleus manufactures so much Hn RNA, most of which does not seem to be used by the cell, although its character is informational. Many molecular biologists are now at work to elucidate this question. Another tricky problem concerns the nuclear short-chain RNA which is different from rRNA and 5S RNA.[67] What is their biologic significance? Where do they come from? Do they have any relationship with interchromatin granules?

One of the main challenges for the specialists of the interphase nucleus will be the localization in ultrathin section of all the known and the hitherto unidentified species of extranucleolar RNA. Is the heterogeneous, messenger-like RNA identical to perichromatin fibrils? Where is the short chain RNA situated? Perhaps the best of the present-day approaches would be to apply the in situ hybridization method as proposed by John et al.[38] and Gall and Pardue,[27] which entails an ingenious and rather complex procedure. These authors were able to localize by means of light microscopic autoradiography the exact site of ribosomal RNA synthesis in the cell nucleus. Everything should now be done to adapt their method to the electron microscopic level. The technical problems which have to be solved seem tremendous, but the use of the now constantly improving method of ultrathin frozen sections might be of great help.

Coiled Bodies

These newly described RNA-carrying constituents occur in the nucleoplasm as loose, generally spherical aggregates of 0.3 to 0.5 μ in diameter. They have been observed as single bodies in the interchromatin space of a variety of cells, and may well be present in many others.[43] High-resolution pictures reveal very fine, twisted fibrils about 50

A thick. Coiled bodies may well represent a universally present, hitherto unknown constituent of the nucleus. Their relationship with the well-known "nuclear bodies" is rather doubtful, but cannot be entirely excluded. At present, nothing is known concerning their function.

The Problem of Nuclear Protein Synthesis

True ribosomes of the cytoplasmic type have not been demonstrated so far in the nucleolus, nor in the extranucleolar nucleoplasm. One may therefore wonder if protein synthesis is possible at all without the classic machinery being present. It was shown that both 60S and 40S ribosomal subunits can be found in the nucleolus, but it is generally admitted that the complete assembly of functionally active ribosomes can only take place in the cytoplasm, in spite of the fact that a series of biochemical[4, 11, 44, 69] and autoradiographic[15, 16, 65] studies have led to the conclusion that protein synthesis can take place within the nucleus. The prevailing opinion of today is that most, if not all, nuclear proteins are synthesized on cytoplasmic ribosomes and are then transported into the nucleus.[19] This is certainly the case for histones,[51] but the origin of residual proteins and of the ribosomal proteins remains uncertain. The problem is technically difficult to solve. If the purification of nuclear fraction is taken to the point where no cytoplasmic ribosomes are sticking to the outer leaflet of the nuclear membrane, many nuclear enzymes may be lost, and such fractions are inactive in in vitro tests. Conversely, insufficiently purified nuclear fractions may still have enough cytoplasmic ribosomes to be active for amino acid incorporation. Positive autoradiographic results, obtained even after a short pulse, might reveal the site of accumulation of the synthesized proteins rather than the actual site of synthesis, if, as it is assumed, their transport is very rapid.

It has to be remembered that about 70 to 80% of the dry weight of nuclei is proteins, and not nucleic acids. Do they really all come from the cytoplasm? Could there not exist some more archaic and still undiscovered way of protein synthesis which does not need typical cytoplasmic ribosomes? This is obviously a very obscure problem which needs much further work to be elucidated. The migration of proteins back and forth from nucleus to cytoplasm has been elegantly demonstrated by Goldstein and Prescott[29] in amoebas, and may well illustrate a very basic and general phenomenon.

The Function of Nuclear Proteins

Nuclear proteins, whether histones or nonhistones, represent the main bulk of the nucleoplasm, where they are present in well-balanced proportions and, therefore, guarantee the maintenance of intranuclear homeostasis.

THE HISTONES

As is well known, histones are closely linked with the DNA double helix, and thus are shielding the genetic material. It is assumed that they have a rather general, nonspecific repressor function. Their removal by enzymic digestion increases the transcription rate in in vitro experiments. Their acetylation also is followed by increased RNA synthesis.[3, 25] However, because they are relatively simple molecules with much less variety than was believed a few years ago, it is unlikely that they are specific repressors.[17, 25, 48, 49] Huang and Bonner[36] and Benjamin et al.[6] suggested that there was a short-chain RNA linked with histones and assumed that this nucleoprotein would act as a specific repressor. However, this work has not been confirmed so far. It may also be assumed that histones have a structural function, in particular the lysine-rich fraction, which is responsible for the degree of contraction of chromatin.[40]

NONHISTONE PROTEINS

Nonhistone proteins are supposed to act as linkers between the DNA molecules[35] and, therefore, are probably the most important elements in the maintenance of chromosomal structures. Frenster found an excess of phosphoproteins in euchromatin which he believed to act as polyanionic derepressors of nucleohistones by local removal of histone molecules.[23, 24] This is a plausible explanation, but it is not known if this mechanism really does play a role in specific gene activation.

Further important functions of nonhistone proteins are enzymatic: DNA polymerase, RNA polymerase first of all, but also other nuclear enzymes such as thymidine kinase, nucleoside triphosphatases,[49] DNase, and RNase.[37, 70] Siebert[58] mentions more than 30 nuclear enzymes in his review. Finally, nuclear proteins are involved in binding to the newly formed RNA, and therefore have a protective function against enzymic degradation. Such proteins may be carriers of rRNA or mRNA for their export into the cytoplasm, or they may play an important role in the storage of genetic information in the nucleoplasm or cytoplasm as "informofers" of Georgiev,[28] building up the "informosomes" of Spirin.[60] At this point, we come back to the above-mentioned problem concerning the influence of nuclear proteins on the regulation of gene expression at the epigenetic level. It is known that messenger complexed with proteins (e.g. in *Acetabularia*) may be stored as long as several months before translation and protein synthesis take place. This is a striking example which demonstrates the importance of cytoplasmic factors in the timing of the release of the message.[33]

The Nuclear Membrane

The double leaflet of the nuclear membrane acts as a barrier separating the nucleoplasm from the cytoplasm, and this serves an important function by guaranteeing that there is a constant ionic environment for chromatin activation. The nucleoplasm always has a higher negative charge than the cytoplasm. The nuclear membrane also has an active function. It originates from the endoplasmic reticulum during mitosis in late anaphase, and maintains permanent or temporary structural contiguity with the latter throughout interphase. It can therefore be expected to have certain similar functions, e.g. transport of water and ions from the cell surface to the proximity of the chromatin.[61] More unusual is that the nuclear membrane is also capable of synthesizing proteins if there are ribosomes present at its outer leaflet. In the case of antibody synthesis, this is the very first site where the antibodies appear, probably because the nuclear membrane ribosomes are the first to receive the message.[39]

The presence of regular nuclear "pores" is certainly of great importance for the passage of macromolecules, especially proteins and RNP.[62] As has been pointed out in many papers, the pores are not simply holes, but locks which have an extremely complex ultrastructure probably directly connected with selective permeability.[1, 22, 26] Another fact which has to be stressed is the presence of enzymes within the perinuclear space. Little is known about them, but glycose 6-phosphatase, APTase,[48] nucleoside diphosphatase, and acetylcholin-esterase[45] have already been visualized, and, according to biochemical data, other enzymes are likely to be localized there.[61] The "membrana nucleum limitans" is likely to influence permeability.[22, 61] Finally, it has been demonstrated by Comings and Kakefuda[18] that the replication of DNA starts along the nuclear membrane. The inner leaflet of the nuclear membrane seems to play the same role in the separation of the DNA strands in eukaryotes as do the bacterial membrane or mesosomes in the replication of bacterial DNA.

The Nucleus of the Cancer Cell

As we have pointed out repeatedly,[8, 9] we must distinguish between early changes and late changes. Early changes in cells transformed in vitro or in very young primary tumors are so minute that they can hardly, if at all, be recognized. The same basic structures and functions of cytoplasm and nucleus are preserved. The only difference may be an increased rate of DNA synthesis, the appearance of new antigens, and a slightly changed cell surface. The chromosome number and the size and shape of the interphase nucleus are not modified. Later, both structure and function may be gradually changed under the selective pressure of the organism by immunologic or other humoral mechanisms. The chromosome number becomes aneuploid, but has a tendency to be increased. Accordingly, the nuclear size becomes bigger and more irregular. As the growth rate is generally increased, the nucleolus, a sensitive indicator of protein synthesis, is mostly hypertrophic and may have an abnormal architecture. Abnormal chromatin distribution is observed, which may be accompanied by an increase in the number of perichromatin granules. However, no truly specific change can be detected. The cancer cell nucleus may become a caricature of the normal, but is still capable of carrying out all the functions described above.[9, 32]

Conclusions

The last 10 years have clarified a considerable number of problems dealing with the interphase nucleus. Among them, we would like to mention its fine structural analyses, with the description of hitherto unknown nuclear components, the discovery of the biologic function of the nucleolus, and the isolation of many different species of nuclear RNA with the understanding of their action in protein synthesis. At present, the role of the nucleus in protein production, although essential, is considered to be rather indirect, by means of the production of various types of RNA and the release of messengers for specific proteins synthesized predominantly, if not exclusively, on cytoplasmic ribosomes. The regulation of transcription within the nucleoplasm appears to be of increasing complexity. Various degrees of chromatin activation exist where physicochemical and enzymatic changes of histones are important, but they are not specific enough for the derepression of single genes. Much further work is needed to explain specific gene activation in eukaryotes. The newly transcribed RNA can now be directly visualized in thin sections with the electron microscope, but we are still far from identifying this visible RNA with the various RNA species isolated and characterized by methods of molecular biology. The discovery of "heterogeneous" or "messenger-like" RNA, which does not leave the nucleus but is rapidly metabolized in situ, is most intriguing. Concerning the nuclear proteins, it is now assumed that most, perhaps all of them originate from the cytoplasm; but there are also reasons to believe that some of them may be synthesized within the nucleoplasm, although typical ribosomes have not been demonstrated there so far. The nuclear membrane is probably a very active organelle rather then a passive barrier, playing a decisive role not only in selective permeability and transport, but also in the initiation of DNA replication and in protein synthesis.

The interphase nucleus not only preserves and replicates the genetic information of the cell, but it also guarantees the regularity of transcription by maintaining nucleoplasmic homeostasis. Furthermore, it plays a role in the storage and transport of the transcribed RNA, whether informational or not, and thus also has a regulator function in protein synthesis. The nucleus has a prospective significance and holds the keys to the past and to the immediate or distant future, whereas the cytoplasm can only act for the present, its functions being carried out and manifested immediately.

References

1. Abelson, H. T., and G. H. Smith: J. Ultrastr. Res., 30:558-588, 1970.
2. Allfrey, V. G.: Exp. Cell Res., Suppl. 9:183-212, 1963.
3. Allfrey, V. G.: Cancer Res., 26:2026-2040, 1966.
4. Beck, J. P., J. M. Guerne, G. Schmidt, F. Stutinsky, and J. P. Ebel: Compt. Rend. Acad. Sci. (Paris) , 266:940-943, 1968.
5. Beermann, W.: Chromosoma, 12:1-25, 1961.
6. Benjamin, W., A. D. Levander, A. Gellhorn, and R. H. De Bellis: Proc. Nat. Acad. Sci. USA, 858-865, 1966.
7. Bernhard, W.: J. Ultrastr. Res., 27:250-265, 1969.
8. Bernhard, W.: In: Handbook of Molecular Cytology (A. Lima-de-Faria, ed.) , North Holland Publishing Co., 1969, Chapt. 28, pp. 687-715.
9. Bernhard, W., and N. Granboulan: Exp. Cell Res., Suppl. 9:19-53, 1963.
10. Bernhard, W., and N. Granboulan: In: The Nucleus (A. J. Dalton, and Fr. Haguenau, eds.) , Academic Press, 1968, pp. 81-149.
11. Birnstiel, M. L., and W. G. Flamm: Science, 145:1435-1437, 1964.
12. Birnstiel, M. L., J. Spiers, I. Purdom, K. Jones, and U. E. Loening: Nature, 219: 454-463, 1968.
13. Britten, R. J., and D. E. Kohne: In: Handbook of Molecular Cytology (A. Lima-de-Faria, ed.) , North Holland Publishing Co., 1969, Chapt. 3, pp. 37-51.
14. Brown, D. D., and J. B. Dawid: Science, 160:272-280, 1968.
15. Carneiro, J., and C. P. Leblond: Science, 129:391-392, 1959.
16. Chouinard, L. A., and C. P. Leblond: J. Cell Sci., 2:473-480, 1967.
17. Comings, D. E.: J. Cell Biol., 35:699-708, 1967.
18. Comings, D. E., and T. Kakefuda: J. Mol. Biol., 33:225-229, 1968.
19. Darnell, J. E.: Bact. Rev., 32:262-290, 1968.
20. Davies, H. G.: J. Cell Sci., 3:129-150, 1968.
21. Fakan, S.: Personal communication.
22. Feldherr, C. M.: J. Cell Biol., 39:49-54, 1968.
23. Frenster, J. H.: Nature, 206:680-683, 1965.
24. Frenster, J. H.: Nature, 206:1269-1270, 1965.
25. Frenster, J. H.: In: Handbook of Molecular Cytology (A. Lima-de-Faria, ed.) , North Holland Publishing Co., 1969, Chapt. 12, pp. 251-276.
26. Gall, J. G.: J. Cell Biol., 32:391-400, 1967.
27. Gall, J. G., and M. L. Pardue: Proc. Nat. Acad. Sci. USA, 63:378-383, 1969.
28. Georgiev, G. P.: J. Theoret. Biol., 25:473-490, 1969.
29. Goldstein, L., and D. M. Prescott: J. Cell Biol., 33:637-644, 1967.
30. Granboulan, N., and K. Scherrer: Europ. J. Biochem., 9:1-20, 1969.
31. Gurdon, J. B., and H. R. Woodland: Biol. Rev., 43:233-267, 1968.
32. Haguenau, Fr.: Ultrastructure of the cancer cell. In: The Biological Basis of Medicine. Academic Press, 1968, Vol. 5, Chapt. 12, pp. 433-486.
33. Harris, H.: Nucleus and Cytoplasm. Clarendon Press, Oxford, 1968, pp. 1-142.
34. Hyde, B. B.: Progr. Biophys. Mol. Biol., 15:129-148, 1965.
35. Hilgartner, C. A.: Exp. Cell Res., 49:520-532, 1968.
36. Huang, R. C., and J. Bonner: Proc. Nat. Acad. Sci. USA, 54:960-967, 1965.
37. Howk, R., and T. Y. Wang: Europ. J. Biochem., 13:455-460, 1970.
38. John, H. A., M. L. Birnstiel, and K. W. Jones: Nature, 223:582-587, 1969.
39. Leduc, E. H., S. Avrameas, and M. Bouteille: J. Exp. Med., 127:109-118, 1968.
40. Littau, V. C., C. J. Burdick, V. G. Allfrey, and A. E. Mirsky: Proc. Nat. Acad. Sci. USA, 54:1204-1212, 1965.
41. Miller, O. L., and B. R. Beatty: Science, 164:955-957, 1969.
42. Monneron, A., and Y. Moule: Exp. Cell Res., 51:531-554, 1968.
43. Monneron, A., and W. Bernhard: J. Ultrastr. Res., 27:266-288, 1969.
44. Mirsky, A. E., and S. Osawa: In: The Cell (J. Brachet, ed.) , Academic Press, Vol. 2, 1961, pp. 677-770.

45. Novikoff, A. B., N. Quintana, H. Villaverde, and R. Forschirm: J. Cell Biol., 29:525-545, 1966.
46. Penman, S.: J. Mol. Biol., 17:117-130, 1966.
47. Perry, R. P.: Nat. Cancer Inst. Monogr., 23:527-545, 1966.
48. Ringertz, N. L.: In: Handbook of Molecular Cytology (A. Lima-de-Faria, ed.), North Holland Publishing Co., 1969, Chapt. 27, pp. 656-684.
49. Ris, H.: In: Handbook of Molecular Cytology (A. Lima-de-Faria, ed.), North Holland Publishing Co., 1969, Chap. 4, pp. 221-250.
50. Ris, H.: In: Interpretation of Ultrastructure. Symp. Inter. Soc. Cell Biol., 1:69-88, 1962.
51. Robbins, E., and T. W. Borun: Proc. Nat. Acad. Sci. USA, 57:409-416, 1967.
52. Sadowski, P. O., and J. A. Howden: J. Cell Biol., 37:163-181, 1968.
53. Samarina, O. P., E. M. Lukanidin, J. Molnar, and G. P. Georgiev: J. Mol. Biol., 33:251-263, 1968.
54. Scherrer, K., H. Latham, and J. E. Darnell: Proc. Nat. Acad. Sci. USA, 49:240-248, 1968.
55. Scherrer, K., and L. Marcaud: J. Cell Physiol., 72 (suppl. 1) :181-212, 1968.
56. Sharma, O. K., E. J. Hidvegi, F. Martes, A. W. Prestayko, K. Smetana, and H. Busch: Physiol. Chem. Phys., 1:185-209, 1969. ˙
57. Shankar Narayan, K., W. J. Steele, K. Smetana, and H. Busch: Exp. Cell Res., 46:65-77, 1967.
58. Siebert, J.: In: Methods in Cancer Research (H. Busch, ed.), vol. 3, 1967, pp. 47-59.
59. Soeiro, R., M. H. Vaughan, J. R. Warner, and J. E. Darnell: J. Cell Biol., 39:112-118, 1968.
60. Spirin, A. S.: Europ. J. Biochem., 10:20-35, 1969.
61. Stevens, B. J., and J. Andre: In: Handbook of Molecular Cytology (A. Lima-de-Faria, ed.), North Holland Publishing Co., 1969, Chapt. 33, pp. 837-871.
62. Stevens, B. J., and H. Swift: J. Cell Biol., 31:55-77, 1966.
63. Swain, F. M.: Ann. Rev. Microbiol., 23:455-472, 1969.
64. Swift, H.: In: Interpretation of Ultrastructure, Symp. Int. Soc. Cell Biol., 1:213-232, 1962.
65. Tixier-Vidal, A., S. Fiske, R. Picart, and Fr. Haguenau: Compt. Rend. Acad. Sci. (Paris), 261:1133-1136, 1965.
66. Watson, M. L.: J. Cell Biol., 13:162-167, 1962.
67. Weinberg, R. A., and S. Penman: J. Mol. Biol., 38:289-304, 1968.
68. Yasuzumi, G., and I. Tsubo: Exp. Cell Res., 43:281, 1966.
69. Zimmerman, E. F., J. Hackney, P. Nelson, and I. M. Arias: Biochemistry, 8:2636-2644, 1969.
70. Zotikov, L., and W. Bernhard: J. Ultrastr. Res., 30:642-663, 1970.

The Nucleolus and Its Function

MASAMI MURAMATSU AND
TORU HIGASHINAKAGAWA

*Department of Chemistry, Cancer Institute, Japanese Foundation for
Cancer Research, Tokyo, Japan*

RECENT PROGRESS IN molecular biology as applied to eukaryotes has accumulated a considerable amount of knowledge concerning the function of the nucleus as well as nucleolus.

At the present time, the main function of the nucleolus can be summarized as the production of the ribosomes.[22] Other functions assigned to the nucleolus in the history of cytology have not been verified; many have been disproved.

The hypertrophy and pleomorphism of the nucleoli of cancer cells were also the subject of interest, and even regarded as pathognomonic. However, since these characteristics can be seen in many other rapidly dividing cells or cells which produce large amounts of proteins, we are not yet certain if nucleolar abnormality is characteristic of or inherent in malignant growth.[11]

In this paper, we would like to concentrate on a well-proved function of the nucleolus, i.e. ribosome formation, rather than to review a variety of speculative functions which may be present in the nucleolus. Even in this area of ribosome biosynthesis, there are a number of problems yet to be solved, some of which may be very important in understanding the malignant nature of cancer cells.[9]

To give a perspective, I shall discuss three aspects of the nucleolar function: (1) nucleolar RNA, (2) nucleolar ribonucleoproteins and (3) some aspects of control of nucleolar RNA synthesis.

Isolation of Nucleoli

In Figure 16-4, a nuclear preparation of rat liver isolated by a modified Chauveau procedure with Mg^{2+} is presented. The nucleolar preparation isolated by our sonication procedure is shown in Figure 16-5. These highly purified nucleoli were the starting material with which the following experiments were carried out. Figures 16-6 and 16-7 show electron micrographs of nuclear and nucleolar preparation, respectively. Figure 16-8 presents a nucleolus in higher magnification, in which nucleolar ultrastructure is seen clearly. The nucleolus is surrounded with darkly stained nucleolus-associated chromatin which penetrates

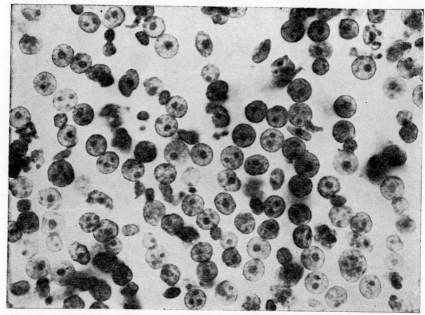

FIG. 16–4.—Isolated nuclei of rat liver, stained with Azure C.

FIG. 16–5.—Isolated nucleoli of rat liver, stained with Azure C.

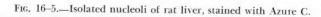

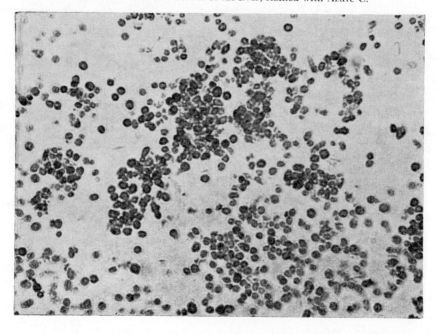

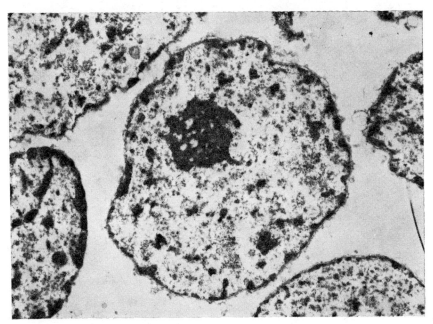

Fig. 16–6.—Electron micrograph of isolated nuclei of rat liver, taken by Dr. H. Sugano, Department of Pathology, Cancer Institute.

Fig. 16–7.—Electron micrograph of isolated nucleoli of rat liver, taken by Dr. H. Sugano, Department of Pathology, Cancer Institute.

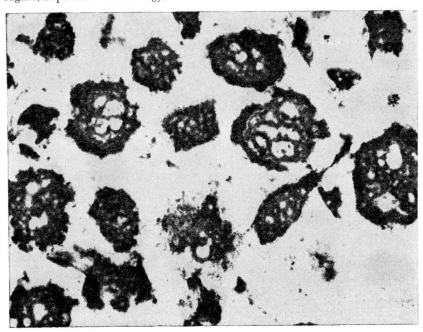

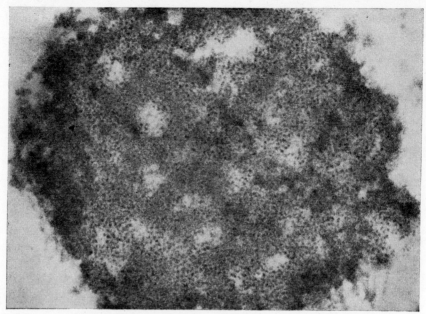

Fig. 16–8.—Electron micrograph of an isolated nucleolus of Morris hepatoma 7316B. Granular and fibrillar components as well as nucleolus-associated chromatin are shown together.[14]

into the nucleolonemas consisting of fibrillar and granular components. The latter is 150 to 200 A in diameter, which is similar to the size of the cytoplasmic ribosomes.

Isolated nuclei can be fractionated into nucleolar and extranucleolar nuclear fractions by sonication followed by differential centrifugation.[10, 18]

Nucleolar RNA

The RNAs extracted with an SDS-hot phenol procedure[12, 23] showed the patterns shown in Figure 16-9. The broken lines indicate the ^{32}P radioactivity at 30 min of injection, which represents the newly synthesized RNA in each fraction. As can be seen, the nucleolar RNA has large optical density peaks of 45S and 35S, which are not present in extranucleolar nuclear RNA. The base composition of RNA sedimenting with different S values is presented in Table 16-1. The nucleolar RNA showed a high GC content everywhere, especially at the 45S region, while the extranucleolar nuclear RNA contained high AU-type RNA species, especially at the 45S and low-molecular-weight regions. Thus the nucleolar RNA is qualitatively distinct from the RNA species in the extranucleolar fractions. The ^{32}P base composition of the whole nuclear fraction was between nucleolar and extranucleolar nuclear RNA, indicating the composite nature of this fraction.[15]

The kinetics of labeling of nucleolar RNA is shown in Figure 16-10. [14C] Orotic acid was injected iv into rats 10 min prior to the injection of actinomycin D, which stops nucleolar RNA synthesis within a minute. The rats were killed at specified time periods shown in the pattern, and the nucleolar RNA was examined on the gradient. As clearly seen, the radioactivity appeared on the 45S peak with 10 min of labeling, moved to the 35S RNA, and then to the 28S RNA peak in the complete absence of new RNA synthesis. At the same time, the optical density peak of 45S decreased rapidly, followed by the 35S peak, indicating a rapid processing of 45S RNA into 28S RNA via the 35S intermediate.[16]

The site of methylation of ribosomal RNA was found to be in the nucleolus.[3, 12, 29] Figure 16-11 shows that at 10 min after injection of [Me3H] methionine, most of the radioactivity was associated with the 45S RNA in the nucleolus. As time proceeded, the radioactivity moved to 35S and then to 28S RNA, again confirming the transition of the 45S RNA as proposed previously.[20, 21] If the rats were treated with actinomycin D before injection of [Me3H] methionine, no radioactivity

Fig. 16–9.—Sedimentation profiles of nuclear, nucleolar, and extranucleolar nuclear RNA. The broken lines show the 32P radioactivity at 30 min of injection (see Table 16-1).

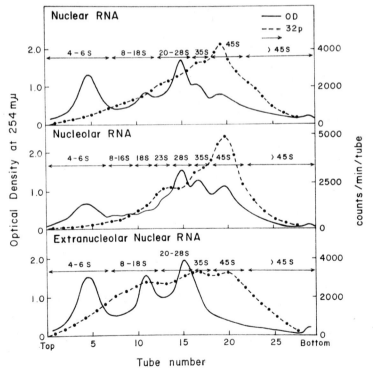

TABLE 16-1.—BASE ANALYSIS (^{32}P) OF SUCROSE DENSITY
GRADIENT FRACTIONS SHOWN IN FIGURE 16-9

FRACTION	APPROXIMATE S	A	U	G	C	(A + U): (G + C)
Nuclear RNA						
1-7	4-6	24.3	24.5	26.2	25.0	0.95
8-11	8-18	25.6	23.9	26.2	24.3	0.98
12-16	20-28	25.2	23.5	27.6	23.7	0.95
17-18	35	24.7	22.1	29.1	24.1	0.88
19-22	45	25.1	22.1	28.5	24.3	0.89
23-28	>45	25.7	23.7	26.3	24.3	0.98
Nucleolar RNA						
1-7	4-6	19.8	20.6	34.0	25.6	0.68
8-9	8-16	20.4	19.2	35.2	25.2	0.66
10-11	18	20.7	16.7	35.8	26.8	0.60
12-13	23	19.9	17.5	35.8	26.8	0.60
14-16	28	20.5	17.2	36.3	26.0	0.61
17-18	35	20.3	17.1	39.1	23.5	0.60
19-22	45	19.3	16.6	39.4	24.7	0.56
23-28	>45	20.3	16.6	37.1	26.0	0.58
Extranucleolar nuclear RNA						
1-7	4-6	25.8	27.0	24.2	23.0	1.12
8-11	8-18	26.8	25.8	23.3	24.1	1.11
12-16	20-28	26.2	25.4	23.7	24.7	1.07
17-18	35	26.9	25.1	23.9	24.1	1.08
18-22	45	26.6	24.9	25.0	23.5	1.06
23-28	>45	28.4	25.4	23.1	23.1	1.16

Abbreviations: A, adenine; C, cytosine; G, guanine; U, uracil.

could be found on any peak of nucleolar RNA at any time points, indicating that methylation occurs as the transcription of 45S RNA proceeds and little or no methyl groups are added to ribosomal RNA during the steps of maturation.

Summarizing the above results, we can picture the processing of the nucleolar RNA as in Figure 16-12. While more steps could be recognized by acrylamide gel electrophoresis,[8, 26] kinetic and hybridization data suggest strongly the following conclusions.[7] The precursor 45S RNA which contains both the 28S and 18S RNA sequences cleaves off the 18S RNA and a considerable length of nonribosomal sequences at the first step to make 35S RNA. This RNA, then, cleaves off a smaller fragment to become 28S RNA, which is the component of the large subunit of the ribosomes. Since the molecular weights estimated for 45S, 35S, 28S, and 18S RNA are 4.6×10^6, 2.7×10^6, 1.6×10^6, and 0.63×10^6, respectively, and also not more than one of each ribosomal sequences were found in the 45S RNA,[1, 6] about half of the 45S RNA must represent nonribosomal sequences. The order of arrangement of these RNAs in the precursor molecules is one of the prime concerns to the investigators in this field, and study is now under way to es-

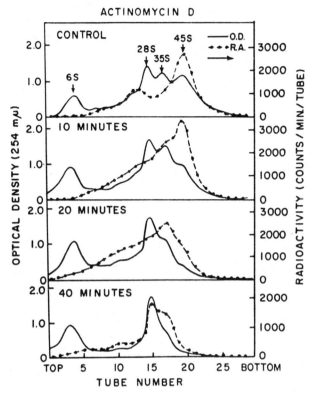

FIG. 16–10.—Effect of actinomycin D on labeling of nucleolar RNA.

tablish these points.[2, 17, 27] The precise mechanisms of cleavage and the functions, if any, of nonribosomal sequences released during transition also remain to be determined.

Next, let us look at the proteins of the nucleolus.

Nucleolar Ribonucleoproteins

When we treat the nucleolar preparation with 67% acetic acid and examine the acid-soluble proteins on an acrylamide gel electrophoresis, the pattern shown in Figure 16-13 is obtained. As can be seen, these proteins consist of 30 or more clearly separated bands which are not demonstrated in total nuclear acid-soluble proteins containing a large amount of histones.[4] When we compare these proteins on split-gel electrophoresis, we can demonstrate that many of these bands coincide with those of the ribosomal proteins, especially with those of large subunit of ribosomes (Figure 16-14). There are, however, several

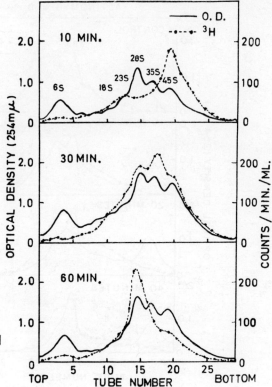

FIG. 16–11.—Labeling patterns of nucleolar RNA after injection of L-[Me-³H] methionine.

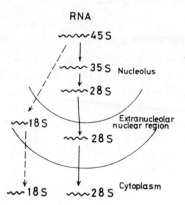

FIG. 16–12.—Processing of the nucleolar RNA during the steps of maturation.

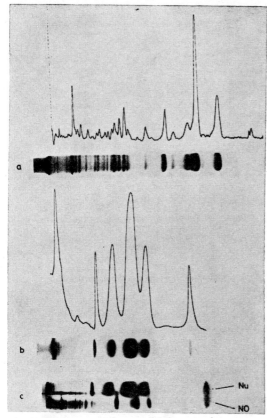

FIG. 16–13.—Polyacrylamide gel electrophoresis patterns (pH 4.3) and densitometric recordings of nuclear and nucleolar acid-soluble proteins: *a*—nuclear acid-soluble proteins; *b*—nucleolar acid-soluble proteins; *c*—split-gel comparison of nuclear and nucleolar proteins. Nu—nuclear proteins, NO—nucleolar proteins.

bands which agree neither with histones nor with ribosomal proteins. The identification and analysis of the function of these proteins will be an interesting subject for future studies.

Evidence from several laboratories indicates that the synthesis of these proteins appears to be localized in the cytoplasm rather than in the nucleolus.[5, 19] However, the nucleoli appear to have a certain pool of these ribosomal proteins, assembling ribosomes as the ribosomal precursor RNA is transcribed.[25] The process of assembly of ribosomes could be followed by extracting ribosomal precursor particles from isolated nucleoli from animals labeled for certain time periods with [14C] orotic acid. Nucleolar ribonucleoprotein particles can be extracted by a mild treatment of nucleolar preparation with DNase and detergents.[4, 8, 24] Figure 16-15 shows that these ribonucleoproteins have a sedimentation constant of approximately 60S and contain solely 28S RNA. The gel pattern of the proteins of these particles resembles closely that of the ribosomes, indicating that these particles represent the precursors of the large subunit of the ribosomes.

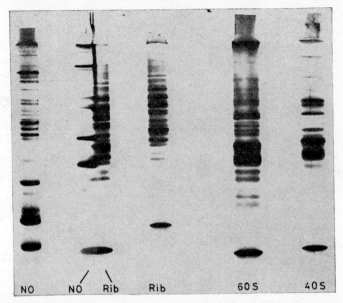

FIG. 16–14.—Split-gel comparison of nucleolar and ribosomal proteins. NO—nucleolar proteins, Rib—total ribosomal proteins, 60S—proteins of larger subunit, 40S—proteins of smaller subunit.

FIG. 16–15.—Sedimentation profiles of nucleolar ribonucleoprotein (RNP) particles and the component RNA. Electrophoretic gels of the proteins of nucleolar RNP are also presented as compared with nucleolar and ribosomal proteins. NO-RNP—proteins of nucleolar RNP particles, NO—nucleolar acid-soluble proteins, Rib—total ribosomal proteins.

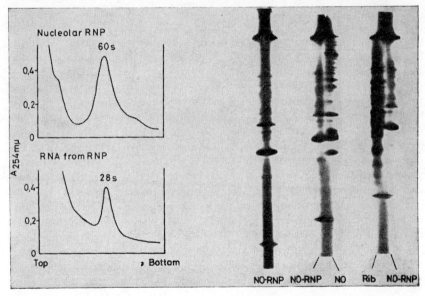

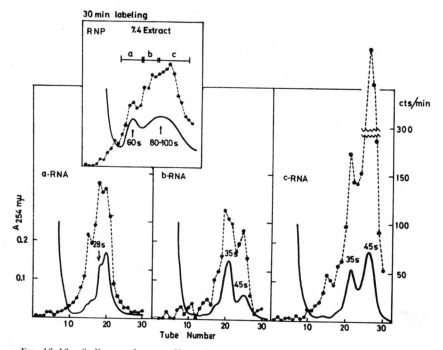

FIG. 16–16.—Sedimentation profiles of nucleolar RNP extracted with the buffer containing polyvinylsulfate (PVS), and the component RNAs. Solid lines show optical density at 254 mμ. Broken lines show the radioactivity at 30 min of injection of [14C] orotic acid.

When the nucleoli were further treated with a buffer containing polyvinylsulfate, other species of ribonucleoprotein particles were extracted as shown in Figure 16-16. In this system, the sucrose density gradient pattern shows two peaks of about 60S and 80-100S. The RNAs present in three regions of the gradient (shown by the bars) are mainly 28S, 35S and 45S RNA, respectively as shown by the radioactivity as well as by the optical density.[4]

The analysis of proteins of these precursor particles is now under way. However, there is some difficulty at the present time since polyvinylsulfate binds tightly to these proteins, preventing the migration of the latter in the gels.

Protein Synthesis and Nucleolar RNA

Last, we would like to comment on the control of nucleolar RNA synthesis. In the course of the study on the maturation of ribosomal precursor particles, we noted a peculiar phenomenon; when rats were treated with a high dose (20 mg/kg) of cycloheximide to stop protein

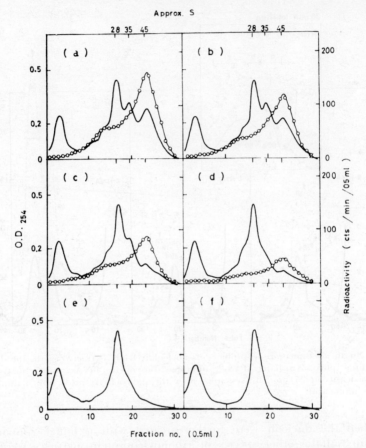

Fraction no. (0.5ml)

FIG. 16–17.—Effect of cycloheximide (CH) on the sedimentation profiles of nucleolar RNA. CH was injected at a dose of 20 mg/kg body weight into rats at specified time periods prior to the termination of the experiments. Five μc of [^{14}C] orotic acid were given iv 10 min prior to sacrifice, as seen in the diagram.

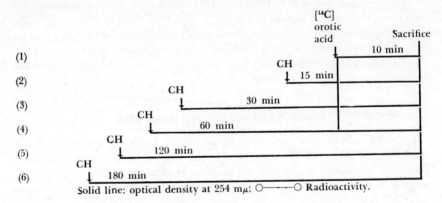

Solid line: optical density at 254 mμ; O————O Radioactivity.

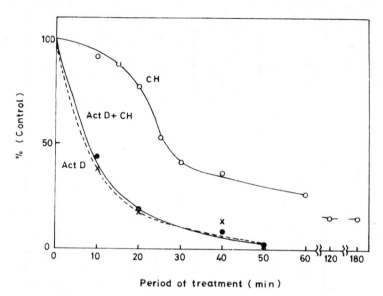

Fig. 16–18.—The decay of 45S RNA in the nucleolus after various treatments. O———O CH treated, X . . . X actinomycin D treated, ●———● treated with both CH and actinomycin D.

synthesis, the nucleolar RNA apparently began to decrease.[13] Figure 16-17 shows the change in the sedimentation profile of nucleolar RNA after cycloheximide injection. The rats were injected with radioactive orotic acid 10 min prior to sacrifice so as to show the synthesis of 45S RNA at respective time points. As can be seen, the size of the 45S RNA peak decreased with the time after cycloheximide treatment, and the radioactivity also decreased gradually to about 30% at one hr. This inhibition was not observed for the extranucleolar nuclear RNA at least for one hr, as shown in Figure 16-18. The inhibition of nucleolar RNA synthesis by cycloheximide also has a short lag, suggesting a different mechanism of inhibition than that of actinomycin D. These phenomena could be repeated in an in vitro system in which isolated nucleoli were incubated with labeled UTP. Figure 16-19 shows the rate of inhibition of in vitro RNA synthetic capacity of isolated nucleoli from cycloheximide-treated animals. The rate of decrease in the incorporation of UMP residues into nucleolar RNA is almost parallel to that found in in vivo experiments. Also remarkable is the relative insensitivity of extranucleolar nuclear fraction to cycloheximide treatment.

It could be concluded from these data that the synthesis of 45S RNA appears to be coupled somehow with the protein synthesis, or in other words, continued protein synthesis is required for the normal transcription of nucleolar genes. The differential effects of cycloheximide on

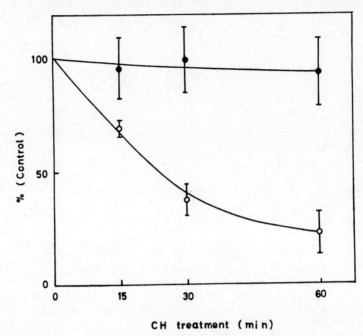

FIG. 16–19.—In vitro RNA synthetic activity of nucleolar and extranucleolar nuclear fraction after CH treatment. O——O nucleolar fraction; ●——● extranucleolar nuclear fraction.

the nucleolar and extranucleolar nuclear RNA may suggest possible differences in the control mechanisms of the synthesis of these two RNA species.

References

1. Amaldi, F., and G. Attardi: J. Mol. Biol., 33:737, 1968.
2. Choi, Y. C., C. M. Mauritzen, C. W. Taylor, and H. Busch: Fed. Proc. In press.
3. Greenberg, H., and S. Penman: J. Mol. Biol., 21:527, 1966.
4. Higashinakagawa, T., and M. Muramatsu: In preparation.
5. Izawa, M., and K. Kawashima: Biochim. Biophys. Acta, 190:139, 1969.
6. Jeanteur, P., F. Amaldi, and G. Attardi: J. Mol. Biol., 33:757, 1968.
7. Jeanteur, P., and G. Attardi: J. Mol. Biol., 45:305, 1969.
8. Liau, M. C., and R. P. Perry: J. Cell Biol., 42:272, 1969.
9. Muramatsu, M.: Gann Monogr., 4:35, 1968.
10. Muramatsu, M., and H. Busch: Cancer Res., 24:1028, 1964.
11. Muramatsu, M., and H. Busch: Meth. Cancer Res., 2:303, 1967.
12. Muramatsu, M., and T. Fujisawa: Biochim. Biophys. Acta, 157:476, 1968.
13. Muramatsu, M., N. Shimada, and T. Higashinakagawa: Submitted for publication.
14. Muramatsu, M., T. Higashinakagawa, T. Ono, and H. Sugano: Cancer Res., 28: 1126, 1968.
15. Muramatsu, M., J. L. Hodnett, and H. Busch: J. Biol. Chem., 241:1544, 1966.
16. Muramatsu, M., J. L. Hodnett, W. J. Steele, and H. Busch: Biochim. Biophys. Acta, 123:116, 1966.
17. Muramatsu, M., K. Sakuma, M. Sugiura, and M. Takanami: Fed. Proc. In press.
18. Muramatsu, M., K. Smetana, and H. Busch: Cancer Res., 23:510, 1963.
19. Ogata, K., K. Terao, and H. Sugano: Biochim. Biophys. Acta, 149:572, 1967.

20. Penman, S., I. Smith, and E. Holtzman: Science, 154:786, 1966.
21. Perry, R. P.: Nat. Cancer Inst. Monogr., 23:527, 1966.
22. Perry, R. P.: Progr. Nucl. Acid Res. Mol. Biol., 6:219, 1967.
23. Scherrer, K., and J. E. Darnell: Biochim. Biophys. Res. Comm., 7:486, 1962.
24. Warner, J. R., and R. Soeiro: Proc. Nat. Acad. Sci. USA, 58:1984, 1967.
25. Warner, J. R., M. Girard, H. Latham, and J. E. Darnell: J. Mol. Biol., 19:373, 1966.
26. Weinberg, R. A., U. Loening, M. Willems, and S. Perman: Proc. Nat. Acad. Sci. USA, 58:1088, 1967.
27. Wikman, J., E. Howard, and H. Busch: J. Biol. Chem., 244:5471, 1969.
28. Zimmerman, E. F., and B. W. Holler: J. Mol. Biol., 23:149, 1967.

Form and Structure of Mitochondrial DNA

DAVID R. WOLSTENHOLME, KATSURO KOIKE, AND HARTMUT C. RENGER

Division of Biology, Kansas State University, Manhattan, Kansas, USA

THERE IS NOW clear evidence that mitochondria contain their own DNA molecules. A study of the size and structure of such molecules is in itself of interest, but has more far-reaching implications when considered as the physical basis of cytoplasmic inheritance. The lengths of the mitochondrial DNA (M-DNA) molecules and the population of different base sequences define the total amount of genetic information which organelle DNA can carry. This in turn sets limits to the autonomy with which this secondary genetic system can influence the functioning of the cell.

A study of the size and structure of M-DNA molecules in phylogenetically diverse organisms might be expected to both indicate the present diversity of the mitochondrial genetic system, and provide some information concerning the evolution of this system.

The purpose of this paper is to describe what we know at the present time concerning the form and structure of M-DNA.

Pure M-DNA has been successfully isolated from a number of animal tissues by the procedure outlined in Table 16-2.

The buoyant density of the M-DNA of many species is distinct from that of the organism's nuclear DNA (Table 16-3), though in *Xenopus*

TABLE 16–2.—Basic Procedure for the Isolation of Pure
Mitochondrial DNA from Animal Tissues

1. Tissue is immersed in buffered 0.3 M sucrose.
2. Break up tissue first in Waring blender and then in Potter-Elvehjem homogenizer.
3. Centrifuge at 500 × g to remove remaining whole cell nuclei.
4. Centrifuge at between 8,000 and 12,000 × g to obtain a crude mitochondrial pellet (monitor by electron microscopy).
5. Resuspend pellet in buffered sucrose and digest with pancreatic DNase to remove contaminating nuclear DNA. (The mitochondria are impermeable to this nuclease[54] and the DNA within the organelles is therefore unaffected.)
6. Wash mitochondria free from DNase by repeated centrifugation and resuspension.
7. Extract M-DNA by chloroform procedure of Marmur[45] or by use of phenol.[36]
8. DNA is finally concentrated and purified either by step elution from a methylated albumin Kieselguhr column or by banding in a cesium chloride preparative gradient.
9. For further details of this whole procedure for the preparation of M-DNA see Kirschner, Wolstenholme and Gross.[36]

Exceptional Tissues
A. The mitochondria of a number of tissues, salamander liver,[70] frog liver[3] and sheep heart[39] seem to be permeable to DNase. In these cases the mitochondria have been freed from nuclear DNA contamination by banding in a sucrose gradient. This latter procedure is also included when it is necessary to ensure the mitochondrial origin of a DNA.
B. M-DNA from oocytes or eggs of the two frogs, *Xenopus laevis,* the South African clawed toad, and *Rana pipiens,* the leopard frog, is in 200- to 500-fold excess to the nuclear DNA,[18, 19] so that for practical purposes, the problem of nuclear DNA contamination is nonexistent.

laevis, Rana pipiens, and the mouse, they appear identical. In mammals, with the exception of man, and in reptiles there is little difference in buoyant density between the two types of DNA. In birds and in fishes, the densities of M-DNAs are consistently higher than the respective nuclear DNAs. The M-DNAs of anuran amphibians are similar in density to the organism's nuclear DNA, but in urodele amphibians the M-DNAs are noticeably less dense than the respective nuclear DNAs.

M-DNA from cells of all metazoan animals studied so far has been found to comprise circular molecules which have a contour length of from 4.5 to 6.0 μ. Such a molecule is shown in Figure 16-20. A similar circular form has been found by various workers for the DNA from mitochondria of a nematode worm,[74] an annelid worm,[21] a fly,[10] a crab,[75] an echinoderm,[53] and a number of fishes, amphibians, reptiles, birds, and mammals (see Table 16-3).

Fresh preparations of M-DNA also contain varying proportions of highly twisted or supercoiled circular molecules (Figure 16-21).

From the results of studies made with M-DNA from the oocytes and eggs of two frogs, *Xenopus laevis* and *Rana pipiens,* Dawid and Wolstenholme[22] concluded that circular M-DNA has a similar structure to that of the smaller circular polyoma viral DNA described by Vinograd and Lebowitz.[68] A similar conclusion has been drawn by a number of workers for the M-DNA of a variety of metazoan animals.[4, 5, 7, 39, 53] The essential experimental data on which Dawid and Wolstenholme[22] based their interpretation were as follows.

When fresh preparations of M-DNA were band-sedimented in 1 M sodium chloride, two components were found which sedimented at 39S and 27S. The proportion of the 39S component (about 65%) was similar to the proportion of the supercoiled circles seen in electron micrographs of the same preparations. In one preparation, upon band sedimentation, only the 27S component could be detected, and examination in the electron microscope revealed only 4% supercoiled circles. The 39S component appeared, therefore, to be the supercoiled circle, and the 27S component, the open circle. Digestion of M-DNA with pancreatic DNase (1.5×10^{-7} µg/ml for five min) resulted in conversion of the 39S component to the 27S component. Correspondingly, it was found by electron microscopy that this treatment resulted in conversion of the supercoiled form to the open circular form.

TABLE 16–3.—BUOYANT DENSITIES AND CONTOUR LENGTHS OF VERTEBRATE CIRCULAR MITOCHONDRIAL DNAs

	BUOYANT DENSITY		CONTOUR LENGTH OF CIRCULAR M-DNA	REFERENCE
	Nuclear	Mitochondrial		
Mammalia				
Man	1.700	1.707	5.1	17, 49
Rat	1.703	1.701	5.0	61, 73
Mouse	1.699	1.699	5.0	76
Guinea-pig	1.702	1.702	5.0	74
Rabbit	1.701	1.703		5
Ox	1.704	1.703	5.1	5, 63
Sheep	1.703	1.703	5.4	39
Dog	1.700	1.703	5.0	77
Aves				
Duck	1.700	1.711	5.1	5, 39
Pigeon	1.700	1.707		5
Chicken	1.698	1.708	5.1	54, 63
Reptilia				
Chuckwalla				
(*Sauromalus ater*)	1.700		5.3	77
Turtle				
(*Terrapene ornata*)	1.702	1.701	5.3	77
Amphibia				
Anura				
Rana pipiens	1.702	1.702	5.8	18, 70
Xenopus laevis	1.700	1.702	5.8	18, 70
Urodela				
Siredon mexicanum	1.704	1.695	4.7	70
Necturus maculosus	1.707	1.695	4.8	70
Pisces				
Channel catfish				
(*Ictalurus punctatus*)	1.699	1.708	5.1	77

FIG. 16–20.—*(Left)* Electron micrograph of molecule of M-DNA prepared by the protein monolayer technique of Kleinschmidt[26] and rotary shadowed with platinum-palladium. (Figure from Wolstenholme et al.[73]) An open circular molecule of contour length 4.9 μ from an Ehrlich mouse ascites tumor. ×47,000.

FIG. 16–21.—*(Right)* Electron micrograph of molecule of M-DNA prepared by the protein monolayer technique of Kleinschmidt[26] and rotary shadowed with platinum-palladium. (Figure from Wolstenholme et al.[73]) A supercoiled circular molecule of contour length 4.9 μ from an Ehrlich mouse ascites tumor. ×47,000.

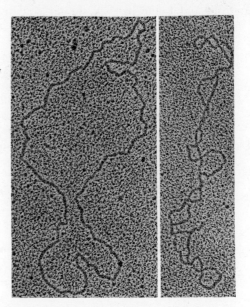

It seems that in the supercoiled forms, the two strands of the DNA double helix are intact; that is, not a single phosphodiester bond in either of the two polynucleotide chains of each molecule is broken. The observed supercoiling is apparently brought about by a deficiency of Watson-Crick turns in the closed molecule, such that in order to complete base pairing, the molecule must twist on itself to the right. If a single phosphodiester bond is broken in just one of the strands, such as by digestion with pancreatic DNase, then a swivel point is created opposite the break, and the supercoil in the molecule is relaxed. Thus, the supercoiled circle is converted to the open circle.

If the supercoiled molecule is a covalently closed circle, then it should be possible to reversibly denature it, as the single polynucleotide strands should not be able to leave each other even if hydrogen bond separation occurs, because of their topologic bonding. That is, such molecules would instantly "snap back" into the native configuration after removing the denaturing agent. This prediction was tested by alkali-denaturing a preparation of M-DNA, neutralizing the solution, and subjecting it to cesium chloride equilibrium centrifugation. Two bands were formed, one at the density of native M-DNA and the other at the density of denatured M-DNA, which is about 14 mg/ml greater than native density. The proportion of DNA banding at native density was similar to the proportion of supercoiled circles in the original preparation. Following neutralization, the preparation was examined in the electron microscope and found to include numerous molecules indistinguishable from native supercoiled circles.

Figure 16-22 summarizes these experiments. When both strands of the double helix were broken simultaneously, which was achieved by digestion with *Escherichia coli* DNase II, a third component which sedimented at 24S was produced. This is assumed to be a linear form of the molecule. Denaturation of the open circular form resulted in a single-stranded circle and a single-stranded linear piece. These latter forms have been observed in electron microscope preparations of denatured open circular rat liver M-DNA.[72]

When M-DNA was band-sedimented in alkaline cesium chloride, which denatures the DNA, two components were found. The slow component is assumed to represent a mixture of the single-stranded

Fig. 16–22.—Schematic presentation of the different forms of M-DNA (modified from Dawid and Wolstenholme, 1967).[22] The covalently closed, supercoiled circle (component I) is converted to the open circle (component II) by breaking one of the strands, and to the linear form (component III) by breaking both strands at the same position. Denaturation of the covalently closed circle proceeds first through an open form (I') which resembles component II, then through a left supercoiled form (II") to the tightly coiled component I_{alk}. Denaturation of component II leads to a mixture of linear and circular single-stranded molecules (II_{alk}).

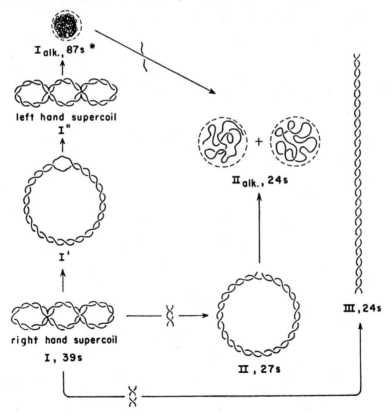

linear and single-stranded circular forms. The fast component which sedimented at 87S is assumed to be the supercoiled form which results from the double-stranded circle first unwinding, then, as denaturation proceeds, collapsing into two interlocked tight single-stranded coils which, as will be recalled, cannot separate from each other because of their topologic interlocking.

The effect of heating covalently closed circular M-DNA from rat liver to various temperatures in the presence of 10% formaldehyde has been studied in the electron microscope.[72] Formaldehyde lowers the melting temperature by about 30 C and has the property of preventing the rejoining of base pairs upon cooling the DNA. By 40 C the supercoiled circles were converted to open circular forms. This is the form I' (Figure 16-22), which we assume is produced by separation of just enough base pairs to allow unwinding of the supercoil. Increase in temperature above 50 C (at about which temperature the two strands of the open circular forms separate) resulted in reappearance of supercoiled circles (I'', Figure 16-22). This supercoiling is presumably to the left, and results from further unwinding of the double helix as more base pairs separate.[24] At temperatures above 70 C, cross-linking of the two polynucleotide chains by formaldehyde prevented useful interpretation of the data.

Resistance to denaturation of covalently closed circular DNA is also indicated by observations of the behavior of this form of DNA upon continuous heating in a spectrophotometer. Covalently closed circular guinea pig liver M-DNA failed to show any increase in absorbancy when heated in 0.05 M sodium phosphate to 98 C.[74] In contrast, open circular DNA underwent a clear thermal transition at 80.6 C. A similar observation has been made for covalently closed circular kinetoplast DNA of *Trypanosoma lewisi* in SSC (0.15 M sodium chloride, 0.015 M sodium citrate)[57] (see below). Covalently closed circular polyoma DNA[68] and mouse L cell M-DNA[49] were both found to show a much lower rate of increase in absorbancy than their respective open circular forms, when continuously heated in SSC.

By observing the amount of DNA associated with mitochondria when the mitochondria were burst open by osmotic shock, Nass[48] determined that each mitochondrion of mouse L cells contains from two to six circular molecules. A question of importance is whether all of the circles of M-DNA of a cell have the same base sequence and, therefore, carry the same genetic message. There is no evidence for more than one size class of circles of M-DNA within a single animal species. This holds true for M-DNA from different organs.[63, 77] Also, for any one species the M-DNA forms a single band upon equilibrium centrifugation in cesium chloride. These observations are consistent with there being only one kind of circle. When open circular M-DNA is denatured, in contrast to nuclear DNA, it can be easily reannealed to such an extent that it returns either completely to, or to within 3 mg/

cm³ of native density;[6, 16, 23] see also Sinclair et al.[64] for yeast M-DNA, and Wolstenholme and Gross[71] for plant M-DNA. From a consideration of the reassociated kinetics of chick M-DNA, Borst, Ruttenberg and Kroon[5] suggested that there is only one kind of M-DNA molecule in this organism.

We have used the denaturation mapping technique of Inman[33] to map and compare individual molecules of M-DNA from rat liver.[72]

The principle of this method is based upon the finding that if DNA is heated in the presence of formaldehyde to specific temperatures within its melting range, the regions of the molecule rich in adenine-

Fig. 16–23.—Denaturation maps of 25 rat liver M-DNA molecules, each containing three regions of strand separation, obtained by heating to 49 C in 0.05 M sodium phosphate and 10% formaldehyde. Each circular molecule was converted to a linear rod. The three regions of strand separation (thick line) were always contained within a segment of the molecule equal to less than half the length of the molecule. The midpoint of this segment in each molecule was taken as the common point by which the molecules were lined up (arrow). The larger of the two regions of native DNA between the three strand separations was placed to the left in each molecule, thus defining direction. The histogram at the bottom of the diagram has been constructed from the 25 maps to show the variation in occurrence of regions of strand separation at intervals of 0.5% (about 250 A) around the molecule. (Data from Wolstenholme, Kirschner and Gross.[72])

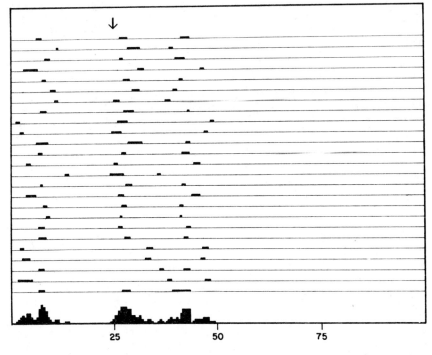

PERCENTAGE   CONTOUR   LENGTH

thymine base pairs tend to melt at temperatures lower than regions rich in guanine-cytosine base pairs.[25, 33] As formaldehyde prevents the rejoining of base pairs upon cooling, regions of strand separation can be detected in the electron microscope, and individual molecules can be mapped with respect to the gross distribution of the different base pairs.

It was determined that in the presence of 10% formaldehyde in 0.05 M sodium phosphate, open circular molecules of rat liver M-DNA melt within the range 44 C to 55 C with a midpoint (T_m) of 49.5 C. A proportion of the molecules heated to 49 C were found to have from one to four regions of strand separation.

We first compared molecules having three regions of strand separation. In a circular molecule, unlike the λ molecules studied by Inman, there is no beginning or natural reference point. Also there is no indication of direction. We therefore converted each circular molecule to a linear rod (Figure 16-23). The three regions of strand separation were always contained within a segment of the molecule equal to less than half the length of the molecule. The midpoint of this segment in each molecule was taken as the common point by which the molecules were lined up. The larger of the two regions of native DNA between the three strand separations was placed to the left in each molecule, thus defining direction. The result of comparing 25 such maps is seen at the bottom of Figure 16-23. There is a distinct indication of three common regions of strand separation in the molecules compared. Also, as mentioned above, the regions of strand separation, which we assume to be adenine-thymine rich regions, are limited to less than 50% of the molecule. A similar situation, where approximately one half of the molecule differs distinctly in average base composition from the other half, has been well documented for λ phage DNA.[28, 33, 34]

For M-DNA molecules with two regions of strand separation, the positions of the separations can be arranged to fit the three strand separation map. When an attempt was made to similarly map the best fit for four strand separations, again three common regions could be discerned but the fourth mapped more or less at random. This latter observation may be an indication of the limitation of the technique. Open circular molecules heated to 50 C had up to 14 regions of strand separations. No clear common groupings were found.

The molecules showing two, three and four strand separations at 49 C represent about 25% of the open circular DNA. Inman[33] found that individual molecules from a known homogeneous population of molecules showed variation in the number of strand separations at given temperatures. Our mapping results for molecules heated to 49 C are, therefore, not inconsistent with the interpretation that M-DNA molecules comprise only one species with respect to their base sequences.

The amount of genetic information that could be carried by a single

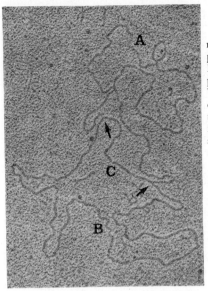

Fig. 16–24.—Electron micrograph of molecule of M-DNA prepared by the protein monolayer technique of Kleinschmidt[28] and rotary shadowed with platinum-palladium. (Figure from Wolstenholme et al.[73]) A partially duplicated circular molecule from a Chang rat solid tumor. The positions of the two forks are indicated by the arrows. Two of the segments (A and B) delimited by the forks are equal in length (4.3 μ), while the third (C) has an odd length (0.7 μ). The sum of the lengths of A or B plus C gives 5.0 μ, which is similar to the lengths of single nonduplicated molecules. Segments A and C are therefore taken to be the products of the portion of the molecule which has replicated, and segment C is taken to be the unreplicated portion. ×48,000.

DNA molecule of 5 μ is obviously severely limited. A DNA molecule of this size has a molecular weight of about 10×10^6 [44] and could, in fact, code for the amino acid sequences of about 25 proteins with an average molecular weight of 20,000, or the equivalent of about three sets of ribosomal RNAs.

There is evidence that mitochondria increase by growth and division,[40–42] and that M-DNA is synthesized in situ rather than being manufactured in the nucleus and transported to the mitochondria.[52, 56] A rather direct indication of the latter was the finding of circular molecules of DNA, isolated from rat liver mitochondria, which had apparently been arrested in the process of replication.[36] Each such molecule had two forks (Figure 16-24). The lengths of two of the segments delimited by the forks were identical; the third was either larger or shorter than the other two. The sum of the length of one of the similar segments plus the length of the odd segment always equaled a length that was within the range of lengths of non-forked circular molecules. Addition of the lengths of the similar segments always gave molecules which were either too long or too short. The similar segments are taken to be the products of the portion of the molecule which has undergone replication, and the odd segment is taken to be the unreplicated portion. This configuration is exactly what would be expected if synthesis of M-DNA proceeds as suggested by Cairns[11] for the large circular DNA molecule of *Escherichia coli*. DNA molecules of λ phage[51] and of polyoma virus[30] which were partially replicated, as indicated by their density after growth in the presence of ^{15}N (λ) or

5-bromodeoxyuridine (polyoma), also have this form. Similar molecules have been claimed as the replicating forms of DNA of *Mycoplasma hominis*.[2]

Of about 10,000 rat liver M-DNA molecules examined, only 21 partially duplicated molecules were found. Rat liver M-DNA has been shown to have a half-life of about nine days.[27] If in fact the partially duplicated molecules are replicative forms, then they should be more frequent in M-DNA from tissues undergoing rapid growth. To test this, we examined the M-DNA from a number of mouse and rat tumors (Table 16-3). In M-DNA from all of the growing tumors examined, partially duplicated molecules occurred with a frequency of from six to 28 times that found in M-DNA of normal rat liver.

Covalently closed circular DNA binds less of the dye ethidium bromide than does open circular or linear DNA and, therefore, bands at a greater density in a cesium chloride gradient.[1, 55] We found that when M-DNA from either the Novikoff tumor or the Chang tumor was centrifuged to equilibrium in a cesium chloride-ethidium bromide gradient, the partially duplicated molecules banded exclusively with the open circular molecules.[37, 38] This confirms that, as might be expected for a molecule in the process of replication, the continuity of the circle is dependent upon a single phosphodiester bond between at least two adjacent nucleotide pairs. It was also observed that the replicative forms came to equilibrium at the denser side of the lighter band. When Novikoff tumor M-DNA was centrifuged to equilibrium in a cesium chloride gradient in which ethidium bromide was absent, the same observation was made (Figure 16-25). This indicates that the replicative molecules are denser than the normal circles, suggesting that the first portion of the molecule to be duplicated is a region rich in guanylic and cytidylic acid.[88] This finding also confirms the results of denaturation mapping of rat liver M-DNA molecules,[72] that one half of the rat M-DNA circle is distinguished from the other half by a substantial difference in average guanylic plus cytidylic acid content.

Clayton and Vinograd[15] found that up to 39% of the M-DNA of human leukemic leukocytes is in the form of double-sized circles. They later showed that this form of molecule was present to varying degrees in a number of human solid tumors. In normal tissues, such forms are usually absent or occur in very low frequency. In M-DNA from rat liver, for example, we found only one molecule in 1,000 with a contour length of 10 μ.[78] A dimeric form consisting of two single circles which are interlocked is much more common in normal tissues. Such forms, together with higher oligomers, were first demonstrated by Hudson and Vinograd in M-DNA isolated from HeLa cells. Since then they have been found to account for up to 10% of the M-DNA of a number of species.[13]

Nass[50] found 8% double-sized molecules in M-DNA from mouse

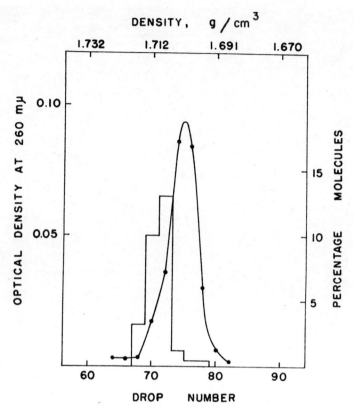

FIG. 16–25.—The distribution of partially duplicated molecules (histogram) in a band of Novikoff ascites tumor M-DNA (curve) formed by centrifugation to equilibrium in a cesium chloride gradient. Each point on the curve represents the OD_{260} of two pooled drops. Estimates of frequencies of partially duplicated molecules were made by examining in the electron microscope at least 200 molecules from each pair of drops. (Data from Koike and Wolstenholme.[38])

L-cells harvested in the logarithmic phase of growth. In contrast, she found that M-DNA molecules of cells in the stationary phase of growth consist of up to 82% dimeric and 11% polymeric forms. Of the dimers, 60% were double-sized circles. M-DNA from cells starved of methionine or phenylalanine, or treated with cycloheximide or chloramphenicol also contained an unusually high number of dimers and, following cycloheximide treatment, a higher number of polymers.

We have made a study of the M-DNA from a number of rat and mouse tumors.[73] An unusually high proportion of the M-DNA of mouse Ehrlich ascites tumor is in the form of interlocked circles. Of this DNA, 22% is in the dimeric form and a further 16% is in the form of higher oligomers comprising as many as six circles (Figure 16-26).

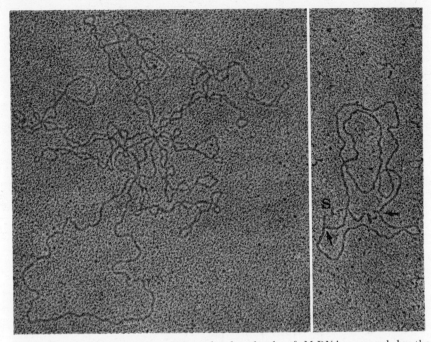

Fig. 16–26.—*(Left)* Electron micrograph of molecule of M-DNA prepared by the protein monolayer technique of Kleinschmidt[26] and rotary shadowed with platinum-palladium. (Figure from Wolstenholme et al.[73]) A molecule apparently comprising five interlocked single-length ($\simeq 5\ \mu$) circles from an Ehrlich mouse ascites tumor. Four of the circles are supercoiled and one is open. ×47,000.

Fig. 16 27.— *(Right)* Electron micrograph of molecule of M-DNA prepared by the protein monolayer technique of Kleinschmidt[26] and rotary shadowed with platinum-palladium. (Figure from Wolstenholme et al.[73]) An apparently partially duplicated molecule in which one of the segments is single-stranded (S), from a Chang rat solid tumor. The arrows indicate the positions of the forks. Under the conditions used to make these preparations, single-stranded DNA either collapses or appears as in this micrograph, as a kinky thread, quite distinct from the more rigid fiber of double-stranded DNA.[23] ×47,000.

Similar results were found for M-DNA from a solid tumor produced by injecting the ascites tumor cells under the skin on the backs of mice. The reality of the interlocking of circles has been demonstrated by the use of special shadowing techniques in the electron microscope, by dilution experiments, and by sedimentation studies.[15, 32] Molecules consisting of three or more interlocked circles are rare or absent in most normal tissues.

In M-DNA of the rat Chang solid hepatoma (originally induced by feeding rats 3-methyl-4-dimethyl aminoazobenzene),[12] dimeric and higher oligomeric forms are found with less frequency than in the mouse tumor M-DNAs, but in higher frequencies than in normal rat liver M-DNA (Table 16-4). In contrast, M-DNA from rat Novikoff ascites tumor did not contain a high number of dimeric forms, compared to normal rat liver M-DNA, and higher oligomeric forms accounted for only 0.6 to 1.6% of the DNA.

As was mentioned earlier, partially duplicated molecules were found in M-DNA of growing tumors in varying frequencies, but always in a considerably higher frequency than in normal rat liver M-DNA. The one exception was in M-DNA from a terminal Chang tumor (removed 15 min post mortem). In this case no replicating molecules were found.

A class of circular molecules, defined by the presence of a single-stranded region somewhere in the molecule, was found in varying proportions in tumor cell M-DNAs. Some molecules appeared as simple circles in which a region was single-stranded. Others had the forms of partially duplicated molecules in which the whole or part of one of the segments was single-stranded (Figure 16-27). In cesium chloride gradients, it was found that such molecules came to equilibrium at a mean density significantly greater than replicating molecules,[38] supporting the view that they are partially duplicated molecules in which one of the strands of the parent double helix has, in whole or in part, failed to replicate. The simple circles which include a single-stranded region would be produced when such molecules finally separate. The frequency of molecules containing a single-stranded segment was greatest in M-DNA from advanced tumors (Table 16-4), suggesting that such forms might result from specific chemical starvations of cells in advanced tumors. In line with this suggestion is the finding that the highest frequency of these molecules was found in advanced solid Chang tumors where cell starvation might be expected to be greatest.

No double-sized circular molecule has been observed in any of the rodent M-DNAs examined by us.

Two things further are clear from our data. A high proportion of dimeric and polymeric forms of M-DNA circles is not a feature common to all tumors. Also, the frequencies of these forms of M-DNA is not positively correlated to the speed of tumor growth. Novikoff ascites

TABLE 16–4.—THE FREQUENCIES OF DIFFERENT MOLECULAR FORMS IN M-DNA FROM NORMAL RAT LIVER AND FROM TWO RAT TUMORS

MOLECULAR FORM	NORMAL LIVER	CHANG SOLID HEPATOMA			NOVIKOFF ASCITES	
		Terminal*	Advanced (70gm)	Early (35gm)	Advanced (7th day)	Early (5th day)
Supercoiled	51.3	71.0	52.0	81.8	74.7	80.5
Dimer	7.3	1.9	16.2	11.1	8.1	8.5
Higher polymer	0.3	0	4.7	4.0	0.1	1.6
Partially duplicated	0.09	0	2.01	0.63	1.75	2.6
Molecules containing single-stranded region	0.09	4.7	15.0	0.18	2.8	0.3

* The terminal Chang tumor was harvested 15 minutes post-mortem.

tumor, the M-DNA of which differs very little from normal rat liver M-DNA with respect to polymeric forms, kills rats in six to eight days, having increased in cell mass by at least 70 times. The highest frequency of polymeric forms was found in M-DNA from mouse Ehrlich ascites tumor, which takes at least twice as long to kill its host, having increased proportionally in cell mass about the same as the Novikoff ascites tumor.

The final point, which is important, is that none of the unusual structures which we observe can be claimed as a basic causal effect in the production of malignant cell growth in rodents. This is worth mentioning, because it has been proposed by Clayton, Smith, and Vinograd[14] that a significant relationship exists between the formation and presence of the double-sized circle and neoplasia in man.

The circular M-DNA molecules of many vertebrates appear to be similar in contour length (Table 16-3), and there is evidence from hybridization studies for some sequence homologies between species even of different phyla.[23] However, the buoyant densities of M-DNAs of species even within the same class may vary greatly (Table 16-2), indicating that such M-DNAs from different species can, in fact, differ in the genetic information they carry. A further indication that the genetic information can differ, either qualitatively or quantitatively, in different species was provided by the findings of Wolstenholme and Dawid[70] that M-DNA molecules from anuran amphibians are longer than those of urodele amphibians. Specifically, it was demonstrated that M-DNA molecules of two frogs, *Xenopus laevis* and *Rana pipiens,* were about equal in length. The M-DNA molecules of two salamanders, *Siredon mexicanum* and *Necturus maculosus,* were equal to each other in length but as much as 19% shorter than the frog M-DNA molecules. This finding has a more general implication. If M-DNA circles do represent more than one molecular species, then equal size changes would have had to occur during evolution in all of the molecules involved.[67]

M-DNA has been isolated from a number of protozoans and fungi. In all cases, the buoyant density of the M-DNA is lower than that of the nuclear DNA, except for *Paramecium aurelia* where the reverse was found.[67]

Up to the present time, the form and size of M-DNA has been studied in comparatively few microorganisms. Suyama and Miura[66] found that the M-DNA which they isolated from the protozoan ciliate *Tetrahymena pyriformis* was linear, and the longer molecules had a modal length of about 17 μ. The M-DNA of the fungus *Neuraspora crassa*[43] and of the slime mold *Physarium polycephalum*[35] appear to be linear. It also was reported first that yeast *(Saccharomyces cerevisiae)* M-DNA was extractable only as linear molecules in the order of 0.1 to 5.5 μ in length.[63] Later, however, Shapiro et al.[62] demonstrated that about 3% of the total M-DNA molecules of yeast are covalently closed

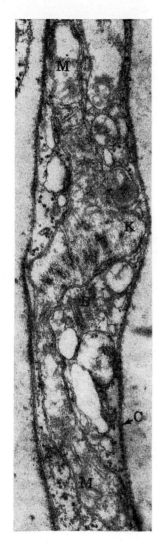

Fig. 16–28.—An electron micrograph of a longitudinal section through the posterior portion of a blood strain *Trypanosoma lewisi*. The kinetoplast (K) is shown, consisting of a mass of DNA-containing fibrils within an enlarged portion of a mitochondrion (M). B, basal body. C, cell wall. × 37,500. The organisms were prepared for electron microscopy by fixation according to Ryter et al.,[60] and embedding in Epon. (Figure from Renger and Wolstenholme.[57])

circles, ranging from 3 to 6 μ in contour length. They also showed that some of the linear molecules possess cohesive termini of the type found for λ phage DNA molecules,[29] which interact to produce hydrogen-bonded circles.

Members of the protozoan order Kinetoplastida,[31] which includes the mammalian blood flagellates of the genera *Trypanosoma* and *Leishmania,* are characterized by the presence of a body known as a kinetoplast. In 1924, Bresslau and Scremin[8] showed by use of the Feulgen reaction that the kinetoplast contains DNA. It was not until 1958,

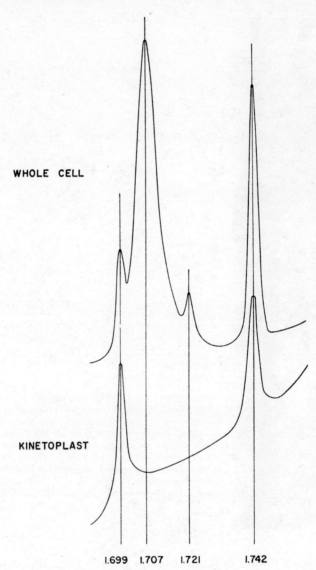

WHOLE CELL

KINETOPLAST

1.699 1.707 1.721   1.742

Fig. 16–29.—Microdensitometer tracings of uv photographs of cesium chloride buoyant density gradients of DNA from whole cells, and from a kinetoplast fraction of
blood strain *Trypanosoma lewisi.* The reference band (1.742) to the right is native
DNA of SPO1. (Data from Renger and Wolstenholme.[57])

however, that, by use of electron microscopy, Meyer, de Oliveira-
Musacchio and de Andrade-Mendonca[47] confirmed earlier cytologic evidence that the kinetoplast DNA is contained within a modified region
of a mitochondrion (Figure 16-28). In effect, this became the first
clear reproducible demonstration of DNA in mitochondria.

We have made a study of the kinetoplast DNA of the rat hemo-flagellate *Trypanosoma lewisi*.[57] Cesium chloride centrifugation of DNA extracted from whole cells revealed a main band with a buoyant density of 1.707, a light satellite, $\rho = 1.699$, and a heavy satellite, $\rho = 1.721$ (Figure 16-29). A cell fraction rich in kinetoplasts was prepared and treated with DNase to remove contaminating nuclear DNA. DNA

Fig. 16–30.—Electron micrographs of rotary shadowed molecules of DNA from a kinetoplast fraction of *Trypanosoma lewisi*. *A* and *B*, Single circular molecules of contour lengths approximately 0.4 μ. ×92,700. *C*, A mass of DNA apparently made up of interlocking circles of approximate contour length 0.4 μ. Seven 0.4 μ circles (arrows) are visible lying free at the edge of the mass. ×56,000. (Figures from Renger and Wolstenholme.[57])

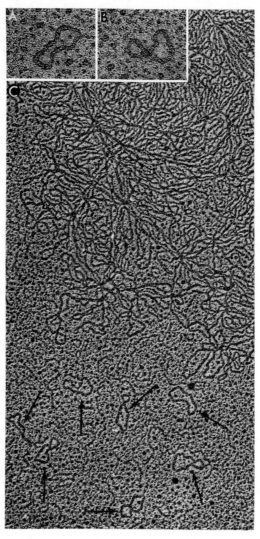

isolated from the kinetoplast fraction consisted only of the light satellite (Figure 16-29). In the electron microscope, this DNA comprised mainly circular molecules with a contour length of only 0.4 μ (Figure 16-30A and B). Large masses of DNA were also found which apparently comprise up to thousands of interlocked 0.4 μ circles (Figure 16-30C). Some long (up to 7 μ) noncircular molecules were also found associated with the large DNA masses. The 0.4 μ circles were found to have the properties of covalently closed circles. They banded at a density greater than noncircular molecules in a cesium chloride-ethidium bromide gradient. When heated in a spectrophotometer, they showed resistance to denaturation, a property which was lost when the circles were first broken by sonication. Interpretation of the large masses of DNA as comprising interlocked covalently closed circles was supported by the findings that they banded with single circular molecules in cesium chloride-ethidium bromide gradients, and following breakage of some circles by mild sonication, they disappeared and were replaced by molecules made up of low numbers of apparently interlocked 0.4 μ circles.

It is not known what genetic information is carried by kinetoplast DNA. A single molecule of DNA with a contour length of 0.4 μ, mol wt 7.7×10^5, could contain the information for determining the sequences of amino acids in only two proteins with an average molecular weight of 20,000. The circles are homogeneous with respect to size, but there is no indication from our data as to whether they all have identical nucleotide sequences and therefore carry the same genetic information. The relatively long linear molecules which are always found in preparations of kinetoplast DNA might carry considerably more information than the circles. It is also possible, however, that the linear molecules comprise tandem repeats of a single 0.4 μ nucleotide sequence.

Riou and Paoletti[59] and Riou and Delain[58] separated a light satellite DNA from whole cells of *Trypanosoma cruzi,* which they presumed was kinetoplast DNA. They also found that this DNA comprised mainly 0.45 μ circles, and masses of interlocked covalently closed 0.45 μ circles with which some linear DNA molecules were associated.

The buoyant density of M-DNA of angiosperm plants has been found to be consistently within the range 1.706 to 1.707, and at least 13 mg/ml denser than the respective organism's nuclear DNA.[65, 71] The form and size of M-DNA has been studied only in one higher plant, the red kidney bean, *Phaseolus vulgaris.*[71] A mitochondrial fraction was prepared from etiolated hypocotyls and digested as usual with DNase to remove contaminating nuclear DNA. The buoyant density of the DNA isolated from this fraction was 1.707, compared to a buoyant density of 1.693 found for the whole cell DNA. A portion of the mitochondrial pellet was digested with pronase, and spread and rotary-shadowed for electron microscopy. Only linear DNA molecules were found. They ranged in size from 1 to 62 μ and had a mean length of about 19.5 μ. The possibility that a small amount of nuclear DNA contamination could account for the longer pieces was ruled unlikely by the finding that the mean length of whole cell DNA from these experiments was never more than 1.8 μ. The possibility that the DNA attributed to mitochondria originated from chloroplasts was also discounted. The DNase treatment completely eliminated DNA from chloroplast preparations. Also, when proplastids which are present in hypocotyls were transformed into chloroplasts before isolation of mitochondria, the range and mean of lengths of M-DNA was not affected. In short, there seems little reason, from the results of Wolstenholme and Gross,[71] to doubt that bean mitochondria do in fact contain DNA molecules as long as 62 μ. Such a molecule has a molecular weight of 121×10^6, and if it is a unique sequence, could carry more than 10 times the genetic information of a single metazoan animal M-DNA circle. Alternately, such a molecule may comprise tandem repeats of a shorter sequence. It is also not known whether the different-sized molecules observed are the product of breakdown of longer molecules, or an expression of heterogeneity of M-DNA molecules in this species. There is no evidence that bean M-DNA molecules exist in situ as circles.

In summary, M-DNA from all metazoan animals examined to date is in the form of a circle about 5 μ in contour length. The circle is found either as a covalently closed structure in which the two strands of the DNA double helix are intact and topologically interlocked, or as an open circular structure in which at least one phosphodiester bond in one of the strands of the helix is broken. The structure of metazoan animal M-DNA is, therefore, similar to the structure of the DNA of a polyoma virus.

One half of the rat M-DNA molecule is distinguished from the other half by a substantial difference in guanylic plus cytidylic acid content.

Partially duplicated circular molecules of M-DNA have been found. They are more common in fast-growing than in slow-growing tissues, supporting the contention that they are replicative forms of M-DNA. Replication of the molecule begins in the region rich in guanylic plus cytidylic acid.

Molecules consisting of two interlocked 5 μ circles are found with a frequency of up to 10% in M-DNA of normal tissues. Interlocked polymeric forms are rare. Some tumor M-DNAs are distinguished by a high frequency of interlocked dimers and polymers, or by the presence of double-sized circles. Circular molecules including a single-stranded region are common in advanced rodent tumors.

It appears from the limited information we have at the present time that the genetic information which the M-DNA of any one animal species can carry may be defined by the length of a single circle of DNA. The genetic information carried by M-DNAs of different metazoan animal species, may, however, vary qualitatively and, within certain limits, quantitatively. A single 5 μ circular M-DNA molecule could code for only about 25 proteins of average molecular weight of 20,000, which sets severe limits to the direct control of M-DNA over mitochondrial functioning.

The kinetoplast DNA of at least two trypanosomes is mainly in the form of 0.4 μ circles. Yeast M-DNA molecules are shorter than metazoan animal M-DNA molecules, and only a small proportion is circular. With these exceptions, the M-DNA molecules of microorganisms and of a higher plant seem to be linear and in many cases longer than in metazoan animals, suggesting at least the possibility that they carry considerably more genetic information.

Acknowledgments

The more recent work cited in this paper was supported by National Institutes of Health, U. S. Public Health Service, Grant GM-16636, American Cancer Society Grant E-531, and National Science Foundation Development Award 0735.

References

1. Bauer, W., and J. Vinograd: J. Mol. Biol., 33:141, 1968.
2. Bode, H. R., and H. J. Morowitz: J. Mol. Biol., 23:191, 1967.
3. Borst, P.: In: Biogenesis of Mitochondria (E. Quagliariello, E. C. Slater, S. Papa, and J. M. Tager, eds.), Adriatica Edtrice, Bari, Italy, 1968.
4. Borst, P., E. F. J. van Bruggen, G. J. C. M. Ruttenberg, and A. M. Kroon: Biochim. Biophys. Acta, 149:156, 1967.
5. Borst, P., A. M. Kroon, and G. J. C. M. Ruttenberg: In: Genetic Elements: Properties and Function (D. Shugar, ed.), Academic Press and P.W.N., London and Warsaw, 1967, p. 81.
6. Borst, P., and G. J. C. M. Ruttenberg: Biochim. Biophys. Acta, 114:645, 1966.
7. Borst, P., G. J. C. M. Ruttenberg, and A. M. Kroon: Biochim. Biophys. Acta, 149:140, 1967.
8. Bresslau, E., and L. Scremin: Arch. Protistenk, 55:509, 1924.
9. van Bruggen, E. F. J., P. Borst, G. J. C. M. Ruttenberg, M. Gruber, and A. M. Kroon: Biochim. Biophys. Acta, 119:437, 1966.
10. van Bruggen, E. F. J., C. M. Runner, P. Borst, G. J. C. M. Ruttenberg, A. M. Kroon, and F. M. A. H. Schuurmans Stekhoven: Biochim. Biophys. Acta, 161:402, 1968.
11. Cairns, J.: Cold Spring Harbor Symp. Quant. Biol., 28:43, 1963.
12. Chang, J. P., C. W. Gibley, and K. Ichinoe: Cancer Res., 27:2065, 1967.
13. Clayton, D. A., C. A. Smith, J. M. Jordan, M. Teplitz, and J. Vinograd: Nature, 220:976, 1968.
14. Clayton, D. A., C. A. Smith, and J. Vinograd: Fed. Proc., 28:532, 1969.
15. Clayton, D. A., and J. Vinograd: Nature, 216:652, 1967.
16. Corneo, G., C. Moore, D. R. Sanadi, L. I. Grossman, and J. Marmur: Science, 151:687, 1966.
17. Corneo, G., L. Zardi, and E. Polli: J. Mol. Biol., 36:419, 1968.
18. Dawid, I. B.: J. Mol. Biol., 12:581, 1965.
19. Dawid, I. B.: Proc. Nat. Acad. Sci. USA, 56:269, 1966.
20. Dawid, I. B.: Discussion. In: Biogenesis of Mitochondria (E. Quagliariello, E. C. Slater, S. Papa, and J. M. Tager, eds.), Adriatica Edtrice, Bari, Italy, 1968.

21. Dawid, I. B., and D. D. Brown: Submitted for publication.
22. Dawid, I. B., and D. R. Wolstenholme: J. Mol. Biol., 28:233, 1967.
23. Dawid, I. B., and D. R. Wolstenholme: Biophys. J., 8:65, 1968.
24. Follett, E. A. C., and L. V. Crawford: J. Mol. Biol., 28:455, 1967.
25. Follett, E. A. C., and L. V. Crawford: J. Mol. Biol., 28:461, 1967.
26. Freifelder, D., and A. K. Kleinschmidt [sic]: J. Mol. Biol., 14:271, 1965.
27. Gross, N. J., G. S. Getz, and M. Rabinowitz: J. Biol. Chem., 244:1552, 1969.
28. Hershey, A. D., and E. Burgi: Proc. Nat. Acad. Sci. USA, 53:325, 1965.
29. Hershey, A. D., E. Burgi, and L. Ingraham: Proc. Nat. Acad. Sci. USA, 49:748, 1963.
30. Hirt, B.: J. Mol. Biol., 40:141, 1969.
31. Honigberg, B. M., W. Balamuth, E. C. Bovee, J. O. Corliss, M. Gojdics, R. P. Hall, R. R. Kudo, N. D. Levine, A. R. Loeblich, J. Weiser, and D. H. Wenrich: J. Protozool., 11:7, 1964.
32. Hudson, B., and J. Vinograd: Nature, 216:647, 1967.
33. Inman, R. B.: J. Mol. Biol., 18:464, 1966.
34. Inman, R. B.: J. Mol. Biol., 28:103, 1967.
35. Kessler, D.: J. Cell Biol., 43:68a, 1969.
36. Kirschner, R. H., D. R. Wolstenholme, and N. J. Gross: Proc. Nat. Acad. Sci. USA, 60:1466, 1968.
37. Koike, K.: In preparation.
38. Koike, K., and D. R. Wolstenholme: In preparation.
39. Kroon, A. M., P. Borst, E. F. J. van Bruggen, and G. J. C. M. Ruttenberg: Proc. Nat. Acad. Sci. USA, 56:1836, 1966.
40. Luck, D. J. L.: J. Cell Biol., 16:483, 1963.
41. Luck, D. J. L.: Amer. Naturalist, 99:241, 1965.
42. Luck, D. J. L.: J. Cell Biol., 24:445, 1965.
43. Luck, D. J. L., and E. Reich: Proc. Nat. Acad. Sci. USA, 52:931, 1964.
44. MacHattie, L. A., and C. A. Thomas: Science, 144:1142, 1964.
45. Marmur, J.: J. Mol. Biol., 3:208, 1961.
46. Meselson, M., F. W. Stahl, and J. Vinograd: Proc. Nat. Acad. Sci. USA, 43:581, 1957.
47. Meyer, H., M. de Oliveira-Musacchio, and I. de Andrade-Mendonca: Parasitology, 48:1, 1958.
48. Nass, M. M. K.: Proc. Nat. Acad. Sci. USA, 56:1215, 1966.
49. Nass, M. M. K.: J. Mol. Biol., 42:529, 1969.
50. Nass, M. M. K.: Nature, 223:1124, 1969.
51. Ogawa, T., J-I. Tomizawa, and M. Fuke: Proc. Nat. Acad. Sci. USA, 60:861, 1968.
52. Parsons, J. A., and R. C. Rustad: J. Cell Biol., 37:683, 1968.
53. Pikó, L., A. Tyler, and J. Vinograd: Biol. Bull., 132:68, 1967.
54. Rabinowitz, M., J. Sinclair, L. DeSalle, R. Haselkorn, and H. H. Swift: Proc. Nat. Acad. Sci. USA, 53:1126, 1965.
55. Radloff, R., W. Bauer, and J. Vinograd: Proc. Nat. Acad. Sci. USA, 57:1514, 1967.
56. Reich, E., and D. J. L. Luck: Proc. Nat. Acad. Sci. USA, 55:1600, 1966.
57. Renger, H. C., and D. R. Wolstenholme: Submitted for publication.
58. Riou, G., and E. Delain: Proc. Nat. Acad. Sci. USA, 62:210, 1960.
59. Riou, G., and C. Paoletti: J. Mol. Biol., 28:377, 1967.
60. Ryter, A., E. Kellenberger, A. Birch-Andersen, and Maaløe: J. Naturf., 13b:597, 1958.
61. Schneider, W. C., and E. L. Kuff: Proc. Nat. Acad. Sci. USA, 54:1650, 1965.
62. Shapiro, L., L. I. Grossmann, J. Marmur, and A. K. Kleinschmidt: J. Mol. Biol., 33:907, 1968.
63. Sinclair, J. H., B. Stevens, N. Gross, and M. Rabinowitz: Biochim. Biophys. Acta, 145:528, 1967.
64. Sinclair, J. H., B. J. Stevens, P. Sanghavi, and M. Rabinowitz: Science, 156:1234, 1967.
65. Suyama, Y., and W. D. Bonner: Proc. Nat. Acad. Sci. USA, 60:235, 1966.

66. Suyama, Y., and K. Miura: Proc. Nat. Acad. Sci. USA, 60:235, 1968.
67. Swift, H., and D. R. Wolstenholme: In: Handbook of Molecular Cytology (A. Lima-de-Faria, ed.), North Holland Publishing Co., Amsterdam, 1969, pp. 972-1046.
68. Vinograd, J., and J. Lebowitz: J. Gen. Physiol., 49:103, 1966.
69. Wolstenholme, D. R., and I. B. Dawid: Chromosoma, 20:445, 1967.
70. Wolstenholme, D. R., and I. B. Dawid: J. Cell Biol., 39:222, 1968.
71. Wolstenholme, D. R., and N. J. Gross: Proc. Nat. Acad. Sci. USA, 61:245, 1968.
72. Wolstenholme, D. R., R. H. Kirschner, and N. J. Gross: In preparation.
73. Wolstenholme, D. R., K. Koike, and J. D. McLaren: In preparation.
74. Wolstenholme, D. R.: Unpublished data.
75. Wolstenholme, D. R., and J. D. McLaren: Unpublished data.
76. Sinclair, J. H., and B. J. Stevens, 1966.
77. Wolstenholme, D. R., J. D. McLaren, H. C. Renger, and Iyer: Unpublished data.
78. Kirschner, R. H., D. R. Wolstenholme, and N. J. Gross. Unpublished data.

The Role of Intracellular Membranes in the Regulation of Genetic Expression

HENRY C. PITOT, M.D., Ph.D.

McArdle Laboratory, Departments of Oncology and Pathology, University of Wisconsin Medical School, Madison, Wisconsin, USA

THAT CELLULAR MEMBRANE systems are involved in the regulation of genetic expression has only recently become apparent from a number of studies. In bacterial systems as well as in eukaryotic cells, the rate of DNA synthesis is regulated in part by an interaction with the cell or nuclear membrane.[1-3] Earlier studies by several authors,[4-6] utilizing bacterial systems, have demonstrated that in several strains of *Bacillus*, RNA associated with cellular membranes was resistant to the effects of actinomycin D, and during sporulation was found to be present in a membrane-bound form. Utilizing DNA-RNA hybridization, this membrane-bound RNA in sporulating bacteria was demonstrated to have the characteristics of messenger RNA (mRNA) and also was shown to be associated with polysomes. The polysome-membrane interaction resulted in an increased stability of the mRNA to exogenous ribonuclease treatment in vitro. Therefore, the evidence is apparent that in microbial systems membranes affect DNA synthesis as well as the regulation of genetic expression through the stabilization of specific mRNA templates.

As our knowledge of neoplasia expands, it is apparent that no single biochemical alteration is common to all neoplasms. Rather, tumors are characterized by their diversities, such as unique transplantation antigens in chemically induced tumors,[7] phenotypes of hepatocellular and mammary carcinomas,[8, 9] in addition to the numerous morphologic and karyologic variation, even within the same neoplasm. In the midst of this extreme confusion, however, one point is rapidly becoming clarified. In all instances studied, no neoplasm exhibited the regulation of the expression of its genome characteristically found in the cell from which it arises. This has now become apparent from studies based on hepatocellular carcinomas, mammary carcinomas, renal cell carcinomas, and many others.[10] A few of these defective mechanisms are listed in Table 16-5 for hepatocellular and mammary carcinomas. In addition to those listed in the hepatomas, the finding of the absence of a feedback of cholesterol on the enzyme, hydroxymethylglutaryl-coenzyme A reductase, appears to be characteristic of all hepatomas thus far studied.[11] In addition to these defects, abnormalities in membrane components of neoplastic cells are now quite well recognized.[12] The lack of contact inhibition, electrophoretic differences, and the appearance of new transplantation antigens present in the plasma membrane of tumor cells are all differences found in many, if not most, neoplastic cells. In addition, several abnormalities have been demonstrated in the endoplasmic reticulum of neoplastic cells, both chemically and virally induced. Several defects in the enzymology of the endoplasmic reticulum of normal and neoplastic hepatocytes have now been described.[11, 13] Earlier studies have also demonstrated[14] that a number of highly

TABLE 16–5.—SOME DEFECTIVE REGULATORY MECHANISMS IN RAT NEOPLASMS IN VIVO

HEPATOCELLULAR CARCINOMAS

Enzyme	Environmental Control	Defect	Ref.
Serine dehydratase induction	Amino acids	Absent or adrenal dependent	(10)
Ornithine transaminase induction	Amino acids	Absent or "hypersensitive"	(34)
Tryptophan pyrrolase induction	Tryptophan or cortisone	Absent or adrenal dependent	(10)
Tyrosine transaminase induction	Cortisone	Hypersensitive or absent	(10)
Thymidine kinase "induction"	Amino acids or hepatectomy	Hypersensitive or absent No response to hepatectomy	(35)

MAMMARY CARCINOMAS

Glucose-6-phosphate dehydrogenase "induction"	Estrogen	Insensitive to actinomycin in tumor	(9)
Malic enzyme "induction"	Estrogen	"Paradoxical effect" of actinomycin in tumor	(9)

differentiated and poorly differentiated murine hepatomas exhibited considerably fewer polysomes bound to membranes of the endoplasmic reticulum than were present in normal liver.

In view of the role of membranes in the regulation of genetic expression in both prokaryotic and eukaryotic cells, coupled with the ubiquitous abnormalities in the regulation of genetic expression seen in neoplastic cells, studies in this laboratory have been directed toward an understanding of the mechanisms of the role of membranes in the regulation of genetic expression. Specifically correlated in this area, as seen in Table 16-6, is the fact that the sensitivity of enzyme synthesis to actinomycin D administration is quite different in the case of those enzymes studied when tumor and cell of origin are compared. Thus, as in the case of serine dehydratase, the actual time during which enzyme synthesis (translation) may occur in the absence of RNA synthesis is about six hr. This has been termed the template lifetime.[15] It can be seen from Table 16-6 that, in general, the template lifetimes of these enzymes are quite different in the tumor than in the normal tissue. That translational regulation of genetic expression may occur has been shown in several laboratories.[16, 17] These studies thus suggest that the neoplastic transformation may be related, if not equated, to an alteration in template stabilities which are maintained in a dividing cell population. The growth advantage seen in most neoplasms may well be caused by a selection of cells having the highest stability for templates of enzymes directly involved in cellular replication, such as thymidine kinase, as seen in Table 16-6.

If one accepts this relationship, then the next step in the sequence of investigations is to be directed at an understanding of the mechanisms of template stability and its alteration in hepatomas as well as in other neoplasms. As had been demonstrated in bacterial systems,[4-6] the presence of mRNA in close association with intracellular membranes became of considerable importance in mammalian systems. However, in

TABLE 16–6.—ESTIMATED mRNA TEMPLATE LIFETIME FOR ENZYMES IN RAT TISSUES IN VIVO

Enzyme	Liver	Hepatocellular Carcinoma
Serine dehydratase	6-8 hrs	H-35 = < 1 hr
		5123 = >2 wks
Ornithine transaminase	18-24 hrs	5123 = > 24 hrs
Tryptophan pyrrolase	> 2 wks	H-35 = < 12 hrs
		5123, etc. = < 30 min (?)
Tyrosine transaminase (induced)	2-3 hrs	H-35 = > 6 hrs
Thymidine kinase (intact)	< 3 hrs	H-35 = > 12 hrs
	Mammary Gland	Mammary Carcinoma (R3230AC)
Glucose-6-phosphate dehydrogenase	< 2 days	> 2 days
Malic enzyme	< 2 days	> 2 days

numerous studies in liver and other tissues, the presence of poly-somes bound to the endoplasmic reticulum in the form of "rough" endoplasmic reticulum is well known. In our laboratory, this RNA may be labeled with ^{32}P or ^{3}H-orotic acid under conditions in which ribosomal RNA is essentially not synthesized.[18] This RNA is in close association with the membrane of the endoplasmic reticulum, and is found in both normal and neoplastic hepatocytes, as one might expect.[19] As in bacterial systems, a component of this RNA is stable to removal by chelating agents and also to treatment with dilute ribonuclease. That such RNA is in fact mRNA has now been shown by dissociation of polysomes into subunits and by fixation with formaldehyde with subsequent banding in equilibrium density gradients of cesium chloride.[20] Therefore, in liver in close association with the membranes of the endoplasmic reticulum, mRNA does occur, and is present in the form of ribonucleoprotein particles which have been described as occurring in both the nucleus and the cytoplasm of mammalian cells.[21, 22]

That such mRNA is functional in the synthesis of enzymes involved in the metabolism of the cell has also been demonstrated.[23] In Figure 16-31 are seen the data from an experiment utilizing pulse labeling with a ^{14}C amino acid in vivo, followed by isolation of the rough endoplasmic reticulum and free polysomes, with subsequent treatment of each fraction with puromycin to obtain the release into the soluble fraction of proteins being synthesized and still associated with tRNA. This puromycin-releasable material was reacted with specific antiserine dehydratase antibody in order to determine the incorporation of label

Fig. 16–31.—Incorporation of labeled valine in vivo into serine dehydratase antigen released in vitro by treatment of the rough endoplasmic reticulum (RER) and free polysomes. Animals were induced with amino acids (induction) and induced with amino acids but given glucose 30 min before initiation of labeling (repression). The label was injected into the portal vein at zero time, and groups of animals were sacrificed thereafter with subsequent isolation of RER and free polysomes, suitably washed, and then treated with puromycin.[34]

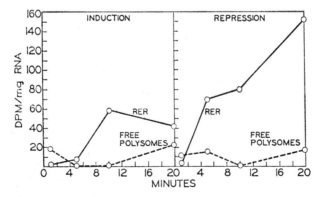

and thus the site of synthesis of this particular enzyme. As can be seen from the data in the figure, the rough endoplasmic reticulum plays a major role in the synthesis of this enzyme. Furthermore, because of the geometry of the experiment, the enzyme is released into what is in vivo the intracellular compartment of the tissue. There is no question that bound polysomes synthesize protein for export. Evidence from these experiments, as well as more recent studies,[23] demonstrates that polysomes bound to the endoplasmic reticulum are also capable of synthesizing enzymes for intracellular metabolism. Furthermore, during periods of increased intracellular enzyme synthesis, such as after the administration of cortisone, studies[24] have demonstrated that the binding of polysomes to membranes is increased.

The association of polysomes with membranes of the endoplasmic reticulum in vitro comprises the third major area of investigation aimed at understanding the mechanism of template stabilization. Utilizing a system previously described,[25, 26] the binding of polysomes to membranes of the endoplasmic reticulum has been studied utilizing a cell-free system. By means of high-speed centrifugation (400,000 × g) over dense sucrose gradients, membrane-bound polysomes may be separated from unbound polysomes. By previously labeling polysomes in vivo and mixing these with membrane preparations in vitro with

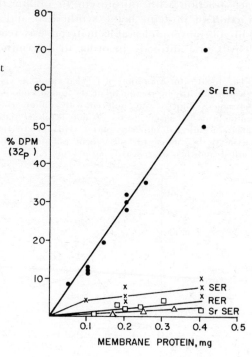

Fig. 16–32.—The in vitro binding of ^{32}P-labeled polyribosomes isolated from rat liver to fractions of the endoplasmic reticulum isolated from the same organ. The technique of the experiment is described in the text and in detail in reference 26.

subsequent centrifugation, one may determine the amount of polysomes associated with the membrane fraction or reconstituted "rough" endoplasmic reticulum in vitro. In Figure 16-32 can be seen the association of polysomes with smooth, rough, and both smooth and rough endoplasmic reticulum which have been previously treated with chelating agents to remove bound ribosomes. It may be seen from this figure that only rough endoplasmic reticulum from which polysomes have previously been removed is capable of binding polysomes in vitro. Conversely, in more recent studies, membranes of the smooth endoplasmic reticulum can be made to bind polysomes by increasing the temperature at which the binding occurs. At 37 C only smooth endoplasmic reticulum binds significant numbers of polysomes. Previous work[27] has demonstrated that the binding of polysomes to membranes of the endoplasmic reticulum is dependent on the presence of an enzyme catalyzing the rearrangement of protein disulfide bonds. This enzyme is native to the membranes of the endoplasmic reticulum. Studies in this laboratory are consistent with this finding in that the treatment of membranes of the endoplasmic reticulum with trypsin completely prevents their association with polysomes in the system described here. That a certain degree of membrane specificity occurs between organs has been shown in the case of membranes isolated from kidney, these membranes having a markedly diminished capacity to bind polysomes from liver. Membranes of the endoplasmic reticulum isolated from several hepatocellular carcinomas also exhibit a decreased capacity to bind polysomes. This decreased capacity, however, appears to be explained on the basis of marked instability of these membranes when compared to comparable preparations from liver.

The MEMBRON Hypothesis

From the studies described above, as well as others reported earlier,[28] we have formulated a working model of the stable template in hepatic cells which is hopefully applicable to template stability in general. The evidence for this model has been presented in this paper and succinctly outlined in a previous publication.[28] The model, termed the MEMBRON, is represented in Figure 16-33. In the figure is seen the pseudohelix of a polysome lying on the surface of the mosaic of the membrane of the endoplasmic reticulum. The pseudohelical configuration of the polysome has been described by others,[29] and is shown with the smaller subunit directed towards the interior of the pseudohelix. Whether the polysome approximates to the membrane with both the large and small subunits in contact with the membrane surface is still open to some question, since some workers[30, 31] have argued that this may not be so. The mosaic pattern of the membrane seen in the background of the figure is postulated to consist of multiple structures, the nature of which is largely unknown, but from arguments presented

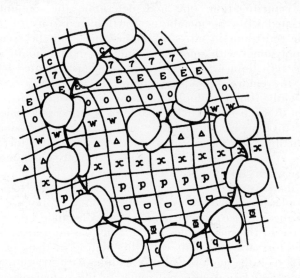

FIG. 16–33.—Proposed structure of the MEMBRON. The background lettered squares represent specific chemical structures in the molecular mosaic of the membrane of the endoplasmic reticulum. The double circles represent the ribosomal subunits with the smaller subunit directed to the interior of the pseudohelix. See reference 28 for further details.

earlier, the protein disulfide interchange enzyme may well be one of these components involved in the close association of the polysome with the membrane. The inheritance of this configuration may be postulated to occur in a manner similar to that described for the inheritance of the surface membrane of protozoa.[32]

Thus, from the model depicted here, the neoplastic transformation may be represented as an alteration of the population of MEMBRONs in the transformed cell as compared to the cell from which it arose. The change in MEMBRON population may be solely a result of an alteration in the mosaic of the membranes of the endoplasmic reticulum, a phenomenon consonant with the altered transplantation antigens which are exceedingly complex, and may, in fact, be attributable to spatial rearrangements rather than specific amino acid sequence alterations.[33] Therefore, as was suggested some years ago by this laboratory, the altered MEMBRON populations seen in neoplasms give rise to a phenotypic "mask" resulting in the altered regulation of genetic expression which we call neoplasia.

Acknowledgments

This work was supported in part by grants from the National Cancer Institute (CA-07175) and the American Cancer Society (P-314).

References

1. Trembleay, G. Y., M. J. Daniels, and M. Schaechter: J. Mol. Biol., 40:65, 1969.
2. Ganesan, A. T., and J. Lederberg: Biochem. Biophys. Res. Comm., 18:824, 1965.
3. Smith, D. W., and P. C. Hanawalt: Biochim. Biophys. Acta, 149:519, 1967.
4. Yudkin, M. D., and B. Davis: J. Mol. Biol., 12:193, 1965.
5. Aronson, A.: J. Mol. Biol., 13:92, 1965.
6. Schlessinger, D., V. T. Marchesi, and B. C. K. Kwan: J. Bacteriol., 90:456, 1965.
7. Prehn, R. T.: Cancer Res., 28:1326, 1968.
8. Potter, V. R., M. Watanabe, H. C. Pitot, and H. P. Morris: Cancer Res., 29:55, 1969.
9. Hilf, R., I. Michel, G. Silverstain, and C. Bell: Cancer Res., 25:1854, 1965.
10. Pitot, H. C.: Cancer Res., 28:1880, 1968.
11. Siperstein, M. D., V. M. Fagan, and H. P. Morris: Cancer Res., 26:7, 1966.
12. Wallach, D. F. H.: N. Eng. J. Med., 280:761, 1969.
13. Adamson, R. H., and J. R. Fouts: Cancer Res., 21:667, 1961.
14. Webb, T. E., G. Blobel, and V. R. Potter: Cancer Res., 24:1229, 1964.
15. Pitot, H. C.: In: Molecular Genetics (J. H. Taylor, ed.), Academic Press, Inc., New York, Vol. 2, 1967, pp. 383-423.
16. Just, J-P., E. A. Khairallah, and H. C. Pitot: J. Biol. Chem., 243:3057, 1968.
17. Berman, M.: Bulletin, Institute of Cellular Biology, University of Connecticut, 8 (No. 6) :1, 1967.
18. Lamar, C., M. Prival, and H. C. Pitot: Cancer Res., 26:1909, 1966.
19. Sladek, N. E., and H. C. Pitot: Cancer Res. In press.
20. Cihak, A., D. Wilkinson, and H. C. Pitot: Arch. Biochem. Biophys. In press.
21. Georgiev, G. P.: In: Regulatory Mechanisms for Protein Synthesis in Mammalian Cells (A. San Pietro, M. R. Lamborg, and F. T. Kenney, eds.), Academic Press, New York, 1968, pp. 25-48.
22. Parsons, J. T. and K. S. McCarty: J. Biol. Chem., 243:5377, 1968.
23. Tata, J. R.: Fed. Proc., 29:604, 1970.
24. Williams, D. J., and B. R. Rabin: FEBS Letters, 4:103, 1969.
25. Suss, R., G. Blobel, and H. C. Pitot: Biochem. Biophys. Res. Comm., 23:299, 1966.
26. Ragland, W. R., T. K. Shires, and H. C. Pitot: J. Cell Biol. In press.
27. Williams, D. J., D. Gurari, and B. R. Rabin: FEBS Letters, 2:133, 1968.
28. Pitot, H. C.: Arch. Path., 87:212, 1969.
29. Shelton, E., and E. L. Kuff: J. Mol. Biol., 22:23, 1966.
30. Sabatini, D. D., Y. Tashiro, and G. E. Palade: J. Mol. Biol., 19:503, 1966.
31. Sabatini, D. D., and G. Blobel: J. Cell Biol., 45:146, 1970.
32. Sonneborn, T. M.: Proc. Nat. Acad. Sci. USA, 51:915, 1964.
33. Haughton, G., and D. B. Amos: Cancer Res., 28:1839, 1968.
34. Peraino, C., and H. C. Pitot: Unpublished data.
35. Gebert, R., V. R. Potter, and H. C. Pitot: Unpublished data.

17

Gene Action: Metabolic Patterns in Normal and Cancerous Cells

Respiration, Glycolysis and Enzyme Alterations in Liver Neoplasms

SIDNEY WEINHOUSE

The Fels Research Institute, Temple University School of Medicine, Philadelphia, Pennsylvania, USA

UNTIL COMPARATIVELY RECENT years it was generally held that the cancer cell is dedifferentiated, a view supported by the observation that functionally active, differentiated cells have distinctive enzyme patterns which make each tissue unique, whereas rapidly proliferating neoplastic cells have largely or completely lost the unique metabolic capabilities of their tissue of origin.[1] The neoplastic cell thus was considered a unique cell type, with a characteristic enzymatic makeup that underlies its biologic behavior. This hypothesis is in accord with and supports the Warburg theory,[2] which proposes that the cancer cell has lost its respiratory capability and survives by developing a mechanism for energy transduction through anaerobic utilization of glucose. Without dwelling on the long-standing, acrimonious controversy which accompanied the Warburg hypothesis, it will suffice to say that although the respiratory incapability of tumors proved to be an untenable hypothesis,[3] it was generally accepted that high aerobic and anaerobic glycolysis is a common feature of all neoplastic cells.

With the development of the series of transplantable hepatic tumors of the rat known as the Morris hepatomas,[4] by Harold P. Morris in

TABLE 17-1.—General Properties of Morris Hepatomas[4, 5]

| PROPERTY | Degree of Differentiation | | |
	High	Well	Poor
Growth rate	Very low	Low	Rapid
Chromosome number	Normal	Nearly normal	Abnormal
Chromosome karyotype	Normal	Nearly normal	Abnormal
Respiration	High	Moderate	Moderately low
Glycolysis	Low	Low	High
Enzyme Pattern	Liver-like	Some deletions	Many deletions

1960, two important concepts arose which were in decided opposition to the above-mentioned conceptions. Studies of these tumors showed: (1) that tumors of a single cell of origin could display a wide diversity in degree of differentiation, paralleled by variations in growth rate and in the retention and loss of hepatic function; and (2) that a high aerobic glycolysis is not necessary for tumor growth. These tumors display a wide spectrum in degree of differentiation as revealed by histologic examination,[4] but we have found it convenient to divide these into three groups; namely, highly differentiated, well differentiated, and poorly differentiated. A summary of their properties is in Table 17-1. Closely correlated with the degree of differentiation is the growth rate, which is very low in the few highly differentiated tumors, extending to nearly a year for a transplant generation. (Growth rate is expressed as the average time between inoculation and transplantation.) Growth rates are considerably faster, at two to six months, for well-differentiated tumors, and are extremely rapid, at two weeks or less, for the poorly differentiated hepatomas.[5] The highly differentiated tumors have the normal liver chromosome number and karyotype, the well-differentiated tumors differ slightly, and the poorly differentiated deviate markedly in chromosome karyotype and number, from those of rat liver.[5] Respiration decreases moderately with loss of differentiation, but the striking feature is the low or negligible glycolysis in the well-differentiated tumors, in contrast with the usual high level of glycolysis in the poorly differentiated ones.[6, 7] These well-differentiated tumors, with their low glycolytic activity, make it clear that high lactic acid production is not an absolute requirement for tumor survival; these low-glycolyzing tumors can grow, albeit slowly, and they can also metastasize, and can ultimately kill their hosts.

In the time available, I should like to describe studies from our laboratory which bear on two aspects of the biochemistry of these tumors: (1) some of the molecular alterations which underlie the varied behavior of these tumors, particularly some striking alterations of isozyme patterns and (2) certain control sites of glycolysis which might explain the peculiar glycolytic properties of these and other tumors.

Hexokinases

The phosphorylation of glucose-6-phosphate is catalyzed by a glucose-ATP phosphotransferase which exists in multiple forms in liver (Table 17-2). The term hexokinase is employed to cover actually three isozymes which have similar properties, and which are present in liver at a very low total activity which does not change with diet or hormonal conditions.[8-11] Conversely, the fourth isozyme, called glucokinase, is highly responsive to dietary and hormonal conditions, being low in fasted normal animals, and high in carbohydrate-fed animals.[8, 9] It is also insulin-dependent, being extremely low in diabetes and restored by insulin injection.[12, 13] This isozyme has an important physiologic function in hepatic glucose utilization. It has a high Km for glucose, and it is this property that is responsible for the fact that the liver takes up glucose only when the blood glucose concentration is high. In a few highly differentiated hepatomas, the isozyme pattern is very similar to that of normal liver, with high glucokinase and low-to-moderate hexokinase. In a large number of well-differentiated tumors, studied over a wide range of transplant generations, the glucokinase drops to very low levels, with essentially no change in hexokinase.[15, 16] This is a striking observation in view of the fact that tumors in general have rather high hexokinase levels. Indeed, when broken-cell preparations of such well-differentiated tumors were incubated aerobically, glucose utilization and lactic acid production were very low; and a rate-limiting role of the low glucose phosphotransferase activity was verified by greatly increased glycolysis when such preparations were fortified with exogenous crystalline yeast hexokinase.[18] In contrast, poorly differentiated hepatocarcinomas exhibit high hexokinase activity with little or no glucokinase, and similar preparations of these tumors invariably have a high glycolytic activity.[17] Thus, loss of differentiation in hepatic tumors is accompanied by virtual loss of a

TABLE 17-2.—ISOZYME PATTERNS IN RAT HEPATOMAS

| ENZYME | STATE OF DIFFERENTIATION | | |
	High	Well	Poor
Glucose ATP Phosphotransferases			
Glucokinase	++++	+	+
Hexokinase(s)	+	+	++++
Aldolases			
Liver Aldolase B	++++	+++	--
Muscle Aldolase A	--	+	++++
Pyruvate Kinase			
PK B (liver)	++++	+	+ (?)
PK A (muscle)	+	+	++++++
Adenylate Kinase			
AK III (liver)	++++	++	+
AK II (muscle)	+	+	+

glucose phosphotransferase which is physiologically functional and under regulation by diet and hormones, and replacement by isozymes which are ordinarily low in normal liver.

Aldolase

Aldolase also exists in multiple forms which, like lactate dehydrogenase,[18] are tetramers of subunits with different primary structures distinguishable by immunologic or kinetic criteria.[19] In normal liver and in highly differentiated tumors, the aldolase is nearly or entirely in the B form. In the well-differentiated tumors, aldolase B is preponderant, though variable quantities of aldolase A also appear. However, in the poorly differentiated tumors, the B form has been essentially completely replaced by the A form.[20]

Pyruvate Kinase

A crucial enzyme in the glycolytic pathway is the transphosphorylase which catalyzes the transfer of phosphate from phosphoenolpyruvate to ADP. This enzyme also exists in multiple forms. Two major forms are found in liver; an A form, similar in kinetic properties to the muscle enzyme, and a B form, which is found as the predominant form in normal liver.[21, 22] The latter is highly responsive to carbohydrate in the diet and has a number of distinctive kinetic properties which differentiate it sharply from the former. It is also low in diabetic rats, and its activity is restored by insulin treatment.[23] Thus it shares in common with other liver "marker" enzymes specific functions that give the liver cells their unique metabolic significance. The highly differentiated tumors have the same isozyme pattern as liver, with predominance of the B type. However, the well-differentiated have very low levels of both isozymes, and striking alteration occurs in the rapidly growing, poorly differentiated tumors; these have extremely high levels of an isozyme which has the properties of the A type, with little or no B type isozyme.

Adenylate Kinase

An ATP-AMP phosphotransferase, responsive to diet and insulin, was reported recently by Adelman et al. to be present in liver cytosol.[24] Since this enzyme catalyzes the equilibrium among the three adenine nucleotides, AMP, ADP, and ATP, substances that are substrates or modulators of many enzymes of great functional significance in liver, its importance can hardly be overestimated. It exists in four distinct forms, the predominant one of which is the adaptive enzyme.[25] Although all four forms are retained in the hepatomas, the activity of the adaptive form which is unique to liver drops sharply with loss of differentiation. Again, we see another example of the loss of a liver "marker" enzyme with loss of differentiation of hepatic tumors.

Pyruvate Kinase in Relation to Glycolysis and Respiration

The high aerobic and anaerobic glycolysis of tumor tissues has been a subject of controversy that burned brightly for many years and is still flickering. The great German biochemist, Otto Warburg, first observed this phenomenon in 1922 and propounded his well-known theory of respiratory impairment in cancer cells.[2] He observed that both normal and neoplastic tissue slices utilized glucose and produced lactic acid when incubated in vitro in a medium of physiologic pH and ionic environment. He made the further significant observation that this process was lowered quantitatively when the incubation was conducted in oxygen rather than in nitrogen. He termed this phenomenon the Pasteur effect, since Pasteur had noted some 60 years earlier that yeast cells placed in an aerobic environment ceased to make alcohol, that is, fermentation stopped. Although the Pasteur effect has not yet been explained satisfactorily, it has been a focal point for much discussion and experiment on regulatory mechanisms of carbohydrate metabolism.

According to Warburg, the Pasteur effect operates in tumors, but is quantitatively deranged in that it does not inhibit glycolysis as efficiently as it does in normal tissues. A generation ago, Johnson[26] and Lynen[27] independently suggested that the Pasteur effect may be mediated by competition for substrates between the transphosphorylating enzymes of glycolysis and the respiratory ADP and P_i acceptor systems for oxidative phosphorylation. The three enzyme sites are at triose phosphate dehydrogenase, where P_i is taken up into organic combination; and at phosphoglycerate kinase and pyruvate kinase, where ADP is converted to ATP. The Johnson and Lynen theory languished for many years without definitive evidence pro or con; in recent years attention has shifted to phosphofructokinase and hexokinase, two irreversible steps at earlier stages in the glycolytic sequence. Although phosphofructokinase is likely to be a control site for the Pasteur effect in muscle, pyruvate kinase seemed to us to be a very good possibility in the Morris hepatomas, since there was an excellent correlation between low pyruvate kinase and the low glycolysis of the well-differentiated tumors, and the high pyruvate kinase and high glycolysis of the poorly differentiated tumors. Without going into details of the experimental procedures, which are described,[28] we were able to show that the addition of fructose diphosphate (FDP) to whole, respiring homogenates of the well-differentiated tumors resulted in only a low production of lactate and a low yield of glycolytic ATP, with no decrease in the high respiratory ATP production. However, when FDP was added to respiring homogenates of the poorly differentiated tumors, glycolysis was very high, accompanied by a high glycolytic ATP production; and the otherwise low respiratory phosphorylation was reduced to zero (Table 17-3). By intermixing experiments in which

TABLE 17–3.—Effect of Fructose-1,6-diphosphate (FDP) on Glycolytic and Respiratory Phosphorylation (Condensed from Ref. 28)

Tissue	Substrate	2-DG Uptake	O₂ Uptake	Lactate	P Resp	P Glyc
Liver	None	19.7	11.5	0.9	19.7	—
	FDP	25.3	10.0	9.1	7.1	18.2
Hepatoma						
5123D	None	18.3	9.5	0	18.3	—
	FDP	23.7	10.0	3.0	17.7	6.0
3683	None	2.6	0.8	0.6	2.6	—
	FDP	28.4	3.5	13.0	2.4	26.0

particulate fractions of one tumor type were mixed with supernatant fractions of the other type (Table 17-4), we observed that the glycolytic activity of the supernatant fraction did, indeed, determine the degree of glycolytic phosphorylation. When FDP was added to a mixture of the poorly differentiated highly glycolyzing tumor supernatant and the well differentiated tumor respiratory system, the respiratory activity was characteristic of that of the well-differentiated tumor homogenates, while the glycolytic activity and resultant glycolytic phosphorylation were greatly decreased below that of the poorly differentiated whole tumor homogenate. When the mixing was reversed, that is, when the well-differentiated tumor supernatant was mixed with the poorly differentiated tumor particles, glycolytic activity was greatly increased, and accounted for a larger proportion of the total phosphorylation than that exhibited by the well-differentiated whole tumor homogenate. Evidently, a powerful glycolytic system can carry on glycolytic phosphorylation at the expense of respiratory phosphorylation, and a normally low glycolytic system can increase greatly when the competition by respiration is removed. Although it would be premature to propose that pyruvate kinase is the site of the Pasteur effect in all tumors, such a possibility suggests itself on the basis of the behavior of this model system.

Competition for ADP between mitochondrial respiration and pyruvate kinase has been demonstrated clearly in another model system by Dr. Gosalvez in our laboratory.[37] He found that when pyruvate kinase

TABLE 17–4.—Effect of Intermixing Supernatants and Particles of Well and Poorly Differentiated Tumors on Glycolytic and Respiratory Phosphorylation with FDP as Substrate (Condensed from Ref. 28)

Supernatant	Particles	2-DG Uptake	O₂ Uptake	Lactate	P Resp	P Glyc
5123	5123	18.6	9.6	1.8	15.0	3.6
3683	3683	36.0	4.2	17.6	0.8	35.2
5123	3683	27.0	4.0	13.5	0	27.0
3683	5123	36.1	9.8	8.2	19.7	16.4

plus phosphoenolpyruvate were added to respiring rat liver mitochondria in state 3, either with excess added ADP or with an ADP-regenerating system consisting of glucose and hexokinase, there was an immediate drop in oxygen uptake to that characteristic of state 4 respiration. That this drop was caused directly by successful competition for ADP by pyruvate kinase was shown by suitable controls, by simultaneous production of pyruvate, and by the complete restoration of respiration by adding the uncoupler, dinitrophenol. This experiment leaves no room for doubt of the ability of pyruvate kinase to compete successfully with mitochondria, but in view of the complexity of glycolysis, it would be an oversimplification to assume that this is the only site of glycolytic control in tumors.

Oxidation of Fatty Acids

The survival and growth of hepatomas that have low glycolytic activity require consideration of their source of metabolic fuel; and studies conducted in our laboratory point to fatty acids.[29] When ^{14}C-labeled palmitate or butyrate was incubated with respiring whole homogenates of well-differentiated tumors, the conversion to [14]CO$_2$, indicative of complete oxidation, was in the same range as in the same preparations of liver. However, their oxidation in homogenates of poorly differentiated tumors was negligible. The same relationships hold also for β-hydroxybutyrate dehydrogenase activity,[30] and recent work of Langan[38] in our laboratory indicates that the levels of fatty-acid activating enzyme (Acyl-CoA synthetase) and mitochondrial ketone body production also are high in well-differentiated and low or absent in poorly differentiated tumors. It would appear from this work that the degree of glucose utilization, bears an inverse relationship to fatty acid utilization; and that with loss of differentiation there is a switch from fatty acids to glucose, accompanied by loss of enzyme activities involved in fatty acid catabolism.

Discussion

The Morris hepatomas illustrate a growing recognition that the neoplastic transformation of a single cell type, the parenchymal liver cell, may give rise to an exceedingly diverse family of tumors. At the one extreme are the few highly differentiated tumors with high respiration and low glycolysis, and with a full complement of enzymes of fatty acid catabolism, making fatty acids their predominant metabolic fuel. At the opposite extreme are the virtually undifferentiated tumors with high glycolysis and low-to-moderate respiration, whose absence of enzymatic equipment for fatty acid catabolism points to glycolysis as their major source of metabolic energy. From the foregoing studies of our own and those of other laboratories, it seems clear that high aerobic glycolysis once thought to be the sine qua non of cancer is, indeed, a resultant of progression rather than initiation of neoplasia.

Tumors whose glycolytic activity has been found to be high are invariably those which, through repeated transplantation, have undergone progression to a virtually undifferentiated state. It is likely that their high aerobic glycolysis, as well as the Pasteur effect, is attributable generally to successful competition for ADP by a high pyruvate kinase activity associated with a low or moderate respiratory system.

The marked alterations in isozyme patterns make it clear that mere comparisons of total enzyme activity between a tumor and its tissue of origin, or among different tumors, are inadequate to disclose profound phenotypic alterations which may accompany the neoplastic condition. Moreover, the continued presence of liver marker isozymes in well-differentiated hepatomas shows that alteration or loss of such enzymes, which is often seen in liver neoplasms, need not relate causally to the initiation of neoplasia, but rather represents the underlying molecular mechanism of tumor progression. This conception does not necessarily discount the significance of such alterations; indeed, they are probably crucial to the growth and development of the tumor. The loss of those enzymes concerned with functional activities of the tissue of origin would conceivably stimulate cell replication by removal of competing energy-requiring processes. The further replacement of isozymes geared to function by other isozymes geared to rapid and efficient utilization of metabolic fuel would possibly impart to such cells advantages of growth rate that would ensure their survival despite the possible existence of host defense mechanisms. The end result of this sequential series of enzyme alterations would be an anaplastic, rapidly growing tumor which, by loss of those distinguishing morphologic and biochemical characteristics of the tissue of origin, would resemble only other tumors similarly derived. One can therefore understand why, according to the so-called Greenstein generalization, the many-times transplanted tumors resemble each other more closely than they resemble their tissue of origin.[1]

It is noteworthy that with the loss of regulation of cell division in the hepatoma, there is a loss or suppression of a number of enzymes whose activity in liver is under regulation by hormones; and it is of further significance that as regulatory control is further lost by decreased differentiation, the new enzymes that appear are not of the adaptive type. A corollary question now emerges, whether those adaptive enzymes that are retained in the well-differentiated tumors are still responsive. Our own studies have shown that neither glucokinase, pyruvate kinase, nor adenylate kinase in well-differentiated liver tumors is responsive to dietary or hormonal manipulation. Furthermore, these enzymes cannot be made to appear by treatments that lead to enhancement of their activity in normal liver. However, a more recent study indicates that hormones such as cortisol and glucagon may affect the activities in certain hepatomas of such enzymes as tyrosine-α-ketoglutarate amino-transferase, serine dehydratase, glucose-6-phosphatase, and glucose-6-phosphate dehydrogenase.

How are the activities of these isozymes switched off and on, and how are such changes related to the process of dedifferentiation? The loss of differentiation would require first a repression of those genes that code for the liver-type isozymes, and as dedifferentiation proceeds, there is a derepression of other genes that code for enzymes that are repressed in the normal liver. Both processes do not occur simultaneously, and it would appear that repression of the liver-specific isozymes has to occur before derepression of the nonhepatic isozyme, since the nonhepatic isozymes have never appeared in high activity in the same tumors having high activity of the liver isozyme. However, there is as yet no clear-cut evidence that differences in the respective activities are attributable to differences in rates of protein synthesis; and even if so, it is not certain that the transcriptional phase is involved.

RESEMBLANCE OF POORLY DIFFERENTIATED TUMORS TO FETAL LIVER

In their isozyme patterns, the poorly differentiated tumors closely resemble the fetal liver. Since the embryonal liver cell only develops the liver-type isozymes at or near parturition, it is perhaps not too surprising that tumors resemble fetal liver, just as poorly differentiated tumors resemble one another. However, there may be more to this similarity than meets the eye, since Abelev[31] has recently found the production of fetal globulins in chemically induced liver tumors, and Gold and his co-workers[32] found a fetal antigen in certain gastrointestinal tumors. These findings support the view that tumor dedifferentiation may, in its basic biochemical mechanism, be a reversal of normal embryonic development and may account for the often noted resemblance of tumors to embryonic tissue.

There is a growing body of evidence to indicate that neoplasia may be associated with bizarre aberrations of protein synthesis, notably reported in the clinical literature. Lipsett[33] has cited over 100 cases of Cushing's syndrome associated with a variety of clinical nonpituitary neoplasms, principally bronchogenic carcinoma, apparently caused by secretion of substances having the hormonal activity of ACTH. Severe hypoglycemia has been frequently reported as an accompaniment of various tumors of nonendocrine origin, and recently Miyabo et al.[34] found evidence of immunoreactive insulin in a gastric tumor associated with hypoglycemia. Goodall[35] and Eliel[36] have also reviewed the clinical literature which points to production and secretion of hormones from a variety of tumors of nonendocrine origin. Evidently the gene readout mechanism can be distorted in certain neoplasms so that genes normally completely repressed in the tissue of origin are unmasked for transcription and translation.

When the Morris hepatomas first appeared, they were hailed as the hope for an eventual understanding of the molecular basis of cancer formation. According to Potter, the availability of liver tumors that are undoubtedly malignant, yet differ in few biochemical parameters from the normal, differentiated liver cell of origin, opens the possibility for identifying the crucial first step of the chemically induced neoplastic transformation. Since this process is a lengthy one, and probably involves several stages of preneoplasia, it is probably too much to hope that it would be explainable on the basis of one or a few enzyme aberrations. At any rate, if this hope has not yet been realized, nonetheless the intensive biochemical studies of these tumors are providing a much clearer picture of the underlying molecular alterations which accompany the spectrum of variations in growth rate and degree of differentiation which characterize neoplasia.

Acknowledgments

Work carried out by the author and his associates was aided by grants CA-07174, CA-10439, AM-05487, and CA-10916 from the National Institutes of Health, U. S. Public Health Service, and P-202 from the American Cancer Society.

All of the work on the Morris hepatomas was done with the active collaboration of H. P. Morris; the following collaborators participated in the work from the author's laboratory: D. L. DiPietro, C. Sharma, R. Manjeshwar, J. Shatton, R. C. Adelman, F. A. Farina, C. H. Lo, W. Criss, G. Litwack, L. Bloch-Frankenthal, J. Langan, and K. Ohe. We are indebted to Dr. David Meranze for histologic examination of these hepatic tumors.

References

1. Greenstein, J. P.: Biochemistry of Cancer. 2nd ed., Academic Press, New York, 1954.
2. Warburg, O.: The Metabolism of Tumors. Arnold Constable, London, 1930.
3. Weinhouse, S.: Oxidative Metabolism of Tumors, 3:269-325, 1955.
4. Morris, H. P.: Studies on the development, biochemistry and biology of experimental hepatomas. Adv. Cancer Res., 9:227-302, 1965.
5. Nowell, P. C., H. P. Morris, and V. R. Potter: Chromosomes of minimal deviation hepatomas. Cancer Res., 27:1561-1579, 1967.
6. Weber, G., G. Banerjee, and H. P. Morris: Comparative biochemistry of hepatomas, I. Carbohydrate enzymes in Morris hepatoma 5123. Cancer Res., 21:933-937, 1961.
7. Aisenberg, A. C., and H. P. Morris: Energy pathways of hepatoma 5123. Nature, 191:1314-1316, 1961.
8. DiPietro, D. L., C. Sharma, and S. Weinhouse: Studies on glucose phosphorylation in rat liver. Biochemistry, 1:455-462, 1962.
9. Vinuela, E., M. Salas, and A. Sols: Glucokinase and hexokinase in rat liver. J. Biol. Chem. 238:1175-1177, 1963.
10. Grossbard, L., and R. T. Schimke: Multiple hexokinase of rat tissues. Purification and comparison of soluble forms. J. Biol. Chem., 241:3546-3560, 1966.
11. Katzen, H. M., and R. T. Schimke: Multiple forms of hexokinase in the rat. Proc. Nat. Acad. Sci. USA, 54:1218-1225, 1965.

12. Salas, M., E. Vinuela, and A. Sols: Insulin dependent synthesis of liver glucokinase in the rat. J. Biol. Chem., 238:3535-3538, 1963.
13. Sharma, C., R. Manjeshwar, and S. Weinhouse: Effects of diet and insulin on glucose-ATP phosphotransferase of rat liver. J. Biol. Chem., 238:3840-3845, 1963.
14. Ballard, F. J., and I. T. Oliver: Kethexokinase isozymes of glucokinase and glycogen synthesis from hexoses in neonatal rat liver. Biochem. J., 90:261-268, 1964.
15. Sharma, R. M., C. Sharma, A. J. Donnelly, H. P. Morris, and S. Weinhouse: Glucose-ATP phosphotransferases during hepatocarcinogenesis. Cancer Res., 25:193-199, 1965.
16. Shatton, J. B., H. P. Morris, and S. Weinhouse: Kinetic, electrophoretic, and chromatographic studies on glucose-ATP phosphotransferases in the rat. Cancer Res., 29:1161-1172, 1969.
17. Elwood, J. C., U. C. Lin, V. J. Cristofalo, S. Weinhouse, and H. P. Morris: Glucose utilization homogenates of the Morris 5123 and related tumors. Cancer Res., 23: 906-913, 1963.
18. Fondy, T. P., and N. O. Kaplan: Structural and functional properties of H and M subunits of lactic dehydrogenase. Ann. N. Y. Acad. Sci., 119:888-904, 1965.
19. Penhoet, E., T. Rajkumar, and W. J. Rutter: Multiple forms of fructose, diphosphate aldolase in mammalian tissues. Proc. Nat. Acad. Sci. USA, 56:1275-1282, 1966.
20. Adelman, R. C., H. P. Morris, and S. Weinhouse: Fructokinase, triokinase, and aldolases in liver tumors of the rat. Cancer Res., 27:2408-2413, 1967.
21. Tanaka, T., Y. Harano, F. Sue, and H. Morimura: Crystallization characterization and metabolic regulation of two types of pyruvate kinase isolated from rat tissues. J. Biochem. (Tokyo), 62:71-91, 1967.
22. Bailey, E., and P. E. Walker: A comparison of the properties of the pyruvate kinase of the fat body and flight muscle of the adult male desert locust. Biochem. J., 111:359-364, 1969.
23. Weber, G., N. B. Stamm, and E. A. Fischer: Insulin: Inducing of pyruvate kinase. Science, 149:65-67, 1965.
24. Adelman, R. C., C. H. Lo, and S. Weinhouse: Dietary and hormonal effects of adenosine triphosphate-adenosine monophosphate phosphotransferase activity in rat liver. J. Biol. Chem., 243:2538-2544, 1968.
25. Criss, W. E., G. Litwack, H. P. Morris, and S. Weinhouse: ATP-AMP phosphotransferase isozymes in rat liver and hepatomas. Cancer Res. In press.
26. Johnson, M. J.: The role of aerobic phosphorylation in the Pasteur Effect. Science, 94:200-202, 1941.
27. Lynen, F.: The aerobic phosphate requirements of yeast: The Pasteur Effect. Ann. Chem., 546:120-141, 1941.
28. Lo, C. H., V. J. Cristofalo, H. P. Morris, and S. Weinhouse: Studies of respiration and glycolysis in transplanted hepatomas on the rat. Cancer Res., 28:1-10, 1968.
29. Bloch-Frankenthal, L., J. Langan, H. P. Morris, and S. Weinhouse: Fatty acid oxidation and ketogenesis in transplantable liver tumors. Cancer Res., 25:732-736, 1965.
30. Ohe, K., H. P. Morris, and S. Weinhouse: β-Hydroxydrate dehydrogenase activity in liver and liver tumors. Cancer Res., 27:1360-1371, 1967.
31. Abelev, G. I., S. V. Assecritova, N. A. Kraevsky, S. D. Perocla, and N. J. Perovodchikova: Embryonal serum α-globulin in cancer patients: Diagnostic value. Internat. J. Cancer, 2:551-558, 1967.
32. von Kleist, S., and P. Burtin: Isolation of a fetal antigen from human colonic tumors. Cancer Res., 29:1961-1964, 1969.
33. Lipsett, M. B.: Humoral syndromes associated with non-endocrine tumors. Ann. Int. Med., 61:733-756, 1964.
34. Miyabo, S., T. Fujimura, and M. Murakami: Gastric cancer containing insulin and associated with hypoglycemia. Diabetes, 17:286-289, 1968.
35. Goodall, C. M.: A review: On para-endocrine cancer syndromes. Int. J. Cancer, 4:1-10, 1969.

36. Eliel, L. P.: Non-endocrine secreting neoplasms: Clinical manifestations. Cancer Bull. 20:37-39, 1968.
37. Gosalvez: Unpublished data.
38. Langan, J.: Unpublished data.

Nucleic Acid Metabolism in Neoplasms

GLYNN P. WHEELER

*Cancer Biochemistry Division, Southern Research Institute,
Birmingham, Alabama, USA*

THERE ARE TWO prominent reasons for biochemically characterizing neoplasms: to better define and understand the neoplastic process, and to find biochemical differences between normal and neoplastic tissues that might be exploited through therapy. Since biochemical characterization of neoplasms is of little value unless comparison with normal tissues is made, much effort has been put into such comparisons.

Very few qualitative differences between nucleic acid metabolism of normal tissues and neoplasms have been found. Differences in the extents of methylation of RNA[1-3] and of DNA[4] have been noted, and the resulting alkylated materials might be qualitatively different. The full significance of these differences is not presently known.

Conversely, numerous quantitative differences in the biosynthesis and catabolism of precursors of nucleic acids and of nucleic acids themselves by normal and cancer tissues have been noted. Assessing the importance of these differences is difficult, however, because of the great ranges of metabolic activity in normal tissues and in cancer tissues. Selection of an appropriate normal tissue as a frame of reference is a problem, and it is a fallacy to assume that the metabolism of even a specified neoplasm is unchanging and that a single set of values satisfactorily or completely characterizes it. We shall now address ourselves to this latter point.

It is well established that the rate of growth of a neoplasm commonly decreases when the tumor becomes large[5] or when the number of ascites cells becomes large.[6-9] If the rate of growth changes, then quantitative aspects of metabolism would most likely change also. The quantities of adenine-^{14}C, formate-^{14}C, thymidine-^{3}H, and leucine-^{3}H fixed in vivo into the acid-insoluble fraction of leukemia L1210 cells harvested from the peritoneal cavity two hr following ip injection of the radioactive substrate decreased between days 6 and 8, during which time the number of cells in the peritoneal cavity and the viability of these cells changed very little. The decreases in specific activity were probably not attributable to an inadequate supply of substrate, because the total quantity of fixed substrates also decreased and because the intracellular quantities of radioactive substrates as intermediates of nucleic acid synthesis were as large, or larger, on day 8 as on days 4 and 6. Figure 17-1 shows that the rates of synthesis of both RNA and DNA decreased between days 6 and 8, and the rate for RNA also decreased between days 4 and 6.

Some commonly espoused reasons for decreases in growth rates are inadequate vascularization and supply of nutrients, stress of crowding of cells, and debilitation of the host. Perhaps each of these factors, as well as others, contributes to the decrease, but the net result is an alteration in the cell and/or tissue kinetics of the neoplasm.

Alterations of the kinetics might include changes in the length of the cell cycle and of the various phases of the cycle, changes in the growth fraction of the cells of the neoplasms, and cell loss from the neoplasm.[10] The data for adenocarcinoma 755 (Table 17-5) indicate that the length of the cell cycle increased and the growth fraction decreased as the tumor became larger. The length of the cell cycle of leukemia

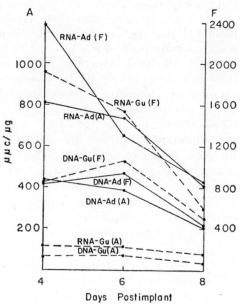

FIG. 17–1.—Specific activities of nucleic acid purines of leukemia L1210 cells harvested from the peritoneal cavity of mice two hr following the ip injection of adenine-8-[14]C (A) or formate-[14]C (F). Scale A is for adenine-8-^{14}C, and scale F is for formate-[14]C.

TABLE 17–5.—KINETIC PARAMETERS OF ADENOCARCINOMA 755[5]

DAYS POST-IMPLANT	MEAN WEIGHT (MG.)	T_{G_1}	T_S	T_{G_2}	T_M	T_C	LABELING INDEX (%)	CALCULATED GROWTH FRACTION
			TIMES OF CELL CYCLE (HOURS)					
4	46	3.5	7.0	0.5	ca 1.0	12	27	0.51
8	378	4.5	6.0	2.5	ca 1.0	14	18	0.45
14	2660	7.5	6.0	1.5	ca 1.0	16	9	0.28
19	3630	3.5	15.5	4.0	ca 1.0	24	9	0.14

L1210 increased greatly on day 7 compared to day 6 (Table 17-6), but the length of the S phase increased relatively little. The extent and rate of cell loss in leukemia L1210 is not known, but it is known that extensive infiltration of L1210 cells into host tissues occurs.[11]

Figure 17-2 gives the results of an experiment in which cultured H. Ep. #2 cells were exposed to the indicated radioactive substrate for 30 min at various times after adding Colcemid to the heterogeneous, exponentially growing culture and the acid-insoluble fraction of the cells were assayed for radioactivity; by 28 hr, 90% of the cells had accumulated at mitosis. The curve for the thymidine index shows the portion of the cell population that is synthesizing DNA at the various times; this curve and that for the quantity of thymidine-C^3H_3 fixed at these times are in good agreement. Adenine-8-^{14}C should be incorporated into both DNA and RNA; formate should be incorporated into DNA, RNA, and protein; and leucine-^3H should be incorporated only into protein. The curves indicate that the rates of synthesis of RNA and protein were greatest during the period when the rate of synthesis of DNA was greatest, as others have also observed.[12, 13] Therefore the portion of the population of cells in S phase at a given time will have a great influence upon the observed mean extent of synthesis of nucleic acids by the cells. An increase in T_C with little change in T_S (as was observed for leukemia L1210 cells, Table 17-6) would give apparently a lower ability to synthesize nucleic acids, since there would be fewer cells in S at a given time.

It is reasonable to assume that nonproliferating cells (those in G_0) would synthesize very little or no DNA and probably very little RNA. Therefore, as the growth fraction decreases, the mean quantity of DNA synthesized by the cells of the population would also decrease.

The influence of cell loss upon the observed metabolic activity of a neoplasm is dependent upon the relative rates of cell proliferation and

TABLE 17–6.—KINETIC PARAMETERS OF LEUKEMIA L1210[14]

DAYS POST-IMPLANT	T_S	$T_{G_2} + T_M + T_{G_1}$	T_C	LABELING INDEX (%)
	TIME OF CELL CYCLE (HOURS)			
6	8.9	2.9	11.8	61.5
7	10.7	10.3	21.0	52.7

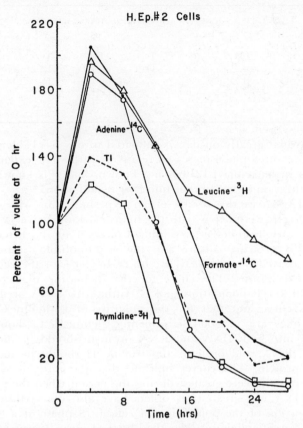

H.Ep.#2 Cells

Percent of value at 0 hr

Time (hrs)

Adenine-^{14}C

TI

Leucine-^{3}H

Formate-^{14}C

Thymidine-^{3}H

FIG. 17–2.—Specific activities (expressed as percentage of the value at zero hr) of the acid-insoluble portion of H.Ep.#2 cells exposed to the indicated radioactive substrates for 30 min at various times after adding Colcemid to heterogeneous, exponentially growing cultures. TI, thymidine index.

cell loss and upon the metabolic activity of the cells just prior to loss. (The loss might be due to cell migration [metastasis] or cell death and lysis.)

Consideration of the facts considered above leads one to conclude that he must be cautious in assigning enzymatic, synthetic, or catabolic activities to experimental neoplasms, since the profile of metabolic activities might be dependent upon the age and size of the neoplasm. This is particularly important, because it is often tempting to use large tumors in experiments in order to have plenty of material with which to work.

The same factors that account for the changing metabolic activity of tumors when the rate of growth changes might, at least partially, account for the observed metabolic differences in tumors of different growth rates and different types. In other words, the observed quantitative aspects of the metabolism of various tumors might be reflections of the cell and tissue kinetics of those tumors and not necessarily indications of the metabolic potential of the individual cells. Since the relative contributions of the various kinetic factors differ from one kind of neoplasm to another, it is not surprising that there are many observed quantitative differences in the metabolism of neoplasms.

These kinetic factors might also contribute to observed differences in the metabolism of neoplasms and normal or host tissues.

In this discussion, it is not intended to imply that there might not be significant qualitative differences between the metabolism of neoplasms and normal tissues nor that all quantitative differences are caused by kinetic factors. Surely there must be differences in gene expression corresponding to differences in degree of differentiation of neoplastic tissues. Since control of cell and tissue kinetics is a manifestation of gene expression, abnormal kinetics result from abnormal gene expression through regulatory mechanisms involving metabolic processes. Thus there is a mutual relation between kinetics and metabolism. Perhaps the changes in metabolism (gene expression) that alter cell kinetics are quite small and difficult to detect, whereas much of the observed difference in metabolism is a normal result of the altered kinetics.

In the past, many studies have been directed toward consideration of whole tissues (neoplasms) without considering the metabolic and kinetic heterogeneity of the population of cells. Perhaps we must now adapt our thinking to consider the individual cells and the factors determining and regulating the metabolism and proliferation of them. It seems likely that the more we know about the events occurring within the various phases of the cell cycle and the control of these events, the better we will understand the alterations existing in neoplastic cells and tissues.

Acknowledgments

The assistance of Mrs. Jo Ann Alexander and Miss Bonnie J. Bowdon in performing the experiments reported here is gratefully acknowledged.

References

1. Borek, E.: Methylation reactions as possible control factors in protein synthesis: A personal essay. In: Exploitable Molecular Mechanisms and Neoplasia (A Collection of Papers Presented at the Twenty-second Annual Symposium on Fundamental Cancer Research, 1968), The Williams and Wilkins Company, 1969, pp. 163-188.
2. Kaye, A. M., and P. S. Leboy: Methylation of RNA by mouse organs and tumors: Ionic stimulation *in vitro*. Biochim. Biophys. Acta, 157:289-302, 1968.
3. Stewart, M. J., and M. H. Corrance: The methylation of transfer RNA *in vitro* by extracts of normal and malignant tissue. Cancer Res., 29:1642-1646, 1969.
4. Silber, R., E. Berman, B. Goldstein, H. Stein, G. Farnham, and J. R. Bertino: Methylation of nucleic acids in normal and leukemic leukocytes. Biochim. Biophys. Acta, 123:638-640, 1966.

5. Simpson-Herren, L., and H. H. Lloyd: Kinetic parameters and growth curves for experimental tumor systems. Cancer Chemother. Rep. In press.
6. Klein, G., and L. Révész: Quantitative studies on the multiplication of neoplastic cells *in vivo*. I. Growth curves of the Ehrlich and MCIM ascites tumors. J. Nat. Cancer Inst., 14:229-278, 1953.
7. Lala, P. K., and H. M. Patt: Cytokinetic analysis of tumor growth. Proc. Nat. Acad. Sci. USA, 56:1735-1742, 1966.
8. Patt, H. M., and M. E. Blackford: Quantitative studies of the growth response of the Krebs ascites tumor. Cancer Res., 14:391-396, 1954.
9. Skipper, H. E., F. M. Schabel, Jr., and W. S. Wilcox: Experimental evaluation of potential anticancer agents. XIII. On the criteria and kinetics associated with "curability" of experimental leukemia. Cancer Chemother. Rep., 35:1-111, 1964.
10. Steel, G. G.: An approach to the analysis of the growth of tumor cell populations. In: The Proliferation and Spread of Neoplastic Cells (A Collection of Papers Presented at the Twenty-first Annual Symposium on Fundamental Cancer Research, 1967), The Williams and Wilkins Company, 1968, pp. 269-278.
11. Skipper, H. E., F. M. Schabel, Jr., W. S. Wilcox, W. R. Laster, Jr., M. W. Trader, and S. A. Thompson: Experimental evaluation of potential anticancer agents. XVIII. Effects of therapy on viability and rate of proliferation of leukemic cells in various anatomic sites. Cancer Chemother. Rep., 47:41-64, 1965.
12. Pfeiffer, S. E., and L. J. Tolmach: RNA synthesis in synchronously growing populations of HeLa S3 cells. I. Rate of total RNA synthesis and its relationship to DNA synthesis. J. Cell. Physiol., 71:77-94, 1968.
13. Stubblefield, E., R. Klevecz, and L. Deaven: Synchronized mammalian cell cultures. I. Cell replication cycle and macromolecular synthesis following brief Colcemid arrest of mitosis. J. Cell. Physiol., 69:345-354, 1967.
14. Yankee, De Vita, and Perry: Cancer Res., 27:2381, 1967.

Mechanisms of Translational Control

G. DAVID NOVELLI

Carcinogenesis Program, Biology Division, Oak Ridge National Laboratory,
Oak Ridge, Tennessee, USA

Introduction

TRANSLATION OF A SPECIFIC messenger RNA (mRNA) is an exceedingly complex reaction in which a large number of macromolecular components participate. Cairns[2] has estimated that over 150 distinct macromolecules are involved in the formation of peptide bonds. Figure 17-3 (which I owe to Dr. Preston Ritter's efforts) illustrates schematically the progression of events from polypeptide chain initiation through chain termination and release. Perhaps at this date the scheme could

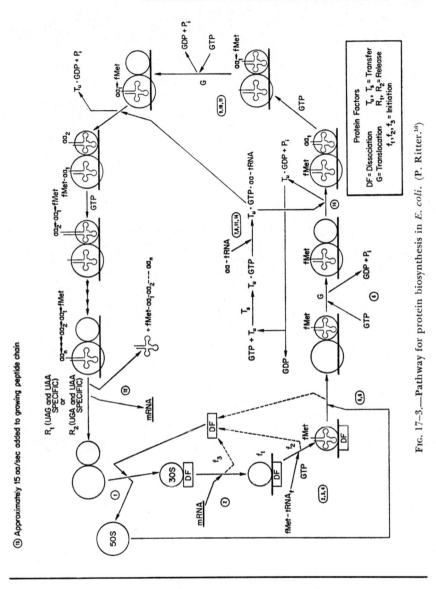

FIG. 17–3.—Pathway for protein biosynthesis in *E. coli.* (P. Ritter.[16])

be updated, but in its present form it is still useful to illustrate the points I want to make. It should be noted that chain initiation involves three protein factors together with formylmethionyl-transfer RNA (fmet-tRNA). Currently there is still some dispute as to whether the "dissociation factor" is part of the cycle. There are two "transfer factors" and one "translocation factor" and, finally, there are two release factors in the *Escherichia coli* scheme. Although no such detailed scheme has emerged from studies with in vitro systems from mammalian cells, what information exists suggests that except for minor details these mammalian systems probably function as this scheme illustrates.

It seems that regulation or control at the level of the ribosome, chain initiation, transfer factors, etc., would be too nonspecific for the differential control of the reading of different mRNAs. However, the synthesis of hemoglobin in the reticulocyte may be an exception. It has long been known that the synchronous synthesis of the α and β chains of hemoglobin is regulated by hemin. It is also well known that globin chains synthesized in its absence are unstable. In a continuation of their study of hemoglobin synthesis in rabbit reticulocytes, Rabinowitz and his colleagues[7] suggest as a working hypothesis that globin molecules, modified in the absence of hemin and thus unable to combine with it, inhibit chain initiation. Their model suggests that hemin plays a single role in hemoglobin synthesis. Its combination with globin is both a step in the formation of hemoglobin and an act in the prevention of the formation of the inhibitor of chain initiation, the modified globin. Since more than 80% of the protein synthesized by the reticulocyte is hemoglobin, in this special case, regulation of chain initiation would be a logical place for translational control to be exerted.

The rapid increase in our knowledge of tRNA because of improved separation methods made it evident that a given amino acid could be carried by one or more structurally different molecules of tRNA (isoaccepting tRNAs) often responding to different codons. In a given set of isoaccepting tRNAs, each individual one can be present as a different fraction of the total in the set. Thus, one of a set, responding to a unique codon, could be rate-limiting for the synthesis of proteins whose mRNAs contained this unique codon.

Itano[4] was the first to recognize the possibility that the rate of synthesis of hemoglobin in different cells could be regulated by a tRNA that is present in rate-limiting amount. This idea was subsequently formalized by Ames and Hartman[1] in their "modulation hypothesis" that states that the translation of mRNA is limited by modulating

Fig. 17–4.—Co-chromatography of leucyl-tRNA, from normal (O) cells of *E. coli* and from cells after 6 min of infection with phage (△) T₂. (From Waters and Novelli.[10])

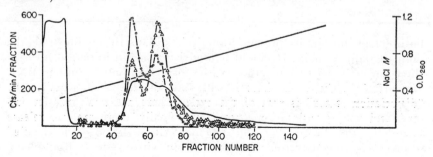

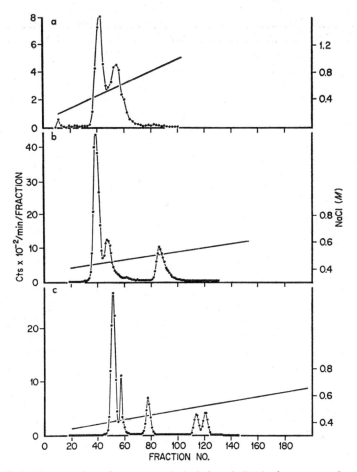

Fig. 17–5.—Comparative chromatography of leucyl-tRNA from normal cells of *E. coli*. Upper frame on MAK. Middle frame on RP-1, bottom frame on RP-2. (From L. C. Waters.[14])

codons that, in turn, correspond to modulating tRNA, i.e., one that is present in rate-limiting amounts.

The quantitative amount of a given isoaccepting tRNA is known to vary between cell types, during the growth cycle, during differentiation, and as a function of nutrition. In addition, qualitative changes in tRNA are known to occur between different cell types, as a result of viral infection, during chemical carcinogenesis, and other upsets in metabolism.

One of the first alterations in tRNA as a result of virus infection was the change in the chromatographic profile of leucyl-tRNA on methylated albumin-keiselguhr (MAK) after infection of *E. coli* with phage T_2 or T_4, as reported by Sueoka and Kano-Sueoka.[8] This is illustrated in Figure 17-4. Phage infection of *E. coli* leads, after three to six min, to an apparent decrease of the first peak of leucyl-tRNA and a corresponding increase in the second peak. This was interpreted at the time as being a phage-induced modification of leucyl-tRNA without any change in the total leucine acceptor activity.

In the meantime, new separations systems were being developed at the Oak Ridge National Laboratory that gave increased resolution of tRNAs.[6] Time does not permit a discussion of these systems, but Figure 17-5 illustrates the comparative resolution of the normal *E. coli* leucyl-tRNA on MAK, reversed phase RP-1 and RP-2. Waters and Novelli[10] examined the effect of phage T_2 infection on the chromatographic profile of *E. coli* leucyl-tRNA on RP-2 and also measured the total leucine acceptor activity six min after phage, relative to seven other amino acids. We found that six min after infection the leucine acceptor activity had decreased to only about 70% of the control. When this fact is taken into account in plotting the data (see Figure 17-6), the early change observed by the Sueokas is the destruction of one of two species of leucyl-tRNA in the first peak. Recently, Kano-Sueoka and Sueoka[5] confirmed our finding of the loss in leucine acceptor activity shortly after phage infection. The leucine tRNA destroyed responds to the codon CUG, and T_2 mRNA rarely contains this codon. This leads them to suggest this as a mechanism for inhibiting host protein synthesis without inhibiting phage-specific protein synthesis.

In another experiment, Waters and Novelli[9] prolonged the phage infection for over two hr by using a high multiplicity of infecting

FIG. 17-6.—Co-chromatography of leucyl-tRNA from the normal cells and from cells six min after T_2 infection. A, normal leucyl-tRNA ([3]H-21,000 count/min) ; B, six min T_2 leucyl-tRNA ([14]C-21,200 count/min); and C, six min T_2 leucyl-tRNA ([14]C-15,000 count/min) on RP-2. (From Waters and Novelli.[10])

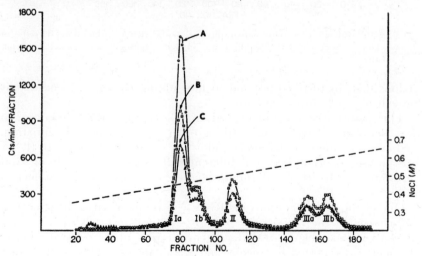

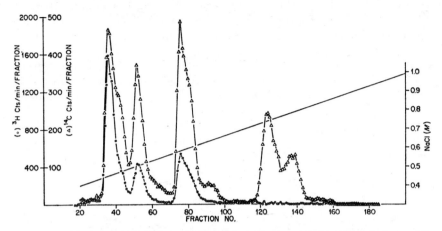

FIG. 17–7.—Co-chromatography of leucyl-tRNA from normal cells and from cells after two hr of infection with phage T_2 on RP-2 leucyl-tRNA from normal cells (O) and after two hr T_2 infection (△). (From L. C. Waters.[14])

phages. We found that near the time for normal lysis, two new leucyl-tRNAs appear that chromatograph in a position different from all other leucyl-tRNAs. The co-chromatography of a sample of tRNA taken two hr after infection is shown in Figure 17-7. Recently Abelson[15] has shown by fingerprinting that these leucine tRNAs were different and that they hybridize to phage DNA, but not to host DNA. What function these new leucine tRNAs have in the phage life cycle

FIG. 17–8.—Co-chromatography of seryl-tRNA from plasma cell tumor MOPC 31 (IgG producer) (△) and MPC 62 (IgA producer) (O). (From Yang and Novelli.[12])

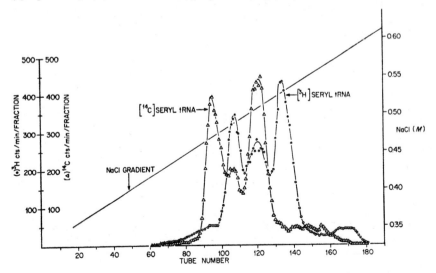

remains to be determined, but it seems that amber mutants that are blocked in some late function, although they bring about the early change in leucyl-tRNA, are incapable of causing the synthesis of these new ones.[14]

This is one example of a virus-induced change in tRNA. Several other such changes have been described, but time does not permit a detailed discussion. Some of these involve cases in which the viral genome codes for a new tRNA; in other cases with RNA viruses, it appears that the virus carries with it some of its own species of tRNA. I suspect that as time goes on we will see an increasing number of these virus-induced changes.

Differences in isoaccepting tRNAs have been observed in the same cell type that are producing different proteins. An example of this has been studied by Dr. Yang,[12] who showed that plasma cell tumors that

FIG. 17–9.—RPC co-chromatography *(a-h)* of eight aminoacyl-tRNAs showing similar to minimally different profiles in the 199 L-M cells in culture and from the same cells growing in the mouse as a tumor. Four aminoacyl-tRNAs *(i-l)* show quantitative differences among the isoaccepting species between the cells in culture as compared with the tumors. (From Yang et al.[13])

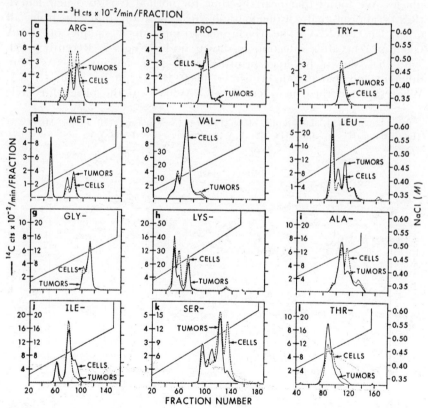

synthesize different myeloma proteins have a different set of isoaccepting seryl-tRNAs. This is shown in Figure 17-8. The plasma cell tumor that produces immunoglobulin G has an early eluting peak that is small or absent in the comparable tumor that produces immunoglobulin A, whereas the latter has a late-eluting species that is absent in the former. The finding of differences in seryl-tRNAs is especially interesting, since serine is one of the few amino acids found to differ significantly in amount in the active fragment of different antibody immunoglobulins. However, it remains to be established whether the present finding of differences in seryl-tRNA is directly related to the synthesis of different myeloma immunoglobulins. It also remains to be determined whether this change in isoaccepting tRNAs is merely a response to the necessity for translating different genetic messages or whether it serves to modify the translation of the genetic code and thus alters the primary structure of the protein.

Another case of differences in isoaccepting tRNAs that should be of particular interest at this meeting are the changes observed when the tRNAs in cultured fibroblasts (L-M cells) are compared with the tRNAs from solid tumors produced by injecting these cells into mice. Dr. Yang[13] has made a detailed comparison of the tRNA profile of these tissues for 16 amino acids using RP-2 column chromatography. These data are presented in Figures 17-9 and 17-10. In general his results can be summarized as follows: (1) For eight of the amino acids, namely arginine, methionine, proline, tryptophan, valine, glycine, leucine, and lysine, there was little or no difference in the chromatographic profile of the tRNAs from the two sources; (2) for alanine, isoleucine, serine, and threonine, there was a significant quantitative difference in the tRNA profiles; and (3) marked differences in aspartyl-, histidyl-, phenylalanyl-, and tyrosyl-tRNA were observed. These results are shown in Figures 17-9 and 17-10. These differences all disappeared when the cells were recultured from the tumor. The transfer of L-M cells from a serum-free medium in vitro to the body of the mouse in vivo, or vice versa, undoubtedly creates a drastic change in their nutritional environment. The appearance of the different isoaccepting tRNA species in the L-M tumors and the disappearance of them upon in vitro culturing of the tumor cells, therefore, may indicate an adaptive response to these nutritional changes.

We have considered three possible cellular mechanisms, which may relate to these findings: (1) selection of L-M cell clones in vivo, (2) viral activation during growth of cells in the serum environment, and (3) development of "differentiated" progeny as a result of in vivo homeostasis. These imply that the different isoaccepting tRNAs observed in the tumors are: (1) gene products of the selected clones, or (2) are induced by the action of a foreign genome, or (3) are related to the expression of different gene functions. I shall return to this subject a little later.

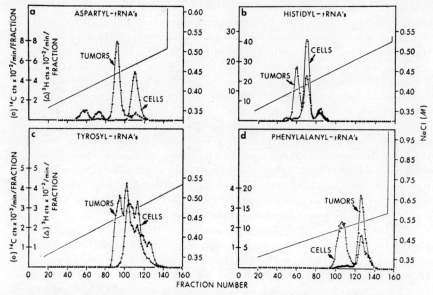

Fig. 17–10.—RP-2 co-chromatography of four aminoacyl-tRNAs showing marked qualitative and quantitative differences in the L-M cells as compared with the tumors. (From Yang et al.[13])

I mentioned earlier that changes in nutrition and other metabolic processes have been shown to cause changes in tRNA. This is because, of all nucleic acids, tRNA is unique in having a large number of modified bases. There have been more than 40 modified bases isolated from various tRNAs. These modifications take place after the primary oligonucleotide structure has been laid down and involve a large number of highly specific enzymes. The enzymes appear to be not only specific with regard to a given position on a specific base, but also to a spe-

Fig. 17–11.—RP-2 co-chromatography of phenylalanyl-tRNA from normal cells (-△-) and from cells after exposure to chloramphenicol for four hr (-○-). (From Waters.[11])

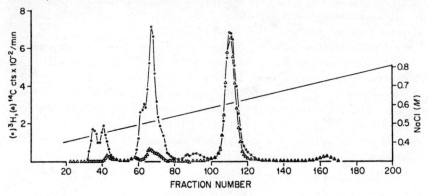

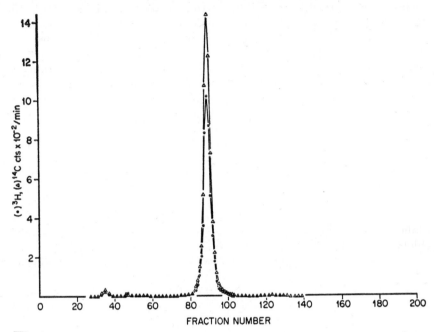

FIG. 17–12.—Reversal of the effect of chloramphenicol on the phenylalanyl-tRNA profile. The cells were first incubated with chloramphenicol for two hr, then washed with fresh medium and reincubated for two and one-half hr in the absence of chloramphenicol. The phenylalanyl-tRNA from such cells was co-chromatographed with phenylalanyl-tRNA from normal cells on RP-2. (From L. C. Waters.[14])

cific base in a given oligonucleotide sequence. For example, an isopentenyl group has been found on the 6 position of the base adenine. This is the only position where this group has been found, and the particular adenine is always located on the 3′ OH side of the anticodon.

Often these base modifications are necessary for the functioning of tRNA, either for recognition by the amino acid activating enzyme, or for binding to the ribosome.

In studying the effect of the inhibition of protein synthesis by chloramphenicol (CAP) on the tRNAs of *E. coli*, Dr. Larry Waters[11] made the surprising observation that the chromatographic profiles of some of the tRNAs are altered. An example of one such alteration can be seen in Figure 17-11. This represents the chromatographic profile of phenylalanyl-tRNA from cells that had been inhibited with chloramphenicol for four hr. Normally, *E. coli* exhibits a single sharp peak of phenylalanyl-tRNA, but after chloramphenicol for four hr there are four and possibly five peaks. This phenomenon is not limited to chloramphenicol, but is related to the inhibition of protein synthesis, whether by puromycin or withholding an essential amino acid. The phenomenon is readily reversible, as can be seen in Figure 17-12. In this case the cells were exposed to chloramphenicol for two hr, then washed and reincubated for two and one-half hr in the absence of chloramphenicol. Our interpretation of these observations is that some of the enzymes that are involved in specific base modification of tRNA have a relatively short half-life, and if their resynthesis is inhibited, the tRNAs, although being synthesized, fail to have some of their usual bases modified. A finding possibly analogous to this was reported by Gefter and Russell.[3] They showed that infection of *E. coli* with bacteriophage Φ80, carrying a gene for a tyrosine tRNA, led to the production of three chromatographically separable forms of tyrosyl-tRNA. They showed that the three forms differed in the relative completion of the adenine base adjacent to the anticodon. Furthermore, the species that had a completely unmodified adenine in this position, although capable of accepting the amino acid, was unable to bind to ribosomes or to participate in protein synthesis. It is quite probable that the multiple forms of tyrosyl-tRNA which they observed were a consequence of their use of chloramphenicol in their manipulation of their cells.

Now to return to the changes in the tRNA from the L-M tumors. Because of the foregoing results, we can suggest that differences in chromatographic profiles of isoaccepting tRNAs from L-M cells and L-M tumors may represent base exchanges, resulting in a different codon recognition, or base modifications, or both. For this distinction, three particular chromatographic features seem helpful. First, L-M tumors have four aspartyl-, four to five tyrosyl-, and three histidyl-tRNA peaks. Each is more than two, which is the number of codons recognized by these aminoacyl tRNAs in *E. coli* as well as in livers of the frog and the guinea pig. Furthermore, the aspartyl-tRNAs can be paired into duplex sets. Second, the tRNAs of the L-M cells tend to elute in the middle of the chromatogram, a feature consistent with what has been found for undermethylated *E. coli* tRNAs. Third, our observation shows that the late-eluting peaks of Ser- and Ile-tRNAs, which are marked in the L-M cells, become relatively obliterated when a reducing agent is omitted from the gradient buffer. These observations suggest that the L-M cells and the tumor may differ in tRNA base modifications involving a methyl group or an oxidizable side chain, or both.

This leads me to conclude that although tRNA may well be the vehicle by which translational control is exercised, the actual molecular control point may be at the level of synthesis and turnover of the enzymes that bring about specific base modifications in tRNA.

Acknowledgments

This research was jointly sponsored by the National Cancer Institute and the U. S. Atomic Energy Commission under contract with Union

Carbide Corporation, and in part by a Scholar grant in Cancer Research by the American Cancer Society.

References

1. Ames, B. N., and P. E. Hartman: Cold Spring Harbor Symp. Quant. Biol., 28:349, 1963.
2. Cairns, J.: Cold Spring Harbor Symp. Quant. Biol., 34: Forward, 1969.
3. Gefter, M. L., and R. L. Russell: J. Mol. Biol., 39:145, 1969.
4. Itano, H. A.: In: Abnormal Hemoglobins in Africa (J. H. P. Jonxis, ed.), Oxford University Press, London and New York, Blackwell, Oxford, 1963, p. 3.
5. Kano-Sueoka, T., and N. Sueoka: Proc. Nat. Acad. Sci. USA, 62:1229, 1969.
6. Kelmers, A. D., H. O. Weeren, J. F. Weiss, R. L. Pearson, M. P. Stulberg, and G. D. Novelli: Methods in Enzymology. Academic Press, New York. In press.
7. Rabinowitz, M., M. L. Freedman, J. M. Fisher, and C. R. Maxwell: Cold Spring Harbor Symp. Quant. Biol., 34:567, 1969.
8. Sueoka, N., and T. Kano-Sueoka: Proc. Nat. Acad. Sci. USA, 52:1535, 1964.
9. Waters, L. C., and G. D. Novelli: Proc. Nat. Acad. Sci. USA, 57:979, 1967.
10. Waters, L. C., and G. D. Novelli: Biochem. Biophys. Res. Comm., 32:971, 1968.
11. Waters, L. C.: Biochem. Biophys. Res. Comm., 37:296, 1969.
12. Yang, W. K., and G. D. Novelli: Biochem. Biophys. Res. Comm., 31:534, 1968.
13. Yang, W. K., A. Hellman, D. H. Martin, K. B. Hellman, and G. D. Novelli: Proc. Nat. Acad. Sci. USA, 64:1411, 1969.
14. Waters, L. C.: Unpublished data.
15. Abelson: Personal communication.
16. Ritter, P.: Unpublished data.

Anomalous Distribution of Glutaminase Isozyme in Various Hepatomas

NOBUHIKO KATUNUMA, YASUHIRO
KURODA, YUKIHIRO SANADA, IKUKO
TOMINO, AND HAROLD P. MORRIS

Department of Enzyme Chemistry, Institute for Enzyme Research,
School of Medicine, Tokushima University, Tokushima, Japan;
Department of Biochemistry, School of Medicine,
Howard University, Washington, D. C., USA

Introduction

WE REPORTED PREVIOUSLY that there are two types of glutaminase (EC 3.5.1.2, L-glutamine amidohydrolase) in various organs. One isozyme requires high concentration of phosphate for activity (phosphate-dependent [PD]), while the other in kidney does not require phosphate either as a cofactor or an activator, and another isozyme in liver is activated by a very low concentration of phosphate (phosphate-independent [PI]), but is activated by maleate or N-acetyl glutamate.[1, 5] By purification of these isozymes to homogeneous states, we found that the PIs in adult kidney and adult liver are entirely different proteins. Since the distribution of these organ-characteristic isozymes poses an important problem, the change in the PI isozyme patterns during development of rats was studied. It has already been reported in the previous papers that no kidney-type PI was observed in adult or regenerating liver, but kidney-type PI was found in fetal liver using antiserum for PI purified from adult kidney.[2-4]

Experimental Grounds for the Existence of Kidney-Type Glutaminase in Fetal Liver

The following were the experimental bases for the existence of the liver-type glutaminase in fetal liver: (1) resistant to heat (50 C, two min) and PCMB (0.75 mM) treatment; (2) tightly bound to a particle fraction in mitochondria; (3) can be purified by the same procedure as for the purification of adult kidney glutaminase; (4) the same effects for activators and inhibitors and the same kinetics as kidney glutaminase are observed; (5) gives clear fusion line with antiserum against adult kidney enzyme; (6) no allosteric polymerization is observed in the presence of substrate; and (7) shows the same sedimentation constant as the purified adult kidney glutaminase.

We propose the following hypothesis for differentiation of organ-specific function. The differentiation of organ-characteristic function is related to the disappearance of the isozyme which is not inherent to the particular organ. It is interesting to see, in this connection, whether there is any relation between the degree of dedifferentiation of some hepatomas and their growth rates. Taking advantage of the organ-characteristic glutaminase isozymes, the following three problems were investigated in the present work. First, is there any relationship between the growth rates of tumors and the quantity or properties of these isozymes? Second, are the patterns of these isozymes related to the growth rates in six kinds of hepatomas? Third, the relation between process of carcinogenesis and appearance of the anomalous isozyme was studied. The results obtained in the present study of the tumors were compared with those obtained previously on the changes in the isozyme patterns during development and regeneration of normal organs.

Materials and Methods

Experimental Animals

All rats employed in studies on normal liver, fetal liver and regenerating liver were male Donryu and Buffalo strains. The activities and properties of the enzyme were the same in both strains. Rats weighing 150 to 200 g were partially hepatectomized by the method of Higgins and Anderson.[6] The tumors used were Morris minimal deviation hepatomas (3924A, 7777, 5123C, 7793, and 9618A), kidney tumors (9789K, 9786K, and 8997K), and Yoshida ascites hepatoma (AH 130). Their growth rates increased in the following order: for hepatomas 9618A< 7793<5123C<7777<3924A<AH 130, and for kidney tumors 8997K, 9786K, 9789K. The hepatomas (7777, 5123C, 7793, and 9618A) and three kidney tumors were grown in Buffalo rats. Hepatoma 3924A and AH 130 were grown in ACL/N and Wistar rats, respectively. Control rats were of the same strain, age, and sex as the tumor-bearing animals.

Glutaminase Assay

Fresh tissues were homogenized for five min with a Potter-Elvehjem Teflon homogenizer in 2 to 5 vol of cold distilled water in ice-cold conditions. Activity in these homogenates was assayed with 3 to 10 mg protein/tube after removing undestroyed cells by centrifugation at $600 \times g$ for 15 min. Enzyme activity was assayed by determining the amount of ammonia liberated during 15 to 30 min incubation (Katunuma et al.[2, 3]). The reaction mixture used for determination of PI contained 40 μmoles of L-glutamine, enzyme at two protein concentrations, 0.1 M tris-HCl buffer (pH 7.4 or 8.6), and 40 μmoles of maleate in a total volume of 2 ml. The reaction mixture used for assay of PD contained the same constituents except that 200 μmoles of phosphate were used instead of maleate. Kidney PI displayed no requirement for phosphate, but liver PI was always assayed in the presence of 10^{-3}M phosphate because the enzyme was extremely labile when incubated in the absence of phosphate. From kidney, PI and PD were isolated and purified to the exclusion of each other, and the activity of PI thus isolated displayed no dependency upon the concentration of phosphate. From liver, PI has been purified free of PD, but the best PD preparations obtained to date have still been contaminated by PI activity. Yet, the property of liver PI has been shown to be clearly different from that of kidney PI by immunoanalysis and the kinetic behavior of the two isozymes with respect to phosphate concentration. Unlike kidney PI, the liver PI is activated by 1/100 concentration of phosphate required for the activation of PD, and this phosphate activation can be substituted by the addition of maleate, N-acetyl glutamate, or citrate. It should be noted that a higher concentration of phosphate strongly inhibits liver PI activity. Liver PD, like kidney PD, was activated by 2×10^{-1}M phosphate, and the activity was not influenced by the addition of organic acids. These relationships are shown in Figure 17-13. The reaction was carried out for 15 or 30 min at 37 C and terminated by the addition of 1 ml of 10% TCA. After centrifugation, 1 ml of the supernatant was introduced into a Selligson-Shibata ammonium diffusion apparatus. The amount of ammonium sulfate obtained was measured colorimetrically by the Nessler method. We previously purified the PI in kidney to a homogeneous protein (820-fold) and the liver PI was purified 470-fold. From the known properties of these isozymes, it is certain that the assay of these enzymes with crude extracts of tumors in this way gives correct representation for the enzyme activity.[3] The reaction proceeded linearly for one hr, and the exact linearity was obtained between the activity and the enzyme amount in the range of 2 to 10 mg of protein. Specific activity is expressed as μmoles of ammonia liberated from glutamine per hour per mg protein. The PI activity was measured with and without maleate as an activator. The PD activity was calculated by subtracting PI activity (without maleate) from the observed activity in 100 mM phosphate. The PD/PI ratio represents PD activity over PI activity (without maleate).

PRODUCT INHIBITION OF GLUTAMINASE BY L-GLUTAMATE

The degree of product inhibition of various glutaminases (PI with maleate) was expressed as percentage of activity remaining after the addition of the same amount of L-glutamate as substrate.

ASSAY OF KIDNEY-TYPE GLUTAMINASE

Since the glutaminase (PI) in adult kidney is resistant to heat (at 50 C for two min) and PCMB treatment (1.5 μmoles/2 ml), while adult liver PI activity is completely lost on these treatments, as reported previously,[2] kidney-type PI was assayed as the activity remaining after both heat treatment and addition of 1.5 μmoles of PCMB. By immunoanalysis and kinetic studies on the purified enzyme, we previously demonstrated that the enzyme activity assayed by this method represented the true kidney-type PI activity.[4]

Preparation of Glucosamine Synthetase

Rat liver was homogenized in a solution containing 0.154 M KCl, 1 mM EDTA, and 3.3 mM F-6-P, and the homogenates were centrifuged for 15 min at 6,000 $\times$ g. The fraction of the supernatant precipitating at 40 to 50% saturation of ammonium sulfate was dissolved in 0.1 M tris-HCl buffer, pH 8.3, and dialyzed for two hr against the same buffer. The particle-bound enzyme was removed by precipitation at 0 to 40% saturation of the salt.

Glucosamine Synthetase Assay

Enzyme activity was assayed by determining the amount of glucosamine produced during incubation. The reaction mixture contained L-glutamine 30 μmoles, cysteine 3 μmoles, F-6-P 30 μmoles, the enzyme preparation in 0.033 M tris-HCl buffer, pH 8.3, in a total volume of 3 ml. The mixture was incubated for 30 min at 37 C and the reaction was terminated by boiling the mixture for seven min. After centrifugation, 2 ml of the supernatant were applied on a Dowex 50 (H-form) column (1 $\times$ 3 cm). The column was washed twice with 4 ml aliquots of water and then eluted with 3 ml of 2 N HCl. This eluate was neutralized with saturated Na_2CO_3. After removing the substrates by these treatments, the amount of glucosamine phosphate formed was determined by Boas' method.[11]

Results

Relation of Glutaminase Activity to Growth Rate

The relationship between the glutaminase isozyme and F-6-P glutamine amidotransferase activities in regenerating rat liver is shown in Table 17-7 and that in developing liver in Table 17-8. Since F-6-P amid transferase and glutaminase are involved respectively in the first anabolism and catabolism of the amido group of glutam' activities of these two enzymes were thought to be i regulation of glutamine metabolism. In the liver tomized rats, the specific activities of the c' abnormally low, and, conversely, F-6-P am abnormally high. The PD/PI ratio increased magnitude of the change being parallel with liver cells. Conversely, no great change in these observed during a three-day period of fasting. I

TABLE 17-7.—CHANGES OF GLUTAMINASE ISOZYME AND F-6-P
AMIDOTRANSFERASE ACTIVITIES IN REGENERATING LIVER

REGENERATING LIVER	GLUTAMINASE NH₃ Formed (μmoles/mg/hr)				F-6-P AMIDO-TRANSFERASE
	PI		PD		
Time After Partial Hepatectomy	Without Maleate	With Maleate (20mM)	100mM of PO₄⁻⁻⁻	PD/PI Ratio	Glucosamine-6-P Formed (mμmoles/mg/hr)
6 hours	0.117	0.424	0.325	2.78	
1 day	0.106	0.296	0.310	2.92	31.5
2.5 days	0.043	0.230	0.406	9.45	23.4
3 days	0.094	0.340	0.457	4.87	12.5
3.5 days	0.104	0.352	0.616	5.92	
7 days	0.304	0.930	0.746	2.45	
Normal liver	0.738 ± 0.190	1.230 ± 0.20	0.642 ± 0.02	0.87	8.1

No differences were observed between the activities in normal liver and the liver of sham operated animals. These enzyme activities fluctuated only ±0.200 (S.D.) in animals on the control diet. Each value represents the average of 4-6 rats.

activities of the glutaminase isozymes in fetal and neonatal livers were very low, and the PD/PI ratio was comparable to the values in the regenerating liver.

In general, rapidly growing tissues, such as fetal liver and regenerating liver, have low glutaminase activity. Glutaminase activity is also low in rapidly growing hepatomas. But comparison of the specific activities of glutaminase in hepatoma tissues involves some technical difficulties because these tissues are not homogeneous, containing necrotic, caseinous masses and blood. Therefore, the PD/PI ratio is now considered to be a better index, since its change parallels the growth rates of the cells. In contrast to the change in glutaminase activity, F-6-P amidotransferase activity is high in rapidly growing cells. The data on Morris hepatomas in Table 17-9 are arranged according to the growth rate of the hepatomas. A clear parallelism was found between the growth rates of these hepatomas and the PD/PI ratios. Knox et al.

TABLE 17-8.—CHANGES IN ACTIVITIES OF GLUTAMINASE
ISOZYMES DURING DEVELOPMENT

	NH₃ FORMED (μMOLES/MG/HR)			
	PI		PD	
	Without Maleate	With Maleate (20mM)	100mM OF PO₄⁻⁻⁻	PD/PI RATIO
neonetal liver (1 day old)	0.195	0.600	0.280	1.44
liver	0.139	0.400	0.361	2.60

values are the averages of 10-20 rats. These enzyme activities fluctuated within ± 0.1 (S.D.).

TABLE 17-9.—Relationship between Growth Rate of Morris Hepatomas and Changes in Glutaminase Isozyme Patterns

| | NH3 Formed (μmoles/mg/hr) | | | |
| | PI | | PD | |
	Without Maleate	With Maleate (20mM)	100mM OF PO$_4$---	PD/PI Ratio
AH 130	0.301 ± 0.062	1.039 ± 0.180	1.713 ± 0.316	5.7
3924A	0.244 ± 0.058	0.665 ± 0.081	1.150 ± 0.187	4.7
7777	0.204 ± 0.049	0.429 ± 0.068	0.551 ± 0.055	2.7
5123C	0.578 ± 0.071	1.560 ± 0.441	0.792 ± 0.272	1.4
7793	0.660 ± 0.155	0.970 ± 0.071	0.565 ± 0.012	0.86
9618A	0.069	0.096	0.076	1.1
Normal liver	0.738 ± 0.190	1.230 ± 0.206	0.642 ± 0.2	0.87

Values are the averages of tumors of 4-6 rats.

also reported recently that the PD/PI ratio in some was higher than that in normal tissues.[8] The activity of glutaminase, a catabolic enzyme of glutamine, decreases with an increase in the growth rate, while the activity of F-6-P amidotransferase which is involved in the anabolic process increases with the growth rate.

Anomalous Distribution of Organ-Specific Isozymes in Tumors

Various glutaminase isozymes were purified to homogeneous proteins, and the properties of the organ-characteristic isozymes were compared, as reported previously.[3] The changes in the PI isozyme pattern during development and in regenerating liver are shown in Figure 17-13. Fetal liver contained both liver and kidney type enzymes. The amount of kidney-type PI, which is not inherent to liver, decreased gradually after birth, disappearing completely within four to five days.[4] It should be noted that no kidney-type enzyme was found in any stages of liver regeneration, although this tissue was growing rapidly. Thus regenerating liver seems to have already completed the differentiation of the isozyme. It should also be noted that the inhibition of enzyme activity by the product (glutamate) was not observed in adult and regenerating liver PI, while the inhibition was clearly recognized in fetal and neonatal liver PI. The degree of this inhibition can be used as a marker of change in isozyme profiles during development. It may be considered that the relationship between the fetal glutaminase which shows product inhibition, and the adult enzyme which does not show product inhibition, is analogous to the change in protein structure of hemoglobin during development. As shown in Figure 17-13, no product inhibition by glutamate was observed in adult liver PI, while fetal liver PI was inhibited 60 to 70%. This inhibition decreased gradually

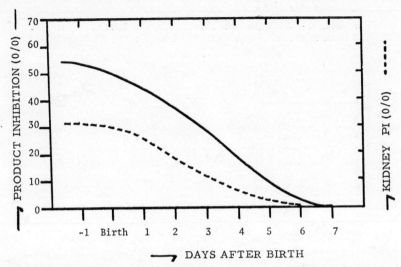

Fig. 17–13.—Changes of product inhibition of liver PI during development from fetus to neonatal rats.

after birth, disappearing completely within one week. No product inhibition was observed at any stages in regenerating liver. Phylogenic and ontogenic significance of the existence of the enzymes which have product inhibition are shown in Table 17-10.

TABLE 17–10.—CORRELATION BETWEEN PRODUCT INHIBITION OF GLUTAMINASE BY GLUTAMATE AND DISPOSAL MECHANISM OF AMMONIA IN ORGANS AND SPECIES

SPECIES	ORGANS		GLU. INHIBITION	DISPOSAL FORM OF AMMONIA
	Brain	(A)	+	Glu-NH$_2$
	Spleen	(A)	+	Glu-NH$_2$
	Lung	(A)	+	Glu-NH$_2$
	Bone M.	(A)	+	Glu-NH$_2$
Rat		(A)	−	NH$_3 \longrightarrow$ urea
	Liver	(F)	+	Glu-NH$_2$
		Regenerat.	−	NH$_3 \longrightarrow$ urea
		Hepatoma	+	Glu-NH$_2$
	Kidney	(A)	−	Glu-NH$_2 \rightarrow$ NH$_3$ salt
		Tumor	+	Glu-NH$_2$
Human	Liver	(A)	−	NH$_3 \longrightarrow$ urea
		(F)	+	Glu-NH$_2$
Bird	Liver	Pigeon	+	Glu-NH$_2 \rightarrow$ uric acid
		Quail	+	Glu-NH$_2 \rightarrow$ uric acid
		Chicken	+	Glu-NH$_2 \rightarrow$ uric acid
Fish	Liver	(Hamachi)	−	Glu-NH$_2 \rightarrow$ NH$_3$ salt

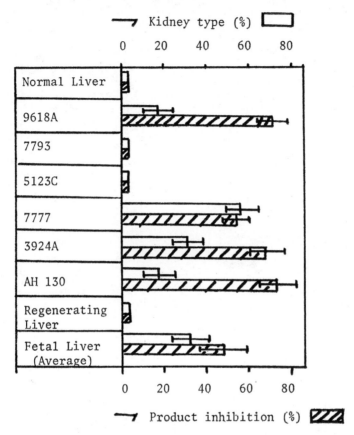

FIG. 17–14.—Existence of kidney type PI and product inhibition in Morris hepatomas.

Figure 17-14 shows the results on the Morris hepatoma obtained with the two indicators of isozyme differentiation during development. The presence of kidney type PI and of product inhibition were observed in some hepatomas, but the content of kidney type PI and the extent of inhibition showed no relationship to the growth rates. Thus, there is no direct relationship between the growth rate and the degree of differentiation of organ-specific isozymes. Hepatoma 7777 contained 50 to 60% kidney type PI, and partially purified kidney-type enzyme from this tumor was neutralized with antiserum from adult kidney PI. Weinhouse et al.[9] also reported recently that the pyruvate kinase isozyme which is not inherent in the particular organ was observed in some Morris hepatomas.

APPEARANCE OF ANOMALOUS ISOZYME DURING
CARCINOGENESIS

The relation between process of carcinogenesis by DAB diet and appearance of the anomalous isozyme was tested. Rats were fed ad libitum on laboratory chow containing 0.06% 3'-DAB. Small hepatoma spots appeared at three months after starting DAB diet. The DAB-induced hepatoma cell itself contains a considerable amount of kidney-type PI, but we could not recognize the appearance of the anomalous isozyme in the so-called precancerous stage. The process is shown in Figure 17-15.

FIG. 17–15.—Appearance of anomalous isozyme (months after starting DAB diet) in hepatoma (kidney type PI) during carcinogenesis.

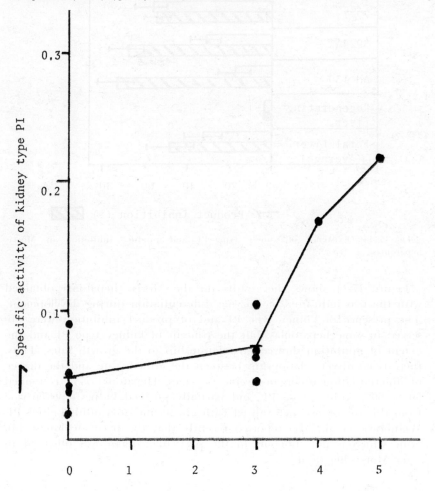

Discussion

METABOLIC ROLE OF ORGAN-SPECIFIC
GLUTAMINASE ISOZYMES

Glutaminase isozymes were used in this study as markers for assessing differentiation of organ-specific function. Therefore, the correlation between the glutaminase isozymes and their metabolic roles should be explained. We found that two isozymes of glutaminase exist in various organs. One of these (PD) requires phosphate, and the other (PI) which we discovered is not activated by phosphate but is strongly activated by maleate or N-acetyl glutamate.[2] The PIs in different organs are now considered to be isozymes. By purification of the isozymes of PI in adult liver and kidney to homogeneous states, we found that they were different proteins.[3, 4] They differed in molecular weight, reactivity with their respective antisera (immunochemical properties), heat stability, sensitivity to PCMB, optimal pH (kidney PI: pH 7.2, and liver PI: pH 8.5), mode of activation by maleate, effects of N-acetyl glutamate and tricarboxylic acids involved in the TCA cycle (these compounds activate liver PI but not kidney PI), polymerization by the substrate, and inducibility by a high protein diet. These differences in organ-characteristic properties seem to be related to organ-specific function.

The glutamine synthesized in various organs is transported in the blood, and most of its nitrogen is converted to urea in the liver, although some of it is excreted as ammonium salts in the urine. Since inorganic ammonia is the substrate for carbamyl phosphate synthetase, the amide of glutamine has to be hydrolyzed to ammonia by liver glutaminase prior to its incorporation into carbamyl phosphate. The most important regulatory mechanism for the control of glutamine metabolism in liver is the allosterism of glutaminase by its substrate, glutamine.[5] At low concentrations of substrate the enzyme activity is rather low, but the presence of a large amount of the substrate causes polymerization of the enzyme molecules, resulting in high activity. This may be considered as one form of positive feedback control. Furthermore, the activators (N-acetyl glutamate and tricarboxylic acids involved in the TCA cycle) facilitate the polymerization of the enzyme and cause a decrease in the K_m value for the substrate. This conformational change by the substrate is an important automatic form of regulation. N-acetyl glutamate and related compounds activate carbamyl phosphate synthetase, as shown by Cohen.[12] These compounds also activate the liver-type PI but not the kidney-type PI. The activation of the two successive reactions in the transfer of amide nitrogen of glutamine to carbamyl phosphate by common activators should provide a highly efficient regulatory mechanism. At the same time, a rich supply of ATP and CO_2 is necessary for the synthesis of urea, and the finding that the carboxylic acids of the TCA cycle activate both glutaminase and the TCA cycle provides another example of an intricate regulatory mechanism. Glutamine is also an important source of amide for the synthesis of purine bases and amino sugars. This is the anabolic pathway of glutamine; i.e. via glutaminase there is reciprocal variation with the activities of the enzymes in the anabolic pathway.

HISTOCHEMICAL ANALYSIS OF MORRIS HEPATOMAS

According to the Karnovsky method, the glutamate formed by the glutaminases from added glutamine was detected using glutamic dehydrogenase and tetrasolium.[7] Glutaminase in tumors was violet colored. The preparations from which glutamine was omitted in the incubation mixture were used as the control. As mentioned before, liver-type PI is inhibited by a low concentration of PCMB while kidney-type PI is not. In histochemical studies, glutaminase in hepatoma 5123C, which contains no kidney-type PI, is not stained in the presence of PCMB, but hepatoma 7777, which contains an appreciable amount of kidney-type PI, is stained extensively and homogeneously even in the presence of a high concentration of PCMB.

COMPARATIVE STUDY ON PRODUCT INHIBITION BY GLUTAMATE

In adult rats, no product inhibition by glutamate was observed with liver and kidney PIs, while the brain enzyme was strongly inhibited by the addition of glutamate.[2, 10] There is no physiologic necessity for product inhibition in the liver or kidney, because these two organs possess the urea cycle and an ammonium excretion system, respectively. There is no system for disposal of ammonia in the brain tissue; instead, the glutaminase activity is controlled by the glutamate level in the tissue so that the other product, ammonia, does not increase beyond a certain level. Strong product inhibition was observed in all kinds of avian livers tested, in which nitrogen is excreted by synthesis of uric acid from glutamine directly, and also in fetal liver of rat which has not yet developed urea cycle enzymes.

DIFFERENTIATION OF ORGAN-CHARACTERISTIC ISOZYME IN HEPATOMAS

There have been various opinions on this problem. Weinhouse indicated the dedifferentiational nature of cancer enzymes at the molecular level on the grounds that muscle-type pyruvate kinase isozyme was detected in some hepatomas. Potter also suggested recently that dedifferentiation of cancer enzymes is caused by a block of ontogenecity.[14] From the study on the distribution of organ-specific aldolase isozyme in hepatomas with different growth rates, Sugimura suggested that the most suitable explanation for the peculiar pattern in these hepatomas was that of "dys-differentiation."[15] We do not consider that there is any direct relationship between the growth rate and the degree of differentiation of an organ-specific isozyme such as glutaminase isozyme, whose pattern changes irreversibly in the course of development. It should be pointed out from our data that the activity of this marker enzyme does not change in regenerating liver or on various hormonal treatments, in contrast to the results on other enzymes used by previous workers.

Acknowledgments

This work was supported by Grant DRG-959 from the Damon Runyon Memorial Fund, the Cancer Special Fund of the Japanese Government and in part by U. S. Public Health Service Grant No. CA-10729.

References

1. Katunuma, N., I. Tomino, and H. Nishino: Glutaminase isozyme in rat kidney. Biochem. Biophys. Res. Comm., 22:321-328, 1966.
2. Katunuma, N., A. Huzino, and I. Tomino: Organ specific control of glutamine metabolism. Adv. Enzyme Reg., 5:55-69, 1967.
3. Katunuma, N., T. Katsunuma, I. Tomino, and Y. Matsuda: Regulation of glutaminase activity and differentiation of the isozyme during development. Adv. Enzyme Reg., 6:227-242, 1968.
4. Katunuma, N., I. Tomino, and Y. Sanada: Differentiation of organ specific glutaminase isozyme during development. Biochem. Biophys. Res. Comm., 32:426-432, 1968.
5. Katsunuma, T., M. Temma, and N. Katunuma: Allosteric nature of a glutaminase isozyme in rat liver. Biochem. Biophys. Res. Comm., 32:433-437, 1968.
6. Higgins, G. H.: Experimental pathology of the liver. Arch. Path., 12:186-202, 1931.
7. Karnovsky, M. J., and S. R. Himmelhoch: Histochemical localization of glutaminase 1 activity in kidney. Amer. J. Physiol., 201:786-890, 1961.
8. Knox, W. E., G. C. Tremblay, B. B. Spanier, and G. H. Friedell: Glutaminase activities in normal and neoplastic tissues of the rat. Cancer Res., 27:1456-1458, 1967.
9. Chai-ho, L., V. J. Cristofalo, H. P. Morris, and S. Weinhouse: Studies on respiration and glycolysis in transplanted hepatic tumors of the rat. Cancer Res., 28:1-10, 1968.
10. Krebs, H. A.: Metabolism of amino acids. Biochem. J., 29:1951-1969, 1935.
11. Boas, N. F.: Method for the determination of hexosamines in tissues. J. Biol. Chem., 204:553-563, 1953.
12. Grisolia, S., and P. P. Cohen: Catalytic role of glutamate derivatives in citrulline biosynthesis. J. Biol. Chem., 204:753-757, 1963.
13. Kishino, Y., T. Matsuzawa, and N. Katunuma: Histochemical study of aspartate transaminase in normal and pathological states using diazonium salt. In: Symposium on Pyridoxal Enzymes, Maruzen Press, 1968, pp. 223-229.
14. Potter, V. R., and M. Watanabe: Some biochemical essentials of malignancy. Personal communication, 1967.
15. Matsushima, T., S. Kawabe, M. Sibuya, and T. Sugimura: Biochem. Biophys. Res. Comm., 30:565, 1968.

18

Regulation of Cell Cycle and Function

Regulatory Genetic Changes in the Origin of Asparaginase-Sensitive Leukemias

J. A. SERRA

Pacific Northwest Research Foundation, Seattle, Washington, USA, and Faculty of Science, Lisbon, Portugal

Introduction

ALTHOUGH THE LIMITATIONS of asparaginase therapy for human leukemia are now well apparent, interest in the study of the antineoplastic action of this enzyme has not abated. Not only does asparaginase alone or in combination with other drugs continue to be employed with some success in remission of some human leukemias (recent reviews in Adamson and Fabro,[1] Burchenal;[9] cf., however, Holland,[15] Young[38]), but it is also possible that clarification of the mode of action of this enzyme will be helpful in our understanding of how leukocytes and possibly other cell types become neoplastic.

The first hypothesis, which may be called metabolic and now appears as an oversimplification, proposed to explain the action of asparaginase in producing remission or cure of some leukemias in experimental animals, stated that asparaginase injected or naturally present in the plasma of some mammals has the effect of depriving susceptible cells of asparagine, with the consequence that such cells will become unable to multiply or will die. In this hypothesis, susceptibility of the cells is imputed to a so-called genetic defect through which asparagine, normally a nonessential amino acid, becomes an essential amino acid. Some more complex variants of the hypothesis impute the consequences of the genetic defect to more than one amino acid as, for example, asparagine and glutamine, or asparagine and glycine.

In the present paper, through analysis of pertinent data, I propose another explanation for the biologic role and connected therapeutic use of asparaginase. The hypothesis here proposed, which may be called genetic-regulatory, interprets the so-called genetic defect associated with asparaginase sensitivity as being produced by genetic changes, of treptional nature, connected with tissue and organ differentiation. This type of genetic change is briefly discussed, having in view its application to neoplastic transformation in general. The physiologic consequences of the genetic changes are also discussed as a part of the proposed hypothesis.

Asparaginase and Asparagine-Synthetase (ASase) in Mammals

Discovery of a plasma antileukemic factor[17] was possible because natural differences in this respect occur between guinea pig serum and the serum of mice and rats in which certain lymphomas had been transplanted. Subsequently, the factor responsible for suppression of these mouse and rat lymphomas was shown to be asparaginase.[7, 8] Asparaginase had been known to be present in guinea pig serum since the work of Clementi in 1922.[12] After the discovery of the antilymphoma effect, this enzyme was detected in the plasma of several other South American rodents of the superfamily Cavioidea, and more recently in the plasma of South American primates of the superfamily Ceboidea (see Table 18-1).

Asparaginase (L-asparagine amidohydrolase) activity in significant concentration in the plasma is incompatible with the continued presence in the plasma of free asparagine, which is converted by the enzyme into asparatic acid according to the reaction:

$$H_2NCO \cdot CH_2 \cdot CH(NH_2) \cdot COOH + H_2O \longrightarrow (Enz) \rightarrow$$
$$HOOC \cdot CH_2 \cdot CH(NH_2) \cdot COOH + NH_3.$$

Asparagine absorbed from the food is rapidly converted into aspartic acid. One point to note in Table 18-1 is the increase of plasma asparaginase concentration with age. This evolution cannot be imputed to differences in diet; even on an asparagine-free synthetic diet, guinea pigs maintain their plasma asparaginase concentration at a remarkably constant level.[37] The same data indicate no appreciable difference between strains. It would not be surprising that a similar evolution with age was also found in primates.

Asparagine nonavailability to the cells caused by the action of plasma asparaginase does not automatically lead to this amino acid being unavailable for protein synthesis in the cell. In active metabolizing or-

TABLE 18–1.—PLASMA ASPARAGINASE ACTIVITY IN MAMMALS*

ORDER AND SUPER-FAMILY	SPECIES†	CIRCULATORY PROTEIN MEAN (g %)	ASPARAGINE (MG %)	ASPARTIC ACID (MG %)	L-ASPARAGINASE ACTIVITY /ML SERUM/HR	L-ASPARAGINASE ACTIVITY (μMOLES NH$_3$) /MG PROT/HR	REF.‡
Rodents:							
Hystricoidea	Coendu	—	—	—	<1	—	1
Cavioidea	Guinea pig	5.1 ± 0.0	—	—	115	—	1
"	" newborn		—	—	119 ± 6	2.3 ± 0.1	2
"	" 2 days		—	—	11.95	1.2	3
"	" 8 days		—	—	20.4	3.3	3
"	" 8 weeks		—	—	46.0	7.7	3
"	" > 1 year		—	—	86.9 ± 5.0	9.7	3
"	(adult)		—	—	130.0	13.6	3
"	Dolichotis		—	—	113	—	1
"	Hydrochoerus		—	—	32§	—	1
"	Cuniculus		—	—	64	—	1
"	Dasyprocta		—	—	583	—	1
Chinchilloidea	Chinchilla		—	—	1	—	1
Octodontoidea	Myocastor		—	—	1	—	1
Primates:							
Ceboidea	Aotes	8.8 ± 0.2	—		113	1.6	2
"	Saimiri	10.0 ± 0.3	0.01	0.49 ± 0.10	177 ± 2	2.0 ± 0.2	2
Cercopithecoidea	Rhesus	8.6 ± 0.3	0.55 ± 0.03	0.22 ± 0.01	<5	<0.05	2
"	Macaque	7.1 ± 0.3	0.53 ± 0.06	0.18 ± 0.02	<5	<0.05	2
"	Cercopithecus	6.8 ± 0.3	1.07 ± 0.16	0.23 ± 0.06	<5	<0.05	2
Hominoidea	Chimpanzee		0.49 ± 0.04	0.08 ± 0.01	<5	<0.05	2
"	Man		0.63 ± 0.004	0.04 ± 0.01	<5	<0.05	2

* Errors when given are standard errors.

† With some reserve because species are not always given the nomenclatural designation in the literature, species in this Table are by the order they are cited: Coendou prehensilis, Cavia porcellus, the Patagonian hare Dolichotis patagona, the capybara Hydrochoerus hydrochaeris, the paca Cuniculus paca, the aguti Dasyprocta aguti, the chinchilla Chinchilla lanigera, the coypu or nutria Myocastor coypus, the night monkey Aotes trivirgatus, the squirrel monkey Saimiri sciureus, the rhesus monkey Macaca mullata, the stump-tail macaque Macaca speciosa, the talapoin Cercopithecus talapoin, the chimpanzee Pan troglodytes.

‡ References 1. Old et al. 1963; 2. Peters et al. 1970; 3. Tower et al. 1963.

§ The Capybara was an immature animal.

ganisms and cells, asparagine may, in this respect, be considered to be distributed in three fractions, which determine the over-all intracellular concentration rate $[C] = dC/dt$ of free asparagine (available for protein synthesis). At any moment $[C]$ is determined by similarly defined concentration rates of plasma asparagine, $[P]$, of asparagine cellularly synthesized, $[S]$, and of asparagine $[A]$ which in the cell is being transformed into other compounds.

Rate fraction $[S]$ is produced from aspartic acid through the action

TABLE 18–2.—Intracellular Asparaginase and Asparagine Synthetase (ASase) Activity in Normal Tissues and Some Neoplasms*

SPECIES	ORGAN OR NEOPLASM	ASPARAGINASE μMOLES NH/MG PROT/HR	ASASE NMOLES ASPARAGINE FORMED/ MG PROT/HR	REF.[†]
Guinea pig	small intestine	—	34 ± 12	1
"	spleen	—	19 ± 6	1
"	liver	—	18 ± 6	1
"	lymph nodes	—	12.5[‡]	1
"	kidney	—	4.5[‡]	1
"	brain	—	3.5[‡]	1
"	testes	—	5[‡]	1
Rat, normal	spleen	0	0.978	2
" "	lung	0	0.614	2
" "	kidney	0.260	0.360	2
" "	liver	0.784	0.110	2
" "	" −3 days[§]	0	8.16	2
" "	" 2 days	0.13	2.49	2
" "	" 22 days	0.18	0.42	2
" "	" ≈ 2 months	0.63	0.16	2
Mouse, normal	spleen	—	2.3	3
" "	lymph n.+thym.#	—	1.6	3
" "	kidney	—	0.3	3
" "	liver	—	1.1	3
" "	brain	—	5.2	3
" "	testes	—	13.6	3
" "	liver,n.diet**	6.40 ± 0.46	—	4
" "	" st.	4.40 ± 0.44	—	4
" "	" asp.i.	5.34 ± 0.18	—	4
Mouse, leukemic	ERLD[††]	—	0.4	3
" "	ERLD-R 1	—	10	3
" "	ERLD-R 2	—	66	3
" "	EARAD 1	—	0.9	3
" "	EARAD 1-R	—	6.4	3
" "	ESL 1 (Res.)	6	2.3	3

* Errors when given are standard errors.
[†] References: 1. Holcenberg 1969; 2. Patterson, Jr. and Orr 1969; 3. Horowitz et al. 1968; 4. Bonetti et al. 1969.
[‡] Mean of two determinations.
[§] Three days before birth. If no reference is made in the Table to age, the animals are supposed to be adults.
Lymph nodes plus thymus.
** Abbreviations: n, normal; st., starvation for 3 days; asp.i., 100 mg asparagine injected i.p. per day for 8 days.
[††] Several other leukemias were studied; of those here mentioned, only ESL 1 (Res.) was spontaneous. R or Res. stands for asparaginase-resistant.

of asparagine synthetase (ASase). Known data have not, to date, revealed other routes for asparagine synthesis, but ASase occurs in more than one variant. One found in mammalian tumor tissue utilizes ATP, and AMP and PP_i are final products: aspartic acid + NH_3 + ATP——(enzyme + Mg^{++})→asparagine + H_2O + AMP + PP_i.[22] Another variant found in microbes produces ADP and P_i from ATP, and Mg^{++} may be partly substituted by Mn^{++}.[1, 16] Both types, probably with isozymes, appear to be able to utilize NH_3 from ammonium compounds or glutamine.

Some data on ASase and intracellular or tissue asparaginase are shown in Table 18-1. It is apparent from this table that in each type of organ, e.g. spleen, ASase tends to be found with higher activity in a species such as the guinea pig, which has plasma asparaginase, than in species devoid of this circulatory enzyme. This is to be expected if non-availability of systemic asparagine is compensated for by the intracellular synthesis of this amino acid.

Some data on the variation of both enzymes with age and with diet are included in Table 18-2. More data on these effects, and also on sex differences (apparent in the rat but not in the mouse), gonadectomy, adrenalectomy, and other conditions are available, principally in references 2 and 4. According to the presence or absence of plasma asparaginase, mammals considered in Tables 18-1 and 18-2 may belong to one of two groups: (1) $[P] + [S] - [A] = [C]$, and (2) $[S] - [A] = [C]$, with the Cavioidea and the studied Ceboidea belonging to group 2 and the other mammals to group 1. Rate fraction $[P]$ of plasma asparagine appears to be relatively constant, being practically nil in group 2 and from about 0.5% to 1% or slightly more, according to the species, in group 1. Fractions $[S]$ and $[A]$ are variable according to physiologic demand and, as shall be discussed in the next section, according to the genetic determination of the tissue.

With respect to variability in ASase activity, the case of leukemias which become transformed from asparaginase-sensitive to asparaginase-resistant, spontaneously or during treatment with asparaginase, is exemplified in Table 18-2. The intracellular asparaginase of these leukemias and that of organs of the animals which bear these neoplasms or others, may also be variable, although probably not so markedly as the ASase necessary for resistance to systemically administered asparaginase.

The Metabolic and the Genetic-Regulatory Hypotheses

The metabolic hypothesis referred to in the Introduction provides an ad hoc explanation of the sensitivity of certain tumors to systemic asparaginase. However, not only does it not encompass the normal difference between groups of mammals with respect to regulation of the three fractions of asparagine, $[P]$, $[S]$, and $[A]$, but also it does not correspond to other data on the effects of administered asparaginase. For example, of the two *Escherichia coli* asparaginases studied, asparaginase-2 acts as a potent antilymphoma agent while asparaginase-1 does not, although both have about the same action on asparagine.

L-Glutaminase activity, which has been suspected of being instrumental in supplementing asparaginase action in leukemia treatment,[39, 40] was found to be 10 times higher in the inactive *E. coli* enzyme. Effects of asparaginase on normal lymphocyte blastogenesis in tissue culture,[3] which could not be counteracted by the addition of asparagine to the medium, also could not be imputed to glutaminase activity.[13] A similar observation has also been made in tissue culture of several human leukemia lymphoblastic cells, the effects not being imputable to general asparaginase "toxicity."[18] It is concluded that the action of administered asparaginase is exerted in more than one manner, not only by the hydrolysis of plasma asparagine, but also in other ways intracellularly.

The principle of the genetic-regulatory hypothesis, as it applies to neoplasms, is that certain leukemias and other malignant conditions are sensitive to asparaginase treatment because this enzyme intervenes in the availability and utilization of asparagine in the tissues, these effects being subject to systemic and local (in the cell, tissue, or organ) regulation, which is basically genetic. In the case of asparagine, the uncovered regulatory agents are the two types of asparaginase, systemic and/or local, and ASase. The metabolic hypothesis imputes the sensitivity of several leukemias to asparaginase treatment to a "genetic defect," presumably a mutation. Because of this "defect," such leukemias would be genetically different, as to asparaginase susceptibility, from the normal tissue from which they derived.

In the genetic-regulatory hypothesis, the genetic constitution of asparaginase-sensitive neoplastic cells is considered to be basically the same, with respect to asparagine regulation, but obviously not with respect to the neoplastic transformation, as that of the normal tissues from which the leukemic cells originated. Differences in function, but not in state, of the genetic constitution may occur between the normal and the neoplastic tissue, or the changes in state, if they occur, are considered not to be essential for the sensitivity to asparaginase.

The two hypotheses also differ in the interpretation of transformation of a neoplastic tissue from asparaginase-sensitive to asparaginase-resistant. In the metabolic hypothesis, this transformation is viewed as in some way the return to a condition similar in asparagine independence to that the tissue had before the "genetic defect" occurred. In the genetic-regulatory hypothesis, the transformation from sensitive to resistant is evaluated as involving a genetic change away from the original constitution of the tissue. Genetic interpretation of the two hypotheses may be diagrammed as follows:

1. (Differentiation ————————→) Normal $\xrightarrow{V_a (V_n?)}$
cells

Sensitive $\xrightarrow{RV_a(V_n?)}$ Resistant
neoplasmic neoplasmic
cells cells

2. Differentiation $\xrightarrow{V_a}$ Normal $\xrightarrow{V_n}$
cells

Sensitive $\xrightarrow{RV_a(V_n)}$ Resistant
neoplastic neoplastic
cells cells.

V stands for genetic variant(s) produced by a process of mutation or treption presently to be discussed. V_a refers to genetic variant(s) which limit asparagine availability within the cell to low $[C]$, thus rendering the cells sensitive to circulatory asparaginase. In the genetic-regulatory hypothesis it is important that this enzyme can enter the cells. V_n stands for genetic variant(s) for the transformation from the normal to a neoplastic state, and R refers to a state of resistance to asparaginase treatment.

Differentiation, not explicitly considered in the metabolic hypothesis and thus indicated in parentheses in alternative 1, is considered explicitly in the genetic-regulatory hypothesis. It is during differentiation that in alternative 2 the V_a genetic changes occur. In formulating alternative 2, it is understood that V_a refers to the genetic part which underlines the phenotypic variation in $[C]$ through physiologic response to adequate stimuli or through physiologic adaptation. For example, enzyme evolution with age and enzyme variation with dietary and other factors are basically determined by the genes, and a temporary physiologic response is involved in the second of these cases.

It has not been explicitly stated by proponents of the metabolic hypothesis whether production of the V_a variant(s) or the "defect" for asparaginase sensitivity involves also production of the neoplastic state. Because of this, V_n is within parentheses in alternative 1. That the transformation from asparaginase sensitivity to resistance does not automatically revert the neoplasm to normal tissue supports the contention that the two properties have distinct genetic determinations. The assumption, which then must be made, of concomitant or concatenated production of two types of independent genetic variants, V_a and V_n, is one of the reasons that alternative 1 is unlikely from the genetic point of view. In the simplest case, if each of the variants was a single mutation with the usual logarithmic probability of occurrence of the order of $-6(\pm2)$, the concomitant or concatenated occurrence of two such independent events would have a vanishing logarithmic probability of the order of $-12(\pm4)$.

The two hypotheses make very different predictions for the frequency of occurrence of asparaginase-sensitive neoplasms from a certain origin (organ and tissue). Since in hypothesis 1, the probability of V_a events is not tied to tissue differentiation, there is no reason why asparaginase sensitivity should be connected with the nature of the tissue from which the neoplasm is originated. Differences in this respect between tissues might lie within the range of about two orders of magnitude, as is the case for the frequency of single mutations. In any case, the probability of occurrence of asparaginase-sensitive neoplasms originating from a certain tissue would remain low. Thus, leukemias or any other type of neoplasm classified as to tissue of origin should have no predilection for asparagine sensitivity, which is not true: among leukemias, about 26% of the spontaneous, 44% of the x-ray induced, and 8% of the chemically produced leukemias are asparaginase-sensitive.[1]

The genetic-regulatory hypothesis explains tissue predilection for asparaginase sensitivity by the course of differentiation. Neoplasms are expected to possess at first the sensitivity of the normal cells from which they derive, but, when they are later surveyed for a property such as asparaginase sensitivity, they may have changed from the tissue of origin because of: (1) physiologic variation of cells which were near the threshold for sensitivity (cells relatively high in ASase activity before the neoplastic change occurred), (2) selective preferential growth of cells which in the cell population that generated the neoplasms were asparaginase-insensitive, or (3) genetic change which occurred between the neoplastic change and the sampling for asparaginase sensitivity.

It is well known that neoplasms usually are heterogeneous as to the cells which form them, a subject further considered in the next section. Since there is no reason to presume that conditions (1) and (3) are different according to the agent which produced the neoplastic transformations, the genetic-regulatory hypothesis predicts that the leukemias which are less frequently asparaginase-sensitive, as, for example, those of chemical and viral origin, will more frequently obey condition (2), their populations of cells being at the origin more greatly or more frequently heterogeneous with respect to genetic endowment than the cell populations of the other leukemias. This prediction may be tested by early observation of the cells of the neoplasm as to their observable characteristics, from chromosome composition to heterogeneity in cloning in different culture media, and the like.

We have yet to learn which tissues in the body undergo V_a genetic changes during their differentiation, but from the data, hematopoietic tissues in spleen and lymph nodes, and possibly the bone marrow lines of white cells, appear to belong to such tissues. Differentiation of blood cells follows a very complex course, involving embryonic events and several stimuli, among them stimuli from the bursa or thymus or both, and from the spleen. It appears that V_a genetic changes are included in one of the steps of white cell differentiation, or in the dichotomy between red and white cells. From the low phenotypic values of ASase activity often found in kidney and liver, some neoplasms originating in these organs could be expected to be asparaginase-sensitive. However, we have yet to know whether in these cases low ASase activity is genetically fixed or physiologically adaptive. Rather marked variability in endogenous ASase and asparaginase, as in the case of liver, favors the hypothesis of physiologic regulation, for which the genetic basis permits variation within wide limits.

Genetic Changes Implicated in Asparagine Regulation and Neoplastic Transformation

Protein synthesis is connected with genetic determination through the process of mRNA translation. It has been largely assumed that the process of messenger transcription established for bacteria is also valid for higher cells. The recent discovery in the cytoplasm of information DNA[4] supports previously postulated direct intervention of cytoplasm DNA as one of the means of gene expression in phenotype realization (Serra, Chapter 12[32]). Enzyme synthesis is ultimately genetically determined directly from cytoplasmic DNA or indirectly from nuclear DNA and transcribed RNA. There is good reason to think that enzyme release from cells by operation of a system or permeases or in the manner of secretion is ultimately also of genetic determination which takes place during differentiation.

In the case of an amino acid such as asparagine, differentiation of the normal tissues includes regulation of input through the $[P]$ and/or $[S]$ fractions and regulation of output through the $[A]$ fraction. From what has been learned of the two groups of mammals in Table 18-1, different enzymes are involved in the regulation of the $[A]$ and $[P]$ fractions, the second including some secretory and/or permease systems.

Two types of genetic changes may be involved in differentiation, changes of function, which have been proposed to be called ergosis, and changes of state, which include mutation and treption.[32] The most discussed type of functional genetic change now is repression-depression, but any other process through which the rate of transcription or translation, or both, could be influenced, such as end-product inhibition, is in the category of ergosis. The type of mutation which could be implicated in differentiation would be somatic mutation which, from known data, does not differ in frequency of occurrence and in incertitude of site and time of occurrence of a particular mutation from germinal mutation whose frequency is low.

To keep the concept of mutation true to these characteristics, another type of genetic change must be postulated for differentiation. This type of change, regulatory in nature as is development, has been proposed to be called treption, from the Greek for turned, changed (with an etymologic preposition such as "around" omitted). Treptional changes are well documented to occur not only during development, but also in virus- and episome-produced genetic changes, in sex determination, in the production of mottling or variegated phenotypes and in several phenomena of virus variation, particularly host cell range.[33]

At the molecular level, treption is a basic property of the nucleic acids, similar in this respect to replication and transcription-translation for phenotype realization, such properties being implemented by interaction with suitable cell proteins.[34] Evidence has been provided for the belief that treption is the main genetic phenomenon behind the great lines which biologic evolution has followed, with mutation playing the role of diversifying the details of the process. Selection will act similarly when either treption or mutation is the source of genetic variation.[31, 33]

In the case under discussion, of production in the course of development of the genetic apparatus for regulation of synthesis of the two main types of enzymes which control the [S], [P], and/or [A] asparagine fractions, it is likely that treption is involved. Study of somatic cell characteristics, with tissue culture cloning and with hybridization techniques, could help reach a conclusion in this respect. In the absence of such a study, operational criteria which can distinguish between mutation and treption or ergosis relate to the concomitant or concatenated occurrence of two or more changes and their reversibility or irreversibility. Concomitant or concatenated mutations are very unlikely, and the easily reversible changes relate to ergosis.

For example, in asparagine regulation, the gradual but irreversible changes with age observed in guinea pig plasma asparaginase must be based on treption, which triggers the adequate physiologic responses. Conversely, the differences in ASase or in intracellular asparaginase with diet are physiologic responses. These responses may involve ergosis if some genes in some cells are turned off or on, or are induced to temporarily change their rates of transcription or translation. Changes attributable to the presence of a neoplasm or which occur in tumor cells may also be of the physiologic type involving ergosis. For example, ASase activity in arbitrary units has been reported to pass in the spleen of normal mice from zero to about 1.1 one day following the injection of asparaginase, and to about 1.5 under the same conditions in the spleen of AKR leukemic mice.[24] In both cases the changes were probably reversible, although those involving presence of leukemia would be difficult to test in this respect.

The differences, produced programmedly during development, between organs such as the spleen and the brain with respect to the enzymes which control asparagine availability and use, obviously must be concatenated, since otherwise the two or three types of enzyme would not work harmoniously in the regulation of this amino acid. A single mutation is unlikely to affect two or three enzymes concomitantly, unless a common operon is involved, which for very different enzymes is unusual. Even if a single operon was involved, it is unlikely that a mutation will occur at just a certain point of the development. So treption must be involved in the genetic changes of this developmental process, since it is precisely characteristic of treptional changes that they are regulatory in nature and that several such changes may take place sequentially or concomitantly.[33]

The operational criterion of the frequency of occurrence may now be employed in trying to distinguish between mutation and treption in the origin of the transformation to asparaginase insensitivity of leukemias or other neoplasms derived as variants from sensitive neoplasms. As may be seen from data in Table 18-2 (and from other data not shown in this table which have a similar interpretation), the property observed to be affected in the change to asparaginase resistance concerns mainly the $[S]$ fraction, although some change in $[A]$ is not excluded. Since the change is not easily counteracted or reversible back to the asparaginase-sensitive state, ergosis is involved in the change from $[S_l]$ to $[S_h]$, from low to high ASase activity. Treption or mutation must be involved. To compare the probability of occurrence of the two types of events with actual data, let us consider briefly the nature of the processes from which the over-all probability of treption, P_t, and of mutation, P_m, may be derived.

Treption is interpreted to consist of the change of genetic nucleic acid, cytoplasmic or nuclear, the change being generally produced through the work of one enzyme or a group of enzymes capable of impinging on nucleic acid. One of the most direct cases of these changes is known as "DNA modification and restriction in viruses," for which methylation of DNA bases has been implicated.[2] Methylases are the enzymes active in this change. In the case of T2 and T6 phages, changed contents of glucose in the DNA, according to the host range to which the phages are induced to adapt by multiplication in certain host strains, are caused by the effect of a phosphorylase.[32-34] Numerous, more complex cases of treption, some involving episomes and viruses, have been found in plants and animals.[33] Enzymes which are able to affect the genetic material are not only the replicases, the repair enzymes, and recombination enzymes such as perhaps the ligases, but also enzymes which, during replication, can modify by changed metabolism some nucleic acid component, the bases by methylation, for example, or the sugar.

The nature of the treptional processes is such that when the right conditions are attained inside the cell, a certain type of treption is then expected to occur with almost unfailing certitude, thus with probability of occurrence $p_t \approx 1$. This probability results from the play of a probability p_{st} for the occurrence of the right state of the cell to undergo treption, and the probability of occurrence of treption in these conditions $p_{ot} \approx 1$. For natural treption it is $p_{st} \approx 1$ and, thus, $p_t = p_{st}$

$\times p_{ot} \approx 1$ for a certain step of differentiation such as that which produces asparagine regulation by V_a changes. But under experimental conditions, as will be presently discussed, the case may be different.

The processes which lead to mutation are basically dependent on the production of active radicals which may attack the nucleic acid directly or through enzymes that otherwise would repair damaged nucleic acid. Several mutagens may also attack the DNA directly. Active radicals are so common in actively metabolizing and multiplying cells that in these cells it seems reasonable to set the probability of occurrence of a state in which the cell is apt to undergo mutation as $p_{sm} \approx 1$. The occurrence of mutation in this state is counteracted by radical scavengers, repair enzymes, and similar processes which lead to a probability of actual occurrence of mutation, p_{om}, much smaller than 1. In conditions of spontaneous mutability, it is $\log p_{om} \approx -6(\pm 2)$, which gives, for the over-all probability of occurrence of a certain mutation at a certain time, $p_m = p_{sm} \times p_{om} \approx 1 \times 10^{-6(\pm 2)}$.

Applying these deductions to the case of transformation of leukemias from asparaginase-sensitive to asparaginase-resistant, to decide from the frequency of the event whether treption or mutation is involved, we have to know which value is attributed to p_{st} in comparison with p_{om} for a given neoplasm. In the case of the Jensen rat sarcoma, the over-all frequency of cells, which were found by cloning to have changed in culture from asparagine-requiring (minimum concentration 0.01 M/ml) to asparagine-independent, was about 10^{-4}.[21] This frequency is near the higher limit expected for mutation, so that only tentatively may it be taken as referring to p_{st} for treption. For a surer conclusion in this respect, a more detailed study of the kinetics of the sarcoma cells, before and after the change to asparagine independence, has to be made.

The kinetics of tumor cells are complicated by the fact that a tumor always comprises heterogeneous cell populations. Leaving aside the possible presence of stem cells with the power to multiply from the normal tissue of origin, and similar cells from reversion of neoplastic to normal, there are the probably neoplastic but nonproliferating cells in the G_0 phase, and proliferating neoplastic cells in several phases from G_1 and S periods to several M mitotic phases.[19, 20] It is likely that only cells in the S phase, and probably only in a well-defined state of this phase, are apt to undergo treption. The probability p_{st} refers to such cells. It is clear that ways to render the cells homogeneous by synchronization, or to reasonably account for their heterogeneity, are needed to provide reliable experimental conditions or reliable kinetics for the study of treption vs. mutation in the reversion of neoplastic cells to a certain state.

The question of treption vs. mutation is also relevant for the origin of cancer in general. Because of the ultimate connection between enzymes or other proteins and genes and from the fact that a neoplastic state corresponds to changed metabolism, with the changes possibly reduced in several cases to the quantitative level of reaction rates, it now appears practically certain that neoplastic changes are ultimately referable to the genetic material. Mutation appears unlikely to explain progression as is often observed in oncogenesis. Moreover, there is no reason to expect that mutations from normal to neoplastic states would be confined to somatic cells. For a germ cell recessive mutation of this type, a simple Mendelian cancer inheritance would be expected in many cases, since the probability of clustered mutation is small. Even allowing for complications involving penetrance and expressivity, simple cancer inheritance would often be found in the mutational hypothesis—which is not the case, inheritance of propensity to cancer being complicated and generally far from the simple Mendelian type.

As just shown in the case of asparagine regulation, treption is free from the objections against mutation when clustering and progression of genetic changes have to be accounted for. Moreover, the case of viruses, now well established as oncogenic agents, is easily encompassed by treption, which is typically caused in many cases by episomes. Viruses behave as episomes or the related plasmids. A detailed discussion of this theory is, however, out of the scope of the present paper.[30]

Conclusions: Biologic Action and Therapeutic Role of Systemic Asparaginase

In the context of the genetic-regulatory hypothesis, some conclusions may now be drawn. As is usual with recently developed lines of work, the problems raised surpass those already solved. Implications of these problems for oncogenesis in general and for the therapeutics of malignancy are rather obvious.

1. One of the actions of asparaginase corresponds to its biochemical property as an enzyme, of rendering unavailable to the cells as much asparagine as it may convert to aspartic acid. This action accounts for only a part of the effects of asparaginase. Other actions are exerted at the cellular level as, for example, the now well-established blastogenesis inhibition[3] and the correlated immune suppression.[5, 11, 28]

2. Intracellular effects may be explained starting from the hypothesis that administered asparaginase intervenes in the asparagine regulatory system of the cells. Besides its role in protein synthesis in general, asparagine control appears to be critical for the synthesis of some specific proteins of certain tissues at certain points of the cell cycle. For example, if data on glycine involvement with asparagine in neoplasms[27] are confirmed, the specific asparagine control role may be exerted through some high-glycine protein. One histone extracted in high yield from cells, which has about 17% glycine residues, might be such a protein. Other possibilities are specific proteins of white blood cells and immune globulins.

3. Critical control of specific proteins would explain, from the biochemical point of view, tissue specificity in asparaginase sensitivity. The pattern of uridine incorporation into certain fractions of cell RNA[35] agrees with a primary effect of asparaginase on proteins. It remains to be seen whether the same applies to DNA synthesis. Incorporation of thymidine in normal mouse liver is delayed by asparaginase, and replicase does not appear to be involved in the delay.[29] These and other effects on cellular syntheses may explain the varied side effects of asparagine therapy which have been repeatedly reported.[14]

4. It remains to be determined which type of mammal with respect to asparagine control, the majority type which includes man or the minority type of the guinea pig, is the primitive one. The systematic position in their orders of the two superfamilies of the minority type suggests that this type is more specialized, but further findings on the distribution of the two types, and especially in lower mammals, may alter the perspective in this respect. Now it seems that homeostatic control of asparagine in plasma of the majority type was substituted in the minority type by homeostatic control of plasma asparaginase. The known advantage of the substitution is freedom from asparaginase-sensitive neoplasms, especially certain leukemias. Whether this will prove to be enough for selection of the minority type to have taken place, or whether some ecologic factors of the South American area where the type evolved may also have been involved remains for future studies. The probable treptional origin of differences of this type is to be kept in mind in such a study.

5. The biochemical and physiologic control is genetically determined through the connections between genes and enzyme synthesis. The ceiling for synthesis, especially ASase intracellular regulation, is determined during development by the treptions a tissue undergoes. This explains basic tissue specificity for asparaginase sensitivity and predicts effects of cell heterogeneity in a neoplasm according to the oncogenic agent employed, or the natural origin of malignancy. Transformation from asparaginase sensitivity to resistance may be similarly accounted for. Combination or sequential therapy of asparaginase and diverse cytostatic or cytolytic agents of S or M cell periods, as is now practiced, is indicated to overcome the effects of cell heterogeneity; or other combinations, including virus nucleic acid segments, for which the case of the LDH virus of the mouse is suggestive[26, 39–41] may be attempted. Until the genetic determination of tissue specificity and cell heterogeneity is better known, empirical in vitro tests for asparaginase sensitivity[1] continue to be needed as a therapeutic guide. Tests for intracellular effects must be included in the probe.

6. Attacks on malignancy will continue to be directed at the manifold manifestations of neoplastic cell characteristics. The case of asparaginase sensitivity is but one of the lines of work which might more fruitfully lead to an attack aimed at the common origin of the several

types of neoplasms, which must be the malignant transformation of the genetic material of the cells of origin. Now it appears likely that this transformation is of treptional nature, produced by episomes and plasmids which include the viruses. If it is so, ultimately it will be through the control of episomal and plasmid elements that the problem of malignancy may be approached in a more general way.

Summary

Based on the analysis of pertinent data, the genetic-regulatory hypothesis of the action of asparaginase is presented and compared with the metabolic hypothesis. Predictions from this hypothesis as to asparaginase sensitivity or resistance and neoplastic cell heterogeneity in relation with the use of asparaginase in combination therapy are discussed. Probable relations of the two types of mammals as to asparagine regulations are considered. A comparison is made between the roles of treptional and mutational genetic changes in asparaginase sensitivity and in the neoplastic transformation in general.

Acknowledgments

The friendly cooperation of Dr. V. Riley, Chairman of the Department of Microbiology, Pacific Northwest Research Foundation, and of Miss Mary-Anne Fitzmaurice is gratefully acknowledged.

References

1. Adamson, R. H., and S. Fabro: Cancer Chemother. Rep. (Part 1), 52:617-626, 1968.
2. Arber, W., and S. Linn: Ann. Rev. Biochem., 38:467-500, 1969.
3. Astaldi, G., D. Micu, A. Astaldi, Jr., and G. R. Burgio: Lancet, 2:1357, 1969.
4. Bell, E.: Nature, 224:326-328, 1969.
5. Bertelli, A., L. Donati, and E. Trabucchi, Jr.: Arch. Ital. Pat. Clin. Tumori, 11:475-479, 1968.
6. Bonetti, E., A. Abbondanza, E. Della Corte, and F. Stirpe: Biochem. J., 115:597-601, 1969.
7. Broome, J. D.: Nature, 191:1114-1115, 1961.
8. Broome, J. D.: J. Exp. Med., 118:99-120; 121-148, 1963.
9. Burchenal, J. H.: Cancer Res., 29:2262-2268, 1969.
10. Busch, H. A., L. T. Mashburn, E. A. Boyse, and L. D. Old: Biochemistry, 6:721-730, 1967.
11. Chakrabarty, A. K., and H. Friedman: Science, 167:869-870, 1970.
12. Clementi, A.: Arch. Intern. Physiol., 19:369-398, 1922.
13. Dartnall, H. A.: Lancet, II:1357-1358, 1969.
14. Haskell, C. M., G. P. Canellos, B. G. Leventhal, P. P. Carbone, A. A. Serpick, and H. H. Hansen: Cancer Res., 29:974-975, 1969.
15. Holland, J. F.: Cancer Res., 29:2262-2268, 1969.
16. Holcenberg, J. S.: Biochim. Biophys. Acta, 185:228-238, 1969.
17. Kidd, J. G.: J. Exp. Med., 98:565-582; 583-585, 1953.
18. Lazarus, H., T. A. McCoy, S. Farber, E. F. Barell, and G. E. Foley: Exp. Cell Res., 57:134-138, 1969.
19. Mendelsohn, M. L.: Cancer Res., 29:2390-2393, 1969.
20. Mueller, G. C.: Cancer Res., 29:2394-2397, 1969.

21. Patterson, M. K., Jr., M. D. Maxwell, and E. Conway: Cancer Res., 29:296-300, 1969.
22. Patterson, M. K., Jr., and G. R. Orr: J. Biol. Chem., 243:376-380, 1968.
23. Patterson, M. K., Jr., and G. R. Orr: Cancer Res., 29:1179-1186, 1969.
24. Prager, M. D., and N. Bachynsky: Arch. Biochem. Biophys., 127:645-654, 1968.
25. Regan, J. D., H. Vodopick, S. Takeda, W. H. Lee, and F. M. Faulcon: Science, 163:1452-1453, 1969.
26. Riley, V.: Proc. Amer. Ass. Cancer Res., 10:73, 1969.
27. Ryan, W. L., and H. C. Sornson: Science, 167:1512-1513, 1970.
28. Schwartz, R. S.: Nature, 224:275-276, 1969.
29. Seeber, S., and U. Weser: Nature, 225:652-653, 1970.
30. Serra, J. A.: J. Theoret. Biol., 6:371-374, 1964.
31. Serra, J. A.: Can. J. Genet. Cytol., 8:165-183, 1966.
32. Serra, J. A.: Modern Genetics. Academic Press, London and New York, Vol. 2, 1966.
33. Serra, J. A.: Modern Genetics. Academic Press, London and New York, Vol. 3, 1968.
34. Serra, J. A.: Revue Roum. Biol. (Hommage N. Teodoreanu). In press.
35. Stevens, J., L. T. Mashburn, and V. P. Hollander: Biochim. Biophys. Acta, 186: 332-339, 1969.
36. Suld, H. M., and P. M. Herbut: J. Biol. Chem., 240:2234-2241, 1965.
37. Tower, D. B., E. L. Peters, and W. C. Curtis: J. Biol. Chem., 238:983-993, 1963.
38. Young, C. W.: Cancer Res., 29:2281-2283, 1969.
39. Riley, V., D. H. Spackman, and M. A. Fitzmaurice: In: Tenth International Cancer Congress Abstracts. Houston, 1970, pp. 445-446.
40. Spackman, D. H., V. Riley, L. Teschner: In: Tenth International Cancer Congress Abstracts. Houston, 1970, pp. 443-444.
41. Santisteban, G. A., V. Riley, and K. Willhight: In: Tenth International Cancer Congress Abstracts. Houston, 1970, p. 302.

Regulation of the Cell Respiration

BRITTON CHANCE

*Johnson Research Foundation, University of Pennsylvania,
Philadelphia, Pennsylvania, USA*

THE MAIN FEATURE which distinguishes eukaryotic cells from bacteria is the control exerted in the former cells by the demand for the cell energy over its supply. This may be largely attributable to the unique properties exhibited by a special cell device, the mitochondrion, which couples the two phenomena (Figure 18-1). The flow of electrons which occurs principally in the mitochondrial membrane and to a

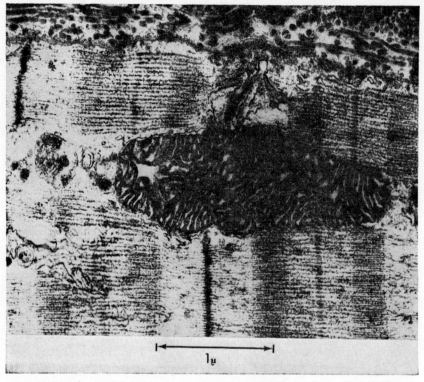

FIG. 18–1.—The mitochondrion—a device for coupling of a supply and demand for cell energy.

small extent in the matrix space is determined by three factors: (1) the need for adenosine triphosphate (ATP), (2) the need for the maintenance of ionic gradients across the membrane, and (3) the need for the maintenance of the redox state of the mitochondrial redox couples. These three energy-requiring functions govern the rate of electron flow and consequently determine the rate of oxygen metabolism of the cell.

The cancer cell, as any other cell, is equipped in the same molecular mechanisms which regulate the electron flow rate.

Therefore I have chosen as the main topic of my presentation, the molecular mechanism for the control of electron flow by the energy demand. This affords a unique example of how biochemical reactions of membrane-bound proteins may involve special control mechanisms which are not necessarily available to protein in solution.

An essential feature in the study of control mechanisms is a purely technical one—that of furnishing us with the information that a control has actually occurred. Two approaches have been used for this purpose. In the first one, mitochondrial pigments themselves serve as the probe of the membrane state. The fact that pigments act as the electron carriers affords a unique possibility in this matter. In the second one, charged anions and cations are introduced which are able to penetrate various regions of the membrane and change their characteristics upon the changes in the membrane environment.[1]

Figure 18-2 is an example of the general appliance of the first technique, now widely developed and commonly used. In the suspension of isolated rat liver mitochondria, it illustrates the response of cytochrome c, one of the membrane pigments, to two types of functional energy demand: adenosine diphosphate (ADP) and calcium ion. The former represents the above-stated need for ATP, the latter, the energy demand for the ion transport. Both factors introduce an energy demand in excess of the energy supply and result in an acceleration of the specific reaction rates between the electron carriers of the mitochondrial membrane. It is apparent that the responses are rapid, that they affect the electron flow as indicated by the increased respiratory activity recorded polarographically, and that they last only as long as the stimulus is present. On the conversion of the added ADP to ATP or on the accumulation of the added Ca^{2+} into the matrix space, the respiration rate slackens, indicative of the completion of the control cycle. Mitochondrial pyridine nucleotides respond to the addition of ADP or Ca^{2+} in a manner which is similar to cytochrome c. The ef-

FIG. 18–2.—An illustration of the use of mitochondrial pigments to readout control phenomena in mitochondrial transitions from the resting to the active states as effected by additions of ADP and then calcium. The top trace represents cytochrome c; the second trace from the top, NADH; the third trace, the rate of oxygen utilization; the fourth trace, the amount of oxygen utilization. Rat liver mitochondria, 4 mM succinate, 5 mM Mg + 3.3 mM P_1.

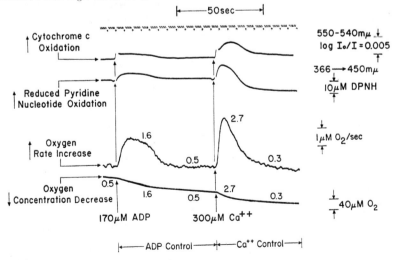

fective oxidoreduction potential of the reduced pyridine nucleotide pool is about 300 mv below that of succinate, which was used as the substrate. Nevertheless, the level of reduced pyridine nucleotides attains a high state of reduction after the addition of ADP or Ca^{2+} because of the expenditure of energy between succinate and NADH in the electron transfer reactions. The same methods are applicable to both cell suspension and to the exposed surfaces of the tissues of various organs, and essentially the same relations as those observed in the isolated mitochondria between the energy supply and the energy demand are found.

Changes in the redox state of the respiratory carriers clearly depict the impact of energy demand upon electron flow; they do not, however, reveal the mechanism of the process, but only indicate that some reaction velocity constants have been altered because of chemical or structural changes in the membranes. Since the energy coupling and electron transfer phenomena can be identified with the conformational states of the electron carriers, an insight into the intimate mechanisms of these reactions seems to be afforded by the introduction of probes into the specific regions of the membrane in which the changes occur.

A variety of such probes are suitable for exploration of the membrane properties (Table 18-3), both of anionic and cationic character. The first class is represented by 1-8-anilinonaphthalene sulfonate (ANS), 1 or 2-ANS-paratoluidino-naphthalene (TNS) 6-sulfonate and n-methyl-2-anilino-6-naphthalene sulfonate (MNS), the second by ethidium bromide. The anionic probes show very similar properties with respect to (1) wavelength shift—an indicator of the degree of hydrophobicity of the membrane, (2) dissociation constant (approximately 50 μM), (3) number of binding sites (from 40 to 80 nmole/mg of protein), and (4) the nature of the fluorescence change on energization. If a cationic probe such as ethidium bromide is employed, the same number of binding sites seems to be involved, but the affinity for ethidium bromide is much higher and the fluorescence change on energization occurs in the opposite direction. Dependence of the direction of fluorescence changes induced by energization on the character

TABLE 18-3.—PROPERTIES OF MEMBRANE PROBES OF SUBMITOCHONDRIAL PARTICLES

PROBE	CHARGE	λ SHIFT (NM)	DISSOCIATION CONSTANT (μM)	NUMBER OF BINDING SITES (NMOLES/MG PROT.)	FLUORESCENCE CHANGE IN RESPONSE TO ENERGY COUPLING
1-8 ANS	Negative	−80	24	80	Increase
2-6 TNS	Negative	−50	46	50-55	Increase
MNS	Negative	−100	29	40-43	Increase
Ethidium Bromide	Positive	<5	9.8	45	Decrease

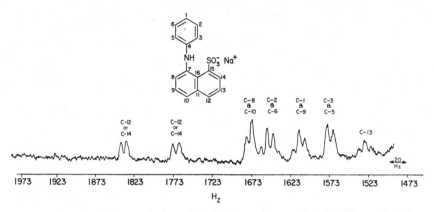

Fig. 18–3.—The high resolution (200 MHz) spectrum of 1-8-anilino-naphthalene sulfonate.

of the probe identifies the controlled region of the membrane as having a positive charge.

The most successfully used probe for the acquisition of the energized and controlled state of mitochondria proved to be ANS,[1, 3, 4] employed previously to identify the hydrophobic regions of protein such as serum albumin and apomyoglobin.[2] Figures 18-3 and 18-4 depict the chemical structure of this probe and elegantly delineate its proton resonances, by the 220 MHz NMR spectrum, in solution and in the membrane environment.

The addition of membrane fragments of mitochondria to the ANS

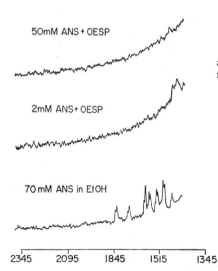

Fig. 18–4.—The effect of membrane addition upon resonances in 1-8-anilino-naphthalene sulfonate.

broadens the proton resonances to the point where they can no longer be detected, which identifies the sequence of the occurring results: penetration of the probe to the region of paramagnetic atoms, presumably the cytochrome itself, its relaxation by the cytochrome magnetic field, and diffusion out again into the medium in times of hundredths or thousandths of a second.

An example of the dramatic effect of membrane energization upon the ANS response is indicated by Figure 18-5, which illustrates the time course of fluorescence changes for fragments of beef heart mitochondria. The addition of the probe itself to the membranes causes a small fluorescence increase. Further increase occurs upon succinate-induced electron flow through the membrane. Energy coupling and control of electron flow is evoked by the addition of appropriate antibiotics, oligomycin or rutamycin, which results in a very large fluorescence enhancement as indicated by the exponential rise of the trace. The membranes have now achieved a state in which energy coupling and controlled electron flow is occurring. Addition of an uncoupling agent destroys energy conservation and controlled electron flow and reverses the fluorescence enhancement.

Table 18-4 summarizes the information obtained on ANS characteristics and identifies the state of the membrane associated with controlled electron flow. Interestingly enough, control and energization do not alter the hydrophobicity of the environment, as indicated by the emission peak of the probe or the number of binding sites for the probe in nmoles/mg protein. As indicated by the degree of fluorescence depolarization, the rotational mobility of the probe is not altered; thus theories suggesting that one of the salient features of membrane function is involved in transition from less mobilized to more mobilized en-

FIG. 18–5.—Illustrations of the transitions from the uncontrolled, unenergized states to the controlled and energized states in membrane fragments following the addition of succinate and an energy coupling factor oligomycin. The reverse transition is effected by an addition of an uncoupler FCCP.

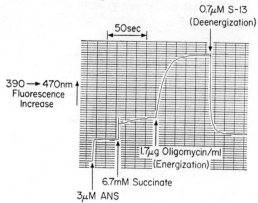

TABLE 18–4.—Parameters of ANS Response in Energized and Nonenergized
Membranes of Submitochondrial Particles

State	λmax (nm)	Kd Dissoc. Const. (M)	N Binding Sites (nmoles/mg prot.)	φ Rel. Quantum Yield	τ Life Time nsec	P Depolari- zation
Nonenergized	470	35×10^{-6}	80	1	5 (9)	0.19
Energized	470	20×10^{-6}	80	2.5	(5) 9	0.19

vironment, as suggested by spin label studies, do not apply to the controlled and energized state.

The significant changes occurring in the membranes would appear to be at the level of small environmental changes of membrane components, which are supported by the changes in the quantum yield fluorescence and the fluorescence lifetime. The quantum yield is increased by 2.5-fold in this type of membranes, and up to five-fold in others. The decay time of the fluorescence (fluorescence lifetime), greatly delayed with respect to that of free ANS, achieves two values for decay time, one at predominantly 5 nsec for the nonenergized and uncontrolled state and 9 nsec for the energized and controlled state. Concomitantly, the dissociation constant decreases so that the membrane will bind more of the probe in the controlled and energized state.

These probe responses are summarized in the two diagrams of Figure 18-6, which may indicate two types of mechanisms for the membrane function. In A, the alteration of the quantum efficiency and the lifetime of the probe are attributed to alterations in the structured water in the vicinity of the probe. Control and energization phenomena according to this mechanism lead to the exclusion of a portion of the water from the part of the membrane which is occupied by the probe. An explanation for the increased affinity of the membrane for ANS in the controlled and energized state is illustrated by diagram B. Negatively charged molecules are not bound in the uncontrolled deenergized state, but are bound in the presence of energy because of the acquisition of positive charge on the membrane. The acquisition of

Fig. 18–6.—Schematic diagram of probe responses in energy coupling and controlled electron flow.

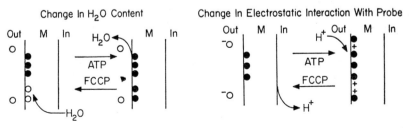

such charges is readily measured by the binding of hydrogen ion to the membrane. These two points of view can be combined into a single one which arises from a generality of experiments on a wide range of biologic membranes capable of energy-coupling mitochondria, chromatophores, and chloroplasts. Our studies of rapid hydrogen ion movement, together with the probe responses, suggest that the salient feature of controlled and energized states involves increased protonation of the membrane together with a state transformation and corresponding movement of structured water. Since hydrogen ions are involved in the membrane structure change, we prefer to use the terminology developed for the interaction of hydrogen ions with liganding of hemoglobin by oxygen or CO; thus, the structural response of the membrane to increased hydrogen ion binding is termed "a membrane Bohr effect."

This brief summary of a molecular approach to the problem of the control of electron flow in membrane systems perhaps gives you more of an idea of our ignorance than of our omnipotence in this area. The study does point to the unique properties of electron-transporting proteins in membranes which can apparently alter their properties so as to control electron flow and to afford a suitable environment for energy coupling.

In the energization of the membrane we find, on a magnified scale, one of the salient features of the active sites of enzymes—a controlled hydrophobic environment required for the formation or breaking down of the chemical bonds involved in oxidative phosphorylation.[5]

The relation of these molecular mechanisms to the cancer problem is possibly as general as the relationship between membrane structure and function and the regulation of the cell function itself. Many parameters are unknown, but a sound structure for the entire regulatory phenomenon may eventually be observed, as molecular mechanisms begin to evolve.

References

1. Azzi, A., B. Chance, G. K. Radda, and C. P. Lee: Proc. Nat. Acad. Sci. USA, 62:612, 1969.
2. Weber, G., and L. B. Young: J. Biol. Chem., 239:1415, 1964.
3. Azzi, A., and H. V. Vainio: Proceedings of the Symposium on Electron Transport and Energy Conservation, Bari. In press.
4. Brocklehurst, J. R., R. B. Freedman, D. J. Hancock, and G. K. Radda: Biochem. J., 116:721, 1970.
5. Chance, B., C. P. Lee, and L. Mela: Fed. Proc., 26:1341, 1967.

Biochemical Perspectives of the Cell Cycle

GERALD C. MUELLER, M.D., Ph.D.

McArdle Laboratory, University of Wisconsin, Madison, Wisconsin, USA

REPLICATION OF AN animal cell is a cyclic process involving the orderly expression of specific genetic information at each step in the cycle.[1-3] The spectacular achievement in this process is that both active and inactive chromatin are replicated exactly and distributed with precision to daughter cells—assuring both phenotypic and genetic continuity. Whereas studies in cell culture demonstrate that the reactions leading to cell replication are programmed from the cell's own genetic system, observation on cell growth in the living animal or in organ culture reveals that the expression of these genes is subject, as well, to control by factors in the extracellular environment; such factors involve nutrients, hormones, and cell-to-cell interaction.[4-8] The result is that cells of a living organism vary vastly in the frequency at which they undergo replication: some cells replicate every 10 to 12 hr, while others wait days, weeks, or months—or even die before replication can ensue. This beautiful interplay of controls is illustrated in normal organ growth where the replication of the various cell types is delicately balanced so as to yield a functioning organ of many cooperating cell types.

Cancer, however, whether induced by viruses or chemical carcinogens, whether it arises through mutation or a spurious differentiation, concerns a derangement in these controls. The cancer cell, amid a population of normal cells, does not sense or respond in a normal way to the signals of its extracellular environment—signals which regulate its life span and tell it when or when not to undergo replication.

A prime interest in our laboratory concerns the biochemical delineation of the steps in the cell cycle and the elucidation of the genetic controls which regulate a cell's progress around the cycle. The target of our research is shown in Figure 18-7. In the terminology of the day the cell cycle is divided grossly into the G_1, S, and G_2 mitotic intervals. Cells entering the S phase have achieved a competency to begin replication of their chromatin, that is, the replication of their DNA and the synthesis of chromosomal proteins. In most cells these processes require six to seven hr for completion. From autoradiographic, biophysical, and genetic studies of synchronized cell cultures, we know that DNA replication amid the chromatin is a multifocal and highly or-

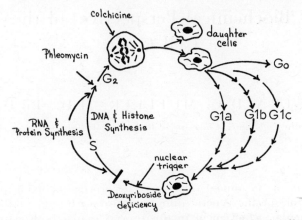

Fig. 18–7.—Diagram of a cell cycle. The replication of animal cells is a highly ordered sequence of molecular events requiring the expression of specific genetic information at certain steps in the cycle. S phase, an interval lasting six to seven hr in many cells, is concerned with the synthesis of a complete complement of DNA and histones; progression through this interval requires the timely synthesis of RNA as well as DNA and proteins. The G_2 interval, mitosis, and cell division require approximately two to three hr, and these stages are concerned with the formation of newly synthesized chromatin into chromosome pairs and the distribution of the condensed chromosomes into the daughter cells. Progression into the G_2 interval requires the completion of DNA synthesis and the antecedent synthesis of RNA and protein. Phleomycin blocks the cell cycle in HeLa cells near the end of the DNA synthesis period. Colchicine and other agents active against the microtubules block the progression of cells through metaphase. Cells with different replication times vary mainly in the duration of the G_1 interval, as indicated in the diagram as G_{1a}, G_{1b}, G_{1c}, and G_0. During this interval the cell expresses the phenotypic character of its particular differentiated state. Depending on intracellular and extracellular factors, cells progress through G_1 and become triggered for nuclear replication; at this point they have achieved the ability to initiate DNA replication and to express the genes for histone synthesis. Cells may be synchronized for DNA replication by gathering cells at this point in the cycle with a reversible inhibitor of DNA synthesis. Cells may also be synchronized for mitosis with colchicine or for entry into G_1 by the mechanical collection of small round cells.

dered process.[3, 9-14] Certain fractions of DNA require the antecedent synthesis of both RNA and protein. Using cultures of HeLa cells, which have been synchronized by a deoxyriboside deficiency, we have shown previously with inhibitor studies[15] that the synthesis of RNA during the first two hr of the S phase is required if cells are to replicate the majority of their late-replicating DNA. We have also learned that some RNA must be synthesized during the last two hr of the S phase in order to prepare the cells to replicate the last 3% of their DNA (i.e. the late-replicating DNA) and to enter into the G_2 interval.[16]

DNA replication is even more dependent on the synthesis of protein during the S phase.[17-21] During this interval histones, in a mass equal to that of the DNA, are synthesized[22] and accumulated while the old histones are conserved.[22, 23] While the inhibition of protein synthesis with agents like puromycin or cycloheximide permits DNA replication to continue for one to two hr,[17] blockade of DNA synthesis results in an immediate cessation in the accumulative synthesis of histones.[22, 24] This is to say that the synthesis of histones is tightly coupled to the continued replication of DNA.

During the final moments of the S phase, the HeLa cell also synthesizes proteins which are needed for the G_2 mitotic interval. Blocking protein synthesis with inhibitors[16] or substituting p-fluorophenyl-alanine[15] for the natural amino acid prevents the cells from entry or progression through the G_2 interval. The peptide antibiotics, phleomycin and bleomycin, act after the completion of S phase to specifically prevent the condensation of the chromatin in preparation for mitosis.[25, 26] This action is antecedent to that of colchicine derivatives or vinca alkaloids, which appear to affect the mitotic apparatus primarily. It is important to note in passing that the biochemistry of chromatin condensation is almost completely unknown. Perhaps these antibiotics, in studies with subcellular preparations from synchronized cell cultures, will open a way to this understanding.

Passing through cell division, again a process which is little understood, the daughter cells enter into the G_1 interval. In this period, cells express their particular phenotypes and carry out the processes which permit us to identify them as a pituitary, liver, kidney, or muscle cell. This interval is of particular interest to cancer scientists since this is the interval in which growth-regulatory mechanisms are largely exercised. The duration of the G_1 interval may be several hours or it may last days, weeks, months, or an infinity. It appears that cells vary vastly in the number of things that they must do in preparation for re-entry into S phase and nuclear replication. Factors such as hormones, nutrients, mitogenic stimuli, and cell contacts have remarkable effects on the duration of this period; agents may act either to lengthen or to abbreviate this interval. Each cell operates in the pattern of its phenotype, which in most cases has been recapitulated during the previous S and G_2 intervals. It would appear that cells proceed through a hierarchy of interlocking genetic controls, whose nature is depicted diagrammatically in Figure 18-8 as the G_1 funnel. For purposes of discussion, one can visualize cells of differing phenotypes as passing through G_1 by different or alternative routes; routes which at the outset of G_1 interval may be quite remote from each other, but as the cell progresses through the G_1 interval, the frequency of cross-over becomes increasingly probable. At the end of this funnel of interlocking genetic events is the activation of the genetic processes which effect the replication of native DNA in its chromosomal setting. The assembly of an active DNA replicase appears to be the final and crowning achievement of the G_1 interval; for the ability to carry out the other S phase reactions, such as the synthesis of histones and other chromosomal proteins, follows readily upon activation of DNA replication.

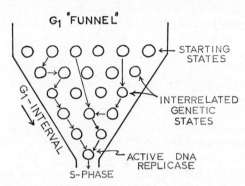

G₁ "FUNNEL"

STARTING
STATES

G₁-INTERVAL

INTERRELATED
GENETIC
STATES

ACTIVE DNA
REPLICASE

S-PHASE

FIG. 18–8.—Interlocking genetic events leading to S phase: The G₁ funnel. Cells, in accord with their particular phenotypes, are depicted as entering the G₁ interval with widely varying patterns of gene activity. From these diverse starting positions, the cells are pictured as progressing toward S phase by independent routes involving the sequential induction and repression of specific genes. It is proposed that, in the course of this progression, certain genes are activated which have an interlocking relationship with the specific genes which give rise to an active DNA replicase for the replication of DNA in native chromatin. This happens with an increasing probability as the G₁ interval progresses.

Something of the complexity of the problem which lies before the cell re-entering S phase is revealed in electron micrographs of nucleo-chromatin. Pictures prepared by Dr. Hans Ris,[27] using the Klein-schmidt technique to disrupt and spread nuclei, show that native chromatin is a complex web of 200 to 250 A nucleoprotein fibers. Treatment with a chelating agent allows these fibers to pull apart and to be stretched out at the air-water interface, yielding 100 A fibers which are highly nodular in appearance. Digestion with the proteolytic enzyme, pronase, removes the nodularity and releases the 25 A fibers of double-stranded DNA. Accordingly, one must conclude that native nucleochromatin is a complex molecular aggregate in which proteins cover the DNA and provide for the extensive cross-bridging seen in the presence of certain metal ions. The challenge that the cell meets on entry into the S phase is to replicate DNA which is covered so extensively with chromosomal proteins; at best, it is a complicated problem in molecular mechanics.[28]

To explore the nature of these processes and to characterize the cell's achievement during G₁, our laboratory has attempted to reconstruct the major S phase reactions in cell-free systems derived from synchronized cells; these are the replication of chromosomal DNA and the synthesis of histones. Using subcellular preparations from synchronized HeLa cells, we have found that nuclei, on entry into S phase, exhibit an active DNA replicase; this is bound to the nucleus. In addition to the usual requirements for deoxynucleoside triphosphates and ions, the nuclear system has a special requirement for ATP and some protein factors in the cytoplasm (CF).[29] Fractionation experiments have revealed the latter to be multiple in character and to vary in type and amounts during the course of the S phase.[16]

Analysis of the DNA made in this subcellular system supports the conclusions presented diagrammatically in Figure 18-9: (1) DNA replication continues in vitro largely at or near the sites of replication which were active in the living cell; (2) the DNA is synthesized in short fragments similar to the Okazaki fragments which have been described in bacteria; these are subsequently ligated to form longer units; (3) ATP is involved in this ligation reaction; and (4) the cytoplasmic protein factors are in some manner concerned with the initiation of DNA synthesis at new sites as well as the continuation of this process at existing sites. Remembering the molecular aggregate character of nucleochromatin and the multifocal ordering of DNA replication in the living nucleus, it is suggested that the CF may recognize specific sites in the chromatin and assist in the exposure of the underlying DNA to the DNA replicase. In this way the ordering of DNA replication can be explained in part by replication-controlled transcriptions.

Fig. 18–9.—A hypothetical view of DNA replication in the nuclei of eukaryotic cells. Once cells have become triggered for nuclear replication, DNA replication begins at multiple sites in the chromatin. In both living cells and isolated nuclei the DNA is synthesized in short segments which are subsequently ligated together to form interphase DNA[29, 32] by an ATP-requiring reaction. Studies in isolated nuclei illustrate that soluble cytoplasmic factors facilitate the initiation of DNA synthesis at new sites. In the diagram the incoming CF units are depicted to modify specific protein DNA associations of the nucleochromatin so as to render contiguous segments of DNA accessible for polymerase and ligase function.

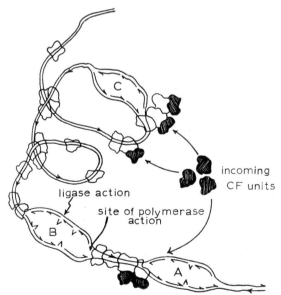

The synthesis of the other chromosomal constituents, the histones and nonbasic proteins, appears to follow in the aftermath of DNA replication. In our laboratory we have demonstrated that isolated cytoplasmic polysomes from S phase cells continue to synthesize histones in vitro in the absence of nuclei.[24, 30] Their competence for histone synthesis, however, is totally dependent on being derived from cells which are in the process of DNA replication. Blockade of DNA synthesis with hydroxyurea results in a very rapid decline of the histone-synthesizing activity of the polysome fraction.[24] Restoration of DNA synthesis on removal of the hydroxyurea is associated with a rapid restoration of histone synthesis in the polysome fraction. Since the return of this activity did not occur if RNA synthesis was blocked during the resumption of DNA synthesis, it is concluded that the coupling between DNA replication and histone synthesis involves the transcription of some histone mRNAs. Recent experiments on the labeling and isolation of intermediate-sized RNA from active polysomes reveals the presence of three RNA species (6 to 8S) which fit the role of presumptive messengers for histone synthesis.[31]

Returning to the summary slide (Figure 18-7), I wish to conclude that the analysis of the S phase reactions in synchronized cell preparations has begun to give us significant insights into the nature of chromosome replication. With continued study, it should be possible to define in molecular terms what is involved in the natural initiation of DNA synthesis in an animal cell, the nature of the active DNA replicase, and, most importantly, the genetic controls which regulate the assembly of the active system. This information appears vital to the design of more effective and physiologic methods for cancer chemotherapy.

Acknowledgment

The author has a Research Career Award from the National Cancer Institute, U. S. Public Health Service.

References

1. Howard, A., and S. R. Pelc: Heredity, 6 (Suppl. 1) :261, 1953.
2. Baserga, R.: Cell Tissue Kinet., 1:167, 1968.
3. Mueller, G. C., and K. Kajiwara: In: Developmental and Metabolic Control Mechanisms and Neoplasia, Baltimore, Williams and Wilkins, 1965, p. 452.
4. Baserga, R., R. D. Estensen, and R. O. Petersen: Proc. Nat. Acad. Sci. USA, 54: 1141, 1965.
5. Leighton, J.: In: Methods in Cancer Research (H. Busch, ed.), Academic Press, New York, Vol. IV, 1968, p. 86.
6. Lockwood, D. H., A. E. Voytovitch, F. E. Stockdale, and Y. J. Topper: Proc. Nat. Acad. Sci. USA, 58:658, 1967.
7. Papaconstantinon, J.: Science, 156:338, 1967.
8. Turkington, R. W.: Curr. Top. Develop. Biol., 3:199, 1968.
9. Cairns, J.: J. Mol. Biol., 15:372, 1966.
10. German, J. L.: Trans. N. Y. Acad. Sci. Ser. 2, 24:395, 1962.

11. Kajiwara, K., and G. C. Mueller: Biochim. Biophys. Acta, 91:486, 1964.
12. Mueller, G. C., and K. Kajiwara: Biochim. Biophys. Acta, 114:118, 1966.
13. Stubblefield, E., and G. C. Mueller: Cancer Res., 22:1091, 1962.
14. Taylor, J. H.: J. Biophys. Biochem. Cytol., 7:455, 1960.
15. Mueller, G. C., and K. Kajiwara: Biochim. Biophys. Acta, 119:557, 1966.
16. Mueller, G. C.: Fed. Proc., 28:1780, 1969.
17. Mueller, G. C., K. Kajiwara, E. Stubblefield, and R. R. Rueckert: Cancer Res., 22:1084, 1962.
18. Terasima, T., and M. Yasukawa: Exp. Cell Res., 44:669, 1966.
19. Kim, J. H., A. S. Gelbard, and A. G. Perez: Exp. Cell Res., 53:478, 1968.
20. Taylor, E. W.: Exp. Cell Res., 40:316, 1965.
21. Young, C. W.: Mol. Pharmacol., 2:50, 1966.
22. Spalding, J., K. Kajiwara, and G. C. Mueller: Proc. Nat. Acad. Sci. USA, 55:1535, 1966.
23. Hancock, R.: J. Mol. Biol., 40:457, 1969.
24. Gallwitz, D., and G. C. Mueller: J. Biol. Chem., 244:5947, 1969.
25. Kajiwara, K., U. H. Kim, and G. C. Mueller: Cancer Res., 26:233, 1966.
26. Wheatley, D., and G. C. Mueller: In preparation.
27. Ris, H.: In: Regulation of Nucleic Acid and Protein Biosynthesis (V. V. Koningsberger and L. Bosch, eds.), Elsevier Publishing Co., Amsterdam, 1967, p. 11.
28. Mueller, G. C.: In: The Cell Cycle and Cancer (R. Baserga, ed.), Marcel Dekker, Inc. In press.
29. Friedman, D. L., and G. C. Mueller: Biochim. Biophys. Acta, 161:455, 1968.
30. Gallwitz, D., and G. C. Mueller: Science, 163:1351, 1969.
31. Gallwitz, D., and G. C. Mueller: FEBS Letters, 6:83, 1970.
32. Kidwell, W. R., and G. C. Mueller: Biochem. Biophys. Res. Commun., 36:756, 1969.

Enzyme Regulation in Cancer Cells

VAN R. POTTER

McArdle Laboratory, University of Wisconsin Medical School, Madison, Wisconsin, USA

ENZYME REGULATION in cancer cells can be discussed in terms of enzymes related to the cell cycle, in which DNA synthesis and related systems are involved, as in the immediately preceding presentation by Dr. G. C. Mueller (see pages 719-725, this volume). It can also be discussed in terms of hormonal or other feedback regulations on enzyme synthesis or activity. My paper is appropriately juxtaposed between Dr. Mueller's report and the report by Dr. Williams-Ashman (see pages 731-732, this volume).

Oncogeny as a Locked-In Ontogeny

Oncogeny is a word that can be appropriately used in parallel with the word ontogeny, if we wish to imply that there is a relationship between the two processes. A number of investigators[1] have related oncogeny (the development of tumors) to ontogeny (the development of an individual being through embryonic stages). Matsushima and Sugimura and co-workers[2] described the process of cancer formation as a "dys-differentiation," while Uriel[3] has described it as a "retrodifferentiation." The entire session on ontogenic defects in oncogenesis (see pages 803-836, this volume), may provide further illumination for the concept. I wish to emphasize that ontogeny does not lead to a fixed program of gene expression, but rather to the capability for an appropriate gene expression in the particular environment in which the cell is found. In my laboratory, we make use of some of the numerous transplantable hepatomas provided by Dr. Harold P. Morris. We challenge the ability of these hepatomas to respond to dietary or hormonal stimuli, and we compare their response to that of adult, fetal, and newborn liver.

Oncogeny as a Composite of Program Errors

I would like to state my present view of the nature of oncogeny, which is simply another word for carcinogenesis or cancer formation. We emphasize that "Ontogeny (the normal process) is an unfolding of 'environmental response systems' for modulating gene expression according to a programmed time schedule." When we look at oncogeny (the abnormal or pathologic process), we have to consider the experimental data that establish the facts of biochemical diversity in the transplantable lines provided by Morris, some of which are minimal deviation by our criteria, and others which are considered to have more extensive deviations. We have no doubt that our description of the normal process (ontogeny) is a legitimate one as far as it goes. We also believe that the description of the pathologic process (oncogeny) will prove to be valid. The simple statement of this cancer theory is that "oncogeny is an accumulation of locked-in gene configurations (available or unavailable) that were scheduled to be unlocked at different times." By that I mean that they were scheduled for different times in the normal process of development, that is, in ontogeny. It seems to me that if there is a normal process which changes genes from available to unavailable and vice versa during development, and if we produce changes in the state of these genes in several loci, then we will obtain a diversity of biochemical patterns that will not coincide with the pattern of liver cells in any normal stage of development. In fact, this is the picture that seems to be emerging from the data on biochemical diversity as experiments progress in our laboratory and in other laboratories that are examining cancer tissue in comparison with embryonic tissue. The amount of experimental data that is available is now quite voluminous; I will present a sketch of the experimental system, establish the fact of diversity, and show our most recent data.

We Can Modulate Gene Expression in Hepatoma Cells

The experimental system that we use can be described as follows: The first point of reference is cell replication or DNA replication, which relates to the report by Dr. Mueller. Our work has involved labeling of DNA by radioactive thymidine and enumeration of labeled nuclei in tissue sections, in cooperation with Dr. Sam Lesher. Second, I wish to emphasize our use of tyrosine aminotransferase (TAT) as an enzyme that appears in the course of normal development or ontogeny, but which is repressed in the embryonic liver cell. Third, I wish to emphasize our findings on amino acid transport as studied by radioactive aminoisobutyric acid (AIB). Fourth, I want to emphasize that we use hydrocortisone, glucagon, and theophylline as well as controlled feeding schedules and dietary variations to perturb the liver plus hepatoma plus body system and to determine the capability of the given hepatoma line to respond like adult liver or in some other way.

Modulation of DNA Synthesis in Morris Hepatoma No. 7793

We emphasize only two time points in a 24-hr cycle to show that the rate of DNA synthesis in hepatoma 7793 is modulated by the physiological controls of the animal in which the hepatoma is found. The maximum rate of DNA labeling was at 0600 and the minimum rate was at 1,800 hr. The rate in the hepatoma oscillated through a 10-fold range and was essentially unaffected by the diet. Intermediate time points fell between these extreme values. Host liver had much less activity and a high variability. In a regenerating liver experiment, these values for host liver would appear very close to the base line. We hope to return to this model experiment, using the methods of perturbation that I will now describe in connection with the other parameters previously mentioned.

TAT in Morris Hepatoma 9618A

The characteristic response of normal liver to the experimental pattern employed[5] was plotted, with each point representing an individual animal and the three curves labeled 60, 30, and 12 to denote the percentage of protein in the diet. The feeding schedule and lighting schedule were controlled, and the enzyme activity rose and fell each day, according to a definite time schedule and in response to dietary protein. These data on hepatoma-bearing host livers are not significantly different from normal liver data.

The data from 30 hepatomas taken from the leg muscle of the same rats whose livers were used for the data just described were also plotted. No matter which diet or what time of day was considered, the hepatomas failed to respond to the stimuli that were able to produce dramatic changes in the liver. We may point out that these stimuli included not only diet but cyclic variations in circulating corticosterone, insulin, glucagon, and epinephrine, and possibly other stimuli that we have failed to consider. We must now emphasize that the response by hepatoma 9618A is not the same as that of other hepatoma lines, and, in fact, this hepatoma lies at one end of a broad spectrum of responses, which will now be described.

Survey of Hepatoma Lines for TAT and AIB

Enzyme data[6] and amino acid transport data[7] were combined, and data on normal liver were inserted. The amino acid transport system was expressed as the ratio between the radioactivity in the tissue and the radioactivity in blood plasma. The data were obtained from the same animals. As noted before, hepatoma 9618A lies at the lower end of the range for both parameters. None of the hepatomas responded identically with normal liver, and the various hepatoma lines were distributed over a range of values in the same order for both parameters. That is, the highest enzyme value was seen in hepatoma line No. 5123C, which had the highest value for amino acid transport, and so on. A number of other enzymes have been studied. The question we now pose is whether the hepatoma values are truly autonomous as these data suggest, or can we modulate the expression of their biochemical capabilities. Here I may say that adrenalectomy lowered the high values shown by 5123C, and hydrocortisone raised the median values shown by line 7800, but hydrocortisone had no effect on the low values shown by line 9618A.[6, 7] Accordingly, other means to elevate the response by 9618A were attempted.

Induction of TAT in Hepatoma 9618A

After several experiments on the modification of the normal liver response, Dr. Watanabe and Dr. Baril succeeded in inducing TAT in hepatoma 9618A; and Dr. Watanabe later developed a more successful protocol.[8] This hepatoma failed to respond to diet or to daily hormone fluctuations,[5] in contrast to rats treated with hydrocortisone two times daily for seven days and then injected twice with low doses of glucagon.[8] This suggests that the steroid modified the relation between the liver plus body system and the injected glucagon.[6, 7, 8] From these experiments, we proceeded to further studies on the liver plus body system with simultaneous measurements of enzyme (TAT) and the amino acid transport system.[9]

Inductions by Glucagon plus Theophylline

We see parallel stimulations of the TAT enzyme and the AIB pump, or transport system in normal liver, as a function of time. Three animals were killed at each time point. All of the rats received 2.5 mg theophylline per 100 g body weight, but one group received 2.0 mg glucagon per 100 g body weight, while another group received only 0.25 mg glucagon per 100 g body weight. There was remarkable parallelism between the enzyme induction and the response of the amino acid transport system. On the basis of this experiment, Dr. Scott selected the four-hr time point for a dose-response study.

Glucagon Dose-Response for Inductions with and without Theophylline

In a demonstration of the parallelism of the enzyme induction and the amino acid transport system, we obtained dose-response curves for the two parameters with glucagon doses from 0 to 2.0 mg glucagon per 100 g body weight, with a family of curves obtained with different doses of theophylline. The responses with 10, 2.5, and 0 mg theophylline, with all animals killed at four hr, based on the previous experiment, were plotted. With these data we could not return to the hepatoma 9618A.[9]

Inductions in Hepatoma 9618A with Glucagon

Suspecting that the glucagon injected ip might be less available to the hepatoma than subcutaneous glucagon, and noting the critical effects of dosage and theophylline, additional experiments were performed with hepatoma 9618A.[10] The animals were killed at four hr, and tests were made on two occasions. A glucagon induction of the enzyme was obtained with subcutaneous glucagon, but theophylline did not modify the response alone or with glucagon. Intraperitoneal glucagon alone was ineffective, but in a previous experiment ip glucagon plus theophylline gave a strong induction in the hepatoma. Normal liver has always given a strong response with theophylline alone. The amino acid transport paralleled the enzyme data.

Summary

We have demonstrated a marked parallelism between amino acid transport, as measured by radioactive AIB ratios, and a wide range of TAT activities and have demonstrated that both of these parameters can be experimentally altered in hepatomas and in normal liver by means of hydrocortisone, glucagon, and theophylline, but the resultant of the factors involved seems to be different in each hepatoma and to differ from adult liver. We conclude from these and other data that each hepatoma represents a different combination of locked-in gene expressions that cannot undergo a further developmental program, but that are nevertheless capable of being hormonally modulated within the locked-in configuration. Further work is being attempted to test whether a sufficient perturbation can be achieved to escape the locked-in configuration of active and inactive genes, and these studies involve simultaneous measurements of the DNA systems mentioned in the first part of this paper.

References

1. Potter, V. R.: Can. Cancer Conf., 8:9, 1969.
2. Matsushima, T., S. Kawabe, M. Shibuya, and T. Sugimura: Biochem. Biophys. Res. Commun., 30:565, 1968.
3. Uriel, J.: Pathol.-Biol., 17:877, 1969.
4. Potter, V. R., R. A. Gebert, H. C. Pitot, C. Peraino, C. Lamar, S. Lesher, and H. P. Morris: Cancer Res., 26:1547, 1966.
5. Potter, V. R., and M. Watanabe: In: Proceedings of the International Conference on Leukemia-Lymphoma (C. J. D. Zarafonetis, ed.), Lea and Febiger, Philadelphia, 1968, pp. 33-46.
6. Watanabe, M., V. R. Potter, H. C. Pitot, and H. P. Morris: Cancer Res., 29:2085, 1969.
7. Baril, E. F., V. R. Potter, and H. P. Morris: Cancer Res., 29:2101, 1969.
8. Potter, V. R., R. D. Reynolds, M. Watanabe, H. C. Pitot, and H. P. Morris: In: Advances in Enzyme Regulation (G. Weber, ed.), Vol. 8, 1970.
9. Scott, D. F., R. D. Reynolds, and V. R. Potter: In preparation.
10. Reynolds, R. D., D. F. Scott, and V. R. Potter: In preparation.

19

Modification of Gene Expression

Hormonal Regulation of Gene Expression and Control of Cancer

H. G. WILLIAMS-ASHMAN

Ben May Laboratory for Cancer Research and Department of Biochemistry, University of Chicago, Chicago, Illinois, USA

THE CONCEPT OF hormone dependence or independence of certain tumors, introduced by Huggins,[1] has had a profound influence on both the understanding of and the treatment for some cancerous diseases. A great deal of research over the last decade has established that androgens and estrogens, which effectively regulate the functional differentiation as well as the growth of secondary sexual tissues, exercise control over ribonucleic acid and protein biosynthetic reactions (gene expression mechanisms) in normal male and female genital organs.[2-5] This may have bearing on recent ideas that neoplasms are essentially the result of disturbances of normal cell differentiation rather than of growth control mechanisms per se;[6] however, experimental examination of the regulation of genetically determined protein-synthesizing apparatus in sex hormone-dependent tumors is still in its infancy.

Recently it has been shown that normal estrogen-responsive tissues are rich in cytoplasmic proteids that tenaciously bind these hormones, and seem to be involved in a two-step mechanism whereby estrogens are retained in cell nuclei in combination with specific macromolecules and without undergoing chemical change.[7, 8] Similarly, androgen-dependent normal tissues selectively accumulate testosterone, but in this case largely in the form of the reduced metabolite 5α-dihydrotestosterone (5α-androstan-17β-ol-3-one). Again, specific cytoplasmic proteids appear to be an integral part of a two-step process by which 5α-dihydrotestosterone is retained in cell nuclei of normal male genital glands.[9, 10] The relationship of these intracellular sex hormone-binding proteids to the stimulation of RNA and protein biosynthesis by these hormones remains obscure.

There are a number of reports[11-14] that the selective uptake and retention of labeled estrogens by hormone-dependent rat dimethyl-benzanthracene-induced mammary cancers is greater than that found in corresponding tumors of the hormone-independent variety. Studies on the accumulation of estrogens and on specific estrogen-binding proteids in human mammary cancer cells are now underway in various laboratories.[15-18]

References

1. Huggins, C.: Cancer Res., 27:1925, 1967.
2. Tata, J. R.: Progr. Nucleic Acid Res. Mol. Biol., 5:191, 1966.
3. Williams-Ashman, H. G.: Cancer Res., 25:1096, 1965.
4. Hechter, O., and I. D. K. Halkerston: Ann. Rev. Physiol., 27:133, 1965.
5. Williams-Ashman, H. G.: In: The Androgens of the Testis (K. B. Eik-Nes, ed.), Marcel Dekker, New York, 1970, pp. 117-143.
6. Markert, C. L.: Cancer Res., 28:1908, 1968.
7. Jensen, E. V., M. Numata, M. Smith, T. Suzuki, and E. R. DeSombre: Develop. Biol., Suppl. 3:151, 1970.
8. Gorski, J., D. Toft, G. Shyamala, D. Smith, and A. Notides: Rec. Progr. Hormone Res., 24:45, 1968.
9. Bruchovsky, N., and J. D. Wilson: J. Biol. Chem., 243:2012, 1968.
10. Fang, S., K. M. Anderson, and S. Liao: J. Biol. Chem., 244:6548, 1969.
11. Terenius, L.: Cancer Res., 28:328, 1968.
12. Mobbs, B. G.: J. Endocrinol., 41:339, 1968.
13. Mobbs, B. G.: J. Endocrinol., 44:463, 1969.
14. Sander, S., and A. Attramadal: Acta Path. Microbiol. Scandinav., 74:169, 1968.
15. Deshpande, N., V. Jensen, R. D. Bulbrook, T. Berne, and F. Ellis: Steroids, 10: 219, 1967.
16. Jensen, E. V., E. R. DeSombre, and P. W. Jungblut: In: Endogenous Factors Influencing Host-Tumor Balance (R. W. Wissler, T. Dao, and S. Wood, Jr., eds.), University of Chicago Press, Chicago, 1967, pp. 15-30.
17. Korenman, S.: J. Clin. Endocrinol., 30:639, 1970.
18. Braunsberg, H., W. T. Irvine, and V. H. T. James: In: Prognostic Factors in Breast Cancer (A. M. P. Forrest and P. B. Kunkler, eds.), Livingston, London, 1968, pp. 363-367.

Interaction of Glucocorticoid Hormones with Rat Liver Chromatin

YU-HUI TSAI and LUBOMIR S. HNILICA

Department of Biochemistry, The University of Texas M. D. Anderson Hospital and Tumor Institute at Houston, Houston, Texas, USA

Introduction

THE ADMINISTRATION OF glucocorticoid hormones to adrenalectomized rats has been known to increase nuclear RNA synthesis in liver.[1] Several enzymes concerned in gluconeogenesis are synthesized at an increased rate as a result of the administration of glucocorticoids.[2] Cortisol has been shown to cause rapid alteration in the distribution of labeled RNA.[3] Peterkofsky and Tomkins[4] have demonstrated that the earliest response of cultured hepatic cells to a synthetic glucocorticoid hormone is the increase of tyrosine aminotransferase synthesis which can be inhibited by actinomycin D. Addition of these hormones to isolated rat liver nuclei causes a substantial increase in RNA synthesis and in the template activity of chromatin in vitro.[5] This indicates that a derepression of chromatin might have occurred at transcriptional level. Sekeris and Lang[6] and Sluyser[7, 8] reported the binding of glucocorticoid hormones to histones in vivo and in vitro. A direct interaction of corticosteroid hormones with histones in chromatin has been suggested as the mechanism by which these hormones induce the increase in RNA synthesis. To test this possibility, in vivo and in vitro interactions of corticosteroid hormones with histones and chromatin were investigated; the results are reported in this paper.

Materials and Methods

MATERIALS

Cortisone and cortisol were purchased from Mann Research Laboratories. Cortisone-1,2-[3]H (51.6 mC/μmole), hydrocortisone-1,2-[3]H (18 mC/μmole, 44 mC/μmole), and tetrahydrocortisol-1,2-[3]H (18 mC/μmole) were obtained from New England Nuclear Corp. Radioactive labeled nucleotides (Schwarz Bio Research Inc.), calf thymus type-1 deoxyribonucleic acid, sodium salt (Sigma Chemical Company), and unfractionated calf thymus histone prepared in this laboratory[9] were used in the in vitro studies. *Micrococcus lysodeikticus* was purchased from Miles Chemical Inc., and Sprague-Dawley male albino rats, either normal or hypophysectomized, were used for all animal experiments.

PREPARATION OF CHROMATIN

Chromatin was isolated according to the procedure described by Bonner et al.[10] After dialysis against 0.01 M tris buffer pH 8.0 for 12 hr, the chromatin was sheared in an Omni Mixer at 100 v for 90 sec, followed by 20 min of centrifugation at 2,000 × g.

ISOLATION OF HISTONES

PROCEDURE A.—Livers were removed from decapitated rats and frozen immediately in dry ice-ethanol mixture. The liver was homogenized in 10 vol of 2.2 M sucrose in a glass homogenizer with a Teflon pestle. The homogenate was strained through six layers of cheesecloth to remove connective tissues, and the filtrate was centrifuged in a Spinco #21 rotor at 19,000 rpm for one hr. The upper layer of cytoplasm and the supernatant were carefully removed, and the tube wall was cleaned with deionized water. The clear nuclear pellet was dispersed in 0.25 M sucrose containing 0.01 M $MgCl_2$ (about 5 to 8 vol), and collected by centrifuging at 1,000 × g for 20 min. The nuclear pellet was suspended in approximately 20 vol of 0.14 M NaCl containing 0.01 M trisodium citrate, and the suspension was centrifuged at 1,600 × g for 20 min in a refrigerated centrifuge. The sediment resulting from this centrifugation was rehomogenized twice in approximately 20 vol of 0.1 M tris buffer pH 7.6 and centrifuged at 1,600 × g for 20 min. The final sediment was washed with 20 vol of cold 95% ethanol. The crude nucleohistone was stored at −20C if left overnight.

The arginine-rich histones F2a and F3 were extracted from the ethanol-washed nucleohistone with 10 vol of absolute ethanol containing 1.25 N HCl (4:1 v/v) as described by Johns et al.[11] The extraction was repeated three times. The combined extract was precipitated with 10 vol of cold acetone, and let stand overnight at 4C. The F1 and F2b fractions were extracted with 0.2 N HCl, three times, from the final sediment after extraction of F2aF3. The precipitate of lysine-rich histones was formed by standing overnight at 4C in 10 vol of acetone. The histone fractions were collected by centrifugation, and dissolved in small volumes of deionized water and filtered through glass wool. The filtrates were dialyzed against deionized water at 4C overnight with one change of dialysate. Finally, the dialyzed fractions were lyophilized.

PROCEDURE B.—This procedure was exactly as used by Sluyser.[12] In brief, crude rat liver nuclei obtained by centrifugation of the homogenate in 0.25 M sucrose were extracted with hot (80C) 0.14 M NaCl. The sediment was used for extraction of lysine-rich histones with 5% perchloric acid, arginine-rich histones with 96% ethanol, and moderately lysine-rich histones with 0.2 N HCl. The individual histone fractions were recovered as was described by the authors.[12]

Procedure C.—Rat liver nuclei were isolated according to the procedure of Blobel and Potter.[13] After centrifugation the nuclear pellet was collected in 1 vol (original volume of liver, v/w) of 0.25 M sucrose in 50 mM tris, 25 mM KCl, and 5 mM $MgCl_2$ pH 7.6, and spun at 16,000 $\times$ g for 20 min. The whole histone was extracted with 0.4 N H_2SO_4 by repeating the extraction procedure three times. The combined extracts were dialyzed against deionized water overnight at 4C, and lyophilized.

Procedure D.—This procedure was based on the method of Sekeris et al.[6] Rat livers were homogenized in 6 vol of 0.25 M sucrose solution pH 7.6, containing 0.05 M tris, 0.025 M KCl and 0.01 M $MgCl_2$. The homogenate was diluted to 20 vol with the same solution, and centrifuged at 1,000 $\times$ g for 20 min. The pellet was resuspended in 10 vol of the same solution with Teflon homogenizer and centrifuged as above. This step was repeated once more. The total histone was extracted with three portions of 0.4 N H_2SO_4 from the final sediment. The combined extracts were dialyzed against deionized water and lyophilized.

Preparation of Hormone-Histone Complex

Ten milliliters of 1% unfractionated calf thymus histone in 0.002 M NaCl were incubated with 54.9 mμmoles of hydrocortisone-1,2-^{3}H, or with cold hydrocortisone, in one ml of ethanol at room temperature for 30 min. One-half volume of the mixture was passed through a Sephadex G-25 column using 0.01 N HCl saturated with chloroform for elution.[14] Every 4 ml of the eluent were collected. The optical density (OD) of the fractions was read at 275 mμ. Hydrocortisone-1,2-^{3}H was determined by applying 100 μl of each fraction to a paper disc and measuring its radioactivity in a Packard scintillation spectrometer.

The other half of the mixture was dialyzed against deionized water for about 20 hr with one change, and lyophilized. A 30 mg portion of the dry sample was dissolved in 5 ml of 0.002 M NaCl, and was passed through a Sephadex G-75 column. Every 2 ml of the eluents (0.01 N HCl saturated with chloroform) were collected. One-milliliter portions and 100 μl portions of each fraction were used for the determination of histones and hydrocortisone-1,2-^{3}H respectively. The fractions were dialyzed and lyophilized.

Starch Gel Electrophoresis

The horizontal system described by Johns et al.[15] was employed. Twelve per cent of starch gel in 0.01 M HCl containing 0.2 mM $AlCl_3$ was used. The details of quantitative modification of this procedure were described by Hnilica et al.[16] The method of Kalberer and Rutschmann[17] was used to determine the radioactivity.

POLYACRYLAMIDE GEL ELECTROPHORESIS

For the analysis of histones, the 15% gel system in urea as described by Bonner et al.[10] was used. For the acidic protein analysis, the 15% gel pH 8.9 as described by Spelsberg and Sarkissian[18] was employed.

ASSAY FOR TEMPLATE ACTIVITY OF ISOLATED LIVER CHROMATIN

An assay based on that described by Bekhor et al.[19] was used in all experiments. Each 0.25 ml of reaction volume contained 10 μmoles tris buffer pH 8.0, 1 μmole $MgCl_2$, 0.25 μmoles $MnCl_2$, 3 μmoles mercaptoethanol, 0.2 μmoles of each nucleotide, and 0.4 μmoles of spermidinephosphate. The reaction was carried at 37C for 10 min or as described. The reaction was stopped by an addition of 0.25 ml of cold 0.1 M sodium pyrophosphate and 0.5 ml of cold 10% trichloracetic acid (TCA). The precipitated RNA was collected on a 0.45 μ Millipore filter followed by several washings with 5% cold TCA containing 1% of sodium pyrophosphate. After immersing in toluene for 20 min, the dried discs were counted in a scintillation mixture consisting of PPO and 0.1 g of dimethyl PPO per liter of toluent solution.

INCUBATION OF RAT LIVER MINCES WITH CORTISOL IN VITRO

Rat liver was removed from the decapitated animal and was placed in cold McCoy's medium. The tissue was cut into 1 × 2 cm pieces in the cold room, and the cut pieces were kept in a fresh McCoy's medium (pH 7.6). The cut pieces were then minced (into 0.2 mm of thickness) with the aid of a tissue sectioner. Equal-weight portions (about 11g) of the minced tissue were put in sterile petri dishes; one served as a control, and 22.5 ml of McCoy's medium (pH 7.6) containing 10 μg of cortisol per ml of medium were added to the other. The minced tissue was incubated in an incubator at 37C for 15, 30, and 60 min. The incubation was stopped by one rinse with regular cold medium and two with cold saline solution pH 7.6. Finally, the minced tissue was placed in a small amount of saline-EDTA, and used for chromatin isolation.

PREPARATION OF RNA POLYMERASE

The enzyme was prepared from *Micrococcus lysodeikticus* as described by Nakamoto et al.[20] The enzyme was first precipitated with 10% of streptomycin sulfate, then extracted with 0.5% solution of streptomycin sulfate in 0.05 M phosphate buffer pH 7.5. The crude enzyme was purified by repeated precipitation with protamine. Further purification was done by adsorption on DEAE cellulose slurry pH 7.5; the enzyme was then eluted with 0.3 M $(NH_4)_2SO_4$–0.001 M mercaptoethanol—0.2 M sucrose pH 7.5. Active fractions were pooled and precipitated with $(NH_4)_2SO_4$ to 40% saturation. The polymerase was stored at −20C in 0.01 M tris pH 7.5 containing an equal volume of glycerol.

EXTRACTION OF CYTOPLASMIC SUPERNATANT AND NUCLEAR EXTRACT

The cytoplasmic supernatant was prepared by homogenizing 5 g of rat liver in 0.25 M sucrose containing 1 mM $MgCl_2$ (10 ml), filtering the homogenate through 12 layers of cheesecloth, and centrifuging the filtrate at 40,000 rpm in a Spinco #40 rotor for one hr. The supernatant was carefully collected and mixed with an equal volume of 0.05 M tris buffer pH 7.6 containing 0.02 M mercaptoethanol, and stored at 0C.

The nuclear extract was prepared by homogenizing 10 g of fresh liver in 0.25 M sucrose containing 1 mM $MgCl_2$, filtering the homogenate through 12 layers of cheesecloth, and centrifuging the filtrate at 1,000 × g for 20 min. The pellet was then resuspended in the same solution and centrifuged as above. This washing procedure was repeated four times. The final pellet was homogenized in 0.05 M tris buffer, pH 7.6, containing 25% glycerol, 0.001 M mercaptoethanol and 0.01 M $MgCl_2$ (10 ml), and spun at 40,000 rpm in a Spinco #40 rotor for one hr. The supernatant was collected and stored at 0C.

CHEMICAL ANALYSIS

Nucleic acids were extracted from chromatin with hot 0.4 M perchloric acid for 15 min in a boiling water bath. The protein in the acid-insoluble pellet was dissolved in 1 N NaOH. The diphenylamine method[21] was used to assay for DNA. The orcinol reaction[22] was used to determine the RNA content. The Lowry method[23] was employed for the analysis of protein content.

AMINO ACID ANALYSIS

A sample weighing 1 mg was dissolved in 1 ml of constant boiling HCl (5.7 N), sealed in evacuated test tubes, and hydrolyzed at 110C for 22 hr. The hydrolysate was evaporated in vacuo and dissolved in citrate buffer pH 2.2, and its amino acid composition was analyzed with the aid of a Beckman automatic amino acid analyzer.

Results

THE EFFECT OF GLUCOCORTICOID HORMONES ON CHROMATIN ACTIVITY IN VITRO

When liver minces were incubated with cortisol (10 μg/ml) at 37C for 15, 30, and 60 min, the templating activity of isolated chromatin

TABLE 19–1.—THE EFFECT OF CORTISOL ON TEMPLATE ACTIVITY OF
CHROMATIN FROM MINCED LIVER

CHROMATIN PREPARATION	TIME OF INCUBATION OF MINCED LIVER WITH CORTISOL	$\mu\mu$MOLE OF UTP-^{3}H INCORPORATION PER REACTION	$\mu\mu$MOLE OF CTP-^{3}H INCORPORATION PER REACTION	% OF INCREASE OVER CONTROL
Control	15 min	—	76.62*	
Cortisol-Treated	15 min	—	79.53*	+3.8%
Control	30 min	50.18†	—	
Cortisol-Treated	30 min	59.64†	—	+18.9%
Control	60 min	36.8‡	—	
Cortisol-Treated	60 min	42.3‡	—	+14.95%

The minced liver was incubated with 10 μg of cortisol per ml of McCoy's media for the intervals as indicated.
* Amount of chromatin used as template contained 9 μg of DNA.
† Amount of chromatin used as template contained 14 μg of DNA.
‡ Amount of chromatin used as template contained 5 μg of DNA.
The amount of RNA polymerase used was capable of incorporating 1,760 $\mu\mu$mole of CTP-^{3}H (5 μc/μmole) per 50 μg of calf thymus DNA for 10 min of incubation at 37C.
Abbreviations: CTP, cytidine 5'-triphosphate; UTP, uridine 5'-triphosphate.

was increased as shown in Table 19-1. The maximum effect (about 20% increase) was observed at 30 min of incubation. After 30 min, no increase of activity was observed. When cortisol (20 μg/0.25 ml) was added to the control chromatin preparation directly, no effect could be seen. Similarly, no direct effect of the corticosteroid hormones on freshly isolated rat liver chromatin was observed.

To consider the possible enzymatic alteration of the hormone or interaction of corticosteroid hormones with some cell components deemed necessary for the activation of chromatin, cytoplasmic supernatant and nuclear extract from rat liver were prepared and added to the assay system. However, neither of these two extracts in combination with the hormone had any effect regarding the activation of chromatin as a template for RNA synthesis in vitro.

THE IN VIVO AND IN VITRO INTERACTION OF HISTONES WITH GLUCOCORTICOID HORMONES

The binding of steroid hormones to histones in vivo and in vitro, as reported from several laboratories,[6, 7, 8, 24, 25] stimulated thoughts that mechanism of the in vivo activation of chromatin is caused by the binding of corticosteroid hormones directly to histones in chromatin. Our studies confirmed the in vitro histone-hormone interaction (Figures 19-1 and 19-2). The two protein peaks resolved on Sephadex G-75 demonstrated that three times as much cortisol-^{3}H is associated with the F1F3 fractions as with the F2aF2b fractions. Further resolu-

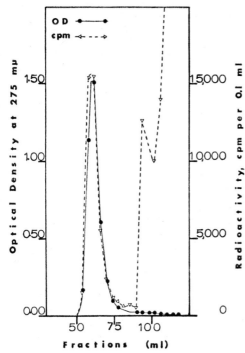

FIG. 19–1.—Interaction of hydrocortisone-1,2-³H with calf thymus histones followed by Sephadex G-25 gel filtration (see text). In this figure counts per minute are not corrected for counting efficiency, which is about 50%; uncorrected 2,000 count/min/vial correspond approximately to 1 $\mu\mu$mole of hydrocortisone-1,2-³H per milliliter of filtrate.

FIG. 19–2.—Fractionation of histone-hydrocortisone-1,2-³H complex on Sephadex G-75 column. Conditions as described in Figure 19-1.

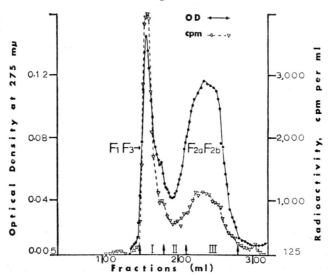

TABLE 19–2.—LOCALIZATION OF HYDROCORTISONE-1,2-^{3}H ON HISTONE FRACTIONS OF CALF THYMUS WHOLE HISTONE IN VITRO

HISTONE FRACTIONS	BAND ON STARCH GEL	TOTAL RADIOACTIVITY (DPM) ON EACH BAND	MG OF PROTEIN ON EACH BAND	SPECIFIC ACTIVITY ($\mu\mu$MOLE ^{3}H-CORTISOL/MG HISTONE)
F3	a Band	2,046 (37.5%)	0.0988 (8.79%)	0.513
	b Band	1,586 (28.3%)	0.1365 (12.15%)	0.287
	a + b Bands	3,632 (65.8%)	0.2353 (20.94%)	0.381
F1	c Band	637 (11.4%)	0.1224 (10.9%)	0.128
F2b	d Band	860 (15.4%)	0.3269 (29.11%)	0.065
F2a	e Band	443 (8%)	0.4383 (39.03%)	0.025

TABLE 19–3.—THE INTERACTION OF HYDROCORTISONE-1,2-^{3}H OR CORTISONE-1,2-^{3}H WITH NUCLEI AND HISTONES IN VIVO

	HYDROCORTISONE-1,2-^{3}H (DPM/MG OF DNA OR PROTEIN)		CORTISONE-1,2-^{3}H (DPM/MG OF DNA OR PROTEIN)	
	Procedure A (Nuclear preparation was washed with saline, tris buffer and ethanol after isolated from hypertonic sucrose soln.)	Procedure B (Nuclear preparation was obtained by sedimentation from 0.25M sucrose soln.) (Sluyser[12])	Procedure C (Nuclei were isolated from hypertonic sucrose soln. in TMK, pH 7.6.) (Blobel et al.[13])	Procedure D (Nuclei were isolated from 0.25M sucrose soln. in TMK, pH 7.6.) (Sekeris et al[6])
Nuclear preparation	390†	—	3,364.3* 841.0†	16,982.86* 1,759.79†
Total histones	—	—	115.37‡	159.86‡
The third extract of total histones contaminated with residue which was hard to spin down	—	—	—	546.03‡
F1F2b	0			
F1		264‡	—	—
F2b		72‡		
F2aF3	0			
F2a		173‡	—	
F3		113‡		

0.97 mμmole of cortisone-1,2-^{3}H (50 μC, 51.6 mC/μmole) was injected per rat (male, weighing 120-130 g) and 1.14 mμmole of hydrocortisone-1,2-^{3}H (50 μC, 44 mC/μmole) was injected per rat (male, weighing 250-300 g) respectively. Ten rats in each group were killed 30 min after injection.
* Assay based on calf thymus DNA (Burton's method).
† Assay based on bovine serum albumin (Lowry method).
‡ Assay based on calf thymus histones (Lowry method).

tion of the cortisol-³H-whole calf thymus histone complex (filtrate on G-25 Sephadex column) on starch gel electrophoresis showed that about 65% of the total radioactivity was associated with the F3 histone which contributed only 20% of the total protein weight (Table 19-2).

However, when 125 μl (6.9 mμmoles) of hydrocortisone-1,2-³H or tetrahydrocortisol-1,2-³H were injected ip into hypophysectomized rats (120 to 130 g), and the animals were sacrificed one hr later, no significant amount of radioactivity was bound to histones. The majority of label was distributed between cytoplasmic and nuclear sap protein fractions. Since Sekeris and Lang[6] and Sluyser[7, 8] reported significant binding of labeled corticosteroid hormone to histones in vivo, a comparative study on the isolation of histones by four various techniques (Procedure A, B, C, and D in Methods) was made. Nuclear preparation isolated by sedimentation in an isotonic sucrose solution (Procedure D) had a higher radioactivity than that isolated from hypertonic sucrose solution (Procedure C). Also, there was more labeled hormone bound to histones from those two nuclear preparations. This indicates that the apparent association of cortisone and cortisol to the histones and nuclei is probably caused by contamination by cytoplasmic proteins. Furthermore, the histone fractions isolated by Procedure A (a method yielding quite clean nuclei) contain no radioactivity (Table 19-3), whereas those prepared by Procedure B contain significant amounts of labeled hormone. As calculated from the binding of cortisol to histones in vitro, there is about one molecule of cortisol for every 3.3×10^4 molecules of histone (based on the average 15,000 mol wt). This can be interpreted that the hormone is bound to a nonhistone protein fraction contaminating the preparations of histones.

THE BINDING OF GLUCOCORTICOID HORMONES TO RAT LIVER CHROMATIN IN VIVO

Liver chromatin of normal rats which were sacrificed 30 min after hydrocortisone-1,2-³H injection showed less than 1 μμmole of hydrocortisone bound per mg of chromatin DNA and no significant binding of hormone per mg of chromatin proteins. More importantly, there was almost no radioactivity in the so-called soluble fraction of active chromatin after shearing (Table 19-4). However, the labeling of chromatin with cortisone-³H prepared from nuclei isolated in isotonic sucrose (0.25 M) (Procedure D) followed by freezing for three weeks was significantly higher. This again indicates that the binding of hormone to chromatin observed in the latter may be caused by the contamination of chromatin by cytoplasmic components or nuclear soluble proteins.

TABLE 19–4.—LABELING OF CHROMATIN FROM TRITIATED HORMONE-INJECTED RAT LIVER

CHROMATIN PREPARATION	CONDITIONS	DPM/MG OF DNA	DPM/MG PROTEIN
Chromatin isolated from hydrocortisone-1,2-³H-treated rat liver directly	Before centrifugation after shearing	42.3	11.2† 8.3‡
	Supernatant after centrifugation	5.1	4.6† 1.0‡
	Pellet after centrifugation	39.84	5.86† 3.78‡
Chromatin isolated from contaminated nuclei* of cortisone-1,2-³H-treated rat liver	Supernatant after centrifugation after shearing	1,764.8	503.16† 414.60‡

* The nuclei were prepared according to Sekeris et al.[6] as described in Procedure D (see Methods) and had been stored at –20C for three weeks until chromatin isolation.
† The pellet of chromatin after nucleic acid extraction was used for protein assay.
‡ Chromatin preparation was used directly for protein assay.

PROTEINS RELEASED FROM CHROMATIN DURING THE TREATMENT WITH GLUCOCORTICOID HORMONES

Since the binding of cortisol in vitro to histone preparations was very stable and did not dissociate in buffer, salt, or ethanol, and was also resistant to dialysis, gel filtration, and electrophoresis, the possibil-

FIG. 19–3.—Electrophoretic analysis of acidic proteins in the supernatant of chromatin preparation after six hr of incubation. Gel 1 and 2, control without incubation; Gel 3 and 4, control after 6 hr of incubation at 37 C; Gel 5 and 6, sample incubated at 37 C for six hr with cortisone; Gel 7 and 8, sample incubated at 37 C for six hr with hydrocortisone. The fast-moving band is the tracer dye band. Anode is at the bottom of the gels.

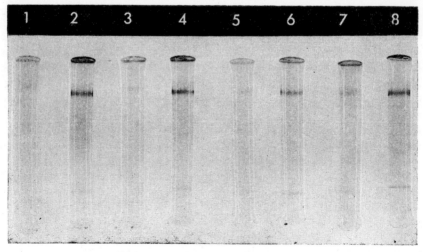

TABLE 19–5.—AMINO ACID COMPOSITIONS OF PROTEINS RELEASED FROM CHROMATIN BY INCUBATION AT 37C

AMINO ACIDS	CONTROL AT 0 HR	CONTROL AT 6 HR OF INCUBATION	TREATED WITH CORTISONE FOR 6 HR	TREATED WITH CORTISOL FOR 6 HR
Lysine	9.58	10.47	9.54	9.84
Histidine	1.43	1.70	1.33	1.62
Arginine	4.79	5.16	5.22	5.07
Aspartic Acid	9.92	8.99	9.53	8.91
Threonine	5.64	5.45	4.98	5.55
Serine (corrected)	7.61	7.29	7.65	6.78
Glutamic Acid	13.85	13.30	13.96	13.00
Proline	6.09	5.97	4.70	6.10
Glycine	9.47	9.64	9.39	9.99
Alanine	9.29	9.79	9.61	10.02
Valine	5.80	5.81	7.27	6.05
Methionine	1.89	1.75	1.76	1.63
Isoleucine	4.56	3.78	3.43	3.83
Leucine	7.25	6.87	7.21	7.56
Tyrosine	1.15	1.76	1.86	1.92
Phenylalanine	1.60	2.14	2.44	2.05
Total Basic Amino Acids	15.80	17.42	16.10	16.63
Total Acidic Amino Acids	23.77	22.29	23.49	21.91
Basic/Acidic	0.66	0.78	0.68	0.75

ity that the histone-hormone complexes were lost during the isolation of nuclei or chromatin is unlikely. The alternate possibility that the hormone may actually remove histones from their sites on chromatin was also investigated by gel electrophoresis and amino acid analysis. No histones were released during incubation of chromatin with hormones in vitro. However, a nonhistone protein was released upon incubation of chromatin at 37C. This protein, represented by a single band in polyacrylamide gel electrophoresis (Figure 19-3), was acidic (a ratio of basic to acidic residues is about 0.7) and relatively rich in glutamic acid (Table 19-5).

Discussion

The effect of glucocorticoid hormones on liver nuclear RNA synthesis has been demonstrated in intact animals,[1, 26] tissue minces (this study), and isolated liver nuclei.[5, 27, 28] In spite of the report of Stackhouse et al.,[29] neither we nor Dahmus et al.[26] nor Beato et al.[5] could demonstrate the association and direct effect of the hormone on isolated chromatin. As long as the nuclei are intact, the action of glucocorticoid hormones can be demonstrated unequivocally. The primary effect of the hormone in nuclei appears to be at the transcriptional level, resulting from the derepression of DNA templates rather than in the activation of RNA polymerase. However, the actual mechanism of action of these hormones is still unknown and requires further investigation.

The steroid hormones, including glucocorticoids, have been found to associate with DNA and histones.[6, 7, 8, 24, 25, 30] The binding of cortisol-^{3}H to arginine-rich histone (F3) in vitro was demonstrated by Sunaga and Koide.[24] Sekeris and Lang[6] reported that rat liver histones had the highest associated radioactivity at 30 min after cortisone-^{3}H injection, and that the level decreased rapidly three hr later. Sluyser[7] also reported the interaction of hydrocortisone-^{3}H with rat liver histones in vivo; the maximum binding occurred to F3 histone and was shown to increase continuously, reaching a maximum approximately two hr after the injection. Therefore, the possible role of steroid-histone interactions in genetic derepression was discussed by several authors. However, our data demonstrate that an increase in the purity of nuclear preparation resulted in lowering the in vivo association of tritiated glucocorticoids with nuclei, chromatin, and histones. Therefore, a conclusion can be drawn that the in vivo binding of glucocorticoid hormones to the histone fraction as reported by Sekeris et al.[6] and Sluyser[7, 8] is the result of the contamination of histones by nonhistone proteins. The biologic role of the contaminating proteins is not clear.

The in vitro experiments described in this paper demonstrate that the binding of hormone to calf thymus whole histone is as low as 1.5 $\mu\mu$mole of cortisol per mg of protein, or 6.6 $\mu\mu$moles of hormone per mg of F1F3 fraction after Sephadex gel filtration, and about 0.5 $\mu\mu$mole of hormone per mg of F3 after the electrophoresis of G-25 filtrate on starch gel. This represents approximately 30 μmoles of cortisol per mole of histone. It is our conclusion that the hormone associated with histone preparations is really bound to a contaminating fraction of acidic proteins, especially in the F3 histone fraction.[31] The binding of hormone to this contaminating protein is very stable. It appears from experiments described herein that the mechanism of action of glucocorticoid hormones as manifested by the increased activity of rat liver chromatin in RNA synthesis is neither through their direct interaction with histones nor through the removal of histones from native chromatin.

Summary

This study confirmed the in vitro interaction of cortisol with calf thymus histone fractions. However, no interaction of glucocorticoid hormones with histones could be detected in vivo. An effect of cortisol on the chromatin activity in minced rat liver was observed, but no direct action of glucocorticoid hormones on isolated chromatin could be demonstrated unequivocally. In addition, no histones were released from chromatin after its exposure to these hormones in vitro. It can be concluded that the increase of nuclear RNA synthesis caused by glucocorticoid hormones in rat liver is attributable to neither direct interaction of hormones with histones nor the removal of histones from chromatin.

Acknowledgments

This investigation was supported by grants from The Robert A. Welch Foundation (G-138), the U. S. Public Health Service (CA-07746), and the American Cancer Society (E-388).

References

1. Kenney, F. T., and F. Kull: Hydrocortisone-stimulate synthesis of nuclear RNA in enzyme induction. Proc. Nat. Acad. Sci. USA, 50:493-498, 1963.
2. Weber, G., R. L. Singhal, and S. K. Srivastava: Regulation of RNA metabolism and amino acid level in hepatomas of different growth rate. Adv. Enzyme Regul., 3:369-387, 1965.
3. Kidson, C., and K. S. Kirby: Selective alterations of mammalian m-RNA synthesis: Evidence for differential action of hormone on gene transcription. Nature, 203: 599-603, 1964.
4. Peterkofsky, B., and G. M. Tomkins: Evidence for the steroid-induced accumulation of tyrosine-amino-transferase messenger RNA in the absence of protein synthesis. Proc. Nat. Acad. Sci. USA, 60:222-228, 1968.
5. Beato, M., J. Homoki, I. Lukacus, and C. E. Sekeris: On the mechanism of hormone action, X. increased template activity for RNA synthesis of rat liver nuclei incubated with cortisol *in vitro*. Hoppe-Seyler's Z. Physiol. Chem., 349:1099-1104, 1968.
6. Sekeris, C. E., and N. Lang: Binding von (^{3}H) Cortison an Histone aus Rattenlever. Hoppe-Seyler's Z. Physiol. Chem., 340:92-94, 1965.
7. Sluyser, M.: Binding of hydrocortisone to rat liver histones. J. Mol. Biol., 19:591-595, 1966.
8. Sluyser, M.: Binding of testosterone and hydrocortisone to rat-tissue histones. J. Mol. Biol., 22:411-414, 1966.
9. Hnilica, L. S.: Studies on nuclear proteins: I. Observation on the tissue and species specificity of the moderately lysine-rich histone 2b. Biochim. Biophys. Acta, 117:163-175, 1966.
10. Bonner, J., G. R. Chalkley, M. Dahmus, D. Fambrough, F. Fujimura, R-C. C. Huang, J. Huberman, R. Jensen, K. Marushige, H. Ohlenbusch, B. Olivera, and J. Widholm: Isolation and purification of nuclear proteins. Methods Enzymol. XII, Part B:3-64, 1968.
11. Johns, E. W., D. M. P. Philips, P. Simson, and J. A. V. Butler: Improved fractionations of arginine-rich histones from calf thymus. Biochem. J., 77:631-636, 1960.
12. Sluyser, M., P. J. Thung, and P. Emmelot: Inhibition of deoxyribonucleic acid synthesis in regulating rat liver by the administration of histone *in vivo*. Biochim. Biophys. Acta, 108:249-258, 1965.
13. Blobel, G., and V. R. Potter: Nuclei from rat liver: Isolation method that combines purity with high yield. Science, 154:1662-1665, 1966.
14. Hnilica, L. S.: The fractionation of arginine-rich histones from calf thymus. Experientia, 21:124-126, 1965.
15. Johns, E. W., D. M. P. Philips, P. Simson, and J. A. V. Butler: The electrophoresis of histones and histone fractions on starch gel. Biochem. J., 80:189-193, 1961.
16. Hnilica, L. S., L. J. Edwards, and A. E. Hey: Studies on nuclear protein II. Quantitative distribution of histone fractions in various tissues. Biochim. Biophys. Acta, 124:109-117, 1966.
17. Kalberer, F., and J. Rutschmann: Eine Schnellmethode zür Bestimmung von Tritium, Radiokohlenstoff und Radioschwefel in Beliebigem Organischem Probenmaterial mittels des Flüssigkeits-Scintillations-Zählers. Helv. Chim. Acta 44:1956-1966, 1961.
18. Spelsberg, T. C., and I. V. Sarkissian: Isolation and electrophoresis of nuclear proteins of bean. Phytochemistry, 7:2083-2088, 1968.

19. Bekhor, I., G. M. Kung, and J. Bonner: Sequence-specific interaction of DNA and chromosomal protein. J. Mol. Biol., 39:351-364, 1969.
20. Nakamoto, T., C. F. Fox, and S. B. Weiss: Enzymatic synthesis of ribonucleic acid. I. Preparation of ribonucleic acid polymerase from extracts of *Micrococcus lysodeikticus*. J. Biol. Chem., 239:167-174, 1964.
21. Burton, K.: A study of the conditions and mechanism of the diphenylamine reaction for the colorimetric estimation of deoxyribonucleic acid. Biochem. J., 62: 315-323, 1956.
22. Hurlbert, R. B., H. Schmitz, A. F. Brumm, and V. R. Potter: Nucleotide metabolism. II. Chromatographic separation of acid soluble nucleotides. J. Biol. Chem., 209:23-39, 1954.
23. Lowry, O. H., N. J. Rosebrough, A. L. Farr, and R. J. Randall: Protein measurement with the folin phenol reagent. J. Biol. Chem., 193:265-275, 1951.
24. Sunaga, K., and S. S. Koide: Interaction of calf thymus histones and DNA with steroids. Steroids, 9:451-456, 1967.
25. Sunaga, K., and S. S. Koide: Structural specificity of the steroids interacting with calf thymus histones. Biochem. Biophys. Res. Commun., 26:342-348, 1967.
26. Dahmus, M. E., and J. Bonner: Increased template activity of liver chromatin, a result of hydrocortisone administration. Proc. Nat. Acad. Sci. USA, 54:1370-1375, 1965.
27. Dukes, P. P., and C. E. Sekeris: Stimulierung des Enbaus von [2-C^{14}] Uracil in Ribonucleinsäure von Rattenleberkernen durch Cortisol *in vitro*. Hoppe-Seyler Z. Physiol. Chem., 341:149-151, 1965.
28. Ohtsuka, E., and S. S. Koide: *In vitro* stimulation of RNA synthesis in isolated rat liver nuclei by glucocorticoids. Biochem. Biophys. Res. Commun., 35:648-652, 1969.
29. Stackhouse, H. L., C. J. Chetsanga, and C. H. Tan: The effect of cortisol on genetic transcription in rat liver chromatin. Biochim. Biophys. Acta, 155:159-168, 1968.
30. Ts'o, P. O. P., and P. Lu: Interaction of nucleic acids. I. Physical binding of thymine, adenine, steroids and aromatic hydrocarbons to nucleic acids. Proc. Nat. Acad. Sci. USA, 51:17-24, 1964.
31. Hnilica, L. S., and L. G. Bess: The heterogeneity of arginine-rich histones. Anal. Biochem., 12:421-436, 1965.

Selective Toxicity by Enzyme Administration: Tumor Inhibitory Actions of a Bacterial Extract with L-Asparaginase and L-Glutaminase Activities

J. D. BROOME

Department of Pathology, New York University School of Medicine, New York, New York, USA

L-ASPARAGINASE HAS BEEN found to be a potent inhibitor of certain tumors in a number of different animal species.[1–3] In examining a bacterial L-asparaginase preparation recently submitted to us, we have found that it is able to inhibit the growth of mouse tumors of two kinds which are resistant to L-asparaginases from *Escherichia coli* and agouti serum and which are not dependent on an external source of L-asparagine for growth in vitro. The effect appears to be caused by an enzyme in the preparation with both L-glutaminase and L-asparaginase activities. This enzyme has properties which differ from those described by Greenberg et al. in a bacterial extract some years ago.[4–6]

Materials and Methods

The bacterial extract, designated CR, was provided by Collaborative Research, Inc., Waltham, Massachusetts. The source was an organism isolated from a soil sample, which, although not yet fully characterized, has properties similar to those of the genus *Pseudomonas*. The organism was cultured aerobically in nutrient broth, cells were collected by centrifugation, lysed, and, after a further centrifugation, the supernatant was fractionated with ammonium sulfate and ethanol. Precipitated proteins were chromatographed on DEAE cellulose, followed by gel exclusion chromatography. Final preparations were desalted and lyophilized. Since only small quantities of the preparations were available, it was necessary to plan all experiments to conserve these to the greatest possible extent. Four fractions examined were derived from different chromatographic cuts and had L-asparaginase activities of 0.33 to 0.67 IU/mg protein when assayed at pH 7.4 and 1×10^{-2} M L-asparagine by our usual method.[7] The fraction with highest specific activity was used in succeeding experiments. Assays of L-glutaminase activity at high substrate concentration were performed in a similar way, substituting L-glutamine for L-asparagine. Assays of L-asparaginase and L-glutaminase at low substrate concentration, and in experiments to measure K_m, were performed using ^{14}C-labeled amino acids (New England Nuclear Corp., Boston, Mass.) as described earlier.[8] 5-Diazo-4-oxo-L-norvaline (DONV) was the gift of Dr. R. E. Handschumacher; 6-diazo-5-oxo-L-norleucine (DON) was the gift of Dr. J. Burchenal.

The principal tumor cell line used was lymphoma 6C3HED (L-asparaginase-sensitive and an L-asparaginase-resistant subline) as described previously,[9] carried in C3H/C57 BL mice. Other lines used were L5147 in AKR mice and L1210 in DBF mice, the latter usually carried as an ascites tumor but carried subcutaneously for two transfer generations before the experiment to be described. In assaying tumor inhibition, mice were implanted with approximately one million lymphoma cells subcutaneously in each flank. Treatment was begun when tumors were small but distinctly palpable nodules of 2 mm or more in diameter. Methods of recording results were similar to those used previously.[2]

Results

The injection of 1 mg of CR on three successive days into mice bearing small asparaginase-sensitive 6C3HED tumors prevented the tumors from increasing in size. Further injections of 2 mg and 3 mg on succeeding days caused the tumors to become soft and then impalpable. Regression was only partial, and 48 hr after the final injection the tumors were obviously regrowing. To conserve material, further and more prolonged treatment was not undertaken.

In another experiment, two daily injections of 3 mg produced com-

TABLE 19–6.—EFFECTS OF CR PREPARATION AND E.COLI L-ASPARAGINASE ON LYMPHOMA 6-C3HED

Type of Tumor	Treatment	Tumor Diameters (mm)						
		Days after Implantation						
		6	7	8	9	10	11	12
6C3HED asparaginase-sensitive	CR 3 mg D6,7	3	3	N	N	3	8	10
	CR 3 mg D6,7	3	2	N	N	3	8	10
	E.coli asparaginase 1.0 I.U. D6,7	4	1	N	N	N	N	2
	Untreated	3	4	6	9	11	14	16
6C3HED asparaginase-resistant	CR 3 mg D6,7	3	N	N	N	5	6	8
	CR 3 mg D6,7	4	N	N	4	6	8	11
	E.coli asparaginase 5.0 I.U. D6,7	4	6	10	11	13	15	16
	Untreated	4	5	7	11	13	15	16

CR–0.67 I.U. asparaginase/mg. Results are from individual mice. Animals were implanted with tumors in each flank. Tumors were usually the same size on each side, but when this was not so measurements were taken from the larger tumor.

TABLE 19–7.—EFFECTS OF CR PREPARATION ON
LYMPHOMA 5147

TREATMENT	TUMOR DIAMETERS (MM)					
	Days after Implantation					
	7	8	9	10	11	12
CR 3 mg D 7,8,9	4	4	4	3	6	8
CR 3 mg D 7,8,9	2	2	2	3	5	7
Untreated	2	5	9	11	12	14

TABLE 19–8.—EFFECTS OF CR PREPARATION
ON LYMPHOMA L1210

TREATMENT	TUMOR DIAMETERS (MM)			
	Days after Implantation			
	4	5	6	7
CR 3 mg D 4,5,6	2	3	4	5
CR 3 mg D 4,5,6	3	4	3	5
Untreated	2	3	4	7

parable results (Table 19-6). In relation to asparaginase assays, *E. coli* asparaginase appeared to be more strongly tumor inhibitory than the present material. Next, mice bearing the asparaginase-resistant variant of lymphoma 6C3HED were treated with CR in a dose of 3 mg daily. A marked degree of tumor inhibition was observed, and cells of the variant seemed to have a degree of sensitivity similar to that of the asparaginase-sensitive line (Table 19-6). But again, recurrence of the tumor was obvious after ending the treatment. Two other kinds of tumors, intrinsically asparaginase-resistant, were tested. Lymphoma 5147 showed slight inhibition, but lymphoma L1210 appeared unaffected (Tables 19-7 and 19-8).

No toxic effect was observed in mice treated with CR preparations. There was no weight loss, and gross and histologic examination of the tissues of treated animals revealed no abnormality.

In view of the unexpected inhibition of asparaginase-resistant tumors by CR, investigations were undertaken to examine the properties of the asparaginase present. The particular objective was to determine whether this enzyme could indeed be responsible for tumor inhibition.

PROPERTIES OF THE L-ASPARAGINASE

Because the rate of disappearance of enzyme from the blood has been associated with tumor-inhibition effectiveness of asparaginases,[7] a clearance test was performed with CR asparaginase. From three hr after iv injection, the enzyme disappeared from the blood of normal mice, with a half-life of 2.7 hr. In mice bearing 6C3HED tumors, the rate of disappearance was considerably slower, and the half-life was approximately 18 hr. These results were very similar to those ob-

TABLE 19–9.—pH DEPENDENCE OF L-ASPARAGINASE AND L-GLUTAMINASE
ACTIVITIES IN CR

pH	5.0	5.6	6.2	6.8	7.4	8.0	8.3	8.6	8.9
Asparaginase*	28	38	47	58	67	76	116	120	160
Glutaminase*	72	78	80	81	84	83	84	84	86

* Enzyme activities: $\times 10^{-8}$ moles/min/mg.
  Substrate concentration 1×10^{-2} M. Buffers: pH 5.0–6.8 0.05 M sodium cacodylate–HCl, pH 7.4–8.9 0.5 M Tris–HCl.

tained with *E. coli* asparaginase,[8] and in themselves could not account for the particular tumor-inhibitory properties of the preparation. Next, experiments were performed to examine substrate specificity. These showed that the enzyme preparation had a strong L-glutaminase activity. Indeed, at pH 7.4 the preparation had even greater glutaminase (by 24%) than asparaginase activity (Table 19-9). At higher pH this relationship was reversed. The high enzyme activities through a wide range of pH values are notable. Lineweaver-Burk plots (Figure 19-4) showed that both asparaginase and glutaminase activities possessed exceedingly low and apparently equal K_m values (3.5×10^{-6} M), considerably lower than for the high affinity *E. coli* asparaginase (1.25×10^{-5} M).[8] However, the plots were not linear throughout. At substrate concentrations of 1×10^{-2} and 1×10^{-3} M, reaction velocity was excessively high. This may be an unusual allosteric effect, but it is possible that the preparation contains an additional enzyme(s) with low substrate affinity. Analogous observations have been made with *E. coli* asparaginase.[9]

Asparaginase and glutaminase activities were destroyed by incuba-

FIG. 19–4.—Lineweaver-Burk plots of L-asparaginase and L-glutaminase activities of CR. Buffer: 0.05 M borate pH 7.4.

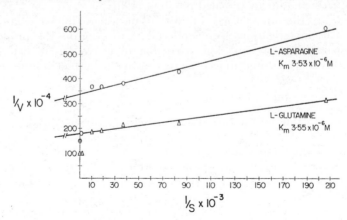

TABLE 19–10.—INACTIVATION OF L-ASPARAGINASE AND L-GLUTAMINASE
ACTIVITIES OF CR PREPARATION

INHIBITOR (1 × 10⁻³M)	SUBSTRATE	RELATIVE ENZYME ACTIVITIES AFTER INCREASING PERIODS OF INCUBATION WITH INHIBITOR			
		0 hr	1 hr	5 hrs	5 hrs and After Injection Into Mice*
DONV	Gln	100	57.1	12.6	20.9
	Asn	100	52.1	0.2	18.9
DON	Gln	100	0.0†		
	Asn	100	0.0†		

* A comparison of blood enzyme activities with mice treated with the same amount of non-inactivated "CR." Samples were removed from animals shown in Figure 19-5, 3 hrs after injection. Figures shown were averages from 2 mice.
† Complete inactivation at 30 minutes.
Incubation at 37° C in 0.05 M Tris pH 7.4. 20 samples removed for enzyme assay.
DONV—1.2 μμmoles/1.0 I.U. L-asparaginase activity.
DON—1.7 μμmoles/1.0 I.U. L-asparaginase activity.

tion with DONV, an analog of asparagine which is known to bind co-valently with asparaginases[10] (Table 19-10). However, inactivation took place slowly and required a higher concentration of the analog than was the case for agouti serum and *E. coli* asparaginases (100% inactivation at 1×10^{-4} M in 30 min in the latter case). No substantial enzymatic breakdown of inhibitor occurred. At five hr, optical density readings at 275 mμ showed that 90 to 95% of the inhibitor remained. By contrast, the glutamine analog DON produced much more rapid inactivation of CR, which was complete in 30 min. Both analogs inhibited asparaginase and glutaminase activities. For DONV, the ratio between residual asparaginase and glutaminase activities remained constant in the first hour. By five hr, however, asparaginase activity was almost completely inhibited, while 12% of the glutaminase activity remained. Partial reactivation, preferentially of asparaginase activity, occurred after injection of the preparations into mice.

A particular purpose of the experiments just described was to obtain preparations of CR in which asparaginase and glutaminase were specifically inactivated, to determine whether the preparations had lost tumor inhibitor activity.

TUMOR INHIBITORY ACTIVITY OF ENZYME-INACTIVATED PREPARATIONS OF CR

Preparations of CR, whose assays are shown in Table 19-10, were injected into groups of mice. It is clear that while the DONV-treated preparations retained some tumor inhibitory activity, this was considerably less than for the uninhibited material (Figure 19-5). Indeed, the degree of in vivo reactivation of the DONV-treated enzyme was consistent with the amount of tumor inhibition which resulted. These results strongly indicate that the tumor-inhibitory activity of

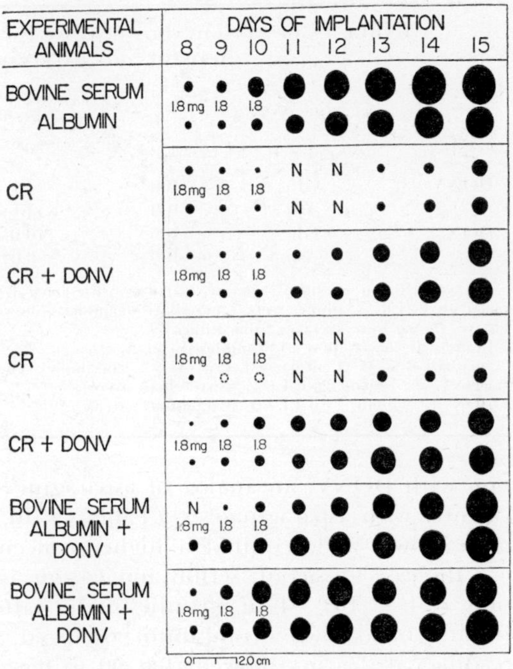

FIG. 19–5.—Effect of DONV incubation on the tumor inhibitory effectiveness of CR preparation. The asparaginase-resistant line of lymphoma 6C3HED was used. Tumors in three additional control animals given bovine serum albumin were essentially the same size as those shown. Assays of asparaginase and glutaminase activities in preparations given to the animals are shown in Table 19-10 (five-hr incubation and five-hr incubation with injection into mice).

the preparation was caused by its asparaginase and/or glutaminase activities, and not to another component.

Discussion

The experimental results described are consistent with the view that asparaginase and glutaminase activities of CR reside in the same enzyme. DON and DONV, which are specific inhibitors for glutaminases and asparaginases, respectively,[10, 11] each inhibit both activities in the present preparation. However, the persistence of a small amount of glutaminase activity after elimination of asparaginase by DONV may indicate that a specific glutaminase is present as a minor component in the preparation. It is also possible that this effect is attributable to the reaction of DONV with sites on the enzyme other than the amido-hydrolase active site,[10] which results in relatively greater loss of asparaginase than glutaminase activity. The marked recovery of asparaginase activity in vivo could be caused by removal of inhibitor from sites of the former kind. Additional evidence that both activities are possessed by the same enzyme is provided by the finding that enzyme activities in different chromatographic fractions are in a constant ratio to each other. Further studies to clarify this point are in progress.

Another question which requires consideration is the mechanism of tumor inhibition by CR. The preparation contains an enzyme with an extremely high affinity for asparagine, and it would be expected to cause a marked depletion of this amino acid from the body fluids of treated animals. This alone could explain the inhibition of asparaginase-sensitive 6C3HED.[8] But cells strongly resistant to *E. coli* asparaginase were also inhibited, and the rather lower K_m of the present enzyme as compared to that of *E. coli* asparaginase seems inadequate to account for its effectiveness. The glutaminase activity now observed would be expected to cause a severe depletion of this amino acid in tissues of treated mice. 6C3HED cells have been reported to possess a relatively low level of glutamine synthetase.[12] Glutamine is a substrate for the asparagine synthetase found in asparaginase-resistant tumor cells.[13] Deprivation of glutamine, therefore, may prevent the formation of adequate amounts of endogenous asparagine by the lymphoma cells, particularly when they are subjected to conditions of severe asparagine depletion such as would be expected during therapy with the present preparation.

Although, like ours, Greenberg's enzyme preparation was tumor inhibitory, the two show notably different enzymologic properties.[4, 5] Both preparations had L-glutaminase and L-asparaginase activities, but glutaminase activity appeared in a higher ratio in the earlier preparation and showed a sharp pH optimum at pH 6.6 which is not now observed. The effect of pH on enzyme activities in the two preparations is greatly different in other ways.[5] Perhaps more significantly in relation to biologic effectiveness, the K_m of the present enzyme is lower than the earlier by a factor of 100. The effect of DON on the two materials differs; in Greenberg's only glutaminase was inactivated, asparaginase was unaffected. This suggests that two enzymes were present. In the present material, inactivation for both substrates took place at a rapid rate. Whatever may be the relationship between the preparations now discussed, it is possible that aminohydrolases of similar kinds are widely distributed among microorganisms, and they may provide useful tumor-inhibitory agents.

Summary

A bacterial extract with L-asparaginase and L-glutaminase activities inhibited both asparaginase-sensitive and asparaginase-resistant lines of lymphoma 6C3HED and lymphoma L5147 but not L1210. At pH 7.4, the preparation possessed 24% more glutaminase than asparaginase activity. Both enzyme activities showed extremely low K_m values (3.5×10^{-6} M). Both activities were inactivated by the asparagine analog DONV, but inactivation was more rapid and complete with the glutamine analog DON. Inactivation of the enzyme activities in vitro led to diminished tumor-inhibitory activity in vivo. The evidence suggests that both asparaginase and glutaminase activities are possessed by the same enzyme. The preparation has notably different properties from that described by Greenberg.

References

1. Broome, J. D.: Evidence that the L-asparaginose activity of guinea pig serum is responsible for its antilymphoma effects. Nature, 191:1114-1115, 1961.
2. Broome, J. D.: Evidence that the L-asparaginase of guinea pig serum is responsible for its antilymphoma effects. I. Properties of the L-asparaginase of guinea pig serum in relation to those of the antilymphoma substance. J. Exp. Med., 118:99-120, 1963.
3. Broome, J. D.: L-Asparaginase: The evolution of a new tumor inhibitory agent. Trans. N. Y. Acad. Sci. 30:690-704, 1968.
4. Ramadan, M. A., F. A. El-Asmar, and D. M. Greenberg: Purification and properties of glutaminase and asparaginase from a Pseudomonad. I. Purification and physical properties. Arch. Biochem. Biophys., 108:143-149, 1964.
5. Ramadan, M. A., F. A. El-Asmar, and D. M. Greenberg: Purification and properties of glutaminase and asparaginase from a Pseudomonad. II. Substrate specificity, kinetics, activation and inhibition. Arch. Biochem. Biophys., 108:150-157, 1964.
6. Greenberg, D. M., G. Blumenthal, and M. A. Ramadan: Effects of administration of the enzyme glutaminase on the growth of cancer cells. Cancer Res., 34:957-963, 1964.
7. Broome, J. D.: Antilymphoma activity of L-asparaginase *in vivo:* Clearance rates of enzyme preparations from guinea pig serum and yeast in relation to their effect on tumor growth. J. Nat. Cancer Inst., 35:967-974, 1965.
8. Broome, J. D.: Factors which may influence the effectiveness of L-asparaginases as tumor inhibitors. Brit. J. Cancer, 22:595-602, 1968.
9. Schwartz, J. H., J. Y. Reeves and J. D. Broome: Two asparaginases from *E. coli* and their actions against tumors. Proc. Nat. Acad. Sci. USA, 56:1516-1519, 1966.
10. Handschumacher, R. E., C. J. Bates, P. K. Chang, A. T. Andrews, and G. A. Fischer: 5-Diazo-4-oxo-L-norvaline: Reactive asparagine analogue with biological specificity. Science, 161:62-63, 1968.
11. Cooney, D. A., and R. E. Handschumacher: L-Asparaginase and L-asparagine metabolism, Ann. Rev. Med., 10, 1970 [sic].
12. Al-Asmar, F. A., and D. M. Greenberg: Studies on the mechanism of tumor growth by the enzyme glutaminase. Cancer Res., 26:116-122, 1966.
13. Broome, J. D.: Studies on the mechanism of tumor inhibition by L-asparaginase. J. Exp. Med., 127:1055-1072, 1968.

Action of Some Antitumor Antibiotics on Gene Transcription and Replication

W. KERSTEN

Physiol.-Chem. Institute, University of Erlangen, Erlangen, FRG

THE NUMBER OF antitumor antibiotics interfering with DNA replication or transcription is steadily increasing. It is beyond the scope of this paper to include even the more recent work within this field. Only a few points of interest should be stressed. As an introduction to this field, it might be useful to review briefly the classification of these drugs into different groups according to their molecular mode of action.

Group I comprises drugs which preferentially inhibit DNA replication. Mainly the mono- or bifunctional alkylating substances are used for the treatment of tumors. The alkylating substances are bound to DNA covalently and irreversibly. Damages at the DNA molecule caused by the alkylating agents can only be repaired by a series of enzymes known as the repair enzymes. Since until now the DNA from tumor cells was not distinguishable from the DNA of normal cells, those drugs will affect the growth of tumors as well as the growth of other tissues. The growth-inhibitory effect is most pronounced in rapidly dividing cell populations. If it would be possible to administer these substances directly into the tumor or into cancer cells with delayed DNA repair, the usefulness of these inhibitors could improve.

Group II includes those drugs which preferentially inhibit DNA transcription by an association with the DNA template. At the right side are the antimalarials. All of them complex with DNA and change the physicochemical properties of the DNA in a way which is characteristic for intercalation. Also, the complexes between DNA and the antitumor antibiotics of the anthracycline group: daunomycin = rubidomycin, adriamycin, nogalamycin, and cinerubin, fit to the intercalation model. The intercalating drugs can easily be removed from the DNA by increasing salt concentration within the solute, which means that electrostatic forces are involved in the interaction with DNA. Actinomycin, which also partially intercalates, is not so easily displaced from the DNA. Probably hydrophobic interactions and stacking forces are responsible for the stronger binding of actinomycin to DNA.

The complex formation of DNA with nogalamycin or daunomycin

is accompanied by changes in the optical properties of the drugs which can be measured by CD spectroscopy. Upon complex formation of DNA with nogalamycin, the CD bands at 343 mμ and at 453 mμ are shifted toward higher wavelengths by about 10 mμ; in addition the amplitudes increase. A new CD band occurs at 315 mμ; the negative maximum at 305 mμ decreases. From these measurements it can be concluded that the anthracyclines, in contrast to actinomycin, apparently do not form dimers in solution. CD spectra of the complexes of nogalamycin with DNA of varying AT content (28% to 66%) were measured. Taking the degree of increase in the amplitude at 400 mμ and the degree of decrease at 305 mμ as indicative of complex formation, we do not find a correlation between the AT content and the amount of drug bound to DNA.[1]

Chromomycin, the closely related mithramycin and olivomycin, as well as luteoskyrin, are bound to the outside of the double helical DNA only in the presence of divalent cations. From the CD spectra of chromomycin and mithramycin in solution, we conclude that in buffer at pH 7 and at a concentration of 1×10^{-4} M both substances form dimers. The association occurs at the chromophores. The CD spectra indicate that at high ratios of DNA-P to drug (24:1) these antibiotics are bound as monomers. The CD spectra of the complexes of chromomycin with DNA of different GC content confirm our earlier observations[2] that the amount of drug which associates with DNA increases with rising GC content. Little is known about the interaction of the other antibiotics with DNA.

Group III comprises substances which inhibit RNA synthesis by binding to the RNA nucleotidyltransferase. The most important observation was that this binding not only was specific for the enzyme but, moreover, that different inhibitors have been found with species specificity: (1) antibiotics which bind to the RNA polymerase of prokaryotes are the rifamycines[3-5] streptovaricin and streptolydigin,[6, 7] and (2) a poison that interacts with RNA polymerase of eukaryotes is α-amanitin.[8-11]

Though these substances do not have carcinostatic properties, these findings encourage us to continue systematically the search for cancer-specific enzymes or proteins and specific inhibitors for these proteins.

Our observation[12] that derivatives of mitomycins, still containing the quinone ring but without the alkylating aziridine ring, preferentially inhibit the synthesis of RNA, and the fact that many of the substances in groups I and II contain quinone ring systems stimulated us to study other quinone antibiotics. Their effect on growth and nucleic acid metabolism was studied in microorganisms and compared with the mode of action of synthetic quinolin quinones or naphthoquinones recently introduced as anticancer drugs.[13] Even though the mode of action of these quinones is not yet fully understood, we may unite them into a IV group: quinones which preferentially inhibit RNA synthesis by an as yet unresolved mechanism.

Granaticin is a new antibiotic isolated from streptomycetes. In the concentration range between 0.1 to 0.8 μg/ml, the effect of granaticin is bacteriostatic; high concentrations are bacteriocidal. At bacteriocidal concentrations, morphologic changes occur which could be demonstrated by electron microscopy. The cell wall and the cytoplasmic membrane are broken up, ribosomes are degraded and lost, and, finally, the whole cell lyses.

At bacteriostatic concentrations, granaticin preferentially inhibits the synthesis of RNA. This effect could not be reversed by the addition of nucleic acids to the culture medium. There was no evidence that granaticin binds to DNA. Granaticin does not cosediment with DNA during ultracentrifugation. The absorption spectrum of granaticin is not changed by the addition of DNA, nor does treatment of *Bacillus subtilis* W 23 with different doses of granaticin affect the transforming activity of the DNA.

A concentration of 0.2 μg/ml granaticin inhibits RNA synthesis in *B. subtilis* nearly totally and DNA synthesis to about 40%, whereas protein synthesis proceeds nearly unaffected for about 20 min. This inhibitory effect on RNA and DNA synthesis decreases on further incubation, and thus is reversible. Similar effects on nucleic acid and protein synthesis can be observed by using quinones of different structures: e.g. the mitomycin derivatives, quinolin quinones, and naphthoquinones. The striking phenomenon is the uncoupling effect of quinones on RNA and protein synthesis at concentrations which, in the case of granaticin, did not affect the respiration of *B. subtilis*.

Granaticin and also other quinones inhibit the synthesis of all types of RNA equally well.[14] The decreased rate of incorporation of radioactive precursors into RNA is not caused by an increased degradation of RNA by RNase, because the activity of RNase in treated cells decreases. Furthermore, when *B. subtilis* cultures were first labeled for 1.5 min with ^{14}C uracil and then treated with the quinones for 15 min, considerable amounts of radioactivity were found within the ribosomal and polysomal fractions. This shows that stable mRNA occurs in the presence of granaticin and other quinones.

To elucidate further the mechanism by which granaticin and synthetic quinolin- or naphthoquinones interfere with RNA synthesis, comparative studies were made with a naphthoquinone-containing antibiotic naphthomycin. The effect of this antibiotic can be antagonized by vitamin K or by cysteine.[15]

The inhibitory effect of granaticin and some other quinones on growth and RNA synthesis in microorganisms could be reversed by cysteine, but not by vitamin K. Our current concept on the mechanism of quinone action is that quinones of different structure might interact with different SH-containing proteins and thus interfere with different steps of cell metabolism. Those quinones which cause the stabilization of polysomes might interfere with an SH-containing protein involved in the regulation of RNA and protein synthesis. Further experiments are in progress along this line to probe this hypothesis. Since several quinone-containing drugs are used in chemotherapy, especially in the treatment for cancer, hopefully other quinones with high specificity against certain proteins will be found which can be used for chemotherapy. The advantage of the quinone inhibitors described here is that DNA itself is not the target molecule, and that the effect of nucleic synthesis, especially on RNA synthesis, is reversible.

References

1. Fey, G., and H. Kersten: Hoppe Seyler's Z. Physiol. Chem., 351:111, 1970.
2. Kersten, W., H. Kersten, and W. Szybalski: Biochemistry, 5:236, 1965.
3. Hartman, G., K. O. Honikel, F. Knüsel, and J. Nuesch: Biochim. Biophys. Acta, 145:843, 1967.
4. Umezawa, H., S. Mizuno, H. Yamazaki, and K. Nitta: J. Antibiot., 21:234, 1968.
5. Wehrli, W., F. Knüsel, K. Schmid, and M. Staehelin: Proc. Nat. Acad. Sci. USA, 61:667, 1968.
6. Mizuno, S., H. Yamazaki, K. Nitta, and H. Umezawa: Biochim. Biophys. Acta, 157:322, 1968.
7. Schleif, R.: Nature, 223:1068, 1969.
8. Seifart, K. H., and C. E. Sekeris: Z. Naturforsch., 24B:1538, 1969.
9. Novello, F., L. Fiume, and F. Stirpe: Biochem. J., 116:177, 1970.
10. Kedinger, C., M. Gniazdowski, J. L. Mandel, Jr., F. Gissinger, and P. Chambon: Biochem. Biophys. Res. Commun., 38:165, 1970.
11. Jacob, S. T., E. M. Sajdel, and H. N. Munro: Nature, 225:60, 1970.
12. Kersten, H., and W. Kersten: In: Inhibitors, Tools in Cell Research. (Th. Bücher and H. Sies, eds.), Springer, New York, 1969.
13. Grundmann, E., L. Jühling, J. Pütter, and H. J. Seidel: Z. Krebsforsch., 72:185, 1969.
14. Kersten, W., H. Kersten, H. Wanke, and A. Ogilvie: Zentralbl. Bakteriol., 212:259, 1970.
15. Balerna, M., W. Keller-Schierlein, C. Martius, H. Wolf, and H. Zähner: Arch. Mikrobiol., 65:303, 1969.

Modification of Gene Expression:
Sustained Remission of Choriocarcinoma

JOHN L. LEWIS, JR., M.D.

Gynecology Service, Memorial Hospital for Cancer and Allied Diseases,
New York, New York, USA

THE PURPOSE OF including this clinical presentation on gestational choriocarcinoma in a session of the Congress devoted to regulation of gene expression is related to a simple but important development: Metastatic gestational choriocarcinoma is curable with chemotherapeutic agents.

This successful treatment for a metastatic cancer in human beings has led to this interesting but ambiguous inclusion in this session. Whereas most of the previous presentations have dealt with studies of gene expression and regulation in normal or neoplastic cells with the goal of attaining knowledge which could lead to a rational approach to cancer therapy, in this paper we will discuss a malignant condition in which the therapeutic goal has been reached, and we must try to determine why.

Since the first report of sustained remissions in patients with metastatic gestational trophoblastic disease receiving methotrexate,[1] it has been shown that therapy with several chemotherapeutic agents can produce complete tumor regression in about three fourths of all patients and that these remissions last many years without further therapy.[2-10] From the experience of Dr. Hertz and his co-workers in Bethesda, it has been calculated that the chances of recurrence after a year of complete remission is less than 1%.

This has been a dramatic change in the clinical course of patients with metastatic gestational choriocarcinoma, for prior to this development most patients with this condition would be dead within a year.

It is appropriate to concentrate on this chemotherapeutic success and to study the disease in which it has taken place in an effort to see what lessons can be learned from this model which might be useful for other malignant diseases in man. Because the tumor is extremely rare in other species and cannot be reliably produced in experimental animals, the observations must be limited to those made in human beings and in heterotransplantation and tissue culture studies.

Aside from the virtually unique responsiveness of this tumor to chemotherapy, there are two other aspects which make it unlike other malignant conditions in human beings. The first is that it arises during pregnancy in a tissue which is fetal in origin, namely, the trophoblastic layer of the placenta. The other unusual characteristic is that when it grows it makes a hormonal substance, human chorionic gonadotropin (HCG), and makes it so consistently that measurements of this hormone are a reliable guide not only for diagnosing the condition but for determining response to therapy. As a manner of organization, we will discuss these three aspects separately.

The responsiveness of gestational choriocarcinoma to methotrexate,[1-3, 5, 6, 8, 10] actinomycin D,[3, 4, 6, 10] 6-mercaptopurine,[5, 7] vincaleukoblastine,[3] 16-diazo-5-oxo-L-norleucine,[9] and other agents has been well documented. When the folic acid antagonist, methotrexate, was the only agent which had produced such responses, this unique response was thought to be caused by the very high folic acid requirements of the normal trophoblastic tissue from which it arose. However, that other agents with different modes of action could also produce remissions made this explanation incomplete.

Hertz[2] has reported that there is early evidence of tumor response to methotrexate in virtually all patients, but that approximately half of the tumors will develop resistance to this drug even though normal tissues retain sensitivity. This induced resistance has no crossover with the other agents which can subsequently be given effectively. Although there is evidence of methotrexate resistance being attributable to cell permeability[11] and induction of folic reductase,[12] there are no reports of such studies in human choriocarcinoma. This area of investigation seems germane to the subject of this conference. Whether this apparent development of resistance is caused by changes in tumor cells or selection of a clone of cells which have been resistant from the start is not established.

An interesting observation made in the National Institute of Health series was that the factors which were related prognostically to a patient's response to therapy were site of metastases, duration of disease prior to onset of chemotherapy, and the level of HCG titer when therapy was begun.[10] Patients who were treated within four months of the onset of disease and whose urinary HCG excretion was less than 100,000 IU/24 hr had a 94% likelihood of having a complete remission. Conversely, those patients whose disease had been present longer than four months before therapy was begun and in whom the HCG excretion was higher than this level had only a 36% complete remission rate. The observation that chemotherapy is more effective in those patients receiving it early, even when corrected for the apparent amount of tumor, raises the question of the mechanism accounting for this difference. Whether this represents a change in the tumor or represents a form of immunologic tolerance is unknown.

In regard to the second unusual characteristic of human trophoblastic tumors, it must be conceded that they are not unique in producing a circulating substance which can be measured as an index of tumor growth. The unusual aspect is that the production of other substances made in normal placental trophoblastic tissue (human placental lactogen, placental alkaline phosphatase, aminopeptidases, diamine oxidase, and others) falls off progressively when measured in the spectrum of benign to malignant hydatidiform moles and finally choriocarcinoma. In other words, the more neoplastic the change in trophoblastic tissue, the less these substances are produced, with the unique exception of HCG. That there is a spectrum of neoplastic change in gestational trophoblastic neoplasms has been shown by histologic studies,[13] chromosome counts[14] and nuclear DNA studies.[15] The significant observation is that in spite of these rather marked differences, the ability to produce HCG remains intact. This ability is still present when the tissue is grown in heterologous animal hosts[16–18] or in tissue culture.[19] Careful measurement of HCG is essential for determining the presence of tumor and its response to a given dose of a chemotherapeutic agent.

It is not yet clear if the HCG made by normal placental tissue and trophoblastic neoplasms is identical. Early work showed that gonadotropin activity was carried in different serum fractions in pregnant women than in women with trophoblastic neoplasms,[20] but efforts to show differences by Ouchterlony techniques have not been successful.[21] Another bit of evidence of heterogeneity has been the observation of a discrepancy of biologic to immunologic activity of HCG obtained from trophoblastic disease patients when compared with HCG from normal pregnancies.[22] The structure of this glycoprotein has not yet been determined, so it is unlikely that the question will be answered until this has been done.

The final area of discussion related to unique aspects of gestational choriocarcinoma is the fact that it arises in a tissue which is not identical in genetic constitution with the host, the fetal placenta. Being fetal in origin, the placenta gets half of its genetic material from the father and half from the mother. To the extent that the paternal contribution carries genes for transplantation antigens not present in the mother, there is the possibility of an immune response to the tumor based on differences in somatic antigens rather than just a response to postulated new tumor-associated transplantation antigens. This makes choriocarcinoma unique in its immunologic relation to the host, but it is not clear that this relation accounts in any way for the tumor's virtually unique responsiveness to chemotherapy.

References

1. Li, M. C., R. Hertz, and D. B. Spencer: Effect of methotrexate therapy upon choriocarcinoma and chorioadenoma. Proc. Soc. Exp. Biol. Med., 93:361-366, 1956.
2. Hertz, R., J. Lewis, Jr., and M. B. Lipsett: Five years' experience with the chemotherapy of metastatic choriocarcinoma and related trophoblastic tumors in women. Amer. J. Obstet. Gynecol., 82:631-640, 1961.

3. Ross, G. T., C. B. Hammond, R. Hertz, M. B. Lipsett, and W. D. Odell: Chemotherapy of metastatic and non-metastatic gestational trophoblastic neoplasms. Texas Rep. Biol. Med., (Suppl.) 24:326-338, 1966.
4. Li, M. C.: Management of choriocarcinoma and related tumors of uterus and testis. Med. Clin. N. Amer., 45:661-676, 1961.
5. Bagshawe, K. D.: Trophoblastic tumours. Chemotherapy and developments. Brit. Med. J., 2:1303-1307, 1963.
6. Brewer, J. I., A. B. Gerbie, R. E. Dolkart, J. H. Skom, R. G. Nagle, and E. E. Torok: Chemotherapy in trophoblastic diseases. Amer. J. Obstet. Gynecol., 90:566-578, 1964.
7. Sung, H. C., T. C. Wu, and T. H. Ho: Treatment of choriocarcinoma and chorioadenoma destruens with 6-mercaptopurine and surgery. Acta Unio Int. Cancr., 20:493-502, 1964.
8. Manahan, C. P., G. Manuel-Limson, and R. Abad: Experience with choriocarcinoma in the Philippines. Ann. N. Y. Acad. Sci., 114:875-880, 1964.
9. Karnofsky, D. A., R. B. Golbey, and M. C. Li: Remissions induced in patients with trophoblastic tumors by 6-diazo-5-oxo-L-norleucine (D.O.N.) . In: Choriocarcinoma, U.I.C.C., Monograph Series (J. F. Holland, and M. M. Hreshchyshyn, eds.) , Springer-Verlag, Berlin and New York, Vol. 3, 1967.
10. Ross, G. T., D. P. Goldstein, R. Hertz, M. B. Lipsett, and W. D. Odell: Sequential use of methotrexate and actinomycin D in the treatment of metastatic choriocarcinoma and related trophoblastic diseases in women. Amer. J. Obstet. Gynecol., 93:223-229, 1965.
11. Werkheiser, W. C.: The biochemical, cellular and pharmacological action and effects of the folic acid antagonists. Cancer Res., 23:1277-1285, 1963.
12. Bertino, J. R.: The mechanism of action of folic acid antagonists in man. Cancer Res., 23:1286-1306, 1963.
13. Hertig, A .T., and W. H. Sheldon: Hydatidiform mole—a pathologico-clinical correlation of 200 cases. Amer. J. Obstet. Gynecol., 53:1-36, 1947.
14. Makino, S., M. S. Sasaki, and T. Fushima: Preliminary notes on the chromosomes of human chorionic lesions. Proc. Jap. Acad., 39:54-58, 1963.
15. Goldfarb, S., R. M. Richart, and T. Okagaki: A cytophotometric study of nuclear DNA content of cyto and syncytiotrophoblast in trophoblastic diseases. Cancer. In press.
16. Hertz, R.: Choriocarcinoma in women maintained in serial passage in hamster and rat. Proc. Soc. Exp. Biol. Med., 102:77-81, 1959.
17. Pierce, G. B., Jr., A. R. Midgley, Jr., and E. L. Verney: Therapy of heterotransplanted choriocarcinoma. Cancer Res., 22:563-567, 1962.
18. Lewis, J. L., Jr., R. C. Davis, and G. T. Ross: Hormonal, immunologic and chemotherapeutic studies of transplantable human choriocarcinoma. Amer. J. Obstet. Gynecol., 104:472-478, 1969.
19. Patillo, R., G. O. Gey, E. Delfs, and R. F. Mattingly: Human hormone production in vitro. Science, 159:1467-1469, 1968.
20. Reisfeld, R. A., D. M. Bergenstal, and R. Hertz: Distribution of gonadotropic hormone activity in the serum proteins of normal pregnant women and patients with trophoblastic tumors. Arch. Biochem. Biophys., 81:456-463, 1959.
21. Lewis, J., Jr., S. Dray, S. Genuth, and H. S. Schwartz: Demonstration of immunological similarities of human pregnancy gonadotropin and choriocarcinoma gonadotropin with antisera prepared in rabbits and monkeys. J. Clin. Endocrinol., 24:197-204, 1964.
22. Wide, L., and B. Hobson: Immunological and biological activity of human chorionic gonadotropin in urine and serum of pregnant women and women with a hydatidiform mole. Acta Endocrinol., 54:105-112, 1967.

20

Replication and Persistence of the RNA Oncogenic Viruses

Historical Perspectives: Avian Tumor Viruses

H. RUBIN

Virus Laboratory and Department of Molecular Biology,
University of California, Berkeley, Berkeley, California, USA

IN A BOOK PUBLISHED in 1931 entitled *The Cause of Cancer*,[1] Gye and Purdy remarked on the commonly encountered difficulty of isolating infectious virus from chicken tumors initiated by the Rous sarcoma virus (RSV). This problem was systematically investigated by Carr in 1943, who found that the amount of virus which could be obtained from Rous sarcomas decreased as the tumors grew older, and concluded that the disappearance of the virus was the result of an immunologic reaction by the host.[2] Similar findings were made by Duran-Reynals[3] and by Rauscher and Groupé,[4] who drew the same conclusion from their data. I confirmed these observations in 1962 using the quantitative focus assay for RSV in tissue culture.[5] The importance of the immunologic response of the host in causing disappearance of RSV from tumors was further confirmed by the finding that tumors in chickens rendered immunologically tolerant to the envelope antigens of RSV always yielded high concentrations of RSV regardless of how old they were. I also showed that the disappearance of virus from tumors was linked to the regression of the tumors (which did not occur in the tolerant chickens), and was caused chiefly by an attack by immune lymphocytes on the tumor cells themselves, rather than by neutralization of virus by circulating antibody.

A novel aspect of the problem was introduced in 1955 by Bryan's observation that tumors induced with very low concentrations of

RSV often yielded no virus whatever.[6] Unlike tumors induced with high concentrations of virus, these were more likely to be noninfective when the tumor first appeared than later in its development, making it most unlikely that an immune response was responsible for the absence of virus.[7] The true explanation for this only became apparent when it was discovered that the Bryan strain of RSV could not code for the production of fully infectious particles unless a helper virus was present.[8] The helper virus had to be a member of the avian leukosis group of viruses, and was found in high concentrations in the Bryan RSV stock. Only when very small amounts of RSV were injected could the situation arise in which no helper virus was included in the inoculum. In such a case, the RSV particle could initiate a tumor, but the new virus particles which emerged were incapable of infecting other cells from that strain of chicken, and therefore the tumors appeared to contain no virus. The persistence of the RSV genome in these tumors could be easily demonstrated by adding a helper virus, which would be followed by the production of large quantities of RSV fully infectious for most strains of chickens.[7]

With the discovery of the apparent defectiveness of the Bryan strain of RSV, the analysis of the persistence of RSV in cells initially transformed by the virus moved almost wholly into the area of tissue culture investigation. There it was found that the apparently defective Bryan RSV actually did produce new particles without a helper virus,[9, 10] but that these particles were only infectious for Japanese quail and for certain uncommon lines of chickens,[11] and even then only with a low efficiency. The picture has become more complex recently with the finding of some RSV variants which produce no new particles, either infectious or otherwise, after they transform cells.[12] All of the indications we have are, however, that the RSV genome persists and multiplies in all the transformed cells.

Another dimension of the problem of persistence of the virus arose when tumors were produced in mammals by infection with certain strains of RSV. Most of the mammalian tumors fail to yield infectious particles. I shall not discuss this aspect of the problem, since it goes beyond the scope of my time and my familiarity. Suffice it to say that the RSV genome can be detected in mammalian cells by fusing them with chicken cells, whereupon infectious viral progeny appear.

In summary then, there appears to be general agreement that the genome of the virus persists in cells transformed by RSV, and it seems likely that its continued presence is required for the expression of the characteristic malignant properties of Rous sarcoma cells. Where infectious virus cannot be detected, its absence can be explained by the immune reaction of the chicken, the defectiveness of the virus, or the foreign nature of the mammalian cell.

We turn now to a related problem in which the areas of general agreement are more restricted. These problems concern the replicative process of the avian tumor viruses as exemplified by RSV, and, in particular, the special nature of their relationship to the host cell.

From the very beginning of modern tissue culture work with RSV, attention was drawn to some similarities to the temperate bacteriophages, which cause the lysogenic state to be established in bacteria.[13] These similarities were: (1) the perpetuation and multiplication of the viral genome through many host cell generations without causing death of the host cell; (2) the relatively low rate of virus production in populations of cells infected by the virus; and (3) the initiation of hereditary changes in the host cell's appearance and behavior as a result of infection. There were, however, some striking differences between the avian tumor viruses and temperate bacteriophages. The most prominent of these is that the avian tumor viruses contain RNA instead of DNA,[14] which lends complexity to any scheme associating the genome of the virus with the genome of the cell. Then, my own early investigation revealed that, under proper conditions, all of the RSV-infected cells were continuously releasing virus while continuing to multiply. This is, of course, in marked contrast to the lysogenic state in which vegetative multiplication of the phage inevitably leads to lysis of the host, and raises the problem of how the RSV genome could be integrated into that of the host cell and at the same time be continuously producing large numbers of infectious particles. There was the further problem that all cells infected with RSV become transformed while the supposedly analogous transduction by temperate bacteriophages occurs at an extremely low frequency. Furthermore, RSV can transform the cells of wholly unrelated species (indeed, even different orders of animals, i.e., birds and mammals), whereas temperate phages are relatively restricted in host range since they must find a specific sequence of nucleotides in DNA with which to recombine.

In the late 1950's and early 1960's there occurred a series of findings which made the lysogeny model again appealing. Temin and I found that unusually small amounts of radiation sufficed to inactivate the capacity of chicken cells to support the early stages of infection with RSV,[15] implying that replication of the host DNA was necessary for infection to be established. Then Temin discovered that chemical inhibitors of DNA-dependent RNA synthesis and of DNA synthesis interfered with the early stages of RSV infection.[16] He also found that infection of chicken cells with low multiplicities of RSV caused a cell transformation which was not accompanied by infectious virus production, and concluded that this was analogous to the integrated state found in lysogeny.[17] This conclusion appeared to be confirmed by his report that the RNA of RSV annealed preferentially to the DNA of RSV-infected chicken cells.[18] From these findings, Temin built a model of infection in which the RNA of RSV is transcribed into DNA (reversing the normal flow of information) which is integrated into the host cell.

There are, however, a number of difficulties with this model. The x-ray inactivation of host cell capacity to support virus multiplication can be overcome by infecting the cells with a high multiplicity of RSV.[19] It remains to be seen what effect high multiplicity infection has on infection in the presence of chemical inhibitors of DNA and RNA infection. The susceptibility of RSV infection to inhibitors of DNA-dependent RNA synthesis is not restricted to tumor viruses. Even poliovirus infection can be inhibited by actinomycin if serum is omitted from the medium.[20] The annealing of RSV-RNA to DNA was found not to be at all specific for infected chicken cells. Indeed, recently, it has been found that RSV-RNA combines as well with plant cell DNA as with Rous sarcoma cell DNA.[21] Furthermore, I have found that the avian leukosis viruses are not transmitted by the sperm, but are transmitted by the egg.[22] Such strict maternal inheritance is classically interpreted as evidence for cytoplasmic factor.

At present the lysogeny interpretation rests on the inhibitor data. There are alternative explanations for these data. It could be, for example, that some host cell function, or even some host cell state, is needed to establish RSV infection, and these are dependent on DNA and RNA synthesis. Alternatively, it is known that these inhibitors cause a marked increase in the soluble nucleases of cells.[23] Since the RNA of RSV is a remarkably unstable molecule (or group of molecules),[24] it may be uniquely vulnerable to increased levels of nucleases.

Whatever the explanation, the problem must be considered unresolved for the present. Recent reports engender optimism about unraveling the replicative scheme. It has been claimed that RNA-dependent RNA replicase[25] as well as double-stranded, replicative intermediates[26] have been isolated from cells infected with RNA tumor viruses. If these claims are substantiated, they will put the RNA tumor viruses into the same replicative schemes as other RNA viruses. This would not, of course, solve the problem of how they cause tumors.

Now that I have accomplished my assigned mission of providing historical perspectives on RNA tumor virus replication in less than 1,500 words, I shall say a few words about the physiologic effects of RSV multiplication on the cells infected by the virus and the normal cells surrounding them. I have shown that cells infected with the Bryan strain of RSV release a substance called "overgrowth stimulating factor" (OSF) which causes normal cells in culture to overcome density-dependent inhibition of growth.[27] OSF can be separated from the virus itself. It is nondialyzable, precipitable by high salt concentrations, and heat labile. It appears in the tissue culture medium of newly infected cells a few days after they undergo the malignant transformation. Material with similar properties can be released from normal cells by disrupting them with sonic oscillation. This cell-associated OSF increases within RSV-infected cells in parallel with the malignant transformation. OSF is a logical candidate for the substance which evokes the blood supply for the tumor and the stromal reaction surrounding the tumor. Its role in perpetuating the growth of the tumor cell itself must also be considered.

Acknowledgment

This investigation was supported by U. S. Public Health Service Research Grant CA 05619 from the National Cancer Institute.

References

1. Gye, W. E., and W. J. Purdy: The Cause of Cancer. Cassell and Co., Ltd., London, England, 1931, 515 pp.
2. Carr, J. G.: The relation between age, structure and agent content of Rous No. 1 sarcomas. Brit. J. Exp. Pathol., 24:133-137, 1943.
3. Duran-Reynals, F., and P. M. Freire: The age of tumor-bearing hosts as a factor conditioning the transmissibility of the Rous sarcoma by filtrates and cells. Cancer Res., 13:376-382, 1953.
4. Rauscher, F., and V. Groupé: Studies on non-infective tumors produced in turkeys by Rous sarcoma virus. J. Nat. Cancer Inst., 25:141-159, 1960.
5. Rubin, H.: The immunological basis for non-infective Rous sarcomas. Cold Spring Harbor Symp. Quant. Biol., 27:441-452, 1962.
6. Bryan, W. R., D. Calnan, and J. B. Moloney: Biological studies on the Rous sarcoma virus. III. The recovery of virus from experimental tumors in relation to initiating dose. J. Nat. Cancer Inst., 16:317-335, 1955.
7. Shimizu, T., and H. Rubin: The dual origin of non-infective Rous sarcomas. J. Nat. Cancer Inst., 33:79-91, 1964.
8. Hanafusa, H., T. Hanafusa, and H. Rubin: The defectiveness of Rous sarcoma virus. Proc. Nat. Acad. Sci. USA, 49:572-580, 1963.
9. Dougherty, R. M., and H. S. Di Stefano: Virus particles associated with "non-producer" Rous sarcoma cells. Virology, 27:351-359, 1965.
10. Robinson, H. Latham: Isolation of noninfectious particles containing Rous sarcoma virus RNA from the medium of Rous sarcoma virus-transformed nonproducer cells. Proc. Nat. Acad. Sci. USA, 57:1655-1662, 1967.
11. Vogt, P. K.: A virus released by "non-producing" Rous sarcoma cells. Proc. Nat. Acad. Sci. USA, 58:801-808, 1967.
    Weiss, R.: Spontaneous virus production from "non-virus producing" Rous sarcoma cells. Virology, 32:719-723, 1967.
12. Hanafusa, H., and T. Hanafusa: Further studies on RSV production from transformed cells. Virology, 34:630-636, 1968.
13. Rubin, H.: Quantitative relations between causative virus and cell in the Rous No. 1 chicken sarcoma. Virology, 1:445-473, 1955.
14. Robinson, W. S., A. Pitkanen, and H. Rubin: The nucleic acid of the Bryan strain of Rous sarcoma virus: Purification of the virus and isolation of the nucleic acid. Proc. Nat. Acad. Sci. USA, 54:137-144, 1965.
15. Rubin, H., and H. M. Temin: A radiological study of cell-virus interaction in the Rous sarcoma. Virology, 7:75-91, 1959.
16. Temin, H. M.: The effects of actinomycin D on growth of Rous sarcoma virus in vitro. Virology, 20:577-582, 1963.
17. Temin, H. M.: Separation of morphological conversion and virus production in Rous sarcoma virus infection. Cold Spring Harbor Symp. Quant. Biol., 27:407-414, 1962.
18. Temin, H. M.: Homology between RNA from Rous sarcoma virus and DNA from Rous sarcoma virus-infected cells. Proc. Nat. Acad. Sci. USA, 52:323-329, 1964.

19. Rubin, H.: Growth of Rous sarcoma virus in chick embryo cells following irradiation of host cells or free virus. Virology, 11:28-47, 1960.
20. Cooper, P. D.: The inhibition of poliovirus growth by actinomycin D and the prevention of the inhibition by pretreatment of the cells with serum or insulin. Virology, 28:663-678, 1966.
21. Yoshikawa-Fukada, M., and J. D. Ebert: Hybridization of RNA from Rous sarcoma virus with cellular and viral DNA's. Proc. Nat. Acad. Sci. USA, 64:870-877, 1969.
22. Rubin, H., L. Fanshier, A. Cornelius, and W. F. Hughes: Tolerance and immunity in chickens after congenital and contact infection with an avian leukosis virus. Virology, 17:143-156, 1962.
23. Erbe, W., J. Preiss, R. Seifert, and H. Hilz: Increase in RNase and DPNase activities in ascites tumor cells induced by various cytostatic agents. Biochem. Biophys. Res. Commun., 23:392-397, 1966.
24. Duesberg, P. H.: Physical properties of Rous sarcoma virus RNA. Proc. Nat. Acad. Sci. USA, 60:1511-1518, 1968.
25. Watson, K. F., and G. S. Beaudreau: Isolation of RNA-dependent RNA polymerase from virus infected myeloblasts. Biochem. Biophys. Res. Commun., 37:925-932, 1969.
26. Biswal, N., and M. Benyesh-Melnick: Complementary nuclear RNA's of murine sarcoma-leukemia virus complex in transformed cells. Proc. Nat. Acad. Sci. USA, 64:1372-1379, 1969.
27. Rubin, H.: Overgrowth stimulating factor released from Rous sarcoma cells. Science, 167:1271-1272, 1970.

Avian Sarcoma Virus: Interaction with a Genetic Factor Present in Normal Cells

HIDESABURO HANAFUSA

*Public Health Research Institute of The City of New York, Inc.,
New York, New York, USA*

STUDIES ON CERTAIN characteristics of avian tumor viruses in the past years have allowed us to classify these viruses into several subgroups according to the properties of their envelopes.[1] Knowledge of these properties and the genetic susceptibility of host cells to these viruses is now a prerequisite in studies on the multiplication of this class of viruses. In addition, since the virus host range is determined by its envelope,[2,3] the interaction of two viruses within the cells leading to the exchange of their envelopes should be taken into consideration in systems where multiplication of two viruses is involved. Although the exchange of envelopes can take place with any combination of viruses,[4] the interaction between the Bryan strain of Rous sarcoma virus (RSV) and avian leukosis virus (ALV) has drawn particular attention, because this strain of RSV made in the absence of ALV is not infectious for most chick embryo cells whereas the exchanged form, RSV (ALV), is infectious.[5] When RSV progeny were found to be produced by transformed cells even in the absence of ALV,[6-10] this virus particle was named RSV (O) to indicate that its envelope is not specified by ALV.[9] Unlike other avian leukosis-sarcoma viruses, RSV (O) had a unique, limited host range for avian cells, but it seemed to multiply by itself in susceptible cells.[9, 10] Thus, one might consider this form a prototype of Bryan RSV with the envelope made by itself.

However, recent studies in our laboratory[11, 12] indicate that such infectious RSV (O) is produced only from certain types of cells which are apparently free of complete virus but which contain genetic material similar to this group of viruses in its function. In other cells, in which the genetic material probably does not exist or its function is totally suppressed, infection with the Bryan strain of RSV results in formation of noninfectious particles.[11, 13] While the possible existence of a cryptic or hidden form of viral genetic material in apparently uninfected normal cells has been suggested by Huebner and Todaro,[14] this would be the first demonstration of this type of agent in avian cells. Therefore, I will present briefly evidence for its presence in chick cells and its nature.

When transformed by RSV (β type), chick cells derived from C/O type embryos, which constitute about 80% of the total embryos studied, produced infectious RSV (O). Cultures derived from the remaining 20% of the embryos, called C/O' type, produced noninfectious RSV. In this system, formation of infectious virus was determined solely by the type of host cell: noninfectious RSV formed in C/O' cells was capable of transforming both C/O and C/O' cells when inoculated into cultures with UV-inactivated Sendai virus, a known fusion agent. The resulting transformants of each cell type produced either infectious or noninfectious particles, respectively.[11] Therefore, superficially, this phenomenon could be regarded as an example of host-controlled modification of virus. However, it became apparent that host-controlled modification was not a proper explanation of the change in RSV, when formation of RSV was thoroughly studied in a special subtype of C/O' cells which were susceptible to RSV (O) and therefore allowed infection with RSV (O) in a higher proportion of cells than that achieved by infection of RSV (O)-resistant C/O' cells with RSV (O) in the presence of UV-Sendai virus.

This RSV (O)-susceptible C/O' type of cells produced noninfectious RSV when infected with low doses of RSV (O), but produced infectious RSV (O) when infected with high doses of RSV (O). This multiplicity effect could be explained if one assumed that the infecting RSV (O) grown in the C/O cells had picked up a viruslike agent in the C/O cells, and that the virus carrying this agent would be the minority in the population, so that only infection with high doses of RSV (O) made it possible for this virus to enter the cells and act as a helper for the majority of RSV (O) which cannot reproduce infectious RSV in C/O' cells. If this explanation is correct, one may expect that the genetic material responsible for RSV (O) replication may also be carried by ALV and be transmitted from C/O to C/O' cells. Experiments proved that this is the case: ALV grown in C/O cells was able to form infectious RSV (O) in addition to RSV (ALV), in C/O' cells transformed by a low dose of RSV, whereas ALV grown in C/O' cells lacked this ability. ALV grown in C/O cells was also shown to contain particles whose host range and antigenicity are identical to that of RSV (O).

The above hypothesis gained further support from the finding of an antigen indistinguishable from the internal group-specific antigen of avian tumor viruses in normal C/O cells but not in C/O' cells.[15] Moreover, a viral envelope antigen of RSV (O) specificity was found in C/O cells.[16] Despite the presence of these antigens, an extensive search for mature virus particles has been unsuccessful. These observations strongly indicate that C/O type cells, though being free of virus, carry a genetic factor which is similar to the avian tumor viruses in the function of synthesizing both envelope and group-specific (GS) antigen of the virus and in acting as a helper for the formation of infectious RSV (O). Apparently infection of C/O cells with RSV or ALV activates the genetic factor to a transmissible form either by incorporation into these viruses or by maturation into a complete virus. Tentatively, we have designated this genetic material in C/O cells as a "chick cell-associated helper factor" (CHF).[12]

One of the intriguing aspects of CHF is its intracellular state. Presence of GS antigen in certain normal chick cells correlates very well with the presence of CHF. It appears, therefore, that the genetic information for CHF is linked to that of GS antigen in the cells, or the gene for the GS antigen is derepressed by CHF. Based on genetic studies with chickens positive and negative for the GS antigen, Payne and Chubb[17] have presented evidence that the GS antigen is an expression of a cellular gene inherited by offspring in a Mendelian manner. If this is applicable to the chick cells used in the studies on CHF, then one may assume that the genetic information of CHF also resides on the cellular chromosomes. Thus, the existence of the genetic factor in apparently normal cells not only provides a satisfactory explanation for the formation of infectious RSV (O), but may also offer a new tool in studies on the interaction of RNA tumor virus with host cells.

References

1. Vogt, P. K.: Adv. Virus Res., 11:293, 1965.
2. Hanafusa, H.: Virology, 25:248, 1965.
3. Vogt, P. K.: Virology, 25:237, 1965.

4. Hanafusa, H., and T. Hanafusa: Proc. Nat. Acad. Sci. USA, 55:532, 1966.
5. Hanafusa, H., T. Hanafusa, and H. Rubin: Proc. Nat. Acad. Sci. USA, 49:572, 1963.
6. Dougherty, R. M., and H. DiStefano: Virology, 27:351, 1965.
7. Robinson, H. L.: Proc. Nat. Acad. Sci. USA, 57:1655, 1967.
8. Weiss, R.: Virology, 32:719, 1967.
9. Vogt, P. K.: Proc. Nat. Acad. Sci. USA, 58:801, 1967.
10. Hanafusa, H., and T. Hanafusa: Virology, 34:630, 1968.
11. Hanafusa, T., T. Miyamoto, and H. Hanafusa: Virology, 40:55, 1970.
12. Hanafusa, H., T. Miyamoto, and T. Hanafusa: Proc. Nat. Acad. Sci. USA, 66:314, 1970.
13. Weiss, R. A.: J. Gen. Virol., 5:511, 1969.
14. Huebner, R. J., and G. J. Todaro: Proc. Nat. Acad. Sci. USA, 64:1087, 1969.
15. Miyamoto, T., E. Fleissner, T. Hanafusa, and H. Hanafusa: Unpublished data.
16. Miyamoto, T., T. Hanafusa, and H. Hanafusa: Unpublished data.
17. Payne, L. N., and R. C. Chubb: J. Gen. Virol., 3:379, 1969.

Persistence and Replication of Murine Leukemia and Sarcoma Viruses

W. H. KIRSTEN AND S. PANEM

Division of Biological Sciences, The University of Chicago, Chicago, Illinois, USA

THIS DISCUSSION WILL be confined to the replication of mouse leukemia-sarcoma viruses, since these fundamental aspects of virus-cell interaction are poorly understood at the present time. The topic will be divided into replication of viral RNA and assembly of viral RNA and proteins into whole virions or their precursors. The "mature" types of mouse leukemia-sarcoma viruses are composed of an electron-dense nucleoid which is assumed to contain the viral RNA and an external lipoprotein envelope which is probably derived from the cell membrane.[1, 2] Certain structural proteins of mouse leukemia-sarcoma viruses can be assigned to either the nucleoid or the whole virion on the basis of distinct migration patterns in the polyacrylamide gels.[3]

Viral RNA

Certain facts should be recalled with regard to the replication of the viral RNA. Mouse leukemia-sarcoma viruses require intact cellular

DNA at the time of infection, and DNA-dependent RNA synthesis is necessary for continuous virus replication.[4, 5] Cellular DNA synthesis is required for the fixation of the transformed state by the mouse sarcoma virus group.[6, 7] The participation of DNA in the replication and transformation of mouse leukemia-sarcoma viruses is derived from experiments using metabolic inhibitors. More direct evidence for the role of cellular DNA in viral RNA replication has been sought by molecular hybridization experiments. Mouse leukemia viruses contain single-stranded, high molecular weight, aggregated (68 to 72S) RNA and a heterogenous, host-derived (4 to 20S) RNA.[8] Separation of the two RNA species is essential for meaningful hybridization results. We have not been able to detect complementarity between the 72S RNA of a mouse leukemia virus and the DNA from infected or uninfected cells.[8] In contrast, Harel et al.[9] have reported partial homology between RNA from Rauscher leukemia virus and cellular DNA. An average of 3.4% of input viral RNA was bound to mouse DNA and, to some extent, to chicken DNA as well. Recently, Biswal and Benyesh-Melnick[10] observed that RNA extracted from a murine leukemia-sarcoma virus is complementary with two heterogenous cellular RNA species (18 to 22S and 31 to 36S). Heated, extracellular viral RNA with sedimentation coefficients of 37S or less was used to detect the complementary strand in nuclear RNA which was isolated from the nuclei of rat embryo fibroblasts transformed by this virus. Approximately 30% of the input viral RNA hybridized with 50 μg of the nuclear RNA from transformed cells, but only 1 to 2% of viral RNA hybridized with cytoplasmic RNA of transformed cells. These findings, if confirmed, are significant in that the RNA synthetic site is being placed in the nucleus. In this context, one may ask whether viral RNA with S values of 36S or less can be isolated from mammalian cells infected with murine leukemia-sarcoma viruses. Recent studies in our laboratory suggest that this may be the case.

Cytoplasmic Virions

The substructure of a mouse leukemia virus after disruption of the envelope with Tween-ether and subsequent purification of the released nucleoids by density gradient centrifugation was first reported by de Thé and O'Connor.[2] The nonionic detergent nonidet P-40 (NP-40) proved a more suitable detergent in our work than Tween-ether. More than 50% of the label could be recovered from ^{3}H-uridine-labeled murine erythroblastosis virus (MEV) following centrifugation in potassium-citrate density gradients (10 to 50%, w/w).[3] Whole MEV harvested from the culture fluids of chronically infected mouse cells has a buoyant density of 1.135 to 1.16 g/cm^2, whereas MEV nucleoids band at a density range of 1.22 to 1.26 g/cm^2 in potassium-citrate. As judged from remaining acid-precipitable counts after enzyme incubation, MEV nucleoids were sensitive to digestion with pronase (0.1 mg/

ml for 30 min) but were resistant to treatment with lipase (1 mg/ml for 30 min) or RNase (10 μg/ml for 30 min). Cytoplasmic extracts were prepared from two mouse cell lines chronically infected with MEV by a method used by Kates and McAuslan[11] for the isolation of poxvirus cores. Gradient centrifugation of ^{3}H-uridine-labeled cytoplasmic extracts from MEV-infected cells consistently revealed acidprecipitable radioactivity in the density regions of whole MEV and MEV nucleoids. In contrast to polysomes or mitochondria from infected or uninfected cells, the radioactive virion and nucleoid peaks from the cytoplasmic extracts were insensitive to digestion with EDTA or RNase.[12] The RNA species extracted from the cytoplasmic density regions of whole MEV and MEV nucleoids revealed two peaks of radioactivity. One sedimented in sucrose velocity gradients at approximately 36S and the other at approximately 20 to 22S in reference to the ribosomal RNA marker. Both RNA peaks could be completely degraded by RNase. The high molecular weight 72S RNA was not detected in any of the cytoplasmic viral peaks, in contrast to the extracellular virions. It therefore appears that MEV RNA is replicated as smaller RNA molecules which are assembled into the virion. The aggregation of low molecular weight RNA to 72S RNA might occur after budding and may represent the molecular basis for the conversion of "immature" into "mature" virions.

FIG. 20–1.—Electrophoresis of proteins solubilized from ^{3}H-glucosamine-labeled MEV. EMS cells were labeled for 24 hr with ^{3}H-glucosamine (10 μc/ml). Culture fluids were clarified, concentrated, and purified by density gradient centrifugation. Lipids were removed from the purified virus by adding to the sample ⅓ volume of dimethylformamide:HCl and dialyzed against this solution for 3 hr. The dialysate was then treated from protein solubilization as samples of MEV labeled with ^{3}H-amino acids. The radioactive protein was electrophoresed on polyacrylamide gels for 17 hr at room temperature with constant voltage (4 volts/cm).

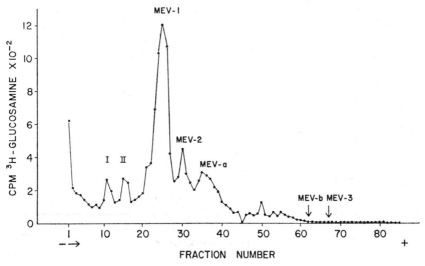

Viral Proteins

The structural proteins of mouse leukemia viruses have recently been analyzed by gel electrophoresis.[13, 14] We have shown that the proteins of MEV can be separated into profiles characteristic for whole virions and those recovered from MEV nucleoids.[3] As a continuation of this work, glucosylation patterns of MEV proteins obtained from extracellular and cytoplasmic virions and their nucleoids were studied. Figure 20-1 represents electropherograms of ^{3}H-glucosamine-labeled

FIG. 20–2.—Electrophoresis of proteins solubilized from cytoplasmic MEV and cytoplasmic MEV nucleoids. EMS cells were labeled for 24 hr with 10 μc/ml ^{3}H-glucosamine, and cytoplasmic extracts were prepared. The density regions of MEV and MEV nucleoids were collected following centrifugation on potassium citrate gradients. Proteins were solubilized and electrophoresed on 10% polyacrylamide gels at 4 volts/cm. A, proteins solubilized from the density region 1.14 to 1.16 gm/cm³. B, proteins solubilized from the density region 1.22 to 1.26 gm/cm³.

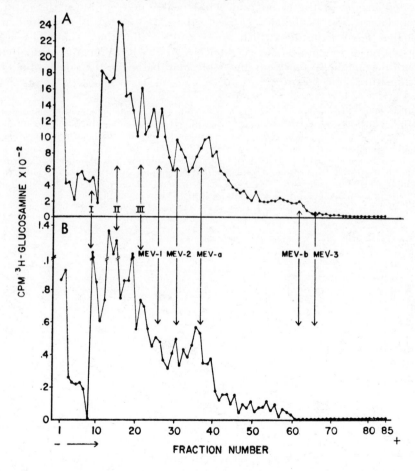

extracellular MEV. Proteins MEV-1, MEV-2, and MEV-a are glucosylated, but in addition, two small peaks of ^{3}H-glucosamine were present in the first quarter of the gel nearest the origin, referred to as proteins I and II. Certain differences became apparent (Figure 20-2) when the electropherograms of MEV proteins from extracellular virions were compared with structural proteins solubilized from cytoplasmic virions. Proteins I and II were more prominent than MEV-1 or MEV-2, and another protein peak (III) appeared in cytoplasmic protein profiles. It was also found that the molecular weight of protein I (95,000) was approximately the additive weight of MEV-1 (74,500) and MEV-3 (15,000) and that protein II (89,000) was the additive weight of MEV-2 (67,500) and MEV-b (19,500).

These data are consistent with the interpretation that cytoplasmic MEV and MEV nucleoids are part of the viral maturation complex. The proteins I and II can be interpreted as precursors of viral structural proteins with distinct glucosylation patterns. Accordingly, a maturation process is suggested: Protein I is cleaved into MEV-1 and MEV-3 and cleavage of protein II would result in MEV-2 and MEV-b. This hypothesis is derived from the ^{3}H-glucosamine-labeling of the proteins and their molecular weight estimates. There is precedence among both nononcogenic viruses for the production of viral structural proteins as larger precursor molecules which cleave into smaller structural proteins during virus assembly.[15] Further studies on the replication of mouse leukemia-sarcoma viruses are needed to answer the more challenging questions of mechanisms of transformation and persistence in transformed cells.

Acknowledgments

This investigation was supported by U. S. Public Health Service Grant CA-04311 and by a grant from the Leukemia Society of Illinois. S. P. was supported by U. S. Public Health Service Training Grant AI 00238. W. H. K. is a National Institutes of Health Career Development Awardee.

References

1. de Harven, E.: Ultrastructural studies on three different types of mouse leukemia; a review. In: Tumors Induced by Viruses: Ultrastructural Studies (A. J. Dalton and F. Haguenau, eds.), Academic Press, New York, 1962, pp. 183-204.
2. de Thé, G., and T. E. O'Connor: Structure of a murine leukemia virus after disruption with Tween-ether and comparison with two myxoviruses. Virology, 28: 713-728, 1966.
3. McDugald, L. V., S. Panem, and W. H. Kirsten: Structural proteins of murine erythroblastosis virus. Int. J. Cancer, 5:64-71, 1970.
4. Bases, R. E., and A. S. King: Inhibition of Rauscher leukemia virus growth by actinomycin D. Virology, 32:175-183, 1967.
5. Duesberg, P., and W. S. Robinson: Inhibition of mouse leukemia virus (MLV) replication by actinomycin D. Virology, 31:742-746, 1967.
6. Nakata, Y., and J. P. Bader: Transformation by murine sarcoma virus: Fixation (deoxyribonucleic acid synthesis) and development. J. Virol., 2:1255-1261, 1968.

7. Hirschman, S., P. J. Fischinger, J. J. Zaccari, and T. E. O'Connor: Effect of cytosine arabinoside on the replication of Moloney sarcoma virus in 3T3 cell cultures. J. Nat. Cancer Inst., 42:399-411, 1969.
8. Wollmann, R. L., and W. H. Kirsten: Cellular origin of a mouse leukemia viral ribonucleic acid. J. Virol., 2:1241-1248, 1968.
9. Harel, L., J. Harel, and J. Huppert: Partial homology between RNA from Rauscher mouse leukemia virus and cellular DNA. Biochem. Biophys. Res. Commun., 28:44-49, 1967.
10. Biswal, N., and M. Benyesh-Melnick: Complementary nuclear RNA's of murine sarcoma-leukemia complex in transformed cells. Proc. Nat. Acad. Sci. USA, 64:1372-1379, 1969.
11. Kates, J. R., and B. R. McAuslan: Poxvirus DNA-dependent RNA polymerase. Proc. Nat. Acad. Sci. USA, 58:134-141, 1967.
12. Attardi, B., B. Cravioto, and G. Attardi: Membrane bound ribosomes in HeLa cells. J. Mol. Biol., 44:47-70, 1969.
13. Duesberg, P. H., H. I. Robinson, W. S. Robinson, R. J. Huebner, and H. C. Turner: Proteins of Rous sarcoma virus. Virology, 36:73-86, 1968.
14. Franker, C. K., and M. Gruca: Structural protein of the Friend virion. Virology, 37:489-493, 1969.
15. Jacobson, M. F., and D. Baltimore: Polypeptide cleavages in the formation of poliovirus proteins. Proc. Nat. Acad. Sci. USA, 61:77-84, 1968.

The DNA Provirus of RNA Sarcoma Viruses

HOWARD M. TEMIN

McArdle Laboratory, University of Wisconsin, Madison, Wisconsin, USA

THE REPLICATION OF RNA sarcoma viruses and the related RNA leukemia viruses appears to differ from that of all other RNA viruses. Infection of a sensitive cell does not lead to cell death, but usually to conversion of the infected cell to a tumor cell. The information for cell conversion and for virus production (either after activation by cell division or fusion with cells permissive for virus production) is carried in the cell in a provirus. There are one or two proviruses per cell. At mitosis they are passed in a regular manner to daughter cells, probably along with the chromosomes.[8, 15] The provirus concept is in contradistinction to the concept of a pool of vegetative virus in an infected cell.[10]

The provirus carries information responsible for transformation.

TABLE 20–1

	at 34°	NUMBER OF FOCI After Shift From 34° to 40°	After Shift From 34° to 40° to 34°
a	45	1	159
b	420	1	170
c	46	7	100
d	>500	33	>200

Secondary cultures of chicken cells were exposed to a mutant stock of Schmidt-Ruppin virus and incubated at 34 C. When foci appeared they were counted, and the cultures were reincubated at 40 C. Two days later the number of foci were counted, the cultures reincubated at 34 C, and the number of foci counted. Foci induced by parental virus were not affected by temperature shifts.

This control is demonstrated most directly by the existence of a class of temperature-sensitive virus mutants which make foci at a permissive temperature which disappear when the cultures are shifted to a higher, nonpermissive temperature (Table 20-1).

The DNA provirus hypothesis states that the replication of RNA sarcoma viruses takes place through a DNA intermediate, rather than through an RNA intermediate as do other RNA viruses. This hypothesis is supported by the sensitivity to actinomycin D of virus production in virus-producing cells[2, 11] and by the results of hybridization studies with RNA from virions and DNA from infected cells.[1, 12]

The DNA provirus hypothesis states that a new virus-specific and virus-coded DNA is made in cells after infection. It is most convenient to study this new DNA synthesis in stationary cultures, since in these cultures normal cellular S-phase DNA synthesis does not occur. If cells in the G_1 stage of the cell cycle as a result of removal of serum[14] are exposed to RSV, they become infected, and provirus is formed. However, virus production and conversion do not occur unless serum is added and the cells divide. If DNA synthesis is blocked soon after exposure to virus, the cells do not become infected, and virus produc-

TABLE 20–2

INHIBITION OF SYNTHESIS OF PROTEIN*	DNA†	AVERAGE NUMBER OF FOCI PER CULTURE	VIRUS YIELD PER CULTURE 2 DAI‡
0	0	88	8.5×10^3
0-12 HAI‡	0	131	15×10^3
0	0-12 HAI	14	1.2×10^3
0	12-24 HAI	47	9×10^3
0-12 HAI	12-24 HAI	42	5×10^3

* Stationary cultures exposed to 0.5 μg/ml cycloheximide.
† Stationary cultures exposed to 5×10^{-5}M cytosine arabinoside
‡ Abbreviations: DAI, days after infection; HAI, hours after infection.

tion and conversion do not occur when serum is added and the cells divide (Table 20-2). Cells are not killed by the inhibition of DNA synthesis, since they are in the G_1 stage of the cell cycle.[7, 13]

David Boettiger, a student in my laboratory, decided it should be possible to label with 5-bromodeoxyuridine (BUdR) the new DNA made in the stationary cells after infection with RSV, and then inactivate the BUdR-labeled DNA by exposure to visible light. (Balduzzi and Morgan independently had the same idea.) The system he developed was as follows: Stationary cultures of chicken cells were exposed to virus, overlaid with medium containing BUdR and no serum, incubated overnight, and exposed to visible light. The cells were then placed in suspension with trypsin and plated on feeder cultures of rat cells in a medium containing serum. Foci developed from cells which contain an active provirus and are able to multiply. The results of a typical experiment show there is inactivation of focus formation by BUdR-treated cells. To distinguish between killing of cells and inactivation of the provirus, control experiments were performed (Table 20-3). It was found that the treatment with light did not cause killing of the stationary cells exposed to BUdR. However, cells exposed to BUdR during S phase DNA synthesis became very sensitive to light. The difference between the slopes of the inactivation curves further demonstrates that cells were not stimulated to DNA synthesis by infection and killed by exposure to light. The BUdR-containing structure which is inactivated by exposure to light could be a small region of the cell genome or could be DNA transcribed from the virus RNA. To distinguish between these alternatives, an experiment using two different multiplicities of infection was performed. The results show that an increased multiplicity of infection makes the ability of an infected cell to form a focus more resistant to inactivation by light and supports the idea that the BUdR-containing structure(s) is transcribed from the infecting viral genomes.

Dr. Satoshi Mizutani then investigated the source of the enzyme for this reverse RNA to DNA transcription. When stationary cultures were exposed to RSV and then overlaid with medium containing enough cycloheximide to inhibit 90% of amino acid incorporation, provirus formation was normal (Table 20-2). Therefore, the enzyme for the DNA synthesis probably was in existence before infection.

TABLE 20–3

| | TREATMENT OF STATIONARY CELLS | |
	BUdR	BUdR AND LIGHT
Relative percent cells capable of DNA synthesis	100	97
Relative percent cells capable of entering mitosis	100	100
Relative plating efficiency of cells infected after exposure to BUdR	100	88

Data from Boettiger and Temin.[3]

TABLE 20-4

System	DPM ³H-TTP Incorporated
Complete with disrupted virions	3032
—Virions	0
with nondisrupted virions	225
with disrupted normal cell supernatant	0
with disrupted virions pretreated with RNase	0
—dATP	369
—dGTP	833
—dCTP	1012
—Mg⁺⁺	0

The complete system contained in 0.125 ml phosphate buffer pH 7.5, deoxynucleotide triphosphates, $MgCl_2$, phosphoenolpyruvate and pyruvate kinase, 10^8 FFU of RSV (5 μg protein) and 2.5 μc of ³H-TTP (12 c/mmole). Acid-soluble counts were determined following incubation at 37 C for one hour.

Since reverse, RNA to DNA, transcription is not normally considered to occur in cells (but see Temin[15]) and polymerases have been found in virions of vaccinia and reovirus,[4–6, 9] we looked in the virion of RSV for an enzyme which could incorporate deoxynucleotide triphosphates using an RNA template. Dr. Mizutani purified Schmidt-Ruppin virus from supernatants of converted cells by differential centrifugation followed by density gradient centrifugation. The virus was disrupted with detergent treatment, mixed with deoxynucleotide triphosphates and labeled TTP, and incubated at 37°, and acid-insoluble counts were measured. TTP was incorporated into an acid-insoluble form. However, if the virus was heated to 80° for 10 min before the incubation, no incorporation was found. Some further characteristics of the system are seen in Table 20-4. Virus must be disrupted to get full activity. Full incorporation is dependent upon the presence of all four deoxyribonucleotide triphosphates. (The partial activity remaining is probably a result of deoxynucleotide triphosphates in the virions. It is known that small molecular weight RNA is trapped in that fashion.[16]) No activity is found in supernatants of normal cells. And most important, the incorporation is completely destroyed by preincubation with RNase (free of active DNase). The results demonstrate that virions of RSV contain an internal enzyme activity that catalyzes the incorporation of deoxyribonucleotide triphosphates into an acid-insoluble structure, and RNase destroys this activity. The simplest interpretation of these results is that there is a new polymerase in virions of RNA sarcoma viruses that forms DNA from an RNA template. If this interpretation is supported by further experiments, it would strongly support the DNA provirus hypothesis that in RNA sarcoma viruses there is transfer of information from RNA to DNA. It would also suggest that this type of information transfer might be operative in other biologic systems.

Acknowledgments

The author is holder of Research Career Development Award 10K3-CA8182 from the National Cancer Institute. The research reported here was supported by Public Health Research Grant CA-07175 from the National Cancer Institute.

References

1. Baluda, M. A.: In: Oncology, 1970: Cellular and Molecular Mechanisms of Carcinogenesis (Proceedings of the 10th International Cancer Congress), Year Book Medical Publishers, Inc., Chicago, Illinois, 1971, pp. 788-793.
2. Baluda, M. B., and D. P. Nayak: J. Virol., 4:554-566, 1969.
3. Boettiger, D., and H. M. Temin: In press.
4. Borsa, J., and A. F. Graham: Biochem. Biophys. Res. Commun., 33:895-901, 1968.
5. Kates, J. R., and B. R. McAuslan: Proc. Nat. Acad. Sci. USA, 57:314-320, 1967.
6. Munyon, W., E. Paoletti, and J. T. Grace: Proc. Nat. Acad. Sci. USA, 58:2280-2287, 1967.
7. Murray, R. K., and H. M. Temin: Int. J. Cancer. In press.
8. Payne, L. N., and R. C. Chubb: J. Gen. Virol., 3:379-391, 1968.
9. Shatkin, A. J., and J. D. Sipe: Proc. Nat. Acad. Sci. USA, 61:1462-1469, 1968.
10. Temin, H. M.: Virol., 13:159-163, 1961.
11. Temin, H. M.: Virol., 20:577-582, 1963.
12. Temin, H. M.: Proc. Nat. Acad. Sci. USA, 52:323-329, 1964.
13. Temin, H. M.: Cancer Res., 28:1835-1839, 1968.
14. Temin, H. M.: Int. J. Cancer, 3:771-787, 1968.
15. Temin, H. M.: Perspect. Biol. Med. In press.
16. Travanicek, M.: Biochim. Biophys. Acta, 182:427-439, 1969.

Virus Induction from Nonpermissive Cells Transformed by RNA Viruses: The RSV Data

PHILIPPE VIGIER

Institut du Radium (Biologie), Faculté des Sciences, Orsay, France

INFECTION OF GENETICALLY susceptible cells of the species of origin with RNA oncogenic viruses—avian or murine—constantly results in the establishment of an endosymbiotic relationship which allows sustained virus production without suppression of the growth capacity of the permissive cells, which may or may not be transformed.[1] Infection of cells of other species may similarly result in the establishment of an endosymbiotic permissive relationship but it also can give rise to cell transformation without virus production. This moderate relationship in which transformed cells are nonpermissive is most frequently encountered in the case of mammalian cells transformed by Rous sarcoma virus (RSV) and is also seen in the case of cells of mammals other than the mouse transformed by murine sarcoma virus (MSV).[1, 2]

In a number of cases, it can be shown that nonpermissive transformed cells retain the complete viral genome, as was first observed by Svoboda in the case of the XC rat sarcoma cell line produced in vivo by RSV: grafting of XC cells to chicken, even after years of serial passages in vivo or in vitro and isolation of clonal lines resulted in the production of chicken sarcomas containing RSV.[3] Similarly, co-cultivation of XC cells and chick embryo fibroblasts resulted in the appearance of RSV in the culture medium. Subsequently RSV could be induced by both methods from a variety of tumor cell lines produced in different mammalian species, in vivo or in vitro.[1, 2]

As shown by Huebner and associates,[5] a second marker of the persistence of the viral genome in nonpermissive transformed cells is the presence of the group-specific (gs) nucleocapsid antigen common to all leukosis and sarcoma viruses of the fowl or the mouse. However, it is not established that gs antigen is virus-coded, and certain data even suggest that it could be coded by the cellular genome.[6]

A third marker is the new nonviral antigen(s) located on the cell surface which can be detected by graft rejection or in vitro methods.[7] Yet, as in the case of the gs antigen, it is not demonstrated that it is coded by the virus.

Therefore, the most reliable proof that the viral genome persists in nonpermissive transformed cells is the capacity of these cells to be induced by association with permissive cells in vivo or in vitro. Moreover, the study of the mechanism of induction by cell association is evidently of importance for understanding the reasons for nonpermissiveness which can be expected to exist also in the case of tumors of men caused by oncogenic RNA viruses, if such tumors and viruses actually exist.

All existing data concerning induction of RNA oncogenic viruses by cell association will not be reviewed but I will only clarify the picture obtained by the study of cells transformed by RSV, which remains the model virus from most viewpoints. I also will present the data obtained recently by myself and by Svoboda and associates, with whom I have been working in close contact for over five years.

In 1964, at the Durham meeting on avian tumor viruses, we discussed the possibility that induction of RSV by association of nonpermissive transformed mammalian cells and permissive normal chicken cells could result from the formation of permissive heterokaryons;[3] our subsequent investigations have shown that this is indeed the case.

The major argument in favor of this model until recently was that fusion of nonpermissive and permissive cells by inactivated Sendai virus increases considerably the recovery of RSV and of RSV-producing infective centers in mixed cultures.[8, 9, 10] This argument has been reinforced since it has been demonstrated that the heterokaryons formed are the first and only infective centers in the days following cell fusion.

However, these findings cannot rule out the possibility that other mechanisms of virus induction could exist in the absence of cell fusion artificially produced by Sendai virus or in addition to the formation of permissive heterokaryons occurring normally in untreated mixed cultures, or following grafting of nonpermissive cells to a permissive host. Therefore, it appeared necessary to test in parallel and in absence of Sendai virus all the plausible models of induction which could be conceived a priori, namely: (1) activation of nonpermissive cells by co-cultivation with permissive cells, (2) transfer of a subviral determinant from nonpermissive to permissive cells, and (3) unmediated formation of permissive heterokaryons.

These three models were first tested four years ago[11] using two clones of nonpermissive BHK 21/13 cells transformed in suspension in agar medium, the first by Schmidt-Ruppin strain RSV (SR-RSV) and the second by Bryan strain RSV (B-RSV). These two clones were found to be absolutely nonpermissive and repeated study of their cells by electron microscopy has never revealed the presence of type-C particles or of eventual precursors of mature virions. They also were shown to differ importantly regarding their inducibility by association with chick embryo cells: whereas the first (RS_2) was constantly inducible by association with the cells of embryos of a Brown Leghorn strain of chicken free of any lymphomatosis virus, the second (RB_{12}) could be induced by association with the same cells only if a lymphomatosis virus able to infect these cells, i.e., RAV_1, was added to the mixed cultures at time of plating or in the first days afterwards, or if the chick embryo cells were preinfected with RAV.[11, 12] The reason for this difference is most probably that whereas activated RS_2 cells produce SR-RSV able to infect the Brown Leghorn cells, which are mainly of the C/O type, the activated RB_{12} cells produce B-RSV (O) unable to infect these cells unless it is phenotypically mixed with a lymphomatosis virus of a type-specificity compatible with the cell phenotype.[13, 14] Consequently, it could be predicted that different results should be obtained in induction experiments depending on the cell clone and the models considered as listed below.

1. *Activation of nonpermissive cells in presence of permissive cells.* Activated cells should retain capacity to multiply, and the number of infective centers and amount of RSV produced should, therefore, increase steadily even in absence of secondary infection of neighboring chick embryo (CE) cells. Further, SR-RSV produced by the RS clone

in absence of any added virus should be able to infect neighboring CE cells and transform them to Rous cells shedding RSV; whereas B-RSV (O) produced in the absence of added virus or B-RSV (RAV) produced in presence of RAV by the RB clone should not be able to infect CE cells since they would be resistant to infection by B-RSV (O) genetically and to infection by B-RSV (RAV) by interference (as they would be initially also infected with RAV).[1] Moreover, addition of anti-SR-RSV type-specific antiserum should prevent infection of the CE cells and appearance of Rous cells, in the case of the RS clone.

2. *Transfer of a subviral determinant.* The first infective centers should be the CE cells infected by transfer (presumably by contact) of the determinant and some of these cells should become Rous cells shedding SR-RSV or B-RSV (O) in absence of added virus, or B-RSV (RAV) if RAV is added, in the case of the RB clone. The transfer should not be prevented by neutralizing antiserum, in the case of the SR clone, nor by the genetic or interference blocks against B-RSV (O) or B-RSV (RAV), in the case of the RB clone, since these blocks operate against the viral envelope.[14]

3. *Formation of permissive heterokaryons.* Heterokaryons formed by fusion of mammalian and chicken cells should not be able to multiply and the initial viruses or infective centers should not increase before and unless neighboring CE cells are infected. This infection should be prevented by antiserum, in the case of the SR clone, and by the genetic or the interference blocks in the case of the RB clone, as in model 1.

Experiments to test these predictions were done both with unirradiated RS and RB cells and with cells preirradiated at 5,000 r with X- or γ-rays, to prevent them from overgrowing the CE cells (irradiation at this dose does not interfere with induction). The results, which have been checked repeatedly, were in agreement with model 3 and ruled out models 1 and 2.[11, 13]

In absence of Sendai virus, the number of infective centers, i.e. of permissive heterokaryons, generally remains low: 1 in 10^5 to 10^6 nonpermissive cells when scored by the count of foci of Rous cells produced by reinfection of chicken cells under an agar overlay.[13, 15] However, this scoring underestimates the actual number of infective centers by a factor of about 10. The number of permissive heterokaryons formed also depends on the ratio of the permissive to the nonpermissive cells and reaches a maximum for a ratio of about five.[13]

Fusion with Sendai virus inactivated with UV-light or β-propiolactone can raise over 100-fold the number of the infective centers and the initial production of RSV.[8, 9, 10, 13, 15] The number of infective centers increases with the amount of Sendai virus added and also with the ratio of permissive to nonpermissive cells, the optimal ratio being in that case about 10 times that in absence of Sendai virus.[16, 17]

Heterokaryons are easily seen in Sendai-fused mixed cultures, and their number correlates with that of the infective centers detected by focus assay.[13, 16] Moreover, in carefully carried out investigations, Machala, Donner, and Svoboda[18] have recently shown by an immunofluorescence test that only the heterokaryons produce RSV. They also observed by transferring single heterokaryons obtained by visually controlled fusion into microdrops of medium under paraffin oil, that each produced virus. The amount of virus produced was found to increase with the number of nuclei of nonpermissive cells (a clone of Chinese hamster fibroblasts transformed in vitro by SR-RSV) in the heterokaryons, i.e. presumably with the number of viral genomes present.

The contribution of each of the partner cells in heterokaryons to the induction of virus is not yet known. However, my recent radiobiologic investigations suggest that the part of the nonpermissive cell may be only to bring the viral genome, the permissive cell's information and constituents which normally intervene in viral synthesis being also entirely responsible for this synthesis in the heterokaryons. Indeed, it has been found that when the nonpermissive cells are irradiated with γ-rays or UV-light before being fused with the permissive cells, the inactivation curve of the capacity of the irradiated cells to form permissive heterokaryons is the same as that of free RSV. This is also found when the nonpermissive cells exposed to UV-light are co-cultivated with CE cells in absence of fusion with Sendai virus, but the capacity of the nonpermissive cells irradiated with γ-rays and co-cultivated with CE cells in absence of Sendai virus-mediated fusion is definitely more radioresistant than free RSV. A tentative explanation for this unexpected finding is that X-irradiation may increase the incidence of spontaneous formation of heterokaryons.[17]

I recently studied the metabolic requirements of induction by cell association by adding inhibitors of DNA synthesis and DNA-dependent RNA synthesis to mixed cultures of RS cells (irradiated at 5,000 r) and CE cells fused in monolayer, one day after seeding, with inactivated Sendai virus. The inhibitors tested have been 5-bromodeoxyuridine (BUDR: 100 μg/ml), cytosine arabinoside (Ara-C:25 μg/ml), mitomycin C(MC:2-3 μg/ml), and actinomycin D(AD:0.1 μg/ml). The inhibitors were added at the end of the fusion period (20 min at 4C and 20-40 min at 37C) and kept in contact with the cells for six to 24 hr (AC, AD, and MC) or 24-72 hr (BUDR). The virus produced in the medium 24, 48, and 72 hr after fusion was assayed on CE cells as described earlier.[cf. 1] Inhibition of induction of RSV was negligible after exposure to BUDR and Ara-C for 24 hr after cell fusion (even 72 hr in the case of BUDR) and to MC for 6 hours (exposure for 24 hr resulting in a pronounced toxic effect). Exposure to AD for 24 hr inhibited about 10-fold the production of RSV in the next 24 hr but it later on returned to the level of production of controls.[17] These results show that the metabolic requirements of the heterokaryons for producing RSV are the same as those of established Rous cells and clearly different from those for initiating infection in CE cells since all inhibitors tested prevent this initiation; inhibition following early addition is not reversible with any one.[cf. 1]

Until recently, it was generally agreed that the effects of inhibitors showed that both DNA synthesis and DNA-dependent RNA synthesis were required for initiation of replication of RNA oncogenic viruses whereas only DNA-dependent RNA synthesis remained necessary for their subsequent production by established virus-producing cells.[cf. 1] However, finding that the inhibitors tested may also raise the level of intracellular ribonucleases suggests an alternative explanation, i.e. the resistance to the inhibitors of the virus-producing capacity of established virus-producing cells as opposed to the sensitivity of that of newly infected cells may reflect increase in the number of viral genomes or their passage to a form or a site less accessible to nucleases, or both. In this case, the findings with heterokaryons would mean either that they contain as many genomes as established Rous cells, these genomes being presumably brought by the nonpermissive cell, or that the viral genomes already are in a protected form or in protected sites before or immediately after cell fusion—the two possibilities being nonexclusive.

A last series of experiments which I wish to report briefly were done with Bataillon, to see whether the capacity of nonpermissive cells to be induced after heterokaryon formation may not depend on their content in gs antigen, assuming this content reflects the number of viral genomes present in the cell. These experiments were made possible by Bataillon's earlier finding that the average content in gs antigen of the RS_2 and RB_{12} cells remained remarkably constant with the passages in vitro; the same was true for subclones of these clones. However, marked differences in gs content existed between subclones, some of which even had no detectable amount of gs antigen (less than one complement-fixing unit in 8.10^6 cells in the COFAL test).[19] Sendai fusion and/or co-cultivation with CE cells of the cells of two RS_2 subclones selected (the first, for its high gs content and, the second, for the absence of any detectable gs antigen) showed that 100-fold more RSV was induced in the high than in the low gs subclone following Sendai-mediated fusion; virus was recovered only in the high gs subclone in absence of Sendai virus. Further, after a certain number of passages, no RSV could be recovered from the low gs subclone even after Sendai-mediated cell fusion, whereas the recovery from the high gs subclone remained constantly high. Virus was constantly recovered, but in a lesser amount, following Sendai-mediated fusion of the cells of the RS clone of origin which contained less gs antigen than the high gs subclone; but virus was not recovered in all experiments from this clone in absence of Sendai virus. In addition, three clones of BHK 21/13 cells presumably transformed by SR-RSV since no transformed colonies appeared in the controls were recently obtained by the agar suspension method and these clones which contained no detectable gs antigen from the start could not be induced following Sendai-mediated fusion with CE cells.

Summarizing these data it may be provisionally concluded that: (1) virus induction by association on nonpermissive transformed cells with permissive cells results from formation of permissive heterokaryons, (2) in at least some cases, all heterokaryons are able to produce virus, the virus production depending on the number of nuclei of nonpermissive cells in each heterokaryon, (3) production of the induced virus presumably depends entirely on the genetic information and functions supplied to each heterokaryon by the permissive cell, (4) permissive heterokaryons exposed to inhibitors of DNA synthesis and DNA-dependent RNA synthesis behave like established virus-producing cells, (5) the capacity of nonpermissive cells to form virus-producing heterokaryons may depend on the number of viral genomes they carry or, alternately, on the degree of expression of these genomes as measured by the cell content in gs antigen, and (6) some nonpermissive cells may not contain gs antigen and not be inducible by any known means. This obliges us to reconsider the generally accepted conclusion or postulate that the viral genome must persist within the cells to maintain the transformed state since, if no other marker of the presence of the viral genome is found in these gs noninducible cells, there is no known way to prove that they actually contain the genome.

Finally if further investigations confirm that viral genomes present in nonpermissive cells can segregate unequally in daughter cells, this would rule out the possibility that the viral genome in these cells may consist of one or more DNA templates integrated as a prophage in the cellular DNA. The possible models remaining would be either the nonintegrated episomes, if the viral genome is a DNA template, or, more simply, nonintegrated viral RNA genomes replicating by orthodox means and expressing their information to various degrees, depending on the cell genotype and phenotype. The data on the replication of RNA of mouse leukemia virus obtained recently by Biswal and Benyesh-Melnick[20] cause me today to be in favor of this last model, which does not exclude the possibility that, in addition, the small part of the viral RNA which is homologous of sites of the cellular DNA could be primed by the cellular genome.

References

1. Vigier, P.: RNA oncogenic viruses: Structure, replication, and oncogenicity. Prog. Med. Virol. In press.
2. Svoboda, J.: Dependence among RNA-containing animal viruses: In: The Molecular Biology of Viruses, 18th Symp. Soc. Gen. Microbiol., Cambridge University Press, 1968, pp. 249-271.
3. Svoboda, J.: Malignant interaction of Rous virus with mammalian cells *in vivo* and *in vitro*. Nat. Cancer Inst. Monogr., 17:277-292, 1968.
4. Simkovic, D.: Interaction between mammalian cells induced by Rous virus and chicken cells. Nat. Cancer Inst. Monogr., 17:351, 1969.

5. Huebner, R. J.: *In vitro* methods for detection and assay of leukemia viruses. In: Carcinogenesis: A Broad Critique, Williams and Wilkins, Baltimore, 1967, pp. 23-45.
6. Payne, L. N., and R. C. Chubb: Studies on the nature and genetic control of an antigen in normal chick embryos which reacts in the COFAL test. J. Gen. Virol., 3:379-391, 1968.
7. Old, L. J., E. Boyse, G. Geering, and H. F. Oettgen: Serologic approaches to the study of cancer in animals and man. Cancer Res., 28:1288-1299, 1968.
8. Svoboda, J., O. Machala, and T. Hlozanek: Influence of Sendai virus on RSV formation in mixed cultures of virogenic mammalian cells and chicken fibroblasts. Folio Biol., 13:155-157, 1967.
9. Vigier, P.: Persistance du génome du virus de Rous dans les cellules du Hamster converties *in vitro*, et action du virus Sendai inactivé sur sa transmission aux cellules de poule. Compt. Rend. Acad. Sci., Paris, 264D:422-425, 1967.
10. Yamaguchi, N., M. Takeuchi, and T. Yamamoto: Rous sarcoma virus production in mixed culture of mouse tumor cells and chicken embryo fibroblasts by the addition of UV-irradiated HVJ. Jap. J. Exp. Med., 37:83-86, 1967.
11. Vigier, P., and L. Montagnier: Persistence and action of the Rous sarcoma virus genome in transformed rodent cells. In: Subviral Carcinogenesis, 1st International Symposium on Tumor Viruses, Aichi Cancer Center, Nagoya, 1967, pp. 156-175.
12. Vigier, P.: Persistance du génome du virus de Rous dans les cellules de hamster converties *in vitro* par un virus non-défectif et un virus défectif. Compt. Rend. Acad. Sci., Paris, 262D:2554-2557, 1966.
13. Vigier, P.: Persistance du génome du virus de Rous dans les cellules de mammifères transformées et mécanisme de sa transmission aux cellules de poule. IIeme Colloque International sur les Virus Oncogenes, Royaumont, 1969, Ed. du C.N.R.S., Paris. In press.
14. Duff, R. G., and P. K. Vogt: Characteristics of two new avian tumor virus subgroups. Virology, 39:18-30, 1969.
15. Svoboda, J., I. Hlozanek, and O. Machala: Rescue of Rous sarcoma virus in mixed cultures of virogenic mammalian and chicken cells, treated and untreated with Sendai virus and detected by focus assay. J. Gen. Virol., 2:461-464, 1968.
16. Svoboda, J. and R. Dourmashkin: Rescue of Rous sarcoma virus from virogenic mammalian cells associated with chicken cells and treated with Sendai virus. J. Gen. Virol., 4:523-529, 1969.
17. Vigier, P.: Unpublished data.
18. Machala, O., L. Donner, and J. Svoboda: A full expression of RSV genome in heterokaryons formed after fusion of virogenic mammalian cells and chicken fibroblasts. J. Gen. Virol. In press.
19. Bataillon, G.: Etude de l'antigène spécifique du groupe des virus oncogènes avaires dans des clones de cellules de hamster transformées par le virus de Rous. Compt. Rend. Acad. Sci., Paris, 269D:2156-2158, 1969.
20. Biswal, N., and M. Benyesh-Melnick: Complementary nuclear RNAs of murine sarcoma-leukemia virus complex in transformed cells. Proc. Nat. Acad. Sci. USA, 64:1372-1379, 1969.

DNA-RNA Hybridization Studies with Avian Myeloblastosis Virus

M. A. BALUDA

Department of Medical Microbiology and Immunology, School of Medicine,
University of California at Los Angeles, Los Angeles, California, USA

Introduction

THE RNA ISOLATED from purified avian myeloblastosis virus (AMV) consists of two single-stranded components.[1, 9] The heavy component represents the viral genome; it has a sedimentation coefficient of 71S, in 10^{-1} M salt-sucrose, possibly as a result of having a considerable degree of tertiary structure. The small component (4 to 5S in 10^{-1} M salt-sucrose) is cellular tRNA and is present either inside the AMV virions, or in cellular micelles contaminating the virus preparation.[2]

Although AMV is an RNA virus, there is much indirect evidence that it replicates via a DNA intermediate.[3] To obtain direct evidence for this hypothesis, virus-producing leukemic cells were investigated to determine whether they contain DNA which is complementary to the 71S viral RNA. For this purpose, DNA-RNA hybridization studies were made according to the procedure of Gillespie and Spiegelman.[5]

Materials and Methods

VIRUS AND CELLS

The BAI strain A of AMV was used and myeloblasts were obtained from leukemic chicks, as previously described.[3]

DNA

Cellular DNA was extracted in the presence of mercaptoethanol (1%) and SDS (1%) at 60C for 10 min, followed by two extractions with chloroform-isoamyl alcohol and three extractions with cold phenol. To eliminate contaminating RNA, the DNA was treated with 0.3N KOH for 16 hr at 30C, neutralized and dialyzed against $0.1 \times$ SSC. Only DNA with an OD 260:OD 280 ratio of 1.8 was used.[3] The DNA was boiled in $0.1 \times$ SSC immediately before fixation on nitrocellulose filters (Millipore HA 0.45 μm) by gravity filtration at a concentration of 4 μg/ml in $4 \times$ SSC. The DNA filters were then washed with 20 ml of $4 \times$ SSC, dried, stored at room temperature, and oven-heated at 70C for four hr just before hybridization.

AMV RNA

[3]H-labeled AMV was prepared using three or four ^{3}H-labeled ribonucleosides and purified as previously described.[3] ^{3}H-labeled 71S RNA and 5S RNA were isolated after velocity sedimentation of RNA extracted from purified virions. ^{3}H-labeled 71S RNA had a specific activity of 3.6 to 4.9×10^5 count/min/μg.

In some experiments, ^{3}H-labeled 71S AMV RNA was treated with DNase (10 μg/ml) in Tris-HCl 10^{-2} M (pH 7.4) and $MgCl_2$ 10^{-2} M at 25C for 30 min. The DNase (Mann Research Laboratories, New York, New York) had been freed of RNase by velocity ultracentrifugation (60 hr at 39K in the Beckman SW-40 rotor) in a 15 to 30% linear glycerol gradient.

DNA-RNA HYBRIDIZATION

DNA-RNA hybridization was done at 70C for 10 hr in $4 \times$ SSC in the presence of 0.05% SDS and 1.5 to 3.0 mg of unlabeled, unfractionated chick embryo RNA (CE-RNA). To eliminate nonspecifically bound radioactivity, the following procedure was finally settled upon. After hybridization, the filters, five to seven at a time, were washed twice in 300 ml of $4 \times$ SSC, heated at 70C for 10 min in 250 ml of $2 \times$ SSC, treated with RNase (Pancreatic fraction A: 25 μg/ml plus T_1: 20 units/ml) in $2 \times$ SSC at 37C for 30 min, washed twice more in 300 ml of $4 \times$ SSC, placed on Millipore filter holders, and each side was washed with 75 ml of $4 \times$ SSC. The rims of the filters were cut off and the centers were dried and counted in a Picker 220 liquid scintillation spectrophotometer. After counting, the amount of DNA trapped on each filter was determined by the diphenylamine test.

Results

HYBRIDIZATION OF 71S AMV RNA WITH LEUKEMIC AND NORMAL CHICK DNA

[3]H-labeled 71S AMV RNA was hybridized with DNA extracted from leukemic myeloblasts, decapitated normal 10-day chick embryos, mouse embryos or *Escherichia coli* K12 (λ). Table 20-5 demonstrates

TABLE 20–5.—HYBRIDIZATION BETWEEN 71S-AMV-RNA AND DNA FROM LEUKEMIC AND NORMAL CELLS*

Expt.	Input RNA (μg/ml)	CPM HYBRIDIZED PER 100 μG DNA FROM			
		Myeloblasts	Chick Embryos	Mouse Embryos	E. Coli
1	2.8	387 ± 8 (8) †	193 ± 13 (8)	27 ± 6 (8)	37 ± 9 (8)
2	5.7	928 ± 63 (3)	510 ± 24 (3)	41 ± 6 (3)	

* Each vial contains 5 filters in 1.5 ml of $4 \times$ -SSC with 0.05% SDS, 3 mg CE-RNA and H[3]-71S-AMV-RNA (specific activity: 3.6×10^5 cpm/μg). Average amount of DNA recovered per filter: 40 μg.
† Cpm ± standard deviation and in parentheses, the numbers of filters used.
Cpm in blank filters treated identically have been subtracted.

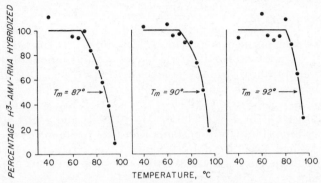

Fig. 20–3.—Melting curves of DNA-RNA hybrids. The melting of DNA-RNA hybrids was performed as previously described.[2] Three separate experiments were performed, and the mean values are plotted as percentages of RNase-resistant ^{3}H AMV RNA vs. heating temperatures. The curve on the left represents the melting of AMV RNA hybridized with normal chick embryo DNA, and the middle curve the melting of AMV RNA hybridized with leukemic DNA. The curve on the right represents the counts/min hybridized to leukemic DNA less the counts/min hybridized to chick embryo DNA, i.e., the melting of hybrids formed between AMV RNA and DNA present exclusively in leukemic cells.

that there is DNA complementary to 71S AMV RNA not only in leukemic cells but also in apparently normal chick embryos. However, leukemic DNA hybridizes 1.9 times as much viral RNA as normal DNA does.

That all the hybridized radioactivity is in viral RNA and not in contaminating DNA was shown in two ways: (1) All of the hybridized radioactivity was rendered soluble in trichloroacetic acid if the filters were treated with 0.3N KOH at 30C for 16 hr, and (2) the [3]H-71S AMV RNA used in experiment two had been treated with DNase as described in Materials and Methods.

It has already been shown that the increased hybridization of AMV RNA by leukemic DNA is not caused by some nonspecific binding.[2] DNA isolated from either leukemic or normal cells hybridized the same amount of ^{3}H-labeled larger than 45S nuclear RNA, 28S or 18S RRNA, or 4S RNA obtained from normal chick embryo fibroblasts. Therefore, the higher degree of binding between leukemic cell DNA and AMV RNA results from specific hybridization.

This specificity was further demonstrated by competitive inhibition with unlabeled 71S AMV RNA. The latter had been prepared in the same manner as the ^{3}H-labeled AMV RNA was. As shown previously,[2] a 16-fold excess of unlabeled viral 71S RNA competed successfully with the hybridization of 4 μg/ml of [3]H-71S AMV RNA, whereas 1,500 μg/ml of cold chick embryo RNA did not. In the presence of cold viral RNA, there was no difference between the amount of [3]H 71S RNA immobilized by leukemic cell DNA and by normal DNA. These results also supported the existence of specific hybridization between AMV RNA and chicken DNA.

To determine the length of the nucleotide sequences involved in the previous experiments, the heat stability of the DNA RNA hybrids was determined. Three separate thermal melting experiments in $2 \times$ SSC were performed as previously described;[2] the average values are plotted in Figure 20-3. The heat stability and high T_m of the DNA-RNA hybrids indicate that long sequences of at least 100 nucleotides are involved.[4, 6-8, 11] The hybrid formed between AMV RNA and normal chicken DNA melts with a sharp profile and a T_m of 88C; that formed between AMV RNA and leukemic DNA has a T_m of 90C. The part of the viral RNA which is complementary to DNA present only in leukemic cells has a higher T_m of 92C. Therefore, extensive homology not dependent on accidental similarities exists between AMV RNA and normal or leukemic DNA.

Hybridization of 71S AMV RNA with DNA from Cells Transformed by B-77 Avian Sarcoma Virus (B-77-SV) or by Schmidt-Ruppin Avian Sarcoma Virus (SR-SV)

The objection might be raised that DNA from whole 10-day chick embryos or from chick embryo fibroblasts is not a rigorous control for DNA from leukemic myeloblasts. This objection was removed in the next experiments. Rat embryonic cells transformed in vitro with B-77-SV and chick embryonic cells transformed in vitro with SR-SV were obtained from Professor H. M. Temin of the University of Wisconsin. The DNA from transformed cells was compared with the DNA from uninfected sister cells for its capacity to hybridize with ^{3}H-labeled AMV RNA. As shown in Table 20-6, the results obtained are even bet-

TABLE 20–6.—Hybridization of H^3-71S-AMV-RNA with DNA from Cells Transformed by B-77-SV or Schmidt Ruppin SV*

Source of DNA[†]	CPM Hybridized per 100 μg DNA[‡]
Rat embryonic fibroblasts —B-77-SV transformed	694 ± 29 (59 μg)
—control	29 ± 9 (69 μg)
Chick embryonic fibroblasts—SR-SV transformed	2739 ± 68 (59 μg)
—control	506 ± 39 (51 μg)
Leukemic myeloblasts (AMV transformed)	939 ± 45 (42 μg)
Chick embryos	565 ± 70 (30 μg)
Mouse embryos	19 ± 17 (59 μg)

* Each hybridization vial contained 5 filters in 1.5 ml of $4 \times$ SSC with 0.05% SDS, 2280 μg/ml CE-RNA and 5.8 μg/ml H^3-71S-AMV-RNA (specific activity: 3.9×10^5 cpm/μg).

† The rat and chick embryonic fibroblasts, control and virus-transformed, were obtained from Dr. H. M. Temin.

‡ Cpm ± standard deviation (average of 5 filters) and in parentheses the average amount of DNA recovered per filter. Cpm bound by blank filters treated identically have been subtracted (82 ± 5 cpm).

ter than those obtained with cells transformed by AMV, despite the fact that AMV and the avian sarcoma strains used do not contain exactly homologous genomes. DNA from normal rat embryonic cells, like that from normal mouse embryonic cells, does not hybridize with AMV RNA. Conversely, DNA from B-77-SV transformed rat cells hybridizes with AMV RNA almost to the same extent as leukemic DNA does, and DNA from SR-SV transformed chick embryo fibroblasts hybridizes three times as much AMV RNA as DNA from leukemic cells does.

Discussion

This study demonstrates that there is DNA complementary to 71S AMV RNA in cells transformed by avian leukosis viruses and in apparently normal chick embryonic cells. The heat stability and high T_m of the DNA-RNA hybrids show that extensive homology not dependent on accidental similarities exists between the two nucleic acids.

There are at least eight copies of the DNA equivalent of the AMV genome in leukemic cells and at least 24 copies in SR-SV transformed cells (assuming a mol wt of 4×10^6 per viral genome). It is not known, however, whether the homologous DNA corresponds to the entire viral genome or to part of it. Analyses of the average base composition of the hybridized viral RNA will resolve this point.

The transformed cell DNA that is complementary to the viral RNA represents either (1) a viral DNA intermediate, or (2) a virus-induced redundancy of normal chicken DNA sequences homologous to the viral RNA.

Since the DNA-RNA hybrid which forms only between AMV RNA and leukemic DNA has a T_m about 4C higher than the T_m of the hybrid formed between AMV RNA and normal DNA, these two hybrids represent nucleic acid sequences which differ by about 10% in G + C content. Therefore, either (1) two different regions of the viral genome are involved, or (2) the two nucleic acids are only partially homologous.

The hybridization of AMV RNA with DNA from normal chick embryos could indicate either (1) a natural homology, or (2) contamination of the chick embryos by some avian leukosis virus DNA which is partially homologous to AMV RNA. The second hypothesis is favored for several reasons: Approximately 10% of the chickens in the White Leghorn strain (Kimber Farms strain K-137) used in these studies develop spontaneous leukotic neoplasias during the first eight months of life. The proportion of infected embryos must be much higher, since only one out of seven chickens which are congenitally infected with avian leukosis viruses is a virus producer and not all the virus-producing birds develop tumors.[10] Second, all of 11 embryos which had been individually tested contained DNA which was complementary to AMV RNA. They were of several classes whose DNA was 35% to 90% homologous to leukemic DNA.[12] Finally, whereas DNA from normal mouse or rat cells does not hybridize with AMV RNA, DNA from rat cells transformed by B-77 virus hybridizes approximately to the same extent as DNA from pooled, apparently normal chick embryos.

Acknowledgments

It is a pleasure to thank Professor H. M. Temin for providing the cells transformed by B-77-SV and by SR-ASV, Mr. P. A. Markham for his help in some experiments and Miss E. A. Matsch for her skillful technical assistance.

This investigation was supported by U. S. Public Health Service Research Grant CA-10197 from the National Cancer Institute. The author is the recipient of American Cancer Society Award (PRA-34) for faculty position support.

References

1. Baluda, M. A.: In: Subviral Carcinogenesis, First International Symposium on Tumor Viruses (Y. Ito, ed.), Maruzen Co. Ltd., Tokyo, 1967, pp. 19-35.
2. Baluda, M. A., and D. P. Nayak: Proc. Nat. Acad. Sci. USA. In press.
3. Baluda, M. A., and D. P. Nayak: In: Biology of Large RNA Viruses (R. D. Barry and B. W. Mahy, eds.), Academic Press, New York, 1970.
4. Chamberlin, J., and P. Berg: J. Mol. Biol., 8:297, 1964.
5. Gillespie, D., and S. Spiegelman: J. Mol. Biol., 12:829, 1965.
6. McCarthy, B. J.: In: Subviral Carcinogenesis, First International Symposium on Tumor Viruses (Y. Ito, ed.), Maruzen Co. Ltd., Tokyo, 1967, pp. 43-61.
7. McCarthy, B. J., and E. T. Bolton: J. Mol. Biol., 8:184, 1964.
8. Niyogi, S. K.: J. Biol. Chem., 244:1576, 1969.
9. Robinson, W. S., and M. A. Baluda: Proc. Nat. Acad. Sci. USA, 54:1686, 1965.
10. Rubin, H., L. Fanshier, A. Cornelius, and W. F. Hughes: Virology, 17:143, 1962.
11. Sinsheimer, R. L., and M. Lawrence: J. Mol. Biol., 8:289, 1964.
12. Baluda, M. A.: Unpublished data.

Analogy of the Mechanism Involved in Polyoma and SV40 Virus-Induced Replication of Mouse Cell Chromosomes

ROGER WEIL, EVELYNE MAY,

AND PIERRE MAY

Swiss Institute for Experimental Cancer Research, Lausanne, Switzerland

IN THIS PAPER, we will present a summary of an extensive comparative study on the sequential events taking place after infection of confluent, "contact-inhibited" primary mouse kidney (MK) cultures with polyoma (Py) or SV40 virus.[29] We will show that the early events of the lytic (Py) and the nonlytic (SV40) infection are analogous and lead in both instances to virus-induced replication of the host-cell chromosomes. We will propose a working hypothesis which attempts to explain the mechanism of virus-induced replication and we will discuss the possible relevance of the experimental observations to virus-induced cell "transformation."

Tissue Culture System Used for Infection with Polyoma or SV40 Virus

For all experiments reported here, primary MK cultures[50] were used one to three days after they had reached confluence.[48] At the time of infection, such cultures consisted mainly of epithelial-like cells most of which (80-90%) were arrested in stage G_1 of the mitotic cycle. Both cells arrested in G_1 and G_2 participated in virus-induced chromosome replication (Haemmerli and Weil, unpublished). In addition, MK cultures contained small, multilayered colonies of fibroblast-like cells which showed decreased contact inhibition and thus continued to undergo DNA synthesis and mitotic division, though at a relatively low rate.

Time Course of Infection with Polyoma Virus (Lytic Infection)

It was shown elsewhere that, in individual cells, the onset of Py-induced DNA synthesis was very asynchronous.[32, 48, 49] Under standard conditions of infection (37C; approximately 10^9 PFU/ml) a small number of cells ($<1\%$) started Py-induced DNA synthesis around 12 hr postinfection. Thereafter the number of the DNA synthesizing cells rapidly increased and reached a maximum of 60-80% around 25-30 hr postinfection, a level maintained during the later stages of infection. Specific activities, in cell-free extracts, of the enzymes of the cellular DNA-synthesizing apparatus increased parallel to the number of DNA synthesizing cells. Several lines of experimental evidence made it appear likely that most or all enzymes analyzed were coded for by the host-cell genome.[1, 48] If Py-induced DNA synthesis was inhibited by the addition of 5-fluorodeoxyuridine (FUdR) to the culture medium immediately after the adsorption of Py virus, little if any capsid protein was synthesized. However, the early metabolic events of the infection which led to the activation of the cellular DNA-synthesizing apparatus took place just as they did in parallel cultures infected without this inhibitor. The results were essentially the same if cytosine arabinoside (Ara-C) were used instead of FUdR (Weil and Kára, unpublished). If the FUdR inhibition was reversed with deoxythymidine (TdR) around 30 hr postinfection when most cells were activated, Py-induced DNA synthesis (cellular and viral) started synchronously in all cells.[32] This synchronized system was of use for analysis of the sequential events of phase 2 of the lytic cycle, i.e. of Py-induced chromosome replication and the actual production of progeny virus.[18, 20] In the lytic infection, Py-induced chromosome replication was never followed by mitosis. These earlier observations led to the working hypothesis that during the apparently silent phase 1, Py virus directs synthesis of a substance which activates the cellular DNA-synthesizing apparatus and, as a consequence, induces the replication of the host cell's chromosomes. For other reasons,[48] we considered the possibility that the Py-specific "tumor antigen" (T antigen) might be this activator. Py-specific T antigen can be detected by immunochemical methods in the nuclei of virus-free cells derived from tumors induced by Py virus and also in cells undergoing lytic infection.[15, 42]

From numerous experimental observations, we concluded that virus-specific T antigen appeared in Py-infected MK cells regularly before activation of the cellular DNA-synthesizing apparatus, and further, that the asynchronous appearance of T antigen was very similar to the subsequent asynchronous onset of Py-induced DNA synthesis, detectable by autoradiography.[49] If Py-induced DNA synthesis was blocked with FUdR or Ara-C immediately after adsorption of the virus, both the appearance of T antigen[17] and the subsequent activation of the cellular DNA-synthesizing apparatus[32] took place essentially as they did in the absence of the inhibitors. These results, considered with those reported below, support the working hypothesis that Py- and SV40-specific T antigen trigger replication of the host-cell chromosomes in "contact-inhibited" MK cells.

Time Course of Infection with SV40

In 1963, it was reported[2] that infection of primary MK cultures with SV40 led to the appearance of "transformed" cells. The findings were confirmed[23] and it was further shown that infection stimulated the synthesis of cellular DNA while little if any viral DNA or progeny virus were produced.

Because of these findings, we did a detailed analysis of the time course of the infection with virus SV40 in confluent primary MK cultures.[29] Under standard conditions of infection (37C; 10^8 PFU/ml) SV40-specific intranuclear T antigen, determined by immunofluorescence,[6, 8, 15, 33, 35] could first be detected in a small number of the cells (<5%) around six to seven hr postinfection. Thereafter, the relative number of positive cells rapidly increased and reached a plateau around 18 hr postinfection when 40-50% of the cells were positive for T antigen. As determined autoradiographically on cultures pulse-labeled for one hr with thymidine-^{3}H, the number of DNA synthesizing cells began to increase around nine to 10 hr postinfection above the level (2-4%) of uninfected control cultures and reached a maximum around 21 hr postinfection when 30-35% of the cells were synthesizing DNA. Even by the use of selective SDS extraction[19] we were unable to detect replicating SV40 DNA, a finding in accordance with the results reported by others.[24] Under all experimental conditions tested, the curve reflecting the increase in the number of T antigen positive cells (plotted as a function of time) preceded the curve corresponding to the increase in the number of DNA-synthesizing cells; in all experiments, the maximum number of cells positive for T antigen exceeded by a few per cent the number of DNA-synthesizing cells. The appearance of SV40-specific T antigen[22, 23, 36] and the subsequent activation of the cellular DNA-synthesizing apparatus[29] proceeded in the presence of inhibitors of DNA synthesis such as FUdR (or Ara-C) as in parallel cultures infected without the inhibitor. Therefore, the onset of SV40-induced DNA synthesis could be synchronized[29] by the method used to synchronize the onset of Py-induced DNA synthesis.[32] Preliminary results obtained from a collaborative study with Dr. Ion Gresser (Paris) showed that pretreatment of confluent MK cultures with mouse-specific interferon for 24 hr before infection with SV40 led to a considerable decrease (over 70%) in the number of cells positive for SV40-specific T antigen and to a comparable reduction in the number of cells participating in virus-induced DNA synthesis. Interferon added after adsorption of SV40 virus exhibited little if any effect on the appearance of T antigen or on subsequent virus-induced DNA synthesis. Oxman and Black[31] reported a similar inhibitory effect of pretreatment with mouse-specific interferon on the appearance of SV40-specific T antigen in 3T3 cultures (mouse fibroblasts). Todaro and Green[45] did not observe any effect of pretreatment with interferon on SV40-induced DNA synthesis in 3T3 cultures. However, they did not determine the effect of interferon on the appearance of T antigen. Lately, Boehlandt et al.[4] reported that pretreatment of primary monkey kidney cell cultures with monkey-specific interferon led to a drastic decrease in the number of T antigen positive cells and to a very marked reduction of SV40-induced synthesis of cellular and viral DNA.

Under standard conditions of infection, a burst of mitoses could be observed in the MK cultures around 24-30 hr postinfection. At this time, up to 20% of the cells positive for T antigen were found in mitosis. The over-all mitotic index of the infected cultures reached a maximum between 24-30 hr postinfection corresponding to about 5%. After 30-35 hr postinfection it decreased but remained always significantly higher than in uninfected control cultures. Most mitotic cells in the SV40-infected MK cultures exhibited a strong immunofluorescence reaction for SV40-specific T antigen with a distribution similar to that found by Defendi et al.[7] in SV40-infected human fibroblasts undergoing virus-induced mitosis. In contrast, mitotic cells in uninfected MK cultures exhibited only a faint, nonspecific fluorescence when reacted under the same conditions. From evidence to be reported elsewhere,[29] we concluded that most or all of cells which underwent SV40-induced mitosis, also had participated in virus-induced replication of their chromosomes and, further that, in most cells, mitosis was followed by cell division. While most epithelial-like cells underwent only one or a limited number of virus-induced cell divisions, a marked and continuous mitotic stimulation could be observed within and around the colonies made up of fibroblast-like cells. In both epithelial- and fibroblast-like cells, many virus-induced mitoses were tri- or multipolar. These abnormalities apparently led to nuclear fragmentation, the appearance of multinucleated cells, and rather often to cell death. The finding that continuous mitotic stimulation was largely confined to fibroblast-like cells, suggests that the physiologic state, at the time of the infection, played a major role in the reaction of the cells toward the virus-induced mitotic stimulus. As a result of the continuous mitotic stimulation many fibroblast-like colonies began to increase in size and, within two to four weeks, appeared as dense colonies visible by the naked eye. Microscopic observations of these colonies revealed, even early after infection, marked virus-induced cytopathic effects and a considerable degree of cellular pleomorphism. Since essentially all cells contained the SV40-specific T antigen, we assume that the dense colonies in the SV40-infected MK cultures corresponded to the colonies of "transformed" cells described by others,[25] though they neither reported cellular pleomorphism nor virus-induced cytopathic effects. When tested by Kit et al.[25] after 26 transfers in vitro (subcultures prepared twice weekly) the "transformed" cells contained the SV40-specific T antigen and, as judged by the fusion technique,[11, 27, 46] "integrated" SV40 DNA. However, when injected into isologous mice, the "transformed" cells did not form tumors and thus were not malignant, as judged by the criterion of transplantability. When cultures were tested again after 71 transfers in vitro, they were malignant and developed into tumors. The possibility has to be considered that the long lag between the initial infection and the development of transplantability might have been sufficient to allow spontaneous malignant conversion of uninfected control cultures.[38]

Conclusions

The results summarized in this paper show that in "contact-inhibited" primary MK cultures the early events of the lytic infection with Py and the nonlytic infection with SV40 virus are analogous: the asynchronous appearance, in individual cells, of Py- or SV40-specific T antigen is followed by a comparable asynchronous onset of virus-induced replication of the host-cell chromosomes. The experimental results are in agreement with the working hypothesis that under the conditions used, Py- or SV40-specific T antigen activates the cellular DNA-synthesizing apparatus and, as a consequence, induces replication of the host-cell chromosomes. They do not rule out, however, the possibility that virus-induced chromosome replication might be triggered or mediated by a yet unknown viral function which would parallel the appearance of T antigen but would not be directly connected with it.

In Py-infected MK cultures, virus-induced chromosome replication was regularly accompanied by the synthesis of Py viral DNA and by the production of progeny virus and was followed by cell death. In contrast, no replicating viral DNA could be detected in MK cultures infected with SV40. This suggests that the appearance of virus-specific T antigen and the subsequent virus-induced replication of the host-cell chromosomes are necessary but insufficient conditions for the onset of viral DNA synthesis. If these results are considered together with those reported by Swetly et al.[41] it appears likely that the onset of viral DNA synthesis requires a specific host-cell factor(s).

In Py-infected MK cultures, virus-induced chromosome replication was not followed by mitosis. In contrast, most cells which participated in SV40-induced chromosome replication subsequently entered normal or abnormal mitosis. While most SV40-infected cells underwent one or at most a limited number of virus-induced cell divisions, the abortive infection stimulated some fibroblast-like cells into continuous cycles of mitotic division. As a result of this continued stimulation, many small colonies of fibroblast-like cells began to increase in size and to develop into large colonies, probably corresponding to the colonies of "transformed" cells observed by Kit et al.[25] From our results,[29] we concluded that the abortive infection with SV40 conferred to a fraction of the MK cells present in the cultures a mitotic stimulus, a decreased dependence on serum factors, an increased potential for growth in vitro and last, but not least, a striking cytogenetic and karyotypic instability. The latter led, already during the first cycle of virus-induced chromosome replication, in many cells to abnormal mitosis, followed by a broad spectrum of nuclear abnormalities, which were closely similar to those observed after the infection with virus SV40 of tissue culture cells derived from several other species.[2, 3, 9, 10, 26, 30, 34, 39, 40, 43] Kit's observation[25] that SV40-"transformed" MK cells became malignant (i.e. able to produce tumors in isologous hosts) only after a prolonged period (several months) of cultivation in vitro is consistent with experimental evidence that "early virus-transformed" tissue culture cells were generally not malignant. Though viral DNA may become covalently linked ("integrated") to chromosomal DNA in the nonlytic[37] and, possibly also early in the lytic infection (Weil, unpublished), the malignant conversion of tissue culture cells by Py or SV40 virus actually exhibits few if any of the characteristics of phage conversion in bacteria. The synonymous use of the terms "transformed," "neoplastic," and "malignant" has led to considerable conceptual confusion. It therefore should be stressed that neither specific phenotypic properties nor malignancy are regularly associated with virus-"transformed" mammalian cells.[13] Though the possibility has to be considered that an abortive infection (mitotic stimulus?) may confer to cells directly a malignant phenotype,[9, 12] the virus-induced oncogenic conversion of tissue culture cells is generally a complex and prolonged process. The experimental evidence presently available is compatible with the following hypothesis: virus-induced mitotic stimulation (T antigen?), combined with the loss of the cytogenetic equilibrium, converts rather rapidly primary cultures or cell strains into established cell lines which have a potential for unlimited growth (cell multiplication) in vitro; soon after infection these established cell lines are not malignant and thus probably correspond to the "early transformed cells" first described by Vogt and Dulbecco.[47] Only during the prolonged propagation in vitro would they acquire malignant properties, possibly by a process of cytogenetic variation and selection (progression)[14] analogous to that postulated for "spontaneous"[38] or chemically induced malignant conversion of tissue culture cells.[28] After establishment of cell lines, virus-specific imprints would no longer be needed, either for the development or, later, for the maintenance of the malignant phenotype, though such imprints might confer to the cells a selective advantage for growth in vitro or in vivo. This hypothesis would also account for the finding that highly malignant (uninfected) tissue culture cells as well as cells "transformed" by another oncogenic virus could be "supertransformed" by Py- or SV40-virus[44] and that this "supertransformation," though accompanied by certain phenotypic alterations, did not lead to a significant change in their malignant potential.[5]

For the reasons outlined above, we concluded that the usefulness of Py and SV40 virus for studies on the mechanism of carcinogenesis may actually be rather limited and that the main potential of these viruses lies in the fact that they are powerful tools to study genetic regulation in mammalian cells.

References

1. Basilico, C., Y. Matsuya, and H. Green: Origin of the thymidine kinase induced by polyoma virus in productively infected cells. J. Virol., 3:140-145, 1969.
2. Black, P. H., and W. P. Rowe: SV40 induced proliferation of tissue culture cells of rabbit, mouse, and porcine origin. Proc. Soc. Exp. Biol. Med., 114:721-727, 1963,a.
3. Black, P. H., and W. P. Rowe: An analysis of SV40-induced transformation of hamster kidney tissue in vitro. I. General characteristics. Proc. Nat. Acad. Sci. USA, 50:1148-1156, 1963,b.
4. Boehlandt, D., G. Brandner, and J. Burger: Inhibition of DNA and RNA synthesis in SV40 infected african green monkey kidney cell cultures by interferon. In press.
5. Defendi, V., J. Lehman, and P. Kraemer: "Morphologically normal" hamster cells with malignant properties. Virology, 19:592-598, 1963.
6. Defendi, V.: Transformation in vitro of mammalian cells by polyoma and simian 40 viruses. In: Progress in Experimental Tumor Research (F. Homburger, ed.), S. Karger, Basel and New York, Vol. 8, 1966, pp. 125-188.
7. Defendi, V., F. Jensen, and G. Sauer: Analysis of some viral functions related to neoplastic transformation. In: The Molecular Biology of Viruses (J. S. Colter and W. Paranchich, eds.), Academic Press, New York, 1967, pp. 645-663.
8. Deichman, G. I.: Immunological aspects of carcinogenesis by deoxyribonucleic acid tumor viruses. In: Advances in Cancer Research (G. Klein, and S. Weinhouse, eds.), Academic Press, New York and London, Vol. 12, 1969, pp. 101-106.
9. Diamandopoulos, G. Th., M. F. Dalton-Tucker, and J. van der Noordaa: Early in-vitro SV40-mediated morphologic transformation of primary hamster cells. Its correlation with the development of the oncogenic state. Amer. J. Pathol., 57:199-213, 1969.
10. Diderholm, H., R. Berg, and T. Wesslén: Transformation of rat and guinea-pig cells in vitro by SV40 and the transplantability of the transformed cells. Int. J. Cancer, 1:139-148, 1966.
11. Dubbs, D. R., S. Kit, R. A. de Torres, and M. Anken: Virogenic properties of bromodeoxyuridine-sensitive and bromodeoxyuridine-resistant simian virus 40-transformed mouse kidney cells. J. Virol., 1:968-979, 1967.
12. Duff, R., and F. Rapp: Quantitative characteristics of the transformation of hamster cells by PARA (defective simian virus 40)-adenovirus 7. J. Virol., 5:568-577, 1970.
13. Eagle, H., G. E. Foley, H. Koprowski, H. Lazarus, E. M. Levine, and R. A. Adams: Growth characteristics of virus-transformed cells. Maximum population density, inhibition by normal cells, serum requirement, growth in soft agar and xenogeneic transplantability. J. Exp. Med., 131:863-879, 1970.
14. Enders, J. F., and G. Th. Diamandopoulos: A study of variation and progression in oncogenicity in an SV40-transformed hamster heart cell line and its clones. Proc. Roy. Soc. B, 171:431-443, 1969.
15. Fogel, M., R. Gilden, and V. Defendi: Polyoma virus-induced "complement-fixing antigen" in tumors and infected cells as detected by immunofluorescence. Proc. Soc. Exp. Biol. Med., 124:1047-1052, 1967.
16. Gilden, R. V., R. I. Carp, F. Taguchi, and V. Defendi: The nature and localization of the SV40-induced complement-fixing antigen. Proc. Nat. Acad. Sci. USA, 53:684-692, 1965.

17. Habel, K.: Virus tumor antigens: specific fingerprints? Cancer Res., 26:2018-2024, 1966.
18. Hancock, R., and R. Weil: Biochemical evidence for induction by polyoma virus of replication of the chromosomes of mouse kidney cells. Proc. Nat. Acad. Sci. USA, 63:1144-1150, 1969.
19. Hirt, B.: Selective extraction of polyoma DNA from infected mouse cell cultures. J. Mol. Biol., 26:365-369, 1967.
20. Hudson, J. B., D. Goldstein, and R. Weil: A study on the transcription of the polyoma viral genome. Proc. Nat. Acad. Sci. USA, 65:226-233, 1970.
21. Kára, J., and R. Weil: Specific activation of the DNA-synthesizing apparatus in contact-inhibited mouse kidney cells by polyoma virus. Proc. Nat. Acad. Sci. USA, 57:63-70, 1967.
22. Kit, S., D. R. Dubbs, P. M. Frearson, and J. L. Melnick: Enzyme induction in SV40-infected green monkey kidney cultures. Virology, 29:69-83, 1966,a.
23. Kit, S., D. R. Dubbs, L. J. Piekarski, R. A. de Torres, and J. L. Melnick: Acquisition of enzyme function by mouse kidney abortively infected with papovavirus SV40. Proc. Nat. Acad. Sci. USA, 56:463-470, 1966,b.
24. Kit, S., R. A. de Torres, D. R. Dubbs, and M. L. Salvi: Induction of cellular deoxyribonucleic acid synthesis by simian virus 40. J. Virol., 1:738-746, 1967.
25. Kit, S., T. Kurimura, and D. R. Dubbs: Transplantable mouse tumor lines induced by injection of SV40-transformed mouse kidney cells. Int. J. Cancer, 4:384-392, 1969.
26. Koprowski, H., J. A. Pontén, F. Jensen, R. G. Ravdin, P. S. Moorhead, and E. Saksela: Transformation of cultures of human tissue infected with simian virus SV40. J. Cell. and Comp. Physiol., 59:281-292, 1962.
27. Koprowski, H., F. C. Jensen, and Steplewski: Activation of production of infectious tumor virus SV40 in heterokaryon cultures. Proc. Nat. Acad. Sci. USA, 58:127-133, 1967.
28. Levan, A.: Chromosome abnormalities and carcinogenesis. In: Handbook of Molecular Cytology (A. Lima de Faria, ed.) , North Holland, 1969, pp. 716-731.
29. May, E., P. May, and R. Weil: In preparation.
30. Moorhead, P. S., and E. Saksela: The sequence of chromosome aberrations during SV40 transformation of a human diploid cell line. Hereditas, 52:271-284, 1965.
31. Oxman, M. N., and P. H. Black: Inhibition of SV40 T-antigen formation by interferon. Proc. Nat. Acad. Sci. USA, 55:1133-1140, 1966.
32. Pétursson, G., and R. Weil: A study on the mechanism of polyoma-induced activation of the cellular DNA-synthesizing apparatus. Synchronization by FUdR of virus-induced DNA synthesis. Arch. Ges. Virusforsch., 24:1-29, 1968.
33. Pope, J. H., and W. P. Rowe: Detection of specific antigen in SV40 transformed cells by immunofluorescence. J. Exp. Med., 120:121-127, 1964.
34. Rabson, A. S., and R. L. Kirschstein: Induction of malignancy in vitro in newborn hamster kidney tissue infected with simian vacuolating virus (SV40) . Proc. Soc. Exp. Biol. Med., 111:323-328, 1962.
35. Rapp, F., T. Kitahara, J. S. Butel, and J. L. Melnick: Synthesis of SV40 tumor antigen during replication of simian papovavirus (SV40) . Proc. Nat. Acad. Sci. USA, 52:1138-1142, 1964.
36. Rapp, F., J. S. Butel, L. A. Feldman, T. Kitahara, and J. L. Melnick: Differential effects of inhibitors on the steps leading to the formation of SV40 tumor and virus antigens. J. Exp. Med., 121:935-944, 1965.
37. Sambrook, J., H. Westphal, P. Sprinivasan, and R. Dulbecco: The integrated state of viral DNA in SV40-transformed cells. Proc. Nat. Acad. Sci. USA, 60:1288-1295, 1968.
38. Sanford, K. K.: Malignant transformation of cells in vitro. In: International Review of Cytology (G. H. Bourne and J. F. Danielli, eds.) , Vol. 18, 1965, pp. 249-311.
39. Shein, H. M., and J. F. Enders: Transformation induced by simian virus 40 in human renal cell cultures, I. Morphology and growth characteristics. Proc. Nat. Acad. Sci. USA, 48:1164-1172, 1962.

40. Shein, H. M., J. F. Enders, J. D. Levinthal, and A. E. Burket: Transformation induced by simian virus 40 in newborn Syrian hamster renal cell cultures. Proc. Nat. Acad. Sci. USA, 49:28-34, 1963.
41. Swetly, P., G. B. Brodano, B. Knowles, and H. Koprowski: Response of simian virus 40-transformed cell lines and cell hybrids to superinfection with simian virus 40 and its deoxyribonucleic acid. J. Virol., 4:348-355, 1969.
42. Takemoto, K. K., R. A. Malmgren, and K. Habel: Immunofluorescent demonstration of polyoma tumor antigen in lytic infection of mouse embryo cells. Virology, 28:485-488, 1966.
43. Todaro, G. J., S. R. Wolman, and H. Green: Rapid transformation of human fibroblasts with low growth potential into established cell lines by SV40. J. Cell. Comp. Physiol., 62:257-266, 1963.
44. Todaro, G. J., K. Habel, and H. Green: Antigenic and cultural properties of cells doubly transformed by polyoma virus and SV40. Virology, 27:179-185, 1965.
45. Todaro, G. J., and H. Green: Interferon resistance of SV40 induced DNA synthesis. Virology, 33:752-754, 1967.
46. Tournier, P., R. Cassingena, R. Wicker, J. Coppey, and H. Suarez: Study of the induction mechanism in Syrian hamster cells transformed by SV40 virus. Int. J. Cancer, 2:117-132, 1967.
47. Vogt, M., and R. Dulbecco: Steps in the neoplastic transformation of hamster embryos cells by polyoma virus. Proc. Nat. Acad. Sci. USA, 49:171-179, 1963.
48. Weil, R., G. Pétursson, J. Kára, and H. Diggelmann: On the interaction of polyoma virus with the genetic apparatus of host cells. In: The Molecular Biology of Viruses (J. S. Colter, and W. Paranchich, eds.), Academic Press, New York, London, 1967, pp. 593-626.
49. Weil, R., and J. Kára: Polyoma "tumor antigen": An activator of chromosome replication? Proc. Nat. Acad. Sci. USA. In press.
50. Winocour, E.: Purification of polyoma virus. Virology, 19:158-168, 1963.

21

Ontogenic Defects in Oncogenesis

Immunologic Abnormalities and Cancer

RICHARD A. GATTI, M.D., AND
ROBERT A. GOOD, M.D., PH.D.

Pediatric Research Laboratories of the Variety Club Heart Hospital,
University of Minnesota, Minneapolis, Minnesota, USA

WE HAVE HEARD about ontogenic defects as they relate to the development of cancer, convincing evidence implicating the genetic predisposition of the host as a prerequisite for a large variety of malignant diseases. Supplementing this genetic approach are our observations supporting the hypothesis that inadequate immunologic host responses also foster carcinogenesis. Whether these two mechanisms influence oncogenesis collectively or independently is not yet understood.

Before attempting to develop the above hypothesis, let us briefly review the immunologic apparatus as we presently interpret it. Two basic types of immunologic responses prevail: (1) a humoral response mediated via circulating antibodies synthesized by plasma cells, and (2) a cell-mediated response mediated by lymphocytes which develop under thymic influence. These dual functions trace their origins to a common precursor stem cell population. This lymphoid stem cell population probably has its ultimate origin in blood islands of the yolk sac and fetal liver and develops later in the bone marrow. Development of the lymphoid system occurs as these precursor cells sequentially migrate through various different microenvironments. Those stem cells which traffic to the thymus proliferate extensively and through a process destroying the great majority of elements derived, a small proportion differentiate into small lymphocytes which then pass into the circulation where they enter a circulating pool of immune competent postthymic lymphocytes which reside preferentially in certain thymus-dependent areas, e.g. in the deep cortical regions of the lymph nodes. These cells have the capacity to react with foreign antigens and initiate responses of delayed hypersensitivity, homograft rejection, rejection of solid tissue malignancies and graft vs. host reactions. Stem cell trafficking, instead, to the bursa of Fabricius in birds differentiate into plasma cells responsible for humoral antibody formation. Anatomic localization of a bursal equivalent in man has not been defined. Lymphoid organs thought to be the bursa have been described in turtles[1] and tadpoles,[2] and evidence has been presented that the appendix and other gut epithelium-associated lymphoid tissues in the rabbit subserve, at least in part, this differentiating function.[3] While in human beings this site is still unknown, it is clear that in certain diseases of man the entire plasma cell system may be absent while the thymus-dependent lymphoid system remains intact. Thus, for man, as well as birds, one must think of two separate immunologic developments.[4, 5] The two-component lymphoid concept is summarized in Figure 21-1.

Probably the most convincing circumstantial evidence linking oncogenesis to inadequate immune function comes from our clinical experience with the patients suffering from immunologic deficiency diseases. Within this group, we have been impressed by the high frequency of malignant diseases in patients with immune deficiency and the association of certain forms of malignant diseases with specific types of immunologic deficiency. For instance, patients with Bruton-type congenital sex-linked agammaglobulinemia who lack immunoglobulins (Igs) and the ability to form antibodies in response to repeated antigenic challenge, yet have normal cell-mediated immune responses, develop leukemia exclusively (Table 21-1). No other forms of malignant diseases have been observed in this group of patients. While it is clear that these patients are extremely susceptible to bacterial infections with such high-grade encapsulated extracellular pyogenic pathogens as pseudomonas, streptococcus, pneumococcus, *H. influenzae* and meningococcus, they seem able to handle many viral infections normally. Hepatitis virus has, however, on several occasions been associated with a fulminating progressive fatal hepatitis.[6] Among some 40 to 50 cases of well-documented Bruton-type agammaglobulinemia, five have had leukemia.[7, 8] Two of these presented with tumors in the thymus gland.[7] These findings are of particular interest since Gorer[10] showed long ago that humoral immune responses seem to play a major role in resistance to oncogenesis of certain mouse leukemias, whereas in other solid tissue malignant diseases of both lymphoid and nonlymphoid origin, cell-mediated immune mechanisms seemed to be the major bulwark of defense. Recently, Dupuy et al.[11] confirmed that immunity to Friend virus-induced leukemia seems to involve primarily humoral immune

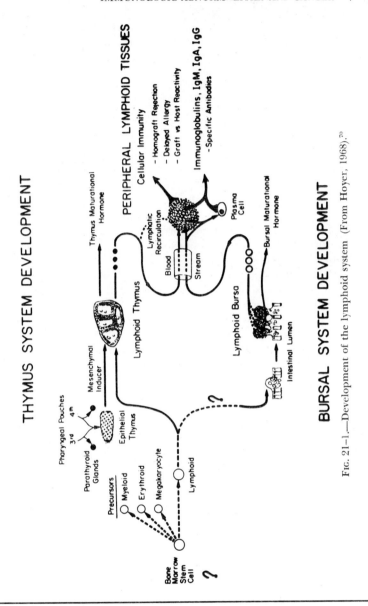

Fig. 21-1.—Development of the lymphoid system (From Hoyer, 1968).[70]

defenses. The Hellströms' recent work[12, 13, 14] with colony inhibition of neuroblastoma cell cultures by sensitized lymphocytes from patients or close contacts of patients with neuroblastoma suggests that cell-mediated and humoral immune responses both play interacting roles in the immune response to cancer.

Early work by Furth et al.[15] showed that mice of a strain which have

TABLE 21–1.—MALIGNANCIES IN BRUTON-TYPE
AGAMMAGLOBULINEMIA

1. Acute lymphocytic leukemia[7]
2. Malignant lymphoma[7]
3.* Chronic monomyelogenous leukemia[8]
4. Thymoma with leukemia[9]
5. Lymphatic leukemia[9]

* Chromosomal abnormalities.

a high incidence of spontaneous leukemia do not develop leukemia if they are thymectomized early in life. Conversely, experiments performed by Peterson et al.,[16, 17] Cooper et al.,[18] and Dent et al.[19] in chickens showed that bursectomy prevents the development of lymphoma induced by the avian leukosis virus. Removal of the thymus does not interfere with development of this lymphoma.

It would appear to us then that the patients with Bruton-type agammaglobulinemia possess the necessary target cell or differentiative site, such as thymus, for successful adaptation of a malignant clone while, conversely, they seem less capable than normal individuals of resisting development of this malignancy. Since the only abnormality so far defined in this group of patients involves an inability to form antibodies and Igs, the extremely high frequency of lymphoma and leukemia seems more than fortuitously related to their immunologic deficit.

A somewhat similar situation occurs in patients with Wiskott-Aldrich disease. Though the immunologic deficit in this group of patients is more variable than in patients with Bruton-type agammaglobulinemia, the type of cancer, i.e. lymphoreticular, is once again almost exclusive of other forms[20–28, 103] (Table 21-2). These children suffer from severe recurrent bacterial infections, eczema, and thrombocytopenia.[29] Immunologically they are unable to form antibody in response to polysaccharide antigens such as blood group substances; they have low IgM levels and often have high IgA and IgE levels. Early in the course of their disease cell-mediated responses are intact; however, with time, these patients develop prolonged homograft rejection responses, weak delayed hypersensitivity reactions and even poor in vitro lymphocyte responses to phytohemagglutinin and allogeneic cells. These children often have marked generalized lymphadenopathy for months before developing lymphoreticular malignant diseases.[30] Though roughly 15% of such patients have developed cancer, it is conceivable that this figure will actually rise as our understanding of this disease and improved pediatric care minimize early deaths from infections and bleeding disorders. Platelet function, size, and metabolism are also abnormal in these patients.[31-33]

Three other groups with primary immunologic deficiency are known to have an inordinately high frequency of malignant diseases: these are the patients with ataxia-telangiectasia and late-onset hypogammaglobulinemia. Both groups have variable deficits of immune function which involve both cell-mediated and humoral immunity and, in both groups, a variety of malignant diseases, representing a very broad range of cellular origins are involved in the malignant adaptation.

Patients with ataxia-telangiectasia may have normal Ig levels and, by present criteria, normal cell-mediated immune responses when tested early in the course of their disease.[34-36] In many patients, however, IgA and IgE are low and cell-mediated responses are depressed.[37] It now seems clear that IgE levels are also abnormal in members of the patients' families.[38] At postmortem examination of children with ataxia-telangiectasia, the thymus is regularly small and lacks Hassall's corpuscles. Malignant lymphoma, various forms of leukemia, reticulum cell sarcoma, Hodgkin's disease, gastric carcinoma, glioma, medulloblastoma and dysgerminoma have been reported in these patients (Table 21-3), bringing the incidence of cancer in this group to about 10%.[30-52, 104-115]

A most striking observation from Table 21-3 is the occurrence of the same form of malignant diseases among the siblings of five families.[40, 46, 50, 51, 113] In the two families where karyotypes were studied, chromosomal breaks were observed, though cytogenetic studies of several of the other patients included in the table were normal. Chromosomal abnormalities have also been observed in a patient with Wiskott-Aldrich disease and lymphosarcoma (Table 21-2)[27] and in a child with Bruton-type agammaglobulinemia and chronic monomyelogenous leukemia (Table 21-1).[8] Chromosomal breaks have been described in karyotypes of other patients with ataxia-telangiectasia without malignant diseases[46, 53, 54] and in an infant with agammaglobulinemia and

---

TABLE 21–2.—MALIGNANCIES IN WISKOTT-ALDRICH
DISEASE

1. Malignant reticuloendotheliosis[20]
2. Malignant reticuloendotheliosis[21]
3. Astrocytoma of brain[22]
4. Malignant lymphoma[23]
5. Lymphoma[23]
6. Myelogenous leukemia[24]
7. Malignant reticuloendotheliosis[24]
8. Thymosarcoma[25]
9. Lymphoma[26]
10.* Reticular lymphosarcoma[27]
11. Histiocytosis-X[28]
12. Leiomyosarcoma, multiple[103]

* Chromosomal abnormality.

TABLE 21–3.—MALIGNANCIES IN ATAXIA-TELANGIECTASIA*

1. Reticulum cell sarcoma[39]
2. Hodgkin's disease[39]
3. Undifferentiated round cell sarcoma[39]
4-6. Malignant lymphoma—3 sibs[40]
7. Glioma[41]
8. Ovarian dysgerminoma[42]
9. Reticulum cell hyperplasia[43]
10. Small cell hyperplasia[43]
11. Reticulum cell sarcoma[44]
12. Lymphoma[105]
13. Cerebellar medulloblastoma[45]
14. Leukemia[106]
15. Lymphosarcomatosis[106]
16-17.† Acute lymphocytic leukemia—2 sibs[46]
18. Lymphosarcoma[47]
19. Reticulum cell lymphoma[107]
20. Hodgkin's lymphoma[108]
21. Lymphosarcoma and tuberous sclerosis[109]
22. Leukemia[110]
23. Malignant lymphoma[111]
24. Malignant lymphoma[48]
25. Hodgkin's disease[49]
26. Reticulum cell lymphoma[112]
27-28.† Gastric adenocarcinoma—2 sibs[50]
29-30. Acute lymphoblastic leukemia—2 sibs[51]
31. Lymphoma[52]
32-33. Lymphosarcoma—2 sibs[113]
34. Acute lymphoblastic leukemia[114]
35. Lymphoma[104]
36. Lymphoma[115]

* Prepared with the assistance of Drs. E. Boder and R. P. Sedgwick.
† Chromosomal breaks.

C'q deficiency.[55] Similar breaks are also commonly found in Bloom's syndrome[56] and Fanconi's anemia;[57] both diseases are associated with a high frequency of cancer and an increased susceptibility of the skin fibroblasts to in vitro malignant transformation by simian virus 40 (SV40) as has been demonstrated by Todaro and Takemoto.[58]

If we assume for a moment that the essential prerequisites for oncogenesis are a carcinogen, a target cell or target gene appropriate for that carcinogen and a deficient immunity, ataxia-telangiectasia may represent Nature's experiment of carcinogenesis resulting in oncogenesis without the mask of the immune responses. It is doubtful that so rare a form of malignant disease as gastric adenocarcinoma in children could develop in two siblings by chance alone. We consider it much more likely that these children were subjected to a common carcinogen resulting in malignant transformation of gastric mucosal cells. (It is also possible that they shared a genetic predisposition to this carcinogen.) In the absence of normal immunologic surveillance or rejection mechanisms, the malignant adaptation was successful in both cases. A similar proposal could be made with regard to the common malignant disease in the other four families.

The frequency of malignant diseases in patients with late-onset hypogammaglobulinemia is again extremely high and includes all types of lymphoreticular malignancies,[26, 59-63] carcinoma of the bowel[26] and stomach[26, 64] and even osteochondromata.[65] There can be no question that in this disease as well, one encounters the inextricable relationship between a propensity to malignant adaptation and immune deficiency. It will be difficult to analyze this association of oncogenesis and immunologic deficiency precisely, however, until we can further dissect and divide the heterogeneous group of patients included under the heading "late-onset hypogammaglobulinemia"; this group currently includes acquired hypogammaglobulinemia, sporadic agammaglobulinemia, the various types of dysgammaglobulinemias, and primary immunologic deficiency of adults.[5, 66] Taken together, this group of patients represents the most common form of immunologic deficiency in the general population. Within the families of these patients, one often finds other individuals with immunoglobulin abnormalities, autoimmune disease and malignant disease.[60] An extraordinary hypertrophy of the lymphoid tissue of the ileum and lower bowel has occasionally been noted in patients with late-onset hypogammaglobulinemia[67-71] and, is in some ways, remindful of the generalized lymphadenopathy seen in Wiskott-Aldrich disease prior to the development of lymphoreticular malignancy.[26, 72]

Last, a word should be said about the incidence of cancer in patients with the lymphopenic forms of agammaglobulinemia.[5, 73] These infants lack both humoral and cell-mediated immunity and almost invariably die within the first two years of life thus allowing little time to develop malignant disease. Nonetheless, in two instances early malignant changes have been noted. In one infant, described by Kadowaki et al.,[74] a second cell line with a mode of 45 emerged at 15 months of age suggesting early acute leukemia. Recently, a centrally placed 2-cm. splenic tumor was found at postmortem examination of a six-month-old Norwegian infant with lymphopenic agammaglobulinemia.[75] Microscopically, the tumor resembled a lymphosarcoma. These experiences suggest that the high frequency with which malignant disease is found in other forms of immunologic deficiency disease would also hold true in these patients if they were to survive other consequences of their immunologic disease.

It has recently become very clear that patients maintained on immunosuppressants for long periods of time develop malignant disease with a frequency much in excess of that in the general population.[76, 77] An analysis of the types of malignant diseases seen in these patients should be separated into two groups: those of donor origin and those of host origin. If viewed from this perspective, we can clearly see that cancers of donor origin include a large variety of malignant diseases such as those of the breast,[78] lung,[79, 80] liver,[81] kidney,[82] thyroid,[83] and larynx.[84] Such cancers may develop as long as three years after transplantation of the malignant cells.[81] When immunosuppression has been discontinued, these cancers have regressed and their absence has been conspicuous at postmortem examination in a number of patients. Cancers of host origin cover a broad spectrum of malignant diseases.[77] The incidence of reticulum cell sarcoma seems to be increased disproportionately. It should be emphasized, however, that in contrast to conclusions of others, these de novo tumors occurring in the immunosuppressed patients are not exclusively lymphoreticular and include carcinomas and solid tissue sarcomas as well. According to Dr. Israel Penn, 37 instances have been recorded of such de novo tumors arising in transplant patients while on immunosuppression; 21 of these were of epithelial origin while only 16 were lymphoreticular.

It is, perhaps, too early to further analyze this group on the basis of specific immunosuppressants received, though Deodhar's report of a reticulum cell sarcoma developing at the site of administration of antilymphocyte globulin after 37 injections over a period of eight weeks[85] certainly points to the antilymphocyte globulin as one agent which can foster the malignant adaptation. Whether different forms of immunosuppression will foster different types of malignant diseases remains to be seen.

Carcinogens are also immunosuppressants. Chemically related compounds which are not carcinogenic are not immunosuppressive.[86–88] While not all immunosuppressants are known to be carcinogenic, such immunosuppressants as corticosteroids have been shown to potentiate chemical carcinogenesis with methyl cholanthrene[89] and to induce metastases of tumors which would not ordinarily metastasize.[90] Indeed, all known immunosuppressants are known to foster the malignant adaptation. It is conceivable that a successful carcinogen must not only be capable of transforming its target cell, it must effectively suppress or misdirect the host's immunologic mechanisms of surveillance and rejection against the transformed clone (Figure 21-2).

ONCOGENESIS

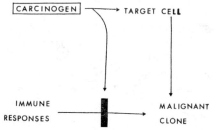

Fig. 21–2.—Schematic representation of oncogenesis depicting the dual effects of a carcinogen in vivo: (1) malignant transformation of an appropriate target cell and (2) blocking of immunologic responses of the host against the malignant clone.

We have discussed the unusually high incidence of malignant diseases among patients with immunologic deficiency diseases; lastly, let us for a moment turn to the converse of this situation and consider the immunologic status of patients with malignant disease of lymphoid and nonlymphoid origin.

In the former group, patients with chronic lymphatic leukemia often have Ig levels resembling those of agammaglobulinemia patients.[91] This deficiency involves all of the Ig classes so far studied and is accompanied by strikingly poor antibody formation following antigenic stimulation. These patients also regularly have marked deficits of delayed hypersensitivity and homograft rejection capacity. When viewed in this light, it is not surprising that 35% of patients with chronic lymphatic leukemia develop a second primary cancer.[92] Indeed, second primaries are not uncommon in cancer patients.

The cell-mediated immune deficit seen in Hodgkin's disease is now well documented.[91] Originally described by Schier et al.[93] with respect to cutaneous responses, this deficit has been confirmed by prolonged homograft rejection[94] and by poor in vitro lymphocyte responses as well.[95, 96] Recently, several investigators have demonstrated a correlation between prognosis in this disease and ability to develop skin reactivity to dinitrofluorobenzene (DNFB), dinitrochlorobenzene, and PPD.[97, 98] An elevation of alpha$_2$ globulins has also been described in this disease. By contrast, these patients have normal Igs and well-preserved antibody responses. The opposite is seen in myeloma where patients have well-preserved cell-mediated immune responses but are lacking in humoral immunities. The different spectra of infections in Hodgkin's disease and myeloma seem to reflect these specific immune deficits.[91]

The finding of immunologic deficiencies in patients suffering from cancers of nonlymphoid origin seems even more pertinent to our hypothesis than the above association of impaired immunologic functions in patients with lymphoid cancers since the latter association very well could be secondary to diversion of specific lymphoid cell populations into malignant proliferation. A number of early investigations noted waning of PPD and DNFB hypersensitivity responses in patients with terminal solid tissue malignant diseases.[99, 100] Following this lead, Garrioch, in our laboratories in Minneapolis, studied the in vitro lymphocyte responses to phytohemagglutinin (PHA) in 46 patients with a large variety of nonlymphoid tumors who were not being treated with chemotherapeutic agents or steroids.[101] Age-matched controls were used since PHA responses have been shown to wane with age. The scattergram best demonstrated the markedly depressed PHA responses among a large number of these patients (Figure 21-3). We next attempted to determine the mechanisms responsible for this depressed lymphocyte activity—a response which has been shown to reflect the integrity of the thymus-dependent immune functions. Incubation of normal lymphocytes with the plasma of cancer patients pro-

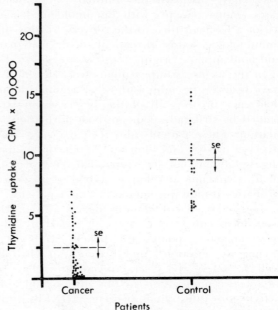

FIG. 21–3.—Tritiated thymidine uptake of PHA-stimulated leukocyte cultures from patients with nonlymphoid malignancies and age-matched controls.

duced a marked depression of PHA responses in 16 of 22 patients while normal plasma had no such effect on normal lymphocytes. We recently repeated these studies in untreated patients, again with a large variety of cancers, and confirmed our original observations that plasma from many cancer patients possesses factors which depress the in vitro lymphocyte response of normal cells to PHA.[102] We are presently focusing on further isolation and characterization of these factors.

In summary, there is much evidence to support a relationship between cancer and immunity. The crucial question we are asking is whether this relationship is a primary one: Is malignant adaptation in the host successful only in the face of deficient immunologic responses? If so, the risk of fostering carcinogenesis should be carefully considered whenever therapy with immunosuppressants is considered. We recognize three important landmarks in oncogenesis: (1) genetic changes as discussed earlier by Conen and by Miller, (2) cell surface changes of permeability and the development of tumor-specific antigens, and (3) host response to the malignant clone. The frequent development of malignant clones apparently is a common phenomenon in all higher species. Perhaps malignant disease per se then should be considered a normal biologic variant whereas successful malignant adaptation is the result of an inappropriate host response. If this hypothesis is correct, the patients with immunologic deficiency diseases are presenting oncogenesis to us in its simplest clinical form.

Acknowledgments

Aided by grants from The National Foundation—March of Dimes, The American Heart Association, the American Cancer Society, and the U. S. Public Health Service (AI-08677, NB-02042, and AI-00292).

References

1. Sidkey, Y. A., and R. Auerbach: Tissue culture analysis of immunological capacity of snapping turtles. J. Exp. Zool., 167:187, 1968.
2. Trach, E., and R. A. Good: Phylogenetic study: The lymphoid organs of the bullfrog Rana catesbeiana: A bursa? In preparation.
3. Cooper, M. D., D. Y. Perey, A. E. Gabrielsen, D. E. R. Sutherland, M. F. Mc-Kneally, and R. A. Good: Production of an antibody deficiency syndrome in rabbits by neonatal removal of organized intestinal lymphoid tissues. Int. Arch. Allergy and Appl. Immunol., 33:65, 1968.
4. Gatti, R. A., O. Stutman, and R. A. Good: The lymphoid system. Ann. Rev. Physiol., 32:529, 1970.
5. Gatti, R. A., and R. A. Good: Immunological deficiency diseases. Med. Clin. North Amer., 54:281, 1970.
6. Good, R. A., and A. R. Page: Fatal complications of virus hepatitis in two agammaglobulinemic patients. Amer. J. Med., 29:804, 1960.
7. Page, A. R., A. E. Hansen, and R. A. Good: Occurrence of leukemia and lymphoma in patients with agammaglobulinemia. Blood, 21:197, 1963.
8. Reisman, L. E., M. Mitani, and W. W. Zuelzer: Chromosome studies in leukemia. I. Evidence for the origin of leukemic stem lines from aneuploid mutants. New Engl. J. Med., 270:591, 1964.
9. Good, R. A.: Unpublished observations.
10. Gorer, P. A.: Some reactions of H-2 antibodies in vitro and in vivo. Ann. N. Y. Acad. Sci., 73:707, 1958.
11. Dupuy, J. M., O. Stutman, and R. A. Good: Unpublished observations.
12. Hellström, I., K. E. Hellström, G. E. Pierce, and A. H. Bill: Demonstration of cell-bound and humoral immunity against neuroblastoma cells. Proc. Nat. Acad. Sci. USA, 60:1231, 1968.
13. Hellström, K. E., and I. Hellström: Cellular immunity against tumor antigens. Advances Cancer Res., 12:167, 1969.
14. Hellström, K. E., and I. Hellström: Immunologic defenses against cancer. Hosp. Prac., 5:45, 1970.
15. McEndy, D. P., M. C. Boon, and J. Furth: On the role of the thymus, spleen and gonads in the development of leukemia in a high-leukemia stock of mice. Cancer Res., 4:377, 1944.
16. Peterson, R. D. A., B. H. Burmester, T. N. Fredrickson, and R. A. Good: The prevention of lymphatic leukemia in the chicken by the surgical removal of the bursa of Fabricius. J. Lab. Clin. Med., 62:1000, 1963.
17. Peterson, R. D. A., B. R. Burmester, T. N. Frederickson, H. G. Purchase, and R. A. Good: The effect of bursectomy and thymectomy on the development of visceral lymphomatosis in the chicken. J. Nat. Cancer Inst., 32:1343, 1964.
18. Cooper, M. D., L. N. Payne, P. B. Dent, B. R. Burmester, and R. A. Good: The pathogenesis of avian lymphoid leukosis. I. Histogenesis. J. Nat. Cancer Inst., 41:373, 1968.
19. Dent, P. B., M. D. Cooper, L. N. Payne, J. Solomon, B. R. Burmester, and R. A. Good: The pathogenesis of avian lymphoid leukosis. II. Immunological reactivity during lymphomagenesis. J. Nat. Cancer Inst., 41:391, 1968.
20. Coleman, A., S. Leikin, and G. H. Guin: Aldrich's syndrome. Clin. Proc. Child. Hosp., 17:22, 1961.

21. Kildeberg, P.: A case of Aldrich's syndrome. Acta Paediat. Suppl., 140:120, 1961.
22. Amiet, A.: Aldrich's syndrome: A report of two cases. Ann. Paediat., 201:315, 1963.
23. Pearson, H. A., N. R. Shulman, F. A. Oski, and D. V. Eitzman: Platelet survival in Wiskott-Aldrich syndrome. J. Pediat., 68:754, 1966.
24. Ten Bensel, R. W., E. M. Stadlan, and W. Krivit: The development of malignancy in the course of the Aldrich syndrome. J. Pediat., 68:761, 1966.
25. Chaptal, J., P. Royer, R. Jean, D. Alagille, H. Bonnet, E. Lagarde, M. Robinet, and D. Rieu: Syndrome de Wiskott-Aldrich avec survie pronlongee (9 ans). Arch. Franc. Pediat., 23:907, 1966.
26. Hermans, P. E., K. A. Huizenga, and H. N. Hoffman: Dysgammaglobulinemia associated with nodular lymphoid hyperplasia of the small intestine. Amer. J. Med., 40:78, 1966.
27. Radl, J., J. Masopust, J. Houstek, and O. Hrodek: Paraproteinaemia and unusual dys-γ-globulinemia in a case of Wiskott-Aldrich syndrome. An immunochemical study. Arch. Dis. Child., 42:608, 1967.
28. Huber, J.: Experience with various immunologic deficiencies in Holland. In: Immunologic Deficiency Diseases in Man (R. A. Good and D. Bergsma, eds.), National Foundation Press, Vol. 4, 1968, pp. 53.
29. Cooper, M. D., H. P. Chase, J. T. Lowman, W. Krivit, and R. A. Good: Immunologic defects in patients with Wiskott-Aldrich syndrome. In: Immunologic Deficiency Diseases in Man, National Foundation Press, Vol. 4, 1968, p. 378.
30. Berglund, G., O. Finnstrom, S. G. Johanson, and K. L. Moller: Wiskott-Aldrich syndrome. A study of 6 cases with determination of Ig's A, D, G, M and ND. Acta Paediat. Scand., 57:89, 1968.
31. Krivit, W., E. Yunis, and J. G. White: Platelet survival studies in Aldrich syndrome. Pediatrics, 37:339, 1966.
32. Gröttum, K. A., T. Hovig, H. Holmsen, A. Foss Abrahamsen, M. Jeremia, and M. Seip: Wiskott-Aldrich syndrome: Qualitative platelet defects and short platelet survival. Brit. J. Haemat., 17:373, 1969.
33. Kuramoto, A., M. Steiner, and M. G. Baldini: Lack of platelet response to stimulation in the Wiskott-Aldrich syndrome. New Engl. J. Med., 282:475, 1970.
34. Boder, E., and R. P. Sedgwick: Ataxia-telangiectasia, a familial syndrome of progressive cerebellar ataxia, oculocutaneous telangiectasia and frequent pulmonary infection. Pediatrics, 21:526, 1958.
35. Boder, E., and R. P. Sedgwick: Ataxia-telangiectasia: A review of 101 cases. In: Cerebellum, Posture and Cerebral Palsy (G. Walsh, ed.), Little Club Clinics in Developmental Medicine, No. 8, 1963, p. 110.
36. Peterson, R. D. A., M. D. Cooper, and R. A. Good: Lymphoid tissue abnormalities associated with ataxia-telangiectasia. Amer. J. Med., 41:342, 1966.
37. Ammann, A. J., W. A. Cain, K. Ishizaka, R. Hong, and R. A. Good: Immunoglobulin E deficiency in ataxia-telangiectasia. New Engl. J. Med., 281:469, 1969.
38. Lapointe, N., et al.: Unpublished data.
39. Boder, E.: In discussion following paper by Peterson et al. J. Pediat., 63:702, 1963.
40. Szanto, P. B.: Personal communication.
41. Young, R. R., K. F. Austen, and H. W. Moser: Abnormalities of serum gamma-1-A globulin and ataxia-telangiectasia. Medicine, 43:423, 1964.
42. Dunn, H. G., H. Meuwissen, C. S. Livingstone, and K. K. Pump: Ataxia-telangiectasia. Canad. Med. Ass. J., 91:1106, 1964.
43. Peterson, R. D. A., W. D. Kelly, and R. A. Good: Ataxia-telangiectasia, its association with defective thymus, immunologic deficiency disease and malignancy. Lancet, 1:1189, 1964.
44. Murphy, M. L. and M. O'Neal: "Malformations observed in children's cancer population." Presented at Annual Meeting of the Teratology Society, San Francisco, May 27, 1965.
45. Shuster, J., Z. Hart, C. W. Stimson, A. J. Brough, and M. D. Poulik: Ataxia-telangiectasia with cerebellar tumor. Pediatrics, 37:776, 1966.

46. Hecht, F., R. D. Koler, D. A. Rigas, G. S. Dahnke, M. D. Case, V. Tisdale, and R. W. Miller: Leukemia and lymphocytes in ataxia-telangiectasia. Lancet, 2:1193, 1966.

47. Smeby, B.: Ataxia-telangiectasia. Acta Paediat., 55:239, 1966.

48. Landing, B. H.: Unpublished data.

49. Morgan, J. L., T. M. Holcomb, and R. W. Morrissey: Radiation reaction in ataxia-telangiectasia. Amer. J. Dis. Child., 116:557, 1968.

50. Haerer, A. F., J. F. Jackson, and C. G. Evers: Ataxia-telangiectasia with gastric adenocarcinoma. J. Amer. Med. Ass., 210:1884, 1969.

51. Lampert, F.: Akute lymphoblastische leukämie bei geschwistern mit progressiver kleinhiruataxie (Louis-Bar syndrom). Deut. Med. Wochensch., 94:217, 1969.

52. Feigen, R. D.: Personal communication.

53. Gropp, A., and G. Flatz: Chromosome breakage and blastic transformation of lymphocytes in ataxia-telangiectasia. Human-Genetik, 5:77, 1967.

54. Lisker, R., and A. Cobo: Chromosome breakage in ataxia-telangiectasia. Lancet, 1:618, 1970.

55. Jacobs, C. J., W. A. Blanc, A. de Capoa, W. C. Heird, E. McGiluray, O. J. Miller, J. H. Morse, R. D. Rossen, J. N. Schullinger, and R. A. Walzer: Complement deficiency and chromosomal breaks in a case of Swiss-type agammaglobulinemia. Lancet, 1:499, 1968.

56. Sawitsky, A., D. Bloom, and J. German: Chromosomal breakage and acute leukemia in congenital telangiectatic erythema and stunted growth. Intern. Med., 65:487, 1966.

57. Bloom, G. E., S. Warner, P. S. Gerald, and L. K. Diamond: Chromosomal abnormalities in constitutional aplastic anemia. New Engl. J. Med., 274:8, 1966.

58. Todaro, G. J., and K. K. Takemoto: "Rescued" SV 40: Increased transforming efficiency in mouse and human cells. Proc. Nat. Acad. Sci., 62:1031, 1969.

59. Fudenberg, H., and A. Solomon: Acquired agammaglobulinemia with autoimmune hemolytic disease: Graft-versus-host reaction? Vox Sang., 6:68, 1961.

60. Wolf, J. K., M. Gokcen, and R. A. Good: Heredo-familial disease of the mesenchymal tissue: Clinical and laboratory study of one family. J. Lab. Clin. Med., 61:230, 1963.

61. Dent, P. B., R. D. A. Peterson, and R. A. Good: The relationship between immunologic function and oncogenesis. In: Immunologic Deficiency Diseases in Man (R. A. Good and D. Bergsma, eds.), National Foundation Press, Vol. 4, 1968, p. 443.

62. Green, I., S. Litivin, R. Adlersberg, and I. Rubin: Hypogammaglobulinemia with late development of lymphosarcoma. Arch. Int. Med., 118:592, 1966.

63. Medical Research Council Working Party: Hypogammaglobulinemia in the United Kingdom. Summary Report. Lancet, 1:163, 1969.

64. Cattan, R., and P. Delavietre: Association d'un cancer gastrique et d'une leucemie lymphoide, accompagnee d'anomalies des proteines seriques. Arch. Mal. Appar. Dig., 47:1226, 1958.

65. Zelman, S., and H. Lewin: Adult agammaglobulinemia associated with multiple congenital anomalies. Amer. J. Med., 25:150, 1958.

66. Seligmann, M. M., H. G. Fudenberg, and R. A. Good: A proposed classification of primary immunological deficiencies. Amer. J. Med., 45:817, 1968.

67. Brem, T. H., and M. E. Morton: Defective serum gamma globulin formation. Ann. Int. Med., 43:465, 1955.

68. Latimer, E. O., E. J. Fitzsimmons, and P. S. Rhoads: Hypogammaglobulinemia associated with a severe wound infection. J. Amer. Med. Ass., 158:1344, 1955.

69. Van Gelder, D. W.: Clinical significance of alterations in gamma globulin levels. Southern Med. J., 50:43, 1957.

70. Good, R. A., S. J. Zak, R. M. Condie, and R. A. Bridges: Clinical investigation of patients with agammaglobulinemia and hypogammaglobulinemia. Pediat. Clin. North Amer., 7:397, 1960.

71. Kirkpatrick, C. H., D. Waxman, O. D. Smith, and R. N. Schimke: Hypogamma-

globulinemia with nodular lymphoid hyperplasia of the small bowel. Arch. Int. Med., 121:273, 1968.

72. Clinicopathological Conference: Rademacher's disease. Amer. J. Med., 32:80, 1962.
73. Hoyer, J. R., M. D. Cooper, A. E. Gabrielsen, and R. A. Good: Lymphopenic forms of congenital immunologic deficiency diseases. Medicine, 47:201, 1968.
74. Kadowaki,, J., R. I. Thompson, W. W. Zuelzer, P. V. Wooley, Jr., A. J. Brough, and D. Gruber: XX/XY lymphoid chimaerism in congenital immunological deficiency syndrome with thymic alymphoplasia. Lancet, 2:1152, 1965.
75. Lamvik, J., and P. J. Moe: Thymic dysplasia with immunological deficiency. Acta Path. Microbiol. Scand., 76:349, 1969.
76. Immunosuppression and cancer. An editorial. Lancet, 1:505, 1969.
77. McKhann, C. F.: Primary malignancy in patients undergoing immunosuppression for renal transplantation. Transplantation, 8:209, 1969.
78. MacLea, L. D., J. B. Dossetor, M. H. Gault, J. A. Oliver, F. G. Inglis, and K. J. Mackinnon: Renal homotransplantation using cadaver donors. Arch. Surg., 91:288, 1965.
79. Martin D. C., M. Rubini, and V. J. Rosen: Cadaveric renal homotransplantation with inadvertent transplantation of carcinoma. J. Amer. Med. Ass. 192:752, 1965.
80. Wilson, R. E., E. B. Hager, C. L. Hampers, J. M. Carson, J. P. Merrill, and J. E. Murray: Immunologic rejection of human carrier transplanted with a renal allograft. New Engl. J. Med., 278:479, 1968.
81. Zukoski, C. F., D. A. Killer, E. Ginn, B. Matter, D. O. Lucas, and H. F. Seigler: Transplanted carcinoma in an immunosuppressed patient. Transplantation, 9:71, 1970.
82. Hume, D. M.: Progress in clinical renal homotransplantation. Advances Surg., 2:419, 1966.
83. Muiznieks, H. W., J. W. Berg, W. Lawrence, and H. T. Randall: Suitability of donor kidneys from patients with cancer. Surgery, 64:871, 1968.
84. McPhaul, J. J., and D. A. McIntosh: Tissue transplantation still vexes. New Engl. J. Med., 272:105, 1965.
85. Deodhar, S. D., A. G. Kuklinca, D. G. Vidt, A. L. Robertson, and J. B. Hazard: Development of reticulum-cell sarcoma at the site of antilymphocyte globulin injection in a patient with renal transplant. New Engl. J. Med., 280:1104, 1969.
86. Malmgran, R. A., B. E. Bennison, and T. W. McKinley, Jr.: Reduced antibody titers in mice treated with carcinogenic and cancer chemotherapeutic agents. Proc. Soc. Exp. Biol. Med., 79:484, 1952.
87. Stjernswärd, J.: Effect of noncarcinogenic and carcinogenic hydrocarbons on antibody-forming cells measured at the cellular level *in vitro*. J. Nat. Cancer Inst., 36:1189, 1966.
88. Stjernswärd, J.: Immunodepressive effect of 3-MC. Antibody formation at the cellular level and reaction against weak antigenic homografts. J. Nat. Cancer Inst., 35:885, 1965.
89. Sulzberger, M. B., F. Herrman, R. Piccagli, and L. Frank: Incidence of epidermal methylcholanthrene tumors in mice after administration of cortisone. Proc. Soc. Exp. Biol. Med., 82:673, 1963.
90. Agosin, M., R. Cristen, O. Badinez, G. Gasic, A. Neghme, O. Pizzaro, and A. Jarpa: Cortisone induced metastases of adenocarcinoma in mice. Proc. Soc. Exp. Biol. Med., 80:128, 1952.
91. Good, R. A., and J. Finstad: The association of lymphoid malignancy and immunologic functions. In: Proceedings of the International Conference on Leukemia-Lymphoma (C. Zarafonetis, ed.), Lea & Febiger, 1968, pp. 175-197.
92. Hyman, G. A.: Increased incidence of neoplasia in association with chronic lymphocytic leukaemia. Scand. J. Hematol., 6:99, 1969.
93. Schier, W. W., A. Roth, G. Ostroff, and M. H. Schrift: Hodgkin's disease and immunity. Amer. J. Med., 20:94, 1956.
94. Kelly, W. D., R. A. Good, and R. L. Varco: Anergy and skin homograft survival in Hodgkin's disease. Surg. Gynecol. Obstet., 107:565, 1958.

95. Aisenberg, A. C.: Quantitative estimation of reactivity of normal and Hodgkin's disease lymphocytes with thymidine-2-^{14}C. Nature, 205:1233, 1965.
96. Hirschhorn, K., R. R. Schreibman, F. H. Bach, and L. E. Sitzbach: In vitro studies of lymphocytes from patients with sarcoidosis and lymphoproliferative disease. Lancet, 2:842, 1964.
97. Sokal, J. E., and C. W. Aungst: Response to BCG vaccination and survival in advanced Hodgkin's Disease. Cancer, 24:128, 1969.
98. Eilber, F. R., and D. L. Morton: Cutaneous anergy and prognosis following cancer surgery. Unpublished data.
99. Logan, J.: The delayed type of allergic reaction in cancer: Altered response to tuberculin and mumps virus. New Zeal. Med. J., 55:408, 1956.
100. Hughes, L. E., and W. D. Mackay: Suppression of the tuberculin response in malignant disease. Brit. Med. J., 2:1346, 1965.
101. Garrioch, D. B., R. A. Good, and R. A. Gatti: Lymphocyte response to PHA in patients with non-lymphoid tumours. Lancet, 1:618, 1970.
102. Gatti, R. A., D. B. Garrioch, and R. A. Good: Depressed PHA responses in patients with non-lymphoid malignancies. (Abstract) Fifth Leukocyte Culture Conference, Ottawa, Canada, June 25-27, 1970.
103. Huff, D., and L. Rupprecht: In preparation.
104. Arey, J. B., and A. DiGeorge: Personal communication.
105. Rosenthal, I. M., A. S. Markowitz, and R. Medenis: Immunologic incompetence in ataxia-telangiectasia. Amer. J. Dis. Child., 110:69, 1965.
106. Fois, A.: Presentazione di 4 casi di atassia teleangectasica. Riv. Clin. Pediat., 77:250, 1966.
107. Miller, D. G.: Association of immune disease and malignant lymphoma. Ann. Int. Med., 66:511, 1967.
108. Dugois, P., P. Ambilard, and R. Imbert. Ataxie telangiectasie et maladie de Hodgkin (A propos d'une observation). Bull. Soc. Franc. Derm. Syph., 74:507, 1967.
109. Gotoff, S. P., E. Amirmokri, and E. J. Liebner: Ataxia-telangiectasia: Neoplasia, untoward response to x-irradiation and tuberous sclerosis. Amer. J. Dis. Child., 114:617, 1967.
110. Harley, R. D., H. W. Baird, and E. A. Muffett: Ataxia-telangiectasia. Report of 7 cases. Read before the Ophthalmology Section, A.M.A. Chicago, June, 1966.
111. Harley, R. D., H. W. Baird, and E. M. Craven: Ataxia-telangiectasia. Report of 7 cases. Arch. Ophthalmol., 77:582, 1967.
112. Aguilar, M. J., S. Kamoshita, B. H. Landing, E. Boder, and R. P. Sedgwick: Pathological observations in ataxia-telangiectasia. A report on 5 cases. J. Neuropathol. Exp. Neurol., 27:659, 1968.
113. Castaigne, P., J. Cambier, and P. Brunet: Ataxie-télangiectasies, désordres immunitaires, lymphosarcomatose terminale chez deux frères. La Presse Med., 77:347, 1969.
114. Taleb, N., S. Tohmé, S. Ghostine, B. Barmada, and S. Nahas: Association d'une ataxie-télangiectasie avec une leucémie aigue lymphoblastique. La Presse Med., 77:345, 1969.
115. Boder, E., and R. P. Sedgwick: Personal communication.

Genetic Conditions Producing Increased Risk of Tumor, with Emphasis on Children

BENJAMIN H. LANDING

Departments of Pathology and Pediatrics, University of Southern California School of Medicine, Los Angeles, California, USA

FURTHER IMPROVEMENT IN survival of patients with malignant tumors depends only in part on improved therapeutic methods (surgery, radiotherapy, chemotherapy, immunotherapy, etc.). It requires also earlier recognition of tumors and perhaps, especially in children, increased recognition of "premalignant conditions." By this term one means conditions present in childhood which produce an increase in risk of tumor, either benign or malignant, in childhood or in later life. Identification of these conditions, and application to each of the diagnostic methods indicated by the nature of the specific process, permit the children at risk to receive the follow-up care, and early or prophylactic treatment, which will minimize the effect of the tumor, when and if it develops, on their well-being or life expectancy.

Table 21-4 presents a modified and extended "Richardson list" of conditions of children generally considered to cause, by a number of different mechanisms, tumors, either benign or malignant, or both. Such a list, of course, also applies to adults, and, in fact, quite a number of additional conditions, resulting particularly from occupational or other exposure to carcinogenic agents, could be added to a list designed to apply to adults. Inspection of the list shows that it includes a number of different types of conditions apparently operating by a variety of different mechanisms, including direct genetic effect, exposure to an environmental factor, genetically determined sensitivity to an environmental factor (e.g., solar radiation), chronic hyperplasia of an endocrine organ, and others. In terms of identification of children at risk, the presence of certain of the conditions on the list (e.g., ulcerative colitis, caustic esophageal stricture, radiated bone, exstrophy of bladder, cryptorchidism, large pigmented nevus, chronic renal insufficiency) is ordinarily known to patients and their physicians, but certain of the older conditions (e.g., past radiation of the thyroid, immunologic deficiency, gonadal dysgenesis and the hereditary intestinal polyposis called Peutz-Jeghers disease) may not be so easily recognizable in childhood. The list is not meant to imply that the neoplasm will necessarily develop during childhood; for example, esophageal carcinomas arising in caustic esophageal strictures, or skin carcinoma arising in burn scars, usually do not appear until middle age. The medical literature contains hints that still other predisposing conditions can be added to Table 21-4. Examples of such hints, presented here to encourage the studies necessary to establish or deny their validity, include the possible association of Turner's gonadal dysgenesis with acidophile cell hyperplasia progressing to adenoma of the an-

---

TABLE 21–4.

"Premalignant" Situations of Children

Polyposis of intestine (3 of 4 hereditary forms) *	—carcinoma of colon, small intestine
Ulcerative colitis	—carcinoma of colon
Caustic esophageal stricture	—carcinoma of esophagus
Congenital lung cyst (? only if genetic*)	—carcinoma of lung
Burn scars	—carcinoma of skin
Radiation dermatitis	—carcinoma of skin
Aberrant breast tissue	—carcinoma of breast
Radiated thyroid	—adenoma, carcinoma of thyroid
Abnormal susceptibility to sunlight (2 diseases) *	—carcinoma of skin
Chronic endocrine hyperplasia, several types* (pituitary, thyroid, parathyroid, adrenal)	—adenoma (carcinoma possible)
Cryptorchidism (especially male pseudohermaphroditism*)	—seminoma, ? other testis tumors, Wilms' tumor
Cirrhosis of liver*	—hepatoma
Exstrophy of bladder	—mucous carcinoma of bladder
Radiated bone	—osteochondroma/sarcoma
Giant pigmented nevus; neurocutaneous melanosis	—malignant melanoma
Immunosuppression, genetic*/iatrogenic/acquired spontaneous	—leukemia, malignant lymphoma
Malabsorption Syndromes* (a) (? only with immune defect)	(a) malignant lymphoma, especially of bowel
(b) chronic hypocalcemia	(b) parathyroid adenoma
Chronic renal insufficiency*	—parathyroid adenoma (tertiary hyperparathyroidism)
Teratoma	—late carcinoma of pancreas, etc. (orchioblastoma embryonal carcinoma, chorio-carcinoma are inherent, and not secondary processes, in teratomas)
Gonadal dysgenesis* (? especially XY/XO Nosaicism)	—gonadoblastoma
Hemihypertrophy	—Wilms' tumor, adrenal cortical and liver tumors
Aniridia	—Wilms' tumor

* See also genetic disease list.

TABLE 21–5.—Genetic Diseases Causing Tumors

A. Specific Genetic Diseases, Malignancy Regular, Inherent (All Dominant)

Retinoblastoma	—retinoblastoma
Trichoepithelioma (Spiegler-Brooke epithelioma adenoides cysticum; cylindromatosis; turban tumors)	—trichoepithelioma (cylindroma)
von Recklinghausen's neurofibromatosis	—neurofibrosarcoma, benign and malignant gliomas, pheochromocytoma
Tuberose sclerosis (epiloia)	—malignant glioma
Basal cell nevus syndrome	—basal cell carcinoma, medulloblastoma
Multiple colonic polyposis #1 (familial polyposis)	—carcinoma of colon
Multiple colonic polyposis #3 (Gardner)	—carcinoma of colon, malignant glioma (called Turcot's Syndrome)
Multiple colonic polyposis #4 (Multiple juvenile polyps)	—? No risk of malignant tumor

B. Specific Genetic Diseases, Endocrine Tumor Inherent (All Dominant)

Regular

Multiple endocrine adenomatosis #1 (Werner)	—adenomas of pituitary parathyroid, pancreatic islet; carcinoid (G.I. tract and lung)
Multiple endocrine adenomatosis #2 (Sipple) (PTC-Syndrome)	—thyroid carcinoma; parathyroid adenoma; pheochromocytoma; ? carcinoid-thyroid carcinoma, pheochromocytoma

Variable

von Hippel-Lindau angiomatosis of cerebellum retina, spinal cord	—pheochromocytoma
Intestinal polyposis #2 (Peutz-Jeghers)	—Sex-cord tumor with annular tubules, ? dysgerminoma, carcinoma of intestine
von Recklinghausen's neurofibromatosis	—pheochromocytoma

C. Specific Genetic Diseases, Tumor Secondary (Variable)*

"Immunosuppression" R,SLR—agammaglobulinemia	—leukemia
R—Wiskott-Aldrich disease	
R—Ataxia-telangiectasia	—lymphoreticular system tumors
R—Chediak-Higashi disease	
Chromosome fragility	
R—Bloom dwarfism disease	—leukemia
R—Fanconi's anemia	—leukemia
Cirrhosis of liver	
R—Type 4 glycogen storage disease (Brancher enzyme deficiency)	
R—Tyrosinosis	hepatoma
D—Hemochromatosis	
?— (Neonatal hepatitis/biliary atresia, familial but ? genetic)	

TABLE 21–5. *(cont.)*

Light sensitivity
  R—Xeroderma pigmentosum (deficient DNA repair) —skin carcinoma, ? leukemia
  R—Porphyria (increased U V sensitivity) —skin carcinoma
Abnormal "growth" control
  R—Hyperplastic fetal visceromegaly (Beckwith)   —Wilms' tumor, adrenal
                                                          cortical tumor, liver tumors
Endocrine hyperplasia
  R—adrenogenital syndrome—adrenal, Leydig cell tumors
  R—goitrous cretinism—thyroid adenoma
  ?— (Chronic thyroiditis—? thyroid carcinoma—? genetic influence)
Various—parathyroid hyperplasia (renal, malabsorptive)   —parathyroid adenoma
  (also non-genetic causes—see Table 21-4)   (tertiary hyperpara-
                                                          thyroidism)

D. SPECIFIC GENETIC DISEASES, TUMOR VARIABLE, ? MECHANISM

D—Multiple exostosis (diaphyseal aclasis)   —chondrosarcoma
?—SLD—Paget's disease—sarcoma of bone
R—Gonadal dysgenesis (some forms) —gonadoblastoma
R—Type I glycogen storage disease (von Gierke) —hepatoma
D—Tylosis palmaris—carcinoma of esophagus
D—Fibrocystic pulmonary dysplasia—carcinoma of lung
R, ?SLR—Male pseudohermaphroditism (feminizing testis syndrome) —seminoma

---

 * R, recessive; SLR, sex-linked recessive; D, dominant; SLD, sex-linked dominant.

---

terior pituitary, of Alport's familial nephritis with renal carcinoma, and of at least one form of polycystic disease of liver and kidneys with thyroid hyperplasia progressing to adenoma.

Table 21-4 contains predominantly conditions which are "premalignant" in the sense that tumors, when they develop, arise in an organ or tissue clinically involved by the basic disease. However, the table also contains some conditions which serve as "signs" that the patient is at risk for development of a tumor, even though the "sign" does not involve the organ where the tumor will develop. Recently emphasized examples of such "signs" are aniridia and hemihypertrophy, both of which identify an increased risk of Wilms' tumor (nephroblastoma), and hemihypertrophy also of tumors of the adrenal cortex and liver.

The genetically determined conditions listed are only a fraction of the specific genetic diseases which can cause tumors, and for which identification of potentially or actually affected persons is aided by the presence of the disorder in members of the family. Table 21-5 lists the more important specific genetic diseases which cause tumors, either regularly or with increased frequency. In considering this table, and its implications for genetic counseling, one must bear in mind that the statement "a genetically determined condition is present in childhood" applies to patients with all genetically determined diseases whether the condition causes clinical disease in childhood and whether a laboratory test for the preclinical state exists. Confusion on this at times results from the similarity of the name of a disease to the name of a lesion. Thus, a person with neurofibromatosis or tuberous sclerosis has the disease from birth, even though neurofibromas or cerebral tubers may not be demonstrable for some years.

Seven disorders are listed in Table 21-5 (Part A), all of which appear to produce malignant tumors by a direct genetic effect, with or without an antecedent "benign" tumor phase, either with high frequency or invariably, and all of which are autosomal dominant disorders—namely, affected persons ordinarily have an affected parent and will, if they live to reproduce, often have affected children themselves. A group of disorders are separated in Table 21-5 (Part B); they again are all autosomal dominant diseases, in which tumors of endocrine organs appear to occur as an inherent feature of the disease, either invariably, as in the multiple endocrine adenomatosis diseases, or occasionally. The importance of this group, and of those secondary endocrine tumors listed in Table 21-5 (Parts C and D), in the context of tumor prophylaxis or early therapy, lies in the possibility of recognizing the presence of the tumor, or of following its behavior, by chemical or hormonal assays. Table 21-5 (Part C) lists a wide variety of specific genetic diseases which dispose patients to tumors of the types listed, and for which a proposal on the mechanism by which the disease causes the tumor can be made, even though the precise nature of the mechanism by which some (e.g. cirrhosis of liver) operate is not known. Table 21-5 (Part D) contains specific genetic diseases which sometimes cause tumors, and for which a mechanism by which the disease leads to tumor can not be proposed with certainty. More detailed analysis of Table 21-5 is precluded by the number of variety of the conditions it contains. However, recognition of one of these conditions in a patient should dictate the appropriate aspects of his medical care and follow-up, as well as appropriate study and genetic counseling of apparently unaffected family members. In the context of this discussion, the latter point applies particularly to children, whether the index case be a parent, a sibling, or other relative (e.g. mother's brother).

A good illustration of the several ways to which factors which increase a person's risk of developing a malignant tumor operate is shown by a list of conditions which cause enhanced risk of leukemia (Table 21-6). Some of these conditions are definitely or presumably genetic, while others are caused by a chromosome abnormality whether inherent or acquired, and still others are caused by exposure (accidental, iatrogenic, or occupational) to leukemogenic environmental factors.

Several local oncogenic effects of radiation (of skin, bone, and thyroid) are listed in Table 21-4, and the ability of both local and whole body radiation to cause leukemia is emphasized in Table 21-6. The follow-up studies of persons exposed to whole body radiation in

TABLE 21–6.—CONDITIONS WITH INCREASED RISK OF LEUKEMIA

CONDITION	RISK
Identical twin of leukemic	1/5
Polycythemia vera (treated by radiation)	1/5
Bloom and Fanconi diseases*	1/5
Severe whole body radiation	1/60
Down syndrome	1/95
Heavy local radiation (e.g., for ankylosing spondylitis)	1/270
Sib of leukemic	? 4 times normal

Agammaglobulinemia,* benzene exposure—risk increased, but risk-figure not available.
? risk increase—Klinefelter (XXY, etc.) Syndrome, trisomy 13-15, trisomy 18

* See also genetic disease list.

Japan in 1945 indicate that both acute and chronic myeloid leukemia, and acute lymphatic leukemia, may result from radiation, but that chronic lymphatic leukemia apparently does not, so that it apparently differs significantly in basic cause from the other major types of leukemia. This difference is emphasized by the fact that chronic lymphatic leukemia is the type of leukemia which most commonly shows familial, and perhaps genetically determined, occurrence (Table 21-7). The evidence from the studies in Japan that carcinoma of the thyroid definitely, and carcinoma of lung and breast possibly, are increased in patients who survive whole body radiation, may suggest new lines of investigation of the general cause of the latter two tumors.

In addition to the variety of situations listed above, where tumors are the lesion of a genetic disease, or where they occur in some way in association with, and apparently as a result of, a genetic disease, familial occurrence has been reported for over 30 types of human tumors (Table 21-7). These obviously provide an important and fruitful field for study of the exact extent of genetic determination of many tumors. Analysis of the available data for the 38 tumor types listed in Table 21-7 suggests that 14 probably are features of specific genetic diseases. Another eight are tumor types which are sometimes, but apparently not always, associated with specific genetic diseases (see Tables 21-4 and 21-5). For at least 16 of the tumor types listed in Table 21-7, the extent of genetic determination is not adequately known. Establishment of the degree to which such tumors are in fact genetically determined will further extend the ability of the physician to provide his patients appropriate prophylactic or prognostic care. An increased risk of tumor in relatives of patients with certain tumors is sometimes presented as not due to specific genetic influence, but it is difficult to propose an alternative for most such associations. An example is the described increased frequency of brain tumors in siblings of a patient with brain tumor (frequency 15 times normal). Table 21-5 contains five specific genetic diseases causing brain tumor,

TABLE 21–7.—Tumors with Reported Familial Occurrence in
Apparent Absence of Other Genetic Disease

Acoustic neuroma (bilateral)	(a)
Adrenal cortical adenoma (macrosomia adiposa congenita)	(a,b)
Angiofibroma of nasopharynx, juvenile	(c)
Carcinoid	(b)
Carcinoma of bladder	(c)
Carcinoma of breast	(c)
Carcinoma of colon (without polyposis)	(b)
Carcinoma of ureter	(c)
Chemodectoma (carotid body and/or jugular glomus tumors)	(a)
Chondrosarcoma	(b)
Chordoma	(c)
Dysgerminoma	(b)
Giant cell tumor of jaws, bilateral (cherubism)	(a)
Glioblastoma multiforme	(b)
Glomus tumor, multiple	(a)
Hodgkin's disease	(c)
Hypernephroma	(c)
Kaposi's sarcoma	(c)
Leiomyomata of vulva and esophagus	(a)
Leiomyomata, multiple cutaneous	(a)
Leukemia (especially chronic lymphatic)	(b)
Lipoma, multiple (3 different forms)	(a)
Malignant melanoma, multiple cutaneous	(c)
Malignant melanoma, ocular	(c)
Meningioma	(b)
Multiple myeloma	(c)
Neuroblastoma	(c)
Oligodendroglioma	(c)
Osteogenic sarcoma	(b)
Papilloma of choroid plexus	(c)
Parathyroid adenoma	(a,b)
Pheochromocytoma	(a,b)
Pineal tumor	(c)
Syringoma, multiple	(a)
Torus of palate and/or mandible	(a)
Wilms' tumor	(b)

(a) Perhaps specific genetic disease.
(b) Tumor of type sometimes associated with specific genetic disease (see Table 21-5).
(c) Importance of genetic factor(s) not known.

which, collectively could go far to explain the association mentioned, as could establishment of the fact that some or all of the six brain tumors listed in Table 21-7 are truly genetically determined. The suggestive association of rhabdomyosarcomas with other tumors in families needs further study before its possible meaning can be analyzed.

The material presented thus far has attempted to demonstrate that physicians caring for children can make a significant contribution toward improving the morbidity and mortality from tumors by giving thought to the increased risk of tumor attached to certain disorders or states, by considering the implications for other family members of the demonstration of certain tumors or genetic diseases in patients, and by appropriately applying the results of their considerations. That the potentialities of such effort are far from exhausted has been pointed out several times. One can emphasize this latter point still further by a brief consideration of a group of disorders which can be grouped under the rubric, "immunologic defect." There is good reason to believe that malignant cells arise in human beings with considerably greater frequency than has thought to be in the past, but that they are prevented from causing clinical malignancies because they are recognized as "foreign," and destroyed by immunologic and phagocytic mechanisms. In addition to acquired (carcinolytic or immunosuppressive drug therapy; spontaneous) "immunologic paralysis," a considerable number of proved or probably genetically determined disorders of immunocyte and/or immunoglobulin production, or of phagocytic capacity, exists: agammaglobulinemia (three or four different diseases), alymphoplasia and "dysgammaglobulinemia" (at least six types), and phagocytosis defects (four major kinds). In practice, the term dysgammaglobulinemia means selective depression of the blood level of one or more of the immunoglobulin classes A, D, E, G, or M, and not that the immunoglobulins are structurally abnormal and nonfunctional. If the immunoglobulins A, D, E, G, and M can each behave as a unit, the theoretical minimum number of dysgammaglobulinemias" is 30—five disorders each with a single immunoglobulin class deficient; five disorders with a single immunoglobulin class normal and the other four deficient; 10 disorders with two types abnormal and three normal; and 10 disorders with three types abnormal and two normal. Since it is already known that selective deficiency of only certain antibodies in an immunoglobulin class exists for immunoglobulins A, G, and M, one can be sure that the true number of "immune defect diseases" is not yet known, that their importance in permitting malignant tumors to develop is necessarily underestimated at present, and that the potential value to physicians of improved ability to demonstrate them can only be conjectured.

Present evidence is that the lymphoreticular system has two major control mechanisms, one thymic, which controls small lymphocytes and delayed hypersensitivity reactions, and one intestinal (the "bursa equivalent"), which controls large lymphocytes, plasma cells, immunoglobulin production and antigen-antibody mediated reactions. The two systems, the thymic control system and the bursal control system, can be defective together or separately, and there are apparently partial abnormalities of the latter. Obviously, also, both require for normal function an inherently normal lymphoreticular system and normal phagocyte (both macrophage and polymorphonuclear cell) systems. Table 21-8 gives a list of described disorders of the "immune phagocyte" system, in terms of the apparent locus of basic defect, and in

TABLE 21–8.—DISORDERS OF THE LYMPHORETICULAR AND MYELOID SYSTEMS CAUSING
DEFECTS OF IMMUNOCYTES, IMMUNOGLOBULINS, OR PHAGOCYTOSIS

LOCUS OF DEFECT	DISORDER	LYMPHORETICULAR MALIGNANCY REPORTED
Lymphoreticular and myeloid cells deficient	reticular dysgenesis (DeVaal)	
Thymic and bursal control	agammaglobulinemia (Swiss type)	leukemia
Systems (deficiency of all immunocytes and immunoglobulins)	a) autosomal recessive b) sex-lined recesive c) Swiss-type agammaglobulinemia with achondroplasia—autosomal recessive	
Thymic control system (small lymphocyte deficiency)	thymic alymphoplasia a) Nezelof type—immunoglobulins normal	lymphoma, reticular cell sarcoma
	b) ataxia-telangiectasia: gamma A often deficient	" "
	c) thymic alymphoplasia with other dysgammaglobulinemias reported (see below)	" "
	d) DiGeorge disease—with hypoparathyroidism	
Bursal control system (large lymphocyte and plasma cell deficiency, with immunoglobulin abnormality)	Agammaglobulinemia, Bruton type ? partial defects a) dysgammaglobulinemia, type I (gamma A and G low; gamma M elevated) b) dysgammaglobulinemia, type II (gamma A and M low; gamma G normal) c) see also b) under thymic alymphoplasia d) selective plasma cell deficiency reported	leukemia
Phagocyte defects Phagocyte number	granulocytopenia—agranulocytosis: different forms include: chronic familial neutropenia (Kostman) (R,D) cydic-neutropenia (D) lethal congenital neutropenia with eosinophilia (R) Fanconi's pancytopenia (R) neutropenia with maturation arrest, low immunoglobulins (Lonsdale) (R) pancreatic insufficiency and pancytopenia (Shwachman) (R) cartilage-hair hypoplasia and neutropenia (R) dyskeratosis congenita and pancytopenia (Zinsser-Cole-Engman-Syndrome) (R) (see also reticular dysgenesis above)	

TABLE 21–8. *(cont.)*

Locus of Defect	Disorder	Lymphoreticular Malignancy Reported
Enzyme abnormality	septic granulomatosis (PLH disease) susceptibility especially to Staphylococcus, gram-negative bacilli, Nocardia)	
Abnormal lysosomes	Myeloperoxidase deficiency (susceptibility especially to Candida) Chediak-Higashi disease	leukemia-like state
Opsonin-defects	Wiskott-Aldrich disease (defect in recognition of polysaccharide antigens— susceptibility especially to Streptococci and Pneumococcus) ? Sickle-cell anemia (? similar defect— susceptibility especially to Pneumococci reported) (at least 2 other types of phagocyte "impotence" described "granulocytasthemia" and deficiency of non-immunoglobulin phagocytosis-promoting serum factor)	lymphoma
? Reticuloendothelial blockade (deficient antigen-processing and phagocytosis)	hemosiderosis (e.g. thalassemia) lipid histiocytosis (e.g. Gaucher and Niemann-Pick diseases)	
? partial R-E blockade	asplenia (Ivemark) syndrome post-splenectomy sepsis	

terms of reported liability of affected patients to develop lymphoreticular malignancies. Experience in recent years with acquired immunosuppression (e.g. by immunosuppressive drugs or antilymphocyte serum) suggests that patients with many of these diseases should have an increased frequency of other types of tumors as well, but data on children are not yet adequate.

The concept of hamartosis or hamartomatosis frequently arises in discussion of familial tumor syndromes. In Albrecht's original usage, hamartoma meant a tumor composed of cells normally present in the site (as opposed to choristoma, a tumor of cells foreign to the site). The term has since acquired the meaning of tumor-like growths, thought to be due to abnormal mixture and/or proportions of tissues, which in some way differ from "conventional" benign and malignant tumors. Neither use specifies the cause of the growth abnormality, nor that all disorders included under the general term have the same or similar causes, so that the concept has, as is usually applied, no obvious operational value.

Table 21-9 (Part A) lists conditions which we can group as genetically determined skin tumors, other than hemangiomata, and Table 21-9

TABLE 21–9

A. Genetically Determined Diseases with Skin Tumors, not Angiomata

Adiposis dolorosa (Dercum's disease)
Basal cell nevus syndrome
Cervical lipomatosis
Gardner syndrome
Multiple cutaneous glomus tumor
Multiple koratodeanthoma
Multiple cutaneous leiomyoma
Multiple lipomatosis
Multiple sebaceous cysts (steatocystoma multiplex)
Multiple syringoma
Neurofibromatosis
Spiegler-Brooke epithelioma adenoides cysticum (trichoepithelioma, cylindromatosis)
Tuberose sclerosis

B. Genetically Determined Angioma Syndromes (Locus of Vascular Component in Parentheses)

Ataxia telangiectasia (skin, conjunctivae, esophagus)
Blue rubber bleb nevus (skin)
Multiple telangiectasis of brain
Rendu-Osler-Weber hereditary hemorrhagic telangiectasia (skin, mucosae, lung)
Riley-Smith macrocephaly, cutaneous angiomata and pseudopapilledema (skin)
von-Hippel-Lindau disease (eye, cerebellum, spinal cord)
(? Juvenile angiofibroma of nasopharynx is genetically determined)

C. Apparently Non-Genetically Determined Tumor-Like States (? Terms Hamartoma, Hamartomatosis, or Hamartosis Should Be Restricted to This Group)

Sturge-Weber (Kalischer-Dimitri) encephalotrigeminal angiomatosis
Brushfield-Wyatt disease (? same as Sturge-Weber disease, but angioma also involves trunk)
Klippel-Trenaunay-Weber angiomatosis with skeletal hypertrophy
Maffucci disease (hemangiomatosis, enchondromatosis, exostosis, other tumors)
McCune-Albright polyostotic fibrous dysplasia, other tumors
Cystic skeletal lymphangiomatosis (disappearing bone disease)
Cronkite-Canada disease (intestinal polyposis, ectodermal lesions)
Ollier's enchondromatosis
Hemangioma of small intestine in Turner's gonadal dysgenesis giant pigmented nevus; neurocutaneous melanosis
Hemihypertrophy (as in Silver syndrome) (may also occur in Klippel-Trenaunay-Weber disease (see above) and in Beckwith syndrome (see Table 21-5)
Mutation to a dominant abnormal gene is the most probable genetic explanation of apparently non-familial disease; some of these disorders may actually be genetic (? suggestion strongest for Ollier's disease)

(Part B) lists the described genetically determined angioma syndromes, not all of which involve the skin. Some disorders in both groups are often included in a list of hamartomatous disorders, as may be the apparently nongenetically determined disorders listed in Table 21-9 (Part C). One can suggest that a concept of hamartomatous disorders can have operational value if restricted to this group of conditions.

References

1. Fraumeni, J. F., and A. G. Glass: Wilms' tumor and congenital aniridia. J. Amer. Med. Ass., 206:825, 1968.
2. Fraumeni, J. F., and F. P. Li: Hodgkin's disease in childhood: An epidemiologic study. J. Nat. Cancer Inst., 42:681, 1969.
3. Fraumeni, J. F., and R. W. Miller: Adrenocortical neoplasms with hemihypertrophy, brain tumors and other disorders. J. Pediat., 70:129, 1967.
4. Hellström, K. E., and I. Hellström: Immunologic defenses against cancer. Hosp. Practice, 5:45-61, 1970.
5. McKusick, V. A.: Mendelian Inheritance in Man. Catalogs of Autosomal Dominant, Autosomal Recessive, and X-Linked Phenotypes. The Johns Hopkins Press, Baltimore, 2nd Edition, 1968, p. 521.
6. Miller, R. W.: Down's syndrome (mongolism), other congenital malformations and cancers among the sites of leukemic children. New Eng. J. Med., 268:383, 1963.
7. Miller, R. W.: Deaths from childhood cancer in sibs. New Eng. J. Med., 279:122, 1968.
8. Miller, R. W.: Relation between cancer and congenital defects in man. New Eng. J. Med., 275:87, 1966.
9. Miller, R. W.: Delayed radiation effects in atomic-bomb survivors: Major observations by the Atomic Bomb Casualty Commission are evaluated. Science, 166:569, 1969.
10. Miller, R. W., J. F. Fraumeni, and M. D. Manning: Association of Wilms' tumor with aniridia, hemihypertrophy and other congenital malformations. New Eng. J. Med., 270:992, 1964.
11. Li, F. P., and J. F. Fraumeni: Rhabdomyosarcoma in children: Epidemiologic study and identification of a familial cancer syndrome. J. Nat. Cancer Inst., 43:1365, 1969.
12. Scully, R. E.: Sex cord tumor with annular tubules. A distinctive ovarian tumor of the Peutz-Jeghers syndrome. Cancer, 25:1107, 1970.
13. Hirschhorn, K. J., and L. Y. Hsu: Sex chromosome mosaicism in individuals with a Y chromosome. In Phenotypic aspects of chromosomal aberration. Birth Defects: Original Article Series 5, 5:19, 1969.
14. Reed, W. B., S. W. Becker, Sr., S. W. Becker, Jr., and W. R. Nickel: Giant pigmented nevi, melanoma and leptomeningeal melanocytosis. Arch. Dermatol., 91:100, 1965.
15. Drash, A., F. Sherman, W. H. Hartmann, and R. M. Blizzard: A syndrome of pseudohermaphroditism, Wilms' tumor, hypertension, and degenerative renal disease. J. Pediat., 76:585-593, 1970.

Genetic Susceptibility of Human Cells to Cancer Viruses

GEORGE TODARO

Molecular Biology Section, Viral Carcinogenesis Branch, National Cancer Institute, National Institutes of Health, Bethesda, Maryland, USA

FROM SKIN PUNCH biopsies, human cells can be grown in tissue culture and the cells tested for their susceptibility to the transforming effect of oncogenic viruses. Methods have been developed that make it possible to measure the relative susceptibility of cells from different individuals to the tumor viruses. The "transformed" cells can be recognized because they lose contact inhibition of cell division and acquire the ability to grow over one another in a random, disorganized fashion. The control mechanisms that regulated normal cells are lost in the cells transformed by the viruses. The changes produced in human cells in tissue culture are identical to the changes produced in cells of many other species, where it is possible to confirm the malignant change by direct inoculation of virus and/or cells into the animals. The viruses that have been used are the small DNA-containing viruses, simian virus 40 (SV40), human adenovirus type 12, and certain strains of mouse sarcoma virus; all are able, under the proper conditions, to transform human cells.

Various factors influence the probability that a given cell, exposed to a cancer virus will be transformed to a malignant cell by that virus. There are genetic factors, both of the virus and of the cell it infects, that influence the outcome (see Table 21-10). There are also important environmental factors; cells that are rapidly dividing are more susceptible than quiescent cells and cells that are damaged by radiation and chemical carcinogens are more susceptible to the tumor viruses than are healthy, undamaged cells. Further, cells from elderly people are more "cancer-prone" than cells from children or young adults. Cells can also be "aged" in tissue culture, so that after several months the cells are more susceptible to the virus than they were initially.

Perhaps the most interesting finding is that the cells derived from individuals with certain genetic diseases that are known to predispose them to cancer are significantly more susceptible to transformation than are cells derived from apparently normal individuals. The two diseases that have been most thoroughly studied are Down's syndrome (mongolism) and an extremely rare disease called Fanconi's anemia. Both diseases are associated with chromosome abnormalities;

TABLE 21–10.—Factors Affecting Human Cell Susceptibility
to Tumor Viruses

I. Viral
    a. Dose—direct proportionality between number of virus particles and number of cells transformed[4]
    b. Genetics—certain strains of tumor viruses transform human cells much more efficiently than other strains[3]

II. Environmental
    a. Chromosome damaging agents such as radiation and certain drugs increase susceptibility to viral transformation[7]
    b. Aging—cells from elderly people and cells that have been "Aged" *in vitro* are more susceptible[5]

III. Cellular
    a. Down's Syndrome cells for example, more susceptible *in vitro*[2] and at greater cancer risk[6]
    b. "Cancer families"—several members of one family show high susceptibility whether or not they have actually developed cancer[9]

in the former case there is an extra chromosome and in the latter case, a high frequency of broken chromosomes. Children with both diseases are much more likely than the general population to develop leukemia and our tests show that their cells are much more likely to be transformed by cancer viruses when compared to skin cells from normal people.

By carrying out the experiments on isolated cells in tissue culture it is possible to rule out other factors—such as the immunologic defense system, hormonal factors, drugs, etc.—that may influence susceptibility in the body. We conclude that in these two diseases the people are "cancer-prone" because their individual cells are. We thus can study in an isolated cell system the "defect" in the susceptible cells that increases its risk of becoming a malignant cell.

It should be emphasized that the various environmental factors, such as radiation and drugs, as well as the genetic susceptibility factors, are not, in themselves, enough to bring about the change from normal human cells to malignant cells in the absence of added viruses. Their effects then appear to be enhancing rather than direct. A common component, we suggest, is that damage to the cell's genetic material, whether extrinsic, as in the case of drugs and radiation, or intrinsic, as in certain genetic diseases, renders a person's cell more susceptible to virus transformation. During the process of damage and repair of host DNA, it may be easier for the genetic information of the virus to become permanently incorporated into the host cells.

In more recent studies of cells from apparently normal individuals we have found that approximately 3-5% have unusually high susceptibility. When the relatives of one of these was checked it was found that three of them also showed high susceptibility, further suggesting an inherited factor. In one family presently being studied at the National Institute of Health Clinical Center, three of six children have developed acute myelogenous leukemia (AML) and three relatives of the mother also have had AML. The mother has cervical carcinoma. The transformation test shows the mother, one of the three unaffected children, and one relative on the maternal side to have strikingly high tumor virus susceptibility. It appears that this family is unusually "cancer-prone" and that some susceptibility factor has been transmitted through the maternal side. Other high-cancer families and other high-risk diseases are presently being studied.

The skin cell transformation test may allow us to recognize individuals that are at "high risk" of developing cancer. While, at the moment, there is no specific preventative treatment, at the time that such preventatives do become available it will be important to be able to identify those people who stand the greatest risk of developing malignant diseases. The test is now being adapted to study cells from a large number of people to see to what extent it can be used as a prognostic indicator of cancer risk in man. Finally, the use of highly susceptible human cells and optimal tissue culture conditions to detect transformation should help in the search for unknown cancer viruses of man.

References

1. Todaro, G., H. Green, and M. Swift: Susceptibility of human diploid fibroblast strains to transformation by SV40. Science, 153:1252, 1967.
2. Todaro, G., and G. Martin: Down's syndrome: Increased susceptibility of fibroblasts in cell culture to transformation by an oncogenic virus. Proc. Soc. Exp. Biol. Med., 124:1232, 1967.
3. Todaro, G., and S. Aaronson: Human adenovirus type 12: Focus formation in human diploid cells. Proc. Nat. Acad. Sci. USA, 61:1272, 1968.
4. Aaronson, S., and G. Todaro: SV40 T-antigen induction and transformation in human fibroblast cells. Virology, 36:254, 1968.
5. Todaro, G.: Variation in susceptibility of human cell strains to SV40 transformation. Nat. Cancer Inst. Monogr., 29:271, 1968.
6. Miller, R., and G. Todaro: Viral transformation and high risk of cancer. Lancet, 1:81, 1969.
7. Pollock, E., and G. Todaro: Radiation enhancement of SV40 transformation in 3T3 and human cells. Nature, 219:520, 1968.
8. Todaro, G., and K. Takemoto: "Rescued SV40: Increased transforming efficiency for mouse and human cells." Proc. Nat. Acad. Sci. USA, 62:1031-1037, 1969.
9. Snyder, A. L., F. P. Li, E. S. Henderson, and G. J. Todaro: Familial acute myelogenous leukemia: Identification of possible inherited leukemogenic factors in a kindred. Lancet, 1:586, 1970.

Redifferentiation of Certain Neoplasms: Growth, Differentiation, and Function of Neuroblastomas In Vitro

MILTON N. GOLDSTEIN, JAMES M. ENGLAND, AND SHIRLEY SILBERT

Departments of Anatomy and Pathology, Washington University School of Medicine, St. Louis, Missouri, USA

NEUROBLASTOMAS OF CHILDREN are of special interest because of the many reported cases of spontaneous regression and because the malignant neuroblast has the potential to mature into a nonmultiplying neuron.[1] One conclusion that can be drawn from these observations is that large ganglioneuromas must at one time have been neuroblastomas.

Previous investigations showed that neuroblastomas of children could be grown for long periods in tissue culture and during this time neuroblasts differentiated and some matured into ganglion cells.[2, 3]

The following report describes further studies of human neuroblastomas, including a cell line NJB which has been in continuous culture for five years. Some comparisons are made with a mouse neuroblastoma C 1300 and with normal immature sympathetic nerve cells grown under similar conditions in vitro.

Cells were dissociated with trypsin as previously described[3, 4] and explanted on glass, plastic, collagen, or in chicken plasma clots. The medium contained 30% calf serum and medium 199. Cells could also be grown in human sera and defined media F 10 or F 12. In some experiments, one to 100 units/ml of purified nerve growth factor (NGF)[5] was added to the medium; 200 units/ml of penicillin were routinely added.

Human neuroblastomas, including those tumors which by bright field observation consist of small round cells devoid of any specific arrangement or differentiation, begin to send out neurites soon after they are explanted in vitro. The outgrowth of new processes occurs more rapidly when cells are embedded in plasma clots but their formation also occurs when tumor cells are explanted on other substrates. Cells without processes begin to send out a single relatively thick growth cone. As the process becomes longer, it begins to taper and frequently may have two or three branches. The endings become expanded and have many fine filopodia and resemble those of normal motor neurons. In time many cells begin to develop multiple processes. This is especially true when there are dense aggregates of cell bodies. In fluid media, differentiation of the tumor cells is influenced by cell density; the longest neurites always develop from multilayered aggregates. In addition to forming many collaterals which intertwine with those of other tumor cells, the neurites develop fine spines. Eventually, many of the terminals make contact with cell bodies or other processes. At these contacts the endings become dilated and resemble synaptic bulbs. At points of contacts between cell bodies and between the endings of neurites there are localized thickenings of the membranes. These membrane specializations are observed in cultures of normal human sympathetic neurons. They are also found along the cell membranes in biopsied specimens of neuroblastomas.[6]

The ultrastructure of neuroblastomas has been described.[7] The organelles in the cell bodies and neurites which characterize these tumor cells are similar to those found in normal cells and are retained by the cells in culture. Frequently, when cells with sparse perikaryia and relatively large nuclei are explanted, the perikaryia enlarge, the rough-surfaced endoplasmic reticulum increases and becomes organized (Nissl) and dense disorganized arrays of microtubules, dense core vesicles, and small mitochondria appear where previously there were only a small number of these organelles. As the neurites begin to grow, many free ribosomes are found in the developing tips. However when the neurites become long, they no longer contain ribosomes. The disappearance of free ribosomes during the development of the process is confirmed by the loss of staining for RNA with acridine orange and by the absence of labeled RNA after a short pulse with ^{3}H-uridine. The axons and some dendrites of most neurites contain little if any RNA. The malignant neuroblast should be a good cell for studying the mechanism which segregates the large mass of easily detected RNA in the perikaryia from its processes.

The mouse neuroblastoma C 1300, a tumor which has been transplanted for over 30 years in A/JAX mice, is composed of large round cells without processes. When these cells are explanted onto a substrate to which they can attach, they differentiate in a manner similar to human neuroblastomas. These aneuploid tumor cells develop organelles which are found in the normal sympathetic nerve cell and retain a number of the enzymatic properties also characteristic of sympathetic neurons. Their detailed morphology and function have recently been described.[8, 9]

Properties of Cells of the Human Neuroblastoma Line NJB

The neuroblastoma line NJB was explanted in January of 1965. A metastatic lymph node from a two-year-old female child was obtained post-mortem and the cells explanted on collagen coated cover slips in a 5% CO_2 and air atmosphere. After 40 days, cells were explanted to glass and grown in sealed flasks.

The tumor has not been cloned. It has two morphologically distinguishable cell types. One is composed of small neuroblasts which pile up as they multiply and grow as tightly packed aggregates. Neurites migrate from the aggregates and they form the same complex networks observed in primary cultures of other neuroblastomas. The other cell type is epithelium-like. It grows in monolayers and also sends out fine neurites. These neuroepithelial cells appear to differentiate from the more primitive neuroblasts. The neuroepithelial cells may be similar to the chromaffin-like cells that Willis and others described in their studies of tumor biopsies.[10]

It has been considered axiomatic that after normal neuroblasts develop processes and especially after the processes make physical and chemical connections with their target cells, they no longer divide.

NJB cells continue to develop long processes, some like the mouse processes, extend for 2 to 4 mm from the cell bodies. NJB cells with long processes and with terminals which make contact with other cells and their processes can divide after short pulse labeling with ^{3}H-thymidine. Grains are seen over nuclei synthesizing DNA and divisions have been observed among these differentiated malignant nerve cells.

Perhaps in the normal neuron factors other than the formation of differentiated neurites are responsible for inhibition of mitosis.

Effect of NGF on Growth and Differentiation of NJB Cells

In a previous paper,[11] we reported that an antiserum to NGF did not inhibit the growth of neuroblastomas growing in fluid media. The factor did not induce obvious changes in the rate of multiplication or differentiation. Normal sympathetic neuroblasts grown under conditions of culture described above require NGF for long-term survival and the dissociated sympathetic ganglion cells of chick embryos have an absolute requirement for this protein if they are to survive for more than 48 hr in vitro. Recently, in the laboratory of Georges Barski, NJB cells were explanted in chicken plasma clots and fed with a fluid medium of fetal calf serum and medium 199. After 48 hr, some of the cultures were refed with heat inactivated fetal calf serum and medium 199 containing 5 to 100 units of purified NGF. Under these conditions there was a marked stimulation of neurite outgrowth in those cultures containing NGF. The controls were also neuroblasts with processes but they were not as long nor were there as many as in the experimental cultures. (These data will be presented in more detail in another paper.) Further studies with neuroblastomas may provide more information of the role of the important NGF protein in survival and differentiation of the sympathetic neuron. Perhaps a good in vitro assay for NGF effect on neuroblastomas will indicate whether an antiserum to the protein would be effective against some tumors. This area needs further exploration.

Finally, recent studies with the analog of dopamine, 6 OH dopamine, show that it selectively destroys the nerve endings of sympathetic neurons. Levi-Montalcini and Angeletti (personal communication) find that the drug completely destroys the sympathetic nervous system of newborn mice and that it inhibits the growth of the C 1300 mouse neuroblastoma. We find that the drug also is toxic for NJB cells growing in vitro. The unusual selective toxicity of this compound for the normal sympathetic nerve cell ending and for tumors derived from them suggest that 6 OH dopamine may prove useful for therapy of neuroblastomas.

The retention of differentiated properties by neuroblastomas and the re-expression of others associated with normal sympathetic nerve cells suggest that further knowledge of the factors inducing redifferentiation will be important in controlling the growth of this tumor.

Acknowledgments

These studies were supported by U.S.P.H.S. grant Ca 10755 and an institutional grant of the American Cancer Society.

I should like to thank Dr. Georges Barski of the Institut Gustave-Roussy for providing facilities in his laboratory for some of the work reported in this paper while on an International Fellowship of the World Health Organization.

References

1. Greenfield, L. J., and W. M. Shelley: J. Nat. Cancer Int., 35:215, 1965.
2. Goldstein, M. N., and D. Pinkel: J. Nat. Cancer Inst., 20:675, 1958.
3. Goldstein, M. N., J. A. Burdman, and L. J. Journey: J. Nat. Cancer Inst., 32:165, 1964.
4. England, J. M., and M. N. Goldstein: J. Cell Sci., 4:677, 1969.
5. Levi-Montalcini, R., and P. U. Angeletti: Develop. Biol., 7:653, 1963.
6. Luse, S. A.: Arch. Neurol., 11:185, 1964.
7. Staley, N. A., H. F. Polesky, and K. G. Bensch: J. Neuropath. Exp. Neurol., 26:634, 1967.
8. Agusti-Tocco, G., and G. Sato: Proc. Nat. Acad. Sci. USA, 64:311, 1969.
9. Schubert, D., S. Humphreys, C. Baroni, and M. Cohn: Proc. Nat. Acad. Sci. USA, 64:316, 1969.
10. Willis, R. A.: The Pathology of the Tumors of Children. Oliver and Byrd, London, 1962.
11. Burdman, J. A., and M. N. Goldstein: J. Nat. Cancer Inst., 33:123, 1964.

22

Regulation of Gene Expression in Normal and Cancer Cells: A Rapporteur Report

Gene Expression—Its Regulation in Normal and Cancer Cells

G. WEBER

Department of Pharmacology, Indiana University School of Medicine, Indianapolis, Indiana, USA

THE TASK I was assigned by the Congress as Rapporteur was "to give your own perspectives and overview of the field covered by the Preliminary Special Session of the Congress as well as some of the highlights of the Conference itself." Since I was also the Chairman of this Symposium and as Member of the Program Committee participated in designing it, and it is the area in which my own research interest lies, it is a special pleasure to carry out this task.

Design of the Conference

This Conference was designed to take the participants through the quest from the molecular biology of the mechanisms of gene expression through the advances in enzyme and metabolic regulation to the achievements of therapy which are the ultimate aim of those scientists whose target is to control cancer in man.

In the first session, the molecular biology of the gene was explored in terms of expression of the genes and the reprogramming of the genome through external influences, including the action of the viral genome on mammalian cells.

The second session was designed to highlight the role subcellular organelles play in the control, expression, and fate of gene readouts and information transfer. The nucleus and the nucleolus, the masters of gene expression and control, the mitochondria and their DNA, and the cell membranes and their function in normal and cancer cells were brought into focus.

In the third session, gene action was examined in the pattern of gene products, the enzymes and isozymes; the chief energy-producing reactions of the cell, glycolysis and respiration; and the chemical basis of cell replication, the nucleic acid metabolism.

Then the fourth session turned to examining the control mechanisms in terms of the regulation of cell cycle and function. Since neoplasia is considered a manifestation of altered control mechanisms specifically affecting replication and rooted in a reprogramming of the genome, the regulatory mechanisms were examined at the level of energy-yielding reactions such as respiratory control and enzyme regulation, and the application of these principles to the control of the cell cycle.

The final session was dedicated to examining the progress made in modifying genic expression at the enzyme level by feedback mechanisms, and to the regulation of gene expression by hormones and drugs, in the therapy for human cancer. These approaches in clinical chemotherapy were achieved through selective toxicity by enzyme administration, and by antitumor antibiotics on the gene transcription and replication of human cancer cells.

As a result of the bedside application of current understanding of gene expression and regulation, chemotherapeutic cure has been achieved for at least two types of cancer in man by the use of actinomycin and methotrexate, and extensive, prolonged remissions have been achieved by hormone treatment and by an array of single and combination chemotherapeutic measures.

Statement of the Problem

The problem to be solved is the cure of cancer in man. Figure 22-1 shows a picture of a fungating mass choriocarcinoma growing and destroying the womb. Much progress has already been made, since with selective chemotherapy 70% or 80% of these women now can be saved (see Figure 22-14).

However, the average cure rate for all tumors with the best of treatment is only about 50%. You will note that this is worse than any cure rate achieved today in the treatment for infectious diseases. I find that yellow fever is now the only infectious disease which, even if treated appropriately, still results in 50% mortality.

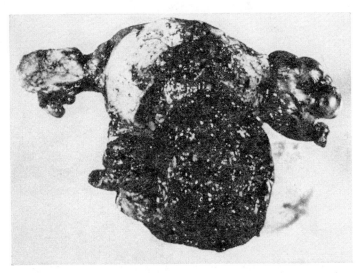

FIG. 22–1.—Fungating mass of choriocarcinoma growing and destroying the uterus. (Courtesy of R. Hertz.)

The altered cell function and cell replication pattern in cancer cells are transferred from generation to generation and thus reside in changes in genic expression. Figure 22-2 shows the encoding and replication of genic information for cell replication and function in the double helical structure of DNA. The expression and the control of this genome are altered by carcinogenic influences, spontaneous or exogenous, resulting in the clinical problem which the physician faces and which the scientist joins him in fighting. The regulation of expression of this genic information and its control by therapeutic means in all cancer patients are the objectives to be achieved.

With this challenge, the first session was opened with a lucid and splendid introduction by Dr. Wendell M. Stanley[1] (see pages 579-586, Volume I) who received the Nobel Prize for his pioneer work for crystallizing the tobacco mosaic virus, which contributed to the birth of the new era called Molecular Biology.

The nature of virus nucleic acid is of great interest, since comparative information on size and estimates of number of genes is available for a number of situations. Subsequently, Wolstenholme[2] (see pages 627-648, Volume I) discussed this subject for the mitochondrial DNA and Bernhard[7] (see pages 600-612, Volume I) for bacterial and mammalian cells. About five to 10 million genes are stored in the nuclei of mammalian cells, but only 2,000 to 4,000 genes are in bacterial cells. The polyoma or SV40 viruses have ring-shaped DNA of a molecular weight of three million, which is equal to about six to 10 genes. The structure of the DNA of the polyoma virus, as pointed out by Wolsten-

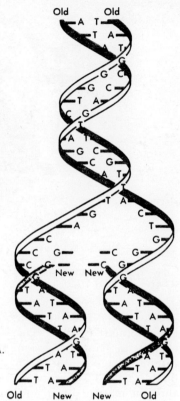

FIG. 22-2.—Double helical structure of DNA. (Courtesy of R. Sinsheimer.)

holme, resembles that of the animal mitochondrial DNA. The mitochondrial DNA could code for only about 25 proteins of average molecular weight of 20,000. Thus a single $5\text{-}\mu$ circular mitochondrial DNA molecule may carry 20 to 25 genes.

In mouse cells transformed by SV40 virus, there are about 20 viral DNA molecular equivalents integrated in the cellular DNA. It is significant that studies on the transcription of this viral DNA indicate that no more than one third of the viral genome is necessary for the neoplastic transformation, hence no more than two or three genes may be involved. One should hope that an understanding of the mechanism involved in the transformation might be close at hand.[1]

Dr. Stanley posed the question, "How soon will it be possible to apply information gained from these model studies to human cancer?" Earlier in his lecture he referred to the discovery of the viral origin of rabbit myxoma in the year 1911, of fowl leukemia in 1908, and of Rous sarcoma in 1911. Dr. Stanley emphasized that "basic biological phenomena generally do not differ strikingly as one goes from one species to another, and I regard the fact, now proved beyond contention, that viruses can cause cancer in animals to be directly pertinent to the human cancer problem." Dr. Stanley concluded with the optimistic tone: "Much remains to be done but potentially productive approaches are clear and the future is indeed rich with promise."

In continuing Session I, the basic problems of gene expression of the cell were confronted. The manifestations of the cell involve replication, cell function, including energy generation, macromolecular synthesis, degradative, and eliminative procedures, and the integration and regulation of these functions.

Dr. P. Lengyel[3] examined the factors required in *Escherichia coli* protein synthesis, the functions of which are summarized in Figure 22-3. The protein factor S_3, active in complex with GTP and activated tRNA, transfers the amino acyl tRNA to the ribosome bearing the nascent peptide chain in an energy-requiring process. The reaction releases an S_3-GDP complex which is acted on by the S_1 protein factor in the presence of GTP and another charged tRNA molecule to regenerate the active tRNA-S_3-GTP complex. The S_2 protein acts in the energy-dependent translocation of the peptide chain regenerating ribosome-message-nascent chain ready for binding of another charged tRNA.

The microbial system involves no less than 130 factors, including tRNA species, ribosomal proteins, and various factors. This type of in-

Fig. 22–3.—Scheme of peptide chain elongation. (Courtesy of P. Lengyel.)

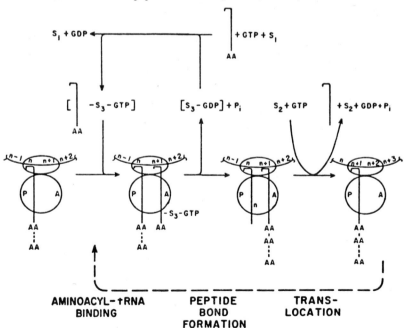

AMINOACYL–tRNA BINDING

PEPTIDE BOND FORMATION

TRANS-LOCATION

formation may appear irrelevant to mammalian cells and cancer; however, the knowledge obtained by examining this pathway in microorganisms has accelerated the progress of similar investigations in higher organisms. The latter should contribute ultimately to the understanding of such diverse phenomena as antibody synthesis, hormone action, and differentiation. In fact, the chemotherapeutic effects of certain new antibiotics are attributed to their action on this mechanism.

In the cancer cell, the outstanding problem that leads to the clinical diagnosis and to the symptoms and eventual outcome of the disease is the apparently uncontrolled replication of the neoplastic cell. Therefore, problems of replication and of gene expression were focused on in the early considerations of Dr. R. Sinsheimer[5] (see pages 586-591, Volume I). A scheme for DNA replication was originally suggested by the complementary double-helical structure for DNA of Watson and Crick, shown in Figure 22-2. The fundamental element of this scheme is the separation of the two parental strands in a semiconservative process, one going to each daughter DNA molecule. The semiconservative nature of DNA replication applies even to single-stranded DNA synthesis.

It is assumed that some of the complicated problems of cell replication of mammalian cells might be understood in a simpler model system, such as the one used by Sinsheimer, which focuses on the manner of replication of the single-stranded DNA of the bacteriophage $\phi x 174$.

The DNA of this virus has a molecular weight of 1.7 million. As soon as it is introduced into the bacterial cell, it is converted to a double-stranded DNA ring in which the parental strand remains integral. This double-stranded DNA, the replicative form, becomes associated with a preexistent site on the bacterial membrane at which it is first transcribed, and subsequently becomes replicated to make daughter double-stranded DNA rings. The replication is such that of the two daughter double-stranded rings, the one with the original parental viral DNA strand remains at the membrane site, while the other progeny ring is released into the cytoplasm. The next important event occurs when some 10 to 15 progeny double-stranded rings have accumulated within the cell. Host DNA synthesis, which has continued unperturbed, is now turned off, and the means by which this is accomplished are unknown. Replication of the membrane site is similarly almost completely turned off. The double-stranded DNA rings which had accumulated in the cytoplasm are now used as templates for the formation of the single-stranded DNAs of the progeny particles.

Even in this comparatively simple system, we do not as yet understand the details of double-stranded DNA replication or the controls of its initiation and termination, further emphasizing the difficulties of the more complex mammalian systems. However, an important beginning has been made with possible relevance to neoplasia.

In the mechanism of gene expression, the flow of biologic information is from DNA through RNA into the translation of protein. The question then arises regarding the mechanism of replication of viruses that contain RNA as their genetic material. Since some RNA viruses, such as the Rous sarcoma and others, are known to cause neoplasms in avian and mammalian organisms, the solution of this problem is of great interest.

The outstanding work of Dr. S. Spiegelman[6] points the way toward an understanding of the mechanism of RNA virus replication. He utilized a comparatively simple system as a model by exploring the replication of an RNA phage, Q beta RNA in *E. coli*. When this phage attacks *E. coli*, the phage RNA is injected into the microorganism. The critical next step is that the phage is capable of inducing a host enzyme called Qβ replicase which carries out the replicative function in the following fashion.

To explain the sequence of reactions required for replication of the single-strand phage RNA, Dr. Spiegelman proposed the following model based on a system of 5' to 3' synthesis (Figure 22-4). As predicted by this model, there is an eclipse of infectivity from the time the orig-

Fig. 22-4.—Replication of single-stranded phage RNA. (Courtesy of S. Spiegelman.)

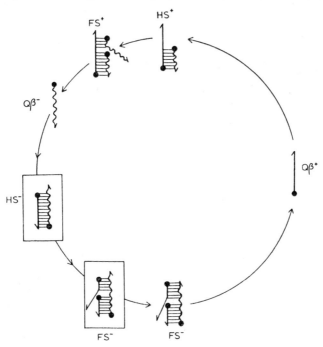

inal $Q\beta+$ strand starts to replicate until the first product $Q\beta+$ strand appears. The chains of the double-strand intermediate are antiparallel. All of the intermediates shown on this slide were separated on polyacrylamide gel electrophoresis. The order of appearance of the intermediates is single-strand to double-strand to multistrand. Pulse-chase experiments show a multiform to be the immediate precursor of the mature $Q\beta+$ strand. Dr. Spiegelman has extended his studies to mammalian virus systems and believes this model may apply to certain of these systems. Modification and extension to mammalian cells of the methods employed so effectively with the viral conditions were discussed.

The techniques used in this $Q\beta$ system and others are the chief contribution of Dr. Spiegelman in this area. They are highly ingenious and effective, and are used with great skill, along with existing techniques. In addition, his method of proposing and proving or disproving in a rigorous manner a model system is especially incisive. The data he presented are from one of his classical studies. It will be very exciting to see the mammalian virus systems brought to this level of sophistication.

It is a special pleasure that some of the mechanisms and structures of gene expression can be visualized through electron microscopy. Dr. W. Bernhard[7] (see pages 600-612, Volume I) presented the brilliant progress achieved in his laboratories and in other centers in visualizing the machinery and elucidating the mechanisms of gene expression in normal and cancer cells.

In the bacterial cell there exist no nuclear membrane, no nucleolus, and no histones as in multicellular organisms and mammals. He pointed out the phylogenetic importance of the acquisition of a nucleus which allows the compartmentation of the carriers of genetic information within the specialized compartment in the nucleus (Figure 22-5). In bacteria where there is no nucleus, transcription is rapidly followed by translation. In contrast, in the mammalian cell there is a complex system of processing of the transcribed RNA and of messages delaying and governing protein synthesis. The pores of the nuclear membrane which are passages for nuclear and cytoplasmic information are probably capable of regulating the flow of information. The maintenance of the chromatin in a separate compartment may provide better homeostasis for gene activation and function. There is more than a quantitative difference between storing the 2,000 to 4,000 genes in bacteria and the five to 10 million in cells of higher organisms.

Dr. Bernhard pointed out that the nucleus appears as the supreme legislator of the cell, with a memory built in and with a degree of executive power to process, accelerate, or delay the information shifted to the cytoplasm. However, the switch of nuclear function appears to be regulated by cytoplasmic signals. With electron microscopic pictures he saw in the interphase nuclei the condensed chromatin (heterochro-

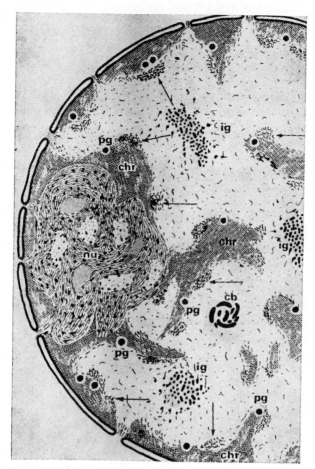

Fig. 22–5.—Nucleus of a liver cell: Schematic drawing. (Courtesy of W. Bernhard.) chr = chromatin, nu = nucleolus, ig = interchromatin granules, pg = perichromatin granules, → = perichromatin fibrils, cb = coiled body.

matin). About 80 to 90% of the nucleohistones are densely packed and probably nonfunctional; they are located along the nuclear membrane and the nucleolus.

The nuclear membrane is a double membrane which acts as a barrier enclosing the genetic material, maintaining constant ionic environment with a higher negative charge than that of the cytoplasm. The nuclear membrane also has an active function in synthesizing proteins, and this is the first site where antibodies appear in the case of antibody synthesis. The occurrence of regulation at the nuclear pores represents active passages showing an extremely complex ultrastructure.

The replication of DNA starts along the nuclear membrane, and the inner leaflet of the membrane may play the same role in the separation of the DNA strands in eukaryotes as does the bacterial membrane in the replication of bacterial DNA.

In early cancerous changes, little if any difference may be recognized in the nucleus except the increased rate of DNA synthesis, the appearance of new antigens, and the slightly changed cell surface. Later, the chromosome number and the nuclear size become bigger and more irregular; the nucleolus, a sensitive indicator of protein synthesis, is hypertrophic and may have abnormal architecture.

Dr. M. Muramatsu[8] (see pages 613-627, Volume I) discussed the nucleolus and singled out the important function of ribosome formation. Much interest centers on the hypertrophy and pleiomorphism exhibited by the nucleoli of cancer cells. These characteristics are also present in other rapidly dividing cells or in cells which produce large amounts of proteins.

With the tools of sucrose density gradient profiles and radioactive labeling of the nuclear, nucleolar, and extranuclear RNA, it was shown that the nucleolar RNA has large density peaks at 45S and 35S which are not present in extranucleolar nuclear RNA. The nucleolar RNA is qualitatively distinct from the RNA in the nucleus. In studying these phenomena, advantage was taken of the fact that intravenous injection of actinomycin D stops nucleolar RNA synthesis within a minute.

Dr. Muramatsu summarized the processing of the nucleolar RNA. At the first step, the precursor 45S RNA which contains both the 28S and the 18S RNA sequences cleaves off the 18S RNA and a considerable length of nonribosomal sequences to make 35S RNA. Then this RNA cleaves off a smaller fragment to become 28S RNA, which is the component of the larger subunit of the ribosomes.

Dr. D. R. Wolstenholme[9] (see pages 627-648, Volume I) presented evidence that mitochondria contain their own DNA molecules. A study of the size and structure of such molecules is of interest, since they may relate to cytoplasmic inheritance.

The M-DNAs from liver are circular molecules which have a contour length of from 4.5 to 6.0 μ. Figure 16-20 of Wolstenholme (see page 630, Volume I) shows such a molecule. Fresh preparations of M-DNA also contain varying proportions of highly twisted or supercoiled circular molecules. The circular M-DNA has a similar structure to that of the smaller circular polyoma viral DNA.

Each mitochondrion of mouse L cells contains from two to six circular molecules. The genetic information that could be carried by a single DNA molecule of 5 μ is obviously severely limited. A DNA molecule of this size has a molecular weight of about 10×10^6,[10] and could code for the amino acid sequences of about 25 proteins with an average molecular weight of 20,000, or the equivalent of about three sets of ribosomal RNAs.

The mitochondria increase by growth and division, and M-DNA is synthesized in situ. A direct indication was the finding of the circular molecules of DNA among the rat liver mitochondria, which were arrested in replication, and they had two forks (see Figure 16-24 of Wolstenholme, page 635, Volume I). The method of reproduction is similar to that suggested for the large circular DNA molecule of *E. coli,* lambda phage, or polyoma virus. Rat liver M-DNA has a half life of about nine days.

Of 10,000 rat liver M-DNAs, only 21 partially duplicated molecules were found. These are replicative forms. In M-DNA from all of the mouse and rat tumors examined, they occurred with a frequency of six to 28 times more than from normal liver.

Wolstenholme and associates observed an unusually high proportion of the M-DNA of mouse Ehrlich ascites tumor in the form of interlocked circles, and 16% is in the form of higher oligomers comprising as many as six circles (Figure 16-26 of Wolstenholme, page 638, Volume I). In contrast, molecules consisting of three or more interlocking circles are rare or absent in most normal tissues.

Several scientists presented concepts, theories, or hypotheses of the mechanism of neoplastic transformation. As you know, theories are of interest if they can be subjected to the rigorous proof of experimental verification and validation. You will be interested in hearing some of these because they have been influencing investigations in a number of laboratories and stimulating research in this area. Such concepts were discussed by Pitot,[13] Potter,[21] Weber,[12] Weinhouse,[14] and others.

In the considerations and experimental approaches of these and other participants, liver tumors played an important role as an experimental model system. A spectrum of liver tumors exhibiting different growth rates, and histologic and biologic characteristics was produced during the past 10 years by Dr. H. P. Morris.[11] These hepatomas were developed in rats by feeding low concentrations of a variety of

TABLE 22–1.—SIGNIFICANT PROPERTIES OF MORRIS HEPATOMA SPECTRUM

PROPERTIES	PARAMETERS	EXTENT OF CHANGE FROM NORMAL		
		SLIGHT	INTERMEDIATE	NORMAL
Biological behavior	Growth rate	Low	Medium	Rapid
Morphology	Differentiation	Near normal	Medium	Poor
Genetic apparatus	Chromosome number	Normal	Increased	High
	Chromosome karyotype	Normal	Nearly normal	Abnormal
Energy generation	Respiration	Normal	Moderate	Moderately low
	Glycolysis	Low	Normal or increased	High
Replication and functions	Imbalance of opposing pathways of synthesis and degradation	Moderate	Pronounced	Extensive

chemicals in the diet. The hepatomas that arose provide a spectrum ranging from well-differentiated neoplasms that closely resemble the liver to tumors that are not well differentiated or are poorly differentiated.[11] Because of the relevance of this model system to the theme of this Conference, I summarized the general properties of these neoplasms in Table 22-1 from the point of view of biologic behavior, growth rate, morphology, genetic apparatus, energy metabolism, replication and functions.[12]

Since the different tumor lines remained, in general, remarkably stable as they were carried by transplantation in inbred strains, there are now some 40 different lines of hepatomas representing different aspects of gene expression and regulation. All the tumors are parenchymal cell neoplasms; thus a spectrum of hepatomas of different growth rates and differentiation is available for study. The various workers utilized this biologic material with different concepts and experimental objectives which I refer to as I discuss their contributions. My own view and utilization of these tumors of different growth rates will also be given below.

Dr. H. C. Pitot[13] (see pages 648-655, Volume I) reviewed the evidence for his model which he termed the Membron. He postulated it on the surface of the endoplasmic reticulum (see page 654, Volume I). The pseudohelical structure of the polysome and the presence of the smaller subunit directed toward the center of the helix are consistent with observations. He postulated that the mosaic pattern of the membrane would determine the tightness or looseness of binding of the polysome to the membrane, forming the Membron. In an electron microscopic picture, he demonstrated the presence of such Membrons in the endoplasmic reticulum and outer nuclear membrane of cells in culture.

Dr. Pitot suggested that the different Membron populations would give rise to the phenotype of the cell, they would be hereditary through membrane replication, and the altered membrane population in neoplasms would become a "phenotypic masque" of neoplasia resulting in an altered regulation of genic expression which we note in cancer cells. This interesting concept should provide a valuable testing ground as it allows experimental verification, and work in this direction is in progress in Dr. Pitot's laboratory and other centers. It has already been shown that, in general, hepatomas have fewer bound polysomes than normal liver.

Dr. S. Weinhouse[14] (see pages 656-667, Volume I) described his valuable studies on the isozyme pattern and on control sites of glycolysis in hepatomas. He showed evidence for the gradual change in isozyme pattern for the glucose phosphorylating enzymes, glucokinase and hexokinase, and for aldolase and pyruvate kinase. In these cases, the liver-specific enzyme decreased and the nonliver type or muscle type increased and replaced the liver-type enzyme.

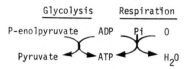

The most important part of Dr. Weinhouse's presentation dealt with his studies which explored the postulate that the high glycolysis in the poorly differentiated, rapidly growing hepatomas could be caused by preferential utilization of ADP by pyruvate kinase over that used for oxydative phosphorylation (Figure 22-6). By intermixing glycolytic systems and mitochondria from well- and poorly-differentiated tumors, it was invariably observed that when a relatively inactive glycolytic system of a well-differentiated (slowly growing) hepatoma was mixed with a low-respiring mitochondrial fraction of a poorly differentiated (rapidly growing) hepatoma, glycolysis was greatly increased, together with glycolytic phosphorylation. Conversely, when a highly active glycolytic system of a poorly differentiated hepatoma was mixed with an active mitochondrial fraction from a well-differentiated hepatoma, glycolysis and glycolytic phosphorylation were greatly decreased while respiratory phosphorylation was greatly increased.

These findings indicate that the high glycolytic capability of poorly differentiated hepatomas has its origin in a high activity level of pyruvate kinase. Since poorly differentiated tumors in general have a high pyruvate kinase activity, it may be speculated that the same mechanism applies to all highly glycolyzing tumors.

The tumors that have high glycolytic activity are invariably those which have undergone progression to a less differentiated state and have a rapid growth rate. It is likely that their high aerobic glycolysis is attributable to successful competition for ADP by high pyruvate kinase activity associated with a low or moderate rate of the respiratory system. Dr. Weinhouse agrees with our conclusion that high aerobic glycolysis is not present in the slowly growing tumors, and that glycolysis correlates with hepatoma growth rate. Dr. Weinhouse concluded that the intensive biochemical studies of the hepatoma spectrum are providing an insight into the underlying molecular alterations which accompany the progression in growth rate and degree of differentiation which characterize neoplasia.

Dr. G. P. Wheeler[15] (see pages 667-672, Volume I) presented evidence that in analyzing the biochemical pattern in neoplastic tissues, it is important to take into consideration the growth fraction and cell kinetics. Through careful analysis of growth rate and growth fraction of several tumors, he showed that as the rate of growth changes, the incorporation of labeled precursors in vivo into DNA and RNA changes with it. Alterations of the cell kinetics in some tumors might include changes in the length of the cell cycle and of the various phases of the cycle, changes in growth fraction and cell loss from the neoplasm. For example, in adenocarcinoma 755, the length of the cell cycle increased and the growth fraction decreased as the tumor became larger. The length of the cell cycle of leukemia L1210 increased greatly on day 7 compared to day 6, but the length of the S phase increased relatively little.

Dr. Wheeler emphasized that one must be cautious in assigning enzymatic or metabolic activities for experimental neoplasms, since metabolic activity might be dependent upon the age and size of the neoplasms. It is possible to minimize the problems this may cause by using tumors of about the same size.

Dr. Wheeler further emphasized his belief that the metabolic differences in gene expression correspond to differences in the degree of differentiation and proliferation rate of neoplastic tissues. Since control of cell kinetics is a manifestation of gene expression, abnormal kinetics result from abnormal gene expression through regulatory mechanisms involving metabolic processes. He concluded by saying that the more we know about the events occurring within the various phases of the cell cycle and the control of these events, the better we will understand the alterations existing in neoplastic cells and tissues.

Dr. G. D. Novelli[16] (see pages 672-683, Volume I) discussed the possibility that control occurs at the translation level. Translation of a specific messenger RNA is an exceedingly complex reaction in which, as Dr. Lengyel pointed out, there are more than 130 distinct macromolecules involved in the formation of peptide bonds producing specific protein products. Because of the complexity of this process, this may well be one of the critical points in gene expression. For this reason, Dr. Novelli examined translation mechanisms in a simple system in *E. coli,* and in mammalian tumor cells. The so-called modulation hypothesis of Ames and Hartman, in which certain tRNA species are present in rate-limiting amounts and thereby act to retard protein synthesis, was discussed. Evidence in support of this model was presented for T_2 phage infection of *E. coli.* On infection, the host tRNA corresponding to CUG, a leucine codon, is destroyed. Since this codon is rare in T_2 message RNA but common in host mRNA, the destruction of this codon may well act to retard host protein synthesis.

A further example of the control possibilities of tRNA was presented in the work on cultured L-M fibroblasts versus the in vivo tumors produced by infecting these cells in mice. Of the 16 tRNA species recognized, eight were identical under in vitro or in vivo conditions. Four more were significantly changed, while another four were drastically altered. All changes from in vitro cultures to in vivo conditions were reversible on reculturing cells from growing tumors.

The results suggest that the differences in these forms may correspond to differences in methylation or other chemical modifications of the preformed base sequences. The enzymes catalyzing these modifications may be the point at which translational control is exerted in various systems, including tumors.

Dr. N. Katunuma[17] (see pages 684-695, Volume I) also took advantage of the hepatoma spectrum to study the relation to growth rate and differentiation of various isozymes involved in glutamine breakdown. He reported that there are two glutaminases in liver; one isozyme requires phosphate for activity (phosphate-dependent: PD), while the kidney is phosphate-independent (PI). The ratio of the isozymes, PD/PI, correlated with tumor growth rate.

In the liver, glutamine is catabolized into glutamate by the enzyme glutaminase; in turn, glutamate can be anabolized into glutamine by an enzyme called amidotransferase. Dr. Katunuma discovered that the activity of glutaminase, the catabolic enzyme of glutamine, decreased, whereas the activity of amidotransferase, the anabolic enzyme, increased parallel with the increase in hepatoma growth rate.

This progressive alteration in the balance of the activities of the opposing enzymes, glutaminase and amidotransferase, again represents a meaningful change in the neoplastic reprogramming of the genome, resulting in the conservation of glutamine which now may be channeled into purine biosynthesis and other biosynthetic pathways vital in nucleic acid synthesis for cell replication.

Dr. G. M. Tomkins[18] discussed the mechanism of steroid induction of the enzyme tyrosine amino transferase in cultured cells of Morris hepatoma 7288-C. Although synthesis of this enzyme may occur at any point in the cell cycle, induction can occur only during the latter part of the G1 phase and during S phase (Figure 22-7). A model explaining the properties of the induction system includes a regulator gene coding for a repressor in addition to a structural gene for tyrosine amino transferase. The repressor is constantly synthesized, and under normal conditions combines with the message from the structural gene, preventing its translation. In this inactive form, the message is degraded. The steroid inducer, when present, blocks the

Fig. 22–7.—Phases of the cell cycle of hepatoma 7288-C in tissue culture. (Courtesy of G. Tomkins.)

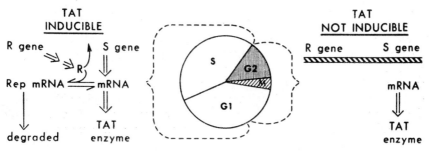

repressor, leaving the message free to be translated into protein. The lack of induction during certain phases of the cell cycle probably relates to the unavailability of the genetic material during this period for new message formation. This model involves control at the translational level. The Jacob-Monod model describing the lactose operon of *E. coli* is a transcriptional control with no message formed under repressing conditions. Although such a transcriptional control may be the most common in microorganisms, several types of translational controls have been proposed for certain mammalian systems.

B. Chance[19] (see pages 711-718, Volume I) discussed regulation of cell respiration. He stated that the main feature which distinguishes eukaryotic cells from bacteria is the control exerted in the former cells by the demand for the cell energy over its supply. This may be largely caused by the unique properties exhibited by a special cell device, the mitochondrion, which couples the two phenomena.

The cancer cell, as any other cell, is equipped in the same molecular mechanism for the control of electron flow. His studies showed in normal cells that the salient features of controlled and energized states involves increased protonation of the membrane, together with a state transformation and corresponding movement of structured water. His studies point to the unique properties of electron-transporting proteins in membranes which can apparently alter their properties so as to control electron flow and to afford a suitable environment for energy coupling.

The relation of these molecular mechanisms to the cancer problem is possibly as general as the relationship between membrane structure and function and the regulation of cell function itself. Many parameters are unknown, but a sound structure for the entire regulatory phenomenon may eventually be observed, as an understanding of molecular mechanisms begins to evolve.

From the clinical point of view, one of the key features of the neoplastic problem lies in the fact that neoplastic cells keep on multiplying, growing, form a mass, and invade and encroach into neighboring, normal tissues. As cells break into the vessels and lymphatics, they settle in various parts of the body, continue replication, and set up secondary deposits, the metastases. This replicating process, which does not usually respond to physiologic control processes and is able to carry out replication in almost any part of the body, focuses attention on the mechanism of replication of the cell.

Dr. G. C. Mueller[20] (see pages 719-725, Volume I) discussed in a beautifully documented presentation some of the biochemical perspectives of the cell cycle. He emphasized that the spectacular achievement in this process is that both active and inactive chromatin are replicated exactly and distributed with precision to daughter cells, thus assuring both genetic and phenotypic continuity. The steps of cell replication are programmed from the cell's own genetic system, but they are subject also to controls by extracellular factors such as hormonal, nutritional, and cell-to-cell interaction effects.

Whereas the replication of various normal cell types is harmoniously balanced, cancer, whether it arises by physical, chemical, or viral carcinogenesis, exhibits different grades of derangement in the control mechanisms. The cancer in the middle of an enormous population of billions of normal cells does not receive, or does not respond in the normal way, to the signals of extracellular environment, and undergoes a replicative cycle which is self-perpetuating and gradually unresponsive or completely unresponsive to normal controls. For this reason, the molecular mechanisms and biochemical basis of cell replication are of prime interest to clinician and basic researcher, and it is an area intimately linked with the cell's replicative expression of the genome.

The excellent summary slide of Dr. Mueller describing in a diagrammatic fashion the cell cycle is shown in his paper (page 720, Volume I). The replication process in animal cells is a highly ordered sequence of molecular events requiring the expression of specific genetic information at the subsequent steps in the cycle.

The S phase, an interval lasting six to seven hours in many cells, accomplishes the synthesis of the complete complement of DNA and histones. Progression through this interval requires the synthesis of RNA, DNA, and proteins.

The G_2 interval, the subsequent mitosis, and cell division require approximately two to three hours. These stages carry out the formation of newly synthesized chromatin into chromosome pairs and the distribution of the condensed chromosomes into the daughter cells. Progression into the G_2 interval requires the completion of DNA synthesis and the antecedent synthesis of RNA and protein.

Phleomycin blocks the cell cycle in HeLa cells near the end of the DNA synthesis period. Colchicine and other agents active against the microtubules block the progression of cells through metaphase.

It is important that cells with different replication times vary mainly in the duration of the G_1 interval, as suggested by his figure. During this interval, the cell expresses the phenotypic character of its particular differentiated state. Conversely, as Dr. Tomkins pointed out, in this phase the cell is resistant to enzyme induction processes.

Depending on intra- and extracellular factors, cells progress through G_1 and become triggered for nuclear replication: at this point they have achieved the ability to initiate DNA replication and to express the genes for histone synthesis. Cells may be synchronized for DNA replication by gathering cells at this point in the cycle with a reversible inhibitor of DNA synthesis. Cells may also be synchronized for mitosis with colchicine.

Dr. Mueller discussed the complexity at the molecular level of these processes, and concluded that the analysis of the S phase reactions in synchronized cell preparations has begun to provide significant insights into the nature of chromosome replication. With continued study, it should be possible to define in molecular terms the factors of the natural initiation of DNA synthesis in animal cells and the genetic controls that regulate it. This information should prove vital in the design of more effective and physiologically sound methods of cancer chemotherapy.

Enzyme regulation in cancer cells was discussed by Van R. Potter[21] (see pages 725-730, Volume I) who also described a hypothesis regarding oncogenesis. Dr. Potter explained his current concept as follows: ". . . The simple statement of this cancer theory is that Oncology is an accumulation of locked-in gene configurations (available or unavailable) that were scheduled to be unlocked at different times." He further explained, " . . . By that I mean that they were scheduled for different times in the normal process of development, that is in ontogeny. It seems to me that if there is a normal process which changes genes from available to unavailable and vice versa during development, and if we produce changes in the state of these genes in several loci, then we will obtain a diversity of biochemical patterns that will not coincide with the pattern of liver cells in any normal state of development. In fact, this is the picture that seems to be emerging from the data on biochemical diversity as experiments progress in our laboratory and in other laboratories that are examining cancer tissue in comparison with embryonic tissue."

Dr. Potter also presented the results of extensive and very interesting experiments on the modulation of gene expression in hepatoma cells carried in rats. These animals were subjected to controlled feeding schedules and dietary variations as well as drug treatments to perturb the liver plus hepatoma plus body system and to determine the capability of the given hepatoma line to respond like adult liver or in some other way.

The incorporation of thymidine into DNA and the behavior of tyrosine aminotransferase were studied. The results indicated a great variety of responses of this enzyme in several well-differentiated, slowly growing hepatomas under the various conditions.

He ". . . concluded from this and other data that each hepatoma represents a different combination of locked-in gene expressions that cannot undergo a further developmental program but that are nevertheless capable of being hormonally modulated within the locked-in configuration."

Dr. M. Siperstein[22] cited the feedback deletion hypothesis proposed by Potter which suggested that in the cancer cell metabolic sequence the ability of an enzyme or enzyme-forming system to respond to negative feedback signals might be decreased or absent. Dr. Siperstein examined the sequence of metabolic reactions leading to the biosynthesis of cholesterol in rat liver. He showed that feeding cholesterol to rats resulted in a decrease in the biosynthesis of cholesterol in the liver.

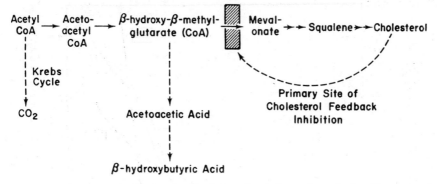

FIG. 22–8.—Site of feedback control of hepatic cholesterol synthesis. (Courtesy of M. D. Siperstein.)

He found that this was attributable to an inhibition of the key enzyme that converts beta-hydroxy-beta-methylglutarate to mevalonate (Figure 22-8). The same feedback inhibition is operative in human liver; with ingenious use of an inhibitory compound, the operation of this feedback was also ascertained in vivo.

Dr. Siperstein examined the Morris hepatomas of different growth rates. He found that cholesterol biosynthesis was high in the slowly growing hepatomas, and it decreased to very low activities in the rapidly growing tumors. The decrease paralleled the growth rate and differentiation of the hepatomas. Feeding of cholesterol failed to turn off cholesterol biosynthesis and revealed the absence of operation of this feedback mechanism in all hepatomas.

The absence of this metabolic regulatory response in all tumors is important. It belongs in Class 2 of Weber's classification where are grouped properties of neoplasms that are decreased in all tumors examined so far.[23] Among these are about 20 parameters, including the decreased feedback inhibition observed for fatty acid synthesis in hepatomas. The failure of cholesterol feedback in neoplasms points to an important change in gene expression and regulation, and its significance and relevance to the core of neoplasia should be elucidated in future work.

In my laboratories, the molecular correlation concept was developed as a conceptual and experimental method in cancer research.[23-25] This concept is based on our postulate that there is a meaningful biochemical pattern in cancer cells which can be correlated with the biologic behavior of tumors and exploited for the design of selective chemotherapy.

With the identification of key enzymes and their role and regulation in opposing biosynthetic and catabolic pathways, it has become possible to recognize the alterations in gene expression and their relation-

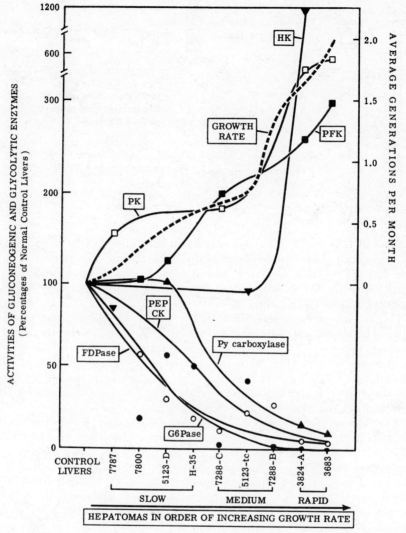

FIG. 22–9.—The key glycolytic enzymes exhibit a positive, the key gluconeogenic enzymes show a negative correlation with hepatoma growth rate. (Courtesy of G. Weber and M. A. Lea.)

ship with tumor proliferation rate. We utilized the spectrum of liver tumors of different growth rates as a biologic model system where the molecular signs of neoplasia and the stages of cancer progression can be examined in terms of biochemical alterations in a graded, quantitative manner.

I have already summarized the significant properties of the hepatoma spectrum (Table 22-1),[12] and from these we have selected growth rate as a comparison with the behavior of metabolic parameters. Without ignoring other important aspects of neoplasia, we have utilized growth rate in these studies because it can be measured with some precision with an array of biologic, cytologic, and biochemical methods; because it enters into clinical diagnosis and prognosis; and because it can be employed in the evaluation of treatment, including chemotherapy.

A study of the relationship of metabolic parameters to growth rate should establish which alterations are essential and which are coincidental,[26] and thus should lead to a rational basis for chemotherapy. With this approach, we demonstrated that the metabolic alterations in tumors can be classified into three groups according to their relation to growth rate. In Class 1 belong biochemical parameters that correlate positively or negatively with growth rate; in Class 2 are those that are increased or decreased in all hepatomas; and in Class 3 are those that show no relation to growth rate.[23–26]

A brief documentation of the use of the molecular correlation concept and the hepatoma spectrum for probing gene expression in analyzing the linkage of enzymatic and metabolic imbalance with cell replication rate is now provided.

FIG. 22–10.—Correlation of ratios of key glycolytic/gluconeogenic enzymes with hepatoma growth rate. (Courtesy of G. Weber, J. A. Ferdinandus, and S. I. F. Queener.)

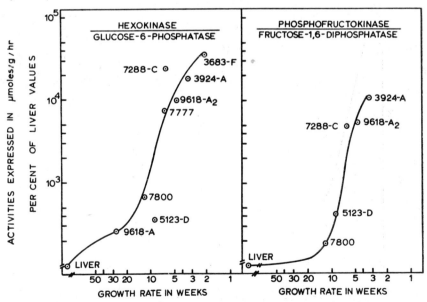

HEPATOMAS: INCREASING GROWTH RATE

Our studies in carbohydrate metabolism suggested that the regulation of opposing pathways of synthesis (gluconeogenesis) and catabolism (glycolysis) is accomplished through control of a quartet of key gluconeogenic and a triad of key glycolytic enzymes.[27] The key gluconeogenic and glycolytic enzymes show an opposing behavior during differentiation and in various nutritional and hormonal conditions. This antagonistic behavior is also manifested by these enzymes in the hepatoma spectrum. Parallel with the increasing growth rate, the key gluconeogenic enzymes decrease and the key glycolytic ones increase (Figure 22-9.)[24] This may be interpreted that the gluconeogenic enzymes are gradually repressed, whereas the glycolytic ones become derepressed parallel with an increase in tumor growth rate. It is important that the ratio of the glycolytic/gluconeogenic enzymes correlates especially closely with the proliferation rate of the different hepatoma cell lines (Figure 22-10). Thus, the cancerous transformation and progression, expressed in the replicative cycle as an increased rate of growth, is expressed concurrently in the extent of progressive imbalance in the ratios of opposing key enzymes of glycolysis and gluconeogenesis. As a result, as first shown in this laboratory, there is a gradual increase in aerobic glycolysis that exhibits a positive correlation with hepatoma growth rate.[28]

FIG. 22-11.—Repression and derepression of synthetic and catabolic pathways of thymidine utilization in liver in differentiation and in induced proliferation. (Courtesy of G. Weber, J. A. Ferdinandus, and S. I. F. Queener.)

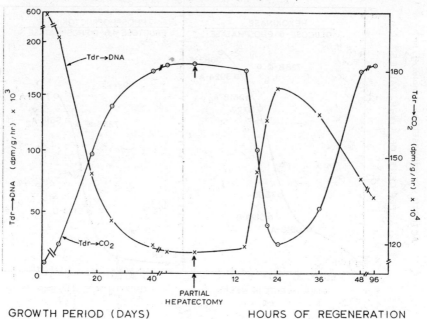

GROWTH PERIOD (DAYS)   HOURS OF REGENERATION

In studying the behavior and regulation of gene expression, particular interest lies in the key enzymes and the opposing biosynthetic and degradative pathways in nucleic acid metabolism. Valuable information was gained from studying the behavior of synthetic and catabolic utilization of thymidine in differentiating, regenerating, and neoplastic liver with a technique developed in my laboratories for the simultaneous assay of thymidine into DNA (biosynthetic utilization) and of thymidine into CO_2 (degradative pathway) in an in vitro system.[12] The data in Figure 22-11 indicate that the biosynthetic utilization of thymidine is high in the liver of newborn rats, whereas the opposing degradative pathway is low. During subsequent differentiation, the biosynthetic pathway decreases to very low levels in the liver of adult rats, whereas the opposing catabolic pathway increases to high activity. These results seem to indicate a sequential derepression of the genes governing the catabolic pathway and the gradual repression of those for the biosynthetic pathway of thymidine during differentiation in rat liver. In consequence, the steady state in the liver of adult rat exhibits a very low ratio of the biosynthetic/catabolic pathway, favoring the degradative utilization of thymidine.

However, the potential of the genome can be unleashed by carrying out partial hepatectomy which results in a decrease in the degradative utilization and a rise in the synthetic utilization of thymidine, leading to an imbalance with a peak about 24 hours after operation (Figure 22-11). Subsequently, the activities of the opposing pathways of thymidine utilization return to the previous adult levels.

Thus differentiation entails the sequential repression and derepression of genes controlling opposing pathways of thymidine utilization. By partial hepatectomy it is possible to unleash the genomic potential, even in the adult rat, resulting in a repression of the derepressed pathway of thymidine degradation and a derepression of the repressed pathway of utilization of thymidine for biosynthesis.[12]

When the opposing pathways of thymidine utilization were examined in the hepatomas, it was found that the opposing behavior of these antagonistic pathways is gradually emphasized with the increasing tumor growth rate. Even in the slowest growing hepatomas, the incorporation of thymidine into DNA increased nearly threefold and the degradation into CO_2 decreased about 50%; the ratio of the two pathways increased sixfold over the value observed in the normal liver of control rats. In the most rapidly growing tumor, the biosynthetic pathway increased about 30-fold, whereas the degradation decreased to a fraction of 0.1% of the normal liver, yielding an increase in the ratio of nearly 14-millionfold.[12] The gradually widening gap between the synthetic and catabolic utilization of thymidine, the resulting preponderance of the synthetic above the degradative pathway, and the correlation with tumor growth rate are shown in Figure 22-12.

The gradually developing imbalance with the increase in tumor

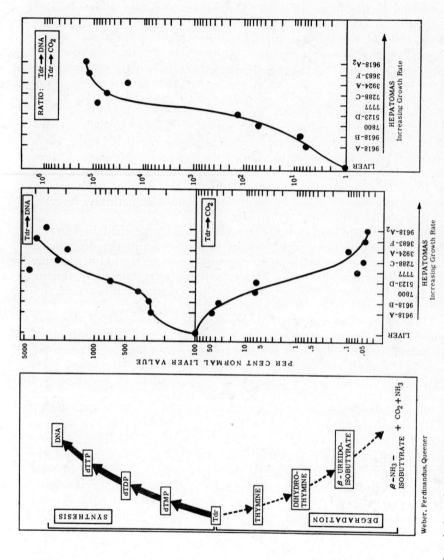

FIG. 22–12.—Correlation of opposing pathways of synthetic and degradative utilization of thymidine with hepatoma growth rate. (Courtesy of G. Weber, J. A. Ferdinandus, and S. I. F. Queener.)

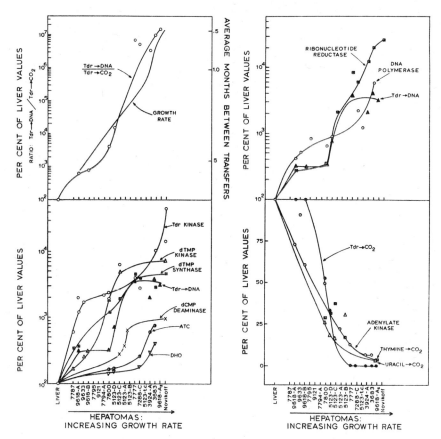

Fig. 22-13.—Correlation of DNA metabolic pathways and enzyme activities with hepatoma growth rate. (Courtesy of G. Weber, J. A. Ferdinandus, and S. I. F. Queener.)

proliferation rate is also linked with a progressive imbalance of synthetic and catabolic pathways and enzymes of pyrimidine and DNA metabolism. In Figure 22-13 we assembled the evidence demonstrating the correlation of DNA metabolic pathways and key enzyme activities with the increase in hepatoma growth rate.[12]

The upper left panel shows the increase in hepatoma growth rate in terms of average months between tumor transfers.[29] The ratios of incorporation of thymidine into DNA/degradation to CO_2 gives a close correlation, indicating good agreement between the biologic and chemical assays of tumor growth rate. The thymidine utilization ratio correlates with growth rate over a millionfold range. Consequently, this is the most sensitive measure for detecting neoplastic alterations and their extent in these tissues.[12]

The upper right panel shows the excellent correlation of ribonucleotide reductase activity[30, 31] and DNA polymerase activity[32] with hepatoma growth rate. For comparison, our data on the incorporation of thymidine into DNA are also given.[12]

The lower left panel illustrates the correlation of aspartate transcarbamylase and dihydroorotase[33] with hepatoma growth rate. In this panel we also present results on other enzymes which we have reorganized and plotted in the order of hepatoma growth rate from results published by Sneider et al.[34] Accordingly, the activities of thymidine kinase, thymidylate kinase, thymidylate synthase, and dCMP deaminase also correlate positively with the growth rate.

The lower right panel indicates the progressive decline in the degradation of thymine, thymidine and uracil into CO_2[12] and the decrease in adenylate kinase[35] activity parallel with the increase in hepatoma growth rate. The decrease in the degradative pathway presents a mirror picture of the progressive increase observed for the biosynthetic pathway.

Thus, the molecular correlation concept provides a powerful tool for probing gene expression in the cancer cells. The presented results indicate to us a close linkage in the expression of the replicative potential of the genome with the extent of the progressive imbalance in the synthetic and catabolic pathways and key enzymes of thymidine, UMP, DNA, and carbohydrate metabolism. The data underline the importance of ratios of opposing key enzymes and metabolic pathways as indicators of the link between replicative and translative and transcriptive expression of the genome in neoplasia.

It is important to emphasize that no imbalance similar to that found in the neoplastic liver has been observed in the regenerating liver. In consequence, the alterations in the progressive metabolic imbalance in hepatomas are specific to and characteristic of neoplasia.

The close linking of cell proliferation rate and biochemical changes reveals gradual shifts in the equilibria of the opposing pathways that are, in essence, not only quantitative, but result in qualitative lesions specific to the cancer cell. The discovery of the correlation of the extent of enzymatic and metabolic imbalance with growth rate now permits the integration of the metabolic changes in a meaningful pattern in cancer cells. Since the correlation of biochemical alterations and growth rate has also been shown to be applicable to a series of kidney[36] and mammary tumors[37] of different growth rates, the approaches of the molecular correlation concept are probably applicable to all neoplastic cells, and should assist in the design of selective chemotherapy.

The final session was designed for the discussion of the modification of gene expression.

Hormonal regulation of gene expression of cancer was discussed by Dr. H. G. Williams-Ashman of the Ben May Laboratory for Cancer Research[39] (see pages 731-732, Volume I). This was fitting, since Professor Charles B. Huggins of that same institute received the Nobel Prize for his contribution on the discovery of hormonal dependence or independence of tumors. This concept was introduced by Huggins in 1945, following his demonstration that human prostatic cancers and their metastases may sometimes regress as a result of altering the hormonal environments by such procedures as orchiectomy and/or treatment with estrogenic substances. This led to prolongation of life in many patients and was an epoch-making breakthrough in the history of the fight against cancer. Dr. Williams-Ashman discussed the modern molecular aspects of the action of androgenic and estrogenic hormones in the light of his own work, and that of Dr. Jensen and their associates.[39]

It may be expected that much further work on this topic will be done over the coming years, and that more investigations on the nature and functions of the sex steroid-binding proteins in the nucleus and cytoplasm of hormone-dependent tumors is likely to be of both clinical and theoretical importance.

A most valuable new approach proved to be the use of enzymes in a way everybody has predicted would be impossible. Of course I am talking about the parenteral use of the enzyme asparaginase in the treatment for certain types of leukemias. This important progress in treatment approach has received much interest clinically and experimentally.

Dr. J. D. Broome[40] (see pages 747-754, Volume I) discussed work on L-asparaginase inhibition of solid tumors in mice. Dr. Broome's work centered on an L-asparaginase preparation from an unknown soil organism, which proved to be inhibitory to the growth of two kinds of mouse tumors which were resistant to L-asparaginases from *E. coli* or agouti serum. The effect appears to be caused by an enzyme which exhibits both L-glutaminase and L-asparaginase activities.

This discovery is also of interest because of the work of Dr. Katunuma that I referred to above, who observed that glutaminase decreased parallel with the increase of hepatoma growth rate.[17] It was also reported recently that glutaminase activity decreased parallel with the growth rate of a number of different types of animal tumors.[37, 38] Thus there might be another application of an enzyme alteration to chemotherapy, and it is hoped that a new beginning has been made.

Professor Walter Kersten discussed his exciting work on the action of some antitumor antibiotics on gene transcription and replication.[4] The two classes of compounds which he reported on relate closely to the central theme of the Conference on regulation of gene expression. For instance, there are antibiotics which interfere with genic expression. I single out here actinomycin D which interferes with transcription and new RNA production. This compound, as you know, proved curative in properly selected cases of choriocarcinoma and Wilms' tumor in children. This topic relates to Figure 22-2 on the structure of DNA; actinomycin intercalates between the strands of the double helix. It has sufficient selectivity to provide the chemotherapeutic effect hoped for in these two types of clinical cancer. This drug is also a splendid tool in molecular biology research.

Another class of compounds are the quinones, among them a recently produced antibiotic called granaticin. Dr. Kersten told us that this compound might affect sulfhydryl proteins, interfering with the stabilization of polysomes and thus interfering with RNA and protein synthesis. The advantage of the quinones is that DNA is not a target, and the effects on RNA proved to be reversible. This he explained in a slide which closely resembles the one Dr. Lengyel showed earlier. There were a number of questions raised as to whether the *E. coli* data have any reference to mammalian systems; the relevance is already becoming evident.

This Conference is designed, as I mentioned, to lead up to the application of basic science to patient care, and to consider the achievements and problems of using the regulation of gene expression in designing selective chemotherapy for clinical cancer.

Dr. J. L. Lewis, Jr. (see pages 759-762, Volume I) presented a most up-to-date picture of the clinical application of chemotherapy for choriocarcinoma, and the news is good.[41] Table 22-2 shows the results of treatment for choriocarcinoma; the cure rate in the 1950's was 48%, but in the 1960's it rose to 76%. The newest statistics he has show that over 80% of these women can be cured with proper application of the chemotherapeutic weapons we now have, namely actinomycin and methotrexate.

Figure 22-14 is a fitting climax to this heroic struggle against an unbelievably difficult problem. This represents a typical case of Dr. Hertz. The patient, after delivering a perfectly normal child, returned for her six weeks' checkup and reported a pain in her chest. She had a high choriogonadotropin level, and X-ray examination showed a typical metastatic lesion in the lungs. The figure shows that with drug treatment the hormone level returned to normal and the metastatic lesion disappeared from the lung. This woman is alive and well now, seven years later, and has no further symptoms.

TABLE 22-2.—RESULTS OF TREATMENT IN 108 CASES OF MTD

| SERIES | NUMBER | COMPLETE REMISSION/TOTAL PATIENTS HISTOPATHOLOGIC DIAGNOSIS ON ADMISSION | |
		Chorioca	Mole, Destruens, Other
A MTX, VLB (1956-1961)	63	21/44 (48%)	9/19 (47%)
B MTX, Actino (1961-1964)	50*	22/29 (76%)	15/21 (73%)

* Includes 5 cases alive with disease from series A.

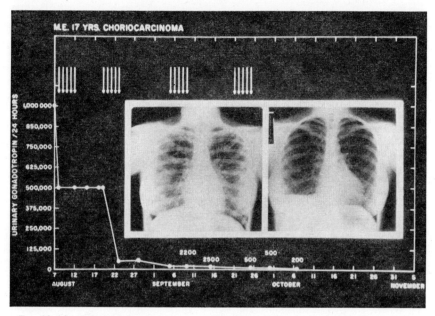

Fig. 22–14.—Effect of chemotherapy on choriogonadotropin level and X-ray findings in a case of choriocarcinoma with lung metastasis. (Courtesy of R. Hertz.)

I have always looked at the physicians and scientists who work against cancer, the basic and the clinical people, as heroes in a great adventure. I wish that when future generations of scientists look back to our generation of cancer researchers, they will say: "They were the ones who fought with Death and won."

Acknowledgments

Supported by grants from the United States Public Health Service (National Cancer Institute Grant No. CA-05034), American Cancer Society, and Damon Runyon Memorial Fund, Inc. The assistance of my associate, Dr. Sherry I. F. Queener, in preparation of this manuscript is gratefully acknowledged.

References

1. Stanley, W. M.: Molecular biology and cancer—historical and perspective. In: Oncology, 1970: A. Cellular and Molecular Mechanisms of Carcinogenesis; B. Regulation of Gene Expression (Proceedings of the 10th International Cancer Congress, Volume I), Year Book Medical Publishers, Inc., Chicago, 1971, pp. 579-586.
2. Wolstenholme, K. Koike, and H. C. Renger: Form and Structure of Mitochondrial DNA. In: Oncology, 1970: Cellular and Molecular Mechanisms of Carcinogenesis (Proceedings of the 10th International Cancer Congress), Year Book Medical Publishers, Inc., Chicago, 1971, pp. 627-648.
3. Lengyel, P.: Presented at the 10th International Cancer Congress, Houston, Texas, 1970.

4. Kersten, W.: Presented at the 10th International Cancer Congress, Houston, Texas, 1970.
5. Sinsheimer, R. L.: Biosynthesis of DNA. In: Oncology, 1970: A. Cellular and Molecular Mechanisms of Carcinogenesis; B. Regulation of Gene Expression (Proceedings of the 10th International Cancer Congress, Volume I), Year Book Medical Publishers, Inc., Chicago, 1971, pp. 586-591.
6. Spiegelman, S.: Presented at the 10th International Cancer Congress at Houston, Texas, 1970.
7. Bernhard, W.: The interphase nucleus: Problems of structure and function in 1970. In: Oncology, 1970: A. Cellular and Molecular Mechanisms of Carcinogenesis; B. Regulation of Gene Expression (Proceedings of the 10th International Cancer Congress, Volume I), Year Book Medical Publishers, Inc., Chicago, 1971, pp. 600-612.
8. Muramatsu, M., and T. Higashinakagawa: The nucleolus, and its function. In: Oncology, 1970: A. Cellular and Molecular Mechanisms of Carcinogenesis; B. Regulation of Gene Expression (Proceedings of the 10th International Cancer Congress, Volume I), Year Book Medical Publishers, Inc., Chicago, 1971, pp. 613-627.
9. Wolstenholme, D. R., K. Koike, and H. C. Renger: Form and structure of mitochondrial DNA. In: Oncology, 1970: A. Cellular and Molecular Mechanisms of Carcinogenesis; B. Regulation of Gene Expression (Proceedings of the 10th International Cancer Congress, Volume I), Year Book Medical Publishers, Inc., Chicago, 1971, pp. 627-648.
10. MacHattie, L. A., and C. A. Thomas: Science, 144:1142, 1964.
11. Morris, H. P.: Adv. Cancer Res., 9:227, 1965.
12. Weber, G., J. A. Ferdinandus, and S. I. F. Queener: Role of metabolic imbalance in neoplasia. In: Oncology, 1970: A. Cellular and Molecular Mechanisms of Carcinogenesis; B. Regulation of Gene Expression (Proceedings of the 10th International Cancer Congress, Volume I), Year Book Medical Publishers, Inc., Chicago, 1971, pp. 510-532.
13. Pitot, H. C.: The role of intracellular membranes in the regulation of genetic expression. In: Oncology, 1970: A. Cellular and Molecular Mechanisms of Carcinogenesis; B. Regulation of Gene Expression (Proceedings of the 10th International Cancer Congress, Volume I), Year Book Medical Publishers, Inc., Chicago, 1971, pp. 648-655.
14. Weinhouse, S.: Respiration, glycolysis and enzyme alterations in liver neoplasms. In: Oncology, 1970: A. Cellular and Molecular Mechanisms of Carcinogenesis; B. Regulation of Gene Expression (Proceedings of the 10th International Cancer Congress, Volume I), Year Book Medical Publishers, Inc., Chicago, 1971, pp. 656-667.
15. Wheeler, G. P.: Nucleic acid metabolism in neoplasms. In: Oncology, 1970: A. Cellular and Molecular Mechanisms of Carcinogenesis; B. Regulation of Gene Expression (Proceedings of the 10th International Cancer Congress, Volume I), Year Book Medical Publishers, Inc., Chicago, 1971, pp. 667-672.
16. Novelli, G. D.: Mechanisms of translational control. In: Oncology, 1970: A. Cellular and Molecular Mechanisms of Carcinogenesis; B. Regulation of Gene Expression (Proceedings of the 10th International Cancer Congress, Volume I), Year Book Medical Publishers, Inc., Chicago, 1971, pp. 672-683.
17. Katunuma, N., Y. Kuroda, Y. Sanada, I. Tomino, and H. P. Morris: Anomalous distribution of glutaminase isozyme in various hepatomas. In: Oncology, 1970: A. Cellular and Molecular Mechanisms of Carcinogenesis; B. Regulation of Gene Expression (Proceedings of the 10th International Cancer Congress, Volume I), Year Book Medical Publishers, Inc., Chicago, 1971, pp. 684-695.
18. Tomkins, G. M.: Presented at the 10th International Cancer Congress at Houston, Texas, 1970.
19. Chance, B.: Regulation of the cell respiration. In: Oncology, 1970: A. Cellular and Molecular Mechanisms of Carcinogenesis; B. Regulation of Gene Expression (Pro-

ceedings of the 10th International Cancer Congress, Volume I), Year Book Medical Publishers, Inc., Chicago, 1971, pp. 711-718.

20. Mueller, G. C.: Biochemical perspectives of the cell cycle. In: Oncology, 1970: A. Cellular and Molecular Mechanisms of Carcinogenesis; B. Regulation of Gene Expression (Proceedings of the 10th International Cancer Congress, Volume I), Year Book Medical Publishers, Inc., 1971, pp. 719-725.

21. Potter, V. R.: Enzyme regulation in cancer cells. In: Oncology, 1970: A. Cellular and Molecular Mechanisms of Carcinogenesis; B. Regulation of Gene Expression (Proceedings of the 10th International Cancer Congress, Volume I), Year Book Medical Publishers, Inc., Chicago, 1971, pp. 725-730.

22. Siperstein, M. D.: Presented at the 10th International Cancer Congress at Houston, Texas, 1970.

23. Weber, G.: Gann Monogr., 1:151, 1966.

24. Weber, G., and M. A. Lea: Meth. Cancer Res., 2:523, 1967.

25. Weber, G.: Naturwissenschaften, 55:418, 1968.

26. Weber, G., and A. Cantero: Cancer Res., 17:995, 1957.

27. Weber, G., R. L. Singhal, N. B. Stamm, M. A. Lea, and E. A. Fisher: Adv. Enzyme Reg., 4:59, 1966.

28. Weber, G.: Adv. Cancer Res., 6:403, 1961.

29. Morris, H. P., and B. P. Wagner: Meth. Cancer Res., 4:125, 1968.

30. Elford, H. L.: Fed. Proc., 27:300, 1968.

31. Elford, H. L., M. Freese, E. Passamani, and H. P. Morris: J. Biol. Chem. Submitted for publication.

32. Ove, P., M. D. Jenkins, and J. Laszlo: Cancer Res., 30:535, 1970.

33. Sweeney, M. J., D. H. Hoffman, and G. A. Poore: Proc. Amer. Ass. Cancer Res., 8:66, 1967.

34. Sneider, T. W., V. R. Potter, and H. P. Morris: Cancer Res., 29:40, 1969.

35. Criss, W. E., G. Litwack, H. P. Morris, and S. Weinhouse: Cancer Res., 30:370, 1970.

36. Lea, M. A., H. P. Morris, and G. Weber: Cancer Res., 28:71, 1968.

37. Knox, W. E., M. L. Horowitz, and G. H. Friedell: Cancer Res., 29:669, 1969.

38. Knox, W. E., M. Linder, and G. H. Friedell: Cancer Res., 30:283, 1970.

39. Williams-Ashman, H. G.: Hormonal regulation of gene expression and control of cancer. In: Oncology, 1970: A. Cellular and Molecular Mechanisms of Carcinogenesis; B. Regulation of Gene Expression (Proceedings of the 10th International Cancer Congress, Volume I), Year Book Medical Publishers, Inc., Chicago, 1971, pp. 731-732.

40. Broome, J. D.: Selective toxicity by enzyme administration: Tumor inhibitory actions of a bacterial extract with L-asparaginase and L-glutaminase activities. In: Oncology, 1970: A. Cellular and Molecular Mechanisms of Carcinogenesis; B. Regulation of Gene Expression (Proceedings of the 10th International Cancer Congress, Volume I), Year Book Medical Publishers, Inc., Chicago, 1971, pp. 747-754.

41. Lewis, J. L., Jr.: Modification of gene expression: Sustained remission of Choriocarcinoma. In: Oncology, 1970: A. Cellular and Molecular Mechanisms of Carcinogenesis; B. Regulation of Gene Expression (Proceedings of the 10th International Cancer Congress, Volume I), Year Book Medical Publishers, Inc., Chicago, 1971, pp. 759-762.

Author Index

Subject Index

Morphology, HeLa cell, effect of Cortisol on, 440–455

Morris hepatoma, *see* Hepatoma, Morris

Mouse, cells of, transformation by defective SV40, 152–153

mRNA, *see* Messenger ribonucleic acid

MTH, *see* Hormones, mammotropic

Multiplication, of cells, 600–655

Murine leukemia, *see* Leukemia, murine

Mutations
DNA-spontaneous, resulting in new antigens, 208
of structural genes, interactions with DNA resulting in, 207–208

Myeloblastosis, avian virus of, DNA-RNA hybridization studies of, 788–793

Myeloma
as biochemical model of cancer, 459–493
clinical studies, 486–493
difference in isoaccepting tRNA among different amino acids, 478
molecular biology of, 476–480
studies
of protein synthesis and secretion in, 477–479
of ribosomal subunits of, 479
of transport and secretion of gamma-globulin in cells of, 479

N

Neoplasia
cell hybridization and, 361–362
cytogenetics of, 358–361
cell hybridization applied to, 358–363
frequency of, and plasma cell differentiation, 486–488
homeostasis of mammary gland and, 293–295
role of metabolic imbalance in, 510–532
unified concept of, 288–289

Neoplasms
cells of
altered surface properties of, 210–225
dormant, 321
nonspecific antigens of, 211–218
specific antigens of, 211
liver, respiration, glycolysis, and enzyme alteration in, 656–667
nucleic acid metabolism in, 667–672
redifferentiation of, 833–836
role of herpesvirus in, 127–132
"spontaneous" transformation of, in vitro, 76–82

Neoplastic transformation, *see* Transformation, neoplastic

Neuroblastomas
growth, differentiation, and function of, in vitro, 833–836
immunity to, in man, 256–257

Neutralization, tests of, for FBJ virus, 429–430

Nitroquinoline-N-oxide, *see* Derivatives, nitroquinoline-N-oxide

Noncytocides, infection with, in cell transformation, 118–119

Nonhistones
chromosomal protein, accumulation of, during chromatin biosynthesis, 506
as proteins, 608

Nuclear membrane, *see* Membrane, nuclear

Nuclear proteins, *see* Proteins, nuclear

Nucleic acid, *see* Acid, nucleic

Nucleolus
function of, 613–627
isolation of, 613–616
protein synthesis in, problems of, 607
ribonucleic acid in, 616–619
and protein synthesis, 623–627
ribonucleoproteins in, 619–623

Nucleoside contrast, 591–599

Nucleus
of cancer cell, 609–610
interphase, problems of structure and function in, 600–612

O

Oligomers, circular dichroism spectra of AAF-modified, 53–54

Oligonucleotides, modification of, with AAF, 50–53

Oncogenesis, ontogenic defects in, 803–836

Oncogeny
as composite of program errors, 726–727
as locked in ontogeny, 726

Ontogeny, locked in, oncogeny as, 726

Organs, cultures of, tests for carcinogenic activity in, 258–287

Organelles, regulatory behavior of, in normal and cancer cells, 600–655

Osteosarcoma, ^{90}Sr, interaction of FBJ osteosarcoma virus with, 422–434

Ovary
experimental tumors of, 313–314
functional tumors of, and hormonal activity, 301–302

Oxidation, of fatty acids, 662

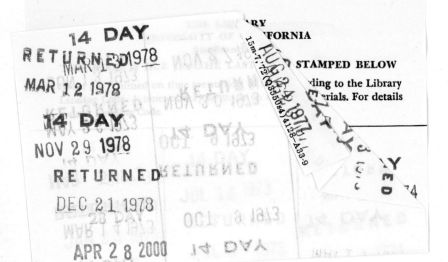